Pediatric Clinical Practice Guidelines & Policies

· ·

A Compendium of Evidence-based Research for Pediatric Practice

5th Edition

American Academy of Pediatrics
141 Northwest Point Blvd
Elk Grove Village, IL 60007-1098
www.aap.org

5th Edition—2005
4th Edition—2004
3rd Edition—2003
2nd Edition—2002
1st Edition—2001

Library of Congress Control Number: 2004116186

ISBN: 1-58110-163-5

MA0305

9-5/0205

The recommendations in this publication do not indicate an exclusive course of treatment or serve as a standard of medical care. Variations, taking into account individual circumstances, may be appropriate.

INTRODUCTION TO
PEDIATRIC CLINICAL PRACTICE GUIDELINES & POLICIES: A COMPENDIUM OF EVIDENCE-BASED RESEARCH FOR PEDIATRIC PRACTICE

Clinical practice guidelines have long provided physicians with evidence-based decision-making tools for managing common pediatric conditions. Policy statements issued and endorsed by the American Academy of Pediatrics (AAP) are developed to provide physicians with a quick reference guide to the AAP position on child health care issues. We have combined these 2 authoritative resources into one comprehensive manual/CD-ROM resource to provide easy access to important clinical and policy information.

This manual contains
- Clinical practice guidelines from the AAP
- Technical report summaries
- Clinical practice guidelines endorsed by the AAP, including abstracts where applicable
- Policy statements, clinical reports, and technical reports issued or endorsed through December 2004, including abstracts where applicable
- Full text of all 2004 AAP policy statements, clinical reports, and technical reports

The CD-ROM, which is located on the inside back cover of this manual, builds on the content of the book and includes full text of
- All AAP clinical practice guidelines
- All AAP policy statements
- All AAP clinical reports
- All AAP technical reports
- All endorsed clinical practice guidelines and policies

We welcome your feedback on *Pediatric Clinical Practice Guidelines & Policies: A Compendium of Evidence-based Research for Pediatric Practice*, 5th edition, and encourage you to fill out the enclosed product evaluation form.

Additional information about AAP policy can be found in a variety of professional publications such as
Guidelines for Perinatal Care, 5th Edition
Pediatric Environmental Health, 2nd Edition
Pediatric Nutrition Handbook, 5th Edition
Red Book®, 26th Edition, and *Red Book Online* (www.aapredbook.org)
School Health: Policy & Practice, 6th Edition

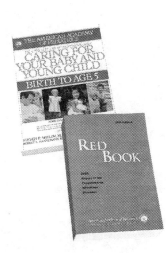

Parenting information consistent with AAP policy is available in a variety of consumer publications such as
ADHD: A Complete and Authoritative Guide
Caring for Your Baby and Young Child: Birth to Age 5
Caring for Your School-Age Child: Ages 5 to 12
Caring for Your Teenager
Guide to Toilet Training
New Mother's Guide to Breastfeeding

For more information on these titles and similar products or for ordering information, please call 888/227-1770 or visit our online Bookstore at www.aap.org/bookstore.

AMERICAN ACADEMY OF PEDIATRICS

The American Academy of Pediatrics (AAP) and its member pediatricians dedicate their efforts and resources to the health, safety, and well-being of infants, children, adolescents, and young adults. The AAP has approximately 60,000 members in the United States, Canada, and Latin America. Members include pediatricians, pediatric medical subspecialists, and pediatric surgical specialists. More than 34,000 members are board certified and called Fellows of the AAP (FAAP).

Core Values. We believe
- In the inherent worth of all children; they are our most enduring and vulnerable legacy.
- Children deserve optimal health and the highest quality health care.
- Pediatricians are the best qualified to provide child health care.

The American Academy of Pediatrics is the organization to advance child health and well-being.

Vision. Children have optimal health and well-being and are valued by society. Academy members practice the highest quality health care and experience professional satisfaction and personal well-being.

Mission. The mission of the American Academy of Pediatrics is to attain optimal physical, mental, and social health and well-being for all infants, children, adolescents, and young adults. To accomplish this mission, the Academy shall support the professional needs of its members.

Table of Contents

SECTION 4

CURRENT POLICIES FROM THE AMERICAN ACADEMY OF PEDIATRICS

SECTION 5

ENDORSED POLICIES

POLICIES BY COMMITTEE

Clinical Practice Guidelines
From the American Academy of Pediatrics
• •

- *Clinical Practice Guidelines*
  EVIDENCE-BASED DECISION-MAKING TOOLS FOR MANAGING COMMON PEDIATRIC CONDITIONS

- *Technical Report Summaries*
  BACKGROUND INFORMATION TO SUPPORT AMERICAN ACADEMY OF PEDIATRICS POLICY

FOREWORD

In response to the growing trend toward the practice of evidence-based medicine, the American Academy of Pediatrics (AAP) created an organizational process and methodology for developing clinical practice guidelines. These guidelines provide physicians with an evidence-based decision-making tool for managing common pediatric conditions.

The evidence-based approach to developing clinical practice guidelines requires carefully defining the problem and identifying interventions and health outcomes. An extensive literature review and data analysis provide the basis for guideline recommendations. The practice guidelines also are subjected to a thorough peer-review process prior to publication and subsequent dissemination, implementation, and evaluation. Clinical practice guidelines are periodically reviewed to ensure that they are based on the most current data available.

American Academy of Pediatrics clinical practice guidelines are designed to provide physicians with an analytic framework for evaluating and treating common childhood conditions and are not intended as an exclusive course of treatment or standard of care. When using AAP practice guidelines, clinicians should continue to consider other sources of information as well as variations in individual circumstances. The AAP recognizes the incompleteness of data and acknowledges the use of expert consensus in cases in which data do not exist. Thus, AAP clinical practice guidelines allow for flexibility and adaptability at the local level and should not replace sound clinical judgment.

This text contains clinical practice guidelines and technical report summaries developed and published by the AAP. Full technical reports are available on the included CD-ROM. The full technical reports contain summaries of the data reviewed, results of data analyses, complete evidence tables, and bibliographies of articles included in the review. This collection of AAP policy also includes abstracts and introductions for evidence-based practice guidelines from other organizations that the AAP has endorsed. Practice guidelines will continually be added to this compendium as they are released or updated. We encourage you to look forward to these future guidelines. This edition also includes the full text of all policy statements, clinical reports, and technical reports published in 2004 by the AAP and abstracts of all active AAP policy statements and reports, as well as those endorsed by the AAP. The full text of all endorsed practice guidelines, as well as all active AAP and endorsed policy statements and reports published prior to 2004, is included on the companion CD-ROM.

If you have any questions about current or future clinical practice guidelines, please contact Caryn Prosansky at the AAP at 800/433-9016, ext 4317. To order copies of the patient education brochures that accompany each guideline, please call the AAP at 888/227-1770 or visit the AAP online Bookstore at www.aap.org/bookstore.

Jay E. Berkelhamer, MD, FAAP
Chairperson, Steering Committee on Quality Improvement and Management

Diagnosis and Evaluation of the Child With Attention-Deficit/Hyperactivity Disorder

- *Clinical Practice Guideline*

AMERICAN ACADEMY OF PEDIATRICS

Committee on Quality Improvement, Subcommittee on Attention-Deficit/Hyperactivity Disorder

Clinical Practice Guideline: Diagnosis and Evaluation of the Child With Attention-Deficit/Hyperactivity Disorder

ABSTRACT. This clinical practice guideline provides recommendations for the assessment and diagnosis of school-aged children with attention-deficit/hyperactivity disorder (ADHD). This guideline, the first of 2 sets of guidelines to provide recommendations on this condition, is intended for use by primary care clinicians working in primary care settings. The second set of guidelines will address the issue of treatment of children with ADHD.

The Committee on Quality Improvement of the American Academy of Pediatrics selected a committee composed of pediatricians and other experts in the fields of neurology, psychology, child psychiatry, development, and education, as well as experts from epidemiology and pediatric practice. In addition, this panel consists of experts in education and family practice. The panel worked with Technical Resources International, Washington, DC, under the auspices of the Agency for Healthcare Research and Quality, to develop the evidence base of literature on this topic. The resulting evidence report was used to formulate recommendations for evaluation of the child with ADHD. Major issues contained within the guideline address child and family assessment; school assessment, including the use of various rating scales; and conditions seen frequently among children with ADHD. Information is also included on the use of current diagnostic coding strategies. The deliberations of the committee were informed by a systematic review of evidence about prevalence, coexisting conditions, and diagnostic tests. Committee decisions were made by consensus where definitive evidence was not available. The committee report underwent review by sections of the American Academy of Pediatrics and external organizations before approval by the Board of Directors.

The guideline contains the following recommendations for diagnosis of ADHD: 1) in a child 6 to 12 years old who presents with inattention, hyperactivity, impulsivity, academic underachievement, or behavior problems, primary care clinicians should initiate an evaluation for ADHD; 2) the diagnosis of ADHD requires that a child meet *Diagnostic and Statistical Manual of Mental Disorders, Fourth Edition* criteria; 3) the assessment of ADHD requires evidence directly obtained from parents or caregivers regarding the core symptoms of ADHD in various settings, the age of onset, duration of symptoms, and degree of functional impairment; 4) the assessment of ADHD requires evidence directly obtained from the classroom teacher (or other school professional) regarding the core symptoms of ADHD, duration of symptoms, degree of functional impairment, and associated conditions; 5) evaluation of the child with ADHD should include assessment for associated (coexisting) conditions; and 6) other diagnostic tests are not routinely indicated to establish the diagnosis of ADHD but may be used for the assessment of other coexisting conditions (eg, learning disabilities and mental retardation).

This clinical practice guideline is not intended as a sole source of guidance in the evaluation of children with ADHD. Rather, it is designed to assist primary care clinicians by providing a framework for diagnostic decisionmaking. It is not intended to replace clinical judgment or to establish a protocol for all children with this condition and may not provide the only appropriate approach to this problem.

ABBREVIATIONS. ADHD, attention-deficit/hyperactivity disorder; DSM-IV, *Diagnostic and Statistical Manual of Mental Disorders, Fourth Edition*; AAP, American Academy of Pediatrics; DSM-PC, *Diagnostic and Statistical Manual for Primary Care*.

Attention-deficit/hyperactivity disorder (ADHD) is the most common neurobehavioral disorder of childhood. ADHD is also among the most prevalent chronic health conditions affecting school-aged children. The core symptoms of ADHD include inattention, hyperactivity, and impulsivity.[1,2] Children with ADHD may experience significant functional problems, such as school difficulties, academic underachievement,[3] troublesome interpersonal relationships with family members[4,5] and peers, and low self-esteem. Individuals with ADHD present in childhood and may continue to show symptoms as they enter adolescence[6] and adult life.[7] Pediatricians and other primary care clinicians frequently are asked by parents and teachers to evaluate a child for ADHD. Early recognition, assessment, and management of this condition can redirect the educational and psychosocial development of most children with ADHD.[8,9]

Recorded prevalence rates for ADHD vary substantially, partly because of changing diagnostic criteria over time,[10–13] and partly because of variations in ascertainment in different settings and the frequent use of referred samples to estimate rates. Practitioners of all types (primary care, subspecialty, psychiatry, and nonphysician mental health providers) vary greatly in the degree to which they use *Diagnostic and Statistical Manual of Mental Health Disorders, Fourth Edition* (DSM-IV) criteria to diagnose ADHD. Reported rates also vary substantially in different geographic areas and across countries.[14]

With increasing epidemiologic and clinical research, diagnostic criteria have been revised on multiple occasions over the past 20 years.[10–13] A recent review of prevalence rates in school-aged community samples (rather than referred samples) indicates rates varying from 4% to 12%, with estimated prevalence based on combining these studies of ~8% to 10%. In the general population,[15–23,24] 9.2% (5.8%–13.6%) of males and 2.9% (1.9%–4.5%) of females are found to have behaviors consistent with ADHD. With the *DSM-IV* criteria (compared with earlier versions), more females have been diagnosed with the predominantly inattentive type.[25,26] Prevalence rates also vary significantly depending on whether they reflect school samples 6.9% (5.5%–8.5%) versus community samples 10.3% (8.2%–12.7%).

Public interest in ADHD has increased along with debate in the media concerning the diagnostic process and treatment strategies.[27] Concern has been expressed about the over-diagnosis of ADHD by pointing to the several-fold increase in prescriptions for stimulant medication among children during the past decade.[28] In addition, there are significant regional variations in the amount of stimulants prescribed by physicians.[29] Practice surveys among primary care pediatricians and family physicians reveal wide variations in practice patterns about diagnostic criteria and methods.[30]

ADHD commonly occurs in association with oppositional defiant disorder, conduct disorder, depression, anxiety disorder,[16] and with many developmental disorders, such as speech and language delays and learning disabilities.

This diagnostic guideline is intended for use by primary care clinicians to evaluate children between 6 and 12 years of age for ADHD, consistent with best available empirical studies. Special attention is given to assessing school performance and behavior, family functioning, and adaptation. In light of the high prevalence of ADHD in pediatric practice, the guideline should assist primary care clinicians in these assessments. The diagnosis usually requires several steps. Clinicians will generally need to carry out the evaluation in more than 1 visit, often indeed 2 to 3 visits. The guideline is not intended for children with mental retardation, pervasive developmental disorder, moderate to severe sensory deficits such as visual and hearing impairment, chronic disorders associated with medications that may affect behavior, and those who have experienced child abuse and sexual abuse. These children too may have ADHD, and this guideline may help clinicians in considering this diagnosis; nonetheless, this guideline primarily reviews evidence relating to the diagnosis of ADHD in relatively uncomplicated cases in primary care settings.

METHODOLOGY

To initiate the development of a practice guideline for the diagnosis and evaluation of children with ADHD directed toward primary care physicians, the American Academy of Pediatrics (AAP) worked with several colleague organizations to organize a working panel representing a wide range of primary care and subspecialty groups. The committee, chaired by 2 general pediatricians (1 with substantial additional experience and training in developmental and behavioral pediatrics), included representatives from the American Academy of Family Physicians, the American Academy of Child and Adolescent Psychiatry, the Child Neurology Society, and the Society for Pediatric Psychology, as well as developmental and behavioral pediatricians and epidemiologists.

This group met over a period of 2 years, during which it reviewed basic literature on current practices in the diagnosis of ADHD and developed a series of questions to direct an evidence-based review of the prevalence of ADHD in community and primary care practice settings, the rates of coexisting conditions, and the utility of several diagnostic methods and devices. The AAP committee collaborated with the Agency for Healthcare Research and Quality in its support of an evidence-based review of several of these key items in the diagnosis of ADHD. David Atkins, MD, provided liaison from the Agency for Healthcare Research and Quality, and Technical Resources International conducted the evidence review.

The Technical Resources International report focused on 4 specific areas for the literature review: the prevalence of ADHD among children 6 to 12 years of age in the general population and the coexisting conditions that may occur with ADHD; the prevalence of ADHD among children in primary care settings and the coexisting conditions that may occur; the accuracy of various screening methods for diagnosis; and the prevalence of abnormal findings on commonly used medical screening tests. The literature search was conducted using Medline and PsycINFO databases, references from review articles, rating scale manuals, and articles identified by the subcommittee. Only articles published in English between 1980 and 1997 were included. The study population was limited to children 6 to 12 years of age, and only studies using general, unselected populations in communities, schools, or the primary clinical setting were used. Data on screening tests were taken from studies conducted in any setting. Articles accepted for analysis were abstracted twice by trained personnel and a clinical specialist. Both abstracts for each article were compared and differences between them resolved. A multiple logistic regression model with random effects was used to analyze simultaneously for age, gender, diagnostic tool, and setting using EGRET software. Results were presented in evidence tables and published in the final evidence report.[24]

The draft practice guideline underwent extensive peer review by committees and sections within the AAP, by numerous outside organizations, and by other individuals identified by the subcommittee. Liaisons to the subcommittee also were invited to distribute the draft to entities within their organizations. The resulting comments were compiled and reviewed by the subcommittee co-chairpersons, and relevant changes were incorporated into the draft based on recommendations from peer reviewers.

The recommendations contained in the practice guideline are based on the best available data (Fig 1).

Where data were lacking, a combination of evidence and expert consensus was used. Strong recommendations were based on high-quality scientific evidence, or, in the absence of high-quality data, strong expert consensus. Fair and weak recommendations were based on lesser quality or limited data and expert consensus. Clinical options were identified as interventions because the subcommittee could not find compelling evidence for or against. These clinical options are interventions that a reasonable health care provider might or might not wish to implement in his or her practice.

RECOMMENDATION 1: In a child 6 to 12 years old who presents with inattention, hyperactivity, impulsivity, academic underachievement, or behavior problems, primary care clinicians should initiate an evaluation for ADHD (strength of evidence: good; strength of recommendation: strong).

The major justification for this recommendation is the high prevalence of ADHD in school-aged populations. School-aged children with a variety of developmental and behavioral concerns present to primary care clinicians.[31] Primary care pediatricians and family physicians recognize behavior problems that may impact academic achievement in 18% of school-aged children seen in their offices and clinics. Hyperactivity or inattention is diagnosed in 9% of children.[32]

Presentations of ADHD in clinical practice vary. In many cases, concerns derive from parents, teachers, other professionals, or nonparental caregivers. Common presentations include referral from school for academic underachievement and failure, disruptive classroom behavior, inattentiveness, problems with social relationships, parental concerns regarding similar phenomena, poor self-esteem, or problems with establishing or maintaining social relationships. Children with core ADHD symptoms of hyperactivity and impulsivity are identified by teachers, because they often disrupt the classroom. Even mild distractibility and motor symptoms, such as fidgetiness, will be apparent to most teachers. In contrast, children with the inattentive subtype of ADHD, where hyperactive and impulsive symptoms are absent or minimal, may not come to the attention of teachers. These children may present with school underachievement.

Symptoms may not be apparent in a structured clinical setting that is free from the demands and distraction of the home and school.[33] Thus, if parents do not bring concerns to the primary clinician, then early detection of ADHD in primary care may not occur. Clinical practices during routine health supervision may assist in early recognition of ADHD.[34,35] Options include direct history from parents and children. The following general questions may be useful at all visits for school-aged children to heighten attention about ADHD and as an initial screening for school performance.

1. How is your child doing in school?
2. Are there any problems with learning that you or the teacher has seen?
3. Is your child happy in school?
4. Are you concerned with any behavioral problems in school, at home, or when your child is playing with friends?
5. Is your child having problems completing classwork or homework?

Alternatively, a previsit questionnaire may be sent to parents or given while the family is waiting in the reception area.[36] When making an appointment for a health supervision visit for a school-aged child, 1 or 2 of these questions may be asked routinely to sensitize parents to the concerns of their child's clinician. For example, "Your child's clinician is interested in how your child is doing in school. You might check with her teacher and discuss any concerns with your child's physician." Wall posters, pamphlets, and books in the waiting area that focus on educational achievements and school-aged behaviors send a message that this is an office or clinic that considers these issues important to a child's development.[37]

RECOMMENDATION 2: The diagnosis of ADHD requires that a child meet DSM-IV criteria (strength of evidence: good; strength of recommendation: strong).

Establishing a diagnosis of ADHD requires a strategy that minimizes over-identification and under-identification. Pediatricians and other primary care health professionals should apply *DSM-IV* criteria in the context of their clinical assessment of a child. The use of specific criteria will help to ensure a more accurate diagnosis and decrease variation in how the diagnosis is made. The *DSM-IV* criteria, developed through several iterations by the American Psychiatric Association, are based on clinical experience and an expanding research foundation.[13] These criteria have more support in the literature than other available diagnostic criteria. The *DSM-IV* specification of behavior items, required numbers of items, and levels of impairment reflect the current consensus among clinicians, particularly psychiatry. The consensus includes increasing research evidence, particularly in the distinctions that the *DSM-IV* makes for the dimensions of attention and hyperactivity-impulsivity.[38]

The *DSM-IV* criteria define 3 subtypes of ADHD (see Table 1 for specific inattention and hyperactive-impulsive items).

- ADHD primarily of the inattentive type (ADHD/I, meeting at least 6 of 9 inattention behaviors)
- ADHD primarily of the hyperactive-impulsive type (ADHD/HI, meeting at least 6 of 9 hyperactive-impulsive behaviors)
- ADHD combined type (ADHD/C, meeting at least 6 of 9 behaviors in both the inattention and hyperactive-impulsive lists)

Children who meet diagnostic criteria for the behavioral symptoms of ADHD but who demonstrate no functional impairment do not meet the diagnostic criteria for ADHD.[13] The symptoms of ADHD should be present in 2 or more settings (eg, at home and in school), and the behaviors must adversely affect

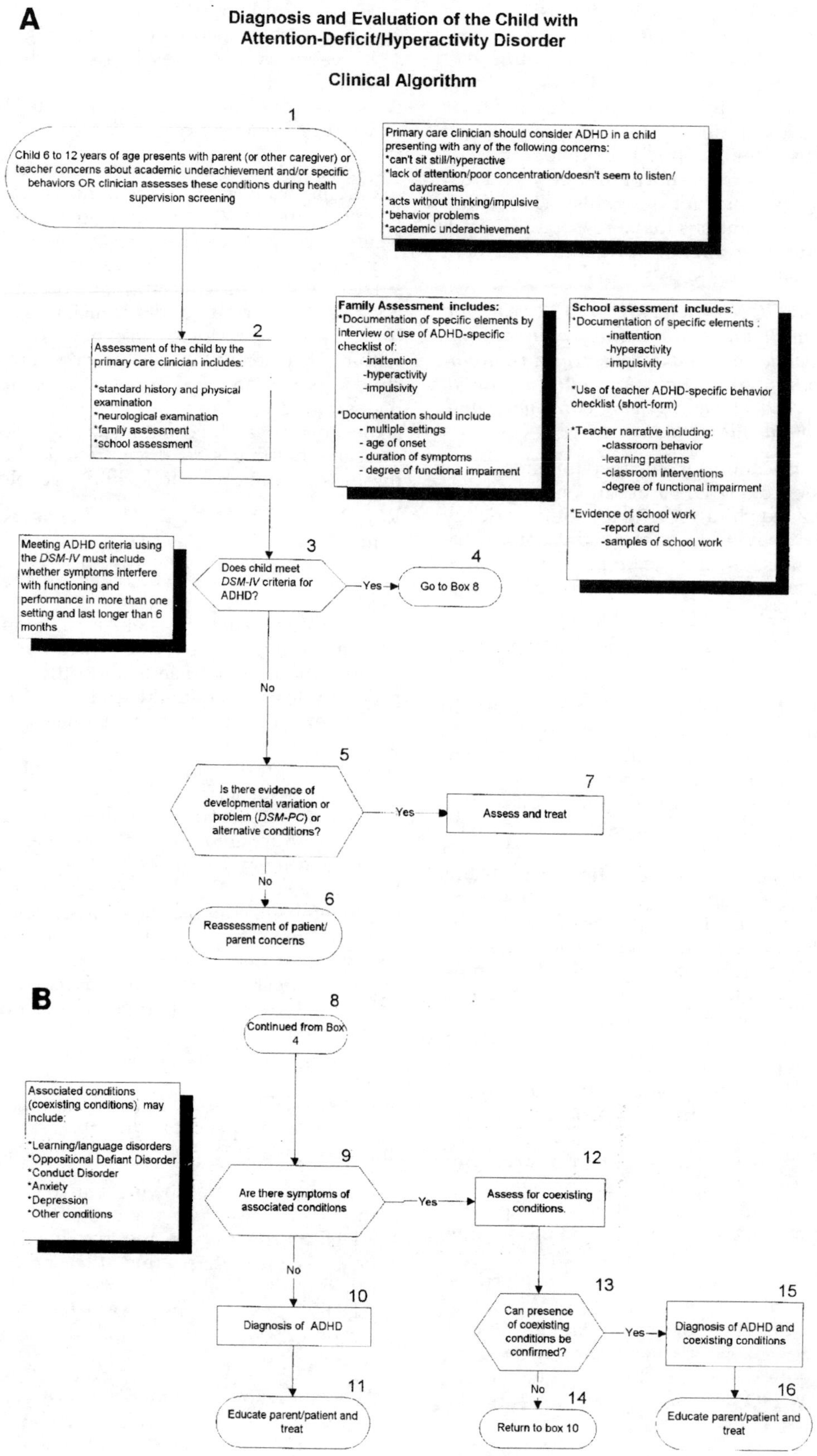

A

Diagnosis and Evaluation of the Child with Attention-Deficit/Hyperactivity Disorder

Clinical Algorithm

Fig 1. Clinical algorithm.

TABLE 1.   Diagnostic Criteria for ADHD

A. Either 1 or 2
    1) Six (or more) of the following symptoms of **inattention** have persisted for at least 6 months to a degree that is maladaptive and inconsistent with developmental level:

Inattention
        a) Often fails to give close attention to details or makes careless mistakes in schoolwork, work, or other activities
        b) Often has difficulty sustaining attention in tasks or play activities
        c) Often does not seem to listen when spoken to directly
        d) Often does not follow through on instructions and fails to finish schoolwork, chores, or duties in the workplace (not due to oppositional behavior or failure to understand instructions)
        e) Often has difficulty organizing tasks and activities
        f) Often avoids, dislikes, or is reluctant to engage in tasks that require sustained mental effort (such as schoolwork or homework)
        g) Often loses things necessary for tasks or activities (eg, toys, school assignments, pencils, books, or tools)
        h) Is often easily distracted by extraneous stimuli
        i) Is often forgetful in daily activities
    2) Six (or more) of the following symptoms of **hyperactivity-impulsivity** have persisted for at least 6 months to a degree that is maladaptive and inconsistent with developmental level:

Hyperactivity
        a) Often fidgets with hands or feet or squirms in seat
        b) Often leaves seat in classroom or in other situations in which remaining seated is expected
        c) Often runs about or climbs excessively in situations in which it is inappropriate (in adolescents or adults, may be limited to subjective feelings of restlessness)
        d) Often has difficulty playing or engaging in leisure activities quietly
        e) Is often "on the go" or often acts as if "driven by a motor"
        f) Often talks excessively

Impulsivity
        g) Often blurts out answers before questions have been completed
        h) Often has difficulty awaiting turn
        i) Often interrupts or intrudes on others (eg, butts into conversations or games)
B. Some hyperactive-impulsive or inattentive symptoms that caused impairment were present before 7 years of age.
C. Some impairment from the symptoms is present in 2 or more settings (eg, at school [or work] or at home).
D. There must be clear evidence of clinically significant impairment in social, academic, or occupational functioning.
E. The symptoms do not occur exclusively during the course of a pervasive developmental disorder, schizophrenia, or other psychotic disorder and are not better accounted for by another mental disorder (eg, mood disorder, anxiety disorder, dissociative disorder, or personality disorder).

Code based on type:
314.01 Attention-Deficit/Hyperactivity Disorder, Combined Type: if both criteria A1 and A2 are met for the past 6 months
314.00 Attention-Deficit/Hyperactivity Disorder, Predominantly Inattentive Type: if criterion A1 is met but criterion A2 is not met for the past 6 months
314.01 Attention-Deficit/Hyperactivity Disorder, Predominantly Hyperactive, Impulsive Type: if criterion A2 is met but criterion A1 is not met for the past 6 months
314.9 Attention-Deficit/Hyperactivity Disorder Not Otherwise Specified

Reprinted with permission from the *Diagnostic and Statistical Manual of Mental Disorders, 4th Ed. (DSM-IV)*. Copyright 1994. American Psychiatric Association.

functioning in school or in a social situation. Reliable and clinically valid measures of dysfunction applicable to the primary care setting have been difficult to develop. The diagnosis comes from a synthesis of information obtained from parents; school reports; mental health care professionals, if they have been involved; and an interview/examination of the child. Current *DSM-IV* criteria require evidence of symptoms before 7 years of age. In some cases, the symptoms of ADHD may not be recognized by parents or teachers until the child is older than 7 years of age, when school tasks become more challenging. Age of onset and duration of symptoms may be obtained from parents in the course of a comprehensive history.

Teachers, parents, and child health professionals typically encounter children with behaviors relating to activity, impulsivity, and attention who may not fully meet *DSM-IV* criteria. The *Diagnostic and Statistical Manual for Primary Care (DSM-PC), Child and Adolescent Version,*[39] provides a guide to the more common behaviors seen in pediatrics. The manual describes common variations in behavior, as well as more problematic behaviors, at levels less than those

specified in the *DSM-IV* (and with less impairment). The behavioral descriptions of the *DSM-PC* have not yet been tested in community studies to determine the prevalence or severity of developmental variations and moderate problems in the areas of inattention and hyperactivity or impulsivity. They do, however, provide guidance to clinicians in the evaluation of children with these symptoms and help to direct clinicians to many elements of treatment for children with problems with attention, hyperactivity, or impulsivity (Tables 2 and 3). The *DSM-PC* also considers environmental influences on a child's behavior and provides information on differential diagnosis with a developmental perspective.

Given the lack of methods to confirm the diagnosis of ADHD through other means, it is important to recognize the limitations of the *DSM-IV* definition. Most of the development and testing of the *DSM-IV* has occurred through studies of children seen in psychiatric settings. Much less is known about its use in other populations, such as those seen in general pediatric or family practice settings. Despite the agreement of many professionals working in this field, the *DSM-IV* criteria remain a consensus with-

TABLE 2.   *DSM-PC: Developmental Variation: Impulsive/Hyperactive Behaviors*

Developmental Variation	Common Developmental Presentations
V65.49 Hyperactive/impulsive variation Young children in infancy and in the preschool years are normally very active and impulsive and may need constant supervision to avoid injury. Their constant activity may be stressful to adults who do not have the energy or patience to tolerate the behavior. During school years and adolescence, activity may be high in play situations and impulsive behaviors may normally occur, especially in peer pressure situations. High levels of hyperactive/impulsive behavior do not indicate a problem or disorder if the behavior does not impair function.	*Early childhood* The child runs in circles, doesn't stop to rest, may bang into objects or people, and asks questions constantly. *Middle childhood* The child plays active games for long periods. The child may occasionally do things impulsively, particularly when excited. *Adolescence* The adolescent engages in active social activities (eg, dancing) for long periods, may engage in risky behaviors with peers.

	Special Information
	Activity should be thought of not only in terms of actual movement, but also in terms of variations in responding to touch, pressure, sound, light, and other sensations. Also, for the infant and young child, activity and attention are related to the interactions between the child and caregiver, eg, when sharing attention and playing together. Activity and impulsivity often normally increase when the child is tired or hungry and decrease when sources of fatigue or hunger are addressed. Activity normally may increase in new situations or when the child may be anxious. Familiarity then reduces activity. Both activity and impulsivity must be judged in the context of the caregiver's expectations and the level of stress experienced by the caregiver. When expectations are unreasonable, the stress level is high, and/or the parent has an emotional disorder (especially depression), the adult may exaggerate the child's level of activity/impulsivity. Activity level is a variable of temperature. The activity level of some children is on the high end of normal from birth and continues to be high throughout their development.

Taken from: American Academy of Pediatrics. *The Classification of Child and Adolescent Mental Diagnoses in Primary Care. Diagnostic and Statistical Manual for Primary Care (DSM-PC), Child and Adolescent Version.* Elk Grove Village, IL: American Academy of Pediatrics; 1996

out clear empirical data supporting the number of items required for the diagnosis. Current criteria do not take into account gender differences or developmental variations in behavior. Furthermore, the behavioral characteristics specified in the *DSM-IV*, despite efforts to standardize them, remain subjective and may be interpreted differently by different observers. Continuing research will likely clarify the validity of the *DSM-IV* criteria (and subsequent modifications) in the diagnosis. These complexities in the diagnosis mean that clinicians using *DSM-IV* criteria must apply them in the context of their clinical judgment.

No instruments used in primary care practice reliably assess the nature or degree of functional impairment of children with ADHD. With information obtained from the parent and school, the clinician can make a clinical judgment about the effect of the core and associated symptoms of ADHD on aca-

demic achievement, classroom performance, family and social relationships, independent functioning, self-esteem, leisure activities, and self-care (such as bathing, toileting, dressing, and eating).

The following 2 recommendations establish the presence of core behavior symptoms in multiple settings.

RECOMMENDATION 3: The assessment of ADHD requires evidence directly obtained from parents or caregivers regarding the core symptoms of ADHD in various settings, the age of onset, duration of symptoms, and degree of functional impairment (strength of evidence: good; strength of recommendation: strong).

Behavior symptoms may be obtained from parents or guardians using 1 or more methods, including open-ended questions (eg, "What are your concerns about your child's behavior in school?"), focused

TABLE 3.   *DSM-PC*: Developmental Variation: Inattentive Behaviors

Developmental Variation	Common Developmental Presentations
V65.49 Inattention variation A young child will have a short attention span that will increase as the child matures. The inattention should be appropriate for the child's level of development and not cause any impairment.	*Early childhood* The preschooler has difficulty attending, except briefly, to a storybook or a quiet task such as coloring or drawing. *Middle childhood* The child may not persist very long with a task the child does not want to do such as read an assigned book, homework, or a task that requires concentration such as cleaning something. *Adolescence* The adolescent is easily distracted from tasks he or she does not desire to perform.

	Special Information
	Infants and preschoolers usually have very short attention spans and normally do not persist with activities for long, so that diagnosing this problem in younger children may be difficult. Some parents may have a low tolerance for developmentally appropriate inattention. Although watching television cartoons for long periods of time appears to reflect a long attention span, it does not reflect longer attention spans because most television segments require short (2- to 3-minute) attention spans and they are very stimulating. Normally, attention span varies greatly depending upon the child's or adolescent's interest and skill in the activity, so much so that a short attention span for a particular task may reflect the child's skill or interest in that task.

Taken from: American Academy of Pediatrics. *The Classification of Child and Adolescent Mental Diagnoses in Primary Care. Diagnostic and Statistical Manual for Primary Care (DSM-PC), Child and Adolescent Version.* Elk Grove Village, IL: American Academy of Pediatrics; 1996

questions about specific behaviors, semi-structured interview schedules, questionnaires, and rating scales. Clinicians who obtain information from open-ended or focused questions must obtain and record the relevant behaviors of inattention, hyperactivity, and impulsivity from the *DSM-IV*. The use of global clinical impressions or general descriptions within the domains of attention and activity is insufficient to diagnose ADHD. As data are gathered about the child's behavior, an opportunity becomes available to evaluate the family environment and parenting style. In this way, behavioral symptoms may be evaluated in the context of the environment that may have important characteristics for a particular child.

Specific questionnaires and rating scales have been developed to review and quantify the behavioral characteristics of ADHD (Table 4). The ADHD-specific questionnaires and rating scales have been shown to have an odds ratio greater than 3.0 (equivalent to sensitivity and specificity greater than 94%) in studies differentiating children with ADHD from normal, age-matched, community controls.[24] Thus, ADHD-specific rating scales accurately distinguish between children with and without the diagnosis of ADHD. Almost all studies of these scales and checklists have taken place under ideal conditions, ie, comparing children in referral sites with apparently healthy children. These instruments may function less well in primary care clinicians' offices than indicated in the tables. In addition, questions on which these rating scales are based are subjective and subject to bias. Thus, their results may convey a false sense of validity and must be interpreted in the context of the overall evaluation of the child. Whether these scales provide additional benefit beyond careful clinical assessment informed by *DSM-IV* criteria is not known. *RECOMMENDA-TION 3A: Use of these scales is a clinical option when evaluating children for ADHD (strength of evidence: strong; strength of recommendation: strong).*

Global, nonspecific questionnaires and rating scales that assess a variety of behavioral conditions, in contrast with the ADHD-specific measures, generally have an odds ratio <2.0 (equivalent to sensitivity and specificity <86%) in studies differentiating children referred to psychiatric practices from children who were not referred to psychiatric practices (Table 5). Thus, these broadband scales do not distinguish well between children with and without ADHD. *RECOMMENDATION 3B: Use of broadband scales is not recommended in the diagnosis of children for ADHD, although they may be useful for other purposes (strength of evidence: strong; strength of recommendation: strong).*

TABLE 4.　　Total ADHD-Specific Checklists: Ability to Detect ADHD vs Normal Controls

Study	Behavior Rating Scale	Age	Gender	Effect Size	95% Confidence Limits
Conners (1997)	CPRS-R:L-ADHD Index (Conners Parent Rating Scale—1997 Revised Version: Long Form, ADHD Index Scale)	6–17	MF	3.1	2.5, 3.7
Conners (1997)	CTRS-R:L-ADHD Index (Conners Teacher Rating Scale— 1997 Revised Version: Long Form, ADHD Index Scale)	6–17	MF	3.3	2.8, 3.8
Conners (1997)	CPRS-R:L-*DSM-IV* Symptoms (Conners Parent Rating Scale—1997 Revised Version: Long Form, *DSM-IV* Symptoms Scale)	6–17	MF	3.4	2.8, 4.0
Conners (1997)	CTRS-R:L-*DSM-IV* Symptoms (Conners Teacher Rating Scale—1997 Revised Version: Long Form, *DSM-IV* Symptoms Scale)	6–17	MF	3.7	3.2, 4.2
Breen (1989)	SSQ-O-I Barkley's School Situations Questionnaire-Original Version, Number of Problem Settings Scale	6–11	F	1.3	0.5, 2.2
Breen (1989)	SSQ-O-II Barkley's School Situations Questionnaire-Original Version, Mean Severity Scale	6–11	F	2.0	1.0, 2.9
Combined				2.9	2.2, 3.5

Taken from: Green M, Wong M, Atkins D, et al. *Diagnosis of Attention Deficit/Hyperactivity Disorder. Technical Review 3.* Rockville, MD: US Department of Health and Human Services, Agency for Health Care Policy and Research; 1999. AHCPR publication 99-0050

TABLE 5.　　Total Scales of Broadband Checklists: Ability to Detect Referred vs Nonreferred

Study	Behavior Rating Scale	Age	Gender	Effect Size	95% Confidence Limits
Achenbach (1991b)	CBCL/4-18-R, Total Problem Scale (Child Behavior Checklist for Ages 4–18, Parent Form)	4–11	M	1.4	1.3, 1.5
Achenbach (1991b)	Same as above	4–11	F	1.3	1.2, 1.4
Achenbach (1991c)	CBCL/TRF-R, Total Problem Scale (Child Behavior Checklist, Teacher Form)	5–11	M	1.2	1.0, 1.4
Achenbach (1991c)	Same as above	5–11	F	1.1	1.0, 1.3
Naglieri, LeBuffe, Pfeiffer (1994)	DSMD-Total Scale (Devereaux Scales of Mental Disorders)	5–12	MF	1.0	0.8, 1.3
Conners (1997)	CPRS-R:L-Global Problem Index (1997 Revision of Conners Parent Rating Scale, Long Version)	—	MF	2.3	1.9, 2.6
Conners (1997)	CTRS-R:L-Global Problem Index (1997 Revision of Conners Teacher Rating Scale, Long Version)	—	MF	2.0	1.7, 2.3
Combined				1.5	1.2, 1.8

Taken from: Green M, Wong M, Atkins D, et al. *Diagnosis of Attention Deficit/Hyperactivity Disorder. Technical Review 3.* Rockville, MD: US Department of Health and Human Services, Agency for Health Care Policy and Research; 1999. AHCPR publication 99-0050.

More research is needed on the use of the ADHD-specific and global rating scales in pediatric practices for the purposes of differentiating children with ADHD from other children with different behavior or school problems.

RECOMMENDATION 4: The assessment of ADHD requires evidence directly obtained from the classroom teacher (or other school professional) regarding the core symptoms of ADHD, the duration of symptoms, the degree of functional impairment, and coexisting conditions. A physician should review any reports from a school-based multidisciplinary evaluation where they exist, which will include assessments from the teacher or other school-based professional (strength of evidence: good; strength of recommendation: strong).

The evaluation of ADHD must establish whether core behavior symptoms of inattention, hyperactivity, and impulsivity are present in >1 setting to meet *DSM-IV* criteria for the condition. Children 6 to 12 years of age generally are students in an elementary school setting, where they spend a substantial proportion of waking hours. Therefore, a description of their behavioral characteristics in the school setting is highly important to the evaluation. With permission from the legal guardian, the clinician should review a report from the child's school. The classroom teacher typically has more information about the child's behavior than do other professionals at the school and, when possible, should provide the report. Alternatively, a school counselor or principal often is helpful in coordinating the teacher's reporting and may be able to provide the required information.

Behavior symptoms may be obtained using 1 or more methods such as verbal narratives, written narratives, questionnaires, or rating scales. Clinicians who obtain information from narratives or interviews must obtain and record the relevant behaviors of inattention, hyperactivity, and impulsivity from the *DSM-IV*. The use of global clinical impressions or general descriptions within the domains of attention and activity is insufficient to diagnose ADHD.

The ADHD-specific questionnaires and rating scales also are available for teachers (Table 4). Teacher ADHD-specific questionnaires and rating scales have been shown to have an odds ratio >3.0 (equivalent to sensitivity and specificity greater than 94%) in studies differentiating children with ADHD from normal peers in the community.[24] Thus, teacher ADHD-specific rating scales accurately distinguish between children with and without the diagnosis of ADHD. Whether these scales provide additional benefit beyond narratives or descriptive interviews informed by *DSM-IV* criteria is not known. *RECOMMENDATION 4A: Use of these scales is a clinical option when diagnosing children for ADHD (strength of evidence: strong; strength of recommendation: strong).*

Teacher global questionnaires and rating scales that assess a variety of behavioral conditions, in contrast with the ADHD-specific measures, generally have an odds ratio <2.0 (equivalent to sensitivity and specificity <86%) in studies differentiating children referred to psychiatric practices from children who were not referred to psychiatric practices (Table 5). Thus, these broadband scales do not distinguish between children with and without ADHD. *RECOMMENDATION 4B: Use of teacher global questionnaires and rating scales is not recommended in the diagnosing of children for ADHD, although they may be useful for other purposes (strength of evidence: strong; strength of recommendation: strong).*

If a child 6 to 12 years of age routinely spends considerable time in other structured environments such as after-school care centers, additional information about core symptoms can be sought from professionals in those settings, contingent on parental permission. The ADHD-specific questionnaires may be used to evaluate the child's behavior in these settings. For children who are educated in their homes by parents, evidence of the presence of core behavior symptoms in settings other than the home should be obtained as an essential part of the evaluation.

Frequently there are significant discrepancies between parent and teacher ratings.[40] These discrepancies may be in either direction; symptoms may be reported by teachers and not parents or vice versa. These discrepancies may be attributable to differences between the home and school in terms of expectations, levels of structure, behavioral management strategies, and/or environmental circumstances. The finding of a discrepancy between the parents and teachers does not preclude the diagnosis of ADHD. A helpful clinical approach for understanding the sources of the discrepancies and whether the child meets *DSM-IV* criteria is to obtain additional information from other informants, such as former teachers, religious leaders, or coaches.

RECOMMENDATION 5: Evaluation of the child with ADHD should include assessment for coexisting conditions (strength of evidence: strong; strength of recommendation: strong).

A variety of other psychological and developmental disorders frequently coexist in children who are being evaluated for ADHD. As many as one third of children with ADHD have 1 or more coexisting conditions (Table 6). Although the primary care clinician may not always be in a position to make a precise diagnosis of coexisting conditions, consideration and examination for such a coexisting condition should be an integral part of the evaluation. A review of all coexisting conditions (such as motor disabilities, problems with parent-child interaction, or family violence) is not possible within the scope of this review. More common psychological disorders include conduct and oppositional defiant disorder, mood disorders, anxiety disorders, and learning disabilities. The pediatrician should also consider ADHD as a coexisting condition when considering these other conditions. Evidence for most of these coexisting disorders may be readily detected by the primary care clinician. For example, frequent sadness and preference for isolated activities may alert the physician to the presence of depressive symptoms, whereas a family history of anxiety disorders coupled with a patient history characterized by frequent fears and difficulties with separation from caregivers may be suggestive of symptoms associated with an anxiety disorder. Several screening tests are available that can detect areas of concern for many of the mental health disorders that coexist with ADHD. Although these scales have not been tested for use in primary care settings and are not diagnostic tests for either ADHD or associated mental health conditions, some clinicians may find them useful to establish high risk for coexisting psychological conditions. Similarly, poor school performance may indicate a learning disability. Testing may be required to determine whether a discrepancy exists between the child's learning potential (intelligence quotient) and his actual academic progress (achievement test scores), indicating the presence of a learning disability. Most studies of rates of coexisting conditions have come from referral populations. The following data generally reflect the relatively small number of studies from community or primary care settings.

TABLE 6. Summary of Prevalence of Selected Coexisting Conditions in Children With ADHD

Comorbid Disorder	Estimated Prevalence (%)	Confidence Limits for Estimated Prevalence (%)
Oppositional defiant disorder	35.2	27.2, 43.8
Conduct disorder	25.7	12.8, 41.3
Anxiety disorder	25.8	17.6, 35.3
Depressive disorder	18.2	11.1, 26.6

Taken from: Green M, Wong M, Atkins D, et al. *Diagnosis of Attention Deficit/Hyperactivity Disorder. Technical Review* 3. Rockville, MD: US Dept of Health and Human Services. Agency for Health Care Policy and Research; 1999. AHCPR publication 99-0050

Conduct Disorder and Oppositional Defiant Disorder

Oppositional defiant or conduct disorders coexist with ADHD in ~35% of children.[24] The diagnostic features of conduct disorder include "a repetitive and persistent pattern of behavior in which the basic rights of others or major age-appropriate social norms or rules are violated."[13] Oppositional defiant disorder (a less severe condition) includes persistent symptoms of "negativistic, defiant, disobedient, and hostile behaviors toward authority figures."[13] Frequently, children and adolescents with persisting oppositional defiant disorder later develop symptoms of sufficient severity to qualify for a diagnosis of conduct disorder. Longitudinal follow-up for children with conduct disorders that coexist with ADHD indicates that these children fare more poorly in adulthood relative to their peers diagnosed with ADHD alone.[41] For example, 1 study has reported the highest rates of police contacts and self-reported delinquency in children with ADHD and coexisting conduct disorder (30.8%) relative to their peers diagnosed with ADHD alone (3.4%) or conduct disorder alone (20.7%). Preliminary studies suggest that these coexisting conditions are more frequent in children with the predominantly hyperactive-impulsive and combined subtypes.[25,26]

Mood Disorders/Depression

The coexistence of ADHD and mood disorders (eg, major depressive disorder and dysthymia) is ~18%.[39] Frequently, the family history of children with ADHD includes other family members with a history of major depressive disorder.[42] In addition, children who have coexisting ADHD and mood disorders also may have a poorer outcome during adolescence relative to their peers who do not have this pattern of co-occurrence.[43] For example, adolescents with coexisting mood disorders and ADHD are at increased risk for suicide attempts.[44] Preliminary studies suggest that these coexisting conditions are more frequent in children with the predominantly inattentive and combined subtypes.[25,26]

Anxiety

The coexisting association between ADHD and anxiety disorders has been estimated to be ~25%.[24] In addition, the risk for anxiety disorders among relatives of children and adolescents diagnosed with ADHD is higher than for typically developing children, although some research suggests that ADHD and anxiety disorders transmit independently from families.[45] In either case, it is important to obtain a careful family history. Preliminary studies suggest that these coexisting conditions are more frequent in children with the predominantly inattentive and combined subtypes.[25,26]

Learning Disabilities

Only 1 published study examined the coexistence of ADHD and learning disabilities in children evaluated in general pediatric settings using *DSM-IV* criteria for the diagnosis of ADHD.[46] The prevalence of learning disabilities as a coexisting condition can-

not be determined in the same manner as other psychological disorders because studies have employed dimensional (looking at the condition on a spectrum) rather than categorical diagnoses. Rates of learning disabilities that coexist with ADHD in settings other than primary care have been reported to range from 12% to 60%.[24]

To date, no definitive data describe the differences among groups of children with different learning disabilities coexisting with ADHD in the areas of sociodemographic characteristics, behavioral and emotional functioning, and response to various interventions. Nonetheless, the subgroup of children with learning disabilities, compared with their ADHD peers who do not have a learning disability, is most in need of special education services. Preliminary studies suggest that these coexisting conditions are more frequent in children with the predominantly inattentive and combined subtypes.[25,26]

***RECOMMENDATION 6:** Other diagnostic tests are not routinely indicated to establish the diagnosis of ADHD (strength of evidence: strong; strength of recommendation: strong).*

Other diagnostic tests contribute little to establishing the diagnosis of ADHD. A few older studies have indicated associations between blood lead levels and child behavior symptoms, although most studies have not.[47–49] Although lead encephalopathy in younger children may predispose to later behavior and developmental problems, very few of these children will have elevated lead levels at school age. Thus, regular screening of children for high lead levels does not aid in the diagnosis of ADHD.

Studies have shown no significant associations between abnormal thyroid hormone levels and the presence of ADHD.[50–52] Children with the rare disorder of generalized resistance to thyroid hormone have higher rates of ADHD than other populations, but these children demonstrate other characteristics of that condition. This association does not argue for routine screening of thyroid function as part of the effort to diagnose ADHD.

Brain imaging studies and electroencephalography do not show reliable differences between children with ADHD and controls. Although some studies have demonstrated variation in brain morphology comparing children with and without ADHD, these findings do not discriminate reliably between children with and without this condition. In other words, although group means may differ significantly, the overlap in findings among children with and without ADHD creates high rates of false-positives and false-negatives.[53–55] Similarly, some studies have indicated higher rates of certain electroencephalogram abnormalities among children with ADHD,[56–58] but again the overlap between children with and without ADHD and the lack of consistent findings among multiple reports indicate that current literature do not support the routine use of electroencephalograms in the diagnosis of ADHD.

Continuous performance tests have been designed to obtain samples of a child's behavior (generally measuring vigilance or distractibility), which may correlate with behaviors associated with ADHD. Several such tests have been developed and tested, but all of these have low odds ratios (all <1.2, equivalent to a sensitivity and specificity <70%) in studies differentiating children with ADHD from normal comparison controls.[24,45,59,60] Therefore, current data do not support the use of any available continuous performance tests in the diagnosis of ADHD.

AREAS FOR FUTURE RESEARCH

The research issues pertaining to the diagnosis of ADHD relate to the diagnostic criteria themselves as well as the methods used to establish the diagnosis. The *DSM-IV* has helped to define behavioral criteria for ADHD more specifically. Although research has established the dimensional concepts of inattention and hyperactivity-impulsivity, further research is required to validate these subtypes. Because most of the existing research has been conducted with referred convenience samples, primarily in psychiatric settings, further research is required to determine whether the findings of previous research are generalizable to the type of children currently diagnosed and treated by primary care clinicians. Although the current *DSM-IV* criteria are appropriate for the age range included in this guideline, there is, as yet, inadequate information about its applicability to individuals younger or older than the age range for this guideline. Further research should clarify the developmental course of ADHD symptomatology. An additional difficulty for primary care is that existing evidence indicates that the behaviors used in making a *DSM-IV* diagnosis of ADHD fall on a spectrum. Currently, decisions about the inappropriateness of the behaviors in children depend on subjective judgments of observers/reporters. There are no data to offer precise estimates of when diagnostic behaviors become inappropriate. This is particularly problematic to primary care clinicians, who care for a number of patients who fit into borderline or gray areas. The inadequacy of research on this aspect is central to the issue of which children should be diagnosed with ADHD and treated with stimulant medication. Further research using normative or community-based samples to develop more valid and precise diagnostic criteria is essential.

The diagnostic process is also an area requiring further research. Because no pathognomonic findings currently establish the diagnosis, further research should examine the utility of existing methods, with the goal of developing a more definitive process. Specific examples include the need for additional information about the reliability and validity of teacher and parent rating scales and the reliability and validity of different interviewing methods. Further, given the prominence of impairment in the current diagnostic requirements, it is imperative to develop and assess better measurements of impairment that can be applied practically in the primary care setting. The research into diagnostic methods also should include those methods helpful in identifying clinically relevant coexisting conditions.

Lastly, research is required to identify more clearly the current practices of primary care physicians beyond using self-report. Such research is critical in determining the practicality of guideline recommendations as a method to determine changes in practice and to determine whether changes have an actual impact on the treatment and outcome of children with the diagnosis of ADHD.

CONCLUSION

This guideline offers recommendations for the diagnosis and evaluation of school-aged children with ADHD in primary care practice. The guideline emphasizes: 1) the use of explicit criteria for the diagnosis using *DSM-IV* criteria; 2) the importance of obtaining information regarding the child's symptoms in more than 1 setting and especially from schools; and 3) the search for coexisting conditions that may make the diagnosis more difficult or complicate treatment planning. The guideline further provides current evidence regarding various diagnostic tests for ADHD. It should help primary care providers in their assessment of a common child health problem.

ACKNOWLEDGMENTS

The Practice Guideline, "Diagnosis and Evaluation of the Child With Attention-Deficit/Hyperactivity Disorder," was reviewed by appropriate committees and sections of the AAP, including the Chapter Review Group, a focus group of office-based pediatricians representing each AAP District: Gene R. Adams, MD; Robert M. Corwin, MD; Diane Fuquay, MD; Barbara M. Harley, MD; Thomas J. Herr, MD, Chair Person; Kenneth E. Mathews, MD; Robert D. Mines, MD; Lawrence C. Pakula, MD; Howard B. Weinblatt, MD; and Delosa A. Young, MD. The Practice Guideline was also reviewed by relevant outside medical organizations as part of the peer review process as well as by several patient advocacy organizations.

REFERENCES

1. Reiff MI, Banez GA, Culbert TP. Children who have attentional disorders: diagnosis and evaluation. *Pediatr Rev.* 1993;14:455–465
2. Barkley RA. *Attention Deficit Hyperactivity Disorder: A Handbook for Diagnosis and Treatment.* 2nd ed. New York, NY: Guilford Press; 1996
3. Zentall SS. Research on the educational implications of attention deficit hyperactivity disorder. *Exceptional Child.* 1993;60:143–153
4. Schachar R, Taylor E, Wieselberg MB, Ghorley G, Rutter M. Changes in family functioning and relationships in children who respond to methylphenidate. *J Am Acad Child Adolesc Psychiatry.* 1987;26:728–732
5. Almond BW Jr, Tanner JL, Goffman HF. *The Family Is the Patient: Using Family Interviews in Children's Medical Care.* 2nd ed. Baltimore, MD: Williams & Wilkins; 1999:307–313
6. Biederman J, Faraone SV, Milberger S, et al. Predictors of persistence and remissions of ADHD into adolescence: results from a four-year prospective follow-up study. *J Am Acad Child Adolesc Psychiatry.* 1996; 35:343–351
7. Biederman J, Faraone SV, Spencer T, et al. Patterns of psychiatric comorbidity, cognition, and psychosocial functioning in adults with attention deficit hyperactivity disorder. *Am J Psychiatry.* 1993;150: 1792–1798
8. Baumgaertel A, Copeland L, Wolraich ML. Attention deficit-hyperactivity disorder. In: *Disorders of Development and Learning: A Practical Guide to Assessment and Management.* 2nd ed. St Louis, MO: Mosby Yearbook, Inc; 1996:424–456
9. Cantwell DP. Attention deficit disorder: a review of the past 10 years. *J Am Acad Child Adolesc Psychiatry.* 1996;35:978–987
10. American Psychiatric Association. *Diagnostic and Statistical Manual for Mental Disorders.* 2nd ed. Washington, DC: American Psychiatric Association; 1967
11. American Psychiatric Association. *Diagnostic and Statistical Manual for Mental Disorders.* 3rd ed. Washington, DC: American Psychiatric Association; 1980
12. American Psychiatric Association. *Diagnostic and Statistical Manual for Mental Disorders-Revised.* 3rd ed. Washington, DC: American Psychiatric Association; 1987
13. American Psychiatric Association. *Diagnostic and Statistical Manual for Mental Disorders.* 4th ed. Washington, DC: American Psychiatric Association; 1994
14. Drug Enforcement Agency. Washington, DC (personal communication)
15. August GJ, Garfinkel BD. Behavioral and cognitive subtypes of ADHD. *J Am Acad Child Adolesc Psychiatry.* 1989;28:739–748
16. August GJ, Realmuto GM, MacDonald AW III, Nugent SM, Crosby R. Prevalence of ADHD and comorbid disorders among elementary school children screened for disruptive behavior. *J Abnorm Child Psychol.* 1996; 24:571–595
17. Bird H, Canino G, Rubio-Stipec M, et al. Estimates of the prevalence of childhood maladjustment in a community survey in Puerto Rico. *Arch Gen Psychiatry.* 1988;45:1120–1126
18. Cohen P, Cohen J, Kasen S, Velez CN. An epidemiological study of disorders in late childhood and adolescence I: age and gender-specific prevalence. *J Child Psychol Psychiatry.* 1993;34:851–867
19. King C, Young RD. Attentional deficits with and without hyperactivity: teacher and peer perceptions. *J Abnorm Child Psychol.* 1982;10:483–495
20. Kuperman S, Johnson B, Arndt S, Lingren S, Wolraich M. Quantitative EEG differences in a nonclinical sample of children with ADHD and undifferentiated ADD. *J Am Acad Child Adolesc Psychiatry.* 1996;35: 1009–1017
21. Newcorn J, Halperin JM, Schwartz S, et al. Parent and teacher ratings of attention-deficit hyperactivity disorder symptoms: implications for case identification. *J Dev Behav Pediatr.* 1994;15:86–91
22. Shaffer D, Fisher P, Dulcan MK, et al. The NIMH Diagnostic Interview Schedule for Children Version 2.3 (DISC-2.3): description, acceptability,

prevalence rates, and performance in the MECA study. Methods for the Epidemiology of Child and Adolescent Mental Disorders Study. *J Am Acad Child Adolesc Psychiatry.* 1996;35:865–877
23. Shekim WO, Kashani J, Beck N, et al. The prevalence of attention deficit disorders in a rural midwestern community sample of nine-year-old children. *J Am Acad Child Adolesc Psychiatry.* 1985;24:765–770
24. Green M, Wong M, Atkins D, et al. *Diagnosis of Attention Deficit/Hyperactivity Disorder: Technical Review 3.* Rockville, MD: US Department of Health and Human Services, Agency for Health Care Policy and Research; 1999. Agency for Health Care Policy and Research publication 99-0050
25. Wolraich ML, Hannah JN, Pinnock TY, Baumgaertel A, Brown J. Comparison of diagnostic criteria for attention deficit/hyperactivity disorder in a county-wide sample. *J Am Acad Child Adolesc Psychiatry.* 1996; 35:319–324
26. Wolraich M, Hannah JN, Baumgaertel A, Pinnock TY, Feurer I. Examination of *DSM-IV* criteria for attention deficit/hyperactivity disorder in a county-wide sample. *J Dev Behav Pediatr.* 1998;19:162–168
27. Gibbs N. Latest on Ritalin. *Time.* 1998;152:86–96
28. Safer DJ, Zito JM, Fine EM. Increased methylphenidate usage for attention deficit disorder in the 1990s. *Pediatrics.* 1996;98:1084–1088
29. Rappley MD, Gardiner JC, Jetton JR, Houang RT. The use of methylphenidate in Michigan. *Arch Pediatr Adolesc Med.* 1995;149:675–679
30. Wolraich ML, Lindgren S, Stromquist A, et al. Stimulant medication use by primary care physicians in the treatment of attention deficit hyperactivity disorder. *Pediatrics.* 1990;86:95–101
31. Mulhern S, Dworkin PH, Bernstein B. Do parental encounters predict a diagnosis of attention deficit hyperactivity disorder? *J Dev Behav Pediatr.* 1994;15:348–352
32. Wasserman R, Kelleher KJ, Bocian A, et al. Identification of attentional and hyperactivity problems in primary care: a report from Pediatric Research in Office Settings and the Ambulatory Sentinel Practice Network. *Pediatrics.* 1999;103(3). URL: http://www.pediatrics.org/cgi/content/full/103/3/e38
33. Sleator EK, Ullmann RK. Can the physician diagnose hyperactivity in the office? *Pediatrics.* 1981;67:13–17
34. American Academy of Pediatrics. *Guidelines for Health Supervision III.* 3rd ed. Elk Grove Village, IL: American Academy of Pediatrics; 1997
35. Green M, ed. National Center for Education in Maternal and Child Health. *Bright Futures: Guidelines for Health Supervision of Infants, Children, and Adolescents.* Arlington, VA: National Center for Education in Maternal and Child Health; 1994
36. Stein MT. Preparing families for the toddler and preschool years. *Contemp Pediatr.* 1998;15:88
37. Dixon S, Stein M. *Encounters With Children: Pediatric Behavior and Development.* 3rd ed. St Louis, MO: Mosby; 1999
38. McBurnett K, Pfiffner LJ, Willcutt E, et al. Experimental cross-validation of *DSM-IV* types of attention-deficit/hyperactivity disorder. *J Am Acad Child Adolesc Psychiatry.* 1999;38:17–24
39. American Academy of Pediatrics. *The Classification of Child and Adolescent Mental Diagnoses in Primary Care: Diagnostic and Statistical Manual for Primary Care (DSM-PC) Child and Adolescent Version.* Elk Grove Village, IL: American Academy of Pediatrics; 1996
40. Lahey BB, McBurnett K, Piacentini JC, et al. Agreement of parent and teacher rating scales with comprehensive clinical assessments of attention deficit disorder with hyperactivity. *J Psychopathol Behav Assess.* 1987;9:429–439
41. Ingrams S, Hechtman L, Morganstern G. Outcome issues in ADHD: adolescent and adult long term outcome. In: *Mental Retardation and Developmental Disabilities.* In press
42. Biederman J, Milberger S, Farone SV, Guite J, Warburton R. Associations between childhood asthma and ADHD: issues of psychiatric comorbidity and familiarity. *J Am Acad Child Adolesc Psychiatry.* 1994;33: 842–848
43. Biederman J, Newcorn PJ, Sprich S. Comorbidity of attention deficit hyperactivity disorder with conduct, depressive, anxiety, and other disorders. *Am J Psychiatry.* 1991;148:564–577
44. Brent DA, Perper JA, Goldstein CE, Kolko DJ, Zelenak JP. Risk factors for adolescent suicide: a comparison of adolescent suicide victims with suicidal inpatients. *Arch Gen Psychiatry.* 1988;45:581–588
45. Faraone SV, Biederman J, Mennin D, Gershon J, Tsuang MT. A prospective four-year follow-up study of children at risk for ADHD: psychiatric, neuropsychological, and psychosocial outcome. *J Am Acad Child Adolesc Psychiatry.* 1996;35:1449–1459
46. August GJ, Garfinkel BD. Behavioral and cognitive subtypes of ADHD. *J Am Acad Child Adolesc Psychiatry.* 1989;28:739–748
47. Kahn CA, Kelly PC, Walker WO Jr. Lead screening in children with

attention deficit hyperactivity disorder and developmental delay. *Clin Pediatr (Phila)*. 1995;34:498–501

48. Tuthill RW. Hair lead levels related to children's classroom attention-deficit behavior. *Arch Environ Health*. 1996;51:214–220

49. Gittelman R, Eskenazi B. Lead and hyperactivity revisited: an investigation of non-disadvantaged children. *Arch Gen Psychiatry*. 1983;40: 827–833

50. Elia J, Gulotta C, Rose SR, Marin G, Rapoport JL. Thyroid function and attention-deficit hyperactivity disorder. *J Am Acad Child Adolesc Psychiatry*. 1994;33:169–172

51. Spencer T, Biederman J, Wilens T, Guite J, Harding M. ADHD and thyroid abnormalities: a research note. *J Child Psychol Psychiatry*. 1995; 36:879–885

52. Weiss RE, Stein MA, Trommer B, Refetoff S. Attention-deficit hyperactivity disorder and thyroid function. *J Pediatr*. 1993;123:539–545

53. Shaywitz BA, Shaywitz SE, Byrne T, Cohen DJ, Rothman S. Attention deficit disorder: quantitative analysis of CT. *Neurology*. 1983;33: 1500–1503

54. Castellanos FX, Giedd JN, Marsh WL, et al. Quantitative brain magnetic resonance imaging in attention-deficit hyperactivity disorder. *Arch Gen Psychiatry*. 1996;53:607–616

55. Lyoo IK, Noam GG, Lee CK, et al. The corpus callosum and lateral ventricles in children with attention-deficit hyperactivity disorder: a brain magnetic resonance imaging study. *Biol Psychiatry*. 1996;40: 1060–1063

56. Matsuura M, Okubo Y, Toru M, et al. A cross-national EEG study of children with emotional and behavioral problems: a WHO collaborative study in the Western Pacific Region. *Biol Psychiatry*. 1993;34:59–65

57. Lahat E, Avital E, Barr J, et al. BAEP studies in children with attention deficit disorder. *Dev Med Child Neurol*. 1995;37:119–123

58. Kuperman S, Johnson B, Arndt S, et al. Quantitative EEG differences in a nonclinical sample of children with ADHD and undifferentiated ADD. *J Am Acad Child Adolesc Psychiatry*. 1996;35:1009–1017

59. Seidel WT, Joschko M. Assessment of attention in children. *Clin Neuropsychology*. 1991;5:53–66

60. Dykman RA, Ackerman PT. Attention deficit disorder and specific reading disability: separate but often overlapping disorders. *J Learn Disabil*. 1991;24:96–103

Treatment of the School-Aged Child With Attention-Deficit/Hyperactivity Disorder

- *Clinical Practice Guideline*

AMERICAN ACADEMY OF PEDIATRICS

Subcommittee on Attention-Deficit/Hyperactivity Disorder

Committee on Quality Improvement

Clinical Practice Guideline: Treatment of the School-Aged Child With Attention-Deficit/Hyperactivity Disorder

ABSTRACT. This clinical practice guideline provides evidence-based recommendations for the treatment of children diagnosed with attention-deficit/hyperactivity disorder (ADHD). This guideline, the second in a set of policies on this condition, is intended for use by clinicians working in primary care settings. The initiation of treatment requires the accurate establishment of a diagnosis of ADHD; the American Academy of Pediatrics (AAP) clinical practice guideline on diagnosis of children with ADHD[1] provides direction in appropriately diagnosing this disorder.

The AAP Committee on Quality Improvement selected a subcommittee composed of primary care and developmental-behavioral pediatricians and other experts in the fields of neurology, psychology, child psychiatry, education, family practice, and epidemiology. The subcommittee partnered with the Agency for Healthcare Research and Quality and the Evidence-based Practice Center at McMaster University, Ontario, Canada, to develop the evidence base of literature on this topic.[2] The resulting systematic review, along with other major studies in this area, was used to formulate recommendations for treatment of children with ADHD. The subcommittee also reviewed the multimodal treatment study of children with ADHD[3] and the Canadian Coordinating Office for Health Technology Assessment report (CCOHTA).[4] Subcommittee decisions were made by consensus where definitive evidence was not available. The subcommittee report underwent extensive review by sections and committees of the AAP as well as by numerous external organizations before approval from the AAP Board of Directors.

The guideline contains the following recommendations for the treatment of a child diagnosed with ADHD:

- Primary care clinicians should establish a treatment program that recognizes ADHD as a chronic condition.
- The treating clinician, parents, and child, in collaboration with school personnel, should specify appropriate target outcomes to guide management.
- The clinician should recommend stimulant medication and/or behavior therapy as appropriate to improve target outcomes in children with ADHD.
- When the selected management for a child with ADHD has not met target outcomes, clinicians should evaluate the original diagnosis, use of all appropriate treatments, adherence to the treatment plan, and presence of coexisting conditions.
- The clinician should periodically provide a systematic follow-up for the child with ADHD. Monitoring should be directed to target outcomes and adverse effects, with information gathered from parents, teachers, and the child.

This guideline is intended for use by primary care clinicians for the management of children between 6 and 12 years of age with ADHD. In light of the high prevalence of ADHD in pediatric practice, the guideline should assist primary care clinicians in treatment. Although many of the recommendations here also may apply to children with coexisting conditions, this guideline primarily addresses children with ADHD but without major coexisting conditions. The guideline is not intended for use in the treatment of children with mental retardation, pervasive developmental disorder, moderate to severe sensory deficits such as visual and hearing impairment, chronic disorders associated with medications that may affect behavior, and those who have experienced child abuse and sexual abuse. This guideline is not intended as a sole source of guidance for the treatment of children with ADHD. Rather, it is designed to assist the primary care clinician by providing a framework for decision-making. It is not intended to replace clinical judgment or to establish a protocol for all children with this condition, and may not provide the only appropriate approach to this problem.

ABBREVIATIONS. AAP, American Academy of Pediatrics; ADHD, attention-deficit/hyperactivity disorder; DSM-IV, Diagnostic and Statistical Manual of Mental Disorders, Fourth Edition; MTA, multimodal treatment study of children with ADHD; CCOHTA, Canadian Coordinating Office for Health Technology Assessment.

The American Academy of Pediatrics (AAP) recognizes the importance of accurate diagnosis and management of children with attention-deficit/hyperactivity disorder (ADHD). The AAP developed a practice guideline for the diagnosis of ADHD among children from 6 to 12 years of age who are evaluated by primary care clinicians.[1] The significant components of the diagnostic guideline include 1) the use of explicit criteria for the diagnosis using the *Diagnostic and Statistical Manual of Mental Health Disorders, Fourth Edition (DSM-IV)* criteria[5]; 2) the importance of obtaining information about the child's symptoms in more than 1 setting (especially from schools); and 3) the search for coexisting conditions that may make the diagnosis more difficult or complicate treatment planning.

This guideline is based on an extensive review of the medical, psychological, and educational literature. The objectives of the literature review were to determine the long- and short-term effectiveness and safety of pharmacological and nonpharmacological interventions for ADHD in children from 6 to 12 years of age, and to compare single treatment methods (eg, medications alone) with combined management strategies. Two systematic, evidence-based reviews were used extensively in the development of this guideline.[2,4] In addition, other resources were used to gather more information.[6,7]

Primary care clinicians cannot work alone in the treatment of school-aged children with ADHD. Ongoing communication with parents, teachers, and other school-based professionals is necessary to monitor the progress and effectiveness of specific interventions. Parents are key partners in the management plan as sources of information and as the child's primary caregiver. Integration of services with psychologists, child psychiatrists, neurologists, educational specialists, developmental-behavioral pediatricians, and other mental health professionals may be appropriate for children with ADHD who have coexisting conditions and may continue to have problems in functioning despite treatment. Attention to the child's social development in community settings other than school requires clinical knowledge of a variety of activities and services in the community.

METHODOLOGY

The AAP collaborated with several organizations to develop a working subcommittee representing a wide range of primary care and subspecialty groups. The subcommittee, chaired by 2 general pediatricians, included representatives from the American Academy of Family Physicians, the American Academy of Child and Adolescent Psychiatry, the Child Neurology Society, the Society for Pediatric Psychology, the Society for Developmental and Behavioral Pediatrics, and the Society for Developmental Pediatrics.

This subcommittee met over a period of 3 years, during which it reviewed basic literature on current practices in the treatment of children with ADHD. The subcommittee developed a series of research questions to direct an extensive evidence-based review, in partnership with the Agency for Healthcare Research and Quality.

In 1997, the McMaster University Evidence-based Practice Center received the contract for reviewing the literature related to treatment of children with ADHD. The McMaster report[2] focused on the evidence from comparative studies on the effectiveness and safety of pharmacological and nonpharmacological interventions for ADHD in children and adults and whether combined interventions are more effective than individual interventions. This resulted in several questions in the following 7 areas: 1) studies with drug-to-drug comparisons of pharmacological interventions; 2) placebo-controlled studies evaluating the effect of tricyclic antidepressants; 3) studies comparing pharmacological and nonpharmacological interventions; 4) studies evaluating the effect of long-term therapies; 5) studies evaluating therapies for ADHD in adults (ie, those older than 18 years of age); 6) studies evaluating therapies given in

combination; and 7) studies evaluating adverse effects of pharmacological interventions.

Several systematic reviews and meta-analyses have examined placebo-controlled trials of stimulant medication and have established the short-term efficacy of these agents for core symptoms. Placebo-controlled trials of stimulant medication were reviewed in the McMaster report only if they met the criteria for inclusion in any of the other 6 areas. The report also focused on head-to-head comparisons of pharmacological interventions and of pharmacological and nonpharmacological interventions because these were identified as of prime interest to clinicians.

The McMaster report of the literature on treatment of ADHD followed current standards for analyzing research evidence.[2] Studies in this report were selected for evaluation if they were randomized, controlled trials that focused on the treatment of ADHD in humans and if they were published in peer-reviewed journals. Nonrandomized, controlled trials were included only if they provided data on adverse effects that were collected for more than 16 weeks. Studies of multiple conditions that included separate analyses for patients with ADHD were also included. The literature search was conducted using MEDLINE (from 1966), CINAHL (from 1982), HEALTHStar (from 1975), PsycINFO (from 1984), and EMBASE (from 1984). The Cochrane Library (issue 4, 1997) was also used in reviewing the literature. A total of 2405 citations were identified by the search strategies, and 92 reports, describing 78 different studies, were identified for further analysis.

In addition to the McMaster report, other sources of data were used to support clinical practice guideline recommendations. Although the McMaster report included results of the multimodal treatment study of children with ADHD (MTA),[3,7] the subcommittee also carefully evaluated the results of this large study separately.[8–16] The subcommittee used data from the Canadian Coordinating Office for Health Technology Assessment (CCOHTA) study.[4] The CCOHTA review addressed the following 3 major issues related to treatment of children with ADHD: 1) a clinical evaluation of the use of methylphenidate for ADHD; 2) the efficacy of stimulant medications and other therapies; and 3) an economic evaluation of the pharmacological and behavioral therapies for ADHD. Many studies of behavioral interventions for ADHD use crossover techniques, where effects were determined on the same children when they did and did not receive treatment.[6,17] The McMaster report excluded these crossover trials.[2]

The draft clinical practice guideline underwent extensive peer review by committees and sections within the AAP, numerous outside organizations, and other individuals identified by the subcommittee. Liaisons to the subcommittee were also invited to distribute the draft to entities within their organizations. Comments were compiled and reviewed by the subcommittee cochairpersons, and relevant changes were incorporated into the guideline.

The recommendations contained in this guideline (see Fig 1) are based on the best available data. For

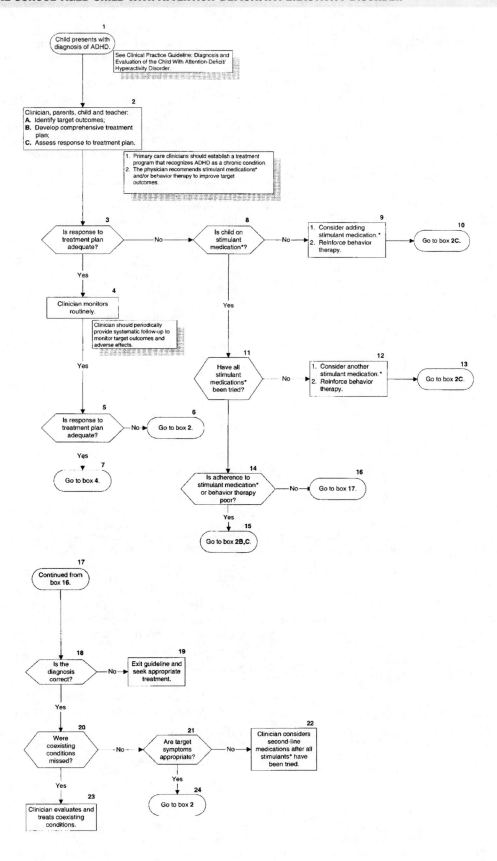

Fig 1. Algorithm for the treatment of the school-aged child with Attention-Deficit/Hyperactivity Disorder.

each recommendation, the subcommittee graded the *quality of evidence* on which the recommendation was based and the *strength* of the recommendation. Grades of evidence were grouped into 3 categories—good, fair, or poor. Recommendations were made at 3 levels. Strong recommendations were based on high-quality scientific evidence or, in the absence of high-quality data, strong expert consensus. Fair and weak recommendations were based on lesser quality or limited data and expert consensus. Clinical options are identified as interventions for which the subcommittee could not find compelling evidence for or against. Clinical options are defined as interventions that a reasonable health care provider might or might not wish to implement in his or her practice.

RECOMMENDATION 1: Primary care clinicians should establish a management program that recognizes ADHD as a chronic condition (strength of evidence: good; strength of recommendation: strong).

Attention-deficit/hyperactivity disorder is one of the more common chronic conditions of childhood. Studies using parent reports indicate persistence of ADHD of 60% to 80% into adolescence.[18–20] Given the high prevalence of ADHD among school-aged children (4% to 12%),[1] primary care clinicians will encounter children with ADHD in their practices regularly and should have a strategy for diagnosis and long-term management of this condition. The primary care of children with ADHD includes attention to the main principles of care for children with any chronic condition, such as

- Providing information about the condition
- Updating and monitoring family knowledge and understanding on a periodic basis
- Counseling about family response to the condition
- Developmentally appropriate education of the child about ADHD, with updates as the child grows
- Availability to answer family questions
- Ensuring coordination of health and other services
- Helping families set specific goals in areas related to the child's condition and its effects on daily activities
- Linking families with other families with children who have similar chronic conditions as needed and available[21–26]

As with other chronic conditions, treatment of ADHD requires the development of child-specific treatment plans that describe methods and goals of treatment and means of monitoring care over time, including specific plans for follow-up (See Recommendation 5.)

Primary care clinicians should educate parents and children about the ways in which ADHD can affect learning, behavior, self-esteem, social skills, and family function. This initial phase of patient education is critical to demystifying the diagnosis and providing parents and children with knowledge about the condition. Education enables parents to work with clinicians, educators, and, in some cases, mental health

professionals to develop an effective treatment plan. A therapeutic alliance among clinicians, parents, and the child is enhanced when attention is directed toward cultural values that affect the child's health and health care. The long-term care of a child with ADHD requires an ongoing partnership among clinicians, parents, teachers, and the child. Other school personnel—nurses, psychologists, and counselors—can also help with developing and monitoring plans.

Studies of children and adults with several chronic conditions indicate better adherence to treatment plans, improved health and disease status measures, and higher levels of satisfaction in the context of a comprehensive treatment plan with specific goals, follow-up activities, and monitoring.[27–28] Thus, careful attention to the key elements of chronic care can lead to improved outcomes for children and families.

Activities specific to the care of children with ADHD include providing current information on the etiology of ADHD, its treatment, long-term outcomes, and effects on daily life and family activities. Thorough family understanding of the problem is essential before discussing treatment options and side effects. What distinguishes this condition from most other chronic conditions managed by primary care clinicians is the important role that the education system plays in the treatment and monitoring of children with ADHD.

Like other chronic conditions, new research on ADHD will change the information available to parents and clinicians over time and fill many gaps in diagnosing and understanding the etiology, treatment, long-term effects, and complications related to ADHD. Families should have access to this information. In addition, national, grassroots, parent-run associations provide support and/or education to caregivers and families of individuals with ADHD (eg, Children and Adults with Attention-Deficit/Hyperactivity Disorder [CHADD]). The clinician should be aware of community resources that provide these services and know how to make referrals. Primary care providers may offer this information directly or collaborate with other providers, especially subspecialists and mental health providers, to ensure families' access to needed information.

RECOMMENDATION 2: The treating clinician, parents, and the child, in collaboration with school personnel, should specify appropriate target outcomes to guide management (strength of evidence: good; strength of recommendation: strong).

The core symptoms of ADHD (ie, inattention, impulsivity, hyperactivity) can result in multiple areas of dysfunction relating to a child's performance in the home, school, or community. The primary goal of treatment should be to maximize function. Desired results include

- improvements in relationships with parents, siblings, teachers, and peers
- decreased disruptive behaviors
- improved academic performance, particularly in volume of work, efficiency, completion, and accuracy

- increased independence in self-care or homework
- improved self-esteem
- enhanced safety in the community, such as in crossing streets or riding bicycles. Target outcomes should follow from the key symptoms the child manifests and the specific impairments these symptoms cause.

The process of developing target outcomes requires input from parents, children, and teachers, as well as other school personnel where available and appropriate.[29] They should agree on at least 3 to 6 key targets and desired changes as prerequisites to constructing the treatment plan. The goals should be realistic, attainable, and measurable. The methods of treatment and of monitoring change will vary as a function of the target outcomes.

RECOMMENDATION 3: The clinician should recommend stimulant medication (strength of evidence: good) and/or behavior therapy (strength of evidence: fair), as appropriate, to improve target outcomes in children with ADHD (strength of recommendation: strong).

The clinician should develop a comprehensive management plan focused on the target outcomes. For most children, stimulant medication is highly effective in the management of the core symptoms of ADHD. For many children, behavioral interventions are valuable as primary treatment or as an adjunct in the management of ADHD, based on the nature of coexisting conditions, specific target outcomes, and family circumstances.

Stimulant Medication

Many studies have documented the efficacy of stimulants in reducing the core symptoms of ADHD. In many cases, stimulant medication also improves the child's ability to follow rules and decreases emotional overreactivity, thereby leading to improved relationships with peers and parents. Three formal meta-analyses[30-32] and 1 review of reviews[33] support the short-term efficacy of stimulant medications in reducing core symptoms of ADHD as well as improving function in a number of domains. The most powerful effects[4] are found on measures of observable social and classroom behaviors and on core symptoms of attention, hyperactivity, and impulsivity.* The effects on intelligence and achievement tests are more modest. Most studies of stimulants have been short-term, demonstrating efficacy over several days or weeks. The MTA study extends the demonstrated efficacy to 14 months.[3] In that study, 579 children 7 to 9.9 years of age with ADHD were randomized to 4 treatment groups: medication management alone, medication and behavior management, behavior management alone, and a standard community care group. The medication management groups followed specific protocols and algorithms in

distinction to routine community practice based on clinicians' best judgments. School-aged children with ADHD showed a marked reduction in core ADHD symptoms over a 14-month period when they were treated with medication management alone or a combination of medication and behavior management. Eighty-five percent of the children treated with medication received a stimulant medication.[3] Despite the efficacy of stimulant medications in improving behaviors, many children who receive them do not demonstrate fully normal behavior (eg, only 38% of medically managed children in the MTA study received scores in the normal range at 1-year follow-up). Although the MTA study demonstrated that efficacy of stimulants lasts at least to 14 months, the longer term effects of stimulants remain unclear, attributable in part to methodologic difficulties in other studies.[35]

Stimulant medications currently available include short-, intermediate-, and long-acting methylphenidate, and short-, intermediate-, and long-acting dextroamphetamine. The latter 2 formulations are mixed amphetamine salts (75% dextroamphetamine and 25% levoamphetamine). Pemoline, a long-acting stimulant, is rarely used now because of its rare but potentially fatal hepatotoxicity.[36] Primary care clinicians should not use it routinely, and this guideline does not include it as a first- or second-line treatment for ADHD. Table 1 indicates available medications and their doses. The McMaster report reviewed 22 studies and showed no differences comparing methylphenidate with dextroamphetamine or among different forms of these stimulants.[2] Each stimulant improved core symptoms equally. Individual children, however, may respond to one of the stimulants but not to another. Recommended stimulants require no serologic, hematologic, or electrocardiogram monitoring. Current evidence supports the use of only 2 other medications for ADHD, tricyclic antidepressants[2] and bupropion.[37] Nine studies carefully evaluated tricyclic antidepressants (6 evaluated desipramine, 3 evaluated imipramine); all indicated positive effects on ADHD symptoms.[2] Four trials comparing tricyclic antidepressants with methylphenidate indicated either no differences in response or slightly better results with stimulant use.[2] The use of nonstimulant medications falls outside this practice guideline, although clinicians should select tricyclic antidepressants after the failure of 2 or 3 stimulants and only if they are familiar with their use. Desipramine use has been associated, in rare cases, with sudden death.[38] Clonidine, one of the antihypertensive drugs occasionally used in the treatment of ADHD, also falls outside the scope of this guideline. Limited studies of clonidine indicate that it is better than placebo in the treatment of core symptoms (although with effect sizes lower than those for stimulants). Its use has been documented mainly in children with ADHD and coexisting conditions, especially sleep disturbances.[39,40]

Detailed instructions for determining the dose and schedule of stimulant medications are beyond the scope of this guideline. However, a few basic principles guide the available clinical options.

---

*The effect size for classroom and social behavior in the CCOHTA meta-analysis averaged 0.81; for core symptoms, 0.78; and for intelligence and achievement, 0.34. The first two of these would be considered a large change, the third, a minor to moderate change.[34]

TABLE 1.　　　Medications Used in the Treatment of Attention-Deficit/Hyperactivity Disorder

Generic Class (Brand Name)	Daily Dosage Schedule	Duration	Prescribing Schedule
Stimulants (First-Line Treatment)			
Methylphenidate			
Short-acting	Twice a day (BID) to 3	3–5 hr	5–20 mg BID to TID
(Ritalin, Metadate, Methylin)	times a day (TID)		
Intermediate-acting	Once a day (QD) to	3–8 hr	20–40 mg QD or 40 mg in the
(Ritalin SR, Metadate ER, Methylin ER)	BID		morning and 20 early afternoon
Extended Release	QD	8–12 hr	18–72 mg QD
(Concerta, Metadate CD, Ritalin LA*)			
Amphetamine			
Short-acting	BID to TID	4–6 hr	5–15 mg BID or 5–10 mg TID
(Dexedrine, Dextrostat)			
Intermediate-acting	QD to BID	6–8 hr	5–30 mg QD or 5–15 mg BID
(Adderall, Dexedrine spansule)			
Extended Release	QD		10–30 mg QD
(Adderall-XR*)			
Antidepressants (Second-Line Treatment)			
Tricyclics (TCAs)	BID to TID		2–5 mg/kg/day†
Imipramine, Desipramine			
Bupropion			
(Wellbutrin)	QD to TID		50–100 mg TID
(Wellbutrin SR)	BID		100–150 mg BID

* Not FDA approved at time of publication.
† Prescribing and monitoring information in *Physicians' Desk Reference.*

Unlike most other medications, stimulant dosages usually are not weight dependent. Clinicians should begin with a low dose of medication and titrate upward because of the marked individual variability in the dose-response relationship. The first dose that a child's symptoms respond to may not be the best dose to improve function. Clinicians should continue to use higher doses to achieve better responses.[3] This strategy may require reducing the dose when a higher dose produces side effects or no further improvement. The best dose of medication for a given child is the one that leads to optimal effects with minimal side effects. The dosing schedules vary depending on target outcomes, although no consistent controlled studies compare different dosing schedules. For example, if there is a need for relief of symptoms only during school, a 5-day schedule may be sufficient. By contrast, a need for relief of symptoms at home and school suggests a 7-day schedule.

Stimulants are generally considered safe medications, with few contraindications to their use. Side effects occur early in treatment and tend to be mild and short-lived.[35] The most common side effects are decreased appetite, stomachache or headache, delayed sleep onset, jitteriness, or social withdrawal. Most of these symptoms can be successfully managed through adjustments in the dosage or schedule of medication. Approximately 15% to 30% of children experience motor tics, most of which are transient, while on stimulant medications. In addition, approximately half of children with Tourette syndrome have ADHD. The effects of medication on tics are unpredictable. The presence of tics before or during medical management of ADHD is not an absolute contraindication to the use of stimulant medications.[41,42] A review of 7 studies comparing stimulants with placebo or with other medications indicated no increase in tics in children treated with stimulants.[2]

According to the *Physicians' Desk Reference*[43] and medication package insert, methylphenidate is contraindicated in children with seizure disorders, a history of seizure disorder, or abnormal electroencephalograms. Studies of the use of methylphenidate have not, however, demonstrated an increase in seizure frequency or severity when it is added to appropriate anticonvulsant medications.[44–46]

Children who receive too high a dose or who are overly sensitive may become overfocused on the medication or appear dull or overly restricted. Many times this side effect can be addressed by lowering the dose. Rarely, with high doses, some children experience psychotic reactions, mood disturbances, or hallucinations.

No consistent reports of behavioral rebound, motor tics, or dose-related growth delays have been found in controlled studies,[47] although they are reported clinically.[33] Appetite suppression and weight loss are common side effects of stimulant medication, with no apparent difference between methylphenidate and dextroamphetamine. Concern for growth delay has been raised, but a prospective follow-up study into adult life[48] has found no significant impairment of height attained. Studies of stimulant use have found little or no decrease in expected height, with any decrease in growth early in treatment compensated for later on.[49–54] Many clinicians recommend drug holidays during summers, although no controlled trials exist to indicate whether holidays have gains or risks, especially related to weight gain.

3A: For children on stimulants, if one stimulant does not work at the highest feasible dose, the clinician should recommend another.

At least 80%[3] of children will respond to one of the stimulants if they are tried in a systematic way. Children who fail to show positive effects or who experience intolerable side effects on one stimulant medication should be tried on another of the recommended stimulant medications. The reasons for this recommendation include the following:

- The finding that most children who fail to respond to one medication will have a positive response to an alternative stimulant
- The safety and efficacy of stimulants in the treatment of ADHD compared with nonstimulant medications
- The numerous crossover trials that indicate the efficacy of different stimulants in the same child[2,4]
- The idiosyncratic responses to medication[55]

Children who fail 2 stimulant medications can be tried on a third type or formulation of stimulant medication for the same reason. (As indicated in Recommendation 4, lack of response to treatment also should lead clinicians to assess the accuracy of the diagnosis and the possibility of undiagnosed co-existing conditions.)

Behavior Therapy

Behavior therapy represents a broad set of specific interventions that have a common goal of modifying the physical and social environment to alter or change behavior. Along with behavior therapy, most clinicians, parents, and schools address a variety of changes in the child's home and school environment, including more structure, closer attention, and limitations of distractions. Such environmental modifications have not undergone careful efficacy assessment, but most treatment plans include them.

Behavior therapy usually is implemented by training parents and teachers in specific techniques of improving behavior. Behavior therapy then involves providing rewards for demonstrating the desired behavior (eg, positive reinforcement) or consequences for failure to meet the goals (eg, punishment). Repetitive application of the rewards and consequences gradually shapes behavior. Although behavior therapy shares a set of principles, it includes different techniques with many of the strategies often combined into a comprehensive program.

Behavior therapy should be differentiated from psychological interventions directed to the child and designed to change the child's emotional status (eg, play therapy) or thought patterns (eg, cognitive therapy or cognitive-behavior therapy). Although these psychological interventions have great intuitive appeal, they have little documented efficacy in the treatment of children with ADHD,[56] and gains achieved in the treatment setting usually do not transfer into the classroom or home. By contrast, parent training in behavior therapy and classroom behavior interventions have successfully changed the behavior of children with ADHD.[6]

Parent training typically begins with 8 to 12 weekly group sessions with a trained therapist. The focus is on the child's behavior problems and difficulties in family relationships. A typical program aims to improve the parents' or caregivers' understanding of the child's behavior and teaching them skills to deal with the behavioral difficulties posed by ADHD. Programs offer specific techniques for giving commands, reinforcing adaptive and positive social behavior, and decreasing or eliminating inappropriate behavior. Programs plan for maintenance and relapse prevention. Parent training improves the child's functioning and decreases disruptive behavior but (as with stimulant medications) does not necessarily bring the behavior of a child with ADHD into the normal range on parent rating scales.[56,57]

Classroom management also focuses on the child's behavior and may be integrated into classroom routines for all students or targeted for a selected child in the classroom. Classroom management often begins with increasing the structure of activities. Systematic rewards and consequences, including point systems or use of token economy (see Table 2), are included to increase appropriate behavior and eliminate inappropriate behavior. A periodic (often daily) report card can record the child's progress or performance with regard to goals and communicate the child's progress to the parents, who then provide reinforcers or consequences based on that day's performance. Classroom behavior management also may improve a child's functioning but may not bring the child's behavior into the normal range on teacher behavior rating scales.[57] Table 2 outlines specific behavior therapies that have been demonstrated as effective for ADHD.[17]

Evidence for the effectiveness of behavior therapy in children with ADHD comes from a variety of studies. The diversity of interventions and outcome

TABLE 2. Effective Behavioral Techniques for Children With Attention-Deficit/Hyperactivity Disorder

Technique	Description	Example
Positive reinforcement	Providing rewards or privileges contingent on the child's performance.	Child completes an assignment and is permitted to play on the computer.
Time-out	Removing access to positive reinforcement contingent on performance of unwanted or problem behavior.	Child hits sibling impulsively and is required to sit for 5 minutes in the corner of the room.
Response cost	Withdrawing rewards or privileges contingent on the performance of unwanted or problem behavior.	Child loses free time privileges for not completing homework.
Token economy	Combining positive reinforcement and response cost. The child earns rewards and privileges contingent on performing desired behaviors and loses the rewards and privileges based on undesirable behavior.	Child earns stars for completing assignments and loses stars for getting out of seat. The child cashes in the sum of stars at the end of the week for a prize.

measures makes meta-analysis of the effects of behavior therapy alone or in association with medications very difficult. Double-blind, randomized, placebo-controlled trials are difficult to perform, in part because of the difficulty of keeping examiners and participants unaware of whether the child is receiving treatment or placebo. Thus, the usual evidence-based medicine searches turn up few studies for review.[2] Alternative experimental methods, such as rigorous single-subject designs, are used frequently in the psychological literature. Studies that compare the behavior of children during periods on and off behavior therapy demonstrate the effectiveness of behavior therapy[17]; however, behavior therapy has been demonstrated to be effective only while it is implemented and maintained.

A number of individual studies indicate positive effects of behavior therapy in addition to medications. Almost all studies comparing behavior therapy with stimulants alone indicate a much stronger effect from stimulants than from behavior therapy. When comparing behavior therapy to stimulant medications, efficacy of their combined treatment could not be demonstrated to be greater than medication alone for the core symptoms of ADHD.[2] The MTA study[3] found that the combined treatment (medication management with behavior therapy), compared with medication alone, offered improved scores on academic measures, measures of conduct, and some specific ADHD symptoms (although not on global ADHD symptom scales). Although these trends were consistent, few reached statistical significance. In addition, parents and teachers of children receiving combined therapy were significantly more satisfied with the treatment plan.[13,14,58-60]

A wide range of clinicians, including psychologists, school personnel, community mental health therapists, or the primary care clinician, can implement behavior therapy directly or train others to implement behavior therapy. Many clinicians prefer to refer to community resources for behavior therapy because behavior therapy with parents is time-consuming and often does not lend itself to the structure and schedule of the primary care office. Schools may provide behavior therapy with teachers in the context of a Rehabilitation Act (Section 504) plan or an individual education plan. Where ADHD has a significant impact on a child's educational abilities, Section 504 requires schools to make classroom adaptations to help children with ADHD function in that setting. Adaptations may include preferential seating, decreased assignment and homework load, and behavior therapy implemented by the teacher.

RECOMMENDATION 4: When the selected management for a child with ADHD has not met target outcomes, clinicians should evaluate the original diagnosis, use of all appropriate treatments, adherence to the treatment plan, and presence of coexisting conditions (strength of evidence: weak; strength of recommendation: strong).

Most school-aged children with ADHD respond to a therapeutic regimen that includes stimulant medications and/or behavioral/environmental interventions. As noted in 3A, when one stimulant medication appears ineffective (despite appropriate titration), clinicians should carry out a trial of a second stimulant medication. Continuing lack of response to treatment may reflect 1) unrealistic target symptoms; 2) lack of information about the child's behavior; 3) an incorrect diagnosis; 4) a coexisting condition affecting the treatment of the ADHD; 5) lack of adherence to the treatment regimen; or 6) a treatment failure. As discussed previously, treatment of ADHD, while decreasing a child's level of impairment, may not fully eliminate the core symptoms of inattention, hyperactivity, and impulsivity. Similarly, children with ADHD may continue to have difficulties with peer relationships despite adequate treatment, and treatment for ADHD frequently shows no association with improvements in academic achievement as measured by standardized instruments.

Evaluation of treatment outcomes requires a careful collection of information from multiple sources, including parents, teachers, other adults in the child's environment (eg, coaches), and the child. If the target symptoms are realistic and the lack of effectiveness is clear, the primary care clinician should reassess the accuracy of the diagnosis of ADHD. This reassessment should include review of the data initially obtained to make the diagnosis, as described in the AAP clinical practice guideline for the diagnosis of children with ADHD.[1] Reassessment usually will require gathering new information from the child, school, and family about the core symptoms of ADHD and their impact on the child's functioning. Clinicians should reconsider other conditions that can mimic ADHD.

As indicated in the diagnostic clinical practice guideline,[1] other conditions commonly accompany ADHD in children, especially oppositional/conduct disorders, anxiety, depression, and learning disorders. These conditions often complicate the treatment of ADHD; clinicians should determine if children who do not respond to treatment have these conditions, either by direct determination in their offices or by referral to appropriate subspecialists (eg, developmental-behavioral pediatricians, child psychiatrists, psychologists, or other mental health clinicians) or the school system (eg, school psychologists for learning disabilities) for further evaluation. These coexisting conditions may not have been fully evaluated initially because of the severity of the ADHD, or the child may have developed another condition with time. Standard psycho-educational testing may clarify the role of learning and language disorders, although other disorders require different assessments.

Treatment plans for ADHD typically require children, families, and schools to enter into a long-term plan that includes a complex medication schedule along with environmental and behavioral interventions. Environmental and behavioral interventions will require ongoing efforts by parents, teachers, and the child. A common cause of nonresponse to treatment is lack of adherence to the treatment plan.

Ongoing monitoring of a child's progress should assess the implementation of the plan and determine key problems with, and barriers to, implementation. The clinician should assess adherence to medication and behavior therapy. Lack of adherence is not the equivalent of treatment failure; clinicians should help families find solutions to adherence problems before considering a plan as a failure.

The following can be considered true treatment failure: 1) lack of response to 2 or 3 stimulant medications at maximum dose without side effects or at any dose with intolerable side effects; 2) inability of behavioral therapy or combination therapy to control the child's behaviors; and 3) the interference of a coexisting condition. In each of these situations, referral to mental health specialists who are knowledgeable about behavioral interventions in children is the next step unless the primary care clinician has expertise and experience in managing these situations.

RECOMMENDATION 5: The clinician should periodically provide a systematic follow-up for the child with ADHD. Monitoring should be directed to target outcomes and adverse effects by obtaining specific information from parents, teachers, and the child (strength of evidence: fair; strength of recommendation: strong).

Clinicians should establish a plan for periodic monitoring of the effects of treatment. Research on adherence to medical regimens in chronic diseases highlights the importance of identifying patient and family concerns and goals and jointly designing a management plan in a way that addresses these concerns and promotes these goals.[61] Plans should include obtaining information about target behaviors, educational output, and medication side effects periodically through office visits, written reports, and phone calls. Monitoring data should include the date of refills, the medication type, dosage, frequency, quantity, and responses to treatment (both medication and behavior therapy). Data can be recorded in a flow sheet, ideally, or in a progress note within each patient's chart. The plan also should include a system for communication among parent, child, and clinician between visits as well as a method for periodic contact with the teacher or other school personnel before a follow-up visit. The monitoring plan should consider normal developmental changes in behavior over time, educational expectations that increase with each grade, and the dynamic nature of a child's home and school environment, because changes in any of these factors may alter target behaviors. All participants should share the plan agenda. Clinicians should provide information and support at frequent intervals in a way that enables the child and family to make informed decisions that promote the child's long-term health and well-being.

Information about target symptoms will continue to come from the parents, child, and teacher. Office interviews, telephone conversations, teacher narratives, and periodic behavior report cards and checklists are among the methods used to obtain needed information. As with the diagnosis of ADHD, clinicians should have active and direct communication with schools. The MTA study indicates the benefit of teacher information over parent-derived information when titrating the medication to maximum benefit.[3,62] Adherence to medication and the behavior therapy program should be reviewed at each encounter.

The frequency of monitoring depends on the degree of dysfunction, complications, and adherence. No controlled trials clearly document the appropriate frequency of follow-up visits. In the MTA trial, children in the medical management groups had better outcomes and more frequent follow-up than those in the standard community category, but whether the frequency of follow-up was a determining factor in outcomes cannot be determined from currently published materials.[3] Once the child is stable, an office visit every 3 to 6 months allows for assessment of learning and behavior. These visits also allow assessment of potential side effects of stimulants, such as decreased appetite and alteration of weight, height, and growth velocity. Periodic requests for medication refills offer an additional opportunity for communication with the family. At the refill request, the family can be asked about the child's functioning in school and interpersonal relationships, as well as updates on communication from the school. If any of the follow-up evaluations reveal a decrease in the targeted outcomes, the clinician must first establish that the family is adhering to the treatment plan.

AREAS FOR FUTURE RESEARCH

Tailoring Treatments to Children and Outcomes

At the present time, the clinician's initial choice of a specific treatment program—the exact stimulant medication and the precise form of behavior therapy—is an area of uncertainty. Research to date has not shown clear advantages of one stimulant medication over others. The process of prescribing an effective and comprehensive plan based on the characteristics of the child and family and tailored in terms of type, intensity, and frequency would help clinicians to improve treatment plans. What is required is information relating specific sociodemographic characteristics (eg, age or sex) or clinical characteristics (eg, subtype of ADHD) to optimal responses to stimulant medication or type of behavior therapy. Moreover, relating treatments to specific behaviors or components of ADHD rather than the whole symptom complex would allow the clinician to better tailor the treatment plan.

Many children with ADHD have coexisting conditions, including anxiety, depression, oppositional defiant disorder, conduct disorder, and learning disabilities. The literature provides minimal information about how to treat these coexisting conditions in conjunction with ADHD and how the conditions affect the effectiveness and safety of treatments. Research on how ADHD and coexisting conditions interact to affect treatment and outcomes will help determine if children require multiple concurrent treatments. Such studies can identify sensible, effective, and comprehensive treatment plans for children with these conditions.

Expanded Treatment Options

A major research challenge pertaining to the treatment of ADHD is the development and evaluation of new treatments for this condition. The 2 current treatments (stimulant medication and behavior therapy) reduce the symptoms and functional consequences of ADHD, but only for as long as they are administered. Treatments with more lasting or even curative effects are needed. A significant number of children do not respond to stimulant medications or have severe side effects. Some families cannot implement behavioral programs. Expanding the available medical and behavioral treatment regimens with additional safe and effective options would be useful for such a prevalent chronic condition where not all children respond to current treatments or adhere to them. Studying common-sense approaches, such as decreasing environmental distraction, should be done. There is also the need for well-designed rigorous studies of currently promoted but less well-established therapies such as occupational therapy, biofeedback, herbs, vitamins, and food supplements. These interventions are not supported by evidence-based studies at the present time.

Long-term Outcomes

Most studies about ADHD and its treatment have been short-term. The long-term outcome of children with ADHD with or without coexisting conditions has not been well studied. Furthermore, there is minimal information about the role of stimulant medication and/or behavior therapy in the natural history of the disorder. Future research should correct these deficits. For this chronic condition, efficacy and safety studies must be extended from weeks or months to years. Long-term outcome studies must be prospective in design and consider changes over time in core symptoms of ADHD, coexisting conditions, and functional outcomes such as occupational successes and long-term relationships.

Service Delivery

Another major research area should address the optimal services and procedures for successful management of ADHD in the real world (ie, in clinical practice and classrooms). Much of the popular controversy over the inappropriate use of stimulant medication relates to how clinicians actually prescribe them. Future research needs to study how medications are actually prescribed and what factors affect physician practice patterns. Research that includes monitoring the outcomes of training will lead to the ability to develop better methods to assist clinicians in using effective treatment practices. Specifically, basic information such as who are the most appropriate clinicians to manage ADHD; the best schedule for follow-up; and the most valid, reliable, sensitive, and cost-effective ways to monitor treatment is essential. Such research must go beyond physician self-reporting and into scrutinizing and evaluating actual practices in clinics and offices. The

most effective and efficient methods for affecting change in clinician practices need to be determined. This determination must be broad, taking into account clinician, practice, family, community, and policy issues that affect treatment. Research also should evaluate the role of school- and community-based professionals, as well as primary care clinicians, in delivering treatment services. Little is known about how short- or long-term effectiveness varies as a function of the school and community-based professional involvement. Further, the studies of service delivery need to include a public health and service system approach. They should consider child and family outcomes and cost-effectiveness of care. Linking outcomes to service parameters is an important step in encouraging practice or system change.

Epidemiology and Etiology

The great growth in the diagnosis of ADHD has led to major new work in the study of treatments. As indicated previously, these efforts should continue and expand. Less investigation has addressed the etiology of ADHD (ie, its biological and socioenvironmental causes) and the opportunities arising from that understanding for prevention. For example, would different social and behavioral arrangements in young families affect the onset of ADHD symptoms? Would early intervention in some way decrease rates of ADHD? A clear need exists for active work in understanding the etiology and prevention of ADHD.

CONCLUSION

This clinical practice guideline offers recommendations for the treatment of school-aged children with ADHD in primary care practice. The guideline emphasizes 1) consideration of ADHD as a chronic condition; 2) explicit negotiations about target symptoms; 3) use of stimulant medication and behavior therapy; and 4) close monitoring of treatment outcomes and failures. The guideline further provides suggestions for pediatric office-based management of ADHD. It should help primary care clinicians in their treatment of a common child health problem.

SUBCOMMITTEE ON
  ATTENTION-DEFICIT/HYPERACTIVITY DISORDER
James M. Perrin, MD, Cochairperson
Martin T. Stein, MD, Cochairperson
Robert W. Amler, MD
Thomas A. Blondis, MD
Heidi M. Feldman, MD, PhD
Bruce P. Meyer, MD
Bennett A. Shaywitz, MD
Mark L. Wolraich, MD

CONSULTANTS
Anthony DeSpirito, MD
Charles J. Homer, MD, MPH
Esther Wender, MD

LIAISON REPRESENTATIVES
Ronald T. Brown, PhD
  Society for Pediatric Psychology

Theodore G. Ganiats, MD
    American Academy of Family Physicians
Brian Grabert, MD
    Child Neurology Society
Karen Pierce, MD
    American Academy of Child and Adolescent
    Psychiatry

STAFF
Carla T. Herrerias, BS, MPH

COMMITTEE ON QUALITY IMPROVEMENT
Charles J. Homer, MD, MPH, Chairperson
Richard D. Baltz, MD
Gerald B. Hickson, MD
Paul V. Miles, MD
Thomas B. Newman, MD, MPH
Joan E. Shook, MD
William M. Zurhellen, MD

LIAISON REPRESENTATIVES
Betty A. Lowe, MD
    National Association of Children's Hospitals
    and Related Institutions
Ellen Schwalenstocker, MBA
    National Association of Children's Hospitals
    and Related Institutions
Michael J. Goldberg, MD
    Council on Sections
Richard Shiffman, MD
    Section on Computers and Other
    Technologies
Jan Ellen Berger, MD
    Committee on Medical Liability
F. Lane France, MD
    Committee on Practice and Ambulatory
    Medicine

ACKNOWLEDGMENTS

The subcommittee wishes to acknowledge the numerous people and groups that made development of this clinical practice guideline possible. The subcommittee would like to thank the Agency for Healthcare Research and Quality and the McMaster University Evidence-based Practice Center for its work in developing the evidence report, and William E. Pelham, Jr, PhD, and Peter Jensen, MD, for their continuous input and insight into the evidence about treatment of ADHD.

REFERENCES

1. American Academy of Pediatrics, Committee on Quality Improvement and Subcommittee on Attention-Deficit/Hyperactivity Disorder. Diagnosis and evaluation of the child with attention-deficit/hyperactivity disorder. *Pediatrics.* 2000;105:1158–1170

2. Jadad AR, Boyle M, Cunningham C, et al. *Treatment of Attention Deficit/ Hyperactivity Disorder. Evidence Report/Technology Assessment No. 11.* Rockville, MD: Agency for Healthcare Research and Quality; 1999. AHRQ Publ. No. 00-E005

3. Jensen P, Arnold L, Richters J, et al. 14-month randomized clinical trial of treatment strategies for attention deficit hyperactivity disorder. *Arch Gen Psychiatry.* 1999;56:1073–1086

4. Miller A, Lee S, Raina P, et al. *A Review of Therapies for Attention-Deficit/ Hyperactivity Disorder.* Ottawa, Ontario: Canadian Coordinating Office for Health Technology Assessment (CCOHTA); 1998

5. American Psychiatric Association. *Diagnostic and Statistical Manual of Mental Disorders.* 4th ed. Washington, DC: American Psychiatric Association; 1994

6. Pelham WE Jr, Wheeler T, Chronis A. Empirically supported psychosocial treatments for attention deficit hyperactivity disorder. *J Clin Child Psychol.* 1998;27:190–205

7. MTA Cooperative Group. Moderators and mediators of treatment response for children with attention-deficit/hyperactivity disorder: the multimodal treatment study of children with ADHD. *Arch Gen Psychiatry.* 1999;56:1088–1096

8. Epstein JN, Conners CK, Erhardt D, et al. Familial aggregation of ADHD characteristics. *J Abnorm Child Psychol.* 2000;28:585–594

9. Hinshaw SP, Owens EB, Wells KC, et al. Family processes and treatment outcomes in the MTA: negative/ineffective parenting practices in relation to multimodal treatment. *J Abnorm Child Psychol.* 2000;28: 555–568

10. Hoza B, Owens JS, Pelham WE Jr, et al. Cognitions as predictors of child treatment response in attention-deficit/hyperactivity disorder. *J Abnorm Child Psychol.* 2000;28:569–583

11. March JS, Swanson JM, Arnold LE, et al. Anxiety as a predictor and outcome variable in the multimodal treatment study of children with ADHD. *J Abnorm Child Psychol.* 2000;28:527–541

12. Pelham WE Jr, Gnagy EM, Greiner AR, et al. Behavioral vs behavioral and pharmacological treatment in ADHD children attending a summer treatment program. *J Abnorm Child Psychol.* 2000;28:507–525

13. Conners CK, Epstein JN, March JS, et al. Multimodal treatment of ADHD (MTA): an alternative outcome analysis. *J Am Acad Child Adolesc Psychiatry.* 2000;40:159–167

14. Wells KC, Epstein JN, Hinshaw SP, et al. Parenting and family stress treatment outcomes in attention deficit hyperactivity disorder (ADHD): an empirical analysis in the MTA study. *J Abnorm Child Psychol.* 2000; 28:543–553

15. Wells KC, Pelham WE Jr, Kotkin RA, et al. Psychosocial treatment strategies in the MTA study. Rationale, methods, and critical issues in design and implementation. *J Abnorm Child Psychol.* 2000;28:483–505

16. Hinshaw SP, March JS, Abikoff H, et al. Comprehensive assessment of childhood attention-deficit hyperactivity disorder in the context of a multisite, multimodal clinical trial. *J Attention Disorders.* 1997;1:217–234

17. Pelham WE Jr, Fabiano G. Behavior modification. *Child Adolesc Psychiatr Clin North Am.* 2001;9:671–688

18. Barkley RA, Fischer M, Edelbrock CS, Smallish L. The adolescent outcome of hyperactive children diagnosed by research criteria: I: an 8-year prospective follow-up study. *J Am Acad Child Adolesc Psychiatry.* 1990; 29:546–557

19. Biederman J, Faraone S, Milberger S, et al. A prospective 4-year follow-up study of attention-deficit hyperactivity and related disorders. *Arch Gen Psychiatry.* 1996;53:437–446

20. Mannuzza S, Klein R, Bessler A, Malloy P, LaPudula M. Adult psychiatric status of hyperactive boys grown up. *Am J Psychiatry.* 1998;155: 493–498

21. American Academy of Pediatrics, Committee on Children With Disabilities. Pediatric services for infants and children with special health care needs. *Pediatrics.* 1993;92:163–165

22. American Academy of Pediatrics, Committee on Children With Disabilities. General principles in the care of children and adolescents with genetic disorders and other chronic health conditions. *Pediatrics.* 1997; 99:643–644

23. American Academy of Pediatrics, Committee on Children With Disabilities. Care coordination: integrating health and related systems of care for children with special health care needs. *Pediatrics.* 1999;104:978–981

24. American Academy of Pediatrics, Committee on Psychosocial Aspects of Child and Family Health and Committee on Children With Disabilities. Psychosocial risks of chronic health conditions in children and adolescents. *Pediatrics.* 1993;92:876–878

25. Perrin JM. Children with chronic illness. In: Behrman RE, ed. *Nelson Textbook of Pediatrics.* 16th ed. Philadelphia, PA: WB Saunders Co; 2000:123–125

26. Perrin JM, Shayne MW, Bloom SR. *Home and Community Care for Chronically Ill Children.* New York, NY: Oxford University Press; 1993

27. Fireman P, Friday GA, Gira C, Vierthaler WA, Michaels L. Teaching self-management skills to asthmatic children and parents in an ambulatory care setting. *Pediatrics.* 1981;68:341–348

28. Jessop DJ, Stein REK. Providing comprehensive health care to children with chronic illness. *Pediatrics.* 1994;93:602–607

29. Nader PR, ed. *School Health: Policy and Practice.* 5th ed. Elk Grove Village, IL: American Academy of Pediatrics; 1993

30. Kavale K. The efficacy of stimulant drug treatment for hyperactivity: a meta-analysis. *J Learn Disabil.* 1982;15:280–289

31. Ottenbacher KJ. Drug treatment of hyperactivity in children. *Dev Med Child Neurol.* 1983;25:358–366

32. Thurber S. Medication and hyperactivity. A meta-analysis. *J Gen Psychol.* 1983;108:79–86

33. Swanson JM, McBurnett K, Wigal T, et al. Effect of stimulant medication on children with attention-deficit disorder—a review of reviews. *Except Child.* 1993;60:154–162

34. Cohen J. *Statistical Power Analysis for the Behavioural Sciences.* New York, NY: Academic Press; 1977

35. Ingram S, Hechtman L, Morgenstern G. Outcomes issues in ADHD: adolescent and adult long-term outcomes. *Ment Retard Dev Disabil Res Rev.* 1999;5:243–250

36. Sheveli M, Schreiber R. Pemoline-associated hepatic failure: a critical analysis of the literature. *Pediatr Neurol.* 1997;16:14–16

37. Connors CK, Casat CD, Guaitieri CT, et al. Bupropion hydrochloride in attention deficit disorder with hyperactivity. *J Am Acad Child Adolesc Psychiatry.* 1996;35:1314–1321

38. Biederman J, Thisted RA, Greenhill LL, Ryan ND. Estimation of the association between desipramine and the risk for sudden death in 5- to 14-year-old children. *J Clin Psychiatry.* 1995;56:87–93

39. Connor DF, Fletcher KE, Swanson JM. A meta-analysis of clonidine for symptoms of attention-deficit hyperactivity disorder. *J Am Acad Child Adolesc Psychiatry.* 1999;38:1551–1559

40. Prince JB, Wilens TE, Biederman J Spencer TJ, Wozniak JR. Clonidine for sleep disturbances associated with attention-deficit hyperactivity disorder: a systematic chart review of 62 cases. *J Am Acad Child Adolesc Psychiatry.* 1996;35:499–605

41. Gadow KD, Sverci J, Sprafkin J, Nolan EE, Grossman S. Long-term methylphenidate therapy in children with co-morbid attention-deficit hyperactivity disorder and chronic multiple tic disorder. *Arch Gen Psychiatry.* 1999;56:330–336

42. Castellanos FX, Giedd JN, Elia J, et al. Controlled stimulant treatment of ADHD and comorbid Tourette's syndrome: effects of stimulant and dose. *J Am Acad Child Adolesc Psychiatry.* 1997;36:589–596

43. PDR Electronic Library. Available at: www.pdrel.com. Accessed March 14, 2001

44. Gross-Tsur V, Manor O, van der Meere J, Joseph A, Shalev RS. Epilepsy and attention deficit hyperactivity disorder: is methylphenidate safe and effective? *J Pediatr.* 1997;130:670–674

45. Wroblewski BA, Leary JM, Phelan AM, Whyte J, Manning K. Methylphenidate and seizure frequency in brain injured patients with seizure disorders. *J Clin Psychiatry.* 1992;53:86–89

46. Feldman H, Crumrine P, Handen BL, Alvin R, Teodori J. Methylphenidate in children with seizures and attention-deficit disorder. *Am J Dis Child.* 1989;143:1081–1086

47. Greenhill LL, Halperin JM, Abikoff H. Stimulant medications. *J Am Acad Child Adolesc Psychiatry.* 1999;38:503–528

48. Mannuzza S, Klein RG, Bonagura N, Malloy P, Giampino TL, Addali KA. Hyperactive boys almost grow up V: replication of psychiatric status. *Arch Gen Psychiatry.* 1991;48:77–83

49. Gross MD. Growth of hyperkinetic children taking methylphenidate, dextroamphetamine or imipramine/desipramine. *Pediatrics.* 1976;58: 423–431

50. Satterfield JH, Cantwell DP, Schell A, Blaschke T. Growth of hyperactive children treated with methylphenidate. *Arch Gen Psychiatry.* 1979; 36:212–217

51. Kent JD, Blader JC, Koplewicz HS, Abikoff H, Foley CA. Effects of late-afternoon methylphenidate administration on behavior and sleep in attention-deficit hyperactivity disorder. *Pediatrics.* 1995;96:320–325

52. Efron D, Jarman F, Barker M. Side effects of methylphenidate and dextroamphetamine in children with attention deficit hyperactivity disorder: a double-blind, crossover trial. *Pediatrics.* 1997;100:662–666

53. Schertz M, Adesman A, Alfieri N, Bienkowski RS. Predictors of weight loss in children with attention deficit hyperactivity disorder treated with stimulant medication. *Pediatrics.* 1996;98:763–769

54. Rappaport JL, Zahn TP, Ludlow C, Mikkelsen EJ. Dextroamphetamine: cognitive and behavioral effects in normal prepubertal boys. *Science.* 1978;199:560–563

55. Arnold LE. Methylphenidate versus amphetamine: a comparative review. In: Greenhill LL, Osman BB, eds. *Ritalin: Theory and Practice.* 2nd ed. Larchmont, NY: Mary Ann Liebert, Inc; 2000:127–140

56. Barkley RA. *Handbook of Attention Deficit Hyperactivity Disorder.* 2nd ed. New York, NY: Guildford; 1998

57. Pelham WE Jr, Hinshaw S. *Handbook of Clinical Behavior Therapy.* Turner S, ed. New York, NY: Wiley; 1992

58. Swanson JM, Kraemer HC, Hinshaw SP, et al. Clinical relevance of the primary findings of the MTA: success rates based on severity of symptoms at the end of treatment. *J Am Acad Child Adolesc Psychiatry.* 2001; 40:168–179

59. Jensen PS, Hinshaw SP, Kraemer HC, et al. ADHD comorbidity findings from the MTA study: comparing comorbid subgroups. *J Am Acad Child Adolesc Psychiatry.* 2001;40:147–158

60. Pelham WE Jr, MTA Cooperative Group. Presented at: Association for the Advancement of Behavioral Therapy. November 2000; New Orleans, LA

61. Clark N, Gong M. Management of chronic disease by practitioners and patients: are we teaching the wrong things? *BMJ.* 2000;320:572–575

62. Greenhill LL, Swanson JM, Vitiello B, et al. Determining the best dose of methylphenidate under controlled conditions: lessons from the MTA titration. *J Am Acad Child Adolesc Psychiatry.* 2001;40:180–198

Early Detection of Developmental Dysplasia of the Hip

- *Clinical Practice Guideline*
- *Technical Report Summary*

Readers of this clinical practice guideline are urged to review the technical report to enhance the evidence-based decision-making process. The full technical report is available on the enclosed CD-ROM.

AMERICAN ACADEMY OF PEDIATRICS

Committee on Quality Improvement, Subcommittee on Developmental Dysplasia of the Hip

Clinical Practice Guideline: Early Detection of Developmental Dysplasia of the Hip

ABSTRACT. *Developmental dysplasia of the hip* is the preferred term to describe the condition in which the femoral head has an abnormal relationship to the acetabulum. Developmental dysplasia of the hip includes frank dislocation (luxation), partial dislocation (subluxation), instability wherein the femoral head comes in and out of the socket, and an array of radiographic abnormalities that reflect inadequate formation of the acetabulum. Because many of these findings may not be present at birth, the term *developmental* more accurately reflects the biologic features than does the term *congenital*. The disorder is uncommon. The earlier a dislocated hip is detected, the simpler and more effective is the treatment. Despite newborn screening programs, dislocated hips continue to be diagnosed later in infancy and childhood,[1-11] in some instances delaying appropriate therapy and leading to a substantial number of malpractice claims. The objective of this guideline is to reduce the number of dislocated hips detected later in infancy and childhood. The target audience is the primary care provider. The target patient is the healthy newborn up to 18 months of age, excluding those with neuromuscular disorders, myelodysplasia, or arthrogryposis.

ABBREVIATIONS. DDH, developmental dysplasia of the hip; AVN, avascular necrosis of the hip.

BIOLOGIC FEATURES AND NATURAL HISTORY

Understanding the developmental nature of developmental dysplasia of the hip (DDH) and the subsequent spectrum of hip abnormalities requires a knowledge of the growth and development of the hip joint.[12] Embryologically, the femoral head and acetabulum develop from the same block of primitive mesenchymal cells. A cleft develops to separate them at 7 to 8 weeks' gestation. By 11 weeks' gestation, development of the hip joint is complete. At birth, the femoral head and the acetabulum are primarily cartilaginous. The acetabulum continues to develop postnatally. The growth of the fibrocartilaginous rim (the labrum) that surrounds

the bony acetabulum deepens the socket. Development of the femoral head and acetabulum are intimately related, and normal adult hip joints depend on further growth of these structures. Hip dysplasia may occur in utero, perinatally, or during infancy and childhood.

The acronym DDH includes hips that are unstable, subluxated, dislocated (luxated), and/or have malformed acetabula. A hip is *unstable* when the tight fit between the femoral head and the acetabulum is lost and the femoral head is able to move within (subluxated) or outside (dislocated) the confines of the acetabulum. A *dislocation* is a complete loss of contact of the femoral head with the acetabulum. Dislocations are divided into 2 types: teratologic and typical.[12] *Teratologic dislocations* occur early in utero and often are associated with neuromuscular disorders, such as arthrogryposis and myelodysplasia, or with various dysmorphic syndromes. The *typical dislocation* occurs in an otherwise healthy infant and may occur prenatally or postnatally.

During the immediate newborn period, laxity of the hip capsule predominates, and, if clinically significant enough, the femoral head may spontaneously dislocate and relocate. If the hip spontaneously relocates and stabilizes within a few days, subsequent hip development usually is normal. If subluxation or dislocation persists, then structural anatomic changes may develop. A deep concentric position of the femoral head in the acetabulum is necessary for normal development of the hip. When not deeply reduced (subluxated), the labrum may become everted and flattened. Because the femoral head is not reduced into the depth of the socket, the acetabulum does not grow and remodel and, therefore, becomes shallow. If the femoral head moves further out of the socket (dislocation), typically superiorly and laterally, the inferior capsule is pulled upward over the now empty socket. Muscles surrounding the hip, especially the adductors, become contracted, limiting abduction of the hip. The hip capsule constricts; once this capsular constriction narrows to less than the diameter of the femoral head, the hip can no longer be reduced by manual manipulative maneuvers, and operative reduction usually is necessary.

The hip is at risk for dislocation during 4 periods: 1) the 12th gestational week, 2) the 18th gestational week, 3) the final 4 weeks of gestation, and 4) the postnatal period. During the 12th gestational week, the hip is at risk as the fetal lower limb rotates medially. A dislocation at this time is termed teratologic. All elements of the hip joint develop abnor-

The recommendations in this statement do not indicate an exclusive course of treatment or serve as a standard of medical care. Variations, taking into account individual circumstances, may be appropriate.

The Practice Guideline, "Early Detection of Developmental Dysplasia of the Hip," was reviewed by appropriate committees and sections of the American Academy of Pediatrics (AAP) including the Chapter Review Group, a focus group of office-based pediatricians representing each AAP District: Gene R. Adams, MD; Robert M. Corwin, MD; Diane Fuquay, MD; Barbara M. Harley, MD; Thomas J. Herr, MD, Chair; Kenneth E. Matthews, MD; Robert D. Mines, MD; Lawrence C. Pakula, MD; Howard B. Weinblatt, MD; and Delosa A. Young, MD. The Practice Guideline was also reviewed by relevant outside medical organizations as part of the peer review process.

mally. The hip muscles develop around the 18th gestational week. Neuromuscular problems at this time, such as myelodysplasia and arthrogryposis, also lead to teratologic dislocations. During the final 4 weeks of pregnancy, mechanical forces have a role. Conditions such as oligohydramnios or breech position predispose to DDH.[13] Breech position occurs in ~3% of births, and DDH occurs more frequently in breech presentations, reportedly in as many as 23%. The frank breech position of hip flexion and knee extension places a newborn or infant at the highest risk. Postnatally, infant positioning such as swaddling, combined with ligamentous laxity, also has a role.

The true incidence of dislocation of the hip can only be presumed. There is no "gold standard" for diagnosis during the newborn period. Physical examination, plane radiography, and ultrasonography all are fraught with false-positive and false-negative results. Arthrography (insertion of contrast medium into the hip joint) and magnetic resonance imaging, although accurate for determining the precise hip anatomy, are inappropriate methods for screening the newborn and infant.

The reported incidence of DDH is influenced by genetic and racial factors, diagnostic criteria, the experience and training of the examiner, and the age of the child at the time of the examination. Wynne-Davies[14] reported an increased risk to subsequent children in the presence of a diagnosed dislocation (6% risk with healthy parents and an affected child, 12% risk with an affected parent, and 36% risk with an affected parent and 1 affected child). DDH is not always detectable at birth, but some newborn screening surveys suggest an incidence as high as 1 in 100 newborns with evidence of instability, and 1 to 1.5 cases of dislocation per 1000 newborns. The incidence of DDH is higher in girls. Girls are especially susceptible to the maternal hormone relaxin, which may contribute to ligamentous laxity with the resultant instability of the hip. The left hip is involved 3 times as commonly as the right hip, perhaps related to the left occiput anterior positioning of most non-breech newborns. In this position, the left hip resides posteriorly against the mother's spine, potentially limiting abduction.

PHYSICAL EXAMINATION

DDH is an evolving process, and its physical findings on clinical examination change.[12,15,16] The newborn must be relaxed and preferably examined on a firm surface. Considerable patience and skill are required. The physical examination changes as the child grows older. No signs are pathognomonic for a dislocated hip. The examiner must look for asymmetry. Indeed, bilateral dislocations are more difficult to diagnose than unilateral dislocations because symmetry is retained. Asymmetrical thigh or gluteal folds, better observed when the child is prone, apparent limb length discrepancy, and restricted motion, especially abduction, are significant, albeit not pathognomonic signs. With the infant supine and the pelvis stabilized, abduction to 75° and adduction to 30° should occur readily under normal circumstances.

The 2 maneuvers for assessing hip stability in the newborn are the Ortolani and Barlow tests. The Ortolani elicits the sensation of the dislocated hip reducing, and the Barlow detects the unstable hip dislocating from the acetabulum. The Ortolani is performed with the newborn supine and the examiner's index and middle fingers placed along the greater trochanter with the thumb placed along the inner thigh. The hip is flexed to 90° but not more, and the leg is held in neutral rotation. The hip is gently abducted while lifting the leg anteriorly. With this maneuver, a "clunk" is felt as the dislocated femoral head reduces into the acetabulum. This is a positive Ortolani sign. The Barlow provocative test is performed with the newborn positioned supine and the hips flexed to 90°. The leg is then gently adducted while posteriorly directed pressure is placed on the knee. A palpable clunk or sensation of movement is felt as the femoral head exits the acetabulum posteriorly. This is a positive Barlow sign. The Ortolani and Barlow maneuvers are performed 1 hip at a time. Little force is required for the performance of either of these tests. The goal is not to prove that the hip can be dislocated. Forceful and repeated examinations can break the seal between the labrum and the femoral head. These strongly positive signs of Ortolani and Barlow are distinguished from a large array of soft or equivocal physical findings present during the newborn period. High-pitched clicks are commonly elicited with flexion and extension and are inconsequential. A dislocatable hip has a rather distinctive clunk, whereas a subluxable hip is characterized by a feeling of looseness, a sliding movement, but without the true Ortolani and Barlow clunks. Separating true dislocations (clunks) from a feeling of instability and from benign adventitial sounds (clicks) takes practice and expertise. This guideline recognizes the broad range of physical findings present in newborns and infants and the confusion of terminology generated in the literature. By 8 to 12 weeks of age, the capsule laxity decreases, muscle tightness increases, and the Barlow and Ortolani maneuvers are no longer positive regardless of the status of the femoral head. In the 3-month-old infant, limitation of abduction is the most reliable sign associated with DDH. Other features that arouse suspicion include asymmetry of thigh folds, a positive Allis or Galeazzi sign (relative shortness of the femur with the hips and knees flexed), and discrepancy of leg lengths. These physical findings alert the examiner that abnormal relationships of the femoral head to the acetabulum (dislocation and subluxation) *may* be present.

Maldevelopments of the acetabulum alone (acetabular dysplasia) can be determined only by imaging techniques. Abnormal physical findings may be absent in an infant with acetabular dysplasia but no subluxation or dislocation. Indeed, because of the confusion, inconsistencies, and misuse of language in the literature (eg, an Ortolani sign called a click by some and a clunk by others), this guideline uses the following definitions.

- A *positive examination* result for DDH is the Barlow or Ortolani sign. This is the clunk of dislocation or reduction.
- An *equivocal examination* or *warning signs* include an array of physical findings that may be found in children with DDH, in children with another orthopaedic disorder, or in children who are completely healthy. These physical findings include asymmetric thigh or buttock creases, an apparent or true short leg, and limited abduction. These signs, used singly or in combination, serve to raise the pediatrician's index of suspicion and act as a threshold for referral. Newborn soft tissue hip clicks are not predictive of DDH[17] but may be confused with the Ortolani and Barlow clunks by some screening physicians and thereby be a reason for referral.

IMAGING

Radiographs of the pelvis and hips have historically been used to assess an infant with suspected DDH. During the first few months of life when the femoral heads are composed entirely of cartilage, radiographs have limited value. Displacement and instability may be undetectable, and evaluation of acetabular development is influenced by the infant's position at the time the radiograph is performed. By 4 to 6 months of age, radiographs become more reliable, particularly when the ossification center develops in the femoral head. Radiographs are readily available and relatively low in cost.

Real-time ultrasonography has been established as an accurate method for imaging the hip during the first few months of life.[15,18–25] With ultrasonography, the cartilage can be visualized and the hip can be viewed while assessing the stability of the hip and the morphologic features of the acetabulum. In some clinical settings, ultrasonography can provide information comparable to arthrography (direct injection of contrast into the hip joint), without the need for sedation, invasion, contrast medium, or ionizing radiation. Although the availability of equipment for ultrasonography is widespread, accurate results in hip sonography require training and experience. Although expertise in pediatric hip ultrasonography is increasing, this examination may not always be available or obtained conveniently. Ultrasonographic techniques include *static evaluation* of the morphologic features of the hip, as popularized in Europe by Graf,[26] and a *dynamic evaluation*, as developed by Harcke[20] that assesses the hip for stability of the femoral head in the socket, as well as static anatomy. Dynamic ultrasonography yields more useful information. With both techniques, there is considerable interobserver variability, especially during the first 3 weeks of life.[7,27]

Experience with ultrasonography has documented its ability to detect abnormal position, instability, and dysplasia not evident on clinical examination. Ultrasonography during the first 4 weeks of life often reveals the presence of minor degrees of instability and acetabular immaturity. Studies[7,28,29] indicate that nearly all these mild early findings, which will not be apparent on physical examination, resolve spontaneously without treatment. Newborn screening with ultrasonography has required a high frequency of reexamination and results in a large number of hips being unnecessarily treated. One study[23] demonstrates that a screening process with higher false-positive results also yields increased prevention of late cases. Ultrasonographic screening of all infants at 4 to 6 weeks of age would be expensive, requiring considerable resources. This practice is yet to be validated by clinical trial. *Consequently, the use of ultrasonography is recommended as an adjunct to the clinical evaluation.* It is the technique of choice for clarifying a physical finding, assessing a high-risk infant, and monitoring DDH as it is observed or treated. Used in this selective capacity, it can guide treatment and may prevent overtreatment.

PRETERM INFANTS

DDH may be unrecognized in prematurely born infants. When the infant has cardiorespiratory problems, the diagnosis and management are focused on providing appropriate ventilatory and cardiovascular support, and careful examination of the hips may be deferred until a later date. The most complete examination the infant receives may occur at the time of discharge from the hospital, and this single examination may not detect subluxation or dislocation. Despite the medical urgencies surrounding the preterm infant, it is critical to examine the entire child.

METHODS FOR GUIDELINE DEVELOPMENT

Our goal was to develop a practice parameter by using a process that would be based whenever possible on available evidence. The methods used a combination of expert panel, decision modeling, and evidence synthesis[30] (see the Technical Report available on *Pediatrics electronic pages* at www.pediatrics.org). The predominant methods recommended for such evidence synthesis are generally of 2 types: a *data-driven* method and a *model-driven*[31,32] method. In data-driven methods, the analyst finds the best data available and induces a conclusion from these data. A model-driven method, in contrast, begins with an effort to define the context for evidence and then searches for the data as defined by that context. Data-driven methods are useful when the quality of evidence is high. A careful review of the medical literature revealed that the published evidence about DDH did not meet the criteria for high quality. There was a paucity of randomized clinical trials.[8] We decided, therefore, to use the model-driven method.

A decision model was constructed based on the perspective of practicing clinicians and determining the best strategy for screening and diagnosis. The target child was a full-term newborn with no obvious orthopaedic abnormalities. We focused on the various options available to the pediatrician* for the detection of DDH, including screening by physical examination, screening by ultrasonography, and episodic screening during health supervision. Because

---

*In this guideline, the term *pediatrician* includes the range of pediatric primary care providers, eg, family practitioners and pediatric nurse practitioners.

the detection of a dislocated hip usually results in referral by the pediatrician, and because management of DDH is not in the purview of the pediatrician's care, treatment options are not included. We also included in our model a wide range of options for detecting DDH during the first year of life if the results of the newborn screen are negative.

The outcomes on which we focused were a dislocated hip at 1 year of age as the major morbidity of the disease and avascular necrosis of the hip (AVN) as the primary complication of DDH treatment. AVN is a loss of blood supply to the femoral head resulting in abnormal hip development, distortion of shape, and, in some instances, substantial morbidity. Ideally, a gold standard would be available to define DDH at any point in time. However, as noted, no gold standard exists except, perhaps, arthrography of the hip, which is an inappropriate standard for use in a detection model. Therefore, we defined outcomes in terms of the *process of care*. We reviewed the literature extensively. The purpose of the literature review was to provide the probabilities required by the decision model since there were no randomized clinical trials. The article or chapter title and the abstracts were reviewed by 2 members of the methodology team and members of the subcommittee. Articles not rejected were reviewed, and data were abstracted that would provide evidence for the probabilities required by the decision model. As part of the literature abstraction process, the evidence quality in each article was assessed. A computer-based literature search, hand review of recent publications, or examination of the reference section for other articles ("ancestor articles") identified 623 articles; 241 underwent detailed review, 118 of which provided some data. Of the 100 ancestor articles, only 17 yielded useful articles, suggesting that our accession process was complete. By traditional epidemiologic standards,[33] the quality of the evidence in this set of articles was uniformly low. There were few controlled trials and few studies of the follow-up of infants for whom the results of newborn examinations were negative. When the evidence was poor or lacking entirely, extensive discussions among members of the committee and the expert opinion of outside consultants were used to arrive at a consensus. No votes were taken. Disagreements were discussed, and consensus was achieved.

The available evidence was distilled in 3 ways.

First, estimates were made of DDH at birth in infants without risk factors. These estimates constituted the baseline risk. Second, estimates were made of the rates of DDH in the children with risk factors. These numbers guide clinical actions: rates that are too high might indicate referral or different follow-up despite negative physical findings. Third, each screening strategy (pediatrician-based, orthopaedist-based, and ultrasonography-based) was scored for the estimated number of children given a diagnosis of DDH at birth, at mid-term (4–12 months of age), and at late-term (12 months of age and older) and for the estimated number of cases of AVN incurred, assuming that all children given a diagnosis of DDH would be treated. These numbers suggest the best strategy, balancing DDH detection with incurring adverse effects.

The baseline estimate of DDH based on orthopaedic screening was 11.5/1000 infants. Estimates from pediatric screening were 8.6/1000 and from ultrasonography were 25/1000. The 11.5/1000 rate translates into a rate for not-at-risk boys of 4.1/1000 boys and a rate for not-at-risk girls of 19/1000 girls. These numbers derive from the facts that the relative risk—the rate in girls divided by the rate in boys across several studies—is 4.6 and because infants are split evenly between boys and girls, so $.5 \times 4.1/1000 + .5 \times 19/1000 = 11.5/1000$.[34,35] We used these baseline rates for calculating the rates in other risk groups. Because the relative risk of DDH for children with a positive family history (first-degree relatives) is 1.7, the rate for boys with a positive family history is $1.7 \times 4.1 = 6.4/1000$ boys, and for girls with a positive family history, $1.7 \times 19 = 32/1000$ girls. Finally, the relative risk of DDH for breech presentation (of all kinds) is 6.3, so the risk for breech boys is $7.0 \times 4.1 = 29/1000$ boys and for breech girls, $7.0 \times 19 = 133/1000$ girls. These numbers are summarized in Table 1.

These numbers suggest that boys without risk or those with a family history have the lowest risk; girls without risk and boys born in a breech presentation have an intermediate risk; and girls with a positive family history, and especially girls born in a breech presentation, have the highest risks. Guidelines, considering the risk factors, should follow these risk profiles. Reports of newborn screening for DDH have included various screening techniques. In some, the screening clinician was an orthopaedist, in

TABLE 1.   Relative and Absolute Risks for Finding a Positive Examination Result at Newborn Screening by Using the Ortolani and Barlow Signs

Newborn Characteristics	Relative Risk of a Positive Examination Result	Absolute Risk of a Positive Examination Result per 1000 Newborns With Risk Factors
All newborns	. . .	11.5
Boys	1.0	4.1
Girls	4.6	19
Positive family history	1.7	
Boys	. . .	6.4
Girls	. . .	32
Breech presentation	7.0	
Boys	. . .	29
Girls	. . .	133

TABLE 2.　　Newborn Strategy*

Outcome	Orthopaedist PE	Pediatrician PE	Ultrasonography
DDH in newborn	12	8.6	25
DDH at ~6 mo of age	.1	.45	.28
DDH at 12 mo of age or more	.16	.33	.1
AVN at 12 mo of age	.06	.1	.1

* PE indicates physical examination. Outcome per 1000 infants initially screened.

others, a pediatrician, and in still others, a physiotherapist. In addition, screening has been performed by ultrasonography. In assessing the expected effect of each strategy, we estimated the newborn DDH rates, the mid-term DDH rates, and the late-term DDH rates for each of the 3 strategies, as shown in Table 2. We also estimated the rate of AVN for DDH treated before 2 months of age (2.5/1000 treated) and after 2 months of age (109/1000 treated). We could not distinguish the AVN rates for children treated between 2 and 12 months of age from those treated later. Table 2 gives these data. The total cases of AVN per strategy are calculated, assuming that all infants with positive examination results are treated.

Table 2 shows that a strategy using pediatricians to screen newborns would give the lowest newborn rate but the highest mid- and late-term DDH rates. To assess how much better an ultrasonography-only screening strategy would be, we could calculate a cost-effectiveness ratio. In this case, the "cost" of ultrasonographic screening is the number of "extra" newborn cases that probably include children who do not need to be treated. (The cost from AVN is the same in the 2 strategies.) By using these cases as the cost and the number of later cases averted as the effect, a ratio is obtained of 71 children treated neonatally because of a positive ultrasonographic screen for each later case averted. Because this number is high, and because the presumption of better late-term efficacy is based on a single study, we do not recommend ultrasonographic screening at this time.

RECOMMENDATIONS AND NOTES TO ALGORITHM (Fig 1)

1. **All newborns are to be screened by physical examination**. The evidence† for this recommendation is good. The expert consensus‡ is strong. Although initial screening by orthopaedists§ would be optimal (Table 2), it is doubtful that if widely practiced, such a strategy would give the same good results as those published from pediatric orthopaedic research centers. **It is recommended that screening be done by a properly trained health care provider** (eg, physician, pediatric nurse practitioner, physician assistant, or physical therapist). (Evidence for this recommendation is strong.) A number of studies performed by properly trained nonphysicians report results

†In this guideline, evidence is listed as good, fair, or poor based on the methodologist's evaluation of the literature quality. (See the Technical Report.)
‡Opinion or consensus is listed as *strong* if opinion of the expert panel was unanimous or *mixed* if there were dissenting points of view.
§In this guideline, the term *orthopaedist* refers to an orthopaedic surgeon with expertise in pediatric orthopaedic conditions.

indistinguishable from those performed by physicians.[36] The examination after discharge from the neonatal intensive care unit should be performed as a newborn examination with appropriate screening. **Ultrasonography of all newborns is not recommended.** (Evidence is fair; consensus is strong.) Although there is indirect evidence to support the use of ultrasonographic screening of all newborns, it is not advocated because it is operator-dependent, availability is questionable, it increases the rate of treatment, and interobserver variability is high. There are probably some increased costs. We considered a strategy of "no newborn screening." This arm is politically indefensible because screening newborns is inherent in pediatrician's care. The technical report details this limb through decision analysis. Regardless of the screening method used for the newborn, DDH is detected in 1 in 5000 infants at 18 months of age.[3] The evidence and consensus for newborn screening remain strong.

Newborn Physical Examination and Treatment

2. **If a positive Ortolani or Barlow sign is found in the newborn examination, the infant should be referred to an orthopaedist**. Orthopaedic referral is recommended when the Ortolani sign is unequivocally positive (a clunk). Orthopaedic referral is not recommended for any softly positive finding in the examination (eg, hip click without dislocation). The precise time frame for the newborn to be evaluated by the orthopaedist cannot be determined from the literature. However, the literature suggests that the majority of "abnormal" physical findings of hip examinations at birth (clicks and clunks) will resolve by 2 weeks; therefore, consultation and possible initiation of treatment are recommended by that time. The data recommending that all those with a positive Ortolani sign be referred to an orthopaedist are limited, but expert panel consensus, nevertheless, was strong, because pediatricians do not have the training to take full responsibility and because true Ortolani clunks are rare and their management is more appropriately performed by the orthopaedist.

If the results of the physical examination at birth are "equivocally" positive (ie, soft click, mild asymmetry, but neither an Ortolani nor a Barlow sign is present), then a follow-up hip examination by the pediatrician in 2 weeks is recommended. (Evidence is good; consensus is strong.) The available data suggest that most clicks resolve by 2 weeks and that these "benign hip clicks" in the newborn period do

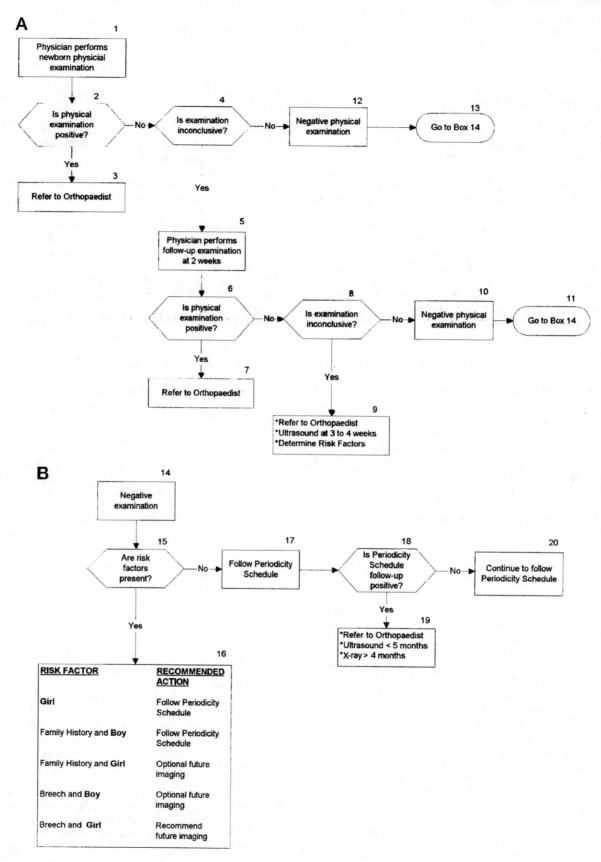

Fig 1. Screening for developmental hip dysplasia—clinical algorithm.

not lead to later hip dysplasia.[9,17,28,37] Thus, for an infant with softly positive signs, the pediatrician should reexamine the hips at 2 weeks before making referrals for orthopaedic care or ultrasonography. We recognize the concern of pediatricians about adherence to follow-up care regimens, but this concern regards all aspects of health maintenance and is not a reason to request ultrasonography or other diagnostic study of the newborn hips.

3. **If the results of the newborn physical examination are positive (ie, presence of an Ortolani or a Barlow sign), ordering an ultrasonographic examination of the newborn is not recommended.** (Evidence is poor; opinion is strong.) Treatment decisions are not influenced by the results of ultrasonography but are based on the results of the physical examination. The treating physician may use a variety of imaging studies during clinical management. **If the results of the newborn physical examination are positive, obtaining a radiograph of the newborn's pelvis and hips is not recommended** (evidence is poor; opinion is strong), because they are of limited value and do not influence treatment decisions.

   The use of triple diapers when abnormal physical signs are detected during the newborn period is not recommended. (Evidence is poor; opinion is strong.) Triple diaper use is common practice despite the lack of data on the effectiveness of triple diaper use; and, in instances of frank dislocation, the use of triple diapers may delay the initiation of more appropriate treatment (such as with the Pavlik harness). Often, the primary care pediatrician may not have performed the newborn examination in the hospital. The importance of communication cannot be overemphasized, and triple diapers may aid in follow-up as a reminder that a possible abnormal physical examination finding was present in the newborn.

2-Week Examination

4. **If the results of the physical examination are positive (eg, positive Ortolani or Barlow sign) at 2 weeks, refer to an orthopaedist.** (Evidence is strong; consensus is strong.) Referral is urgent but is not an emergency. Consensus is strong that, as in the newborn, the presence of an Ortolani or Barlow sign at 2 weeks warrants referral to an orthopaedist. An Ortolani sign at 2 weeks may be a new finding or a finding that was not apparent at the time of the newborn examination.

5. **If at the 2-week examination the Ortolani and Barlow signs are absent but physical findings raise suspicions, consider referral to an orthopaedist or request ultrasonography at age 3 to 4 weeks.** Consensus is mixed about the follow-up for softly positive or equivocal findings at 2 weeks of age (eg, adventitial click, thigh asymmetry, and apparent leg length difference). Because it is necessary to confirm the status of the hip joint, the pediatrician can consider referral to an orthopaedist or for ultrasonography if the constellation of physical findings raises a high level of suspicion.

However, if the physical findings are minimal, continuing follow-up by the periodicity schedule with focused hip examinations is also an option, provided risk factors are considered. (See "Recommendations" 7 and 8.)

6. **If the results of the physical examination are negative at 2 weeks, follow-up is recommended at the scheduled well-baby periodic examinations.** (Evidence is good; consensus is strong.)

7. **Risk factors.** If the results of the newborn examination are negative (or equivocally positive), risk factors may be considered.[13,21,38–41] Risk factors are a study of thresholds to act.[42] Table 1 gives the risk of finding a positive Ortolani or Barlow sign at the time of the initial newborn screening. If this examination is negative, the absolute risk of there being a true dislocated hip is greatly reduced. Nevertheless, the data in Table 1 may influence the pediatrician to perform confirmatory evaluations. Action will vary based on the individual clinician. The following recommendations are made (evidence is strong; opinion is strong):
   * **Girl** (newborn risk of 19/1000). When the results of the newborn examination are negative or equivocally positive, hips should be reevaluated at 2 weeks of age. If negative, continue according to the periodicity schedule; if positive, refer to an orthopaedist or for ultrasonography at 3 weeks of age.
   * **Infants with a positive family history of DDH** (newborn risk for boys of 9.4/1000 and for girls, 44/1000). When the results of the newborn examination in boys are negative or equivocally positive, hips should be reevaluated at 2 weeks of age. If negative, continue according to the periodicity schedule; if positive, refer to an orthopaedist or for ultrasonography at 3 weeks of age. In girls, the absolute risk of 44/1000 may exceed the pediatrician's threshold to act, and imaging with an ultrasonographic examination at 6 weeks of age or a radiograph of the pelvis at 4 months of age is recommended.
   * **Breech presentation** (newborn risk for boys of 26/1000 and for girls, 120/1000). **For negative or equivocally positive newborn examinations, the infant should be reevaluated at regular intervals (according to the periodicity schedule) if the examination results remain negative.** Because an absolute risk of 120/1000 (12%) probably exceeds most pediatricians' threshold to act, imaging with an ultrasonographic examination at 6 weeks of age or with a radiograph of the pelvis and hips at 4 months of age is recommended. In addition, because some reports show a high incidence of hip abnormalities detected at an older age in children born breech, this imaging strategy remains an option for all children born breech, not just girls. These hip abnormalities are, for the most part, inadequate development of the acetabulum. Acetabular dysplasia is best found by a radiographic examination at 6 months of age or older. A

suggestion of poorly formed acetabula may be observed at 6 weeks of age by ultrasonography, but the best study remains a radiograph performed closer to 6 months of age. Ultrasonographic newborn screening of all breech infants will not eliminate the possibility of later acetabular dysplasia.

8. **Periodicity. The hips must be examined at every well-baby visit according to the recommended periodicity schedule for well-baby examinations (2–4 days for newborns discharged in less than 48 hours after delivery, by 1 month, 2 months, 4 months, 6 months, 9 months, and 12 months of age).** If at any time during the follow-up period DDH is suspected because of an abnormal physical examination or by a parental complaint of difficulty diapering or abnormal appearing legs, the pediatrician must confirm that the hips are stable, in the sockets, and developing normally. Confirmation can be made by a focused physical examination when the infant is calm and relaxed, by consultation with another primary care pediatrician, by consultation with an orthopaedist, by ultrasonography if the infant is younger than 5 months of age, or by radiography if the infant is older than 4 months of age. (Between 4 and 6 months of age, ultrasonography and radiography seem to be equally effective diagnostic imaging studies.)

DISCUSSION

DDH is an important term because it accurately reflects the biologic features of the disorder and the susceptibility of the hip to become dislocated at various times. Dislocated hips always will be diagnosed later in infancy and childhood because not every dislocated hip is detectable at birth, and hips continue to dislocate throughout the first year of life. Thus, this guideline requires that the pediatrician follow *a process of care for the detection of DDH*. The process recommended for early detection of DDH includes the following:

- Screen all newborns' hips by physical examination.
- Examine all infants' hips according to a periodicity schedule and follow-up until the child is an established walker.
- Record and document physical findings.
- Be aware of the changing physical examination for DDH.
- If physical findings raise suspicion of DDH, or if parental concerns suggest hip disease, confirmation is required by expert physical examination, referral to an orthopaedist, or by an age-appropriate imaging study.

When this process of care is followed, the number of dislocated hips diagnosed at 1 year of age should be minimized. However, the problem of late detection of dislocated hips will not be eliminated. The results of screening programs have indicated that 1 in 5000 children have a dislocated hip detected at 18 months of age or older.[3]

TECHNICAL REPORT

The Technical Report is available from the American Academy of Pediatrics from several sources. The Technical Report is published in full-text on *Pediatrics electronic pages*. It is also available in a compendium of practice guidelines that contains guidelines and evidence reports together. The objective was to create a recommendation to pediatricians and other primary care providers about their role as screeners for detecting DDH. The patients are a theoretical cohort of newborns. A model-based method using decision analysis was the foundation. Components of the approach include:

- Perspective: primary care provider
- Outcomes: DDH and AVN
- Preferences: expected rates of outcomes
- Model: influence diagram assessed from the subcommittee and from the methodology team with critical feedback from the subcommittee
- Evidence sources: Medline and EMBase (detailed in "Methods" section)
- Evidence quality: assessed on a custom, subjective scale, based primarily on the fit of the evidence in the decision model

The results are detailed in the "Methods" section. Based on the raw evidence and Bayesian hierarchical meta-analysis,[34,35] estimates for the incidence of DDH based on the type of screener (orthopaedist vs pediatrician); the odds ratio for DDH given risk factors of sex, family history, and breech presentation; and estimates for late detection and AVN were determined and are detailed in the "Methods" section and in Tables 1 and 2.

The decision model (reduced based on available evidence) suggests that orthopaedic screening is optimal, but because orthopaedists in the published studies and in practice would differ in pediatric expertise, the supply of pediatric orthopaedists is relatively limited, and the difference between orthopaedists and pediatricians is statistically insignificant, we conclude that pediatric screening is to be recommended. The place for ultrasonography in the screening process remains to be defined because of the limited data available regarding late diagnosis in ultrasonography screening to permit definitive recommendations.

These data could be used by others to refine the conclusion based on costs, parental preferences, or physician style. Areas for research are well defined by our model-based method. All references are in the Technical Report.

RESEARCH QUESTIONS

The quality of the literature suggests many areas for research, because there is a paucity of randomized clinical trials and case-controlled studies. The following is a list of possibilities:

1. Minimum diagnostic abilities of a screener. Although there are data for pediatricians in general, few, if any, studies evaluated the abilities of an individual examiner. What should the minimum

sensitivity and specificity be, and how should they be assessed?

2. Intercurrent screening. There were few studies on systemic processes for screening after the newborn period.[2,43,44] Although several studies assessed postneonatal DDH, the data did not specify how many examinations were performed on each child before the abnormal result was found.

3. Trade-offs. Screening always results in false-positive results, and these patients suffer the adverse effects of therapy. How many unnecessary AVNs are we—families, physicians, and society—willing to tolerate from a screening program for every appropriately treated infant in whom late DDH was averted? This assessment depends on people's values and preferences and is not strictly an epidemiologic issue.

4. Postneonatal DDH after ultrasonographic screening. Although we concluded that ultrasonographic screening did not result in fewer diagnoses of postneonatal DDH, that conclusion was based on only 1 study.[36] Further study is needed.

5. Cost-effectiveness. If ultrasonographic screening reduces the number of postneonatal DDH diagnoses, then there will be a cost trade-off between the resources spent up front to screen everyone with an expensive technology, as in the case of ultrasonography, and the resources spent later to treat an expensive adverse event, as in the case of physical examination-based screening. The level at which the cost per case of postneonatal DDH averted is no longer acceptable is a matter of social preference, not of epidemiology.

ACKNOWLEDGMENTS

We acknowledge and appreciate the help of our methodology team, Richard Hinton, MD, Paola Morello, MD, and Jeanne Santoli, MD, who diligently participated in the literature review and abstracting the articles into evidence tables, and the subcommittee on evidence analysis.

We would also like to thank Robert Sebring, PhD, for assisting in the management of this process; Bonnie Cosner for managing the workflow; and Chris Kwiat, MLS, from the American Academy of Pediatrics Bakwin Library, who performed the literature searches.

COMMITTEE ON QUALITY IMPROVEMENT, 1999–2000
Charles J. Homer, MD, MPH, Chairperson
Richard D. Baltz, MD
Gerald B. Hickson, MD
Paul V. Miles, MD
Thomas B. Newman, MD, MPH
Joan E. Shook, MD
William M. Zurhellen, MD

Betty A. Lowe, MD, Liaison, National Association of Children's Hospitals and Related Institutions (NACHRI)
Ellen Schwalenstocker, MBA, Liaison, NACHRI
Michael J. Goldberg, MD, Liaison, Council on Sections
Richard Shiffman, MD, Liaison, Section on Computers and Other Technology
Jan Ellen Berger, MD, Liaison, Committee on Medical Liability
F. Lane France, MD, Committee on Practice and Ambulatory Medicine

SUBCOMMITTEE ON DEVELOPMENTAL DYSPLASIA OF THE HIP, 1999–2000
Michael J. Goldberg, MD, Chairperson
    Section on Orthopaedics
Theodore H. Harcke, MD
    Section on Radiology
Anthony Hirsch, MD
    Practitioner
Harold Lehmann, MD, PhD
    Section on Epidemiology
Dennis R. Roy, MD
    Section on Orthopaedics
Philip Sunshine, MD
    Section on Perinatology

CONSULTANT
Carol Dezateux, MB, MPH

REFERENCES

1. Bjerkreim I, Hagen O, Ikonomou N, Kase T, Kristiansen T, Arseth P. Late diagnosis of developmental dislocation of the hip in Norway during the years 1980–1989. *J Pediatr Orthop B*. 1993;2:112–114
2. Clarke N, Clegg J, Al-Chalabi A. Ultrasound screening of hips at risk for CDH: failure to reduce the incidence of late cases. *J Bone Joint Surg Br*. 1989;71:9–12
3. Dezateux C, Godward C. Evaluating the national screening programme for congenital dislocation of the hip. *J Med Screen*. 1995;2:200–206
4. Hadlow V. Neonatal screening for congenital dislocation of the hip: a prospective 21-year survey. *J Bone Joint Surg Br*. 1988;70:740–743
5. Krikler S, Dwyer N. Comparison of results of two approaches to hip screening in infants. *J Bone Joint Surg Br*. 1992;74:701–703
6. Macnicol M. Results of a 25-year screening programme for neonatal hip instability. *J Bone Joint Surg Br*. 1990;72:1057–1060
7. Marks DS, Clegg J, Al-Chalabi A. Routine ultrasound screening for neonatal hip instability: can it abolish late-presenting congenital dislocation of the hip? *J Bone Joint Surg Br*. 1994;76:534–538
8. Rosendahl K, Markestad T, Lie R. Congenital dislocation of the hip: a prospective study comparing ultrasound and clinical examination. *Acta Paediatr*. 1992;81:177–181
9. Sanfridson J, Redlund-Johnell I, Uden A. Why is congenital dislocation of the hip still missed? Analysis of 96,891 infants screened in Malmo 1956–1987. *Acta Orthop Scand*. 1991;62:87–91
10. Tredwell S, Bell H. Efficacy of neonatal hip examination. *J Pediatr Orthop*. 1981;1:61–65
11. Yngve D, Gross R. Late diagnosis of hip dislocation in infants. *J Pediatr Orthop*. 1990;10:777–779
12. Aronsson DD, Goldberg MJ, Kling TF, Roy DR. Developmental dysplasia of the hip. *Pediatrics*. 1994;94:201–212
13. Hinderaker T, Daltveit AK, Irgens LM, Uden A, Reikeras O. The impact of intra-uterine factors on neonatal hip instability: an analysis of 1,059,479 children in Norway. *Acta Orthop Scand*. 1994;65:239–242
14. Wynne-Davies R. Acetabular dysplasia and familial joint laxity: two etiological factors in congenital dislocation of the hip: a review of 589 patients and their families. *J Bone Joint Surg Br*. 1970;52:704–716
15. De Pellegrin M. Ultrasound screening for congenital dislocation of the hip: results and correlations between clinical and ultrasound findings. *Ital J Orthop Traumatol*. 1991;17:547–553
16. Stoffelen D, Urlus M, Molenaers G, Fabry G. Ultrasound, radiographs, and clinical symptoms in developmental dislocation of the hip: a study of 170 patients. *J Pediatr Orthop B*. 1995;4:194–199
17. Bond CD, Hennrikus WL, Della Maggiore E. Prospective evaluation of newborn soft tissue hip clicks with ultrasound. *J Pediatr Orthop*. 1997;17:199–201
18. Bialik V, Wiener F, Benderly A. Ultrasonography and screening in developmental displacement of the hip. *J Pediatr Orthop B*. 1992;1:51–54
19. Castelein R, Sauter A. Ultrasound screening for congenital dysplasia of the hip in newborns: its value. *J Pediatr Orthop*. 1988;8:666–670
20. Clarke NMP, Harcke HT, McHugh P, Lee MS, Borns PF, MacEwen GP. Real-time ultrasound in the diagnosis of congenital dislocation and dysplasia of the hip. *J Bone Joint Surg Br*. 1985;67:406–412
21. Garvey M, Donoghue V, Gorman W, O'Brien N, Murphy J. Radiographic screening at four months of infants at risk for congenital hip dislocation. *J Bone Joint Surg Br*. 1992;74:704–707
22. Langer R. Ultrasonic investigation of the hip in newborns in the diagnosis of congenital hip dislocation: classification and results of a screening program. *Skeletal Radiol*. 1987;16:275–279

23. Rosendahl K, Markestad T, Lie RT. Ultrasound screening for developmental dysplasia of the hip in the neonate: the effect on treatment rate and prevalence of late cases. *Pediatrics*. 1994;94:47–52

24. Terjesen T. Ultrasound as the primary imaging method in the diagnosis of hip dysplasia in children aged <2 years. *J Pediatr Orthop B*. 1996;5:123–128

25. Vedantam R, Bell M. Dynamic ultrasound assessment for monitoring of treatment of congenital dislocation of the hip. *J Pediatr Orthop*. 1995;15:725–728

26. Graf R. Classification of hip joint dysplasia by means of sonography. *Arch Orthop Trauma Surg*. 1984;102:248–255

27. Berman L, Klenerman L. Ultrasound screening for hip abnormalities: preliminary findings in 1001 neonates. *Br Med J (Clin Res Ed)*. 1986;293:719–722

28. Castelein R, Sauter A, de Vlieger M, van Linge B. Natural history of ultrasound hip abnormalities in clinically normal newborns. *J Pediatr Orthop*. 1992;12:423–427

29. Clarke N. Sonographic clarification of the problems of neonatal hip stability. *J Pediatr Orthop*. 1986;6:527–532

30. Eddy DM. The confidence profile method: a Bayesian method for assessing health technologies. *Operations Res*. 1989;37:210–228

31. Howard RA, Matheson JE. Influence diagrams. In: Matheson JE, ed. *Readings on the Principles and Applications of Decision Analysis*. Menlo Park, CA: Strategic Decisions Group; 1981:720–762

32. Nease RF, Owen DK. Use of influence diagrams to structure medical decisions. *Med Decis Making*. 1997;17:265–275

33. Guyatt GH, Sackett DL, Sinclair JC, Hayward R, Cook DJ, Cook RJ. Users' guide to the medical literature, IX: a method for grading health care recommendations. *JAMA*. 1995;274:1800–1804

34. Gelman A, Carlin JB, Stern HS, Rubin DB. *Bayesian Data Analysis*. London, UK: Chapman and Hall; 1997

35. Spiegelhalter D, Thomas A, Best N, Gilks W. *BUGS 0.5: Bayesian Inference Using Gibbs Sampling Manual, II*. Cambridge, MA: MRC Biostatistics Unit, Institute of Public Health; 1996. Available at: http://www.mrc-bsu.cam.ac.uk/bugs/software/software.html

36. Fiddian NJ, Gardiner JC. Screening for congenital dislocation of the hip by physiotherapists: results of a ten-year study. *J Bone Joint Surg Br*. 1994;76:458–459

37. Dunn P, Evans R, Thearle M, Griffiths H, Witherow P. Congenital dislocation of the hip: early and late diagnosis and management compared. *Arch Dis Child*. 1992;60:407–414

38. Holen KJ, Tegnander A, Terjesen T, Johansen OJ, Eik-Nes SH. Ultrasonographic evaluation of breech presentation as a risk factor for hip dysplasia. *Acta Paediatr*. 1996;85:225–229

39. Jones D, Powell N. Ultrasound and neonatal hip screening: a prospective study of "high risk" babies. *J Bone Joint Surg Br*. 1990;72:457–459

40. Teanby DN, Paton RW. Ultrasound screening for congenital dislocation of the hip: a limited targeted programme. *J Pediatr Orthop*. 1997;17:202–204

41. Tonnis D, Storch K, Ulbrich H. Results of newborn screening for CDH with and without sonography and correlation of risk factors. *J Pediatr Orthop*. 1990;10:145–152

42. Pauker SG, Kassirer JP. The threshold approach to clinical decision making. *N Engl J Med*. 1980;302:1109–1117

43. Bower C, Stanley F, Morgan B, Slattery H, Stanton C. Screening for congenital dislocation of the hip by child-health nurses in western Australia. *Med J Aust*. 1989;150:61–65

44. Franchin F, Lacalendola G, Molfetta L, Mascolo V, Quagliarella L. Ultrasound for early diagnosis of hip dysplasia. *Ital J Orthop Traumatol*. 1992;18:261–269

ADDENDUM TO REFERENCES FOR THE DDH GUIDELINE

New information is generated constantly. Specific details of this report must be changed over time.

New articles (additional articles 1–7) have been published since the completion of our literature search and construction of this Guideline. These articles taken alone might seem to contradict some of the Guideline's estimates as detailed in the article and in the Technical Report. However, taken in context with the literature synthesis carried out for the construction of this Guideline, our estimates remain intact and no conclusions are obviated.

ADDITIONAL ARTICLES

1. Bialik V, Bialik GM, Blazer S, Sujov P, Wiener F, Berant M. Developmental dysplasia of the hip: a new approach to incidence. *Pediatrics*. 1999;103:93–99

2. Clegg J, Bache CE, Raut VV. Financial justification for routine ultrasound screening of the neonatal hip. *J Bone Joint Surg*. 1999;81-B:852–857

3. Holen KJ, Tegnander A, Eik-Nes SH, Terjesen T. The use of ultrasound in determining the initiation in treatment in instability of the hips in neonates. *J Bone Joint Surg*. 1999;81-B:846–851

4. Lewis K, Jones DA, Powell N. Ultrasound and neonatal hip screening: the five-year results of a prospective study in high risk babies. *J Pediatr Orthop*. 1999;19:760–762

5. Paton RW, Srinivasan MS, Shah B, Hollis S. Ultrasound screening for hips at risk in developmental dysplasia: is it worth it? *J Bone Joint Surg*. 1999;81-B:255–258

6. Sucato DJ, Johnston CE, Birch JG, Herring JA, Mack P. Outcomes of ultrasonographic hip abnormalities in clinically stable hips. *J Pediatr Orthop*. 1999;19:754–759

7. Williams PR, Jones DA, Bishay M. Avascular necrosis and the aberdeen splint in developmental dysplasia of the hip. *J Bone Joint Surg*. 1999;81-B:1023–1028

Technical Report Summary:
Developmental Dysplasia of the Hip Practice Guideline

Authors:

Harold P. Lehmann, MD, PhD; Richard Hinton, MD, MPH;
Paola Morello, MD; and Jeanne Santoli, MD
in conjunction with the
American Academy of Pediatrics
Subcommittee on Developmental
Dysplasia of the Hip

American Academy of Pediatrics
PO Box 927, 141 Northwest Point Blvd
Elk Grove Village, IL 60009-0927

For the complete technical report, including tables, figures, and references, please see the companion CD-ROM.

ABSTRACT

Objective. To create a recommendation for pediatricians and other primary care providers about their role as screeners for detecting developmental dysplasia of the hip (DDH) in children.

Patients. Theoretical cohorts of newborns.

Method. Model-based approach using decision analysis as the foundation. Components of the approach include the following:

Perspective: Primary care provider.

Outcomes: DDH, avascular necrosis of the hip (AVN).

Options: Newborn screening by pediatric examination; orthopaedic examination; ultrasonographic examination; orthopaedic or ultrasonographic examination by risk factors. Intercurrent health supervision-based screening.

Preferences: 0 for bad outcomes, 1 for best outcomes.

Model: Influence diagram assessed by the Subcommittee and by the methodology team, with critical feedback from the Subcommittee.

Evidence Sources: Medline and EMBASE search of the research literature through June 1996. Hand search of sentinel journals from June 1996 through March 1997. Ancestor search of accepted articles.

Evidence Quality: Assessed on a custom subjective scale, based primarily on the fit of the evidence to the decision model.

Results. After discussion, explicit modeling, and critique, an influence diagram of 31 nodes was created. The computer-based and the hand literature searches found 534 articles, 101 of which were reviewed by 2 or more readers. Ancestor searches of these yielded a further 17 articles for evidence abstraction. Articles came from around the globe, although primarily Europe, British Isles, Scandinavia, and their descendants. There were 5 controlled trials, each with a sample size less than 40. The remainder were case series. Evidence was available for 17 of the desired 30 probabilities. Evidence quality ranged primarily between one third and two thirds of the maximum attainable score (median: 10–21; interquartile range: 8–14).

Based on the raw evidence and Bayesian hierarchical meta-analyses, our estimate for the incidence of DDH revealed by physical examination performed by pediatricians is 8.6 per 1000; for orthopaedic screening, 11.5; for ultrasonography, 25. The odds ratio for DDH, given breech delivery, is 5.5; for female sex, 4.1; for positive family history, 1.7, although this last factor is not statistically significant. Postneonatal cases of DDH were divided into mid-term (younger than 6 months of age) and late-term (older than 6 months of age). Our estimates for the mid-term rate for screening by pediatricians is 0.34/1000 children screened; for orthopaedists, 0.1; and for ultrasonography, 0.28. Our estimates for late-term DDH rates are 0.21/1000 newborns screened by pediatricians; 0.08, by orthopaedists; and 0.2 for ultrasonography. The rates of AVN for children referred before 6 months of age is estimated at 2.5/1000 infants referred. For those referred after 6 months of age, our estimate is 109/1000 referred infants.

The decision model (reduced, based on available evidence) suggests that orthopaedic screening is optimal, but because orthopaedists in the published studies and in practice would differ, the supply of orthopaedists is relatively limited, and the difference between orthopaedists and pediatricians is statistically insignificant, we conclude that pediatric screening is to be recommended. The place of ultrasonography in the screening process remains to be defined because there are too few data about postneonatal diagnosis by ultrasonographic screening to permit definitive recommendations. These data could be used by others to refine the conclusions based on costs, parental preferences, or physician style. Areas for research are well defined by our model-based approach. *Pediatrics* 2000;105(4). URL: http://www.pediatrics.org/cgi/content/full/105/4/e57; keywords: *developmental dysplasia of the hip, avascular necrosis of the hip, newborn.*

I. GUIDELINE METHODS

A. Decision Model

The steps required to build the model were taken with the Subcommittee as a whole, with individuals in the group, and with members of the methodology team. Agreement on the model was sought from the Subcommittee as a whole during face-to-face meetings.

1. Perspective

Although there are a number of perspectives to take in this problem (parental, child's, societal, and payer's), we opted for the view of the practicing clinician: What are the clinician's obligations, and what is the best strategy for the clinician? This choice of perspective meant that the focus would be on screening for developmental dysplasia of the hip (DDH) and obviated the need to review the evidence for efficacy or effectiveness of specific strategies.

2. Context

The target child is a full-term newborn with no obvious orthopaedic abnormalities. Children with such findings would be referred to an orthopaedist, obviating the need for a practice parameter.

3. Options

We focused on the following options: screening by physical examination (PE) at birth by a pediatrician, orthopaedist, or other care provider; ultrasonographic screening at birth; and episodic screening during health supervision. Treatment options are not included.

We also included in our model a wide range of options for managing the screening process during the first year of life when the newborn screening was negative.

4. Outcomes

Our focus is on dislocated hips at 1 year of age as the major morbidity of the disease and on avascular necrosis of the hip (AVN), as the primary sentinel complication of DDH therapy.

Ideally, we would have a "gold standard" that would define DDH at any point in time, much as cardiac output can be obtained from a pulmonary-artery catheter. However, no gold standard exists. Therefore, we defined our outcomes in terms of the process of care: a pediatrician and an ultrasonographer perform initial or confirmatory examinations and refer the patient, whereas the orthopaedist treats the patient. It is the treatment that has the greatest effect on postneonatal DDH or on complications, so we focus on that intermediate outcome, rather than the orthopaedist's stated diagnosis. We operationalized the definitions of these outcomes for use in abstracting the data from articles. A statement that a "click" was found on PE was considered to refer to an intermediate result, unless the authors defined their "click" in terms of our definition of a positive examination. Dynamic ultrasonographic examinations include those of Harcke et al, and static refers primarily to that of Graf. The radiologic focus switches from ultrasonography to plain radiographs after 4 months of age, in keeping with the development of the femoral head.

5. Decision Structure

We used an influence diagram to represent the decision model. In this representation, nodes refer to actions to be taken or to states of the world (the patient) about which we are uncertain. We devoted substantial effort to the construction of a model that balanced the need to represent the rich array of possible screening pathways with the need to be parsimonious. We constructed the master influence diagram and determined its construct validity through consensus by the Subcommittee before data abstraction. However, the available evidence could specify only a portion of the diagram. The missing components suggest research questions that need to be posed.

6. Probabilities

The purpose of the literature review was to provide the probabilities required by the decision model. The initial number of individual probabilities was 55. (Sensitivity and specificity for a single truth-indicator pair are counted as a single probability because they are garnered from the same table.) Although this is a large number of parameters, the structure of the model helped the team of readers. As 1 reader said, referring to the influence diagram, "Because we did the picture together, it was easy to find the parameters." What follows are some operational rules for matching the data to our parameters. The list is not complete. If an orthopaedic clinic worked at case finding, we used our judgment to determine whether to accept such reports as representing a population incidence.

Risk factors were included generally only if a true control group was used for comparison. For postneonatal diagnoses, no study we reviewed included the examination of all children without DDH, say, 1 year of age, so there is always the possibility of missed cases (false-negative diagnoses) in the screen,

which leads to a falsely elevated estimate of the denominator. For studies originating in referral clinics, the data on the reasons for referrals were not usable for our purposes.

7. Preferences

Ideally, we would have cost data for the options, as well as patient data on the human burden of therapy and of DDH itself. We have deferred these assessments to later research. Therefore, we assigned a preference score of 0 to DDH at 1 year of age and 1 to its absence; for AVN, we assigned 0 for presence at 1 year of age and 1 for absence at 1 year of age.

B. Literature Review

For the literature through May 1995, the following sources were searched: Books in Print, CAT-LINE, Current Contents, EMBASE, Federal Research in Progress, Health Care Standards, Health Devices Alerts, Health Planning and Administration, Health Services/Technology Assessment, International Health Technology Assessment, and Medline. Medline and EMBASE were searched through June 1996. The search terms used in all databases included the following: hip dislocation, congenital; hip dysplasia; congenital hip dislocation; developmental dysplasia; ultrasonography/adverse effects; and osteonecrosis. Hand searches of leading orthopaedic journals were performed for the issues from June 1996 to March 1997. The bibliographies of journals accepted for use in formulating the practice parameter also were perused.

The titles and the abstracts were then reviewed by 2 members of the methodology team to determine whether to accept or reject the articles for use. Decisions were reviewed by the Subcommittee, and conflicts were adjudicated. Similarly, articles were read by pairs of reviewers; conflicts were resolved in discussion.

The focus of the data abstraction process was on data that would provide evidence for the probabilities required by the decision model.

As part of the literature abstraction process, the evidence quality in each article was assessed. The scoring process was based on our decision model and involved traditional epidemiologic concerns, like outcome definition and bias of ascertainment, as well as influence–diagram-based concerns, such as how well the data fit into the model.

Cohort definition: Does the cohort represented by the denominator in the study match a node in our influence diagram? Does the cohort represented by the numerator match a node in our influence diagram? The closer the match, the more confident we are that the reported data provide good evidence of the conditional probability implied by the arrow between the corresponding nodes in the influence diagram.

Path: Does the implied path from denominator to numerator lead through 1 or more nodes of the influence diagram? The longer the path, the more likely that uncontrolled biases entered into the study, making us less confident about accepting the raw data as a conditional probability in our model. Assignment and comparison: Was there a control group? How was assignment made to experimental or control arms? A randomized, controlled study provides the best quality evidence.

Follow-up: Were patients with positive and negative initial findings followed up? The best studies should have data on both.

Outcome definition: Did the language of the outcome definitions (PE, orthopaedic examination, ultrasonography, and radiography) match ours, and, in particular, were PE findings divided into 3 categories or 2? The closer the definition to ours, the more we could pool the data. Studies with only 2 categories do not help to distinguish clicks from "clunks."

Ascertainment: When the denominator represented more than 1 node, to what degree was the denominator a mix of nodes? The smaller the contamination, the more confident we were that the raw data represented a desired conditional probability.

Results: Did the results fill an entire table or were data missing? This is related to the follow-up category but is more general.

C. Synthesis of Evidence

There are 3 levels of evidence synthesis.

1. Listing evidence for individual probabilities
2. Summarizing evidence across probabilities
3. Integrating the pooled evidence for individual probabilities into the decision model

A list of evidence for an individual probability (or arc) is called an *evidence table* and provides the reader a look at the individual pieces of data. The probabilities are summarized in 3 ways: by averaging, by averaging weighted by sample size (pooled), and by meta-analysis. We chose Bayesian meta-analytic techniques, which allow the representation of *prior belief* in the evidence and provide an explicit portrayal of the uncertainty of our conclusions. The framework we used was that of a hierarchical Bayesian model, similar to the random effects model in traditional meta-analysis. In this hierarchical model, each study has its own parameter, which, in turn, is sampled from a wider population parameter. Because there are 2 stages (ie, population to sample and sample to observation), and, therefore, the population parameter of interest is more distant from the data, the computed estimates in the population parameters are, in general, less certain (wider confidence interval) than simply pooling the data across studies. This lower certainty is appropriate in the DDH content area because the studies vary so widely in their raw estimates because of the range in time and geography over which they were performed. In the Bayesian model, the observations were assumed to be Poisson distributed, given the study DDH rates. Those rates, in turn, were assumed to be Gamma distributed, given the population rate. The prior belief on that rate was set as Gamma $(\propto, \text{ß})$, with mean $\propto/\text{ß}$, and variance $\propto/\text{ß}^2$ (as defined in the BUGS software). In this parameterization, $\propto$ has the semantics closest to that of location, and ß has the semantics of certainty: the higher its value, the narrower the distribution and the more certain we are of the estimate. The parameter, $\propto$, was modeled as Exponential (1), and ß, as Gamma (0.01, 1), with a mean of 0.01. Together, these correspond to a prior belief in the rate of a mean of 100 per 1000, and a standard deviation (SD) of 100, representing ignorance of the true rate.

As an example of interpretation, for pediatric newborn screening, the posterior $\propto$ was 1.46, and the posterior ß was 0.17, to give a posterior rate of 8.6/1000, with a variance of 50, or an SD of 7.1. The value of ß rose from 0.01 to 0.17, indicating a higher level of certainty.

The Bayesian confidence interval is the narrowest interval that contains 95% of the area under the posterior-belief curve. The confidence interval for the prior curve is 2.53 to 370. The confidence interval for the posterior curve is 0.25 to 27.5, a significant shrinking and increase in certainty but still broad.

The model for the odds ratios is more complicated and is based on the Oxford data set and analysis in the BUGS manual.

D. Thresholds

In the course of discussions about results, the Subcommittee was surveyed about the acceptable risks of DDH for different levels of interventions.

E. Recommendations

Once the evidence and thresholds were obtained, a decision tree was created from the evidence available and was reviewed by the Subcommittee. In parallel, a consensus guideline (flowchart) was created. The Subcommittee evaluated whether evidence was available for links within the guidelines, as well as their strength of consensus. The decision tree was evaluated to check consistency of the evidence with the conclusions.

F. "Cost"-Effectiveness Ratios

To integrate the results, we defined cost-effectiveness ratios, in which cost was excess neonatal referrals or excess cases of AVNs, and *effectiveness* was a decrease in the number of later cases. The decision tree from section E ("Recommendations") was used to calculate the expected outcomes for each of pediatric, orthopaedic, and ultrasonographic strategies. Pediatric strategy was used as the baseline, because its neonatal screening rate was the lowest. The cost-effectiveness ratios then were calculated as the quotient of the difference in cost and the difference in effect.

RESULTS

A. Articles

The peak number of articles is for 1992, with 10 articles. The articles are from sites all over the world, although the Nordic, Anglo-Saxon, and European communities and their descendants are the most represented.

B. Evidence

By traditional epidemiologic standards, the quality of evidence in this set of articles is uniformly low. There are few controlled trials and few studies in which infants with negative results on their newborn examinations are followed up. (A number of studies attempted to cover all possible places where an affected child might have been ascertained.)

We found data on all chance nodes, for a total of 298 distinct tables. *Decision* nodes were poorly represented: beyond the neonatal strategy, there were almost no data clarifying the paths for the diagnosis children after the newborn period. Thus, although communities like those in southeast Norway have a postnewborn screening program, it is unclear what the program was, and it was unclear how many examination results were normal before a child was referred to an orthopaedist.

The mode is a score of 10, achieved in 16 articles. The median is 9.9, with an interquartile range of 8 to 14, suggesting that articles with scores below 8 are poor sources of evidence. Note that the maximum achievable quality score is 21, so half the articles do not achieve half the maximum quality score.

Graphing evidence quality against publication year suggests an improvement in quality over time, as shown in Fig 9, but the linear fit through the data is statistically indistinguishable from a flat line. (A nonparametric procedure yields the same conclusion).

The studies include 5 in which a comparative arm was designed into the study. The remainder are divided between prospective and retrospective studies. Surprisingly, the evidence quality is not higher in the former than in the latter (data not shown).

Of the 298 data tables, half the data tables relate to the following:
- probabilities of DDH in different screening strategies
- relative risk of DDH, given risk factors
- the incidence of postneonatal DDH, and
- the incidence of AVN.

The remainder of our discussion will focus on these probabilities.

C. Evidence Tables

The evidence table details are found in the appendix of the full technical report.

1. Newborn Screening

a. Pediatric Screening

There were 51 studies, providing 57 arms, for pediatric screening. However, of these, 17 were unclear on how the intermediate examinations were handled, and, unsurprisingly, their observed rates of positivity (clicks) were much higher than the studies that distinguished 3 categories, as we had specified. Therefore, we included only the 34 studies that used 3 categories.

For pediatric screening, the rate is about 8 positive cases per 1000 examinations. The rates are distributed almost uniformly between 0 and 20 per 1000. All studies represent a large experience: a total   of 2 149 972 subjects. Although their methods may not have been the best, the studies demand attention simply because of their size.

In looking for covariates or confounding variables, we studied the relationship between positivity rate and the independent variables, year of publication, evidence quality, and sample size. Year and evidence quality show a positive effect: the higher the year (slope: 0.2; P 5 .018) or evidence quality (slope: 0.6; P 5 .046), the higher the observed rate. A model with both factors has evidence that suggests that most of the effect is in the factor, year (slope for year: 0.08; P 5 .038; slope for quality of evidence: 0.49; P 5 .09). Note that a regression using evidence quality is improper, because our evidence scale is not properly ratio (eg, the distance between 6 and 7 is not necessarily equivalent to the distance between 14 and 15), but the regression is a useful exploratory device.

b. Orthopaedic Screening

Evidence was found in 25 studies. Three studies provided 2 arms each.

The positivity rate for orthopaedic screening is between 7 and 11/1000. One outlier study, with an observed rate of more than 300/1000, skews the unweighted and meta-analytic averages. The estimate (between 7.1 and 11) is just below that of pediatric screening and is statistically indistinguishable. Note, however, that a fair number of studies have rates near 22/1000 or higher.

Unlike with pediatric screening, there are no correlations with other factors.

c. Ultrasonographic Screening

Evidence was found in 17 studies, each providing a single arm.

The rate for ultrasonographic screening is 20/1000 or more. Although the estimates are sensitive to pooling and to the outlier, the positivity rate is clearly higher than in either PE strategy. There are no correlating factors. In particular, studies that use the Graf method 2 or those that use the method of Harcke et al show comparable rates.

2. Postneonatal Cases

We initially were interested in all postneonatal diagnoses of DDH. However, the literature did not provide data within the narrow time frames initially specified for our model. Based on the data that were available, we considered 3 classes of postneonatal DDH: DDH diagnosed after 12 months of age ("late-term"), DDH diagnosed between 6 and 12 months of age ("mid-term"), and DDH diagnosed before 6 months of age. There were few data for the latter group, which often was combined with the newborn screening programs. Therefore, we collected data on only the first 2 groups.

a. After Pediatric Screening

Evidence was found in 24 studies. The study by Dunn and O'Riordan provided 2 arms. It is difficult to discern an estimate rate for mid-term DDH, because the study by Czeizel et al is such an outlier, with a rate of 3.73/1000, and because the weighted and unweighted averages also differ greatly. The meta-analytic estimate of 0.55/1000 seems to be an upper limit.

The late-term rate is easier to estimate at ~0.3/1000. Although it is intuitive that the late-term rate should be lower than the mid-term rate, our data do not allow us to draw that conclusion.

b. After Orthopaedic Screening

There were only 4 studies. The rates were comparable for mid- and late-term: 0.1/1000 newborns. A meta-analytic estimate was not calculated.

c. After Ultrasonographic Screening

Only 1 study, by Rosendahl et al is available; it reported rates for infants with and without initial risk factors (eg, family history and breech presentation). The mid-term rate was 0.28/1000 newborns in the non-risk group, and the late-term rate was 0/1000 in the same group.

3. AVN After Treatment

For these estimates, we grouped together all treatments, because from the viewpoint of the referring primary care provider, orthopaedic treatment is a "black box:" A literature synthesis that teased apart the success and complications of particular *therapeutic* strategies is beyond the scope of the present study.

The complication rate should depend only on the age of the patient at time of orthopaedic referral and on the type of treatment received. We report on the complication rates for children treated before and after 12 months of age.

a. After Early Referral

There were 17 studies providing evidence. Infants were referred to orthopaedists during the newborn period in each study except 2. In the study by Pool et al, infants were referred during the newborn period and before 2 months of age; in the study by Sochart and Paton, infants were referred between 2 weeks and 2 months of age.

The range of AVN rates per 1000 infants referred was huge, from 0 to 123. The largest rate occurred in the study by Pool et al, a sample-based study that included later referrals. Its evidence quality was 8, within the 7 to 13 interquartile range of the other studies in this group. As in earlier tables, the meta-analytic estimate lies between the average and weighted (pooled) average of the studies.

b. After Later Referral

Evidence was obtained from 6 studies. Some of the studies included children referred during the newborn period or during the 2-week to 2-month period, but even in these, the majority of infants were referred later during the first year of life.

There were no outlier rates, although the highest rate (216/1000 referred children) occurred in the study with the oldest referred children in the sample with children referred who were older than 12 months of age. One study contributed 5700 patients to the analysis, more than half of the 9270 total, so its AVN rate of 27/1000 brought the unweighted rate of 116/1000 to 54. A meta-analytic estimate was not computed.

4. Risk Factors

A number of factors are known to predispose infants to DDH. We sought evidence for 3 of these: sex, obstetrical position at birth, and family history.

Studies were included in these analyses only if a control group could be ascertained from the available study data.

The key measure is the odds ratio, an estimate of the relative risk. The meaning of the odds ratio is that if the DDH rate for the control group is known, then the DDH rate for the at-risk group is the product of the control-group DDH rate and the odds ratio for the risk factor. An odds ratio statistically significantly greater than 1 indicates that the factor is a risk factor.

The Bayesian meta-analysis produces estimates between the average of the odds ratios and the pooled odds ratio and is, therefore, the estimate we used in our later analyses.

a. Female

The studies were uniform in discerning a risk to girls ~4 times that of boys for being diagnosed with DDH. This risk was seen in all 3 screening environments.

b. Breech

The studies for breech also were confident in finding a risk for breech presentation, on the order of fivefold. One study found breech presentation to be protective, but the study was relatively small and used ultrasonography rather than PE as its outcome measure.

c. Family History

Although some studies found family history to be a risk factor, the range was wide. The confidence intervals for the pooled odds ratio and for the Bayesian analysis contained 1.0, suggesting that family history is *not* an independent risk factor for DDH. However, because of traditional concern with this risk factor, we kept it in our further considerations.

D. Evidence Summary and Risk Implications

To bring all evidence tables together, we constructed a summary table, which contains the estimates we chose for our recommendations. The intervals are asymmetric, in keeping with the intuition that rates near zero cannot be negative, but certainly can be very positive.

Risk factors are based on the pediatrician population rate of 8.6 labeled cases of DDH per 1000 infants screened. In the Subcommittee's discussion, 50/1000 was a cutoff for automatic referral during the newborn period. Hence, girls born in the breech position are classified in a separate category for newborn strategies than infants with other risk factors.

If we use the orthopaedists' rate as our baseline, numbers suggest that boys without risks or those with a family history have the lowest risk; girls without risks and boys born in the breech presentation have an intermediate risk; and girls with a positive family history, and especially girls born in the breech presentation, have the highest risks. Guidelines that consider risk factors should follow these risk profiles.

E. Decision Recommendations

With the evidence synthesized, we can estimate the expected results of the target newborn strategies for postneonatal DDH and AVN.

If a case of DDH is observed in an infant with an initially negative result of screening by an orthopaedist in a newborn screening program, that case is "counted" against the orthopaedist strategy.

The numbers are combined using a simple decision tree, which is not the final tree represented by our influence diagram but is a tree that is supported by our evidence. The results show that pediatricians diagnose fewer newborns with DDH and perhaps have a higher postneonatal DDH rate than orthopaedists but one that is comparable to ultrasonography (acknowledging that our knowledge of postneonatal DDH revealed by ultrasonographic screening is limited). The AVN rates are comparable with pediatrician and ultrasonographic screening and less than with orthopaedist screening.

F. Cost-Effectiveness Ratios

In terms of excess neonatal referrals, the ratios suggest that there is a trade-off: for every case that these strategies detect beyond the pediatric strategy, they require more than 7000 or 16 000 extra referrals, respectively.

DISCUSSION

A. Summary

We derived 298 evidence tables from 118 studies culled from a larger set of 624 articles. Our literature review captured most in our model-based approach, if not all, of the past literature on DDH that was usable. The decision model (reduced based on available evidence) suggests that orthopaedic screening is optimal, but because orthopaedists in the published studies and in practice would differ, the supply of orthopaedists is relatively limited, and the difference between orthopaedists and pediatricians is relatively small, we conclude that pediatric screening is to be recommended. The place of ultrasonography in the screening process remains to be defined because there are too few data about postneonatal diagnosis by ultrasonographic screening to permit definitive recommendations.

Our conclusions are tempered by the uncertainties resulting from the wide range of the evidence. The confidence intervals are wide for the primary parameters. The uncertainties mean that, even with all the evidence collected from the literature, we are left with large doubts about the values of the different parameters.

Our data do not bear directly on the issue about the earliest point that any patient destined to have DDH will show signs of the disease. Our use of the terms *mid-term* and *late-term* DDH addresses that ignorance.

Our conclusions about other areas of the full decision model are more tentative because of the paucity of data about the effectiveness of periodicity examinations. Even the studies that gave data on mid-term and late-term case findings by pediatricians were sparse in their details about how the screening was instituted, maintained, or followed up.

Our literature search was weakest in addressing the European literature, where results about ultrasonography are more prevalent. We found, however, that many of the seminal articles were republished in English or in a form that we could assess.

B. Specific Issues

1. Evidence Quality

Our measure of evidence quality is unique, although it is based on solid principles of study design and decision modeling. In particular, our measure was based on the notion that if the data conform poorly to how we need to use it, we downgrade its value.

However, throughout the analyses, there was never a correlation with the results of a study (in terms of the values of outcomes) and with evidence quality, so we never needed to use the measure for weighting the values of the outcome or for culling articles from our review. Had this been so, the measures would have needed further scrutiny and validation.

2. Outliers

Perhaps the true surrogates for study quality were the outlying values of outcomes. In general, however, there were few cases in which the outliers were clearly the result of poor-quality studies. One example is that of the outcomes of pediatric screening ($1\rightarrow3$), in which the DDH rates in studies using only 2 categories were generally higher than those that explicitly specified 3 levels of outcomes.

Our general justification for using estimates that excluded outliers is that the outliers so much drove the results that they dominated the conclusion out of proportion to their sample sizes. As it is, our estimates have wide ranges.

3. Newborn Screening

The set of studies labeled "pediatrician screening" includes studies with a variety of examiners. We could not estimate the sensitivity and specificity of pediatricians' examinations versus those of other primary care providers versus orthopaedists. There are techniques for extracting these measures from agreement studies, but they are beyond the scope of the present study. It is intuitive that the more cases that one examines, the better an examiner one will be, regardless of professional title.

We were surprised that the results did not show a clear difference in results between the Graf and Harcke et al ultrasonographic examinations. Our data make no statement about the relative advantages of these methods for following up children or in addressing treatment.

4. Postneonatal Cases

As mentioned, our data cannot say when a postneonatal case is established or, therefore, the best time to screen children. We established our initial age categories for postneonatal cases based on biology, treatment changes, and optimal imaging and examination strategies. It is frustrating that the data in the literature are not organized to match this pathophysiological way of thinking about DDH. Similarly, as mentioned, the lack of details by authors on the methods of intercurrent screening means that we cannot recommend a preferred method for mid-term or late-term screening.

5. AVN

We used AVN as our primary marker for treatment morbidity. We acknowledge that the studies we grouped together may reflect different philosophies and results of orthopaedic practice. The hierarchical meta-analysis treats every study as an individual case, and the wide range in our confidence intervals reflects the uncertainty that results in grouping disparate studies together.

C. Comments on Methods

This study is unique in its strong use of decision modeling at each step in the process. In the end, our results are couched in traditional terms (estimated rates of disease or morbidity outcomes), although the context is relatively nontraditional: attaching the estimates to strategies rather than to treatments. In this, our study is typical of an *effectiveness* study, which studied results in the real world, rather than of an *efficacy* study, which examines the biological effects of a treatment.

We made strong and recurrent use of the Bayesian hierarchical meta-analysis. A review of the tables will confirm that the Bayesian results were in the same "ballpark" as the average and pooled average estimates and had a more solid grounding.

The usual criticism of using Bayesian methods is that they depend on prior belief. The usual response is to show that the final estimates are relatively insensitive to the prior belief. In fact, for the screening strategies, a wide range of prior beliefs had no effect on the estimate. However, the prior belief used for the screening strategies—with a mean of 100 cases/1000 with a variance of 100—was too broad for the postneonatal case and AVN analyses; when data were sparse, the prior belief overwhelmed the data. For instance, in late-term DDH revealed by orthopaedic screening (53 30), in an analysis not shown, the posterior estimate from the 4 studies was a rate of 0.345 cases per 1000, despite an average and a pooled average on the order of 0.08. Four studies were insufficient to overpower a prior belief of 100.

D. Research Issues

The place of ultrasonography in DDH screening needs more attention, as does the issue of intercurrent pediatrician screening. In the latter case, society and health care systems must assess the effectiveness of education and the "return on investment" for educational programs. The place of preferences—of the parents, of the clinician—must be established.

We hope that the framework we have delineated—of a decision model and of data—can be useful in these future research endeavors.

Long-term Treatment of the Child With Simple Febrile Seizures

- *Clinical Practice Guideline*
- *Technical Report Summary*

Readers of this clinical practice guideline are urged to review the technical report to enhance the evidence-based decision-making process. The full technical report is available on the enclosed CD-ROM.

AMERICAN ACADEMY OF PEDIATRICS

Committee on Quality Improvement, Subcommittee on Febrile Seizures

Practice Parameter: Long-term Treatment of the Child With Simple Febrile Seizures

ABSTRACT. The Committee on Quality Improvement, Subcommittee on Febrile Seizures, of the American Academy of Pediatrics, in collaboration with experts from the Section on Neurology, general pediatricians, consultants in the fields of child neurology and epilepsy, and research methodologists, developed this practice parameter. This guideline provides recommendations for the treatment of a child with simple febrile seizures. These recommendations are derived from a thorough search and analysis of the literature. The methods and results of the literature review can be found in the accompanying technical report. This guideline is designed to assist pediatricians by providing an analytic framework for the treatment of children with simple febrile seizures. It is not intended to replace clinical judgment or establish a protocol for all patients with this condition. It rarely will be the only appropriate approach to the problem.

The technical report entitled "Treatment of the Child With Simple Febrile Seizures" provides in-depth information on the studies used to form guideline recommendations. A complete bibliography is included as well as evidence tables that summarize data extracted from scientific studies. This report also provides pertinent evidence on the individual therapeutic agents studied including study results and dosing information. Readers of this clinical practice guideline are urged to review the technical report to enhance the evidence-based decision-making process. The report is available on the *Pediatrics electronic pages* website at the following URL: http://www.pediatrics.org/cgi/content/full/103/6/e86.

DEFINITION OF THE PROBLEM

This practice parameter provides recommendations for therapeutic intervention in neurologically healthy infants and children between 6 months and 5 years of age who have had one or more simple febrile seizures. A simple febrile seizure is defined as a brief (<15 minutes) generalized seizure that occurs only once during a 24-hour period in a febrile child who does not have an intracranial infec-

tion or severe metabolic disturbance. This practice parameter is not intended for patients who have had complex febrile seizures (prolonged, ie, >15 minutes, focal, or recurrent in 24 hours), nor does it pertain to children with previous neurologic insults, known central nervous system abnormalities, or a history of afebrile seizures.

TARGET AUDIENCE AND PRACTICE SETTING

This practice parameter is intended for use by pediatricians, family physicians, child neurologists, neurologists, emergency physicians, and other health care professionals who treat children with febrile seizures.

POSSIBLE THERAPEUTIC INTERVENTIONS

Possible therapeutic approaches to a child with simple febrile seizures include continuous anticonvulsant therapy with agents such as phenobarbital, valproic acid, carbamazepine, or phenytoin; intermittent therapy with antipyretic agents or diazepam; or no anticonvulsant therapy.

BACKGROUND

For a child who has experienced a simple febrile seizure, there are potentially 2 major adverse outcomes that may theoretically be altered by an effective therapeutic agent. These are the occurrence of subsequent febrile seizures or afebrile seizures, including epilepsy. The risk of having recurrent simple febrile seizures varies, depending on age. Children younger than 12 months at the time of their first simple febrile seizure have approximately a 50% probability of having recurrent febrile seizures. Children older than 12 months at the time of their first event have approximately a 30% probability of a second febrile seizure; of those that do have a second febrile seizure, 50% have a chance of having at least 1 additional recurrence.[1]

Children with simple febrile seizures have only a slightly greater risk for developing epilepsy by the age of 7 years than the 1% risk of the general population.[2,3] Children who have had multiple simple febrile seizures and are younger than 12 months at the time of the first febrile seizure are at the highest risk, but, even in this group, generalized afebrile seizures develop by age 25 in only 2.4%.[4] No study has demonstrated that treatment for simple febrile seizures can prevent the later development of epilepsy. Furthermore, there is no evidence that simple febrile seizures cause structural damage and no evi-

The recommendations in this statement do not indicate an exclusive course of treatment or serve as a standard of medical care. Variations, taking into account individual circumstances, may be appropriate.

This clinical practice guideline was reviewed by the appropriate councils, committees and sections of the American Academy of Pediatrics including the Committee on Practice and Ambulatory Medicine, the Committee on Pediatric Emergency Medicine, the Committee on Drugs and sections on Emergency Medicine, Clinical Pharmacology, and Neurology. It was also reviewed by the Chapter Review Group, a focus group of practicing pediatricians representing each AAP district: Thomas J. Herr, MD, Gene R. Adams, MD, Charles S. Ball, MD, Diane E. Fuquay, MD, Michael J. Heimerl, MD, Donald T. Miller, MD, Lawrence C. Pakula, MD, William R. Sexson, MD, and Howard B. Weinblatt, MD.

PEDIATRICS (ISSN 0031 4005). Copyright © 1999 by the American Academy of Pediatrics.

dence that children with simple febrile seizures are at risk for cognitive decline.[5]

Despite the frequency of febrile seizures (approximately 3%), there is no unanimity of opinion about therapeutic interventions.[3] The following recommendations are based on an analysis of the risks and benefits of continuous or intermittent therapy in children with simple febrile seizures. The recommendations reflect an awareness of the very low risk that a simple febrile seizure poses to the individual child and the large number of children who have this type of seizure at some time in early life.[1,3-5] To be commensurate, a proposed therapy would need to be exceedingly low in risks and adverse effects, inexpensive, and highly effective.

The expected outcomes of this practice parameter include the following:

1. Optimize practitioner understanding of the scientific basis for using or avoiding various proposed treatments for children with simple febrile seizures.
2. Improve the health of children with simple febrile seizures by avoiding therapies with high potential for side effects and no demonstrated ability to improve children's eventual outcomes.
3. Reduce costs by avoiding therapies that will not demonstrably improve children's long-term outcomes.
4. Help the practitioner educate caregivers about the low risks associated with simple febrile seizures.

METHODOLOGY

More than 300 medical journal articles reporting studies of the natural history of simple febrile seizures or the therapy of these seizures were reviewed and abstracted. Emphasis was placed on articles that differentiated simple febrile seizures from other types of febrile seizures, articles that carefully matched treatment and control groups, and articles that described adherence to the drug regimen. Tables were constructed from 62 articles that best fit these criteria. A more comprehensive review of the literature on which this report is based can be found in the technical report. The technical report also contains dosing information.

BENEFITS AND RISKS OF CONTINUOUS ANTICONVULSANT THERAPY

Phenobarbital

Phenobarbital is effective in preventing the recurrence of simple febrile seizures.[6-8] In a controlled, double-blind study, daily therapy with phenobarbital reduced the rate of subsequent febrile seizures from 25 per 100 subjects per year to 5 per 100 subjects per year.[6]

The adverse effects of phenobarbital include behavioral problems such as hyperactivity and hypersensitivity reactions.[6,9-11]

Valproic Acid

In randomized, controlled studies, only 4% of children taking valproate as opposed to 35% of control subjects had a subsequent febrile seizure. Therefore, valproic acid seems to be at least as effective in preventing recurrent, simple febrile seizures as phenobarbital and significantly more effective than placebo.[7,12,13] Drawbacks to therapy with valproic acid include its rare association with fatal hepatotoxicity (especially in children younger than 3 years who also are at greatest risk for febrile seizures), thrombocytopenia, weight loss and gain, gastrointestinal disturbances, and pancreatitis.[14]

Carbamazepine

Carbamazepine has not been shown to be effective in preventing the recurrence of simple febrile seizures.[9]

Phenytoin

Phenytoin has not been shown to be effective in preventing the recurrence of simple febrile seizures.[15]

BENEFITS AND RISKS OF INTERMITTENT ORAL THERAPY

Antipyretic Agents

Antipyretic agents, in the absence of anticonvulsants, are not effective in preventing recurrent febrile seizures.[6,16]

Diazepam

A double-blind, controlled study in patients with a history of febrile seizures demonstrated that administration of oral diazepam (given at the time of a fever) could reduce the recurrence of febrile seizures. Children with a history of febrile seizures were given oral diazepam or a placebo at the time of fever. There was a 44% reduction in the risk of febrile seizures per person-year with diazepam.[17] A potential drawback to intermittent medication is that a seizure could occur before a fever is noticed. Adverse effects of oral diazepam include lethargy, drowsiness, and ataxia.[17] The sedation associated with this therapy could mask evolving signs of a central nervous system infection.

SUMMARY

The Subcommittee has determined that a simple febrile seizure is a benign and common event in children between the ages of 6 months and 5 years. Most children have an excellent prognosis. Although there are effective therapies that could prevent the occurrence of additional simple febrile seizures, the potential adverse effects of such therapy are not commensurate with the benefit. In situations in which parental anxiety associated with febrile seizures is severe, intermittent oral diazepam at the onset of febrile illness may be effective in preventing recurrence. There is no convincing evidence, however, that any therapy will alleviate the possibility of future epilepsy (a relatively unlikely event). Antipyretics, although they may improve the comfort of the child, will not prevent febrile seizures.

RECOMMENDATION

Based on the risks and benefits of the effective therapies, neither continuous nor intermittent anti-

convulsant therapy is recommended for children with 1 or more simple febrile seizures. The American Academy of Pediatrics recognizes that recurrent episodes of febrile seizures can create anxiety in some parents and their children, and, as such, appropriate education and emotional support should be provided.

ACKNOWLEDGMENTS

The Committee on Quality Improvement and Subcommittee on Febrile Seizures appreciate the expertise of Richard N. Shiffman, MD, Center for Medical Informatics, Yale School of Medicine, for his input and analysis in development of this practice guideline. Comments were also solicited and received from organizations such as the American Academy of Family Physicians, the American Academy of Neurology, the Child Neurology Society, and the American College of Emergency Physicians.

COMMITTEE ON QUALITY IMPROVEMENT, 1998–1999
David A. Bergman, MD, Chairperson
Richard D. Baltz, MD
James R. Cooley, MD
Gerald B. Hickson, MD
Paul V. Miles, MD
Joan E. Shook, MD
William M. Zurhellen, MD

LIAISONS
Betty A. Lowe, MD
    National Association for Childrens Hospitals and Related Institutions
Shirley Girouard, PhD, RN
    National Association for Children's Hospitals and Related Institutions
Michael J. Goldberg, MD
    AAP Sections
Charles J. Homer, MD
    AAP Section on Epidemiology
Jan E. Berger, MD
    AAP Committee on Medical Liability
Jack T. Swanson, MD
    AAP Committee on Practice and Ambulatory Medicine

SUBCOMMITTEE ON FEBRILE SEIZURES, 1998–1999
Patricia K. Duffner, MD, Chairperson
Robert J. Baumann, MD, Methodologist
Peter Berman, MD
John L. Green, MD
Sanford Schneider, MD

CONSULTANTS
Carole S. Camfield, MD, FRCP(C)
Peter R. Camfield, MD, FRCP(C)
David L. Coulter, MD

Patricia K. Crumrine, MD
W. Edwin Dodson, MD
John M. Freeman, MD
Arnold P. Gold, MD
Gregory L. Holmes, MD
Michael Kohrman, MD
Karin B. Nelson, MD
N. Paul Rosman, MD
Shlomo Shinnar, MD

REFERENCES

1. Nelson KB, Ellenberg JH. Prognosis in children with febrile seizures. *Pediatrics*. 1978;61:720–727
2. Nelson KB, Ellenberg JH. Predictors of epilepsy in children who have experienced febrile seizures. *N Engl J Med*. 1976;295:1029–1033
3. Verity CM, Golding J. Risk of epilepsy after febrile convulsions: a national cohort study. *Br Med J*. 1991;303:1373–1376
4. Annegers JF, Hauser WA, Shirts SB, Kurland LT. Factors prognostic of unprovoked seizures after febrile convulsions. *N Engl J Med*. 1987;316: 493–498
5. Ellenberg JH, Nelson KB. Febrile seizures and later intellectual performance. *Arch Neurol*. 1978;35:17–21
6. Camfield PR, Camfield CS, Shapiro SH, Cummings C. The first febrile seizure: antipyretic instruction plus either phenobarbital or placebo to prevent recurrence. *J Pediatr*. 1980;97:16–21
7. Wallace SJ, Smith JA. Successful prophylaxis against febrile convulsions with valproic acid or phenobarbitone. *Br Med J*. 1980;280:353–380
8. Wolf SM. The effectiveness of phenobarbital in the prevention of recurrent febrile convulsions in children with and without a history of pre-, peri-, and postnatal abnormalities. *Acta Paediatr Scand*. 1977;66:585–587
9. Antony JH, Hawke S. Phenobarbital compared with carbamazepine in prevention of recurrent febrile convulsions. *Am J Dis Child*. 1983;137: 892–895
10. Knudsen FU, Vestermark S. Prophylactic diazepam or phenobarbitone in febrile convulsions: a prospective, controlled study. *Arch Dis Child*. 1978;53:660–663
11. Vining EPG, Mellits ED, Dorsen MM, et al. Psychologic and behavioral effects of antiepileptic drugs in children: a double-blind comparison between phenobarbital and valproic acid. *Pediatrics*. 1987;80:165–174
12. Marmelle NM, Plasse JC, Revol M, Gilly R. Prevention of recurrent febrile convulsions: a randomized therapeutic assay: sodium valproate, phenobarbital and placebo. *Neuropediatrics*. 1984;:15:37–42
13. Ngwane E, Bower B. Continuous sodium valproate or phenobarbitone in the prevention of "simple" febrile convulsions. *Arch Dis Child*. 1980; 55:171–174
14. Dreifuss FE. Valproic acid toxicity. In: Levy RH, Mattson RH, Meldrum BS, eds. *Antiepileptic Drugs*. New York, NY: Raven Press; 1995:641–648
15. Bacon CJ, Hierons AM, Mucklow JC, Webb J, Rawlins MD, Weightman D. Placebo-controlled study of phenobarbitone and phenytoin in the prophylaxis in febrile convulsions. *Lancet*. 1981;2:600–604
16. Uhari M, Rantala, H, Vainionpaa L, Kurttila R. Effect of acetaminophen and of low intermittent doses of diazepam on prevention of recurrence of febrile seizures. *J Pediatr*. 1995;126:991–995
17. Rosman NP, Colton T, Labazzo J, et al. A controlled trial of diazepam administered during febrile illnesses to prevent recurrence of febrile seizures. *N Engl J Med*. 1993;329:79–84

Technical Report Summary: Treatment of the Child With Simple Febrile Seizures

Author:

Robert J. Baumann, MD

American Academy of Pediatrics
PO Box 927, 141 Northwest Point Blvd
Elk Grove Village, IL 60009-0927

For the complete technical report, including tables, figures, and references, please see the companion CD-ROM.

ABSTRACT

Overview

Simple febrile seizures that occur in children ages 6 months to 5 years are common events with few adverse outcomes. Those who advocate therapy for this disorder have been concerned that such seizures lead to additional febrile seizures, to epilepsy, and perhaps even to brain injury. Moreover, they note the potential for such seizures to cause parental anxiety. We examined the literature to determine whether there was demonstrable benefit to the treatment of simple febrile seizures and whether such benefits exceeded the potential side effects and risks of therapy. The therapeutic approaches considered included continuous anticonvulsant therapies, intermittent therapy, or no anticonvulsant therapy.

Methods

This analysis focused on the neurologically healthy child between 6 months and 5 years of age whose seizure is brief (<15 minutes), generalized, and occurs only once during a 24-hour period during a fever. Children whose seizures are attributable to a central nervous system infection and those who have had a previous afebrile seizure or central nervous system abnormality were excluded. A review of the current literature was conducted using articles obtained through searches in MEDLINE and additional databases. Articles were obtained following defined criteria and data abstracted using a standardized literature review form. Abstracted data were summarized into evidence tables.

Results

Epidemiologic studies demonstrate a high risk of recurrent febrile seizures but a low, though increased, risk of epilepsy. Other adverse outcomes either don't occur or occur so infrequently that their presence is not convincingly demonstrated by the available studies. Although daily anticonvulsant therapy with phenobarbital or valproic acid is effective in decreasing recurrent febrile seizures, the risks and potential side effects of these medications outweigh this benefit. No medication has been shown to prevent the future onset of recurrent afebrile seizures (epilepsy). The use of intermittent diazepam with fever after an initial febrile seizure is likely to decrease the risk of another febrile seizure, but the rate of side effects is high although most families find the perceived benefits to be low. Although antipyretic therapy has other benefits, it does not prevent additional simple febrile seizures.

Conclusions

The Febrile Seizures Subcommittee of the American Academy of Pediatrics' Committee on Quality Improvement used the results of this analysis to derive evidence-based recommendations for the treatment of simple febrile seizures. The outcomes anticipated as a result of the analysis and development of the practice guideline include: 1) to optimize practitioner understanding of the scientific basis for using or avoiding various proposed treatments for children with simple febrile seizures; 2) to improve the health of children with simple febrile seizures by avoiding therapies with high potential for side effects and no demonstrated ability to improve children's eventual outcomes; 3) to reduce costs by avoiding therapies that will not demonstrably improve children's long-term outcomes; and 4) to help the practitioner educate caregivers about the low risks associated with simple febrile seizures. *Key words: febrile seizures, epilepsy, valproic acid, carbamazepine, phenytoin, diazepam, phenobarbital, sodium valproate, pyridoxine.*

The debate over whether children with recurrent febrile seizures benefit from anticonvulsant therapy began early in this century. An important advance was the identification of the subgroup of children with simple febrile seizures; a subgroup that is large, remarkably homogeneous, and healthy at 7- and 10-year follow-ups. Furthermore, the recognition of such favorable outcomes has accentuated the need to balance the risk of any treatment with an expected benefit. Epidemiologic studies helped to identify this subgroup, demonstrated their predominantly favorable outcomes, and confirmed what has long been known: febrile seizures are common events. Of youngsters in a British birth cohort, 2.7% had febrile seizures, 88% of whom had simple febrile seizures.

DEFINITION OF THE PROBLEM

This parameter is limited to children with simple febrile seizures defined as neurologically healthy infants and children between 6 months and 5 years of age whose seizure is brief (<15 minutes), generalized, and occurs only once during a 24-hour period in a febrile child. This definition is easily applied in the usual clinical circumstances and has the additional advantages of encompassing most children with febrile seizures and defining a relatively homogeneous group of patients. This practice parameter excludes children whose seizures are attributable to a central nervous system infection (symptomatic febrile seizures) and those who have had a previous afebrile seizure or central nervous system abnormality (secondary febrile seizures).

BACKGROUND

Proponents of therapy for simple febrile seizures have worried that repeated simple febrile seizures will lead to more febrile seizures and possibly to afebrile seizures (epilepsy). They also have been apprehensive that these seizures will cause brain injury and thus diminish intelligence or impair motor coordination.

A child who has experienced a single simple febrile seizure is likely to experience another. As epidemiologic data indicate, this recurrence rate is strongly age-related. The younger the child at the time of the first event, the more likely there will be subsequent events. In the National Collaborative Perinatal Project (NCPP), half the subjects with onset of febrile seizures during the first year versus approximately 30% with onset after the first year had one or more additional febrile seizures. This project included 1706 prospectively studied children with febrile seizures from approximately 54 000 pregnancies.

The risk of experiencing a single afebrile seizure or two or more afebrile seizures (defined as epilepsy) is elevated when comparing children with simple febrile seizures with the general age-matched population. In the NCPP, the risk factors for epilepsy after a febrile seizure were a positive family history of afebrile seizures, preexisting neurologic abnormality, and a complicated initial febrile seizure. Interestingly, the age at first febrile seizure and the number of febrile seizures did not alter this risk. At age 7 years, only 1.9% of children with simple febrile seizures and negative family histories of epilepsy had experienced a single afebrile seizure, and epilepsy had developed in 0.9%. The comparable figures for study children who never experienced a febrile seizure were 0.9% for a single afebrile seizure and 0.5% for epilepsy. Similar rates were seen in the large British cohort study that included all surviving neonates born in the United Kingdom during 1 week in April 1970. These children were followed until age 10 years, and 305 had an initial simple febrile seizure. Of the 305 children, 8 (2.6%) subsequently had an afebrile seizure and epilepsy eventually developed in 5 (1.6%). The comparable number with epilepsy among the 14 278 children who never had febrile seizures was 53 (0.4%).

Although the risk of epilepsy among children with simple febrile seizures is elevated, the rate is still low, and the number of children in any given study is small. These numbers provide some understanding of the difficulty of designing a population-based study to determine if any treatment for the prevention of simple febrile seizures would subsequently prevent the development of epilepsy.

Investigators have attempted to look at this issue. The Kaiser Foundation Hospitals in Southern California studied 400 children who had febrile seizures (identified from lumbar puncture reports). They divided the children into three study groups: those who received phenobarbital daily, those who received phenobarbital only with fever, and those who received no therapy. Follow-up lasted a mean of 6.3 years. No difference was found in the rate of afebrile seizures. This study included children with complex as well as simple febrile seizures, many children did not receive the prescribed medication (approximately one third), and the study was small and could have missed a statistically valid effect.

In another study, 289 children with febrile seizures were randomized to rectal diazepam prophylaxis at the onset of any fever or rectal diazepam therapy during any febrile seizure. At age 14 years, there was no difference in intelligence, coordination, or occurrence of epilepsy between the two groups. The number of study patients was small, there are questions regarding compliance, and patients with complex and simple febrile seizures were included.

Evidence for adverse outcomes other than epilepsy has been sought. The NCPP had the benefit of longitudinal examination of a predefined group of children. No evidence of death in relation to asymptomatic febrile seizures was found, and examination of the children revealed no evidence for the development of motor deficits. There also has been concern about cognitive deficits in relation to febrile seizures. The NCPP found no effect on intelligence among 431 children with febrile seizures who were compared with their siblings. Comparisons of children with simple febrile seizures with the general population also have found no adverse effect. Smith and Wallace believed that they found an adverse effect of repeated febrile seizures on intelligence as measured by the Griffith Mental Development Scale. Because they studied children

with simple and complex febrile seizures, it is possible that underlying neurologic disease predisposed to further seizures and to lower scores on retesting.

METHODS

Pertinent articles previously obtained by a medline search and a search of the Epilepsy Foundation of America database 4 were reviewed and supplemented by references suggested by members of the Committee and the Committee's consultants. More than 300 articles were reviewed.

The goal of the review was to identify articles that met the following criteria:
- The study children had simple febrile seizures that were convincingly differentiated from afebrile seizures and other types of febrile seizures.
- The subjects with simple febrile seizures were reasonably representative of children with simple febrile seizures.
- A suitable control group was included in the study. Preference was given to blinded protocols.

CONTINUOUS ANTICONVULSANT THERAPY

Phenobarbital

There are several studies in which phenobarbital administered daily successfully prevented recurrent febrile seizures. Camfield and associates randomized 79 children who had had a first simple febrile seizure to receive phenobarbital at 5 mg/kg per day in a single dose or a placebo. Compliance was monitored by use of the urine fluorescence of a riboflavin additive and by measurements of serum phenobarbital levels. There was a significant difference in the incidence of recurrent febrile seizures between the phenobarbital recipients (2/39 [5%]) and the placebo group (10/40 [25%]). Neither parents nor investigators knew which subjects received the active drug. Investigators found no significant difference in IQ (using Stanford-Binet or Bayley Scales) between the placebo and phenobarbital groups after 8 to 12 months of therapy. Nevertheless, phenobarbital was demonstrated to decrease memory and concentration in proportion to higher serum phenobarbital levels. Transient sleep disturbances and daytime fussiness were more common among phenobarbital recipients, but by 1 year, the two groups were indistinguishable. This was partially accounted for by 4 children receiving phenobarbital whose side effects resolved after the dosage was reduced.

In a controlled trial comparing phenobarbital (5 mg/kg per day) with phenytoin (8 mg/kg per day) and placebo, Bacon and associates also found phenobarbital to be effective. In younger children, the febrile seizure recurrence rate was 9% (2/22) for phenobarbital recipients versus 44% (12/27) placebo recipients. This trial included subjects with complicated febrile seizures who were stratified proportionally into the three groups. The study had major problems with compliance. All phenobarbital-treated children with a recurrence for whom drug levels were obtained at the time of recurrence had a plasma level <15 mg/L. Interestingly the reported behavioral changes were similar in the subjects treated with phenobarbital and a placebo.

Mamelle et al compared phenobarbital (3 to 4 mg/kg per day), valproate (30 to 40 mg/kg per day in 2 doses), and placebo in a randomized single-blind study of infants with a first simple febrile seizure. They found significantly fewer recurrences in the valproate (1/22 [4.5%]) and phenobarbital (4/21 [19%]) groups compared with the placebo group (9/26 [35%]). Compliance was measured by serum drug levels. Only 5 subjects were removed from therapy because of side effects; all were described as having agitation and all were receiving phenobarbital. Other studies, some with designs that were less rigorous, also found phenobarbital to be effective, including the previously mentioned Kaiser Foundation study.

Not all studies have found phenobarbital to be effective. Heckmatt et al found recurrent febrile seizures in 14 (19%) of 73 control subjects, 10 (11%) of 88 children for whom phenobarbital was prescribed, and 4 (8%) of 49 who actually took the prescribed phenobarbital (4 to 5 mg/kg per day in divided doses). These last 4 subjects had plasma phenobarbital levels >16 mg/L at the time of recurrence. Although the differences between the treatment groups are not statistically important, they seem to suggest that an effect favoring phenobarbital might have been evident had the numbers been larger or the duration of the study longer.

Children who had complicated febrile seizures analyzed by intention to treat experienced no difference in recurrence rate between phenobarbital-treated subjects and controls. The study described a poor rate of compliance and seemed to show that a medication is not effective if parents are unable to administer it. Early in the study when compliance was high, 56% of phenobarbital recipients (4 to 5 mg/kg once per day) and 35% of placebo recipients were reported to have side effects. The study found that the mean IQ was 8.4 points lower in the phenobarbital group than in the placebo group (95% CI: −3.3 − −3.5, $P = .0057$) at the end of the 2-year study, with an IQ differential that persisted 6 months after the taper of medication had begun. The analysis of these data was complicated by the low compliance rates, the fact that 24 (26%) of 94 placebo recipients and 53 (64%) of 83 phenobarbital recipients were prescribed phenobarbital after the study ended, and the inclusion of subjects with complicated febrile seizures.

Phenobarbital is associated with impairment of short-term memory and concentration and worsening of behavior. Most data on the effects of phenobarbital have been obtained from adults or from children with epilepsy. The drug's effect seems most prominent at the onset of therapy. The reported effect in children with simple febrile seizures varies among studies. In the study by Camfield et al, parents were only aware of side effects early in the study, but higher serum levels were associated with decreased memory concentration. Smith and Wallace found no effect of therapy but believed that repeated seizures in children with complicated febrile seizures were associated with lower mental development scores. Wolf and Forsythe reported hyperactivity in 46 (42%) of 109 children treated with phenobarbital (initial dose, 3 to 4 mg/kg per day, adjusted to give a serum level of 10 to 15 μg/mL) for febrile seizures compared with 21 (17.5%) of 120 not receiving phenobarbital. As in other studies, a sub-stantial rate of improvement was noted in both groups with time. When 25 children from each group were extensively tested, no cognitive differences could be detected.

Valproic Acid

A number of studies have demonstrated the effectiveness of this agent in preventing recurrent febrile seizures. The study by Mamelle et al typifies the studies that found valproic acid to be more effective than phenobarbital. Although no severe adverse effects are described among the children participating in the febrile seizure trials, the numbers in these trials are small. Valproic acid therapy is associated with fatal hepatotoxicity, pancreatitis, renal toxicity, hematopoietic disturbances, and other problems.

Carbamazepine

Carbamazepine was not effective for febrile seizures in preliminary trials and, thus, has not been studied widely. In a double-blind trial of carbamazepine (20 mg/kg per day in twice daily doses) vs phenobarbital (4 to 5 mg/kg per day) involving children with complicated febrile seizures, Antony and Hawke reported recurrent febrile seizures in 9 (47%) of 19 carbamazepine recipients and 2 (10%) of 21 phenobarbital recipients.

Phenytoin

As with carbamazepine, preliminary studies showed no evidence that phenytoin was effective for febrile seizures, so it has not been studied extensively. In a randomized, controlled study of children with simple and complex febrile seizures, the recurrence rate in the phenytoin group (8 mg/kg per day) of younger children was 33% (9/27) compared with 9% (2/22) for the phenobarbital group (5 mg/kg per day) and 44% (12/27) for the equivalent placebo group.

INTERMITTENT THERAPY

Antipyretic Agents

Because simple febrile seizures occur only in conjunction with a fever, it has seemed logical to try to prevent these seizures by using aggressive antipyretic therapy. In the randomized, double-blind study by Camfield and associates, all subjects received detailed instruction about temperature control, including antipyretic use with any rectal temperature higher than 37.2°C (99°F). Ten (25%) of 40 subjects using only temperature control had recurrences compared with 2 (5%) of 39 receiving continuous phenobarbital. A randomized, controlled trial using a complicated study design with placebo, low-dose diazepam, and acetaminophen also found no evidence that acetaminophen prevented recurrent febrile seizures. In this protocol, the diazepam-treated children who had previously experienced a febrile seizure received a rectal diazepam solution (if they weighed <7 kg, they received 2.5 mg; if 7 to 15 kg, 5 mg; and if >15 kg, 10 mg) followed in 6 hours by 0.2 mg/kg three times a day whenever they were febrile. The antipyretic treatment group received 10 mg/kg of acetaminophen four times per day.

In children hospitalized after a simple febrile seizure, Schnaiderman et al found that acetaminophen (15 to 20 mg/kg per dose) given every 4 hours did not prevent a second febrile seizure during that admission any better than giving acetaminophen sporadically. The two groups also had the same frequency, duration, and height of temperature elevations. There is no evidence that aggressive antipyretic therapy prevents recurrent febrile seizures.

Diazepam

The use of intermittent diazepam prophylaxis for febrile seizures is well-reported in the literature. Autret and colleagues, in a randomized, controlled multicenter study, found that oral diazepam (0.5 mg/kg initially, then 0.2 mg/kg every 12 hours) was no more effective than a placebo in preventing recurrent febrile seizures. Most of the children had simple febrile seizures, and the data were analyzed by intention to treat. Recurrence was experienced by 15 (16%) of 93 children in the diazepam group compared with 18 (20%) of 92 children in the placebo group. Although parents "were instructed verbally, in writing, and by demonstration," there were major problems with compliance. In children with recurrences, only 1 (7%) of 15 diazepam recipients and 7 (39%) of 18 placebo recipients received the medication or placebo as prescribed. The difference between these two groups is significant. The reasons that the subjects did not receive their assigned treatment included the following: 1) 7 in each group had a seizure as the first sign of illness, 2) 5 parents in the diazepam group and 4 in the placebo group did not give the medication, and 3) 2 children in the diazepam group would not take their medication. Because 14 (93%) of the 15 children for whom diazepam was prescribed who had a recurrence had not received their prescribed medication, these data demonstrate that a treatment is not effective if parents cannot or will not administer it before the febrile seizure occurs. The only noted side effect was hyperactivity, which was significantly more frequent in the diazepam group (138 vs 34 days).

By contrast, in a similarly well-designed, randomized, double-blind, placebo-controlled trial, Rosman et al found oral diazepam to be significantly more effective than placebo when analyzed by intention to treat. A 44% reduction in the risk of febrile seizures per person-year occurred with diazepam. Children in the diazepam group had 675 febrile episodes and 41 febrile seizures, of which 7 occurred while receiving the study medication. Comparable figures for the placebo group were 526 febrile episodes and 72 febrile seizures, of which 38 occurred while receiving the placebo. These investigators describe febrile seizures as "highly upsetting" to the parent population, which may have influenced adherence. Not surprisingly, they found that a higher rate of side effects accompanied their subjects' better compliance. Of the diazepam recipients, 59 (39%) had at least one "moderate" side effect and a similar number had a "mild" side effect.

The Neurodiagnostic Evaluation of the Child With a First Simple Febrile Seizure

- *Clinical Practice Guideline*
- *Technical Report Summary*

Readers of this clinical practice guideline are urged to review the technical report to enhance the evidence-based decision-making process. The full technical report is available on the enclosed CD-ROM.

Practice Parameter: The Neurodiagnostic Evaluation of the Child With a First Simple Febrile Seizure

Provisional Committee on Quality Improvement, Subcommittee on Febrile Seizures

ABSTRACT. The American Academy of Pediatrics and its Provisional Committee on Quality Improvement, in collaboration with experts from the Section on Neurology, general pediatricians, consultants in the fields of neurology and epilepsy, and research methodologists, developed this practice parameter. This parameter provides recommendations for the neurodiagnostic evaluation of a child with a first simple febrile seizure. These recommendations derive from both a thorough review of the literature and expert consensus. Interventions of direct interest include lumbar puncture, electroencephalography, blood studies, and neuroimaging. The methods and results of the literature review and data analyses can be found in the technical report that is available from the Publications Department of the American Academy of Pediatrics. This parameter is designed to assist pediatricians by providing an analytic framework for the evaluation and treatment of this condition. It is not intended to replace clinical judgment or establish a protocol for all patients with this condition. It rarely will be the only appropriate approach to the problem.

DEFINITION OF THE PROBLEM

This practice parameter provides recommendations for the neurodiagnostic evaluation of neurologically healthy infants and children between 6 months and 5 years of age who have had their first simple febrile seizures and present within 12 hours of the event. This practice parameter is not intended for patients who have had complex febrile seizures (prolonged, focal, and/or recurrent), nor does it pertain to those children with previous neurologic insults, known central nervous system abnormalities, or histories of afebrile seizures.

TARGET AUDIENCE AND PRACTICE SETTING

This practice parameter is intended for use by pediatricians, family physicians, child neurologists, neurologists, emergency physicians, and other providers who treat children for febrile seizures.

INTERVENTIONS OF DIRECT INTEREST

1. Lumbar puncture;
2. Electroencephalography (EEG);
3. Blood studies—serum electrolytes, calcium, phosphorus, magnesium, and blood glucose, and a complete blood count (CBC); and

4. Neuroimaging—skull radiographs, computed tomography (CT), and magnetic resonance imaging.

BACKGROUND

A febrile seizure is broadly defined as a seizure accompanied by fever without central nervous system infection, occurring in infants and children between 6 months and 5 years of age. Febrile seizures occur in 2% to 5% of all children and, as such, make up the most common convulsive event in children younger than 5 years of age. In 1976, Nelson and Ellenberg,[1] using data from the National Collaborative Perinatal Project, further defined febrile seizures as being either simple or complex. Simple febrile seizures were defined as primary generalized seizures lasting less than 15 minutes and not recurring within 24 hours. Complex febrile seizures were defined as focal, prolonged (>15 minutes), and/or occurring in a flurry. Those children who had simple febrile seizures had no evidence of increased mortality, hemiplegia, or mental retardation. During follow-up evaluation, the risk of epilepsy after a simple febrile seizure was shown to be only slightly higher than that of the general population, whereas the chief risk associated with simple febrile seizures was recurrence in one third of the children. The report concluded that simple febrile seizures are benign events with excellent prognoses, a conclusion reaffirmed in the 1980 National Institutes of Health Consensus Statement.[2]

Despite progress in understanding febrile seizures and the development of consensus statements about their diagnostic evaluation and management, a review of practice patterns of pediatricians indicates that a wide variation persists in physician interpretation, evaluation, and treatment of children with febrile seizures.[3]

This parameter is not intended for the evaluation of patients who have had complex febrile seizures, previous neurologic insults, or known brain abnormalities. The parameter also does not address treatment.

The expected outcomes of this practice parameter include the following.

1. Optimizing practitioner understanding of the scientific basis for the neurodiagnostic evaluation of children with simple febrile seizures;
2. Using a structured framework to aid the practitioner in decision making;
3. Optimizing evaluation of the child who has had a simple febrile seizure by ensuring that underlying

diseases such as meningitis are detected, minimizing morbidity, and enabling the practitioner to reassure the anxious parents and child; and

4. Reducing costs of physician and emergency department visits, hospitalizations, and unnecessary testing.

METHODOLOGY

Two hundred three medical journal articles addressing the diagnosis and evaluation of febrile seizures were identified. Each article was subjected to formal, semistructured review by committee members. These completed reviews, as well as the original articles, were then reexamined by epidemiologic consultants to identify those population-based studies limited to children with simple febrile seizures that examined the usefulness of specific diagnostic studies. Given the scarcity of such studies, data from hospital-based studies and comparable groups were also reviewed. Tables were constructed using data from 28 articles. A second literature search failed to disclose pertinent articles containing data on brain imaging in children with febrile seizures.

A summary of the technical report describing the analyses used to prepare this parameter begins on page 773.

RECOMMENDATIONS

Lumbar Puncture

Recommendation. **The American Academy of Pediatrics (AAP) recommends, on the basis of the published evidence and consensus, that after the first seizures with fever in infants younger than 12 months, performance of a lumbar puncture be strongly considered, because the clinical signs and symptoms associated with meningitis may be minimal or absent in this age group. In a child between 12 and 18 months of age, a lumbar puncture should be considered, because clinical signs and symptoms of meningitis may be subtle. In a child older than 18 months, although a lumbar puncture is not routinely warranted, it is recommended in the presence of meningeal signs and symptoms (ie, neck stiffness and Kernig and Brudzinski signs), which are usually present with meningitis, or for any child whose history or examination result suggests the presence of intracranial infection. In infants and children who have had febrile seizures and have received prior antibiotic treatment, clinicians should be aware that treatment can mask the signs and symptoms of meningitis. As such, a lumbar puncture should be strongly considered.**

The clinical evaluation of young febrile children requires skills that vary among examiners. Moreover, published data do not address the quantification of such skills adequately. Because this practice parameter is for practitioners with a wide range of training and experience, the committee chose a conservative approach with an emphasis on the value of lumbar puncture in diagnosing meningitis.

The committee recognizes the diversity of opinion regarding the need for routine lumbar puncture in children younger than 18 to 24 months with first

febrile seizures. In approximately 13% to 16% of children with meningitis, seizures are the presenting sign of disease, and in approximately 30% to 35% of these children (primarily children younger than 18 months), meningeal signs and symptoms may be lacking.[4,5] On the basis of published evidence, cerebrospinal fluid is more likely to be abnormal in children initially seen with fevers and seizures who have had: (1) suspicious findings on physical and/or neurologic examinations (particularly meningeal signs); (2) complex febrile seizures; (3) physician visits within 48 hours before the seizures; (4) seizures on arrival to emergency departments; (5) prolonged postictal states (typically most children with simple febrile seizures recover quickly); and (6) initial seizures after 3 years of age.[6,7] An increased risk of failure to diagnose meningitis occurs in children: (1) younger than 18 months who may show no signs and symptoms of meningitis; (2) who are evaluated by a less-experienced health care provider; or (3) who may be unavailable for follow-up.[5-8] A recognized source of fever, eg, otitis media, does not exclude the presence of meningitis. All recommendations, including those for lumbar puncture, are also given in the Algorithm.

EEG

Recommendation. **The AAP recommends, based on the published evidence and consensus, that EEG not be performed in the evaluation of a neurologically healthy child with a first simple febrile seizure.**

No published study demonstrates that EEG performed either at the time of presentation after a simple febrile seizure or within the following month will predict the occurrence of future afebrile seizures. Although the incidence of abnormal EEGs increases over time after a simple febrile seizure, no evidence exists that abnormal EEGs after the first febrile seizure are predictive for either the risk of recurrence of febrile seizures or the development of epilepsy. Even studies that have included children with complex febrile seizures and/or those with preexisting neurologic disease (a group at higher risk of having epilepsy develop) have not shown EEG to be predictive of the development of epilepsy.[9-10]

Blood Studies

Recommendation. **On the basis of published evidence,[7,8,11] the AAP recommends that the following determinations not be performed routinely in the evaluation of a child with a first simple febrile seizure: serum electrolytes, calcium, phosphorus, magnesium, CBC, or blood glucose.**

There is no evidence to suggest that routine blood studies are of benefit in the evaluation of the child with a first febrile seizure. Although some children initially seen with febrile seizures are dehydrated and have abnormal serum electrolyte values, their conditions should be identifiable by obtaining appropriate histories and performing careful physical examinations. A blood glucose determination, although not routinely needed, should be obtained if the child has a prolonged period of postictal obtundation. CBCs may be useful in the evaluation of fever, particularly in young children, because the incidence of bacteremia in children younger than 2 years of age with or without febrile seizures is the same.[12]

When fever is present, the decision regarding the need for laboratory testing should be directed toward identifying the source of the fever rather than as part of the routine evaluation of the seizure itself.

Neuroimaging

Recommendation. **On the basis of the available evidence and consensus, the AAP recommends that neuroimaging not be performed in the routine evaluation of the child with a first simple febrile seizure.**

The literature does not support the use of skull films in the evaluation of the child with a first febrile seizure.[7,13] Although no data have been published that either support or negate the need for CT or magnetic resonance imaging in the evaluation of children with simple febrile seizures, extrapolation of data from the literature on the use of CT in children who have generalized epilepsy has shown that clinically important intracranial structural abnormalities in this patient population are uncommon.[14,15]

CONCLUSION

Physicians evaluating infants or young children after first simple febrile seizures should direct their evaluations toward the diagnosis of the causes of the children's fevers. A lumbar puncture should be strongly considered in a child younger than 12 months and should be considered in children between 12 and 18 months of age. In children older than 18 months, the decision to do a lumbar puncture rests on the clinical suspicion of meningitis. The seizure usually does not require further evaluation—specifically EEG, blood studies, or neuroimaging.

The practice parameter, "The Neurodiagnostic Evaluation of the Child With a First Simple Febrile Seizure," was reviewed by the appropriate committees and sections of the AAP, including the Chapter Review Group, a focus group of office-based pediatricians representing each AAP district: Gene R. Adams, MD; Robert M. Corwin, MD; Lawrence C. Pakula, MD; Barbara M. Harley, MD; Howard B. Weinblatt, MD; Thomas J. Herr, MD; Kenneth E. Matthews, MD; Diane Fuquay, MD; Robert D. Mines, MD; and Delosa A Young, MD. Comments were also solicited from relevant outside organizations. The clinical algorithm was developed by Michael Kohrman, MD, Buffalo Children's Hospital, and James R. Cooley, MD, Harvard Community Health Plan.

The supporting data analyses are contained in the summary of the technical report, which begins on page 773.

REFERENCES

1. Nelson KB, Ellenberg JH. Predictors of epilepsy in children who have experienced febrile seizures. *N Engl J Med.* 1976;295:1029–1033
2. Consensus statement. Febrile seizures: long-term management of children with fever-associated seizures. *Pediatrics.* 1980;66:1009–1012
3. Hirtz DG, Lee YJ, Ellenberg JH, Nelson KB. Survey on the management of febrile seizures. *Am J Dis Child.* 1986;140:909–914
4. Ratcliffe JC, Wolf SM. Febrile convulsions caused by meningitis in young children. *Ann Neurol.* 1977;1:285–286
5. Rutter N, Smales OR. Role of routine investigations in children presenting with their first febrile convulsion. *Arch Dis Child.* 1977;52:188–191
6. Joffe A, McCormick M, DeAngelis C. Which children with febrile seizures need lumbar puncture? A decision analysis approach. *Am J Dis Child.* 1983;137:1153–1156
7. Jaffe M, Bar-Joseph G, Tirosh E. Fever and convulsions—indications for laboratory investigations. *Pediatrics.* 1981;57:729–731
8. Gerber MA, Berliner BC. The child with a "simple" febrile seizure: appropriate diagnostic evaluation. *Am J Dis Child.* 1981;135:431–433
9. Frantzen E, Lennox-Butchthal M, Nygaard A. Longitudinal EEG and clinical study of children with febrile convulsions. *Electroencephalogr Clin Neurophysiol.* 1968;24:197–212
10. Thorn I. The significance of electroencephalography in febrile convulsions. In: Akimoto H, Kazamatsuri H, Seino M, Ward A, eds. *Advances in Epileptology: XIIIth Epilepsy International Symposium.* New York, NY: Raven Press; 1982:93–95
11. Heijbel J, Blom S, Bergfors PG. Simple febrile convulsions: a prospective incidence study and an evaluation of investigations initially needed. *Neuropaediatrie.* 1980;11:45–56
12. Chamberlain JM, Gorman RL. Occult bacteremia in children with simple febrile seizures. *Am J Dis Child.* 1988;142:1073–1076
13. Nealis GT, McFadden SW, Asnes RA, Ouellette EM. Routine skull roentgenograms in the management of simple febrile seizures. *J Pediatr.* 1977;90:595–596
14. Yang PJ, Berger PE, Cohen ME, Duffner PK. Computed tomography and childhood seizure disorders. *Neurology.* 1979;29:1084–1088
15. Bachman DS, Hodges FJ, Freeman JM. Computerized axial tomography in chronic seizure disorders of childhood. *Pediatrics.* 1976;58:828–832

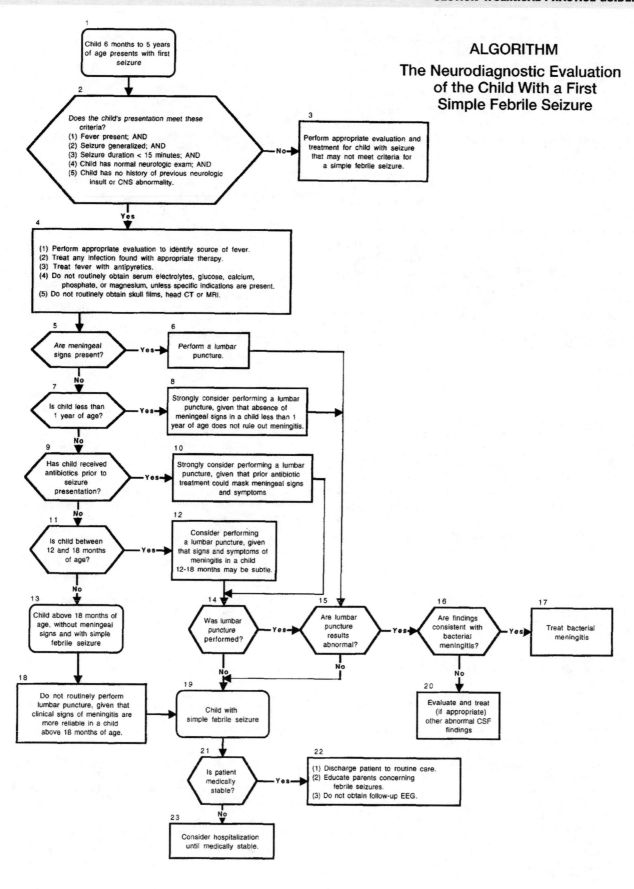

ALGORITHM
The Neurodiagnostic Evaluation
of the Child With a First
Simple Febrile Seizure

1 Child 6 months to 5 years of age presents with first seizure

2 Does the child's presentation meet these criteria?
(1) Fever present; AND
(2) Seizure generalized; AND
(3) Seizure duration < 15 minutes; AND
(4) Child has normal neurologic exam; AND
(5) Child has no history of previous neurologic insult or CNS abnormality.

No →

3 Perform appropriate evaluation and treatment for child with seizure that may not meet criteria for a simple febrile seizure.

Yes ↓

4
(1) Perform appropriate evaluation to identify source of fever.
(2) Treat any infection found with appropriate therapy.
(3) Treat fever with antipyretics.
(4) Do not routinely obtain serum electrolytes, glucose, calcium, phosphate, or magnesium, unless specific indications are present.
(5) Do not routinely obtain skull films, head CT or MRI.

5 Are meningeal signs present?   Yes →   **6** Perform a lumbar puncture.

No ↓

7 Is child less than 1 year of age?   Yes →   **8** Strongly consider performing a lumbar puncture, given that absence of meningeal signs in a child less than 1 year of age does not rule out meningitis.

No ↓

9 Has child received antibiotics prior to seizure presentation?   Yes →   **10** Strongly consider performing a lumbar puncture, given that prior antibiotic treatment could mask meningeal signs and symptoms

No ↓

11 Is child between 12 and 18 months of age?   Yes →   **12** Consider performing a lumbar puncture, given that signs and symptoms of meningitis in a child 12-18 months may be subtle.

No ↓

13 Child above 18 months of age, without meningeal signs and with simple febrile seizure

14 Was lumbar puncture performed?   Yes →   **15** Are lumbar puncture results abnormal?   Yes →   **16** Are findings consistent with bacterial meningitis?   Yes →   **17** Treat bacterial meningitis

No ↓ (14)   No ↓ (15)   No ↓ (16)

18 Do not routinely perform lumbar puncture, given that clinical signs of meningitis are more reliable in a child above 18 months of age.

19 Child with simple febrile seizure

20 Evaluate and treat (if appropriate) other abnormal CSF findings

21 Is patient medically stable?   Yes →   **22**
(1) Discharge patient to routine care.
(2) Educate parents concerning febrile seizures.
(3) Do not obtain follow-up EEG.

No ↓

23 Consider hospitalization until medically stable.

Technical Report Summary:
The Neurodiagnostic Evaluation of the Child
With a First Simple Febrile Seizure

Authors:

Robert J. Baumann, MD
Sandra L. D'Angelo, PhD

University of Kentucky
Lexington, Kentucky

consultants to the Subcommittee on Simple Febrile Seizures

American Academy of Pediatrics
PO Box 927, 141 Northwest Point Blvd
Elk Grove Village, IL 60009-0927

For the complete technical report, including tables, figures, and references, please see the companion CD-ROM.

SUBCOMMITTEE ON DIAGNOSIS AND
TREATMENT OF FEBRILE SEIZURES
1992 – 1995

Thomas A. Riemenschneider, MD, Chairman

Robert J. Baumann, MD

Patricia K. Duffner, MD

John L. Green, MD

Sanford Schneider, MD

In Consultation With:

David L. Coulter, MD

Patricia K. Crumrine, MD

Sandra D'Angelo, PhD (methodology consultant)

W. Edwin Dodson, MD

John M. Freeman, MD

Michael Kohrman, MD

James O. McNamara, MD

Karin B. Nelson, MD

N. Paul Rosman, MD

Shlomo Shinnar, MD

PROVISIONAL COMMITTEE ON QUALITY IMPROVEMENT
1993 – 1995

David A. Bergman, MD, Chairman

Richard D. Baltz, MD

James R. Cooley, MD

John B. Coombs, MD

Michael J. Goldberg, MD
  Sections Liaison

Charles J. Homer, MD, MPH
  Section on Epidemiology Liaison

Lawrence F. Nazarian, MD

Thomas A. Riemenschneider, MD

Kenneth B. Roberts, MD

Daniel W. Shea, MD

Thomas F. Tonniges, MD
  AAP Board of Directors Liaison

INTRODUCTION

The scope of the practice parameter that is supported by this technical report was limited to the initial neurodiagnostic evaluation (within 12 hours of the event) of neurologically normal children with simple febrile seizures. Febrile seizures are a common problem in clinical practice, occurring in 2.7% of children in the British Birth Cohort study. Febrile seizures are also the most common epileptic events in children younger than 5 years. The subcommittee's efforts were focused on the large subgroup of children (88%)[1] who have simple febrile seizures because in the view of most clinicians and on the basis of the epidemiologic evidence, this is a relatively homogeneous clinical grouping in terms of age, clinical presentation, course, and outcome. It is appropriate, therefore, to help clinicians develop a common neurodiagnostic approach for their evaluation.

DEFINITION OF THE PROBLEM

Children younger than 5 years who experience their first seizure in association with a fever are commonly divided into three groups. Children with simple febrile seizures make up the largest group. The second group includes children whose seizures are secondary to a central nervous system (CNS) infection (symptomatic febrile seizures). In the third group, children whose seizures are neither simple nor secondary to CNS infection are classified as having complex febrile seizures.

The practice parameter supported by this technical report contains recommendations for the initial neurodiagnostic evaluation of a child who has experienced a simple febrile seizure. The parameter requires all of the following factors for inclusion: Children who were between 6 months and 5 years at the time of the seizure. Seizures were single, isolated, and generalized; associated with a fever in the absence of a CNS infection; and lasted less than 15 minutes. The study excluded any children experiencing focal or complex seizures or flurries of seizures, or children who had experienced a previous neurologic insult or who were not neurologically normal on examination.

This definition of a simple febrile seizure corresponds to that in usual clinical practice and is also supported by the analysis of data from the Collaborative Perinatal Project of the National Institute of Neurological and Communicative Disorders and Stroke. In that project, Nelson and Ellenberg analyzed the data of 1706 children aged 7 years who had had one or more febrile seizures. The risk of epilepsy (afebrile seizures) was significantly higher for children whose neurological development was not normal before the seizure, whose seizure occurred before 6 months of age, whose seizure lasted longer than 15 minutes, or who had more than one febrile seizure per day. Most recently Verity and Golding examined the records for 398 children who had had at least one febrile seizure. Follow-up continued until age 10 years. They found a higher rate of epilepsy after a complex febrile convulsion (lasting longer than 15 minutes, focal or multiple seizures) than after a simple febrile convulsion. The available data indicated that these children experienced adverse neurologic outcomes (such as early mortality or mental retardation) at rates similar to those of their peers. Nevertheless, their rate for single or repeated afebrile seizures (epilepsy is defined as having two or more afebrile seizures) exceeded that of the general age-matched population. The study concluded that children with simple febrile seizures demonstrated a higher rate for afebrile seizures than that seen in the base population but had a lower rate than subjects who experienced complex febrile seizures.

The Commission on Epidemiology and Prognosis of the International League Against Epilepsy, which published a "Guidelines for Epidemiologic Studies on Epilepsy," suggested that the definition of febrile seizure include "childhood after age 1 month." No maximum age or definition of the duration of childhood was given. This Panel agreed that epidemiologic studies should examine the outcomes of febrile seizures among infants younger than 6 months as well as children older than 5 years. Nevertheless, existing studies as well as common clinical practice suggest that the practice parameter be limited to patients older than 6 months and younger than 5 years of age.

SELECTION OF INTERVENTIONS

The subcommittee further limited the parameter to the study of commonly used neurodiagnostic tests. These tests were evaluated on their potential to help the clinician decide whether children: had experienced a simple febrile seizure (as opposed to a complex or symptomatic febrile seizure) or were likely to have subsequent afebrile seizures or other adverse outcomes.

The following tests were included:
1. Lumbar puncture (to diagnose CNS infection).
2. Electroencephalography (EEG [to predict the likelihood of future afebrile seizures]).
3. Blood chemistries (to discover potential metabolic etiologies for the seizure).
4. Imaging studies of the head and brain, including skull x-ray films, computed tomography (CT), and magnetic resonance imaging (MRI) (to identify brain lesions).

METHODS

In an attempt to discover all pertinent articles, a Medline search was performed by staff of the American Academy of Pediatrics. An additional search from the Epilepsy Foundation of America using their database was also performed. Other articles that were obtained from bibliographies were suggested by subcommittee members; 203 articles were identified. Each article was reviewed by a subcommittee member using a semistructured review form. The completed forms and the articles were reviewed again by the epidemiologic consultants with the assistance of a graduate student.

The goal of this search was to identify population-based studies limited to patients with well-defined simple febrile seizures and in which neurodiagnostic tests were employed. The subcommittee attempted to use the method of Eddy and Woolf to develop these guidelines. Such a rigorous analysis requires well-designed population-based or case-comparison studies. The studies must adhere to a consistent definition of the study group, in this instance children with simple febrile seizures (as previously defined). The diagnostic test of interest must be applied in a standard way to all eligible subjects. The subjects must then be followed up for a sufficient period of time to discover important outcomes.

None of the previously cited population-based studies were designed to investigate the utility of neurodiagnostic testing. In all three studies, tests were selectively requested based on the physician's clinical judgment. Further retrospective analysis is unlikely to be fruitful.

Given the scarcity of population-based studies, data from hospital and clinic series were also analyzed. These studies had the following methodological problems.

Subject Selection. Most studies recruited subjects from clinics, emergency departments, or hospital admissions. The selection factors that influenced the constitution of these patient groups were difficult, if not impossible, to characterize. Moreover children from these patient groups usually have substantially higher rates of adverse outcomes than do children in population-based studies.

Disease Definition. Many studies either failed to define their criteria for febrile seizures, used a definition different from that used in the practice parameter, or did not rigorously follow any specific definition. Often there was no attempt to exclude (or at least identify) children with preexisting neurological disease.

Uniformity of Neurodiagnostic Testing. Many studies failed to apply the test(s) to all eligible subjects, raising serious questions about subject selection. An excess of positive tests and adverse outcomes could be expected based on physicians who exempt "healthier" children from testing.

Duration of Follow-up. Few studies had an extended follow-up period. The number of subjects experiencing afebrile seizures increases with age. Although the optimal duration of follow-up is uncertain, in the Rochester, Minnesota study most subjects were found to have experienced a seizure by age 9 years.

The consultants presented the abstracted data from 28 articles in tabular form, subsequently eliminating nine of them. These do not contain studies suitable for meta-analysis.

The subcommittee was concerned with the use of MRI and CT in evaluating children with febrile seizures. Because the initial literature search did not discover any suitable articles using these technologies, another literature search was conducted using MRI and CT MeSH terms, but again no pertinent articles were located.

Many articles not included in the study were reviews, commentaries, or editorials that lacked original data. Some of these articles reported disorders other than simple febrile seizures or intermingled children with simple seizures with children who were not neurologically normal or who had had complex febrile seizures. An additional 13 studies were eliminated because they did not define "febrile seizure" or used a definition different from that of the subcommittee.

SUBCOMMITTEE RECOMMENDATIONS AND LEVELS OF EVIDENCE

Recommendations were made based on the quality of scientific evidence. In the absence of high-quality scientific evidence, subcommittee consensus or a combination of evidence and consensus was used as the basis for recommendations.

Clinical options are actions for which the Panel failed to find compelling evidence for or against. A health care provider may or may not wish to implement clinical options, depending on the child.

No recommendation was made when scientific evidence was lacking and there was no compelling reason to make an expert judgment.

PANEL RECOMMENDATIONS

Lumbar Puncture

The goal of lumbar puncture is to identify children with CNS infection. A positive spinal fluid examination can have obvious treatment implications. In addition if the seizure is associated with an intracranial infection, the child is considered to have a symptomatic febrile seizure. Lumbar puncture with spinal fluid examination is not an effective neurodiagnostic technique for evaluating the febrile seizure per se.

An important concern is the number of children presenting with fever and seizures who have meningitis (for example, 4/119, or 3.4% [Heijbel et al], 28/562, or 5% [Jaffe et al], 13/241, or 5.4% [Joffe et al], 21/878, or 2.4% [Rossi et al], 6/328, or 1.8% [Rutter and Smales]). In the study by Jaffe et al, children with simple febrile seizures were less likely (2/323) to have meningitis than those with complex febrile seizures (26/239). None of the subjects with simple febrile seizures and 6 subjects with complex febrile seizures had bacterial meningitis. The previously described rates of meningitis (except those for the study by Heijbel et al) include children admitted to emergency departments or the hospital and thus are unlikely to typify the populations from which they come and are likely to vary with the factors that influence emergency department and hospital utilization.

Reviewing the emergency room records for 241 children who had a first seizure with fever and underwent lumbar puncture, Joffe et al found that the following five items were important in determining those with and without meningitis: 1) visiting a physician within 48 hours of the seizure, 2) seizure activity at the time of arrival in the emergency room, 3) a focal seizure, 4) suspicious findings on physical examination (rash or petechiae, cyanosis, hypotension, or grunting respirations), and 5) abnormal neurological examination results (stiff neck, increased tone, deviated eyes, ataxia, no response to voice, inability to fix and follow, no response to painful stimuli, positive doll's eye sign, floppy muscle tone, nystagmus, or bulging or tense fontanel).

Clearly the clinical evaluation of young febrile children requires skills that vary between examiners. Moreover, published data do not adequately address the quantification of such skills. Therefore the subcommittee relied on expert opinion and Panel consensus. Since this practice parameter is for practitioners with a wide range of training and experience, the committee chose a conserva-tive approach with an emphasis on the value of lumbar puncture in diagnosing meningitis. This was not intended to ignore the occurrence of false-negative results (for example, Rutter and Smales found 2/310 false-negative spinal fluid examinations).

In the absence of other data, the Panel reviewed studies in which children with fever and seizures presented to medical institutions. The study of Heijbel et al was population-based, but lumbar puncture was performed selectively in 47 of 107 subjects.

EEG

The primary purpose of EEG in the evaluation of the children with simple febrile seizures is to predict the risk of future afebrile seizures. The subcommittee searched for but could not find a definitive study. In such a population-based study, EEGs would be obtained on children shortly after they experience their first simple seizure, with the EEG pattern being correlated with subsequent seizure occurrence. The study from Macedonia by Sofijanov et al seems to approximate this pattern. Initial EEG data were published; follow-up data, however, are not yet available. In this study 18% of 376 subjects with first febrile seizures had paroxysmal abnormalities on EEG, which were more likely when the seizure was either focal or lasted longer than 15 minutes (not a simple febrile seizure).

Given the high rate of simple febrile seizures and the low rate of subsequent afebrile seizures, obtaining routine EEGs would require a large number of tests to identify a small number of children destined to have these seizures. For example, in the British Birth Cohort study, only 2.6% of children who had experienced their first simple febrile seizure subsequently had a single afebrile seizure before their 10th birthday. Only 1.6% of the children had two or more afebrile seizures (ie, epilepsy). A number of well-known studies included patients with both simple and focal febrile seizures and did not exclude subjects with preexisting neurological disability. The results for subjects with simple febrile seizures from the published data could not be isolated. Heijbel et al limited their study to simple febrile seizures. Their two subjects who subsequently developed epilepsy had normal initial EEGs. Interpretation of their data is complicated by the small number of subjects (n=107) and the elimination of 5 potential subjects because they had epileptiform EEG activity interictally. These 5 subjects were not characterized further so it is unknown whether they fit the clinical criteria for having experienced simple febrile seizures. No follow-up data were given for these 5 children and follow-up was limited to 3 years for the other subjects. Koyama et al evaluated 133 subjects from a population of 490 children with a history of febrile seizures. It is unclear if the 133 subjects are typical of the 490. Moreover, the EEGs were obtained months after the initial seizure; 32% of the subjects had abnormal EEGs—in 9% of the subjects the abnormalities were paroxysmal compared with 7% of the control group (who had had EEGs for "other medical reasons"). Follow-up data were not available.

The study of Heijbel is population-based. Some of its limitations are discussed above. Without other population-based data, the Panel reviewed studies in which relatively large numbers of children with fever and seizures presented to medical institutions. In some studies only a subset of subjects had EEGs, introducing the additional issue of selection bias.

BLOOD CHEMISTRIES

In a population-based study that included 107 children with simple febrile seizures, Heijbel et al retrospectively reviewed the routine blood chemistries requested by the treating physicians. They found no clinically important abnormalities in serum calcium (n=92), phosphorus (n=85), or glucose (n=56) levels. One child with a low glucose level was reportedly asymptomatic on follow-up.

Other studies were hospital-based. For 100 consecutive admissions Gerber and Berliner reported normal values of serum glucose (n=82), calcium (n=58), electrolytes, and urea nitrogen.[7] The five children with elevated glucose levels were asymptomatic. Thirteen children had minimally reduced calcium levels (8.3 to 8.9 mg/dL) and were asymptomatic. Jaffe et al reviewed 323 records of children with simple febrile seizures. Three children had abnormalities (one each hyponatremia, hypocalcemia, and hypokalemia) and the authors thought that the abnormalities could have been anticipated on clinical grounds independent of the occurrence of the simple febrile seizure. One child was a compulsive water drinker, one had "florid" rickets, and one had dehydration due to gastroenteritis. Rutter and Smales[9] reviewed 328 children admitted to the hospital after their first febrile convulsion and found that determinations for serum sugar, calcium, urea, electrolytes, and blood counts were "commonly performed but were unhelpful." Among 269 subjects who had blood glucose measurements they found hyperglycemia to be common (14%) but clinically unimportant. The child who was hypoglycemic on admission (glucose level, 30 mg/dL) subsequently had a normal fasting blood glucose level; of the 232 children who had serum calcium determinations, three of the four children with levels below 8.0 mg/dL were normal on further evaluation and the fourth child was lost to follow-up.

Four authors determined that in their subjects with simple febrile seizures, the routine blood chemistries performed did not alter patient management in an important way. The child's clinical condition and underlying illness determined the need for routine blood chemistries. Otherwise, the management of a child after a simple febrile seizure was not improved.

NEUROIMAGING

To our knowledge, no study has been done in which children with simple febrile seizures have undergone imaging. We also searched (without success) for a related imaging study involving otherwise normal children after a first seizure. Three studies reviewing skull x-ray films in children with febrile seizures concluded that skull x-ray films were not of value.

The Management of Minor Closed Head Injury in Children

- *Clinical Practice Guideline*
- *Technical Report Summary*

Readers of this clinical practice guideline are urged to review the technical report to enhance the evidence-based decision-making process. The full technical report is available on the enclosed CD-ROM.

AMERICAN ACADEMY OF PEDIATRICS

The Management of Minor Closed Head Injury in Children

Committee on Quality Improvement, American Academy of Pediatrics

Commission on Clinical Policies and Research, American Academy of Family Physicians

ABSTRACT. The American Academy of Pediatrics (AAP) and its Committee on Quality Improvement in collaboration with the American Academy of Family Physicians (AAFP) and its Commission on Clinical Policies and Research, and in conjunction with experts in neurology, emergency medicine and critical care, research methodologists, and practicing physicians have developed this practice parameter. This parameter provides recommendations for the management of a previously neurologically healthy child with a minor closed head injury who, at the time of injury, may have experienced temporary loss of consciousness, experienced an impact seizure, vomited, or experienced other signs and symptoms. These recommendations derive from a thorough review of the literature and expert consensus. The methods and results of the literature review and data analyses including evidence tables can be found in the technical report. This practice parameter is not intended as a sole source of guidance for the management of children with minor closed head injuries. Rather, it is designed to assist physicians by providing an analytic framework for the evaluation and management of this condition. It is not intended to replace clinical judgment or establish a protocol for all patients with a minor head injury, and rarely will provide the only appropriate approach to the problem.

The practice parameter, "The Management of Minor Closed Head Injury in Children," was reviewed by the AAFP Commission on Clinical Policies and Research and individuals appointed by the AAFP and appropriate committees and sections of the AAP including the Chapter Review Group, a focus group of office-based pediatricians representing each AAP District: Gene R. Adams, MD; Robert M. Corwin, MD; Diane Fuquay, MD; Barbara M. Harley, MD; Thomas J. Herr, MD, Chair; Kenneth E. Matthews, MD; Robert D. Mines, MD; Lawrence C. Pakula, MD; Howard B. Weinblatt, MD; and Delosa A. Young, MD.

The supporting data are contained in a technical report available at http://www.pediatrics.org/cgi/content/full/104/6/e78.

ABBREVIATIONS. AAP, American Academy of Pediatrics; AAFP, American Academy of Family Physicians; CT, cranial computed tomography; MRI, magnetic resonance imaging.

Minor closed head injury is one of the most frequent reasons for visits to a physician.[1] Although >95 000 children experience a traumatic brain injury each year in the United States,[2] consensus is lacking about the acute care of children with minor closed head injury. The evaluation and management of injured children may be influenced by local practice customs, settings where children are evaluated, the type and extent of financial coverage, and the availability of technology and medical staffing.

Because of the magnitude of the problem and the potential seriousness of closed head injury among children, the AAP and the American Academy of Family Physicians (AAFP) undertook the development of an evidence-based parameter for health care professionals who care for children with minor closed head injury. In this document, the term Subcommittee is used to denote the Subcommittee on Minor Closed Head Injury, which reports to the AAP Committee on Quality Improvement, and the AAFP Commission on Clinical Policies, Research, and Scientific Affairs.

While developing this practice parameter, the Subcommittee attempted to find evidence of benefits resulting from 1 or more patient management options. However, at many points, adequate data were not available from the medical literature to provide guidance for the management of children with mild head injury. When such data were unavailable, we did not make specific recommendations for physicians and other professionals but instead we presented a range of practice options deemed acceptable by the Subcommittee.

An algorithm at the end of this parameter presents recommendations and options in the context of direct patient care. Management is discussed for the initial evaluation of a child with minor closed head injury, and the disposition after evaluation. These recommendations and options may be modified to fit the needs of individual patients.

PURPOSE AND SCOPE

This practice parameter is specifically intended for previously neurologically healthy children of either sex 2 through 20 years of age, with isolated minor closed head injury.

The parameter defines children with minor closed head injury as those who have normal mental status at the initial examination, who have no abnormal or focal findings on neurologic (including fundoscopic) examination, and who have no physical evidence of skull fracture (such as hemotympanum, Battle's sign, or palpable bone depression).

This parameter also is intended to address children who may have experienced temporary loss of consciousness (duration <1 minute) with injury, may have had a seizure immediately after injury, may have vomited after injury, or may have exhibited signs and symptoms such as headache and lethargy. The treatment of these children is addressed by this parameter, provided that they seem to be normal as described in the preceding paragraph at the time of evaluation.

This parameter is not intended for victims of multiple trauma, for children with unobserved loss of consciousness, or for patients with known or suspected cervical spine injury. Children who may otherwise fulfill the criteria for minor closed head injury, but for whom this parameter is not intended include patients with a history of bleeding diatheses or neurologic disorders potentially aggravated by trauma (such as arteriovenous malformations or shunts), patients with suspected intentional head trauma (eg, suspected child abuse), or patients with a language barrier.

The term brief loss of consciousness in this parameter refers to a duration of loss of consciousness of 1 minute or less. This parameter does not make any inference that the risk for intracranial injury changes with any specific length of unconsciousness lasting <1 minute. The treatment of children with loss of consciousness of longer duration is not addressed by this parameter.

Finally, this parameter refers only to the management of children evaluated by a health care professional immediately or shortly after (within 24 hours) injury. This parameter is not intended for the management of children who are initially evaluated >24 hours after injury.

METHODS FOR PARAMETER DEVELOPMENT

The literature review encompassed original research on minor closed head trauma in children, including studies on the prevalence of intracranial injury, the sensitivity and specificity of different imaging modalities, the utility of early diagnosis of intracranial injury, the effectiveness of various patient management strategies, and the impact of minor closed head injury on subsequent child health. Research was included if it had data exclusively on children or identifiable child-specific data, if cases were comparable with the case definition in the parameter, and if the data were published in a peer-reviewed journal. Review articles and articles based solely on expert opinion were excluded.

An initial search was performed on several computerized databases including Medline (1966–1993) using the terms head trauma and head injury. The search was restricted to infants, children, and adolescents, and to English-language articles published after 1966. A total of 422 articles were identified. Titles and abstracts were reviewed by the Subcommittee and articles were reviewed if any reviewer considered the title relevant. This process identified 168 articles that were sent to Subcommittee members

with a literature review form to categorize study design, identify study questions, and abstract pertinent data. In addition, reference lists in the articles were reviewed for additional sources, and 125 additional articles were identified. After excluding review articles and other studies not meeting entry criteria, a total of 64 articles were included for review. All articles were reabstracted by the methodologists and the data summarized on evidence tables. Differences in case definition, outcome definition, and study samples precluded pooling of data among studies.

The published data proved extremely limited for a number of study questions, and direct queries were placed to several authors for child-specific data. Because these data have not been formally published, the Subcommittee does not rest strong conclusions on them; however, they are included in the Technical Report. The Technical Report produced along with this practice parameter contains supporting scientific data and analysis including evidence tables and is available at http://www.pediatrics.org/cgi/content/full/104/6/e78.

SUMMARY

Initial Evaluation and Management of the Child With Minor Closed Head Injury and No Loss of Consciousness

Observation

For children with minor closed head injury and no loss of consciousness, a thorough history and appropriate physical and neurologic examination should be performed. Observation in the clinic, office, emergency department, or at home, under the care of a competent caregiver is recommended for children with minor closed head injury and no loss of consciousness. Observation implies regular monitoring by a competent adult who would be able to recognize abnormalities and to seek appropriate assistance. The use of cranial computed tomography (CT) scan, skull radiograph, or magnetic resonance imaging (MRI) is not recommended for the initial evaluation and management of the child with minor closed head injury and no loss of consciousness.

Initial Evaluation of the Child With Minor Closed Head Injury With Brief Loss of Consciousness

Observation or Cranial CT Scan

For children with minor closed head injury and brief loss of consciousness (<1 minute), a thorough history and an appropriate physical and neurologic examination should be performed. Observation, in the office, clinic, emergency department, hospital, or home under the care of a competent caregiver, may be used to evaluate children with minor closed head injury with brief loss of consciousness. Cranial CT scanning may also be used, in addition to observation, in the initial evaluation and management of children with minor closed head injury with loss of consciousness.

The use of skull radiographs or MRI in the initial management of children with minor closed head injury and loss of consciousness is not recommended. However, there are limited situations in which MRI and skull radiography are options (see sections on skull radiographs and on MRI).

Patient Management Considerations

Many factors may influence how management strategies influence outcomes for children with minor closed head injury. These factors include: 1) the prevalence of intracranial injury, 2) the percentage of intracranial injuries that need medical or neurosurgical intervention (ie, the percentage of these injuries that, if left undiagnosed or untreated, leads to disability or death), 3) the relative accuracy of clinical examination, skull radiographs, and CT scans as diagnostic tools to detect such intracranial injuries that benefit from medical or neurosurgical intervention, 4) the efficacy of treatment for intracranial injuries, and 5) the detrimental effect on outcome, if any, of delay from the time of injury to the time of diagnosis and intervention.

This last factor, delay of diagnosis and intervention, is particularly relevant when trying to decide between a clinical strategy of immediate CT scanning of all patients as opposed to a strategy that relies primarily on patient observation, with CT scanning reserved for rare patients whose conditions change. To our knowledge, no published studies were available for review that compared clinically meaningful outcomes (ie, morbidity or mortality) between children receiving different management regimens such as immediate neuroimaging, or observation. Although some studies were able to demonstrate the presence of intracranial abnormalities on CT scans or MRIs among children with minor head injury, no known evidence suggested that immediate neuroimaging of asymptomatic children improved outcomes for these children, compared with the outcomes for children managed primarily with examination and observation.

Initial Management of the Child With Minor Closed Head Injury and No Loss of Consciousness

Minor closed head injury without loss of consciousness is a common occurrence in childhood. Available data suggest that the risk of intracranial injury is negligible in this situation. Population-based studies have found that fewer than 1 in 5000 patients with minor closed head injury and no loss of consciousness have intracranial injuries that require medical or neurosurgical intervention. In 1 study of 5252 low-risk patients, mostly adults, none were found to have an intracranial injury after minor head injury.[3] Comparably sized studies do not exist for children. In 2 much smaller studies of children with minor head injury, among those with normal neurologic examination findings and no loss of consciousness, amnesia, vomiting, headache, or mental status abnormalities, no children had abnormal CT scan findings.[4,5]

Observation

Among children with minor closed head injury and no loss of consciousness, a thorough history and appropriate physical and neurologic examination should be performed. Subcommittee consensus was that observation, in the clinic, office, emergency department, or home under the care of a competent observer, be used as the primary management strategy. If on examination the patient's condition appears normal (as outlined earlier), no additional tests are needed and the child can be safely discharged to the care of a responsible caregiver. The recommended duration of observation is discussed in the section titled "Disposition of the Child With Minor Head Injury."

CT Scan/MRI

With such a low prevalence of intracranial injury, the Subcommittee believed that the marginal benefits of early detection of intracranial injury afforded by routine brain imaging studies such as CT or MRI were outweighed by considerations of cost, inconvenience, resource allocation, and possible side effects attributable to sedation or inappropriate interventions (eg, medical, surgical, or other interventions based on incidental CT findings in asymptomatic children).

Skull Radiographs

Skull radiographs have only a very limited role in the evaluation of children with minor closed head injury, no loss of consciousness, and no signs of skull fracture (ie, no palpable depression, hemotympanum, or Battle's sign). The substantial rate of false-positive results provided by skull radiographs (ie, a skull fracture detected on skull radiographs in the absence of intracranial injury) along with the low prevalence of intracranial injury among this specific subset of patients, leads to a low predictive value of skull radiographs. Most children with abnormal skull radiographs will not harbor significant intracranial lesions and conversely intracranial injury occurs in the absence of a skull fracture detected on skull radiographs.

There may be some clinical scenarios in which a practitioner desires imaging such as the case of a child with a scalp hematoma over the course of the meningeal artery. In situations such as these, the Subcommittee believes that clinical judgment should prevail. However, given the relatively low predictive value of skull radiographs, the Subcommittee believes that, if imaging is desired, cranial CT scan is the more satisfactory imaging modality.

Initial Management of the Child With Minor Closed Head Injury and Brief Loss of Consciousness

Among children with minor closed head injury, loss of consciousness is uncommon but is associated with an increased risk for intracranial injury. Studies performed since the advent of CT scanning suggest that children with loss of consciousness, or who demonstrate amnesia at the time of evaluation, or who have headache or vomiting at the time of evaluation, have a prevalence of intracranial injury detectable on CT that ranges from 0% to 7%.[5-8] Although most of these intracranial lesions will remain clinically insignificant, a substantial proportion of children, between 2% and 5% of those with minor head injury and loss of consciousness, may require neurosurgical intervention.[6-8] The differences in findings among studies are likely attributable to differences in selection criteria, along with random variation among studies with limited sample size. Although these findings might have been biased somewhat if more seriously injured patients were preferentially selected for CT scans, even studies in which patients were explicitly stated to be neurologically normal and asymptomatic found children with clinically significant injuries that required intervention.[6]

In past studies of children with minor head injury, patient selection may have led to overestimates of the prevalence of intracranial injury. Many of these studies looked at patients referred to emergency departments or trauma centers, patients brought to emergency departments after examination in the field by emergency personnel, or patients for whom the reason for obtaining CT scans was not clearly stated. These factors may have led to the selection of a patient population at higher risk for intracranial injury than the patients specifically addressed in this practice parameter.

As evidence of this, population-based studies before the widespread availability of CT scanning found the prevalence of clinically significant intracranial injury after minor closed head injury to be far less than estimated by the aforementioned studies. One study found a prevalence of intracranial injury that required neurosurgery to be as low as .02%.[9] This discrepancy is consistent also with the fact that many lesions currently identified with cranial CT were not recognized before the availability of this technology. Because most of these lesions do not progress or require neurosurgical intervention, most would not have been diagnosed in studies before the availability of CT scan.

Observation

As discussed earlier, the Subcommittee did not find evidence to show that immediate neuroimaging of asymptomatic children produced demonstrable benefits compared with a management strategy of initial observation alone. In light of these considerations, there was Subcommittee consensus based on limited evidence that for children who are neurologically normal after minor closed head injury with loss of consciousness, patient observation was an acceptable management option.

If the health care practitioner chooses observation alone, it may be performed in the clinic, office, emergency department, hospital, or at home under the care of a competent observer, typically a parent or suitable guardian. If the observer seems unable to follow or comply with the instructions for home observation, observation under the supervision of a health care practitioner is to be considered.

CT Scan

Data that support the routine use of CT scanning of children with minor head injury and loss of consciousness indicate that children with intracranial lesions after minor closed head injury are not easily distinguishable clinically from the large majority with no intracranial injury.[10,11] Children with nonspecific signs such as headache, vomiting, or lethargy after minor closed head injury may be more likely to have intracranial injury than children without such signs. However, these clinical signs are of limited predictive value, and most children with headache, lethargy, or vomiting after minor closed head injury do not have demonstrable intracranial injury. In addition, some children with intracranial injury do not have any signs or symptoms. Because of these findings, many investigators have concluded that the physical and neurologic examination are inadequate predictors of intracranial injury, and that cranial CT is more sensitive than physical and neurologic examinations for the diagnosis of intracranial injury.

The most accurate and rapid means of detecting intracranial injury would be with a clinical protocol that routinely obtained intracranial imaging for all children after head injury. Rapid diagnosis and treatment of subdural hematomas was found in 1 study to significantly reduce morbidity and mortality among severely injured adults.[12] However, this result was not replicated in other studies of subdural or epidural hematomas[13-15] and similar studies have not addressed less severely head injured children, or children with minor closed head injury.

CT itself is a safe procedure. However, some healthy children require sedation or anesthesia, and the benefits gained from cranial CT should be carefully weighed against the possible harm of sedating and/or anesthetizing a large number of children. In addition, CT scans obtained for asymptomatic children may show incidental findings that lead to subsequent unnecessary medical or surgical interventions. To our knowledge, no data are available that demonstrate that children who undergo CT scanning early after minor closed head injury with loss of consciousness have different outcomes compared with children who receive observation alone after injury. A clinical trial comparing the risks and benefits of immediate CT scanning with simple monitored observation for children with minor closed head injury has not been performed, primarily because intracranial injury after minor closed head injury is so rare that the cost and logistics of such a study would be prohibitive. As a result, the risk–benefit ratio for the evaluation and management modalities of CT scanning or observation is unknown.

Simple observation by a reliable parent or guardian is the management option with the least initial costs, while CT scans typically cost less than observation performed in the hospital. A study that compares costs of CT and observation strategies would need data on the cost of following up children with positive CT scans, as well as the potential costs associated with late detection and emergency therapy among those managed by observation alone.

Because of these considerations, there was Subcommittee consensus based on limited evidence that for children who are neurologically normal after minor closed head injury with loss of consciousness, cranial CT scanning along with observation was also an acceptable management option.

Skull Radiographs

Before the availability of CT imaging, skull radiographs were a common means to evaluate children with head injury. Skull radiographs may identify skull fractures, but they do not directly show brain injury or other intracranial trauma. Although intracranial injury is more common in the presence of a skull fracture, many studies have demonstrated that intracranial lesions are not always associated with skull fractures and that skull fractures do not always indicate an underlying intracranial lesion.[7,8,16]

Large studies of children and adults have shown that the sensitivity of skull radiographs for identifying intracranial injury in children is quite low (~25% in some studies). More recent studies limited to children have reported sensitivities between 50% and 100%, with the latter higher figure reported from studies of adolescent patients.[7,8,15,16] The specificity of skull radiographs for intracranial injury (the proportion of patients without intracranial injury who have normal radiographs) has been reported as between 53% and 97% in these same studies. Given the limited specificity of skull radiographs and the low prevalence of intracranial injury, the skull radiographs would likely be interpreted as abnormal for a substantial proportion of patients without intracranial injury. Furthermore, the low sensitivity of the radiographs will result in the interpretation of skull radiographs as normal for some patients with intracranial injury.

The Subcommittee consensus was that skull radiographs have only a limited role in the management of the child with loss of consciousness. If imaging is desired by the health care practitioner and if CT and skull radiographs are available, the Subcommittee believes that CT scanning is the imaging modality of choice, based on the increased sensitivity and specificity of CT scans. When CT scanning is not readily available, skull radiographs may assist the practitioner to define the extent of injury and risk for intracranial injury. In this situation, there was Subcommittee consensus that, for a child who has suffered minor closed head injury with loss of consciousness, skull radiographs are an acceptable management option. However, as noted, skull fractures may be detected on skull radiographs in the absence of intracranial injury, and intracranial injury may be present when no skull fracture is detected on skull radiographs. These limitations should be considered carefully by physicians who elect to use skull radiographs. Regardless of findings on skull films (should the physician elect to obtain them) close observation, as described previously, remains a cornerstone of patient management.

MRI

MRI is another available modality for neuroimaging. Although MRI has been shown to be more sensitive than cranial CT in detecting certain types of intracranial abnormalities, CT is more sensitive for hyperacute and acute intracranial hemorrhage (especially subarachnoid hemorrhage). CT is more quickly and easily performed than MRI, and costs for CT scans generally are less than those for MRI. The consensus of the Subcommittee was that cranial CT offered substantial advantages over MRI in the acute care of children with minor closed head injury.

As is the case with skull radiographs, there may be situations in which CT scanning is not readily available and the health care professional desires to obtain imaging studies. There was Subcommittee consensus that, for a child who has experienced minor closed head injury with loss of consciousness, MRI to evaluate the intracranial status of the child was an acceptable management option.

Disposition of Children With Minor Closed Head Injury

Children Managed by Observation Alone

Children who appear neurologically normal after minor closed head injury are at very low risk for subsequent deterioration in their condition and are unlikely to require medical intervention. Therefore, although observation is recommended for patients after the initial evaluation is completed, such observation may take place in many different settings. The strategy chosen by the health care practitioner may depend on the resources available for observation. Other factors, such as the distance and time it would take to reach appropriate care if the patient's clinical status worsened, may influence where observation occurs.

Historically, when hospitalization has been used to observe children after head injury, the length of stay averaged 12 to 48 hours. This practice was based on the reasoning that most life-threatening complications occur within 24 hours after head injury. The Subcommittee believes that a prudent duration of observation would extend at least 24 hours, and could be accomplished in any combination of locations, including the emergency department, hospital, clinic, office, or home. However, it is important for physicians, parents, and other guardians to have a high index of suspicion about any change in the patient's clinical status for several days after the injury. Parents or guardians require careful instruction to seek medical attention if the patient's condition worsens at any time during the first several days after injury.

In all cases, the health care professional is to make a careful assessment of the parent or guardian's anticipated compliance with the instructions to monitor the patient. If the caregiver is incompetent, unavailable, intoxicated, or otherwise incapacitated, other provisions must be made to ensure adequate observation of the child. These provisions may differ based on the characteristics of each case.

The physician has an important role in educating the parents or guardians of children with minor closed head injury. Understandable, printed instructions should be given to the parent or guardian detailing how to monitor the patient and including information on how and when to seek medical attention if necessary. All children discharged should be released to the care of a reliable parent or guardian who has adequate transportation and who has the capability to seek medical attention if the child's condition worsens.

Children Evaluated by Cranial CT

Neurologically normal patients with normal cranial CT scans are at extremely low risk for subsequent problems. Although there are many reports of patients with head injuries in whom extradural or intracerebral bleeding developed after an initial stable clinical period,[18–22] there are only a few reports of patients in whom extradural or intracerebral bleeding developed after a postinjury CT scan was interpreted as normal.[23–25] Most often when such cases have been described, the patients had sustained a more severe initial head injury than the patient for whom this parameter is intended, and the neurologic status of the patients was not intact at the initial examination following the injury. A number of studies have demonstrated the safety of using cranial CT as a triage instrument for neurologically normal and clinically stable patients after minor closed head injury.[26–31]

Patients may be discharged from the hospital for observation by a reliable observer if the postinjury CT scan is interpreted as normal. The length of observation should be similar to that described in the preceding section. If the cranial CT reveals abnormalities, proper disposition depends on a thorough consideration of the abnormalities and, when warranted, consultations with appropriate subspecialists.

Research Issues

Classification of Head Injury in Children and Prognostic Features

Much remains to be learned about minor closed head injury in children. The implications of clinical events such as loss of consciousness and signs or symptoms such as seizures, nausea, vomiting, and headache remain unclear. Data on patients with low-risk head injuries but with loss of consciousness, such as the data provided on a primarily adult population, are not available for children. Moreover, this practice parameter deals with clinically normal patients who did not lose consciousness at the time of injury and with patients who did lose consciousness with injury. Children with minor head injury, who have experienced loss of consciousness, vomiting or seizures have been found to have a prevalence of intracranial injury ranging from 2% to 5%. Questions remain about the selection of patients for many of these studies, and there is considerable uncertainty about the generalizability of these results to patients within this parameter.

Future studies on minor closed head injury should assess the relationship between characteristics such as these and the risk for intracranial injury among children who are clinically asymptomatic. Specifically, studies should address the question of whether such a history of loss of consciousness is associated with an increased risk for clinically significant intracranial abnormalities. Such studies should not be limited to patients seen in referral settings, but instead should cover patients from a wide range of settings, including those managed in clinics and offices, and if possible, those managed over the phone.

These studies should also address the independent prognostic value of other signs and symptoms for which the clinical significance in children is uncertain. In particular, practitioners are often faced with managing patients who are asymptomatic except for episodes of repeated vomiting or moderate to severe headache. The Subcommittee did not find evidence in the literature that helped differentiate the risk status of children with such symptoms from children without such symptoms. If studies are performed on this population, information should be collected on the presence of signs or symptoms including posttraumatic seizures, nausea with or without vomiting, posttraumatic amnesia, scalp lacerations and hematomas, headache, and dizziness, and their relationship to intracranial injury.

The Benefit of Early Detection of, and Intervention for, Intracranial Lesions in Asymptomatic Children

The outcome for asymptomatic patients found to have intracranial hematomas is of particular interest. Additional studies are needed to determine whether a strategy of immediate CT scan provides measurably improved outcomes for children with minor closed head injury compared with a strategy of observation followed by CT scan for children whose clinical status changes. Although rapid detection and neurosurgical intervention for intracranial injuries such as subdural hematomas has been shown to improve outcome in some studies of patients with more serious head injuries, it is unclear whether the same benefit would accrue to asymptomatic neurologically normal children.

A randomized, controlled trial would provide the most direct information on the risks and benefits of each management strategy. However, such a study would be extremely difficult and expensive to perform because of the rarity of adverse outcomes. Retrospective observational studies among children with minor head injury could be performed more easily and at less cost. However, correct characterization of the patient's clinical status before any treatment strategy or diagnostic procedure would be essential to eliminate bias in the evaluation of the comparison groups.

Finally, if such studies are performed to compare different diagnostic and management strategies, the outcomes should include not only mortality and short-term morbidity, but also long-term outcomes such as persistent psychological problems or learning disorders.

The Management of the Asymptomatic Patient With Intracranial Hemorrhage

The optimal management and prognosis for asymptomatic patients with intracranial hemorrhage is unknown. Because surgery is not always indicated or beneficial, some neurosurgeons and neurologists now advocate an expectant approach of close observation for small intracranial and extradural hemato-

Evaluation and Triage of Children and Adolescents With Minor Head Trauma

Algorithm

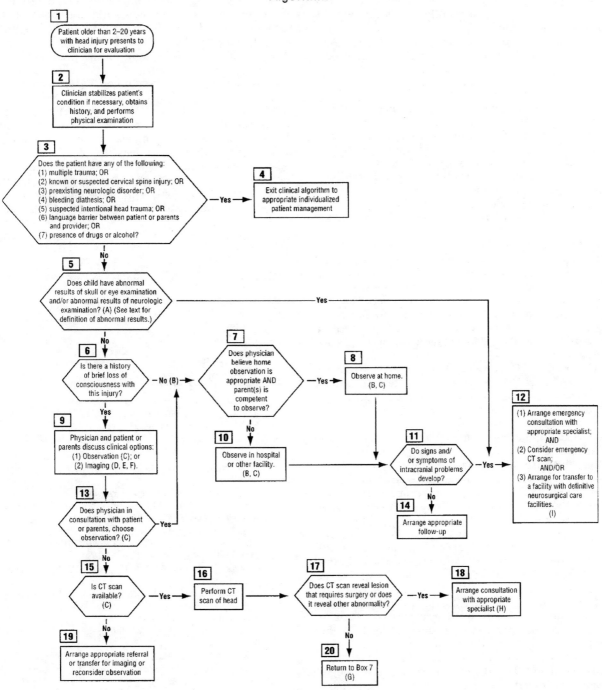

mas, considering hematoma size, shift of intracranial structures, and other factors.

If all asymptomatic children with minor head injury undergo cranial CT scanning, a substantial number of patients with an abnormal result on CT may undergo surgery that is unnecessary or even harmful. Additional research is needed to determine the proper management of asymptomatic children with intracranial hemorrhage. Outcome measures should include mortality and morbidity outcomes such as seizures, learning disabilities, and behavioral disabilities.

Research Into Other Imaging Modalities

As newer modalities for neuroimaging are developed and disseminated, careful evaluation of their relative utility is necessary before they are used for patients with minor closed head injury. Although such new modalities frequently provide new and different types of information to the health care professional, it is important that they be submitted to scientific study to assess their effect on patient outcome.

Algorithm

The notes below are integral to the algorithm. The letters in parentheses correspond to the algorithm.

A. This parameter addresses the management of previously neurologically healthy children with minor closed head injury who have normal mental status on presentation, no abnormal or focal findings on neurologic (including fundoscopic) examination, and no physical evidence of skull fracture (such as hemotympanum, Battle's sign, or palpable depression).

B. Observation in the clinic, office, emergency department, or home, under the care of a competent caregiver is recommended for children with minor closed head injury and no loss of consciousness.

C. Observation in the office, clinic, emergency department, hospital, or home under the care of a competent caregiver may be used to manage children with minor closed head injury with loss of consciousness.

D. Cranial CT scanning along with observation may also be used in the initial evaluation and management of children with minor closed head injury with brief loss of consciousness.

E. If imaging is desired by the health care practitioner and if both CT and skull radiography are available, CT scanning is the imaging modality of choice, because of its increased sensitivity and specificity. When CT scanning is not readily available, skull radiographs may assist the practitioner to define the risk for intracranial injury. However skull fractures may be detected on skull radiographs in the absence of intracranial injury, and occasionally intracranial injury is present despite the absence of a skull fracture detected on skull radiographs. These limitations should be considered by physicians who elect to use skull radiographs. Whether the changed probabilities for harboring an intracranial injury based on the results of the skull radiographs is sufficient to alter the management strategy may depend on the preferences of the family and physician.

F. In some studies MRI has been shown to be more sensitive than CT in diagnosing certain intracranial lesions. However, there is currently no appreciable difference between CT and MRI in the diagnosis of clinically significant acute intracranial injury and bleeding that requires neurosurgical intervention. CT is more quickly and easily performed than MRI, and the costs for CT scans generally are less than those for MRI. Because of this, the consensus among the Subcommittee was that cranial CT offered advantages over MRI in the acute care of children with minor closed head injury.

G. Neurologically normal patients with a normal cranial CT scan are at very low risk for subsequent deterioration. Patients may be discharged from the hospital for observation by a reliable observer if the postinjury CT scan is normal. The decision to observe at home takes into consideration the delay that would ensue if the child had to return to the hospital as well as the reliability of the parents or other caregivers. Otherwise, depending on the preferences of the patient and physician, observation also may take place in the office, clinic, emergency department, or hospital.

H. If the cranial CT reveals abnormalities, proper disposition depends on a thorough consideration of the abnormalities and, when warranted, consultation with appropriate subspecialists.

I. If the child's neurologic condition worsens during observation, a thorough neurologic examination is to be performed, along with immediate cranial CT after the patient's condition is stabilized. If a repeat CT scan shows new intracranial pathologic abnormalities, consultation with the appropriate subspecialist is warranted.

Richard K. Zimmerman, MD, MPH
Lee A. Green, MD, MPH
Jonathan E. Rodnick, MD
Barbara P. Yawn, MD, MSc
Linda L. Barrett, MD, Resident Representative,
1997
Enrico G. Jones, MD, Resident Representative,
1996
Theresa-Ann Clark, Student Representative
Ross R. Black, MD, Liaison, Commission on
Quality and Scope of Practice
Leah Raye Mabry, MD, Liaison, Commision on
Public Health
Herbert F. Young, MD, MA, Staff Executive
Hanan S. Bell, PhD, Assistant Staff Executive

REFERENCES

1. Levin HS, Mattis S, Ruff RM, et al. Neurobehavioral outcome following minor head injury: a three-center study. *J Neurosurg.* 1987;66:234–243
2. Krauss JF, Black MA, Hessol N, et al. The incidence of acute brain injury and serious impairment in a defined population. *Am J Epidemiol.* 1984;119:186–201
3. Masters SJ, McClean PM, Arcarese JS, et al. Skull radiograph examinations after head trauma: recommendations by a multidisciplinary panel and validation study. *N Engl J Med.* 1987;316:84–91
4. Hennes H, Lee M, Smith D, Sty JR, Losek J. Clinical predictors of severe head trauma in children. *Am J Dis Child.* 1988;142:1045–1047
5. Dietrich AM, Bowman MJ, Ginn-Pease ME, Kusnick E, King DR. Pediatric head injuries: can clinical factors reliably predict an abnormality on computed tomography? *Ann Emerg Med.* 1993;22:1535–1540
6. Dacey RG Jr, Alves WM, Rimel RW, Winn HR, Jane JA. Neurosurgical complications after apparently minor head injury: assessment of risk in a series of 610 patients. *J Neurosurg.* 1986;65:203–210
7. Hahn YS, McLone DG. Risk factors in the outcome of children with minor head injury. *Pediatr Neurosurg.* 1993;19:135–142
8. Rosenthal BW, Bergman I. Intracranial injury after moderate head trauma in children. *J Pediatr.* 1989;115:346–350
9. Teasdale GM, Murray G, Anderson E, et al. Risks of acute traumatic intracranial complications in hematoma in children and adults: implications for head injuries. *Br Med J.* 1990;300:363–367
10. Rivara F, Taniguchi D, Parish RA, et al. Poor prediction of positive computed tomographic scans by clinical criteria in symptomatic pediatric head trauma. *Pediatrics.* 1987;80:579–584
11. Davis RL, Mullen N, Makela M, Taylor JA, Cohen W, Rivara FP. Cranial computed tomography scans in children after minimal head injury with loss of consciousness. *Ann Emerg Med.* 1994;24:640–645
12. Seelig JM, Becker DP, Miller JD, Greenberg RP, Ward JD, Choi SC. Traumatic acute subdural hematoma: major mortality reduction in comatose patients treated within four hours. *N Engl J Med.* 1981;304:1511–1518
13. Chen TY, Wong CW, Chang CN, et al. The expectant treatment of asymptomatic supratentorial epidural hematomas. *Neurosurgery.* 1993;32:176–179
14. Hatashita S, Koga N, Hosaka Y, Takagi S. Acute subdural hematoma: severity of injury, surgical intervention, and mortality. *Neurol Med Chir (Tokyo).* 1993;33:13–18
15. Lobato RD, Rivas JJ, Gomez PA, et al. Head injured patients who talk and deteriorate into coma. *J Neurosurg.* 1991;75:256–261
16. Zimmerman RA, Bilaniuk LT, Gennarelli T, Bruce D, Dolinskas C, Uzzell B. Cranial computed tomography in diagnosis and management of acute head trauma. *AJR Am J Roentgenol.* 1978;131:27–34
17. Borovich B, Braun J, Guilburd JN, et al. Delayed onset of traumatic extradural hematoma. *J Neurosurg.* 1985;63:30–34
18. Miller JD, Murray LS, Teasdale GM. Development of a traumatic intracranial hematoma after a "minor" head injury. *Neurosurgery.* 1990;27:669–673
19. Rosenthal BW, Bergman I. Intracranial injury after moderate head trauma in children. *J Pediatr.* 1989;115:346–350
20. Dacey RG, Alves WM, Rimel RW, Winn HR, Jane JA. Neurosurgical complications after apparently minor head injury. *J Neurosurg.* 1986;65:203–210
21. Deitch D, Kirshner HS. Subdural hematoma after normal CT. *Neurology.* 1989;39:985–987
22. Poon WS, Rehman SU, Poon CY, Li AK. Traumatic extradural hematoma of delayed onset is not a rarity. *Neurosurgery.* 1992;30:681–686
23. Brown FD, Mullan S, Duda EE. Delayed traumatic intracerebral hematomas. *J Neurosurg.* 1978;48:1019–1022
24. Lipper MH, Kishore PR, Girevendulis AK, Miller JD, Becker DP. Delayed intracranial hematoma in patients with severe head injury. *Radiology.* 1979;133:645–649
25. Diaz FG, Yock DH Jr, Larson D, Rockswold GL. Early diagnosis of delayed posttraumatic intracerebral hematomas. *J Neurosurg.* 1979;50:217–223
26. Stein SC, Ross SE. The value of computed tomographic scans in patients with low-risk head injuries. *Neurosurgery.* 1990;29:638–640
27. Stein SC, Ross SE. Mild head injury: a plea for routine early CT scanning. *J Trauma.* 1992;33:11–13
28. Harad FT, Kerstein MD. Inadequacy of bedside clinical indicators in identifying significant intracranial injury in trauma patients. *J Trauma.* 1992;32:359–363
29. Livingston DH, Loder PA, Koziol J, Hunt CD. The use of CT scanning to triage patients requiring admission following minimal head injury. *J Trauma.* 1991;31:483–489
30. Feurman T, Wackym PA, Gade GF, Becker DP. Value of skull radiography, head computed tomographic scanning, and admission for observation in cases of minor head injury. *Neurosurgery.* 1988;22:449–453
31. Livingston DH, Loder PA, Hunt CD. Minimal head injury: is admission necessary? *Am Surg.* 1991;57:14–17

Technical Report Summary:
Minor Head Injury in Children

Authors:

Charles J. Homer, MD, MPH
Lawrence Kleinmen, MD, MPH

American Academy of Pediatrics
PO Box 927, 141 Northwest Point Blvd
Elk Grove Village, IL 60009-0927

For the complete technical report, including tables, figures, and references, please see the companion CD-ROM

ABSTRACT

Minor head trauma affecting children is a common reason for medical consultation and evaluation. In order to provide evidence on which to base a clinical practice guideline for the American Academy of Pediatrics, we undertook a systematic review of the literature on minor head trauma in children.

Methods. **Medline and Health databases were searched for articles published between 1966 and 1993 on head trauma or head injury, limited to infants, children, and adolescents. Abstracts were reviewed for relevance to mild head trauma consistent with the index case defined by the AAP subcommittee. Relevant articles were identified, reviewed, and abstracted. Additional citations were identified by review of references and expert suggestions. Unpublished data were also identified through contact with authors highlighting child-specific information. Abstracted data were summarized in evidence tables. The process was repeated in 1998, updating the review for articles published between 1993 and 1997.**

Results. **A total of 108 articles were abstracted from 1033 abstracts and articles identified through the various search strategies. Variation in definitions precluded any pooling of data from different studies. Prevalence of intracranial injury in children with mild head trauma varied from 0% to 7%. Children with no clinical risk characteristics are at lower risk than are children with such characteristics; the magnitude of increased risk was inconsistent across studies. Computed tomography scan is most sensitive and specific for detection of intracranial abnormalities; sensitivity and specificity of skull radiographs ranged from 21% to 100% and 53% to 97%, respectively. No high quality studies tested alternative strategies for management of such children. Outcome studies are inconclusive as to the impact of minor head trauma on long-term cognitive function.**

Conclusions. **The literature on mild head trauma does not provide a sufficient scientific basis for evidence-based recommendations about most of the key issues in clinical management. More consistent definitions and multisite assessments are needed to clarify this field. Pediatrics 1999;104(6). URL:http://www.pediatrics.org/cgi/content/full/104/6/ e78. *Keywords: head trauma, imaging, literature review.***

Minor head trauma affecting a child is a common reason for medical consultation and evaluation. No consensus exists concerning the appropriate diagnostic assessment of such children. Previous surveys of physicians indicated significant variation in practice, and examination of hospitalization rates shows substantial regional variation for this condition. The American Academy of Pediatrics, in coordination with the American Academy of Family Physicians, launched an initiative to develop a clinical practice guideline to reduce variation and improve the quality of care of children with minor head trauma.

This report provides the technical information on the literature concerning minor head trauma in children that was used by the American Academy of Pediatrics/American Academy of Family Physicians' subcommittee in formulating this guideline.

METHODS

The literature review included the following salient aspects of minor head trauma in children:

- Prevalence of intracranial injury
- Sensitivity and specificity of different imaging modalities in detecting intracranial injury, including skull radiography, computed tomography (CT), and magnetic resonance imaging (MRI)
- Utility of early diagnosis of intracranial injury
- Effectiveness of alternative management strategies, and
- Impact of minor head injury on subsequent child health.

The data included for review met the following criteria:

1. publication in a peer-reviewed journal,
2. data related exclusively to children or was identifiable as being specifically related to children, and
3. assurance that cases described in the article were comparable with the case described in the practice guideline. Review articles and expert opinion were excluded.

A medical librarian undertook an initial search of several computerized databases, including Medline (1966–1993) and Health, searching terms of head trauma and head injury, restricted to infancy, children, and adolescents. Four hundred twenty-two articles were identified. Titles and abstracts were reviewed by 4 initial reviewers, including the subcommittee chairperson, American Academy of Pediatrics staff, and methodologic consultants, and articles were obtained when reviewers considered the title to be relevant. Through this process, 168 articles were identified.

Articles were sent to subcommittee members with an article review form, which asked reviewers to categorize the study design, identify the study question, and abstract the data to enable data pooling and meta-analysis. In addition, reviewers were asked to check the article references to see whether additional sources could be found.

Of the initial 168 articles sent out, reviewers excluded 134 papers and included 34 papers in their reviews.

An additional 125 references were identified through bibliography tracing, of which 30 were included for review by the epidemiologist/pediatrician consultants.

All articles included were then abstracted again by the epidemiologist/pediatrician consultants, and the data were compiled using summary tables and evidence tables. Differences in case definition, outcome definition, and study samples precluded pooling of data to arrive at common estimates.

Because the published data proved extremely limited for a number of study questions, direct queries were given to several authors for child-specific data. Because these data have not been formally published, we did not rest strong conclusions on them; when available, however, they are presented with this report.

Because of the lengthy period between the initial review of the literature and final approval of the guideline, a second literature review was performed to assure that the literature review was current. This literature review used the same search headings and targeted the period between January 1, 1993, and July 1, 1997. For this review, only an electronic search was performed. The review identified an additional 486 abstracts, of which 44 were selected for detailed review by the epidemiologist and 11 included in the evidence tables.

RESULTS

In general, interpretation of clinical studies of head trauma was complicated by several characteristics of the literature. Specifically, the head trauma literature suffers by the nonstandardized ways of categorizing head injury, clinical examinations, radiologic outcomes, and clinical outcomes, and by the inconsistent reporting of the subjects included in a study population.

The results of the literature review are presented by each area for which evidence was sought.

Risk of Intracranial Injury

Ten published articles were identified that provided estimates of the prevalence of intracranial injury in children with mild head injury, with CT scans used as the "gold standard". Among these articles, however, 3 included patients with more severe symptoms or findings than specified by the guideline case description (including Glasgow coma scale [GCS] scores as low as 13), and 1 included trivial abnormalities on CT as the principal outcome measure. Among those studies restricting their subjects to GCS scores of 15, and considering abnormal findings to be subdural, extradural, or intracerebral hematomas, ranges of the prevalence of intracranial injury ranged from 0% to 7%. The high estimate of 7% comes from a study in which both initial and delayed (24-hour) CT scans were obtained for most patients; how many patients were referred for care at this institution because of clinical deterioration was not noted.

Three unpublished studies provided prevalence estimates of intracranial injuries ranging from 4% to 10% among patients with a GCS score of 15, without focal neurologic findings, but with either a history of (brief) loss of consciousness or amnesia (J. Finkelstein, 1994; S. C. Stein, 1994; S. C. Stein, 1994).

We sought to determine within these articles whether any clinical characteristics were associated with the presence or absence of significant CT scan abnormalities. Two studies indicated that among patients with a GCS score of 15, normal neurologic examinations, no history of loss of consciousness or amnesia, no vomiting, headache, or subtle changes in mental status, there were no abnormal CT scan findings. One additional case series (49 children) found that no child with a GCS of 15, a completely normal neurologic examination, and no trauma aside from the head injury experienced an intracranial lesion, even with a history of loss of consciousness or amnesia. The upper limits for the 95% confidene interval for this estimate is 6%, and the analysis that identified this group of predictors is exploratory; no confirmatory analyses were undertaken in a second dataset.

One pediatric study used surgery for intracranial bleeding as an indicator of intracranial injury. This study found that .017% of cases with a GCS score of 15 required surgery.

We conclude from these data that:

- the true prevalence of intracranial injury following mild head injury is not clearly known;
- the population as defined by the head trauma task force is likely heterogeneous in its risk;
- children with clinically trivial head injury—no loss of consciousness or amnesia, normal examinations, no vomiting, headache, and a GCS score of 15—are at substantially <1% risk of having an intracranial abnormality of immediate clinical significance;
- children with mild head injury but who have experienced loss of consciousness, amnesia, vomiting, or seizures are at higher risk of having an intracranial injury detected using CT, likely in the 1% to 5% range, with a significantly lower amount requiring any intervention (see below).

We extended this section of the literature review to examine the significance of the abnormalities detected by CT scanning in such patients. No studies randomly assigned patients with abnormal CT scans to receive or not receive surgery. Rather, several reports on the management decisions among those children found to have abnormal CT scans. These studies, and the unpublished data provided to us, indicated that between 20% and 80% of children with abnormal CT scans underwent a neurosurgical procedure, a proportion of which was intracranial pressure monitoring only.

Imaging Modalities

Through the 1970s and early 1980s, controversy raged concerning the role of skull radiography in the assessment of acute head trauma. Although fewer articles are now being written on this topic, the lack of access to CT scanners in some practice settings prompted review of this literature.

We identified 5 studies that examined the sensitivity and specificity of skull radiographs for the detection of intracranial injury, using intracranial abnormality or bleeding as determined by CT scanning as the gold standard. These studies found that the sensitivity of skull films varied from 50% to 100%; 1 of the studies showing 100% sensitivity was restricted to adolescents. The specificity of skull films for intracranial injury (ie, the proportion of patients without intracranial injury who have normal films) has been reported to be between 53% and 97%. Thus, a substantial proportion of patients without intracranial injury will have abnormal skull films.

A few studies have examined the role of MRI in head trauma. These studies indicate that although subtle forms of neural injury can be better detected by MRI, and that isodense subdural collections (as may be found in chronic subdural injuries in adults) also may be more readily identified, in acute settings with children MRI offers no advantage in detecting lesions of clinical concern.

We conclude from this literature that 1) although an abnormal skull film increases the likelihood of a significant intracranial lesion, the test is not of sufficient sensitivity or specificity to be clinically useful in most settings, and 2) CT is sufficiently sensitive and specific as the imaging modality of choice at this time; in most cases, a normal CT scan in a child who meets the case definition provides assurance that subsequent adverse outcomes are very unlikely. A cohort of 399 such children (GCS .12 and normal CT scan) found 3 patients who were readmitted within 1 month, 1 of whom had an intercranial contusion, but none required neurosurgical intervention. Rarely, cases are reported in the literature of children with normal CT scans who subsequently develop "flash edema," or, even more rarely, intracranial (especially epidural) hematomas.

Utility of Early Diagnosis

In the course of the literature review, because the reviewers identified several papers and unpublished reports that noted a higher frequency of intracranial abnormalities than the subcommittee members had anticipated, the subcommittee requested that literature examining the utility of the early diagnosis of these abnormalities be examined. Little child-specific data are available that relate to this question, ie, "Are children with apparently mild head trauma who are discovered to have an intracranial injury better off if the discovery is made sooner rather than later?" Although a classic and often cited study of comatose adults with subdural hematoma showed a dramatic benefit associated with rapid diagnosis and treatment, subsequent study has not replicated that report for either subdural or epidural bleeding. Small case series have similarly not found a correlation between delay in diagnosis of intracranial bleeding and outcome in children. The extreme limitations of these reports in their sample size, and the appropriately nonrandom allocation of time to diagnosis and treatment make any inferences from this work extremely limited.

Effectiveness of Alternative Management Strategies

An ideal study seeking to determine the relative effectiveness of alternative management strategies would initially define a homogeneous population of children with mild head trauma, and randomly assign such children to 1 of 2 or more potential approaches. Such approaches might include inpatient observation for a defined period of time without initial imaging, outpatient observation without imaging, or CT scanning followed by outpatient observation if scans are normal. No such study has been identified in the pediatric literature. The rarity of adverse outcomes would make such a study difficult to perform, and would require careful collaboration across multiple institutions.

One decision analysis has been published that assesses the cost-effectiveness of a particular strategy for the evaluation of head trauma. This analysis, although not limited to children, utilized much pediatric data in developing the probabilities required for the analysis. The authors recommend immediate CT scanning for patients with abnormal clinical signs; for patients who are otherwise normal, these authors recommend skull radiography, with CT if radiographs are abnormal. If such a strategy were followed for 10 000 persons presenting with mild head trauma, of 10 000 individuals with head injuries, the 9900 additional

skull films and 250 CT scans would identify 6 or 7 additional cases of early intracranial hemorrhage.

Outcome of Mild Head Trauma

In an idealized decision analytic framework, the "utilities" to patients of the various clinical outcomes are incorporated in assessing the value of each potential treatment arm. We sought to identify through the literature the long-term outcome for the index case, assuming no significant intracranial abnormalities were identified.

Several studies did not specifically report on outcomes for pediatric patients, although authors typically commented that outcomes for children were better than those for adults. Four studies, however, did specifically examine outcomes for children. One large cohort study of children with "minimal" (or "trivial") head injury, ie, excluding children with skull fracture, loss of consciousness, or having been admitted to an inpatient unit, found physical health 1 month after injury to be identical to that of a normal population, but that role limitations, eg, school absenteeism, was substantially increased. Unfortunately, this study could not distinguish whether this effect was the result of the head injury, or associated either with the use of the emergency department or with whatever factors led to the injury. A smaller study of children with mild injury including "concussion" found a slight increase in teacher-reported hyperactivity (activity and inattentiveness) 10 years after the injury, with no other differences in school performance, cognitive ability, or behavioral symptoms. In this relatively small cohort, no differences in these outcomes between those patients who had been observed in inpatient or out-patient settings were identified. Two more recent studies also suggested some possible long-term impact of head injury. Comparing a cohort of 95 children followed up 1 year after hospitalization for head trauma of varying degree with population norms, investigators found that the children with head injuries had higher levels of physical and behavioral impairment; this investigation did not control for preexisting morbidity leading to the injury. Only patients at the most severe end of the spectrum (Abbreviated Injury Scale level 5) had demonstrably worse outcomes than those with milder injuries (Abbreviated Injury Scale level 2). A more compelling study from New Zealand compared children ages 2½ to 3½ years of age with mild head trauma (evaluated in an emergency department but not admitted to the hospital) with injury date-matched children with other forms of mild trauma 1, 6, and 12 months after the injury and when the children were 6½ years of age. The investigators found specific deficits in solving visual puzzles beginning 6 months after injury and persisting throughout the observation; these children were also more likely to have reading disabilities. We conclude from these investigations that children who present with head injuries or other types of injuries are different from the general population and more likely to have some functional impairment unrelated to the injury per se; at the same time, children with mild or minimal head injury may be more likely to experience subtle abnormalities in specific cognitive functions.

CONCLUSION

The literature on mild head trauma does not provide a sufficient scientific basis on which clinical management decisions can be made with certainty. The field remains burdened by inconsistent definitions of case severity, inadequate specification of the population base, and varied and incomplete definition of outcome. Nonetheless, the published data do indicate that 1) a small proportion of children with minimal and mild head injury will have significant intracranial injury; 2) the presence of either loss of consciousness or amnesia increases the probability that an injury is present in many, but not all studies; 3) CT scanning is the most sensitive, specific, and clinically safe mode of identifying such injury, whereas plain radiographs in this pediatric age group have neither sufficient sensitivity nor specificity to recommend their general use; 4) extremely rare children with normal examinations and CT scans will experience delayed bleeding or edema; and 5) long-term outcomes for children with minimal or mild head injury, in the absence of significant intracranial hemorrhage, are generally very good, with a suggestion of a small increase in risk for subtle specific deficits in particular cognitive skills.

The confusion in this field mandates that multicenter, collaborative investigations be performed that will begin to address the limited information base on which such a large volume of clinical care rests.

Management of Hyperbilirubinemia in the Newborn Infant 35 or More Weeks of Gestation

- *Clinical Practice Guideline*
- *Technical Report Summary*

Readers of this clinical practice guideline are urged to review the technical report to enhance the evidence-based decision-making process. The full technical report is available on the enclosed CD-ROM.

AMERICAN ACADEMY OF PEDIATRICS

CLINICAL PRACTICE GUIDELINE

Subcommittee on Hyperbilirubinemia

Management of Hyperbilirubinemia in the Newborn Infant 35 or More Weeks of Gestation

ABSTRACT. Jaundice occurs in most newborn infants. Most jaundice is benign, but because of the potential toxicity of bilirubin, newborn infants must be monitored to identify those who might develop severe hyperbilirubinemia and, in rare cases, acute bilirubin encephalopathy or kernicterus. The focus of this guideline is to reduce the incidence of severe hyperbilirubinemia and bilirubin encephalopathy while minimizing the risks of unintended harm such as maternal anxiety, decreased breastfeeding, and unnecessary costs or treatment. Although kernicterus should almost always be preventable, cases continue to occur. These guidelines provide a framework for the prevention and management of hyperbilirubinemia in newborn infants of 35 or more weeks of gestation. In every infant, we recommend that clinicians 1) promote and support successful breastfeeding; 2) perform a systematic assessment before discharge for the risk of severe hyperbilirubinemia; 3) provide early and focused follow-up based on the risk assessment; and 4) when indicated, treat newborns with phototherapy or exchange transfusion to prevent the development of severe hyperbilirubinemia and, possibly, bilirubin encephalopathy (kernicterus). *Pediatrics* 2004; 114:297–316; *hyperbilirubinemia, newborn, kernicterus, bilirubin encephalopathy, phototherapy.*

ABBREVIATIONS. AAP, American Academy of Pediatrics; TSB, total serum bilirubin; TcB, transcutaneous bilirubin; G6PD, glucose-6-phosphate dehydrogenase; ETCO$_c$, end-tidal carbon monoxide corrected for ambient carbon monoxide; B/A, bilirubin/albumin; UB, unbound bilirubin.

BACKGROUND

In October 1994, the Provisional Committee for Quality Improvement and Subcommittee on Hyperbilirubinemia of the American Academy of Pediatrics (AAP) produced a practice parameter dealing with the management of hyperbilirubinemia in the healthy term newborn.[1] The current guideline represents a consensus of the committee charged by the AAP with reviewing and updating the existing guideline and is based on a careful review of the evidence, including a comprehensive literature review by the New England Medical Center Evidence-Based Practice Center.[2] (See "An Evidence-Based Review of Important Issues Concerning Neonatal

Hyperbilirubinemia"[3] for a description of the methodology, questions addressed, and conclusions of this report.) This guideline is intended for use by hospitals and pediatricians, neonatologists, family physicians, physician assistants, and advanced practice nurses who treat newborn infants in the hospital and as outpatients. A list of frequently asked questions and answers for parents is available in English and Spanish at www.aap.org/family/jaundicefaq. htm.

DEFINITION OF RECOMMENDATIONS

The evidence-based approach to guideline development requires that the evidence in support of a policy be identified, appraised, and summarized and that an explicit link between evidence and recommendations be defined. Evidence-based recommendations are based on the quality of evidence and the balance of benefits and harms that is anticipated when the recommendation is followed. This guideline uses the definitions for quality of evidence and balance of benefits and harms established by the AAP Steering Committee on Quality Improvement Management.[4] See Appendix 1 for these definitions.

The draft practice guideline underwent extensive peer review by committees and sections within the AAP, outside organizations, and other individuals identified by the subcommittee as experts in the field. Liaison representatives to the subcommittee were invited to distribute the draft to other representatives and committees within their specialty organizations. The resulting comments were reviewed by the subcommittee and, when appropriate, incorporated into the guideline.

BILIRUBIN ENCEPHALOPATHY AND KERNICTERUS

Although originally a pathologic diagnosis characterized by bilirubin staining of the brainstem nuclei and cerebellum, the term "kernicterus" has come to be used interchangeably with both the acute and chronic findings of bilirubin encephalopathy. Bilirubin encephalopathy describes the clinical central nervous system findings caused by bilirubin toxicity to the basal ganglia and various brainstem nuclei. To avoid confusion and encourage greater consistency in the literature, the committee recommends that in infants the term "acute bilirubin encephalopathy" be used to describe the acute manifestations of bilirubin toxicity seen in the first weeks after birth and that the term "kernicterus" be reserved for the chronic and permanent clinical sequelae of bilirubin toxicity.

See Appendix 1 for the clinical manifestations of acute bilirubin encephalopathy and kernicterus.

FOCUS OF GUIDELINE

The overall aim of this guideline is to promote an approach that will reduce the frequency of severe neonatal hyperbilirubinemia and bilirubin encephalopathy and minimize the risk of unintended harm such as increased anxiety, decreased breastfeeding, or unnecessary treatment for the general population and excessive cost and waste. Recent reports of kernicterus indicate that this condition, although rare, is still occurring.[2,5–10]

Analysis of these reported cases of kernicterus suggests that if health care personnel follow the recommendations listed in this guideline, kernicterus would be largely preventable.

These guidelines emphasize the importance of universal systematic assessment for the risk of severe hyperbilirubinemia, close follow-up, and prompt intervention when indicated. The recommendations apply to the care of infants at 35 or more weeks of gestation. These recommendations seek to further the aims defined by the Institute of Medicine as appropriate for health care:[11] safety, effectiveness, efficiency, timeliness, patient-centeredness, and equity. They specifically emphasize the principles of patient safety and the key role of timeliness of interventions to prevent adverse outcomes resulting from neonatal hyperbilirubinemia.

The following are the key elements of the recommendations provided by this guideline. Clinicians should:

1. Promote and support successful breastfeeding.
2. Establish nursery protocols for the identification and evaluation of hyperbilirubinemia.
3. Measure the total serum bilirubin (TSB) or transcutaneous bilirubin (TcB) level on infants jaundiced in the first 24 hours.
4. Recognize that visual estimation of the degree of jaundice can lead to errors, particularly in darkly pigmented infants.
5. Interpret all bilirubin levels according to the infant's age in hours.
6. Recognize that infants at less than 38 weeks' gestation, particularly those who are breastfed, are at higher risk of developing hyperbilirubinemia and require closer surveillance and monitoring.
7. Perform a systematic assessment on all infants before discharge for the risk of severe hyperbilirubinemia.
8. Provide parents with written and verbal information about newborn jaundice.
9. Provide appropriate follow-up based on the time of discharge and the risk assessment.
10. Treat newborns, when indicated, with phototherapy or exchange transfusion.

PRIMARY PREVENTION

In numerous policy statements, the AAP recommends breastfeeding for all healthy term and near-term newborns. This guideline strongly supports this general recommendation.

RECOMMENDATION 1.0: Clinicians should advise mothers to nurse their infants at least 8 to 12 times per day for the first several days[12] (evidence quality C: benefits exceed harms).

Poor caloric intake and/or dehydration associated with inadequate breastfeeding may contribute to the development of hyperbilirubinemia.[6,13,14] Increasing the frequency of nursing decreases the likelihood of subsequent significant hyperbilirubinemia in breastfed infants.[15–17] Providing appropriate support and advice to breastfeeding mothers increases the likelihood that breastfeeding will be successful.

Additional information on how to assess the adequacy of intake in a breastfed newborn is provided in Appendix 1.

RECOMMENDATION 1.1: The AAP recommends against routine supplementation of nondehydrated breastfed infants with water or dextrose water (evidence quality B and C: harms exceed benefits).

Supplementation with water or dextrose water will not prevent hyperbilirubinemia or decrease TSB levels.[18,19]

SECONDARY PREVENTION

RECOMMENDATION 2.0: Clinicians should perform ongoing systematic assessments during the neonatal period for the risk of an infant developing severe hyperbilirubinemia.

Blood Typing

RECOMMENDATION 2.1: All pregnant women should be tested for ABO and Rh (D) blood types and have a serum screen for unusual isoimmune antibodies (evidence quality B: benefits exceed harms).

RECOMMENDATION 2.1.1: If a mother has not had prenatal blood grouping or is Rh-negative, a direct antibody test (or Coombs' test), blood type, and an Rh (D) type on the infant's (cord) blood are strongly recommended (evidence quality B: benefits exceed harms).

RECOMMENDATION 2.1.2: If the maternal blood is group O, Rh-positive, it is an option to test the cord blood for the infant's blood type and direct antibody test, but it is not required provided that there is appropriate surveillance, risk assessment before discharge, and follow-up[20] (evidence quality C: benefits exceed harms).

Clinical Assessment

RECOMMENDATION 2.2: Clinicians should ensure that all infants are routinely monitored for the development of jaundice, and nurseries should have established protocols for the assessment of jaundice. Jaundice should be assessed whenever the infant's vital signs are measured but no less than every 8 to 12 hours (evidence quality D: benefits versus harms exceptional).

In newborn infants, jaundice can be detected by blanching the skin with digital pressure, revealing the underlying color of the skin and subcutaneous tissue. The assessment of jaundice must be per-

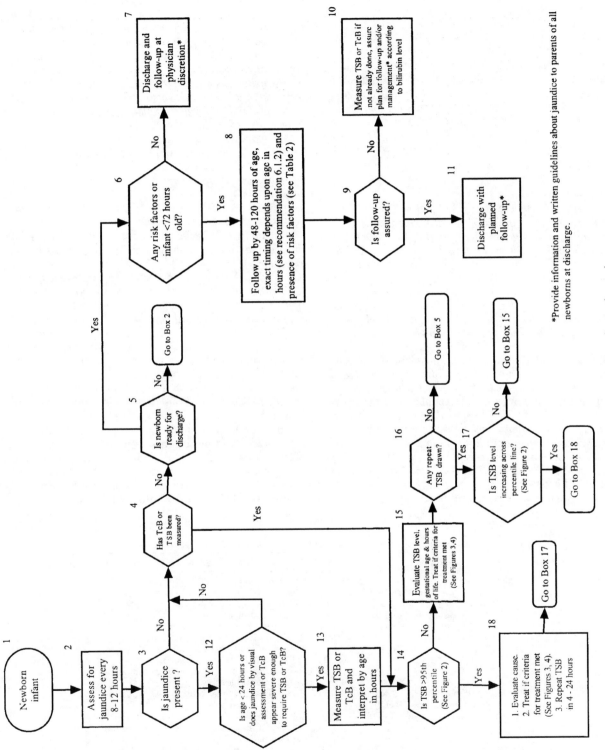

Fig 1. Algorithm for the management of jaundice in the newborn nursery.

*Provide information and written guidelines about jaundice to parents of all newborns at discharge.

1 Newborn infant

2 Assess for jaundice every 8-12 hours

3 Is jaundice present?

12 Is age < 24 hours or does jaundice by visual assessment or TcB appear severe enough to require TSB or TcB?

13 Measure TSB or TcB and interpret by age in hours

14 Is TSB >95th percentile (See Figure 2)

18 1. Evaluate cause. 2. Treat if criteria for treatment met (See Figures 3, 4). 3. Repeat TSB in 4 - 24 hours

Go to Box 17

4 Has TcB or TSB been measured?

5 Is newborn ready for discharge?

Go to Box 2

6 Any risk factors or infant <72 hours old?

7 Discharge and follow-up at physician discretion*

8 Follow up by 48-120 hours of age, exact timing depends upon age in hours (see recommendation 6.1.2) and presence of risk factors (see Table 2)

9 Is follow-up assured?

10 Measure TSB or TcB if not already done, assure plan for follow-up and/or management* according to bilirubin level

11 Discharge with planned follow-up*

15 Evaluate TSB level, gestational age & hours of life. Treat if criteria met (See Figures 3,4)

16 Any repeat TSB drawn?

Go to Box 5

17 Is TSB level increasing across percentile line? (See Figure 2)

Go to Box 15

Go to Box 18

formed in a well-lit room or, preferably, in daylight at a window. Jaundice is usually seen first in the face and progresses caudally to the trunk and extremities,[21] but visual estimation of bilirubin levels from the degree of jaundice can lead to errors.[22–24] In most infants with TSB levels of less than 15 mg/dL (257 μmol/L), noninvasive TcB-measurement devices can provide a valid estimate of the TSB level.[2,25–29] See Appendix 1 for additional information on the clinical evaluation of jaundice and the use of TcB measurements.

RECOMMENDATION 2.2.1: Protocols for the assessment of jaundice should include the circumstances in which nursing staff can obtain a TcB level or order a TSB measurement (evidence quality D: benefits versus harms exceptional).

Laboratory Evaluation

RECOMMENDATION 3.0: A TcB and/or TSB measurement should be performed on every infant who is jaundiced in the first 24 hours after birth (Fig 1 and Table 1)[30] (evidence quality C: benefits exceed harms). The need for and timing of a repeat TcB or TSB measurement will depend on the zone in which the TSB falls (Fig 2),[25,31] the age of the infant, and the evolution of the hyperbilirubinemia. Recommendations for TSB measurements after the age of 24 hours are provided in Fig 1 and Table 1.

See Appendix 1 for capillary versus venous bilirubin levels.

RECOMMENDATION 3.1: A TcB and/or TSB measurement should be performed if the jaundice appears excessive for the infant's age (evidence quality D: benefits versus harms exceptional). If there is any doubt about the degree of jaundice, the TSB or TcB should be measured. Visual estimation of bilirubin levels from the degree of jaundice can lead to errors, particularly in darkly pigmented infants (evidence quality C: benefits exceed harms).

RECOMMENDATION 3.2: All bilirubin levels should be interpreted according to the infant's age in hours (Fig 2) (evidence quality C: benefits exceed harms).

Cause of Jaundice

RECOMMENDATION 4.1: The possible cause of jaundice should be sought in an infant receiving phototherapy or whose TSB level is rising rapidly (ie, crossing percentiles [Fig 2]) and is not explained by the history and physical examination (evidence quality D: benefits versus harms exceptional).

RECOMMENDATION 4.1.1: Infants who have an elevation of direct-reacting or conjugated bilirubin should have a urinalysis and urine culture.[32] Additional laboratory evaluation for sepsis should be performed if indicated by history and physical examination (evidence quality C: benefits exceed harms).

See Appendix 1 for definitions of abnormal levels of direct-reacting and conjugated bilirubin.

RECOMMENDATION 4.1.2: Sick infants and those who are jaundiced at or beyond 3 weeks should have a measurement of total and direct or conjugated bilirubin to identify cholestasis (Table 1) (evidence quality D: benefit versus harms exceptional). The results of the newborn thyroid and galactosemia screen should also be checked in these infants (evidence quality D: benefits versus harms exceptional).

RECOMMENDATION 4.1.3: If the direct-reacting or conjugated bilirubin level is elevated, additional evaluation for the causes of cholestasis is recommended (evidence quality C: benefits exceed harms).

RECOMMENDATION 4.1.4: Measurement of the glucose-6-phosphate dehydrogenase (G6PD) level is recommended for a jaundiced infant who is receiving phototherapy and whose family history or ethnic or geographic origin suggest the likelihood of G6PD deficiency or for an infant in whom the response to phototherapy is poor (Fig 3) (evidence quality C: benefits exceed harms).

G6PD deficiency is widespread and frequently unrecognized, and although it is more common in the populations around the Mediterranean and in the Middle East, Arabian peninsula, Southeast Asia, and Africa, immigration and intermarriage have transformed G6PD deficiency into a global problem.[33,34]

TABLE 1.   Laboratory Evaluation of the Jaundiced Infant of 35 or More Weeks' Gestation

Indications	Assessments
Jaundice in first 24 h	Measure TcB and/or TSB
Jaundice appears excessive for infant's age	Measure TcB and/or TSB
Infant receiving phototherapy or TSB rising rapidly (ie, crossing percentiles [Fig 2]) and unexplained by history and physical examination	Blood type and Coombs' test, if not obtained with cord blood
	Complete blood count and smear
	Measure direct or conjugated bilirubin
	It is an option to perform reticulocyte count, G6PD, and ETCO$_c$, if available
	Repeat TSB in 4–24 h depending on infant's age and TSB level
TSB concentration approaching exchange levels or not responding to phototherapy	Perform reticulocyte count, G6PD, albumin, ETCO$_c$, if available
Elevated direct (or conjugated) bilirubin level	Do urinalysis and urine culture. Evaluate for sepsis if indicated by history and physical examination
Jaundice present at or beyond age 3 wk, or sick infant	Total and direct (or conjugated) bilirubin level
	If direct bilirubin elevated, evaluate for causes of cholestasis
	Check results of newborn thyroid and galactosemia screen, and evaluate infant for signs or symptoms of hypothyroidism

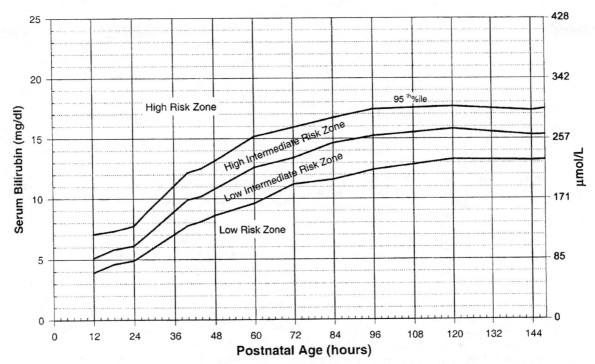

Fig 2. Nomogram for designation of risk in 2840 well newborns at 36 or more weeks' gestational age with birth weight of 2000 g or more or 35 or more weeks' gestational age and birth weight of 2500 g or more based on the hour-specific serum bilirubin values. The serum bilirubin level was obtained before discharge, and the zone in which the value fell predicted the likelihood of a subsequent bilirubin level exceeding the 95th percentile (high-risk zone) as shown in Appendix 1, Table 4. Used with permission from Bhutani et al.[31] See Appendix 1 for additional information about this nomogram, which should not be used to represent the natural history of neonatal hyperbilirubinemia.

Furthermore, G6PD deficiency occurs in 11% to 13% of African Americans, and kernicterus has occurred in some of these infants.[5,33] In a recent report, G6PD deficiency was considered to be the cause of hyperbilirubinemia in 19 of 61 (31.5%) infants who developed kernicterus.[5] (See Appendix 1 for additional information on G6PD deficiency.)

Risk Assessment Before Discharge

RECOMMENDATION 5.1: Before discharge, every newborn should be assessed for the risk of developing severe hyperbilirubinemia, and all nurseries should establish protocols for assessing this risk. Such assessment is particularly important in infants who are discharged before the age of 72 hours (evidence quality C: benefits exceed harms).

RECOMMENDATION 5.1.1: The AAP recommends 2 clinical options used individually or in combination for the systematic assessment of risk: predischarge measurement of the bilirubin level using TSB or TcB and/or assessment of clinical risk factors. Whether either or both options are used, appropriate follow-up after discharge is essential (evidence quality C: benefits exceed harms).

The best documented method for assessing the risk of subsequent hyperbilirubinemia is to measure the TSB or TcB level[25,31,35–38] and plot the results on a nomogram (Fig 2). A TSB level can be obtained at the time of the routine metabolic screen, thus obviating the need for an additional blood sample. Some authors have suggested that a TSB measurement should be part of the routine screening of all newborns.[5,31] An infant whose predischarge TSB is in the

low-risk zone (Fig 2) is at very low risk of developing severe hyperbilirubinemia.[5,38]

Table 2 lists those factors that are clinically signif-

TABLE 2. Risk Factors for Development of Severe Hyperbilirubinemia in Infants of 35 or More Weeks' Gestation (in Approximate Order of Importance)

Major risk factors
　Predischarge TSB or TcB level in the high-risk zone (Fig 2)[25,31]
　Jaundice observed in the first 24 h[30]
　Blood group incompatibility with positive direct antiglobulin test, other known hemolytic disease (eg, G6PD deficiency), elevated ETCO$_c$
　Gestational age 35–36 wk[39,40]
　Previous sibling received phototherapy[40,41]
　Cephalohematoma or significant bruising[39]
　Exclusive breastfeeding, particularly if nursing is not going well and weight loss is excessive[39,40]
　East Asian race[39]*
Minor risk factors
　Predischarge TSB or TcB level in the high intermediate-risk zone[25,31]
　Gestational age 37–38 wk[39,40]
　Jaundice observed before discharge[40]
　Previous sibling with jaundice[40,41]
　Macrosomic infant of a diabetic mother[42,43]
　Maternal age ≥25 y[39]
　Male gender[39,40]
Decreased risk (these factors are associated with decreased risk of significant jaundice, listed in order of decreasing importance)
　TSB or TcB level in the low-risk zone (Fig 2)[25,31]
　Gestational age ≥41 wk[39]
　Exclusive bottle feeding[39,40]
　Black race[38]*
　Discharge from hospital after 72 h[40,44]

* Race as defined by mother's description.

icant and most frequently associated with an increase in the risk of severe hyperbilirubinemia. But, because these risk factors are common and the risk of hyperbilirubinemia is small, individually the factors are of limited use as predictors of significant hyperbilirubinemia.[39] Nevertheless, if no risk factors are present, the risk of severe hyperbilirubinemia is extremely low, and the more risk factors present, the greater the risk of severe hyperbilirubinemia.[39] The important risk factors most frequently associated with severe hyperbilirubinemia are breastfeeding, gestation below 38 weeks, significant jaundice in a previous sibling, and jaundice noted before discharge.[39,40] A formula-fed infant of 40 or more weeks' gestation is at very low risk of developing severe hyperbilirubinemia.[39]

Hospital Policies and Procedures

RECOMMENDATION 6.1: All hospitals should provide written and verbal information for parents at the time of discharge, which should include an explanation of jaundice, the need to monitor infants for jaundice, and advice on how monitoring should be done (evidence quality D: benefits versus harms exceptional).

An example of a parent-information handout is available in English and Spanish at www.aap.org/family/jaundicefaq.htm.

Follow-up

RECOMMENDATION 6.1.1: All infants should be examined by a qualified health care professional in the first few days after discharge to assess infant well-being and the presence or absence of jaundice. The timing and location of this assessment will be determined by the length of stay in the nursery, presence or absence of risk factors for hyperbilirubinemia (Table 2 and Fig 2), and risk of other neonatal problems (evidence quality C: benefits exceed harms).

Timing of Follow-up

RECOMMENDATION 6.1.2: Follow-up should be provided as follows:

Infant Discharged	Should Be Seen by Age
Before age 24 h	72 h
Between 24 and 47.9 h	96 h
Between 48 and 72 h	120 h

For some newborns discharged before 48 hours, 2 follow-up visits may be required, the first visit between 24 and 72 hours and the second between 72 and 120 hours. Clinical judgment should be used in determining follow-up. Earlier or more frequent follow-up should be provided for those who have risk factors for hyperbilirubinemia (Table 2), whereas those discharged with few or no risk factors can be seen after longer intervals (evidence quality C: benefits exceed harms).

RECOMMENDATION 6.1.3: If appropriate follow-up cannot be ensured in the presence of elevated risk for developing severe hyperbilirubinemia, it may be necessary to delay discharge either until appropriate follow-up can be ensured or the period of greatest risk has passed (72-96 hours) (evidence quality D: benefits versus harms exceptional).

Follow-up Assessment

RECOMMENDATION 6.1.4: The follow-up assessment should include the infant's weight and percent change from birth weight, adequacy of intake, the pattern of voiding and stooling, and the presence or absence of jaundice (evidence quality C: benefits exceed harms). Clinical judgment should be used to determine the need for a bilirubin measurement. If there is any doubt about the degree of jaundice, the TSB or TcB level should be measured. Visual estimation of bilirubin levels can lead to errors, particularly in darkly pigmented infants (evidence quality C: benefits exceed harms).

See Appendix 1 for assessment of the adequacy of intake in breastfeeding infants.

TREATMENT

Phototherapy and Exchange Transfusion

RECOMMENDATION 7.1: Recommendations for treatment are given in Table 3 and Figs 3 and 4 (evidence quality C: benefits exceed harms). If the TSB does not fall or continues to rise despite intensive phototherapy, it is very likely that hemolysis is occurring. The committee's recommendations for discontinuing phototherapy can be found in Appendix 2.

RECOMMENDATION 7.1.1: In using the guidelines for phototherapy and exchange transfusion (Figs 3 and 4), the direct-reacting (or conjugated) bilirubin level should not be subtracted from the total (evidence quality D: benefits versus harms exceptional).

In unusual situations in which the direct bilirubin level is 50% or more of the total bilirubin, there are no good data to provide guidance for therapy, and consultation with an expert in the field is recommended.

RECOMMENDATION 7.1.2: If the TSB is at a level at which exchange transfusion is recommended (Fig 4) or if the TSB level is 25 mg/dL (428 μmol/L) or higher at any time, it is a medical emergency and the infant should be admitted immediately and directly to a hospital pediatric service for intensive phototherapy. These infants should not be referred to the emergency department, because it delays the initiation of treatment[54] (evidence quality C: benefits exceed harms).

RECOMMENDATION 7.1.3: Exchange transfusions should be performed only by trained personnel in a neonatal intensive care unit with full monitoring and resuscitation capabilities (evidence quality D: benefits versus harms exceptional).

RECOMMENDATION 7.1.4: In isoimmune hemolytic disease, administration of intravenous γ-globulin (0.5-1 g/kg over 2 hours) is recommended if the TSB is rising despite intensive phototherapy or the TSB level is within 2 to 3 mg/dL (34-51 μmol/L) of the exchange level (Fig 4).[55] If necessary, this dose can be repeated in 12 hours (evidence quality B: benefits exceed harms).

Intravenous γ-globulin has been shown to reduce the need for exchange transfusions in Rh and ABO hemolytic disease.[55–58] Although data are limited, it is reasonable to assume that intravenous γ-globulin will also be helpful in the other types of Rh hemolytic disease such as anti-C and anti-E.

TABLE 3.   Example of a Clinical Pathway for Management of the Newborn Infant Readmitted for Phototherapy or Exchange Transfusion

Treatment
    Use intensive phototherapy and/or exchange transfusion as indicated in Figs 3 and 4 (see Appendix 2 for details of phototherapy use)
Laboratory tests
    TSB and direct bilirubin levels
    Blood type (ABO, Rh)
    Direct antibody test (Coombs')
    Serum albumin
    Complete blood cell count with differential and smear for red cell morphology
    Reticulocyte count
    ETCO$_c$ (if available)
    G6PD if suggested by ethnic or geographic origin or if poor response to phototherapy
    Urine for reducing substances
    If history and/or presentation suggest sepsis, perform blood culture, urine culture, and cerebrospinal fluid for protein, glucose, cell count, and culture
Interventions
    If TSB ≥25 mg/dL (428 μmol/L) or ≥20 mg/dL (342 μmol/L) in a sick infant or infant <38 wk gestation, obtain a type and crossmatch, and request blood in case an exchange transfusion is necessary
    In infants with isoimmune hemolytic disease and TSB level rising in spite of intensive phototherapy or within 2–3 mg/dL (34–51 μmol/L) of exchange level (Fig 4), administer intravenous immunoglobulin 0.5–1 g/kg over 2 h and repeat in 12 h if necessary
    If infant's weight loss from birth is >12% or there is clinical or biochemical evidence of dehydration, recommend formula or expressed breast milk. If oral intake is in question, give intravenous fluids.
For infants receiving intensive phototherapy
    Breastfeed or bottle-feed (formula or expressed breast milk) every 2–3 h
    If TSB ≥25 mg/dL (428 μmol/L), repeat TSB within 2–3 h
    If TSB 20–25 mg/dL (342–428 μmol/L), repeat within 3–4 h. If TSB <20 mg/dL (342 μmol/L), repeat in 4–6 h. If TSB continues to fall, repeat in 8–12 h
    If TSB is not decreasing or is moving closer to level for exchange transfusion or the TSB/albumin ratio exceeds levels shown in Fig 4, consider exchange transfusion (see Fig 4 for exchange transfusion recommendations)
    When TSB is <13–14 mg/dL (239 μmol/L), discontinue phototherapy
    Depending on the cause of the hyperbilirubinemia, it is an option to measure TSB 24 h after discharge to check for rebound

Serum Albumin Levels and the Bilirubin/Albumin Ratio

RECOMMENDATION 7.1.5: *It is an option to measure the serum albumin level and consider an albumin level of less than 3.0 g/dL as one risk factor for lowering the threshold for phototherapy use (see Fig 3) (evidence quality D: benefits versus risks exceptional.).*

RECOMMENDATION 7.1.6: *If an exchange transfusion is being considered, the serum albumin level should be measured and the bilirubin/albumin (B/A) ratio used in conjunction with the TSB level and other factors in determining the need for exchange transfusion (see Fig 4) (evidence quality D: benefits versus harms exceptional).*

The recommendations shown above for treating hyperbilirubinemia are based primarily on TSB levels and other factors that affect the risk of bilirubin encephalopathy. This risk might be increased by a prolonged (rather than a brief) exposure to a certain TSB level.[59,60] Because the published data that address this issue are limited, however, it is not possible to provide specific recommendations for intervention based on the duration of hyperbilirubinemia.

See Appendix 1 for the basis for recommendations 7.1 through 7.1.6 and for the recommendations provided in Figs 3 and 4. Appendix 1 also contains a discussion of the risks of exchange transfusion and the use of B/A binding.

Acute Bilirubin Encephalopathy

RECOMMENDATION 7.1.7: *Immediate exchange transfusion is recommended in any infant who is jaun-diced and manifests the signs of the intermediate to advanced stages of acute bilirubin encephalopathy[61,62] (hypertonia, arching, retrocollis, opisthotonos, fever, high-pitched cry) even if the TSB is falling (evidence quality D: benefits versus risks exceptional).*

Phototherapy

RECOMMENDATION 7.2: *All nurseries and services treating infants should have the necessary equipment to provide intensive phototherapy (see Appendix 2) (evidence quality D: benefits exceed risks).*

Outpatient Management of the Jaundiced Breastfed Infant

RECOMMENDATION 7.3: *In breastfed infants who require phototherapy (Fig 3), the AAP recommends that, if possible, breastfeeding should be continued (evidence quality C: benefits exceed harms). It is also an option to interrupt temporarily breastfeeding and substitute formula. This can reduce bilirubin levels and/or enhance the efficacy of phototherapy[63–65] (evidence quality B: benefits exceed harms). In breastfed infants receiving phototherapy, supplementation with expressed breast milk or formula is appropriate if the infant's intake seems inadequate, weight loss is excessive, or the infant seems dehydrated.*

IMPLEMENTATION STRATEGIES

The Institute of Medicine[11] recommends a dramatic change in the way the US health care system

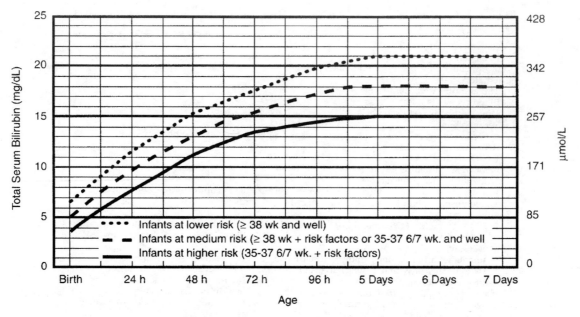

- Use total bilirubin. Do not subtract direct reacting or conjugated bilirubin.
- Risk factors = isoimmune hemolytic disease, G6PD deficiency, asphyxia, significant lethargy, temperature instability, sepsis, acidosis, or albumin < 3.0g/dL (if measured)
- For well infants 35-37 6/7 wk can adjust TSB levels for intervention around the medium risk line. It is an option to intervene at lower TSB levels for infants closer to 35 wks and at higher TSB levels for those closer to 37 6/7 wk.
- It is an option to provide conventional phototherapy in hospital or at home at TSB levels 2-3 mg/dL (35-50mmol/L) below those shown but home phototherapy should not be used in any infant with risk factors.

Fig 3. Guidelines for phototherapy in hospitalized infants of 35 or more weeks' gestation.

Note: These guidelines are based on limited evidence and the levels shown are approximations. The guidelines refer to the use of intensive phototherapy which should be used when the TSB exceeds the line indicated for each category. Infants are designated as "higher risk" because of the potential negative effects of the conditions listed on albumin binding of bilirubin,[45–47] the blood-brain barrier,[48] and the susceptibility of the brain cells to damage by bilirubin.[48]

"Intensive phototherapy" implies irradiance in the blue-green spectrum (wavelengths of approximately 430–490 nm) of at least 30 μW/cm^2 per nm (measured at the infant's skin directly below the center of the phototherapy unit) and delivered to as much of the infant's surface area as possible. Note that irradiance measured below the center of the light source is much greater than that measured at the periphery. Measurements should be made with a radiometer specified by the manufacturer of the phototherapy system.

See Appendix 2 for additional information on measuring the dose of phototherapy, a description of intensive phototherapy, and of light sources used. If total serum bilirubin levels approach or exceed the exchange transfusion line (Fig 4), the sides of the bassinet, incubator, or warmer should be lined with aluminum foil or white material.[50] This will increase the surface area of the infant exposed and increase the efficacy of phototherapy.[51]

If the total serum bilirubin does not decrease or continues to rise in an infant who is receiving intensive phototherapy, this strongly suggests the presence of hemolysis.

Infants who receive phototherapy and have an elevated direct-reacting or conjugated bilirubin level (cholestatic jaundice) may develop the bronze-baby syndrome. See Appendix 2 for the use of phototherapy in these infants.

ensures the safety of patients. The perspective of safety as a purely individual responsibility must be replaced by the concept of safety as a property of systems. Safe systems are characterized by a shared knowledge of the goal, a culture emphasizing safety, the ability of each person within the system to act in a manner that promotes safety, minimizing the use of memory, and emphasizing the use of standard procedures (such as checklists), and the involvement of patients/families as partners in the process of care.

These principles can be applied to the challenge of preventing severe hyperbilirubinemia and kernicterus. A systematic approach to the implementation of these guidelines should result in greater safety. Such approaches might include

- The establishment of standing protocols for nursing assessment of jaundice, including testing TcB and TSB levels, without requiring physician orders.

- Checklists or reminders associated with risk factors, age at discharge, and laboratory test results that provide guidance for appropriate follow-up.
- Explicit educational materials for parents (a key component of all AAP guidelines) concerning the identification of newborns with jaundice.

FUTURE RESEARCH

Epidemiology of Bilirubin-Induced Central Nervous System Damage

There is a need for appropriate epidemiologic data to document the incidence of kernicterus in the newborn population, the incidence of other adverse effects attributable to hyperbilirubinemia and its management, and the number of infants whose TSB levels exceed 25 or 30 mg/dL (428-513 μmol/L). Organizations such as the Centers for Disease Control and Prevention should implement strategies for appropriate data gathering to identify the number of

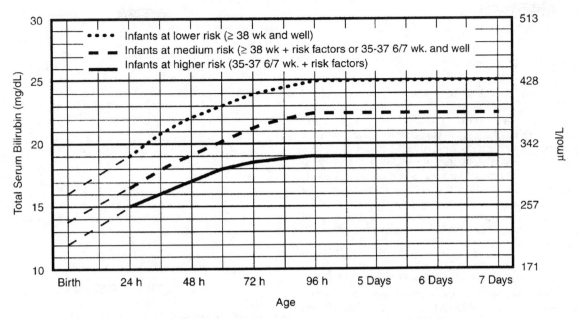

- The dashed lines for the first 24 hours indicate uncertainty due to a wide range of clinical circumstances and a range of responses to phototherapy.
- Immediate exchange transfusion is recommended if infant shows signs of acute bilirubin encephalopathy (hypertonia, arching, retrocollis, opisthotonos, fever, high pitched cry) or if TSB is ≥5 mg/dL (85 μmol/L) above these lines.
- Risk factors - isoimmune hemolytic disease, G6PD deficiency, asphyxia, significant lethargy, temperature instability, sepsis, acidosis.
- Measure serum albumin and calculate B/A ratio (See legend)
- Use total bilirubin. Do not subtract direct reacting or conjugated bilirubin
- If infant is well and 35-37 6/7 wk (median risk) can individualize TSB levels for exchange based on actual gestational age.

Fig 4. Guidelines for exchange transfusion in infants 35 or more weeks' gestation.

Note that these suggested levels represent a consensus of most of the committee but are based on limited evidence, and the levels shown are approximations. See ref. 3 for risks and complications of exchange transfusion. During birth hospitalization, exchange transfusion is recommended if the TSB rises to these levels despite intensive phototherapy. For readmitted infants, if the TSB level is above the exchange level, repeat TSB measurement every 2 to 3 hours and consider exchange if the TSB remains above the levels indicated after intensive phototherapy for 6 hours.

The following B/A ratios can be used together with but in not in lieu of the TSB level as an additional factor in determining the need for exchange transfusion[52]:

Risk Category	B/A Ratio at Which Exchange Transfusion Should be Considered	
	TSB mg/dL/Alb, g/dL	TSB μmol/L/Alb, μmol/L
Infants ≥38 0/7 wk	8.0	0.94
Infants 35 0/7–36 6/7 wk and well or ≥38 0/7 wk if higher risk or isoimmune hemolytic disease or G6PD deficiency	7.2	0.84
Infants 35 0/7–37 6/7 wk if higher risk or isoimmune hemolytic disease or G6PD deficiency	6.8	0.80

If the TSB is at or approaching the exchange level, send blood for immediate type and crossmatch. Blood for exchange transfusion is modified whole blood (red cells and plasma) crossmatched against the mother and compatible with the infant.[53]

infants who develop serum bilirubin levels above 25 or 30 mg/dL (428-513 μmol/L) and those who develop acute and chronic bilirubin encephalopathy. This information will help to identify the magnitude of the problem; the number of infants who need to be screened and treated to prevent 1 case of kernicterus; and the risks, costs, and benefits of different strategies for prevention and treatment of hyperbilirubinemia. In the absence of these data, recommendations for intervention cannot be considered definitive.

Effect of Bilirubin on the Central Nervous System

The serum bilirubin level by itself, except when it is extremely high and associated with bilirubin encephalopathy, is an imprecise indicator of long-term neurodevelopmental outcome.[2] Additional studies are needed on the relationship between central nervous system damage and the duration of hyperbilirubinemia, the binding of bilirubin to albumin, and changes seen in the brainstem auditory evoked response. These studies could help to better identify risk, clarify the effect of bilirubin on the central nervous system, and guide intervention.

Identification of Hemolysis

Because of their poor specificity and sensitivity, the standard laboratory tests for hemolysis (Table 1) are frequently unhelpful.[66,67] However, end-tidal carbon monoxide, corrected for ambient carbon monoxide (ETCO$_c$), levels can confirm the presence or absence of hemolysis, and measurement of ETCO$_c$ is the only clinical test that provides a direct measurement of the rate of heme catabolism and the rate of bilirubin production.[68,69] Thus, ETCO$_c$ may be helpful in determining the degree of surveillance needed and the timing of intervention. It is not yet known, however, how ETCO$_c$ measurements will affect management.

Nomograms and the Measurement of Serum and TcB

It would be useful to develop an age-specific (by hour) nomogram for TSB in populations of newborns that differ with regard to risk factors for hyperbilirubinemia. There is also an urgent need to improve the precision and accuracy of the measurement of TSB in the clinical laboratory.[70,71] Additional studies are also needed to develop and validate noninvasive (transcutaneous) measurements of serum bilirubin and to understand the factors that affect these measurements. These studies should also assess the cost-effectiveness and reproducibility of TcB measurements in clinical practice.[2]

Pharmacologic Therapy

There is now evidence that hyperbilirubinemia can be effectively prevented or treated with tin-mesoporphyrin,[72–75] a drug that inhibits the production of heme oxygenase. Tin-mesoporphyrin is not approved by the US Food and Drug Administration. If approved, tin-mesoporphyrin could find immediate application in preventing the need for exchange transfusion in infants who are not responding to phototherapy.[75]

Dissemination and Monitoring

Research should be directed toward methods for disseminating the information contained in this guideline to increase awareness on the part of physicians, residents, nurses, and parents concerning the issues of neonatal hyperbilirubinemia and strategies for its management. In addition, monitoring systems should be established to identify the impact of these guidelines on the incidence of acute bilirubin encephalopathy and kernicterus and the use of phototherapy and exchange transfusions.

CONCLUSIONS

Kernicterus is still occurring but should be largely preventable if health care personnel follow the recommendations listed in this guideline. These recommendations emphasize the importance of universal, systematic assessment for the risk of severe hyperbilirubinemia, close follow-up, and prompt intervention, when necessary.

SUBCOMMITTEE ON HYPERBILIRUBINEMIA
M. Jeffrey Maisels, MB, BCh, Chairperson
Richard D. Baltz, MD
Vinod K. Bhutani, MD
Thomas B. Newman, MD, MPH
Heather Palmer, MB, BCh
Warren Rosenfeld, MD
David K. Stevenson, MD
Howard B. Weinblatt, MD

CONSULTANT
Charles J. Homer, MD, MPH, Chairperson
   American Academy of Pediatrics Steering
   Committee on Quality Improvement and
   Management

STAFF
Carla T. Herrerias, MPH

ACKNOWLEDGMENTS

M.J.M. received grant support from Natus Medical, Inc, for multinational study of ambient carbon monoxide; WellSpring Pharmaceutical Corporation for study of Stannsoporfin (tin-mesoporphyrin); and Minolta, Inc, for study of the Minolta/Hill-Rom Air-Shields transcutaneous jaundice meter model JM-103. V.K.B. received grant support from WellSpring Pharmaceutical Corporation for study of Stannsoporfin (tin-mesoporphyrin) and Natus Medical, Inc, for multinational study of ambient carbon monoxide and is a consultant (volunteer) to SpectrX (BiliChek transcutaneous bilirubinometer). D.K.S. is a consultant to and holds stock options through Natus Medical, Inc.

The American Academy of Pediatrics Subcommittee on Hyperbilirubinemia gratefully acknowledges the help of the following organizations, committees, and individuals who reviewed drafts of this guideline and provided valuable criticisms and commentary: American Academy of Pediatrics Committee on Nutrition; American Academy of Pediatrics Committee on Practice and Ambulatory Medicine; American Academy of Pediatrics Committee on Child Health Financing; American Academy of Pediatrics Committee on Medical Liability; American Academy of Pediatrics Committee on Fetus and Newborn; American Academy of Pediatrics Section on Perinatal Pediatrics; Centers for Disease Control and Prevention; Parents of Infants and Children With Kernicterus (PICK); Charles Ahlfors, MD; Daniel Batton, MD; Thomas Bojko, MD; Sarah Clune, MD; Sudhakar Ezhuthachan, MD; Lawrence Gartner, MD; Cathy Hammerman, MD; Thor Hansen, MD; Lois Johnson, MD; Michael Kaplan, MB, ChB; Tony McDonagh, PhD; Gerald Merenstein, MD; Mary O'Shea, MD; Max Perlman, MD; Ronald Poland, MD; Alex Robertson, MD; Firmino Rubaltelli, MD; Steven Shapiro, MD; Stanford Singer, MD; Ann Stark, MD; Gautham Suresh, MD; Margot VandeBor, MD; Hank Vreman, PhD; Philip Walson, MD; Jon Watchko, MD; Richard Wennberg, MD; and Chap-Yung Yeung, MD.

REFERENCES

1. American Academy of Pediatrics, Provisional Committee for Quality Improvement and Subcommittee on Hyperbilirubinemia. Practice parameter: management of hyperbilirubinemia in the healthy term newborn. *Pediatrics.* 1994;94:558–562
2. Ip S, Glicken S, Kulig J, Obrien R, Sege R, Lau J. *Management of Neonatal Hyperbilirubinemia.* Rockville, MD: US Department of Health and Human Services, Agency for Healthcare Research and Quality; 2003. AHRQ Publication 03-E011
3. Ip S, Chung M, Kulig J. et al. An evidence-based review of important issues concerning neonatal hyperbilirubinemia. *Pediatrics.* 2004;113(6). Available at: www.pediatrics.org/cgi/content/full/113/6/e644
4. American Academy of Pediatrics, Steering Committee on Quality Improvement and Management. A taxonomy of recommendations. *Pediatrics.* 2004; In press
5. Johnson LH, Bhutani VK, Brown AK. System-based approach to management of neonatal jaundice and prevention of kernicterus. *J Pediatr.* 2002;140:396–403

6. Maisels MJ, Newman TB. Kernicterus in otherwise healthy, breast-fed term newborns. *Pediatrics*. 1995;96:730–733

7. MacDonald M. Hidden risks: early discharge and bilirubin toxicity due to glucose-6-phosphate dehydrogenase deficiency. *Pediatrics*. 1995;96:734–738

8. Penn AA, Enzman DR, Hahn JS, Stevenson DK. Kernicterus in a full term infant. *Pediatrics*. 1994;93:1003–1006

9. Washington EC, Ector W, Abboud M, Ohning B, Holden K. Hemolytic jaundice due to G6PD deficiency causing kernicterus in a female newborn. *South Med J*. 1995;88:776–779

10. Ebbesen F. Recurrence of kernicterus in term and near-term infants in Denmark. *Acta Paediatr*. 2000;89:1213–1217

11. Institue of Medicine. *Crossing the Quality Chasm: A New Health System for the 21st Century*. Washington, DC: National Academy Press; 2001

12. American Academy of Pediatrics, American College of Obstetricians and Gynecologists. *Guidelines for Perinatal Care*. 5th ed. Elk Grove Village, IL: American Academy of Pediatrics; 2002:220–224

13. Bertini G, Dani C, Trochin M, Rubaltelli F. Is breastfeeding really favoring early neonatal jaundice? *Pediatrics*. 2001;107(3). Available at: www.pediatrics.org/cgi/content/full/107/3/e41

14. Maisels MJ, Gifford K. Normal serum bilirubin levels in the newborn and the effect of breast-feeding. *Pediatrics*. 1986;78:837–843

15. Yamauchi Y, Yamanouchi I. Breast-feeding frequency during the first 24 hours after birth in full-term neonates. *Pediatrics*. 1990;86:171–175

16. De Carvalho M, Klaus MH, Merkatz RB. Frequency of breastfeeding and serum bilirubin concentration. *Am J Dis Child*. 1982;136:737–738

17. Varimo P, Similä S, Wendt L, Kolvisto M. Frequency of breast feeding and hyperbilirubinemia [letter]. *Clin Pediatr (Phila)*. 1986;25:112

18. De Carvalho M, Holl M, Harvey D. Effects of water supplementation on physiological jaundice in breast-fed babies. *Arch Dis Child*. 1981;56:568–569

19. Nicoll A, Ginsburg R, Tripp JH. Supplementary feeding and jaundice in newborns. *Acta Paediatr Scand*. 1982;71:759–761

20. Madlon-Kay DJ. Identifying ABO incompatibility in newborns: selective vs automatic testing. *J Fam Pract*. 1992;35:278–280

21. Kramer LI. Advancement of dermal icterus in the jaundiced newborn. *Am J Dis Child*. 1969;118:454–458

22. Moyer VA, Ahn C, Sneed S. Accuracy of clinical judgment in neonatal jaundice. *Arch Pediatr Adolesc Med*. 2000;154:391–394

23. Davidson LT, Merritt KK, Weech AA. Hyperbilirubinemia in the newborn. *Am J Dis Child*. 1941;61:958–980

24. Tayaba R, Gribetz D, Gribetz I, Holzman IR. Noninvasive estimation of serum bilirubin. *Pediatrics*. 1998;102(3). Available at: www.pediatrics.org/cgi/content/full/102/3/e28

25. Bhutani V, Gourley GR, Adler S, Kreamer B, Dalman C, Johnson LH. Noninvasive measurement of total serum bilirubin in a multiracial predischarge newborn population to assess the risk of severe hyperbilirubinemia. *Pediatrics*. 2000;106(2). Available at: www.pediatrics.org/cgi/content/full/106/2/e17

26. Yasuda S, Itoh S, Isobe K, et al. New transcutaneous jaundice device with two optical paths. *J Perinat Med*. 2003;31:81–88

27. Maisels MJ, Ostrea EJ Jr, Touch S, et al. Evaluation of a new transcutaneous bilirubinometer. *Pediatrics*. 2004;113:1638–1645

28. Ebbesen F, Rasmussen LM, Wimberley PD. A new transcutaneous bilirubinometer, bilicheck, used in the neonatal intensive care unit and the maternity ward. *Acta Paediatr*. 2002;91:203–211

29. Rubaltelli FF, Gourley GR, Loskamp N, et al. Transcutaneous bilirubin measurement: a multicenter evaluation of a new device. *Pediatrics*. 2001;107:1264–1271

30. Newman TB, Liljestrand P, Escobar GJ. Jaundice noted in the first 24 hours after birth in a managed care organization. *Arch Pediatr Adolesc Med*. 2002;156:1244–1250

31. Bhutani VK, Johnson L, Sivieri EM. Predictive ability of a predischarge hour-specific serum bilirubin for subsequent significant hyperbilirubinemia in healthy term and near-term newborns. *Pediatrics*. 1999;103:6–14

32. Garcia FJ, Nager AL. Jaundice as an early diagnostic sign of urinary tract infection in infancy. *Pediatrics*. 2002;109:846–851

33. Kaplan M, Hammerman C. Severe neonatal hyperbilirubinemia: a potential complication of glucose-6-phosphate dehydrogenase deficiency. *Clin Perinatol*. 1998;25:575–590

34. Valaes T. Severe neonatal jaundice associated with glucose-6-phosphate dehydrogenase deficiency: pathogenesis and global epidemiology. *Acta Paediatr Suppl*. 1994;394:58–76

35. Alpay F, Sarici S, Tosuncuk HD, Serdar MA, Inanç N, Gökçay E. The value of first-day bilirubin measurement in predicting the development of significant hyperbilirubinemia in healthy term newborns. *Pediatrics*.

2000;106(2). Available at: www.pediatrics.org/cgi/content/full/106/2/e16

36. Carbonell X, Botet F, Figueras J, Riu-Godo A. Prediction of hyperbilirubinaemia in the healthy term newborn. *Acta Paediatr*. 2001;90:166–170

37. Kaplan M, Hammerman C, Feldman R, Brisk R. Predischarge bilirubin screening in glucose-6-phosphate dehydrogenase-deficient neonates. *Pediatrics*. 2000;105:533–537

38. Stevenson DK, Fanaroff AA, Maisels MJ, et al. Prediction of hyperbilirubinemia in near-term and term infants. *Pediatrics*. 2001;108:31–39

39. Newman TB, Xiong B, Gonzales VM, Escobar GJ. Prediction and prevention of extreme neonatal hyperbilirubinemia in a mature health maintenance organization. *Arch Pediatr Adolesc Med*. 2000;154:1140–1147

40. Maisels MJ, Kring EA. Length of stay, jaundice, and hospital readmission. *Pediatrics*. 1998;101:995–998

41. Gale R, Seidman DS, Dollberg S, Stevenson DK. Epidemiology of neonatal jaundice in the Jerusalem population. *J Pediatr Gastroenterol Nutr*. 1990;10:82–86

42. Berk MA, Mimouni F, Miodovnik M, Hertzberg V, Valuck J. Macrosomia in infants of insulin-dependent diabetic mothers. *Pediatrics*. 1989;83:1029–1034

43. Peevy KJ, Landaw SA, Gross SJ. Hyperbilirubinemia in infants of diabetic mothers. *Pediatrics*. 1980;66:417–419

44. Soskolne El, Schumacher R, Fyock C, Young ML, Schork A. The effect of early discharge and other factors on readmission rates of newborns. *Arch Pediatr Adolesc Med*. 1996;150:373–379

45. Ebbesen F, Brodersen R. Risk of bilirubin acid precipitation in preterm infants with respiratory distress syndrome: considerations of blood/brain bilirubin transfer equilibrium. *Early Hum Dev*. 1982;6:341–355

46. Cashore WJ, Oh W, Brodersen R. Reserve albumin and bilirubin toxicity index in infant serum. *Acta Paediatr Scand*. 1983;72:415–419

47. Cashore WJ. Free bilirubin concentrations and bilirubin-binding affinity in term and preterm infants. *J Pediatr*. 1980;96:521–527

48. Bratlid D. How bilirubin gets into the brain. *Clin Perinatol*. 1990;17:449–465

49. Wennberg RP. Cellular basis of bilirubin toxicity. *N Y State J Med*. 1991;91:493–496

50. Eggert P, Stick C, Schroder H. On the distribution of irradiation intensity in phototherapy. Measurements of effective irradiance in an incubator. *Eur J Pediatr*. 1984;142:58–61

51. Maisels MJ. Why use homeopathic doses of phototherapy? *Pediatrics*. 1996;98:283–287

52. Ahlfors CE. Criteria for exchange transfusion in jaundiced newborns. *Pediatrics*. 1994;93:488–494

53. American Association of Blood Banks Technical Manual Committee. Perinatal issues in transfusion practice. In: Brecher M, ed. *Technical Manual*. Bethesda, MD: American Association of Blood Banks; 2002:497–515

54. Garland JS, Alex C, Deacon JS, Raab K. Treatment of infants with indirect hyperbilirubinemia. Readmission to birth hospital vs nonbirth hospital. *Arch Pediatr Adolesc Med*. 1994;148:1317–1321

55. Gottstein R, Cooke R. Systematic review of intravenous immunoglobulin in haemolytic disease of the newborn. *Arch Dis Child Fetal Neonatal Ed*. 2003;88:F6–F10

56. Sato K, Hara T, Kondo T, Iwao H, Honda S, Ueda K. High-dose intravenous gammaglobulin therapy for neonatal immune haemolytic jaundice due to blood group incompatibility. *Acta Paediatr Scand*. 1991;80:163–166

57. Rubo J, Albrecht K, Lasch P, et al. High-dose intravenous immune globulin therapy for hyperbilirubinemia caused by Rh hemolytic disease. *J Pediatr*. 1992;121:93–97

58. Hammerman C, Kaplan M, Vreman HJ, Stevenson DK. Intravenous immune globulin in neonatal ABO isoimmunization: factors associated with clinical efficacy. *Biol Neonate*. 1996;70:69–74

59. Johnson L, Boggs TR. Bilirubin-dependent brain damage: incidence and indications for treatment. In: Odell GB, Schaffer R, Simopoulos AP, eds. *Phototherapy in the Newborn: An Overview*. Washington, DC: National Academy of Sciences; 1974:122–149

60. Ozmert E, Erdem G, Topcu M. Long-term follow-up of indirect hyperbilirubinemia in full-term Turkish infants. *Acta Paediatr*. 1996;85:1440–1444

61. Volpe JJ. *Neurology of the Newborn*. 4th ed. Philadelphia, PA: W. B. Saunders; 2001

62. Harris M, Bernbaum J, Polin J, Zimmerman R, Polin RA. Developmental follow-up of breastfed term and near-term infants with marked hyperbilirubinemia. *Pediatrics*. 2001;107:1075–1080

63. Osborn LM, Bolus R. Breast feeding and jaundice in the first week of life. *J Fam Pract*. 1985;20:475–480

64. Martinez JC, Maisels MJ, Otheguy L, et al. Hyperbilirubinemia in the breast-fed newborn: a controlled trial of four interventions. *Pediatrics.* 1993;91:470–473

65. Amato M, Howald H, von Muralt G. Interruption of breast-feeding versus phototherapy as treatment of hyperbilirubinemia in full-term infants. *Helv Paediatr Acta.* 1985;40:127–131

66. Maisels MJ, Gifford K, Antle CE, Leib GR. Jaundice in the healthy newborn infant: a new approach to an old problem. *Pediatrics.* 1988;81: 505–511

67. Newman TB, Easterling MJ. Yield of reticulocyte counts and blood smears in term infants. *Clin Pediatr (Phila).* 1994;33:71–76

68. Herschel M, Karrison T, Wen M, Caldarelli L, Baron B. Evaluation of the direct antiglobulin (Coombs') test for identifying newborns at risk for hemolysis as determined by end-tidal carbon monoxide concentration (ETCOc); and comparison of the Coombs' test with ETCOc for detecting significant jaundice. *J Perinatol.* 2002;22:341–347

69. Stevenson DK, Vreman HJ. Carbon monoxide and bilirubin production in neonates. *Pediatrics.* 1997;100:252–254

70. Vreman HJ, Verter J, Oh W, et al. Interlaboratory variability of bilirubin measurements. *Clin Chem.* 1996;42:869–873

71. Lo S, Doumas BT, Ashwood E. Performance of bilirubin determinations in US laboratories—revisited. *Clin Chem.* 2004;50:190–194

72. Kappas A, Drummond GS, Henschke C, Valaes T. Direct comparison of Sn-mesoporphyrin, an inhibitor of bilirubin production, and phototherapy in controlling hyperbilirubinemia in term and near-term newborns. *Pediatrics.* 1995;95:468–474

73. Martinez JC, Garcia HO, Otheguy L, Drummond GS, Kappas A. Control of severe hyperbilirubinemia in full-term newborns with the inhibitor of bilirubin production Sn-mesoporphyrin. *Pediatrics.* 1999;103:1–5

74. Suresh G, Martin CL, Soll R. Metalloporphyrins for treatment of unconjugated hyperbilirubinemia in neonates. *Cochrane Database Syst Rev.* 2003;2:CD004207

75. Kappas A, Drummond GS, Munson DP, Marshall JR. Sn-mesoporphyrin interdiction of severe hyperbilirubinemia in Jehovah's Witness newborns as an alternative to exchange transfusion. *Pediatrics.* 2001;108: 1374–1377

APPENDIX 1: Additional Notes

Definitions of Quality of Evidence and Balance of Benefits and Harms

The Steering Committee on Quality Improvement and Management categorizes evidence quality in 4 levels:

1. Well-designed, randomized, controlled trials or diagnostic studies on relevant populations
2. Randomized, controlled trials or diagnostic studies with minor limitations; overwhelming, consistent evidence from observational studies
3. Observational studies (case-control and cohort design)
4. Expert opinion, case reports, reasoning from first principles

The AAP defines evidence-based recommendations as follows:[1]

- Strong recommendation: the committee believes that the benefits of the recommended approach clearly exceed the harms of that approach and that the quality of the supporting evidence is either excellent or impossible to obtain. Clinicians should follow these recommendations unless a clear and compelling rationale for an alternative approach is present.
- Recommendation: the committee believes that the benefits exceed the harms, but the quality of evidence on which this recommendation is based is not as strong. Clinicians should also generally follow these recommendations but should be alert to new information and sensitive to patient prefer-

ences. In this guideline, the term "should" implies a recommendation by the committee.
- Option: either the quality of the evidence that exists is suspect or well-performed studies have shown little clear advantage to one approach over another. Patient preference should have a substantial role in influencing clinical decision-making when a policy is described as an option.
- No recommendation: there is a lack of pertinent evidence and the anticipated balance of benefits and harms is unclear.

Anticipated Balance Between Benefits and Harms

The presence of clear benefits or harms supports stronger statements for or against a course of action. In some cases, however, recommendations are made when analysis of the balance of benefits and harms provides an exceptional dysequilibrium and it would be unethical or impossible to perform clinical trials to "prove" the point. In these cases the balance of benefit and harm is termed "exceptional."

Clinical Manifestations of Acute Bilirubin Encephalopathy and Kernicterus

Acute Bilirubin Encephalopathy

In the early phase of acute bilirubin encephalopathy, severely jaundiced infants become lethargic and hypotonic and suck poorly.[2,3] The intermediate phase is characterized by moderate stupor, irritability, and hypertonia. The infant may develop a fever and high-pitched cry, which may alternate with drowsiness and hypotonia. The hypertonia is manifested by backward arching of the neck (retrocollis) and trunk (opisthotonos). There is anecdotal evidence that an emergent exchange transfusion at this stage, in some cases, might reverse the central nervous system changes.[4] The advanced phase, in which central nervous system damage is probably irreversible, is characterized by pronounced retrocollis-opisthotonos, shrill cry, no feeding, apnea, fever, deep stupor to coma, sometimes seizures, and death.[2,3,5]

Kernicterus

In the chronic form of bilirubin encephalopathy, surviving infants may develop a severe form of athetoid cerebral palsy, auditory dysfunction, dental-enamel dysplasia, paralysis of upward gaze, and, less often, intellectual and other handicaps. Most infants who develop kernicterus have manifested some or all of the signs listed above in the acute phase of bilirubin encephalopathy. However, occasionally there are infants who have developed very high bilirubin levels and, subsequently, the signs of kernicterus but have exhibited few, if any, antecedent clinical signs of acute bilirubin encephalopathy.[3,5,6]

Clinical Evaluation of Jaundice and TcB Measurements

Jaundice is usually seen in the face first and progresses caudally to the trunk and extremities,[7] but because visual estimation of bilirubin levels from the degree of jaundice can lead to errors,[8–10] a low threshold should be used for measuring the TSB.

Devices that provide a noninvasive TcB measurement have proven very useful as screening tools,[11] and newer instruments give measurements that provide a valid estimate of the TSB level.[12–17] Studies using the new TcB-measurement instruments are limited, but the data published thus far suggest that in most newborn populations, these instruments generally provide measurements within 2 to 3 mg/dL (34–51 μmol/L) of the TSB and can replace a measurement of serum bilirubin in many circumstances, particularly for TSB levels less than 15 mg/dL (257 μmol/L).[12–17] Because phototherapy "bleaches" the skin, both visual assessment of jaundice and TcB measurements in infants undergoing phototherapy are not reliable. In addition, the ability of transcutaneous instruments to provide accurate measurements in different racial groups requires additional study.[18,19] The limitations of the accuracy and reproducibility of TSB measurements in the clinical laboratory[20–22] must also be recognized and are discussed in the technical report.[23]

Capillary Versus Venous Serum Bilirubin Measurement

Almost all published data regarding the relationship of TSB levels to kernicterus or developmental outcome are based on capillary blood TSB levels. Data regarding the differences between capillary and venous TSB levels are conflicting.[24,25] In 1 study the capillary TSB levels were higher, but in another they were lower than venous TSB levels.[24,25] Thus, obtaining a venous sample to "confirm" an elevated capillary TSB level is not recommended, because it will delay the initiation of treatment.

Direct-Reacting and Conjugated Bilirubin

Although commonly used interchangeably, direct-reacting bilirubin is not the same as conjugated bilirubin. Direct-reacting bilirubin is the bilirubin that reacts directly (without the addition of an accelerating agent) with diazotized sulfanilic acid. Conjugated bilirubin is bilirubin made water soluble by binding with glucuronic acid in the liver. Depending on the technique used, the clinical laboratory will report total and direct-reacting or unconjugated and conjugated bilirubin levels. In this guideline and for clinical purposes, the terms may be used interchangeably.

Abnormal Direct and Conjugated Bilirubin Levels

Laboratory measurement of direct bilirubin is not precise,[26] and values between laboratories can vary widely. If the TSB is at or below 5 mg/dL (85 μmol/L), a direct or conjugated bilirubin of more than 1.0 mg/dL (17.1 μmol/L) is generally considered abnormal. For TSB values higher than 5 mg/dL (85 μmol/L), a direct bilirubin of more than 20% of the TSB is considered abnormal. If the hospital laboratory measures conjugated bilirubin using the Vitros (formerly Ektachem) system (Ortho-Clinical Diagnostics, Raritan, NJ), any value higher than 1 mg/dL is considered abnormal.

Assessment of Adequacy of Intake in Breastfeeding Infants

The data from a number of studies[27–34] indicate that unsupplemented, breastfed infants experience their maximum weight loss by day 3 and, on average, lose 6.1% ± 2.5% (SD) of their birth weight. Thus, ~5% to 10% of fully breastfed infants lose 10% or more of their birth weight by day 3, suggesting that adequacy of intake should be evaluated and the infant monitored if weight loss is more than 10%.[35] Evidence of adequate intake in breastfed infants also includes 4 to 6 thoroughly wet diapers in 24 hours and the passage of 3 to 4 stools per day by the fourth day. By the third to fourth day, the stools in adequately breastfed infants should have changed from meconium to a mustard yellow, mushy stool.[36] The above assessment will also help to identify breastfed infants who are at risk for dehydration because of inadequate intake.

Nomogram for Designation of Risk

Note that this nomogram (Fig 2) does not describe the natural history of neonatal hyperbilirubinemia, particularly after 48 to 72 hours, for which, because of sampling bias, the lower zones are spuriously elevated.[37] This bias, however, will have much less effect on the high-risk zone (95th percentile in the study).[38]

G6PD Dehydrogenase Deficiency

It is important to look for G6PD deficiency in infants with significant hyperbilirubinemia, because some may develop a sudden increase in the TSB. In addition, G6PD-deficient infants require intervention at lower TSB levels (Figs 3 and 4). It should be noted also that in the presence of hemolysis, G6PD levels can be elevated, which may obscure the diagnosis in the newborn period so that a normal level in a hemolyzing neonate does not rule out G6PD deficiency.[39] If G6PD deficiency is strongly suspected, a repeat level should be measured when the infant is 3 months old. It is also recognized that immediate laboratory determination of G6PD is generally not available in most US hospitals, and thus translating the above information into clinical practice is cur-

TABLE 4.   Risk Zone as a Predictor of Hyperbilirubinemia[39]

TSB Before Discharge	Newborns (Total = 2840), n (%)	Newborns Who Subsequently Developed a TSB Level >95th Percentile, n (%)
High-risk zone (>95th percentile)	172 (6.0)	68 (39.5)
High intermediate-risk zone	356 (12.5)	46 (12.9)
Low intermediate-risk zone	556 (19.6)	12 (2.26)
Low-risk zone	1756 (61.8)	0

rently difficult. Nevertheless, practitioners are reminded to consider the diagnosis of G6PD deficiency in infants with severe hyperbilirubinemia, particularly if they belong to the population groups in which this condition is prevalent. This is important in the African American population, because these infants, as a group, have much lower TSB levels than white or Asian infants.[40,41] Thus, severe hyperbilirubinemia in an African American infant should always raise the possibility of G6PD deficiency.

Basis for the Recommendations 7.1.1 Through 7.1.6 and Provided in Figs 3 and 4

Ideally, recommendations for when to implement phototherapy and exchange transfusions should be based on estimates of when the benefits of these interventions exceed their risks and cost. The evidence for these estimates should come from randomized trials or systematic observational studies. Unfortunately, there is little such evidence on which to base these recommendations. As a result, treatment guidelines must necessarily rely on more uncertain estimates and extrapolations. For a detailed discussion of this question, please see "An Evidence-Based Review of Important Issues Concerning Neonatal Hyperbilirubinemia."[23]

The recommendations for phototherapy and exchange transfusion are based on the following principles:

- The main demonstrated value of phototherapy is that it reduces the risk that TSB levels will reach a level at which exchange transfusion is recommended.[42-44] Approximately 5 to 10 infants with TSB levels between 15 and 20 mg/dL (257–342 μmol/L) will receive phototherapy to prevent the TSB in 1 infant from reaching 20 mg/dL (the number needed to treat).[12] Thus, 8 to 9 of every 10 infants with these TSB levels will not reach 20 mg/dL (342 μmol/L) even if they are not treated. Phototherapy has proven to be a generally safe procedure, although rare complications can occur (see Appendix 2).
- Recommended TSB levels for exchange transfusion (Fig 4) are based largely on the goal of keeping TSB levels below those at which kernicterus has been reported.[12,45-48] In almost all cases, exchange transfusion is recommended only after phototherapy has failed to keep the TSB level below the exchange transfusion level (Fig 4).
- The recommendations to use phototherapy and exchange transfusion at lower TSB levels for infants of lower gestation and those who are sick are based on limited observations suggesting that sick infants (particularly those with the risk factors listed in Figs 3 and 4)[49-51] and those of lower gestation[51-54] are at greater risk for developing kernicterus at lower bilirubin levels than are well infants of more than 38 6/7 weeks' gestation. Nevertheless, other studies have not confirmed all of these associations.[52,55,56] There is no doubt, however, that infants at 35 to 37 6/7 weeks' gestation are at a much greater risk of developing very high

TSB levels.[57,58] Intervention for these infants is based on this risk as well as extrapolations from more premature, lower birth-weight infants who do have a higher risk of bilirubin toxicity.[52,53]

- For all newborns, treatment is recommended at lower TSB levels at younger ages because one of the primary goals of treatment is to prevent additional increases in the TSB level.

Subtle Neurologic Abnormalities Associated With Hyperbilirubinemia

There are several studies demonstrating measurable transient changes in brainstem-evoked potentials, behavioral patterns, and the infant's cry[59-63] associated with TSB levels of 15 to 25 mg/dL (257–428 μmol/L). In these studies, the abnormalities identified were transient and disappeared when the serum bilirubin levels returned to normal with or without treatment.[59,60,62,63]

A few cohort studies have found an association between hyperbilirubinemia and long-term adverse neurodevelopmental effects that are more subtle than kernicterus.[64-67] Current studies, however, suggest that although phototherapy lowers the TSB levels, it has no effect on these long-term neurodevelopmental outcomes.[68-70]

Risks of Exchange Transfusion

Because exchange transfusions are now rarely performed, the risks of morbidity and mortality associated with the procedure are difficult to quantify. In addition, the complication rates listed below may not be generalizable to the current era if, like most procedures, frequency of performance is an important determinant of risk. Death associated with exchange transfusion has been reported in approximately 3 in 1000 procedures,[71,72] although in otherwise well infants of 35 or more weeks' gestation, the risk is probably much lower.[71-73] Significant morbidity (apnea, bradycardia, cyanosis, vasospasm, thrombosis, necrotizing enterocolitis) occurs in as many as 5% of exchange transfusions,[71] and the risks associated with the use of blood products must always be considered.[74] Hypoxic-ischemic encephalopathy and acquired immunodeficiency syndrome have occurred in otherwise healthy infants receiving exchange transfusions.[73,75]

Serum Albumin Levels and the B/A Ratio

The legends to Figs 3 and 4 and recommendations 7.1.5 and 7.1.6 contain references to the serum albumin level and the B/A ratio as factors that can be considered in the decision to initiate phototherapy (Fig 3) or perform an exchange transfusion (Fig 4). Bilirubin is transported in the plasma tightly bound to albumin, and the portion that is unbound or loosely bound can more readily leave the intravascular space and cross the intact blood-brain barrier.[76] Elevations of unbound bilirubin (UB) have been associated with kernicterus in sick preterm newborns.[77,78] In addition, elevated UB concentrations are more closely associated than TSB levels with transient abnormalities in the audiometric brainstem response in term[79] and preterm[80] infants. Long-term studies relating B/A binding in infants to developmental outcome are limited and conflicting.[69,81,82] In addition, clinical laboratory measurement of UB is not currently available in the United States.

The ratio of bilirubin (mg/dL) to albumin (g/dL) does correlate with measured UB in newborns[83] and can be used as an approximate surrogate for the measurement of UB. It must be recognized, however, that both albumin levels and the ability of albumin to bind bilirubin vary significantly between newborns.[83,84] Albumin binding of bilirubin is impaired in sick infants,[84–86] and some studies show an increase in binding with increasing gestational[86,87] and postnatal[87,88] age, but others have not found a significant effect of gestational age on binding.[89] Furthermore, the risk of bilirubin encephalopathy is unlikely to be a simple function of the TSB level or the concentration of UB but is more likely a combination of both (ie, the total amount of bilirubin available [the miscible pool of bilirubin] as well as the tendency of bilirubin to enter the tissues [the UB concentration]).[83] An additional factor is the possible susceptibility of the cells of the central nervous system to damage by bilirubin.[90] It is therefore a clinical option to use the B/A ratio together with, but not in lieu of, the TSB level as an additional factor in determining the need for exchange transfusion[83] (Fig 4).

REFERENCES

1. American Academy of Pediatrics, Steering Committee on Quality Improvement and Management. Classification of recommendations for clinical practice guidelines. *Pediatrics.* 2004; In press
2. Johnson LH, Bhutani VK, Brown AK. System-based approach to management of neonatal jaundice and prevention of kernicterus. *J Pediatr.* 2002;140:396–403
3. Volpe JJ. *Neurology of the Newborn.* 4th ed. Philadelphia, PA: W. B. Saunders; 2001
4. Harris M, Bernbaum J, Polin J, Zimmerman R, Polin RA. Developmental follow-up of breastfed term and near-term infants with marked hyperbilirubinemia. *Pediatrics.* 2001;107:1075–1080
5. Van Praagh R. Diagnosis of kernicterus in the neonatal period. *Pediatrics.* 1961;28:870–876
6. Jones MH, Sands R, Hyman CB, Sturgeon P, Koch FP. Longitudinal study of incidence of central nervous system damage following erythroblastosis fetalis. *Pediatrics.* 1954;14:346–350
7. Kramer LI. Advancement of dermal icterus in the jaundiced newborn. *Am J Dis Child.* 1969;118:454–458
8. Moyer VA, Ahn C, Sneed S. Accuracy of clinical judgment in neonatal jaundice. *Arch Pediatr Adolesc Med.* 2000;154:391–394
9. Davidson LT, Merritt KK, Weech AA. Hyperbilirubinemia in the newborn. *Am J Dis Child.* 1941;61:958–980
10. Tayaba R, Gribetz D, Gribetz I, Holzman IR. Noninvasive estimation of serum bilirubin. *Pediatrics.* 1998;102(3). Available at: www.pediatrics.org/cgi/content/full/102/3/e28
11. Maisels MJ, Kring E. Transcutaneous bilirubinometry decreases the need for serum bilirubin measurements and saves money. *Pediatrics.* 1997;99:599–601
12. Ip S, Glicken S, Kulig J, Obrien R, Sege R, Lau J. *Management of Neonatal Hyperbilirubinemia.* Rockville, MD: US Department of Health and Human Services, Agency for Healthcare Research and Quality; 2003. AHRQ Publication 03-E011
13. Bhutani V, Gourley GR, Adler S, Kreamer B, Dalman C, Johnson LH. Noninvasive measurement of total serum bilirubin in a multiracial predischarge newborn population to assess the risk of severe hyperbilirubinemia. *Pediatrics.* 2000;106(2). Available at: www.pediatrics.org/cgi/content/full/106/2/e17
14. Yasuda S, Itoh S, Isobe K, et al. New transcutaneous jaundice device with two optical paths. *J Perinat Med.* 2003;31:81–88
15. Maisels MJ, Ostrea EJ Jr, Touch S, et al. Evaluation of a new transcutaneous bilirubinometer. *Pediatrics.* 2004;113:1638–1645

16. Ebbesen F, Rasmussen LM, Wimberley PD. A new transcutaneous bilirubinometer, bilicheck, used in the neonatal intensive care unit and the maternity ward. *Acta Paediatr.* 2002;91:203–211
17. Rubaltelli FF, Gourley GR, Loskamp N, et al. Transcutaneous bilirubin measurement: a multicenter evaluation of a new device. *Pediatrics.* 2001;107:1264–1271
18. Engle WD, Jackson GL, Sendelbach D, Manning D, Frawley W. Assessment of a transcutaneous device in the evaluation of neonatal hyperbilirubinemia in a primarily Hispanic population. *Pediatrics.* 2002;110:61–67
19. Schumacher R. Transcutaneous bilirubinometry and diagnostic tests: "the right job for the tool." *Pediatrics.* 2002;110:407–408
20. Vreman HJ, Verter J, Oh W, et al. Interlaboratory variability of bilirubin measurements. *Clin Chem.* 1996;42:869–873
21. Doumas BT, Eckfeldt JH. Errors in measurement of total bilirubin: a perennial problem. *Clin Chem.* 1996;42:845–848
22. Lo S, Doumas BT, Ashwood E. Performance of bilirubin determinations in US laboratories—revisited. *Clin Chem.* 2004;50:190–194
23. Ip S, Chung M, Kulig J. et al. An evidence-based review of important issues concerning neonatal hyperbilirubinemia. *Pediatrics.* 2004;113(6). Available at: www.pediatrics.org/cgi/content/full/113/6/e644
24. Leslie GI, Philips JB, Cassady G. Capillary and venous bilirubin values: are they really different? *Am J Dis Child.* 1987;141:1199–1200
25. Eidelman AI, Schimmel MS, Algur N, Eylath U. Capillary and venous bilirubin values: they are different—and how [letter]! *Am J Dis Child.* 1989;143:642
26. Watkinson LR, St John A, Penberthy LA. Investigation into paediatric bilirubin analyses in Australia and New Zealand. *J Clin Pathol.* 1982;35:52–58
27. Bertini G, Dani C, Trochin M, Rubaltelli F. Is breastfeeding really favoring early neonatal jaundice? *Pediatrics.* 2001;107(3). Available at: www.pediatrics.org/cgi/content/full/107/3/e41
28. De Carvalho M, Klaus MH, Merkatz RB. Frequency of breastfeeding and serum bilirubin concentration. *Am J Dis Child.* 1982;136:737–738
29. De Carvalho M, Holl M, Harvey D. Effects of water supplementation on physiological jaundice in breast-fed babies. *Arch Dis Child.* 1981;56:568–569
30. Nicoll A, Ginsburg R, Tripp JH. Supplementary feeding and jaundice in newborns. *Acta Paediatr Scand.* 1982;71:759–761
31. Butler DA, MacMillan JP. Relationship of breast feeding and weight loss to jaundice in the newborn period: review of the literature and results of a study. *Cleve Clin Q.* 1983;50:263–268
32. De Carvalho M, Robertson S, Klaus M. Fecal bilirubin excretion and serum bilirubin concentration in breast-fed and bottle-fed infants. *J Pediatr.* 1985;107:786–790
33. Gourley GR, Kreamer B, Arend R. The effect of diet on feces and jaundice during the first three weeks of life. *Gastroenterology.* 1992;103:660–667
34. Maisels MJ, Gifford K. Breast-feeding, weight loss, and jaundice. *J Pediatr.* 1983;102:117–118
35. Laing IA, Wong CM. Hypernatraemia in the first few days: is the incidence rising? *Arch Dis Child Fetal Neonatal Ed.* 2002;87:F158–F162
36. Lawrence RA. Management of the mother-infant nursing couple. In: *A Breastfeeding Guide for the Medical Profession.* 4th ed. St Louis, MO: Mosby-Year Book, Inc; 1994:215–277
37. Maisels MJ, Newman TB. Predicting hyperbilirubinemia in newborns: the importance of timing. *Pediatrics.* 1999;103:493–495
38. Bhutani VK, Johnson L, Sivieri EM. Predictive ability of a predischarge hour-specific serum bilirubin for subsequent significant hyperbilirubinemia in healthy term and near-term newborns. *Pediatrics.* 1999;103:6–14
39. Beutler E. Glucose-6-phosphate dehydrogenase deficiency. *Blood.* 1994;84:3613–3636
40. Linn S, Schoenbaum SC, Monson RR, Rosner B, Stubblefield PG, Ryan KJ. Epidemiology of neonatal hyperbilirubinemia. *Pediatrics.* 1985;75:770–774
41. Newman TB, Easterling MJ, Goldman ES, Stevenson DK. Laboratory evaluation of jaundiced newborns: frequency, cost and yield. *Am J Dis Child.* 1990;144:364–368
42. Martinez JC, Maisels MJ, Otheguy L, et al. Hyperbilirubinemia in the breast-fed newborn: a controlled trial of four interventions. *Pediatrics.* 1993;91:470–473
43. Maisels MJ. Phototherapy—traditional and nontraditional. *J Perinatol.* 2001;21(suppl 1):S93–S97
44. Brown AK, Kim MH, Wu PY, Bryla DA. Efficacy of phototherapy in prevention and management of neonatal hyperbilirubinemia. *Pediatrics.* 1985;75:393–400

45. Armitage P, Mollison PL. Further analysis of controlled trials of treatment of hemolytic disease of the newborn. *J Obstet Gynaecol Br Emp.* 1953;60:602–605

46. Mollison PL, Walker W. Controlled trials of the treatment of haemolytic disease of the newborn. *Lancet.* 1952;1:429–433

47. Hsia DYY, Allen FH, Gellis SS, Diamond LK. Erythroblastosis fetalis. VIII. Studies of serum bilirubin in relation to kernicterus. *N Engl J Med.* 1952;247:668–671

48. Newman TB, Maisels MJ. Does hyperbilirubinemia damage the brain of healthy full-term infants? *Clin Perinatol.* 1990;17:331–358

49. Ozmert E, Erdem G, Topcu M. Long-term follow-up of indirect hyperbilirubinemia in full-term Turkish infants. *Acta Paediatr.* 1996;85:1440–1444

50. Perlman JM, Rogers B, Burns D. Kernicterus findings at autopsy in 2 sick near-term infants. *Pediatrics.* 1997;99:612–615

51. Gartner LM, Snyder RN, Chabon RS, Bernstein J. Kernicterus: high incidence in premature infants with low serum bilirubin concentration. *Pediatrics.* 1970;45:906–917

52. Watchko JF, Oski FA. Kernicterus in preterm newborns: past, present, and future. *Pediatrics.* 1992;90:707–715

53. Watchko J, Claassen D. Kernicterus in premature infants: current prevalence and relationship to NICHD Phototherapy Study exchange criteria. *Pediatrics.* 1994;93(6 Pt 1):996–999

54. Stern L, Denton RL. Kernicterus in small, premature infants. *Pediatrics.* 1965;35:486–485

55. Turkel SB, Guttenberg ME, Moynes DR, Hodgman JE. Lack of identifiable risk factors for kernicterus. *Pediatrics.* 1980;66:502–506

56. Kim MH, Yoon JJ, Sher J, Brown AK. Lack of predictive indices in kernicterus. A comparison of clinical and pathologic factors in infants with or without kernicterus. *Pediatrics.* 1980;66:852–858

57. Newman TB, Xiong B, Gonzales VM, Escobar GJ. Prediction and prevention of extreme neonatal hyperbilirubinemia in a mature health maintenance organization. *Arch Pediatr Adolesc Med.* 2000;154:1140–1147

58. Newman TB, Escobar GJ, Gonzales VM, Armstrong MA, Gardner MN, Folck BF. Frequency of neonatal bilirubin testing and hyperbilirubinemia in a large health maintenance organization. *Pediatrics.* 1999;104:1198–1203

59. Vohr BR. New approaches to assessing the risks of hyperbilirubinemia. *Clin Perinatol.* 1990;17:293–306

60. Perlman M, Fainmesser P, Sohmer H, Tamari H, Wax Y, Pevsmer B. Auditory nerve-brainstem evoked responses in hyperbilirubinemic neonates. *Pediatrics.* 1983;72:658–664

61. Nakamura H, Takada S, Shimabuku R, Matsuo M, Matsuo T, Negishi H. Auditory and brainstem responses in newborn infants with hyperbilirubinemia. *Pediatrics.* 1985;75:703–708

62. Nwaesei CG, Van Aerde J, Boyden M, Perlman M. Changes in auditory brainstem responses in hyperbilirubinemic infants before and after exchange transfusion. *Pediatrics.* 1984;74:800–803

63. Wennberg RP, Ahlfors CE, Bickers R, McMurtry CA, Shetter JL. Abnormal auditory brainstem response in a newborn infant with hyperbilirubinemia: improvement with exchange transfusion. *J Pediatr.* 1982;100:624–626

64. Soorani-Lunsing I, Woltil H, Hadders-Algra M. Are moderate degrees of hyperbilirubinemia in healthy term neonates really safe for the brain? *Pediatr Res.* 2001;50:701–705

65. Grimmer I, Berger-Jones K, Buhrer C, Brandl U, Obladen M. Late neurological sequelae of non-hemolytic hyperbilirubinemia of healthy term neonates. *Acta Paediatr.* 1999;88:661–663

66. Seidman DS, Paz I, Stevenson DK, Laor A, Danon YL, Gale R. Neonatal hyperbilirubinemia and physical and cognitive performance at 17 years of age. *Pediatrics.* 1991;88:828–833

67. Newman TB, Klebanoff MA. Neonatal hyperbilirubinemia and long-term outcome: another look at the collaborative perinatal project. *Pediatrics.* 1993;92:651–657

68. Scheidt PC, Bryla DA, Nelson KB, Hirtz DG, Hoffman HJ. Phototherapy for neonatal hyperbilirubinemia: six-year follow-up of the National Institute of Child Health and Human Development clinical trial. *Pediatrics.* 1990;85:455–463

69. Scheidt PC, Graubard BI, Nelson KB, et al. Intelligence at six years in relation to neonatal bilirubin levels: follow-up of the National Institute of Child Health and Human Development Clinical Trial of Phototherapy. *Pediatrics.* 1991;87:797–805

70. Seidman DS, Paz I, Stevenson DK, Laor A, Danon YL, Gale R. Effect of phototherapy for neonatal jaundice on cognitive performance. *J Perinatol.* 1994;14:23–28

71. Keenan WJ, Novak KK, Sutherland JM, Bryla DA, Fetterly KL. Morbidity and mortality associated with exchange transfusion. *Pediatrics.* 1985;75:417–421

72. Hovi L, Siimes MA. Exchange transfusion with fresh heparinized blood is a safe procedure: Experiences from 1069 newborns. *Acta Paediatr Scand.* 1985;74:360–365

73. Jackson JC. Adverse events associated with exchange transfusion in healthy and ill newborns. *Pediatrics.* 1997;99(5):e7. Available at: www.pediatrics.org/cgi/content/full/99/5/e7

74. Schreiber GB, Busch MP, Kleinman SH, Korelitz JJ. The risk of transfusion-transmitted viral infections. *N Engl J Med.* 1996;334:1685–1690

75. Maisels MJ, Newman TB. Kernicterus in otherwise healthy, breast-fed term newborns. *Pediatrics.* 1995;96:730–733

76. Bratlid D. How bilirubin gets into the brain. *Clin Perinatol.* 1990;17:449–465

77. Cashore WJ, Oh W. Unbound bilirubin and kernicterus in low-birth-weight infants. *Pediatrics.* 1982;69:481–485

78. Nakamura H, Yonetani M, Uetani Y, Funato M, Lee Y. Determination of serum unbound bilirubin for prediction of kernicterus in low birth-weight infants. *Acta Paediatr Jpn.* 1992;34:642–647

79. Funato M, Tamai H, Shimada S, Nakamura H. Vigintiphobia, unbound bilirubin, and auditory brainstem responses. *Pediatrics.* 1994;93:50–53

80. Amin SB, Ahlfors CE, Orlando MS, Dalzell LE, Merle KS, Guillet R. Bilirubin and serial auditory brainstem responses in premature infants. *Pediatrics.* 2001;107:664–670

81. Johnson L, Boggs TR. Bilirubin-dependent brain damage: incidence and indications for treatment. In: Odell GB, Schaffer R, Simopoulos AP, eds. *Phototherapy in the Newborn: An Overview.* Washington, DC: National Academy of Sciences; 1974:122–149

82. Odell GB, Storey GNB, Rosenberg LA. Studies in kernicterus. 3. The saturation of serum proteins with bilirubin during neonatal life and its relationship to brain damage at five years. *J Pediatr.* 1970;76:12–21

83. Ahlfors CE. Criteria for exchange transfusion in jaundiced newborns. *Pediatrics.* 1994;93:488–494

84. Cashore WJ. Free bilirubin concentrations and bilirubin-binding affinity in term and preterm infants. *J Pediatr.* 1980;96:521–527

85. Ebbesen F, Brodersen R. Risk of bilirubin acid precipitation in preterm infants with respiratory distress syndrome: considerations of blood/brain bilirubin transfer equilibrium. *Early Hum Dev.* 1982;6:341–355

86. Cashore WJ, Oh W, Brodersen R. Reserve albumin and bilirubin toxicity index in infant serum. *Acta Paediatr Scand.* 1983;72:415–419

87. Ebbesen F, Nyboe J. Postnatal changes in the ability of plasma albumin to bind bilirubin. *Acta Paediatr Scand.* 1983;72:665–670

88. Esbjorner E. Albumin binding properties in relation to bilirubin and albumin concentrations during the first week of life. *Acta Paediatr Scand.* 1991;80:400–405

89. Robertson A, Sharp C, Karp W. The relationship of gestational age to reserve albumin concentration for binding of bilirubin. *J Perinatol.* 1988;8:17–18

90. Wennberg RP. Cellular basis of bilirubin toxicity. *N Y State J Med.* 1991;91:493–496

APPENDIX 2: Phototherapy

There is no standardized method for delivering phototherapy. Phototherapy units vary widely, as do the types of lamps used in the units. The efficacy of phototherapy depends on the dose of phototherapy administered as well as a number of clinical factors (Table 5).[1]

Measuring the Dose of Phototherapy

Table 5 shows the radiometric quantities used in measuring the phototherapy dose. The quantity most commonly reported in the literature is the spectral irradiance. In the nursery, spectral irradiance can be measured by using commercially available radiometers. These instruments take a single measurement across a band of wavelengths, typically 425 to 475 or 400 to 480 nm. Unfortunately, there is no standardized method for reporting phototherapy dosages in the clinical literature, so it is difficult to compare published studies on the efficacy of phototherapy and manufacturers' data for the irradiance produced by different systems.[2] Measurements of irradiance from the same system, using different radiometers,

TABLE 5.   Factors That Affect the Dose and Efficacy of Phototherapy

Factor	Mechanism/Clinical Relevance	Implementation and Rationale	Clinical Application
Spectrum of light emitted	Blue-green spectrum is most effective. At these wavelengths, light penetrates skin well and is absorbed maximally by bilirubin.	Special blue fluorescent tubes or other light sources that have most output in the blue-green spectrum and are most effective in lowering TSB.	Use special blue tubes or LED light source with output in blue-green spectrum for intensive PT.
Spectral irradiance (irradiance in certain wavelength band) delivered to surface of infant	↑ irradiance → ↑ rate of decline in TSB	Irradiance is measured with a radiometer as $\mu W/cm^2$ per nm. Standard PT units deliver 8–10 $\mu W/cm^2$ per nm (Fig 6). Intensive PT requires >30 $\mu W/cm^2$ per nm.	If special blue fluorescent tubes are used, bring tubes as close to infant as possible to increase irradiance (Fig 6). Note: This cannot be done with halogen lamps because of the danger of burn. Special blue tubes 10–15 cm above the infant will produce an irradiance of at least 35 $\mu W/cm^2$ per nm.
Spectral power (average spectral irradiance across surface area)	↑ surface area exposed → ↑ rate of decline in TSB	For intensive PT, expose maximum surface area of infant to PT.	Place lights above and fiber-optic pad or special blue fluorescent tubes* below the infant. For maximum exposure, line sides of bassinet, warmer bed, or incubator with aluminum foil.
Cause of jaundice	PT is likely to be less effective if jaundice is due to hemolysis or if cholestasis is present. (↑ direct bilirubin)		When hemolysis is present, start PT at lower TSB levels. Use intensive PT. Failure of PT suggests that hemolysis is the cause of jaundice. If ↑ direct bilirubin, watch for bronze baby syndrome or blistering.
TSB level at start of PT	The higher the TSB, the more rapid the decline in TSB with PT.		Use intensive PT for higher TSB levels. Anticipate a more rapid decrease in TSB when TSB >20 mg/dL (342 $\mu mol/L$).

PT indicates phototherapy; LED, light-emitting diode.
* Available in the Olympic BiliBassinet (Olympic Medical, Seattle, WA).

can also produce significantly different results. The width of the phototherapy lamp's emissions spectrum (narrow versus broad) will affect the measured irradiance. Measurements under lights with a very focused emission spectrum (eg, blue light-emitting diode) will vary significantly from one radiometer to another, because the response spectra of the radiometers vary from manufacturer to manufacturer. Broader-spectrum lights (fluorescent and halogen) have fewer variations among radiometers. Manufacturers of phototherapy systems generally recommend the specific radiometer to be used in measuring the dose of phototherapy when their system is used.

It is important also to recognize that the measured irradiance will vary widely depending on where the measurement is taken. Irradiance measured below the center of the light source can be more than double that measured at the periphery, and this dropoff at the periphery will vary with different phototherapy units. Ideally, irradiance should be measured at multiple sites under the area illuminated by the unit and the measurements averaged. The International Electrotechnical Commission[3] defines the "effective surface area" as the intended treatment surface that is illuminated by the phototherapy light. The commission uses 60 × 30 cm as the standard-sized surface.

Is It Necessary to Measure Phototherapy Doses Routinely?

Although it is not necessary to measure spectral irradiance before each use of phototherapy, it is important to perform periodic checks of phototherapy units to make sure that an adequate irradiance is being delivered.

The Dose-Response Relationship of Phototherapy

Figure 5 shows that there is a direct relationship between the irradiance used and the rate at which the serum bilirubin declines under phototherapy.[4] The data in Fig 5 suggest that there is a saturation point beyond which an increase in the irradiance produces no added efficacy. We do not know, however, that a saturation point exists. Because the conversion of bilirubin to excretable photoproducts is partly irreversible and follows first-order kinetics, there may not be a saturation point, so we do not know the maximum effective dose of phototherapy.

Effect on Irradiance of the Light Spectrum and the Distance Between the Infant and the Light Source

Figure 6 shows that as the distance between the light source and the infant decreases, there is a corresponding increase in the spectral irradiance.[5] Fig 6 also demonstrates the dramatic difference in irradi-

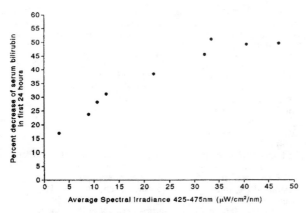

Fig 5. Relationship between average spectral irradiance and decrease in serum bilirubin concentration. Term infants with nonhemolytic hyperbilirubinemia were exposed to special blue lights (Phillips TL 52/20W) of different intensities. Spectral irradiance was measured as the average of readings at the head, trunk, and knees. Drawn from the data of Tan.[4] Source: *Pediatrics*. 1996;98:283-287.

ance produced within the important 425- to 475-nm band by different types of fluorescent tubes.

What is Intensive Phototherapy?

Intensive phototherapy implies the use of high levels of irradiance in the 430- to 490-nm band (usually 30 μW/cm² per nm or higher) delivered to as much of the infant's surface area as possible. How this can be achieved is described below.

Using Phototherapy Effectively

Light Source

The spectrum of light delivered by a phototherapy unit is determined by the type of light source and

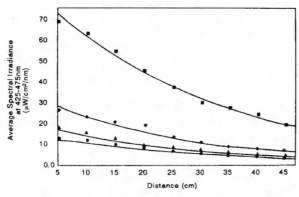

Fig 6. Effect of light source and distance from the light source to the infant on average spectral irradiance. Measurements were made across the 425- to 475-nm band by using a commercial radiometer (Olympic Bilimeter Mark II) and are the average of measurements taken at different locations at each distance (irradiance at the center of the light is much higher than at the periphery). The phototherapy unit was fitted with eight 24-in fluorescent tubes. ■ indicates special blue, General Electric 20-W F20T12/BB tube; ◆, blue, General Electric 20-W F20T12/B tube; ▲, daylight blue, 4 General Electric 20-W F20T12/B blue tubes and 4 Sylvania 20-W F20T12/D daylight tubes; ●, daylight, Sylvania 20-W F20T12/D daylight tube. Curves were plotted by using linear curve fitting (True Epistat, Epistat Services, Richardson, TX). The best fit is described by the equation $y = Ae^{Bx}$. Source: *Pediatrics*. 1996;98:283-287.

any filters used. Commonly used phototherapy units contain daylight, cool white, blue, or "special blue" fluorescent tubes. Other units use tungsten-halogen lamps in different configurations, either free-standing or as part of a radiant warming device. Recently, a system using high-intensity gallium nitride light-emitting diodes has been introduced.[6] Fiber-optic systems deliver light from a high-intensity lamp to a fiber-optic blanket. Most of these devices deliver enough output in the blue-green region of the visible spectrum to be effective for standard phototherapy use. However, when bilirubin levels approach the range at which intensive phototherapy is recommended, maximal efficiency must be sought. The most effective light sources currently commercially available for phototherapy are those that use special blue fluorescent tubes[7] or a specially designed light-emitting diode light (Natus Inc, San Carlos, CA).[6] The special blue fluorescent tubes are labeled F20T12/BB (General Electric, Westinghouse, Sylvania) or TL52/20W (Phillips, Eindhoven, The Netherlands). It is important to note that special blue tubes provide much greater irradiance than regular blue tubes (labeled F20T12/B) (Fig 6). Special blue tubes are most effective because they provide light predominantly in the blue-green spectrum. At these wavelengths, light penetrates skin well and is absorbed maximally by bilirubin.[7]

There is a common misconception that ultraviolet light is used for phototherapy. The light systems used do not emit significant ultraviolet radiation, and the small amount of ultraviolet light that is emitted by fluorescent tubes and halogen bulbs is in longer wavelengths than those that cause erythema. In addition, almost all ultraviolet light is absorbed by the glass wall of the fluorescent tube and the Plexiglas cover of the phototherapy unit.

Distance From the Light

As can be seen in Fig 6, the distance of the light source from the infant has a dramatic effect on the spectral irradiance, and this effect is most significant when special blue tubes are used. To take advantage of this effect, the fluorescent tubes should be placed as close to the infant as possible. To do this, the infant should be in a bassinet, not an incubator, because the top of the incubator prevents the light from being brought sufficiently close to the infant. In a bassinet, it is possible to bring the fluorescent tubes within approximately 10 cm of the infant. Naked term infants do not become overheated under these lights. It is important to note, however, that the halogen spot phototherapy lamps cannot be positioned closer to the infant than recommended by the manufacturers without incurring the risk of a burn. When halogen lamps are used, manufacturers recommendations should be followed. The reflectors, light source, and transparent light filters (if any) should be kept clean.

Surface Area

A number of systems have been developed to provide phototherapy above and below the infant.[8,9] One commercially available system that does this is the BiliBassinet (Olympic Medical, Seattle, WA). This unit provides special blue fluorescent tubes above and below the infant. An alternative is to place fiber-optic pads below an infant with phototherapy lamps above. One disadvantage of fiber-optic pads is that they cover a relatively small surface area so that 2 or 3 pads may be needed.[5] When bilirubin levels are extremely high and must be lowered as rapidly as possible, it is essential to expose as much of the infant's surface area to phototherapy as possible. In these situations, additional surface-area exposure can be achieved by lining the sides of the bassinet with aluminum foil or a white cloth.[10]

In most circumstances, it is not necessary to remove the infant's diaper, but when bilirubin levels approach the exchange transfusion range, the diaper should be removed until there is clear evidence of a significant decline in the bilirubin level.

What Decline in the Serum Bilirubin Can You Expect?

The rate at which the bilirubin declines depends on the factors listed in Table 5, and different responses can be expected depending on the clinical circumstances. When bilirubin levels are extremely high (more than 30 mg/dL [513 μmol/L]), and intensive phototherapy is used, a decline of as much as 10 mg/dL (171 μmol/L) can occur within a few hours,[11] and a decrease of at least 0.5 to 1 mg/dL per hour can be expected in the first 4 to 8 hours.[12] On average, for infants of more than 35 weeks' gestation readmitted for phototherapy, intensive phototherapy can produce a decrement of 30% to 40% in the initial bilirubin level by 24 hours after initiation of phototherapy.[13] The most significant decline will occur in the first 4 to 6 hours. With standard phototherapy systems, a decrease of 6% to 20% of the initial bilirubin level can be expected in the first 24 hours.[8,14]

Intermittent Versus Continuous Phototherapy

Clinical studies comparing intermittent with continuous phototherapy have produced conflicting results.[15–17] Because all light exposure increases bilirubin excretion (compared with darkness), no plausible scientific rationale exists for using intermittent phototherapy. In most circumstances, however, phototherapy does not need to be continuous. Phototherapy may be interrupted during feeding or brief parental visits. Individual judgment should be exercised. If the infant's bilirubin level is approaching the exchange transfusion zone (Fig 4), phototherapy should be administered continuously until a satisfactory decline in the serum bilirubin level occurs or exchange transfusion is initiated.

Hydration

There is no evidence that excessive fluid administration affects the serum bilirubin concentration. Some infants who are admitted with high bilirubin levels are also mildly dehydrated and may need supplemental fluid intake to correct their dehydration. Because these infants are almost always breast-fed, the best fluid to use in these circumstances is a milk-based formula, because it inhibits the enterohepatic circulation of bilirubin and should help to lower the serum bilirubin level. Because the photo-

products responsible for the decline in serum bilirubin are excreted in urine and bile,[18] maintaining adequate hydration and good urine output should help to improve the efficacy of phototherapy. Unless there is evidence of dehydration, however, routine intravenous fluid or other supplementation (eg, with dextrose water) of term and near-term infants receiving phototherapy is not necessary.

When Should Phototherapy Be Stopped?

There is no standard for discontinuing phototherapy. The TSB level for discontinuing phototherapy depends on the age at which phototherapy is initiated and the cause of the hyperbilirubinemia.[13] For infants who are readmitted after their birth hospitalization (usually for TSB levels of 18 mg/dL [308 μmol/L] or higher), phototherapy may be discontinued when the serum bilirubin level falls below 13 to 14 mg/dL (239-239 μmol/L). Discharge from the hospital need not be delayed to observe the infant for rebound.[13,19,20] If phototherapy is used for infants with hemolytic diseases or is initiated early and discontinued before the infant is 3 to 4 days old, a follow-up bilirubin measurement within 24 hours after discharge is recommended.[13] For infants who are readmitted with hyperbilirubinemia and then discharged, significant rebound is rare, but a repeat TSB measurement or clinical follow-up 24 hours after discharge is a clinical option.[13]

Home Phototherapy

Because the devices available for home phototherapy may not provide the same degree of irradiance or surface-area exposure as those available in the hospital, home phototherapy should be used only in infants whose bilirubin levels are in the "optional phototherapy" range (Fig 3); it is not appropriate for infants with higher bilirubin concentrations. As with hospitalized infants, it is essential that serum bilirubin levels be monitored regularly.

Sunlight Exposure

In their original description of phototherapy, Cremer et al[21] demonstrated that exposure of newborns to sunlight would lower the serum bilirubin level. Although sunlight provides sufficient irradiance in the 425- to 475-nm band to provide phototherapy, the practical difficulties involved in safely exposing a naked newborn to the sun either inside or outside (and avoiding sunburn) preclude the use of sunlight as a reliable therapeutic tool, and it therefore is not recommended.

Complications

Phototherapy has been used in millions of infants for more than 30 years, and reports of significant toxicity are exceptionally rare. Nevertheless, phototherapy in hospital separates mother and infant, and eye patching is disturbing to parents. The most important, but uncommon, clinical complication occurs in infants with cholestatic jaundice. When these infants are exposed to phototherapy, they may develop a dark, grayish-brown discoloration of the skin, serum, and urine (the bronze infant syndrome).[22] The pathogenesis of this syndrome is unknown, but it may be related to an accumulation of porphyrins and other metabolites in the plasma of infants who develop cholestasis.[22,23] Although it occurs exclusively in infants with cholestasis, not all infants with cholestatic jaundice develop the syndrome.

This syndrome generally has had few deleterious consequences, and if there is a need for phototherapy, the presence of direct hyperbilirubinemia should not be considered a contraindication to its use. This is particularly important in sick neonates. Because the products of phototherapy are excreted in the bile, the presence of cholestasis will decrease the efficacy of phototherapy. Nevertheless, infants with direct hyperbilirubinemia often show some response to phototherapy. In infants receiving phototherapy who develop the bronze infant syndrome, exchange transfusion should be considered if the TSB is in the intensive phototherapy range and phototherapy does not promptly lower the TSB. Because of the paucity of data, firm recommendations cannot be made. Note, however, that the direct serum bilirubin should not be subtracted from the TSB concentration in making decisions about exchange transfusions (see Fig 4).

Rarely, purpura and bullous eruptions have been described in infants with severe cholestatic jaundice receiving phototherapy,[24,25] and severe blistering and photosensitivity during phototherapy have occurred in infants with congenital erythropoietic porphyria.[26,27] Congenital porphyria or a family history of porphyria is an absolute contraindication to the use of phototherapy, as is the concomitant use of drugs or agents that are photosensitizers.[28]

REFERENCES

1. Maisels MJ. Phototherapy—traditional and nontraditional. *J Perinatol.* 2001;21(suppl 1):S93–S97
2. Fiberoptic phototherapy systems. *Health Devices.* 1995;24:132–153
3. International Electrotechnical Commission. Medical electrical equipment—part 2-50: particular requirements for the safety of infant phototherapy equipment. 2000. IEC 60601-2-50. Available at www.iec.ch. Accessed June 7, 2004
4. Tan KL. The pattern of bilirubin response to phototherapy for neonatal hyperbilirubinemia. *Pediatr Res.* 1982;16:670–674
5. Maisels MJ. Why use homeopathic doses of phototherapy? *Pediatrics.* 1996;98:283–287
6. Seidman DS, Moise J, Ergaz Z, et al. A new blue light-emitting phototherapy device: a prospective randomized controlled study. *J Pediatr.* 2000;136:771–774
7. Ennever JF. Blue light, green light, white light, more light: treatment of neonatal jaundice. *Clin Perinatol.* 1990;17:467–481
8. Garg AK, Prasad RS, Hifzi IA. A controlled trial of high-intensity double-surface phototherapy on a fluid bed versus conventional phototherapy in neonatal jaundice. *Pediatrics.* 1995;95:914–916
9. Tan KL. Phototherapy for neonatal jaundice. *Clin Perinatol.* 1991;18: 423–439
10. Eggert P, Stick C, Schroder H. On the distribution of irradiation intensity in phototherapy. Measurements of effective irradiance in an incubator. *Eur J Pediatr.* 1984;142:58–61
11. Hansen TW. Acute management of extreme neonatal jaundice—the potential benefits of intensified phototherapy and interruption of enterohepatic bilirubin circulation. *Acta Paediatr.* 1997;86:843–846
12. Newman TB, Liljestrand P, Escobar GJ. Infants with bilirubin levels of 30 mg/dL or more in a large managed care organization. *Pediatrics.* 2003;111(6 Pt 1):1303–1311
13. Maisels MJ, Kring E. Bilirubin rebound following intensive phototherapy. *Arch Pediatr Adolesc Med.* 2002;156:669–672
14. Tan KL. Comparison of the efficacy of fiberoptic and conventional phototherapy for neonatal hyperbilirubinemia. *J Pediatr.* 1994;125: 607–612
15. Rubaltelli FF, Zanardo V, Granati B. Effect of various phototherapy regimens on bilirubin decrement. *Pediatrics.* 1978;61:838–841
16. Maurer HM, Shumway CN, Draper DA, Hossaini AA. Controlled trial comparing agar, intermittent phototherapy, and continuous phototherapy for reducing neonatal hyperbilirubinemia. *J Pediatr.* 1973;82:73–76
17. Lau SP, Fung KP. Serum bilirubin kinetics in intermittent phototherapy of physiological jaundice. *Arch Dis Child.* 1984;59:892–894
18. McDonagh AF, Lightner DA. 'Like a shrivelled blood orange'—bilirubin, jaundice, and phototherapy. *Pediatrics.* 1985;75:443–455
19. Yetman RJ, Parks DK, Huseby V, Mistry K, Garcia J. Rebound bilirubin levels in infants receiving phototherapy. *J Pediatr.* 1998;133:705–707
20. Lazar L, Litwin A, Merlob P. Phototherapy for neonatal nonhemolytic hyperbilirubinemia. Analysis of rebound and indications for discontinuing therapy. *Clin Pediatr (Phila).* 1993;32:264–267
21. Cremer RJ, Perryman PW, Richards DH. Influence of light on the hyperbilirubinemia of infants. *Lancet.* 1958;1(7030):1094–1097
22. Rubaltelli FF, Jori G, Reddi E. Bronze baby syndrome: a new porphyrin-related disorder. *Pediatr Res.* 1983;17:327–330
23. Meisel P, Jahrig D, Theel L, Ordt A, Jahrig K. The bronze baby syndrome: consequence of impaired excretion of photobilirubin? *Photobiochem Photobiophys.* 1982;3:345–352
24. Mallon E, Wojnarowska F, Hope P, Elder G. Neonatal bullous eruption as a result of transient porphyrinemia in a premature infant with hemolytic disease of the newborn. *J Am Acad Dermatol.* 1995;33:333–336
25. Paller AS, Eramo LR, Farrell EE, Millard DD, Honig PJ, Cunningham BB. Purpuric phototherapy-induced eruption in transfused neonates: relation to transient porphyrinemia. *Pediatrics.* 1997;100:360–364
26. Tonz O, Vogt J, Filippini L, Simmler F, Wachsmuth ED, Winterhalter KH. Severe light dermatosis following phototherapy in a newborn infant with congenital erythropoietic urophyria [in German]. *Helv Paediatr Acta.* 1975;30:47–56
27. Soylu A, Kavukcu S, Turkmen M. Phototherapy sequela in a child with congenital erythropoietic porphyria. *Eur J Pediatr.* 1999;158:526–527
28. Kearns GL, Williams BJ, Timmons OD. Fluorescein phototoxicity in a premature infant. *J Pediatr.* 1985;107:796–798

All clinical practice guidelines from the American Academy of Pediatrics automatically expire 5 years after publication unless reaffirmed, revised, or retired at or before that time.

ERRATUM

Two errors appeared in the American Academy of Pediatrics clinical practice guideline, titled "Management of Hyperbilirubinemia in the Newborn Infant 35 or More Weeks of Gestation," that was published in the July 2004 issue of *Pediatrics* (2004;114:297–316). On page 107, Background section, first paragraph, the second sentence should read: "The current guideline represents a consensus of the committee charged by the AAP with reviewing and updating the existing guideline and is based on a careful review of the evidence, including a comprehensive literature review by the Agency for Healthcare Research and Quality and the New England Medical Center Evidence-Based Practice Center.[2]" On page 118, Appendix 1, first paragraph, the 4 levels of evidence quality should have been labeled A, B, C, and D rather than 1, 2, 3, and 4, respectively. The American Academy of Pediatrics regrets these errors.

Technical Report Summary:
An Evidence-Based Review of Important Issues Concerning Neonatal Hyperbilirubinemia

Authors:

Stanley Ip, MD; Mei Chung, MPH; John Kulig, MD, MPH; Rebecca O'Brien, MD; Robert Sege, MD, PhD; Stephan Glicken, MD; M. Jeffrey Maisels, MB, BCh; and Joseph Lau, MD, and the Subcommittee on Hyperbilirubinemia

American Academy of Pediatrics
PO Box 927, 141 Northwest Point Blvd
Elk Grove Village, IL 60009-0927

For the complete technical report, including tables, figures, and references, please see the companion CD-ROM

ABSTRACT. This article is adapted from a published evidence report concerning neonatal hyperbilirubinemia with an added section on the risk of blood exchange transfusion (BET). Based on a summary of multiple case reports that spanned more than 30 years, we conclude that kernicterus, although infrequent, has at least 10% mortality and at least 70% long-term morbidity. It is evident that the preponderance of kernicterus cases occurred in infants with a bilirubin level higher than 20 mg/dL. Given the diversity of conclusions on the relationship between peak bilirubin levels and behavioral and neurodevelopmental outcomes, it is apparent that the use of a single total serum bilirubin level to predict long-term outcomes is inadequate and will lead to conflicting results. Evidence for efficacy of treatments for neonatal hyperbilirubinemia was limited. Overall, the 4 qualifying studies showed that phototherapy had an absolute risk-reduction rate of 10% to 17% for prevention of serum bilirubin levels higher than 20 mg/dL in healthy infants with jaundice. There is no evidence to suggest that phototherapy for neonatal hyperbilirubinemia has any long-term adverse neurodevelopmental effects. Transcutaneous measurements of bilirubin have a linear correlation to total serum bilirubin and may be useful as screening devices to detect clinically significant jaundice and decrease the need for serum bilirubin determinations. Based on our review of the risks associated with BETs from 15 studies consisting mainly of infants born before 1970, we conclude that the mortality within 6 hours of BET ranged from 3 per 1000 to 4 per 1000 exchanged infants who were term and without serious hemolytic diseases. Regardless of the definitions and rates of BET-associated morbidity and the various pre-ex-change clinical states of the exchanged infants, in many cases the morbidity was minor (eg, postexchange anemia). Based on the results from the most recent study to report BET morbidity, the overall risk of permanent sequelae in 25 sick infants who survived BET was from 5% to 10%.

The American Academy of Pediatrics (AAP) requested an evidence report from the Agency for Healthcare Research and Quality (AHRQ) that would critically examine the available evidence regarding the effect of high levels of bilirubin on behavioral and neurodevelopmental outcomes, role of various comorbid effect modifiers (eg, sepsis and hemolysis) on neurodevelopment, efficacy of phototherapy, reliability of various strategies in predicting significant hyperbilirubinemia, and accuracy of transcutaneous bilirubin (TcB) measurements. The report was used by the AAP to update the 1994 AAP guidelines for the management of neonatal hyperbilirubinemia. This review focuses on otherwise healthy term or near-term (at least 34 weeks' estimated gestational age [EGA] or at least 2500 g birth weight) infants with hyperbilirubinemia. This article is adapted from that published report with an added section on the risk of blood exchange transfusion (BET).

Neither hyperbilirubinemia nor kernicterus are reportable diseases, and there are no reliable sources of information providing national annual estimates. Since the advent of effective prevention of rhesus (Rh) incompatibility and treatment of elevated bilirubin levels with phototherapy, kernicterus has become uncommon. When laboratory records of a 1995–1996 birth cohort of more than 50 000 California infants were examined, Newman et al reported that 2% had total serum bilirubin (TSB) levels higher than 20 mg/dL, 0.15% had levels higher than 25 mg/dL, and only 0.01% had levels higher than 30 mg/dL. (These data were from infants with clinically identified hyperbilirubinemia and, as such, represent a minimum estimate of the true incidence of extreme hyperbilirubinemia.) This is undoubtedly the result of successful prevention of hemolytic anemia and the application of effective treatment of elevated serum bilirubin levels in accordance with currently accepted medical practice. Projecting the California estimates to the national birth rate of 4 million per year, one can predict 80 000, 6000, and 400 newborns per year with bilirubin levels of more than 20, 25, and 30 mg/dL, respectively.

Recently, concern has been expressed that the increase in early hospital discharges, coupled with a rise in breast-feeding rates, has led to a rise in the rate of preventable kernicterus resulting from "unattended to" hyperbilirubinemia. However, a report published in 2002, based on a national registry established since 1992, reported only 90 cases of kernicterus, although the efficiency of case ascertainment is not clear. Thus, there are no data to establish incidence trends reliably for either hyperbilirubinemia or kernicterus.

Despite these constraints, there has been substantial research on the neurodevelopmental outcomes of hyperbilirubinemia and its prediction and treatment. Subsequent sections of this review describe in more detail the precise study questions and the existing published work in this area.

METHODOLOGY

This evidence report is based on a systematic review of the medical literature. Our Evidence-Based Practice Center formed a review team consisting of pediatricians and Evidence-Based Practice Center methodologic staff to review the literature and perform data abstraction and analysis. For details regarding methodology, please see the original AHRQ report.

Key Questions

Question 1: What is the relationship between peak bilirubin levels and/or duration of hyperbilirubinemia and neurodevelopmental outcome?

Question 2: What is the evidence for effect modification of the results in question 1 by GA, hemolysis, serum albumin, and other factors?

Question 3: What are the quantitative estimates of efficacy of treatment for 1) reducing peak bilirubin levels (eg, number needed to treat [NNT] at 20 mg/dL to keep TSB from rising); 2) reducing the duration of hyperbilirubinemia (eg, average number of hours by which time TSB is higher than 20 mg/dL may be shortened by treatment); and 3) improving neurodevelopmental outcomes?

Question 4: What is the efficacy of various strategies for predicting hyperbilirubinemia, including hour-specific bilirubin percentiles?

Question 5: What is the accuracy of TcB measurements?

Search Strategies

We searched the Medline database on September 25, 2001, for publications from 1966 to the present using relevant medical subject heading terms ("hyperbilirubinemia"; "hyperbilirubinemia, hereditary"; "bilirubin"; "jaundice, neonatal"; and "kernicterus") and text words ("bilirubin," "hyperbilirubinemia," "jaundice," "kernicterus," and "neonatal"). The abstracts were limited to human subjects and English-language studies focusing on newborns between birth and 1 month of age. In addition, the same text words used for the Medline search were used to search the Pre-Medline database. The strategy yielded 4280 Medline and 45 PreMedline abstracts. We consulted domain experts and examined relevant review articles for additional studies. A supplemental search for case reports of kernicterus in reference lists of relevant articles and reviews was performed also.

Screening and Selection Process

In our preliminary screening of abstracts, we identified more than 600 potentially relevant articles in total for questions 1, 2, and 3. To handle this large number of articles, we devised the following scheme to address the key questions and ensure that the report was completed within the time and resource constraints. We included only studies that measured neurodevelopmental or behavioral outcomes (except for question 3, part 1, for which we evaluated all studies addressing the efficacy of treatment). For the specific question of quantitative estimates of efficacy of treatment, all studies concerning therapies designed to prevent hyperbilirubinemia (generally bilirubin greater than or equal to 20 mg/dL) were included in the review.

Inclusion Criteria

The target population of this review was healthy, term infants. For the purpose of this review, we included articles concerning infants who were at least 34 weeks' EGA at the time of birth. From studies that reported birth weight rather than age, infants whose birth weight was greater than or equal to 2500 g were included. This cutoff was derived from findings of the National Institute of Child Health and Human Development (NICHD) hyperbilirubinemia study, in which none of the 1339 infants weighing greater than or equal to 2500 g were less than 34 weeks' EGA. Articles were selected for inclusion in the systematic review based on the following additional criteria:

Question 1 or 2 (Risk Association)

- Population: infants greater than or equal to 34 weeks' EGA or birth weight greater than or equal to 2500 g.
- Sample size: more than 5 subjects per arm
- Predictors: jaundice or hyperbilirubinemia
- Outcomes: at least 1 behavioral/neurodevelopmental outcome reported in the article
- Study design: prospective cohorts (more than 2 arms), prospective cross-sectional study, prospective longitudinal study, prospective single-arm study, or retrospective cohorts (more than 2 arms)

Case Reports of Kernicterus

- Population: kernicterus case
- Study design: case reports with kernicterus as a predictor or an outcome

Kernicterus, as defined by authors, included any of the following: acute phase of kernicterus (poor feeding, lethargy, high-pitched cry, increased tone, opisthotonos, or seizures), kernicterus sequelae (motor delay, sensorineural hearing loss, gaze palsy, dental dysplasia, cerebral palsy, or mental retardation), necropsy finding of yellow staining in the brain nuclei.

Question 3 (Efficacy of Treatment at Reducing Serum Bilirubin)

- Population: infants greater than or equal to 34 weeks' EGA or birth weight greater than or equal to 2500 g
- Sample size: more than 10 subjects per arm
- Treatments: any treatment for neonatal hyperbilirubinemia
- Outcomes: serum bilirubin level higher than or equal to 20 mg/dL or frequency of BET specifically for bilirubin level higher than or equal to 20 mg/dL
- Study design: randomized or nonrandomized, controlled trials

For All Other Issues

- Population: infants greater than or equal to 34 weeks' EGA or birth weight greater than or equal to 2500 g
- Sample size: more than 10 subjects per arm for phototherapy; any sample size for other treatments
- Treatments: any treatment for neonatal hyperbilirubinemia
- Outcomes: at least 1 neurodevelopmental outcome was reported in the article

Question 4 or 5 (Diagnosis)

- Population: infants greater than or equal to 34 weeks' EGA or birth weight greater than or equal to 2500 g
- Sample size: more than 10 subjects
- Reference standard: laboratory-based TSB

Exclusion Criteria

Case reports of kernicterus were excluded if they did not report serum bilirubin level or GA and birth weight.

Results of Screening of Titles and Abstracts

There were 158, 174, 99, 153, and 79 abstracts for questions 1, 2, 3, 4, and 5, respectively. Some articles were relevant to more than 1 question.

Results of Screening of Full-Text Articles

After full-text screening (according to the inclusion and exclusion criteria described previously), 138 retrieved articles were included in this report. There were 35 articles in the correlation section (questions 1 and 2), 28 articles of kernicterus case reports, 21 articles in the treatment section (question 3), and 54 articles in the diagnosis section (questions 4 and 5). There were inevitable overlaps, because treatment effects and assessment of neurodevelopmental outcomes were inherent in many study designs.

Reporting the Results

Articles that passed the full-text screening were grouped according to topic and analyzed in their entirety. Extracted data were synthesized into evidence tables.

Summarizing the Evidence of Individual Studies

Grading of the evidence can be useful for indicating the overall methodologic quality of a study. The evidence-grading scheme used here assesses 4 dimensions that are important for the proper interpretation of the evidence: study size, applicability, summary of results, and methodologic quality.

Definitions of Terminology

- Confounders (for question 1 only): 1) An ideal study design to answer question 1 would follow 2 groups, jaundiced and normal infants, without treating any infant for a current or consequent jaundice condition and observe their neurodevelopmental outcomes. Therefore, any treatment received by the subjects in the study was defined as a confounder. 2) If subjects had known risk factors for jaundice such as prematurity, breastfeeding, or low birth weight, the risk factors were defined as confounders. 3) Any disease condition other than jaundice was defined as a confounder. 4) Because bilirubin level is the essential predictor, if the study did not report or measure bilirubin levels for the subjects, lack of bilirubin measurements was defined as a confounder.
- Acute phase of kernicterus: poor feeding, lethargy, high-pitched cry, increased tone, opisthotonos, or seizures.
- Chronic kernicterus sequelae: motor delay, sensorineural hearing loss, gaze palsy, dental dysplasia, cerebral palsy, or mental retardation.

Statistical Analyses

In this report, 2 statistical analyses were performed in which there were sufficient data: the NNT and receiver operating characteristics (ROC) curve.

NNT

The NNT can be a clinically meaningful metric to assess the benefits of clinical trials. It is calculated by taking the inverse of the absolute risk difference. The absolute risk difference is the difference between the event rates between the treatment and control groups. For example, if the event rate is 15% in the control group and 10% in the treatment group, the absolute risk difference is 5% (an absolute risk reduction of 5%). The NNT then would be 20 (1 divided by 0.05), meaning that 20 patients will need to be treated to see 1 fewer event. In the setting of neonatal hyperbilirubinemia, NNT might be interpreted as the number of newborns needed to be treated (with phototherapy) at 13 to 15 mg/dL to prevent 1 newborn from reaching 20 mg/dL.

ROC Curve

ROC curves were developed for individual studies in question 4 if multiple thresholds of a diagnostic technology were reported. The areas under the curves (AUCs) were calculated to provide an assessment of the overall accuracy of the tests.

Meta-analyses of Diagnostic Test Performance

Meta-analyses were performed to quantify the TcB measurements for which the data were sufficient. We used 3 complementary methods for assessing diagnostic test performance: summary ROC analysis, independently combined sensitivity and specificity values, and meta-analysis of correlation coefficients.

RESULTS

Question 1. What Is the Relationship Between Peak Bilirubin Levels and/or Duration of Hyperbilirubinemia and Neurodevelopmental Outcome?

The first part of the results for this question deals with kernicterus; the second part deals with otherwise healthy term or near-term infants who had hyperbilirubinemia.

Case Reports of Kernicterus

Our literature search identified 28 case-report articles of infants with kernicterus that reported sufficient data for analysis. (The largest case series of 90 healthy term and near-term infants with kernicterus was reported by Johnson et al in 2002, but no individual data were available and therefore were not included in this analysis. Those cases with available individual data previously reported were included in this analysis.) Most of the articles were identified in Medline and published since 1966. We retrieved additional articles published before 1966 based on review of references in articles published since 1966. Our report focuses on term and near-term infants (greater than or equal to 34 weeks' EGA). Only infants with measured peak bilirubin level and known GA or birth weight or with clinical or autop-sy-diagnosed kernicterus were included in the analysis. It is important to note that some of these peak levels were obtained more than 7 days after birth and therefore may not have represented true peak levels. Similarly, some of the diagnoses of kernicterus were made only at autopsies, and the measured bilirubin levels were obtained more than 24 hours before the infants died, and therefore the reported bilirubin levels may not have reported the true peak levels. Because of the small number of subjects, none of the following comparisons are statistically significant. Furthermore, because case reports in this section represent highly selected cases, interpreting these data must be done cautiously.

Demographics of Kernicterus Cases

Articles identified through the search strategy span from 1955 to 2001 with a total of 123 cases of kernicterus. Twelve cases in 2 studies were reported before 1960; however, some studies reported cases that spanned almost 2 decades. Data on subjects' birth years were reported in only 55 cases. Feeding status, gender, racial background, and ethnicity were not noted in most of the reports. Of those that were reported, almost all the subjects were breastfed and most were males.

Geographic Distribution of Reported Kernicterus Cases

The 28 case reports with a total of 123 cases are from 14 different countries. They are the United States, Singapore, Turkey, Greece, Taiwan, Denmark, Canada, Japan, United Kingdom, France, Jamaica, Norway, Scotland, and Germany. The number of kernicterus cases in each study ranged from 1 to 12.

Kernicterus has been defined by pathologic findings, acute clinical findings, and chronic sequelae (such as deafness or athetoid cerebral palsy). Because of the small number of subjects, all definitions of kernicterus have been included in the analysis. Exceptions will be noted in the following discussion.

Kernicterus Cases With Unknown Etiology

Among infants at greater than or equal to 34 weeks' GA or who weighed 2500 g or more at birth and had no known explanation for kernicterus, there were 35 infants with peak bilirubin ranging from 22.5 to 54 mg/dL. Fifteen had no information on gender, 14 were males, and 6 were females. Fourteen had no information on feeding,

20 were breastfed, and 1 was formula-fed. More than 90% of the infants with kernicterus had bilirubin higher than 25 mg/dL: 25% of the kernicterus cases had peak TSB levels up to 29.9 mg/dL, and 50% had peak TSB levels up to 34.9 mg/dL (Fig 2). There was no association between bilirubin level and birth weight.

Four infants died. Four infants who had acute clinical kernicterus had normal follow-up at 3 to 6 years by telephone. One infant with a peak bilirubin level of 44 mg/dL had a flat brainstem auditory evoked response (BAER) initially but normalized at 2 months of age; this infant had normal neurologic and developmental examinations at 6 months of age. Ten infants had chronic sequelae of kernicterus when followed up between 6 months and 7 years of age. Seven infants were noted to have neurologic findings consistent with kernicterus; however, the age at diagnosis was not provided. Nine infants had a diagnosis of kernicterus with no follow-up information provided. To summarize, 11% of this group of infants died, 14% survived with no sequelae, and at least 46% had chronic sequelae. The distribution of peak TSB levels was higher when only infants who died or had chronic sequelae were included.

Kernicterus Cases With Comorbid Factors

In the 88 term and near-term infants diagnosed with kernicterus and who had hemolysis, sepsis, and other neonatal complications, bilirubin levels ranged from 4.0 to 51.0 mg/dL (as previously mentioned, these may not represent true peak levels; the bilirubin level of 4 mg/dL was measured more than 24 hours before the infant died, the diagnosis of kernicterus was made by autopsy). Forty-two cases provided no information on gender, 25 were males, and 21 were females. Seventy-two cases had no information on feeding, 15 were breastfed, and 1 was formula-fed. Most infants with kernicterus had bilirubin levels higher than 20 mg/dL: 25% of the kernicterus cases had peak TSB levels up to 24.9 mg/dL, and 50% had peak TSB levels up to 29.9 mg/dL (Fig 4). In this group, there was no association between the bilirubin levels and birth weight.

Five infants without clinical signs of kernicterus were diagnosed with kernicterus by autopsy. Eight infants died of kernicterus. One infant was found to have a normal neurologic examination at 4 months of age. Another infant with galactosemia and a bilirubin level of 43.6 mg/dL who had acute kernicterus was normal at 5 months of age. Forty-nine patients had chronic sequelae ranging from hearing loss to athetoid cerebral palsy; the follow-up age reported ranged from 4 months to 14 years. Twenty-one patients were diagnosed with kernicterus, with no follow-up information. Not including the autopsy-diagnosed kernicterus, 10% of these infants died (8/82), 2% were found to be normal at 4 to 5 months of age, and

at least 60% had chronic sequelae. The distribution of peak TSB levels was slightly higher when only infants who died or had chronic sequelae were included.

Evidence Associating Bilirubin Exposures With Neurodevelopmental Outcomes in Healthy Term or Near-Term Infants

This section examines the evidence associating bilirubin exposures with neurodevelopmental outcomes primarily in subjects without kernicterus. Studies that were designed specifically to address the behavioral and neurodevelopmental outcomes in healthy infants at more than or equal to 34 weeks' GA will be discussed first. With the exception of the results from the Collaborative Perinatal Project (CPP) (CPP, with 54 795 subjects, has generated many follow-up studies with a smaller number of subjects, and those studies were discussed together in a separate section in the AHRQ summary report), the remainder of the studies that include mixed subjects (preterm and term, diseased and nondiseased) were categorized and discussed by outcome measures. These measures include behavioral and neurologic outcomes; hearing impairment, including sensorineural hearing loss; and intelligence measurements.

The CPP, with 54 795 live births between 1959 and 1966 from 12 centers in the United States, produced the largest database for the study of hyperbilirubinemia. Newman and Klebanoff, focusing only on black and white infants weighing 2500 g or more at birth, did a comprehensive analysis of 7-year outcome in 33 272 subjects. All causes of jaundice were included in the analysis. The study found no consistent association between peak bilirubin level and intelligence quotient (IQ). Sensorineural hearing loss was not related to bilirubin level. Only the frequency of abnormal or suspicious neurologic examinations was associated with bilirubin level. The specific neurologic examination items most associated with bilirubin levels were mild and nonspecific motor abnormalities.

In other studies stemming from the CPP population, there was no consistent evidence to suggest neurologic abnormalities in children with neonatal bilirubin higher than 20 mg/dL when followed up to 7 years of age.

A question that has concerned pediatricians for many years is whether moderate hyperbilirubinemia is associated with abnormalities in neurodevelopmental outcome in term healthy infants without perinatal or neonatal problems. Only 4 prospective studies and 1 retrospective study have the requisite subject characteristics to address this issue. Although there were some short-term (less than 12 months) abnormal neurologic or behavioral characteristics noted in infants with high bilirubin, the studies had methodologic problems and did not show consistent results.

Evidence Associating Bilirubin Exposures With Neurodevelopmental Outcomes in All Infants

These studies consist of subjects who, in addition to healthy term newborns, might include newborns less than 34 weeks' GA and neonatal complications such as sepsis, respiratory distress, hemolytic disorders, and other factors. Nevertheless, some of the conclusions drawn might be applicable to a healthy term population. In these studies, greater emphasis will be placed on the reported results for the group of infants who were at greater than or equal to 34 weeks' EGA or weighed 2500 g or more at birth.

Studies Measuring Behavioral and Neurologic Outcomes in Infants With Hyperbilirubinemia

A total of 9 studies in 11 publications examined primarily behavioral and neurologic outcomes in patients with hyperbilirubinemia. Of these 9 studies, 3 were of high methodologic quality. One short-term study showed a correlation between bilirubin level and decreased scores on newborn behavioral measurements. One study found no difference in prevalence of central nervous system abnormalities at 4 years old if bilirubin levels were less than 20 mg/dL, but infants with bilirubin levels higher than 20 mg/dL had a higher prevalence of central nervous system abnormalities. Another study that followed infants with bilirubin levels higher than 16 mg/dL found no relationship between bilirubin and neurovisuomotor testing at 61 to 82 months of age. Although data reported in the remainder of the studies are of lower methodologic quality, there is a suggestion of abnormalities in neurodevelopmental screening tests in infants with bilirubin levels higher than 20 mg/dL, at least by the Denver Developmental Screening Test, when infants were followed up at 1 year of age. It seems that bilirubin levels higher than 20 mg/dL may have short-term (up to 1 year of age) adverse effects at least by the Denver Developmental Screening Test, but there is no strong evidence to suggest neurologic abnormalities in children with neonatal bilirubin levels higher than 20 mg/dL when followed up to 7 years of age.

Effect of Bilirubin on Brainstem Auditory Evoked Potential (BAEP)

The following group of studies, in 14 publications, primarily examined the effect of bilirubin on BAEP or hearing impairment. Eight high-quality studies showed a significant relationship between abnormalities in BAEP and high bilirubin levels. Most reported resolution of abnormalities with treatment. Three studies reported hearing impairment associated with elevated bilirubin (higher than 16–20 mg/dL).

Effect of Bilirubin on Intelligence Outcomes

Eight studies looked primarily at the effect of bilirubin on intelligence outcomes. Four high-quality studies with follow-up ranging from 6.5 to 17 years reported no association between IQ and bilirubin level.

Question 2. What Is the Evidence for Effect Modification of the Results in Question 1 by GA, Hemolysis, Serum Albumin, and Other Factors?

There is only 1 article that directly addressed this question. Naeye, using the CPP population, found that at 4 years old the frequency of low IQ with increasing bilirubin levels increased more rapidly in infants with infected amniotic fluid. At 7 years old, neurologic abnormalities also were more prevalent in that subgroup of infants.

When comparing the group of term and near-term infants with comorbid factors who had kernicterus to the group of infants with idiopathic hyperbilirubinemia and kernicterus, the overall mean bilirubin was 31.6 ± 9 mg/dL in the former, versus 35.4 ± 8 mg/dL in the latter (difference not significant). Infants with glucose-6-phosphate dehydrogenase deficiency, sepsis, ABO incompatibility, or Rh incompatibility had similar mean bilirubin levels. Infants with more than 1 comorbid factor had a slightly lower mean bilirubin level of 29.1 ± 16.1 mg/dL.

Eighteen of 23 (78%) term infants with idiopathic hyperbilirubinemia and who developed acute kernicterus survived the neonatal period with chronic sequelae. Thirty-nine of 41 (95%) term infants with kernicterus and ABO or Rh incompatibility had chronic sequelae. Four of 5 (80%) infants with sepsis and kernicterus had chronic sequelae. All 4 infants with multiple comorbid factors had sequelae.

No firm conclusions can be drawn regarding co-morbid factors and kernicterus, because this is a small number of patients from a variety of case reports.

There was no direct study concerning serum albumin level as an effect modifier of neurodevelopmental outcome in infants with hyperbilirubinemia. One report found a significant association between reserve albumin concentration and latency to wave V in BAEP studies.

In addition, Ozmert et al noted that exchange transfusion and the duration that the infant's serum indirect bilirubin level remained higher than 20 mg/dL were important risk factors for prominent neurologic abnormalities.

Question 3. What Are the Quantitative Estimates of Efficacy of Treatment at 1) Reducing Peak Bilirubin Levels (eg, NNT at 20 mg/dL to Keep TSB From Rising); 2) Reducing the Duration of Hyperbilirubinemia (eg, Average Number of Hours by Which Time TSB Levels Higher Than 20 mg/dL May Be Shortened by Treatment); and 3) Improving Neurodevelopmental Outcomes?

Studies on phototherapy efficacy in terms of preventing TSB rising to the level that would require BET (and therefore would be considered "failure of phototherapy") were reviewed for the quantitative estimates of efficacy of phototherapy. Because trials evaluating the efficacy of phototherapy at improving neurodevelopmental outcomes by comparing 1 group of infants with treatment to an untreated group do not exist, the effects of treatment on neurodevelopmental outcomes could only be reviewed descriptively. Furthermore, all the reports primarily examined the efficacy of treatment at 15 mg/dL to prevent TSB from exceeding 20 mg/dL. There is no study to examine the efficacy of treatment at 20 mg/dL to prevent the TSB from rising.

Efficacy of Phototherapy for Prevention of TSB Levels Higher Than 20 mg/dL

Four publications examined the clinical efficacy of phototherapy for prevention of TSB levels higher than 20 mg/dL.

Two studies evaluated the same sample of infants. Both reports were derived from a randomized, controlled trial of phototherapy for neonatal hyperbilirubinemia commissioned by the NICHD between 1974 and 1976.

Because the phototherapy protocols differed significantly in the remaining studies, their results could not be statistically combined and are reported here separately. A total of 893 term or near-term jaundiced infants (325 in the treatment group and 568 in the control group) were evaluated in the current review.

The development, design, and sample composition of NICHD phototherapy trial were reported in detail elsewhere. The NICHD controlled trial of phototherapy for neonatal hyperbilirubinemia consisted of 672 infants who received phototherapy and 667 control infants. Brown et al evaluated the efficacy of phototherapy for prevention of the need for BET in the NICHD study population. For the purpose of current review, only the subgroup of 140 infants in the treatment groups and 136 in the control groups with birth weights 2500 g or more and greater than or equal to 34 weeks' GA were evaluated. The serum bilirubin level as criterion for BET in infants with birth weights of 2500 g or more was 20 mg/dL at standard risk and 18 mg/dL at high risk. It was found that infants with hyperbilirubinemia secondary to nonhemolytic causes who received phototherapy had a 14.3% risk reduction of BET than infants in no treatment group. NNT for prevention of the need for BET or for TSB levels higher than 20 mg/dL was 7 (95% confidence interval [CI]: 6–8). However, phototherapy did not reduce the need for BET for infants with hemolytic diseases or in the high-risk group. No therapeutic effect on reducing the BET rate in infants at greater than or equal to 34 weeks' GA with hemolytic disease was observed.

The same group of infants, 140 subjects in the treatment group and 136 controls with birth weights 2500 g or more and greater than or equal to 34 weeks' GA, were evaluated for the effect of phototherapy on the hyperbilirubinemia of Coombs' positive hemolytic disease in the study of Maurer et al. Of the 276 infants whose birth weights were 2500 g or more, 64 (23%) had positive Coombs' tests: 58 secondary to ABO incompatibility and 6 secondary to Rh incompatibility. Thirty-four of 64 in this group received phototherapy. The other 30 were placed in the control group. Of the 212 subjects who had negative Coombs' tests, 106 were in the treatment group and the same number was in the control group. No therapeutic effect on reducing the BET rate was observed in infants with Coombs' positive hemolytic disease, but there was a 9.4% absolute risk reduction in infants who had negative Coombs' tests. In this group of infants, the NNT for prevention of the need for BET, or a TSB higher than 20 mg/dL, was 11 (95% CI: 10–12).

A more recent randomized, controlled trial compared the effect of 4 different interventions on hyperbilirubinemia (serum bilirubin concentration greater than or equal to 291 µmol/L or 17 mg/dL) in 125 term breastfed infants. Infants with any congenital anomalies, neonatal complications, hematocrit more than 65%, significant bruising or large cephalohematomas, or hemolytic disease were excluded. The 4 interventions in the study were 1) continue breastfeeding and observe (N = 25); 2) discontinue breastfeeding and substitute formula (N = 26); 3) discontinue breastfeeding, substitute formula, and administer phototherapy (N = 38); and 4) continue breastfeeding and administer phototherapy (N = 36). The interventions were considered failures if serum bilirubin levels reached 324 µmol/L or 20 mg/dL. For the purpose of the current review, we regrouped the subjects into treatment group or phototherapy group and control group or no-phototherapy group. Therefore, the original groups 4 and 3 became the treatment groups I and II, and the original groups 1 and 2 were the corresponding control groups I and II. It was found that treatment I, phototherapy with continuation of breastfeeding, had a 10% absolute risk-reduction rate, and the NNT for prevention of a serum bilirubin level higher than 20 mg/dL was 10 (95% CI: 9–12). Compared with treatment I, treatment II (phototherapy with discontinuation of breastfeeding) was significantly more efficacious. The absolute risk-reduction rate was 17%, and the NNT for prevention of a serum bilirubin level exceeding 20 mg/dL was 6 (95% CI: 5–7).

John reported the effect of phototherapy in 492 term neonates born during 1971 and 1972 who developed unexplained jaundice with bilirubin levels higher than 15 mg/dL. One hundred eleven infants received phototherapy, and 381 did not. The author stated: "The choice of therapy was, in effect, random since two pediatricians approved of the treatment and two did not." The results showed that phototherapy had an 11% risk reduction of BET, performed in treatment and control groups when serum bilirubin levels exceeded 20 mg/dL. Therefore, the NNT for prevention of a serum bilirubin level higher than 20 mg/dL was 9 (95% CI: 8–10).

Regardless of different protocols for phototherapy, the NNT for prevention of serum bilirubin levels higher than 20 mg/dL ranged from 6 to 10 in healthy term or near-term infants. Evidence for the efficacy of treatments for neonatal hyperbilirubinemia was limited. Overall, the 4 qualifying studies showed that phototherapy had an absolute risk-reduction rate of 10% to 17% for prevention of serum bilirubin exceeding 20 mg/dL in healthy and jaundiced infants (TSB levels higher than or equal to 13 mg/dL) born at greater than or equal to 34 weeks' GA. Phototherapy combined with cessation of breastfeeding and substitution with formula was found to be the most efficient treatment protocol for healthy term or near-term infants with jaundice.

Effectiveness of Reduction in Bilirubin Level on BAER in Jaundiced Infants With Greater Than or Equal to 34 Weeks' EGA

Eight studies that compared BAER before and after treatments for neonatal hyperbilirubinemia are discussed in this section. Of the 8 studies, 3 studies treated jaundiced infants by administering phototherapy followed by BET according to different guidelines, 4 studies treated jaundiced infants with BET only, and 1 study did not specify what treatments jaundiced infants received. All the studies consistently showed that treatments for neonatal hyperbilirubinemia significantly improved abnormal BAERs in healthy jaundiced infants and jaundiced infants with hemolytic disease.

Effect of Phototherapy on Behavioral and Neurologic Outcomes and IQ

Five studies looked at the effect of hyperbilirubinemia and phototherapy on behavior. Of the 5 studies, 4 used the Brazelton Neonatal Behavioral Assessment Scale and 1 used the Vineland Social Maturity Scale. Three studies reported lower scores in the orientation cluster of the Brazelton Neonatal Behavioral Assessment Scale in the infants treated with phototherapy. The other 2 studies did not find behavioral changes in the phototherapy group. One study evaluated IQ at the age of 17 years. In 42 term infants with severe hyperbilirubinemia who were treated with phototherapy, 31 were also treated with BET. Forty-two infants who did not receive phototherapy were selected as controls. No significant difference in IQ between the 2 groups was found.

Effect of Phototherapy on Visual Outcomes

Three studies were identified that studied the effect of serum bilirubin and treatment on visual outcomes. All showed no short-or long-term (up to 36 months) effect on vision as a result of phototherapy when infants' eyes are protected properly during treatment.

Question 4. What Is the Accuracy of Various Strategies for Predicting Hyperbilirubinemia, Including Hour-Specific Bilirubin Percentiles?

Ten qualifying studies published from 1977 to 2001 examining 5 prediction methods of neonatal hyperbilirubinemia were included. A total of 8167 neonates, most healthy near-term or term infants, were subjects. These studies were conducted among multiple racial groups in multiple countries including China, Denmark, India, Israel, Japan, Spain, and the United States. Some studies included subjects with ABO incompatibility, and some did not. Four studies examined the accuracy of cord bilirubin level as a test for predicting the development of clinically significant neonatal jaundice. Four studies investigated the test performance of serum bilirubin levels before 48 hours of life to predict hyperbilirubinemia. Two studies further compared the test performances of cord bilirubin with that of early serum bilirubin levels. The accuracy of end-tidal carbon monoxide concentration as a predictor of the development of hyperbilirubinemia was examined in Okuyama et al and Stevenson et al. The study by Stevenson et al also examined the test performance of a combined strategy of end-tidal carbon monoxide concentration and early serum bilirubin levels. Finally, 2 studies tested the efficacy of predischarge risk assessment, determined by a risk index model and hour-specific bilirubin percentile, respectively, for predicting neonatal hyperbilirubinemia.

ROC curves were developed for 3 of the predictive strategies. The AUCs were calculated to provide an assessment of the overall accuracy of the tests. Hour-specific bilirubin percentiles had an AUC of 0.93, cord bilirubin levels had an AUC of 0.74, and predischarge risk index had an AUC of 0.80. These numbers should not be compared directly with each other, because the studies had different population characteristics and different defining parameters for hyperbilirubinemia.

Question 5. What Is the Accuracy of TcB Measurements?

A total of 47 qualifying studies in 50 publications examining the test performance of TcB measurements and/or the correlation of TcB measurements to serum bilirubin levels was reviewed in this section. Of the 47 studies, the Minolta Air-Shields jaundice meter (Air-Shields, Hatboro, PA) was used in 41 studies, the BiliCheck (SpectRx Inc, Norcross, GA) was used in 3 studies, the Ingram icterometer (Thomas A. Ingram and Co, Birmingham, England; distributed in the United States by Cascade Health Care Products, Salem, OR) was used in 4 studies, and the ColorMate III (Chromatics Color Sciences International Inc, New York, NY) was used in 1 study.

Based on the evidence from the systematic review, TcB measurements by each of the 4 devices described in the literature (the Minolta Air-Shields jaundice meter, Ingram icterometer, BiliCheck, and Chromatics ColorMate III) have a linear correlation to TSB and may be useful as screening devices to detect clinically significant jaundice and decrease the need for serum bilirubin determinations.

Minolta Air-Shields Jaundice Meter

Generally, TcB readings from the forehead or sternum have correlated well with TSB but with a wide range of correlation coefficients, from a low of 0.52 for subgroup of infants less than 37 weeks' GA to as high as 0.96. Comparison of correlations across studies is difficult because of differences in study design and selection procedures. TcB indices that correspond to various TSB levels vary from institution to institution but seem to be internally consistent. Different TSB threshold levels were used across studies; therefore, there is limited ability to combine data across the studies. Most of the studies used TcB measurements taken at the forehead, several studies used multiple sites and combined results, 1 study used only the midsternum site, and 3 studies took the TcB measurement at multiple sites.

The Minolta Air-Shields jaundice meter seems to perform less well in black infants, compared with white infants, performs best when measurements are made at the sternum, and performs less well when infants have been exposed to phototherapy. This instrument requires daily calibration, and each institution must develop its own correlation curves of TcB to TSB. Eleven studies of the test performance of the Minolta Air-Shields jaundice meter measuring at forehead to predict a serum bilirubin threshold of higher than or equal to 13 mg/dL were included in the following analysis. A total of 1560 paired TcB and serum bilirubin measurements were evaluated. The cutoff points of Minolta AirShields TcB measurements (TcB index) ranged from 13 to 24 for predicting a serum bilirubin level higher than or equal to 13 mg/dL. As a screening test, it does not perform consistently across studies, as evidenced by the heterogeneity in the summary ROC curves not explained by threshold effect. The overall unweighted pooled estimates of sensitivity and specificity were 0.85 (0.77–0.91) and 0.77 (0.66–0.85).

Ingram Icterometer

The Ingram icterometer consists of a strip of transparent Plexiglas on which 5 yellow transverse stripes of precise and graded hue are painted. The correlation coefficients (r) in the 4 studies ranged from 0.63 to 0.97. The icterometer has the added limitation of lacking the objectivity of the other methods, because it depends on observer visualization of depth of yellow color of the skin.

BiliCheck

The recently introduced BiliCheck device, which uses reflectance data from multiple wavelengths, seems to be a significant improvement over the older devices (the Ingram icterometer and the Minolta Air-Shields jaundice

meter) because of its ability to determine correction factors for the effect of melanin and hemoglobin. Three studies examined the accuracy of the BiliCheck TcB measurements to predict TSB ("gold standard"). All studies were rated as high quality. The correlation coefficient ranged from 0.83 to 0.91. In 1 study, the BiliCheck was shown to be as accurate as the laboratory measurement of TSB when compared with the reference gold-standard high-performance liquid chromatography (HPLC) measurement of TSB. Analysis of covariance found no differences in test performance by postnatal age, GA, birth weight, or race; however, 66.7% were white and only 4.3% were black.

Chromatics ColorMate III

One study that evaluated the performance of the ColorMate III transcutaneous bilirubinometer was reviewed. The correlation coefficient for the whole study group was 0.9563, and accuracy was not affected by race, weight, or phototherapy. The accuracy of the device is increased by the determination of an infant's underlying skin type before the onset of visual jaundice; thus, a drawback to the method when used as a screening device is that all infants would require an initial baseline measurement.

CONCLUSIONS AND DISCUSSION

Summarizing case reports of kernicterus from different investigators in different countries from different periods is problematic. First, definitions of kernicterus used in these reports varied greatly. They included gross yellow staining of the brain, microscopic neuronal degeneration, acute clinical neuromotor impairment, neuroauditory impairment, and chronic neuromotor impairment. In some cases, the diagnoses were not established until months or years after birth. Second, case reports without controls makes interpretation difficult, especially in infants with comorbid factors, and could very well lead to misinterpretation of the role of bilirubin in neurodevelopmental outcomes. Third, different reports used different outcome measures. "Normal at follow-up" may be based on parental reporting, physician assessment, or formal neuropsychologic testing. Fourth, time of reported follow-up ranged from days to years. Fifth, cases were reported from different countries at different periods and with different standards of practice managing hyperbilirubinemia. Some countries have a high prevalence of glucose-6-phosphate dehydrogenase deficiency. Some have cultural practices that predispose their infants to agents that cause hyperbilirubinemia (such as clothing stored in dressers with naphthalene moth balls). The effect of the differences on outcomes cannot be known for certain. Finally, it is difficult to infer from case reports the true incidence of this uncommon disorder.

To recap our findings, based on a summary of multiple case reports that spanned more than 30 years, we conclude that kernicterus, although infrequent, has significant mortality (at least 10%) and long-term morbidity (at least 70%). It is evident that the preponderance of kernicterus cases occurred in infants with high bilirubin (more than 20 mg/dL).

Of 26 (19%) term or near-term infants with acute manifestations of kernicterus and reported follow-up data, 5 survived without sequelae, whereas only 3 of 63 (5%) infants with acute kernicterus and comorbid factors were reported to be normal at follow-up. This result suggests the importance of comorbid factors in determining long-term outcome in infants initially diagnosed with kernicterus.

For future research, reaching a national consensus in defining this entity, as in the model suggested by Johnson et al, will help in formulating a valid comparison of different databases. It is also apparent that, without good prevalence and incidence data on hyperbilirubinemia and kernicterus, one would not be able to estimate the risk of kernicterus at a given bilirubin level. Making severe hyperbilirubinemia (eg, greater than or equal to 25 mg/dL) and kernicterus reportable conditions would be a first step in that direction. Also, because kernicterus is infrequent, doing a multicenter case-control study with kernicterus may help to delineate the role of bilirubin in the development of kernicterus.

Hyperbilirubinemia, in most cases, is a necessary but not sufficient condition to explain kernicterus. Factors acting in concert with bilirubin must be studied to seek a satisfactory explanation. Information from duration of exposure to bilirubin and albumin binding of bilirubin may yield a more useful profile of the risk of kernicterus.

Only a few prospective controlled studies looked specifically at behavioral and neurodevelopmental outcomes in healthy term infants with hyperbilirubinemia. Most of these studies have a small number of subjects. Two short-term studies with well-defined measurement of newborn behavioral organization and physiologic measurement of cry are of high methodologic quality; however, the significance of long-term abnormalities in newborn behavior scales and variations in cry formant frequencies are unknown. There remains little information on the long-term effects of hyperbilirubinemia in healthy term infants.

Among the mixed studies (combined term and preterm, nonhemolytic and hemolytic, nondiseased and diseased), the following observations can be made:

- Nine of 15 studies (excluding the CPP) addressing neuroauditory development and bilirubin level were of high quality. Six of them showed BAER abnormalities correlated with high bilirubin levels. Most reported resolution with treatment. Three studies reported hearing impairment associated with elevated bilirubin (more than 16 to more than 20 mg/dL). We conclude that a high bilirubin level does have an adverse effect on neuroauditory function, but the adverse effect on BAER is reversible.

- Of the 8 studies reporting intelligence outcomes in subjects with hyperbilirubinemia, 4 studies were considered high quality. These 4 studies reported no association between IQ and bilirubin level, with follow-up ranging from 6.5 to 17 years. We conclude that there is no evidence to suggest a linear association of bilirubin level and IQ.

- The analysis of the CPP population found no consistent association between peak bilirubin level and IQ. Sensorineural hearing loss was not related to bilirubin level. Only the frequency of abnormal or suspicious neurologic examinations was associated with bilirubin level. In the rest of the studies from the CPP population, there was no consistent evidence to suggest neurologic abnormalities in children with neonatal bilirubin levels more than 20 mg/dL when followed up to 7 years of age.

A large prospective study comprising healthy infants greater than or equal to 34 weeks' GA with hyperbilirubinemia, specifically looking at long-term neurodevelopmental outcomes, has yet to be done. The report of Newman and Klebanoff came closest to that ideal because of the large number of subjects and the study's analytic approach. However, a population born from 1959 to 1966 is no longer representative of present-day newborns: 1) there is now increased ethnic diversity in our newborn population; 2) breast milk jaundice has become more common than hemolytic jaundice; 3) phototherapy for hyperbilirubinemia has become standard therapy; and 4) hospital stays are shorter. These changes in biologic, cultural, and health care characteristics make it difficult to apply the conclusions from the CPP population to present-day newborns.

Although short-term studies, in general, have good methodologic quality, they use tools that have unknown long-term predictive abilities. Long-term studies suffer from high attrition rates of the study population and a nonuniform approach to defining "normal neurodevelopmental outcomes." The total bilirubin levels reported in all the studies mentioned were measured anywhere from the first day of life to more than 2 weeks of life. Definitions of significant hyperbilirubinemia ranged from greater than or equal to 12 mg/dL to greater than or equal to 20 mg/dL.

Given the diversity of conclusions reported, except in cases of kernicterus with sequelae, it is evident that the use of a single TSB level (within the range described in this review) to predict long-term behavioral or neurodevelopmental outcomes is inadequate and will lead to conflicting results.

Evidence for the efficacy of treatments for neonatal hyperbilirubinemia was limited. Overall, the 4 qualifying studies showed that phototherapy had an absolute risk-reduction rate of 10% to 17% for prevention of serum bilirubin exceeding 20 mg/dL in healthy jaundiced infants

(TSB higher than or equal to 13 mg/dL) of greater than or equal to 34 weeks' GA. Phototherapy combined with cessation of breastfeeding and substitution with formula was found to be the most efficient treatment protocol for healthy term or near-term infants with jaundice. There is no evidence to suggest that phototherapy for neonatal hyperbilirubinemia has any long-term adverse neuro-developmental effects in either healthy jaundiced infants or infants with hemolytic disease. It is also noted that in all the studies listed, none of the infants received what is currently known as "intensive phototherapy." Although phototherapy did not reduce the need for BET in infants with hemolytic disease in the NICHD phototherapy trial, it could be attributable to the low dose of phototherapy used. Proper application of "intensive phototherapy" should decrease the need for BET further.

It is difficult to draw conclusions regarding the accuracy of various strategies for prediction of neonatal hyper-bilirubinemia. The first challenge is the lack of consistency in defining clinically significant neonatal hyperbilirubine-mia. Not only did multiple studies use different levels of TSB to define neonatal hyperbilirubinemia, but the levels of TSB defined as significant also varied by age, but age at TSB determination varied by study as well. For example, significant levels of TSB were defined as more than 11.7, more than or equal to 15, more than 15, more than 16, more than 17, and more than or equal to 25 mg/dL.

A second challenge is the heterogeneity of the study populations. The studies were conducted in many racial groups in different countries including China, Denmark, India, Israel, Japan, Spain, and the United States. Although infants were defined as healthy term and near-term newborns, these studies included neonates with potential for hemolysis from ABO-incompatible pregnan-cies as well as breastfed and bottle-fed infants (often not specified). Therefore, it is not possible to directly compare the different predicting strategies. However, all the strate-gies provided strong evidence that early jaundice predicts late jaundice.

Hour-specific bilirubin percentiles had an AUC of 0.93, implying great accuracy of this strategy. In that study, 2976 of 13 003 eligible infants had a postdischarge TSB measurement, as discussed by Maisels and Newman. Because of the large number of infants who did not have a postdischarge TSB, the actual study sample would be defi-cient in study participants with low predischarge bilirubin levels, leading to false high-sensitivity estimates and false low-specificity estimates. Moreover, the population in the study is not representative of the entire US population. The strategy of using early hour-specific bilirubin per-centiles to predict late jaundice looks promising, but a large multicenter study (with evaluation of potential dif-ferences by race and ethnicity as well as prenatal, natal, and postnatal factors) may need to be undertaken to pro-duce more applicable data.

TcB measurements by each of the 3 devices described in the literature, the Minolta Air-Shields jaundice meter, the Ingram icterometer, and the Bili-Check, have a linear correlation to TSB and may be useful as screening devices to detect clinically significant jaundice and decrease the need for serum bilirubin determinations.

The recently introduced BiliCheck device, which uses reflectance data from multiple wavelengths, seems to be a significant improvement over the older devices (the Ingram icterometer and the Minolta Air-Shields jaundice meter) because of its ability to determine correction factors for the effect of melanin and hemoglobin. In 1 study, the BiliCheck was shown to be as accurate as laboratory measures of TSB when compared with the reference gold-standard HPLC measurement of TSB.

Future research should confirm these findings in larger samples of diverse populations and address issues that might affect performance, such as race, GA, age at meas-urement, phototherapy, sunlight exposure, feeding and accuracy as screening instruments, performance at higher levels of bilirubin, and ongoing monitoring of jaundice. Additionally, studies should address cost-effectiveness and reproducibility in actual clinical practice. Given the interlaboratory variability of measurements of TSB, future studies of noninvasive measures of bilirubin should use HPLC and routine laboratory methods of TSB as reference standards, because the transcutaneous measures may prove to be as accurate as the laboratory measurement when compared with HPLC as the gold standard.

Using correlation coefficients to determine the accuracy of TcB measurements should be interpreted carefully because of several limitations:

- The correlation coefficient does not provide any infor-mation about the clinical utility of the diagnostic test.
- Although correlation coefficients measure the as-sociation between TcB and "standard" serum bilirubin measurements, the correlation coefficient is highly dependent on the distribution of serum bilirubin in the study population selected.
- Correlation measures ignore bias and measure relative rather than absolute agreement.

ADDENDUM: THE RISK OF BET

At the suggestion of AAP technical experts, a review of the risks associated with BET was also undertaken after the original AHRQ report was published. Articles were obtained from an informal survey of studies published since 1960 dealing with large populations that permitted calculations of the risks of morbidity and mortality. Of 15 studies, 8 consisted of subjects born before 1970. One article published in 1997 consisted of subjects born in 1994 and 1995.

Fifteen studies that reported data on BET-related mor-tality and/or morbidity were included in this review. Three categories were created to describe the percentage of subjects who met the criteria of the target population of our evidence report (ie, term idiopathic jaundice infants). Category I indicates that more than 50% of the study subjects were term infants whose pre-exchange clinical state was vigorous or stable and without disease conditions other than jaundice. Category II indicates that between 10% and 50% of the study subjects had category I characteristics. Category III indicates that more than 90% of the study subjects were preterm infants and/or term infants whose pre-exchange clinical state was not stable or was critically ill and with other disease conditions.

BET Subject and Study Characteristics

Because BET is no longer the mainstay of treatment for hyperbilirubinemia, most infants who underwent BETs were born in the 1950s to 1970s. Two recent studies reported BET-related mortality and morbidity for infants born from 1981 to 1995. After 1970, there were more infants who were premature, low birth weight or very low birth weight, and/or had a clinical condition(s) other than jaundice who received BETs than those born in earlier years. Not all infants in this review received BETs for hyperbilirubinemia. Because of limited data on subjects' bilirubin levels when the BETs were performed, we could not exclude those nonjaundiced infants.

BET-Associated Mortality

For all infants, the reported BET-related mortality ranged from 0% to 7%. There were no consistent definitions for BET-related mortality in the studies. An infant who died within 6 hours after the BET was the first used to define a BET-related death by Boggs and Westphal in 1960. Including the study from Boggs and Westphal, there were 3 studies reporting the 6-hour mortality, and they ranged from 0% to 1.9%. It is difficult to isolate BET as the sole factor in explaining mortality, because most of the subjects have significant associated pre-exchange disease morbidities. Most of the infants who died from BET had blood incompatibility and sepsis or were premature, had kernicterus, and/or were critically ill before undergoing BET. When only term infants were counted, the 6-hour mortality ranged from 3 to 19 per 1000 exchanged. When those term infants with serious hemolytic diseases (such as Rh incompatibility) were excluded, the 6-hour mortality ranged from 3 to 4 per 1000 exchanged infants. All these infants were born before 1970, and their jaundice was primarily due to ABO incompatibility.

BET-Associated Morbidity

There is an extensive list of complications that have been associated with BETs. Complications include those related to the use of blood products (infection, hemolysis of transfused blood, thromboembolization, graft versus host reactions), metabolic derangements (acidosis and perturbation of the serum concentrations of potassium, sodium, glucose, and calcium), cardiorespiratory reactions (including arrhythmias, apnea, and cardiac arrest), complications related to umbilical venous and arterial catheterization, and other miscellaneous complications. As noted previously, the pre-exchange clinical state of the infants studied varied widely, as did the definitions and rates of BET-associated morbidity. In many cases, however, the morbidity was minor (eg, postexchange anemia).

In the NICHD cooperative phototherapy study, morbidity (apnea, bradycardia, cyanosis, vasospasm, thrombosis) was observed in 22 of 328 (6.7%) patients in whom BETs were performed (no data available in 3 BETs). Of the 22 adverse events, 6 were mild episodes of bradycardia associated with calcium infusion. If those infants are excluded, as well as 2 who experienced transient arterial spasm, the incidence of "serious morbidity" associated with the procedure itself was 5.22%.

The most recent study to report BET morbidity in the era of contemporary neonatal care provides data on infants cared for from 1980 to 1995 at the Children's Hospital and University of Washington Medical Center in Seattle. Of 106 infants receiving BET, 81 were healthy and there were no deaths; however, 1 healthy infant developed severe necrotizing enterocolitis requiring surgery. Of 25 sick infants (12 required mechanical ventilation), there were 5 deaths, and 3 developed permanent sequelae, including chronic aortic obstruction from BET via the umbilical artery, intraventricular hemorrhage with subsequent developmental delay, and sudden respiratory deterioration from a pulmonary hemorrhage and subsequent global developmental delay. The author classified the deaths as "possibly" ($n = 3$) or "probably" ($n = 2$) and the complications as "possibly" ($n = 2$) or "probably" ($n = 1$) resulting from the BET. Thus in 25 sick infants, the overall risk of death or permanent sequelae ranged from 3 of 25 to 8 of 25 (12%–32%) and of permanent sequelae in survivors from 1 of 20 to 2 of 20 (5%–10%).

Most of the mortality and morbidity rates reported date from a time at which BET was a common procedure in nurseries. This is no longer the case, and newer phototherapy techniques are likely to reduce the need for BETs even further. Because the frequency of performance of any procedure is an important determinant of risk, the fact that BET is so rarely performed today could result in higher mortality and morbidity rates. However, none of the reports before 1986 included contemporary monitoring capabilities such as pulse oximetry, which should provide earlier identification of potential problems and might decrease morbidity and mortality. In addition, current standards for the monitoring of transfused blood products has significantly reduced the risk of transfusion-transmitted viral infections.

Diagnosis and Management of Acute Otitis Media

- *Clinical Practice Guideline*

AMERICAN ACADEMY OF PEDIATRICS AND AMERICAN ACADEMY OF FAMILY PHYSICIANS

CLINICAL PRACTICE GUIDELINE

Subcommittee on Management of Acute Otitis Media

Diagnosis and Management of Acute Otitis Media

ABSTRACT. This evidence-based clinical practice guideline provides recommendations to primary care clinicians for the management of children from 2 months through 12 years of age with uncomplicated acute otitis media (AOM).

The American Academy of Pediatrics and American Academy of Family Physicians convened a committee composed of primary care physicians and experts in the fields of otolaryngology, epidemiology, and infectious disease. The subcommittee partnered with the Agency for Healthcare Research and Quality and the Southern California Evidence-Based Practice Center to develop a comprehensive review of the evidence-based literature related to AOM. The resulting evidence report and other sources of data were used to formulate the practice guideline recommendations. The focus of this practice guideline is the appropriate diagnosis and initial treatment of a child presenting with AOM.

The guideline provides a specific definition of AOM. It addresses pain management, initial observation versus antibacterial treatment, appropriate choices of antibacterials, and preventive measures. Decisions were made based on a systematic grading of the quality of evidence and strength of recommendations, as well as expert consensus when definitive data were not available. The practice guideline underwent comprehensive peer review before formal approval by the partnering organizations.

This clinical practice guideline is not intended as a sole source of guidance in the management of children with AOM. Rather, it is intended to assist primary care clinicians by providing a framework for clinical decision-making. It is not intended to replace clinical judgment or establish a protocol for all children with this condition. These recommendations may not provide the only appropriate approach to the management of this problem.

ABBREVIATIONS. AOM, acute otitis media; OME, otitis media with effusion; AAP, American Academy of Pediatrics; AAFP, American Academy of Family Physicians; AHRQ, Agency for Healthcare Research and Quality; MEE, middle-ear effusion; CAM, complementary and alternative medicine.

Acute otitis media (AOM) is the most common infection for which antibacterial agents are prescribed for children in the United States. As such, the diagnosis and management of AOM has

a significant impact on the health of children, cost of providing care, and overall use of antibacterial agents. The illness also generates a significant social burden and indirect cost due to time lost from school and work. The estimated direct cost of AOM was $1.96 billion in 1995. In addition, the indirect cost was estimated to be $1.02 billion.[1] During 1990 there were almost 25 million visits made to office-based physicians in the United States for otitis media, with 809 antibacterial prescriptions per 1000 visits, for a total of more than 20 million prescriptions for otitis media–related antibacterials. Although the total number of office visits for otitis media decreased to 16 million in 2000, the rate of antibacterial prescribing was approximately the same (802 antibacterial prescriptions per 1000 visits for a total of more than 13 million prescriptions).[2–4] An individual course of antibacterial therapy can range in cost from $10 to more than $100.

There has been much discussion recently as to the necessity for the use of antibacterial agents at the time of diagnosis in children with uncomplicated AOM. Although in the United States the use of antibacterial agents in the management of AOM has been routine, in some countries in Europe it is common practice to treat the symptoms of AOM initially and only institute antibacterial therapy if clinical improvement does not occur. For the clinician, the choice of a specific antibacterial agent has become a key aspect of management. Concerns about the rising rates of antibacterial resistance and the growing costs of antibacterial prescriptions have focused the attention of the medical community and the general public on the need for judicious use of antibacterial agents. Greater resistance among many of the pathogens that cause AOM has fueled an increase in the use of broader-spectrum and generally more expensive antibacterial agents.

It is the intent of this guideline to evaluate the published evidence on the natural history and management of uncomplicated AOM and to make recommendations based on that evidence to primary care clinicians including pediatricians, family physicians, physician assistants, nurse practitioners, and emergency department physicians as well as otolaryngologists. The scope of the guideline is the diagnosis and management of uncomplicated AOM in children from 2 months through 12 years of age without signs or symptoms of systemic illness unrelated to the middle ear. It applies only to the otherwise healthy child without underlying conditions that may alter the natural course of AOM. These conditions include, but are not limited to, anatomic abnormalities such as cleft palate, genetic conditions such as Down syndrome, immunodeficiencies, and the presence of cochlear implants. Also excluded are children with a clinical recurrence of AOM within 30 days or AOM with underlying chronic otitis media with effusion (OME).

METHODS

To develop the clinical practice guideline on the management of AOM, the American Academy of Pediatrics (AAP) and American Academy of Family Physicians (AAFP) convened the Subcommittee on Management of Acute Otitis Media, a working panel composed of primary care and subspecialty physicians. The subcommittee was cochaired by a primary care pediatrician and a family physician and included experts in the fields of general pediatrics, family medicine, otolaryngology, epidemiology, infectious disease, and medical informatics. All panel members reviewed the AAP policy on conflict of interest and voluntary disclosure and were given an opportunity to present any potential conflicts with the subcommittee's work.

The AAP and AAFP partnered with the Agency for Healthcare Research and Quality (AHRQ) and the Southern California Evidence-Based Practice Center to develop the evidence report, which served as a major source of data for these practice guideline recommendations.[1] Specific clinical issues addressed in the AHRQ evidence report were the 1) definition of AOM, 2) natural history of AOM without antibacterial treatment, 3) effectiveness of antibacterial agents in preventing clinical failure, and 4) relative effectiveness of specific antibacterial regimens. The AHRQ report focused on children between 4 weeks and 18 years of age with uncomplicated AOM seeking initial treatment. Outcomes included the presence or absence of signs and symptoms within 48 hours, at 3 to 7 days, 8 to 14 days, 15 days to 3 months, and more than 3 months and the presence of adverse effects from antibacterial treatment. Southern California Evidence-Based Practice Center project staff searched Medline (1966 through March 1999), the Cochrane Library (through March 1999), HealthSTAR (1975 through March 1999), International Pharmaceutical Abstracts (1970 through March 1999), CINAHL (1982 through March 1999), BIOSIS (1970 through March 1999), and Embase (1980 through March 1999). Additional articles were identified by review of reference lists in proceedings, published articles, reports, and

guidelines. Studies relevant to treatment questions were limited to randomized, controlled trials. For natural history, prospective and retrospective comparative cohort studies were included also. A total of 3461 titles were identified initially for additional review. Of these, 2701 were excluded, and 760 required article review. Finally, 72 English-language and 2 foreign-language articles were reviewed fully. Results of the literature review were presented in evidence tables and published in the final evidence report.

New literature about otitis media is being published constantly. Although the systematic review done by the AHRQ could not be replicated with new literature, members of the Subcommittee on Management of Acute Otitis Media reviewed additional articles published through September 2003. Articles were nonsystematically evaluated for quality of methodology and importance of results. Articles used in the AHRQ review also were reevaluated for their quality. Conclusions were based on the consensus of the subcommittee after the review of newer literature and reevaluation of the AHRQ evidence. Of significance is that the literature includes relatively few cases of uncomplicated AOM in children older than 12 years. The subcommittee therefore limited this guideline to children from 2 months through 12 years of age.

The evidence-based approach to guideline development requires that the evidence in support of a policy be identified, appraised, and summarized and that an explicit link between evidence and recommendations be defined. Evidence-based recommendations reflect the quality of evidence and the balance of benefit and harm that is anticipated when the recommendation is followed. The AAP definitions of evidence-based recommendations are shown in Table 1.

A draft version of this practice guideline underwent extensive peer review by committees and sections within the AAP, reviewers appointed by the AAFP, outside organizations, and other individuals identified by the subcommittee as experts in the field. Members of the subcommittee were invited to distribute the draft to other representatives and committees within their specialty organizations. The resulting comments were reviewed by the subcommittee and, when appropriate, incorporated into the guideline.

RECOMMENDATION 1

To diagnose AOM the clinician should confirm a history of acute onset, identify signs of middle-ear effusion (MEE), and evaluate for the presence of signs and symptoms of middle-ear inflammation. (This recommendation is based on observational studies and a preponderance of benefit over risk; see Table 2.)

TABLE 1. Guideline Definitions for Evidence-Based Statements

Statement	Definition	Implication
Strong recommendation	A strong recommendation in favor of a particular action is made when the anticipated benefits of the recommended intervention clearly exceed the harms (as a strong recommendation against an action is made when the anticipated harms clearly exceed the benefits) and the quality of the supporting evidence is excellent. In some clearly identified circumstances, strong recommendations may be made when high-quality evidence is impossible to obtain and the anticipated benefits strongly outweigh the harms.	Clinicians should follow a strong recommendation unless a clear and compelling rationale for an alternative approach is present.
Recommendation	A recommendation in favor of a particular action is made when the anticipated benefits exceed the harms, but the quality of evidence is not as strong. Again, in some clearly identified circumstances, recommendations may be made when high-quality evidence is impossible to obtain but the anticipated benefits outweigh the harms.	Clinicians would be prudent to follow a recommendation but should remain alert to new information and sensitive to patient preferences.
Option	Options define courses that may be taken when either the quality of evidence is suspect or carefully performed studies have shown little clear advantage to one approach over another.	Clinicians should consider the option in their decision-making, and patient preference may play a substantial role.
No recommendation	No recommendation indicates that there is a lack of pertinent published evidence and that the anticipated balance of benefits and harms is unclear.	Clinicians should be alert to new published evidence that clarifies the balance of benefit versus harm.

TABLE 2. Definition of AOM

TABLE 2. Definition of AOM

A diagnosis of AOM requires 1) a history of acute onset of signs and symptoms, 2) the presence of MEE, and 3) signs and symptoms of middle-ear inflammation.

Elements of the definition of AOM are all of the following:
1. Recent, usually abrupt, onset of signs and symptoms of middle-ear inflammation and MEE
2. The presence of MEE that is indicated by any of the following:
   a. Bulging of the tympanic membrane
   b. Limited or absent mobility of the tympanic membrane
   c. Air-fluid level behind the tympanic membrane
   d. Otorrhea
3. Signs or symptoms of middle-ear inflammation as indicated by either
   a. Distinct erythema of the tympanic membrane or
   b. Distinct otalgia (discomfort clearly referable to the ear[s] that results in interference with or precludes normal activity or sleep)

Children with AOM usually present with a history of rapid onset of signs and symptoms such as otalgia (or pulling of the ear in an infant), irritability in an infant or toddler, otorrhea, and/or fever. These findings, other than otorrhea, are nonspecific and frequently overlap those of an uncomplicated viral upper respiratory infection.[5,6] In a prospective survey among 354 children who visited a physician for acute respiratory illness, fever, earache, and excessive crying were present frequently (90%) in those with AOM. However, these symptoms also were prominent among children without AOM (72%). Other symptoms of a viral upper respiratory infection, such as cough and nasal discharge or stuffiness, often precede or accompany AOM and are nonspecific also. Accordingly, clinical history alone is poorly predictive of the presence of AOM, especially in younger children.[5]

The presence of MEE is commonly confirmed with the use of pneumatic otoscopy[7] but can be supplemented by tympanometry[8] and/or acoustic reflectometry.[9–12] MEE also can be demonstrated directly by tympanocentesis or the presence of fluid in the external auditory canal as a result of tympanic membrane perforation.

Visualization of the tympanic membrane with identification of an MEE and inflammatory changes is necessary to establish the diagnosis with certainty. To visualize the tympanic membrane adequately it is essential that cerumen obscuring the tympanic membrane be removed and that lighting is adequate. For pneumatic otoscopy, a speculum of proper shape and diameter must be selected to permit a seal in the external auditory canal. Appropriate restraint of the child to permit adequate examination may be necessary also.

The findings on otoscopy indicating the presence of MEE and inflammation associated with AOM have been well defined. Fullness or bulging of the tympanic membrane is often present and has the highest predictive value for the presence of MEE. When combined with color and mobility, bulging is also the best predictor of AOM.[7,13,14] Reduced or absent mobility of the tympanic membrane during performance of pneumatic otoscopy is additional evidence of fluid in the middle ear. Opacification or cloudiness, other than that caused by scarring, is also a consistent finding and is caused by edema of the tympanic membrane. Redness of the tympanic membrane caused by inflammation may be present and must be distinguished from the pink erythematous flush evoked by crying or high fever, which is usually less intense and remits as the child quiets down. In bullous myringitis, blisters may be seen on the tympanic membrane.[15] When the presence of middle-ear fluid is difficult to determine, the use of tympanometry or acoustic reflectometry[16] can be helpful in establishing a diagnosis.

A major challenge for the practitioner is to discriminate between OME and AOM.[17,18] OME is more common than AOM. OME may accompany viral upper respiratory infections, be a prelude to AOM, or be a sequela of AOM.[19] When OME is identified mistakenly as AOM, antibacterial agents may be prescribed unnecessarily.[20,21] Clinicians should strive to avoid a false-positive diagnosis in children with middle-ear discomfort caused by eustachian tube dysfunction and retraction of the tympanic membrane or when acute viral respiratory infection is superimposed on chronic preexisting MEE.

The diagnosis of AOM, particularly in infants and young children, is often made with a degree of uncertainty. Common factors that may increase uncertainty include the inability to sufficiently clear the external auditory canal of cerumen, a narrow ear canal, or inability to maintain an adequate seal for successful pneumatic otoscopy or tympanometry. An uncertain diagnosis of AOM is caused most often by inability to confirm the presence of MEE.[22] Acoustic reflectometry can be helpful, because it requires no seal of the canal and can determine the presence of middle-ear fluid through only a small opening in the cerumen.[10,11] When the presence of middle-ear fluid is questionable or uncertain, a diagnosis of AOM may be considered but cannot be confirmed. Although every effort should be made by the clinician to differentiate AOM from OME or a normal ear, it must be acknowledged that, using all available tools, uncertainty will remain in some cases. Efforts to improve clinician education must be increased to improve diagnostic skills and thereby decrease the frequency of an uncertain diagnosis. Ideally, instruction in the proper examination of the child's ear should begin with the first pediatric rotation in medical school and continue throughout postgraduate training.[18] Continuing medical education should reinforce the importance of and retrain the clinician in the use of pneumatic otoscopy. By including the degree of certainty into the formation of a management plan, the everyday challenge of pediatric examinations is incorporated into decision-making.

A certain diagnosis of AOM meets all 3 of the criteria: rapid onset, presence of MEE, and signs and symptoms of middle-ear inflammation. The clinician should maximize diagnostic strategies, particularly to establish the presence of MEE, and should consider the certainty of diagnosis in determining management. Clinicians may wish to discuss the degree of diagnostic certainty with parents/caregivers at the time of initial AOM management.

TABLE 3.   Treatments for Otalgia in AOM

Modality	Comments
Acetaminophen, ibuprofen[26]	Effective analgesia for mild to moderate pain, readily available, mainstay of pain management for AOM
Home remedies (no controlled studies that directly address effectiveness) Distraction External application of heat or cold Oil	May have limited effectiveness
Topical agents Benzocaine (Auralgan, Americaine Otic)[27]	Additional but brief benefit over acetaminophen in patients >5 y
Naturopathic agents (Otikon Otic Solution)[28]	Comparable with ametocaine/phenazone drops (Anaesthetic) in patients >6 y
Homeopathic agents[29,30]	No controlled studies that directly address pain
Narcotic analgesia with codeine or analogs	Effective for moderate or severe pain; requires prescription; risk of respiratory depression, altered mental status, gastrointestinal upset, and constipation
Tympanostomy/myringotomy[31]	Requires skill and entails potential risk

RECOMMENDATION 2

The management of AOM should include an assessment of pain. *If pain is present, the clinician should recommend treatment to reduce pain. (This is a strong recommendation based on randomized, clinical trials with limitations and a preponderance of benefit over risk.)*

Many episodes of AOM are associated with pain.[23] Although pain is an integral part of the illness, clinicians often see otalgia as a peripheral concern not requiring direct attention.[24] The AAP published the policy statement "The Assessment and Management of Acute Pain in Infants, Children, and Adolescents"[25] to assist the clinician in addressing pain in the context of illness. The management of pain, especially during the first 24 hours of an episode of AOM, should be addressed regardless of the use of antibacterial agents.

Various treatments of otalgia have been used, but none has been well studied. The clinician should select a treatment based on a consideration of benefits and risks and, wherever possible, incorporate parent/caregiver and patient preference (Table 3).

RECOMMENDATION 3A

Observation without use of antibacterial agents in a child with uncomplicated AOM is an option for selected children based on diagnostic certainty, age, illness severity, and assurance of follow-up. (This option is based on randomized, controlled trials with limitations and a relative balance of benefit and risk.)

The "observation option" for AOM refers to deferring antibacterial treatment of selected children for 48 to 72 hours and limiting management to symptomatic relief. The decision to observe or treat is based on the child's age, diagnostic certainty, and illness severity. To observe a child without initial antibacterial therapy, it is important that the parent/caregiver has a ready means of communicating with the clinician. There also must be a system in place that permits reevaluation of the child. If necessary, the parent/caregiver also must be able to obtain medication conveniently.

This option should be limited to otherwise healthy children 6 months to 2 years of age with nonsevere illness at presentation *and* an uncertain diagnosis *and* to children 2 years of age and older without severe symptoms at presentation *or* with an uncertain diagnosis. In these situations, observation provides an opportunity for the patient to improve without antibacterial treatment. The association of age younger than 2 years with increased risk of failure of watchful waiting and the concern for serious infection among children younger than 6 months influence the decision for immediate antibacterial therapy. Consequently, the panel recommends an age-stratified approach that incorporates these clinical considerations along with the certainty of diagnosis (Table 4).

Placebo-controlled trials of AOM over the past 30 years have shown consistently that most children do well, without adverse sequelae, even without antibacterial therapy. Between 7 and 20 children must be treated with antibacterial agents for 1 child to derive benefit.[34–36] By 24 hours, 61% of children have decreased symptoms whether they receive placebo or

TABLE 4.   Criteria for Initial Antibacterial-Agent Treatment or Observation in Children With AOM

Age	Certain Diagnosis	Uncertain Diagnosis
<6 mo	Antibacterial therapy	Antibacterial therapy
6 mo to 2 y	Antibacterial therapy	Antibacterial therapy if severe illness; observation option* if nonsevere illness
≥2 y	Antibacterial therapy if severe illness; observation option* if nonsevere illness	Observation option*

This table was modified with permission from the New York State Department of Health and the New York Region Otitis Project Committee.[32,33]

* Observation is an appropriate option only when follow-up can be ensured and antibacterial agents started if symptoms persist or worsen. Nonsevere illness is mild otalgia and fever <39°C in the past 24 hours. Severe illness is moderate to severe otalgia or fever ≥39°C. A certain diagnosis of AOM meets all 3 criteria: 1) rapid onset, 2) signs of MEE, and 3) signs and symptoms of middle-ear inflammation.

antibacterial agents. By 7 days, approximately 75% of children have resolution of symptoms.[37] The AHRQ evidence-report meta-analysis showed a 12.3% reduction in the clinical failure rate within 2 to 7 days of diagnosis when ampicillin or amoxicillin was prescribed, compared with initial use of placebo or observation (number needed to treat: 8).[1]

In 1990 the Dutch College of General Practitioners adopted a guideline for the management of AOM that recommended treating symptoms without antibacterial agents for 24 hours (for those 6–24 months old) or 72 hours (for those more than 24 months) and adding antibacterial agents if no improvement is evident at reassessment. A 1999 revision to this early guideline does not distinguish the younger age group for special consideration.[38] Although this guideline has been widely adopted in The Netherlands, its use in other countries requires consideration of the availability of access to care for follow-up and the presence of an adult who can adequately monitor the child's course. Although there are no controlled studies that address the question of whether the Dutch guideline has resulted in more complications after AOM, van Buchem et al[39,136] found that only 2.7% of 4860 Dutch children older than 2 years given only symptomatic treatment developed severe illness, defined by persistent fever, pain, or discharge after 3 to 4 days. Only 2 children developed mastoiditis. One case of mastoiditis was present at initial assessment, and the other developed within the first week and resolved promptly with oral antibacterial agents.

Randomized trials of observation with symptomatic treatment have been few. A recent randomized trial in general practice in the United Kingdom compared providing immediate antibacterial therapy with delaying antibacterial agents for 72 hours in children aged 6 months to 10 years.[40] Seventy-six percent of children in the delayed-treatment group never required antibacterial agents. Seventy percent of the delayed-antibacterial group were symptomatically better at 3 days, whereas 86% of the immediate-treatment group were better. Immediate use of antibacterial agents was associated with approximately 1-day-shorter illness and one-half teaspoon a day less acetaminophen consumption but no difference in school absence, pain, or distress scores. Among children with fever or vomiting on day 1, those receiving immediate antibacterial agents were 21% less likely to have distress on day 3. In children without fever or vomiting, immediate antibacterial agents decreased distress on day 3 by only 4%.[41] This study, however, was limited because of the use of imprecise criteria for the diagnosis of AOM and the use of low doses of amoxicillin (125 mg, 3 times a day, for 7 days for all patients regardless of weight) in the treatment group.

The likelihood of recovery without antibacterial therapy differs depending on the severity of signs and symptoms at initial examination. Kaleida et al[42] divided patients into severe and nonsevere groups based on degree of fever, a scoring system based on duration and severity of pain or apparent discomfort, and estimated parental anxiety. In the nonse-

vere group, initial treatment failure occurred in 3.8% more children who received placebo rather than amoxicillin. In the severe group of children, the initial failure rate on placebo plus myringotomy was 23.5% versus an initial failure rate of 9.6% on amoxicillin alone (a difference of 13.9%).

Several investigators report poorer outcomes in younger children. A greater number of penicillin-resistant strains of pneumococci are isolated in those younger than 18 months, compared with older children,[43] and are associated with an increased bacteriologic failure rate in children younger than 2 years.[44–47] The study by Kaleida et al[42] also shows a greater initial clinical failure rate (9.8%) in children younger than 2 years than in those older than 2 years (5.5%) who were in the placebo group.

Routine antibacterial therapy for AOM is often cited as the main reason for the decrease in the incidence of mastoiditis in the antibacterial era.[48,49] By the 1950s, mastoiditis (frequent in the pre–antibacterial-agent era[48]) had decreased dramatically. Although some have expressed concern about a possible resurgence,[50,51] such concern is not supported by published data.

The AHRQ evidence report on AOM concluded that mastoiditis is not increased with initial observation, provided that children are followed closely and antibacterial therapy is initiated in those who do not improve. Pooled data from 6 randomized trials and 2 cohort studies showed comparable rates of mastoiditis in children (0.59%) who received initial antibacterial therapy and children (0.17%) who received placebo or observation (P = .212). External validity might be limited, however, because some trials excluded very young children or those with severe illness.[1]

Recently published case series of pediatric mastoiditis show that acute mastoiditis is most common in infants and young children and can be the presenting sign of AOM in a patient with no prior middle-ear disease.[50–60] Routine antibacterial therapy of AOM is not an absolute safeguard against mastoiditis and other complications, because most cases (36%–87%) have received prior antibacterial-agent therapy.[50,53,57–59,61–63]

Van Zuijlen et al[64] compared national differences in acute mastoiditis rates from 1991 to 1998 for children 14 years of age or younger. Incidence rates were higher in The Netherlands, Norway, and Denmark (in which antibacterial agents are not necessarily given on initial diagnosis of AOM) than in the United Kingdom, Canada, Australia, and the United States (in which antibacterial agents are prescribed in more than 96% of cases). However, despite initial use of antibacterial agents more than twice as often in Norway and Denmark than in The Netherlands, mastoiditis rates in all 3 countries were comparable.

Thus current evidence does not suggest a clinically important increased risk of mastoiditis in children when AOM is managed only with initial symptomatic treatment without antibacterial agents. Clinicians should remain aware that antibacterial-agent treatment might mask mastoiditis signs and symptoms, producing a subtle presentation that can delay diagnosis.[56,59,61]

Although bacteremia may accompany AOM, particularly in children with a temperature higher than 39°C,[65] there is little evidence that routine antibacterial treatment for otitis media prevents bacterial meningitis. In a study of 4860 children with AOM who did not receive antibacterial therapy, no cases of bacterial meningitis were observed.[39] However, in a study involving 240 children between 6 and 24 months of age, 1 child in the placebo group was subsequently diagnosed as having meningitis.[66] In another report, positive blood cultures were equally common in children with bacterial meningitis regardless of whether they received preadmission treatment with antibacterials for AOM (77% and 78%).[67] Thus, as with mastoiditis, the incidence of meningitis in those with AOM is unlikely to be influenced by initial treatment of AOM with antibacterial agents.

The incidence of invasive pneumococcal disease has decreased since the introduction of the protein-polysaccharide conjugate vaccine (PPV7). There has been a 69% decline in children younger than 2 years between 1998–1999 and 2001. The decline in this age group for invasive disease caused by vaccine serotypes during that period was 78%.[68] How this will affect the risk of AOM-associated invasive pneumococcal disease is not known yet.

As noted by Dagan and McCracken,[69] studies comparing efficacy of different antibacterial agents or placebo compared with antibacterial therapy often have significant design flaws that may influence the outcome of the studies. Methodologic considerations include enrollment criteria, sample size, diagnostic criteria, dosing regimens, definition and timing of outcome criteria, age, severity of symptoms, race, immune system, compliance, virulence and resistance of the infecting organism, duration of antibacterial therapy, and the presence of an underlying respiratory infection. One of the most important issues among the design characteristics of the studies of otitis media is the definition of AOM used in the individual investigations. If studies that evaluate the impact of antibacterial therapy on the clinical course of children with AOM have weak definitions of AOM (that allow the inclusion of children who are more likely to have OME than AOM), recipients of placebo will not respond significantly differently from those who receive antibacterial therapy.

Given the sum of the available evidence, clinicians may consider observation with symptomatic treatment as an option for initial management of selected children with AOM. If the "observation option" is used, the clinician should share with parents/caregivers the degree of diagnostic certainty and consider their preference. The potential of antibacterial therapy at the initial visit to shorten symptoms by 1 day in 5% to 14% of children can be compared with the avoidance of common antibacterial side effects in 5% to 10% of children, infrequent serious side effects, and the adverse effects of antibacterial resistance. When considering this option, the clinician should verify the presence of an adult who will reliably observe the child, recognize signs of serious illness, and be able to provide prompt access to medical care if improvement does not occur. If there is worsening of illness or if there is no improvement in 48 to 72 hours while a child is under observation, institution of antibacterial therapy should be considered. Reexamination may be warranted if discussion with the parents raises concern as to the degree of illness.

Strategies for following children being managed with initial observation include a parent-initiated visit and/or phone contact for worsening condition or no improvement at 48 to 72 hours, a scheduled follow-up appointment in 48 to 72 hours, routine follow-up phone contact, or use of a safety-net antibiotic prescription to be filled if illness does not improve in 48 to 72 hours.[70,71] Clinicians should determine the most appropriate strategy for their practice setting, taking into account the availability and reliability of the reporting parent/caregiver, available office resources, cost to the health care system and the family, and the convenience of the family. An assessment of the potential risk of inappropriate use of an antibacterial agent in a patient who may be worsening or may have a condition other than AOM must also be made. Table 5 summarizes the data on initial observation versus initial antibacterial-agent treatment of AOM.

RECOMMENDATION 3B

If a decision is made to treat with an antibacterial agent, the clinician should prescribe amoxicillin for most children. (This recommendation is based on randomized, clinical trials with limitations and a preponderance of benefit over risk.)

When amoxicillin is used, the dose should be 80 to 90 mg/kg per day. (This option is based on extrapolation from microbiologic studies and expert opinion, with a preponderance of benefit over risk.)

If a decision is made to treat with antibacterial agents, there are numerous medications that are clinically effective. The choice of first-line treatment should be based on the anticipated clinical response as well as the microbiologic flora likely to be present. The justification to use amoxicillin as first-line therapy in most patients with AOM relates to its general effectiveness when used in sufficient doses against susceptible and intermediate resistant pneumococci as well as its safety, low cost, acceptable taste, and narrow microbiologic spectrum.[75]

In patients who have severe illness (moderate to severe otalgia or fever of 39°C or higher[42]) and in those for whom additional coverage for β-lactamase–positive *Haemophilus influenzae* and *Moraxella catarrhalis* is desired, therapy should be initiated with high-dose amoxicillin-clavulanate (90 mg/kg per day of amoxicillin component, with 6.4 mg/kg per day of clavulanate in 2 divided doses).[76] This dose has sufficient potassium clavulanate to inhibit all β-lactamase–producing *H influenzae* and *M catarrhalis*.

Many clinical studies comparing the effectiveness of various antibacterial agents in the treatment of AOM do not carefully define standard criteria for diagnosis of AOM at entry or for improvement or

TABLE 5. Comparative AOM Outcomes for Initial Observation Versus Antibacterial Agent*

AOM Outcome	Initial Antibacterial Therapy	Initial Observation	P Value
Symptomatic relief at 24 hours[37,72]	60%	59%	NS
Symptomatic relief at 2–3 days[72]	91%	87%	NS
Symptomatic relief at 4–7 days[72]	79%	71%	NS
Clinical resolution at 7–14 days[72]	82%	72%	NS
Pain duration, mean days[73]	2.8	3.3	NS
Crying duration, mean days[73]	0.5	1.4	<.001
Analgesic use, mean doses[66]	2.3	4.1	.004
Fever duration, median days[66]	2.0	3.0	.004
Incidence of mastoiditis or suppurative complications[1]	0.59%	0.17%	NS
Persistent MEE at 4–6 weeks[72]	45%	48%	NS
Persistent MEE at 3 months[72]	21%	26%	NS
Antibacterial-agent–induced diarrhea or vomiting[74]	16%	—	—
Antibacterial-agent–induced skin rash[74]	2%	—	—

* NS indicates not significant.

cure at follow-up.[69] Another way to measure the outcome of treatment of AOM with various antibacterial agents is to assess bacteriologic efficacy. Although this does not provide a one-to-one correlation with clinical effectiveness, there is a definite concordance between the two.[77–79] Children who experience a bacteriologic cure improve more rapidly and more often than children who experience bacteriologic failure. Carlin et al[79] showed an 86% agreement between clinical and bacteriologic response. Dagan et al[77] showed that 91% of clinical failures at or before day 10 were culture-positive at days 4 to 5. If we use bacteriologic cure as a surrogate for clinical efficacy, there is strong evidence that drugs that achieve antibacterial concentrations that are able to eradicate pathogens from the middle-ear fluid are the preferred selection.[80,81]

Numerous studies have shown that the common pathogens in AOM are *Streptococcus pneumoniae*, nontypeable *H influenzae*, and *M catarrhalis*.[82,83] *S pneumoniae* has been recovered from the middle-ear fluid of approximately 25% to 50% of children with AOM, *H influenzae* from 15% to 30%, and *M catarrhalis* from approximately 3% to 20%.[83] There is some evidence that the microbiology of AOM may be changing as a result of routine use of the heptavalent pneumococcal vaccine. Block et al[84] showed an increase in *H Influenzae* from 39% to 52% of isolates in children 7 to 24 months of age with AOM and a decrease in *S pneumoniae* from 49% to 34% between 1992–1998 and 2000–2003. Viruses, including respiratory syncytial virus, rhinovirus, coronavirus, parainfluenza, adenovirus, and enterovirus, have been found in respiratory secretions and/or MEE in 40% to 75% of AOM cases and in MEE without bacteria in 5% to 22% of cases and may be responsible for many cases of apparent antibacterial agent "failure." In approximately 16% to 25% of cases of AOM, no bacterial or viral pathogen can be detected in MEE.[19,85,86]

Currently approximately 50% of isolates of *H influenzae* and 100% of *M catarrhalis* derived from the upper respiratory tract are likely to be β-lactamase–positive nationwide.[87] Between 15% and 50% (average: 30%) of upper respiratory tract isolates of *S pneumoniae* are also not susceptible to penicillin; approximately 50% of these are highly resistant to penicillin (minimum inhibitory concentration: 2.0 μg/mL or higher), and the remaining 50% are intermediate in resistance (minimum inhibitory concentration: between 0.1 and 1.0 μg/mL).[88–91] The mechanism of penicillin resistance among isolates of *S pneumoniae* is not associated with β-lactamase production but rather an alteration of penicillin-binding proteins. This phenomenon, which varies considerably according to geographic location, results in resistance to penicillins and cephalosporins.

Data from early studies of patients with AOM show that 19% of children with *S pneumoniae* and 48% with *H influenzae* cultured on initial tympanocentesis who were not treated with antibacterial agents cleared the bacteria at the time of a second tympanocentesis 2 to 7 days later.[92] Estimates are that approximately 75% of children infected with *M catarrhalis* also experience bacteriologic cure, based on resolution after treatment with an antibacterial agent to which it is not susceptible (amoxicillin).[93,94] Only *S pneumoniae* that are highly resistant to penicillin will not respond to conventional doses of amoxicillin.[95] Accordingly, approximately 80% of children with AOM will respond to treatment with high-dose amoxicillin, including many caused by resistant pneumococci. The higher dose will yield middle-ear fluid levels that exceed the minimum inhibitory concentration of all *S pneumoniae* that are intermediate in resistance to penicillin and many, but not all, highly resistant *S pneumoniae*.[76] Risk factors for the presence of bacterial species likely to be resistant to amoxicillin include attendance at child care, recent receipt (less than 30 days) of antibacterial treatment, and age younger than 2 years.[96,97]

If the patient is allergic to amoxicillin and the allergic reaction was not a type I hypersensitivity reaction (urticaria or anaphylaxis), cefdinir (14 mg/kg per day in 1 or 2 doses), cefpodoxime (10 mg/kg per day, once daily), or cefuroxime (30 mg/kg per day in 2 divided doses) can be used. In cases of type I reactions, azithromycin (10 mg/kg per day on day 1 followed by 5 mg/kg per day for 4 days as a single daily dose) or clarithromycin (15 mg/kg per day in 2 divided doses) can be used in an effort to select an antibacterial agent of an entirely different class. Other possibilities include erythromycin-sulfisoxazole (50 mg/kg per day of erythromycin) or sulfamethoxazole-trimethoprim (6–10 mg/kg per day of trimethoprim). Alternative therapy in the penicillin-allergic patient who is being treated for infection that is known or presumed to be caused by penicillin-resistant S pneumoniae is clindamycin at 30 to 40 mg/kg per day in 3 divided doses. In the patient who is vomiting or cannot otherwise tolerate oral medication, a single dose of parenteral ceftriaxone (50 mg/kg) has been shown to be effective for the initial treatment of AOM.[98,99]

The optimal duration of therapy for patients with AOM is uncertain. Studies comparing standard duration of treatment (10 days) to short-duration treatment (1–7 days) were often characterized by limitations including inadequate sample size (therefore having low or limited statistical power), few or no children younger than 2 years, exclusion of otitis-prone children, lack of standardized or stringent criteria for the diagnosis of AOM or for improvement or cure, use of an antibacterial medication that had less than optimal efficacy against common middle-ear pathogens, use of lower than recommended dosage of a medication, and lack of analysis of outcome by age.[100] Not surprisingly, the results of these studies were variable. Several more recent studies have been reported that addressed the issue of duration of therapy.[101–105] The results favoring standard 10-day therapy have been most significant in children younger than 2 years and suggestive of increased efficacy in those 2 to 5 years of age. Thus, for younger children and for children with severe disease, a standard 10-day course is recommended.[106] For children 6 years of age and older with mild to moderate disease, a 5- to 7-day course is appropriate.

RECOMMENDATION 4

If the patient fails to respond to the initial management option within 48 to 72 hours, the clinician must reassess the patient to confirm AOM and exclude other causes of illness. If AOM is confirmed in the patient initially managed with observation, the clinician should begin antibacterial therapy. If the patient was initially managed with an antibacterial agent, the clinician should change the antibacterial agent. (This recommendation is based on observational studies and a preponderance of benefit over risk.)

When antibacterial agents are prescribed for AOM, the time course of clinical response should be 48 to 72 hours. With few exceptions, the first 24 hours of therapy are characterized by a stabilization of the clinical condition. Early during this period the patient may actually worsen slightly. In the second 24 hours, the patient should begin to improve. If initially febrile, the patient is expected to defervesce within 48 to 72 hours. Irritability should improve, and sleeping and eating patterns should begin to normalize.[37] If the patient is not improved by 48 to 72 hours, either another disease is present or the therapy that has been chosen was not adequate. When

observation has been the chosen management and spontaneous improvement has not been noted by 48 to 72 hours, antibacterial therapy is indicated to limit the duration of further illness.

The patient should be given clear instructions at the initial visit as to when and how to communicate continuation or worsening of signs and symptoms to the clinician to expedite a change in treatment.

Antibacterial-agent choice after initial failure of observation or first-line antibacterial therapy should be based on the likely pathogen(s) present and on clinical experience. If the patient was treated with initial observation, amoxicillin should be started at a dose of 80 to 90 mg/kg per day. For patients who have severe illness (moderate to severe otalgia or temperature of 39°C or higher[42]), in those for whom additional coverage for β-lactamase–positive H influenzae and M catarrhalis is desired, and for those who had been treated initially with amoxicillin and did not improve, high-dose amoxicillin-clavulanate (90 mg/kg per day of amoxicillin component, with 6.4 mg/kg per day of clavulanate in 2 divided doses)[76] should be used. Alternatives in patients with a history of a non–type I allergic reaction to penicillins are cefdinir, cefpodoxime, or cefuroxime.[88] In cases of type I reactions, alternatives are azithromycin, clarithromycin, erythromycin-sulfisoxazole, or sulfamethoxazole-trimethoprim. Ceftriaxone (50 mg/kg per day), given for 3 consecutive days either intravenously or intramuscularly, can be used in children with vomiting or in other situations that preclude administration of oral antibacterial agents. In the treatment of AOM unresponsive to initial antibacterial therapy, a 3-day course of ceftriaxone has been shown to be better than a 1-day regimen.[99] Although trimethoprim-sulfamethoxazole and erythromycin-sulfisoxazole have traditionally been useful as first- and second-line therapy for patients with AOM, recent pneumococcal surveillance studies indicate that resistance to these 2 combination agents is substantial.[90,95] Therefore, when patients fail to improve while receiving amoxicillin, neither trimethoprim-sulfamethoxazole[107] nor erythromycin-sulfisoxazole is optimal for antibacterial therapy.

A patient who fails amoxicillin-potassium clavulanate should be treated with a 3-day course of parenteral ceftriaxone because of its superior efficacy against S pneumoniae, compared with alternative oral antibacterials.[91,99] If AOM persists, tympanocentesis should be recommended to make a bacteriologic diagnosis. If tympanocentesis is not available, a course of clindamycin may be considered for the rare case of penicillin-resistant pneumococcal infection not responding to the previous regimens. If the patient still does not improve, tympanocentesis with Gram-stain, culture, and antibacterial-agent sensitivity studies of the fluid is essential to guide additional therapy. Table 6 summarizes antibacterial options.

Once the patient has shown clinical improvement, follow-up is based on the usual clinical course of AOM. Persistent MEE after resolution of acute symptoms is common and should not be viewed as a need for active therapy. Two weeks after an episode of AOM, 60% to 70% of children have MEE, decreasing

TABLE 6. Recommended Antibacterial Agents for Patients Who Are Being Treated Initially With Antibacterial Agents or Have Failed 48 to 72 Hours of Observation or Initial Management With Antibacterial Agents

Temperature ≥ 39°C and/or Severe Otalgia	At Diagnosis for Patients Being Treated Initially With Antibacterial Agents		Clinically Defined Treatment Failure at 48–72 Hours After Initial Management With Observation Option		Clinically Defined Treatment Failure at 48–72 Hours After Initial Management With Antibacterial Agents	
	Recommended	Alternative for Penicillin Allergy	Recommended	Alternative for Penicillin Allergy	Recommended	Alternative for Penicillin Allergy
No	Amoxicillin, 80–90 mg/kg per day	Non-type I: cefdinir, cefuroxime, cefpodoxime; type I: azithromycin, clarithromycin	Amoxicillin, 80–90 mg/kg per day	Non-type I: cefdinir, cefuroxime, cefpodoxime; type I: azithromycin, clarithromycin	Amoxicillin-clavulanate, 90 mg/kg per day of amoxicillin component, with 6.4 mg/kg per day of clavulanate	Non-type I: ceftriaxone, 3 days; type I: clindamycin
Yes	Amoxicillin-clavulanate, 90 mg/kg per day of amoxicillin, with 6.4 mg/kg per day of clavulanate	Ceftriaxone, 1 or 3 days	Amoxicillin, clavulanate, 90 mg/kg per day of amoxicillin, with 6.4 mg/kg per day of clavulanate	Ceftriaxone, 1 or 3 days	Ceftriaxone, 3 days	Tympanocentesis, clindamycin

to 40% at 1 month and 10% to 25% after 3 months.[37(161–162)] OME must be differentiated clinically from AOM and requires additional monitoring but not antibacterial therapy. Assurance that OME resolves is particularly important for children with cognitive or developmental delays that may be impacted adversely by transient hearing loss associated with MEE.

RECOMMENDATION 5

Clinicians should encourage the prevention of AOM through reduction of risk factors. (This recommendation is based on strong observational studies and a preponderance of benefits over risks.)

A number of factors associated with early or recurrent AOM are not amenable to change, for example, genetic predisposition, premature birth, male gender, Native American/Inuit ethnicity, family history of recurrent otitis media, presence of siblings in the household, and low socioeconomic status.[108–113]

During infancy and early childhood, reducing the incidence of respiratory tract infections by altering child care center attendance patterns can reduce the incidence of recurrent AOM significantly.[108,114] The implementation of breastfeeding for at least the first 6 months also seems to be helpful against the development of early episodes of AOM.[108,109] Avoiding supine bottle feeding ("bottle propping"),[115] reducing or eliminating pacifier use in the second 6 months of life,[116] and eliminating exposure to passive tobacco smoke[117,118] have been postulated to reduce the incidence of AOM in infancy; however, the utility of these interventions is unclear.[108,109,114,119,120]

Immunoprophylaxis with killed[121] and live-attenuated intranasal[122] influenza vaccines has demonstrated more than 30% efficacy in prevention of AOM during the respiratory illness season. Most of the children in these studies were older than 2 years. A controlled study among infants and toddlers 6 to 23 months of age failed to demonstrate any efficacy of killed vaccine in preventing AOM.[123] Pneumococcal conjugate vaccines have proven effective in preventing vaccine-serotype pneumococcal otitis media, but their overall benefit is small, with only a 6% reduction in the incidence of AOM.[124–126] Medical office visits for otitis were reduced by 7.8% and antibiotic prescriptions by 5.7% in a large clinical practice after introduction of the pneumococcal conjugate vaccine.[127] Respiratory syncytial virus, parainfluenza virus, and adenovirus vaccines currently under development hold additional promise for prevention of ear infections.

RECOMMENDATION 6

No recommendations for complementary and alternative medicine (CAM) for treatment of AOM are made based on limited and controversial data.

Increasing numbers of parents/caregivers are using various forms of nonconventional treatment for their children.[128,129] The types of treatments used can differ depending on the ethnic background and belief system of the family and the availability of alternative medicine in a particular community. Treat-

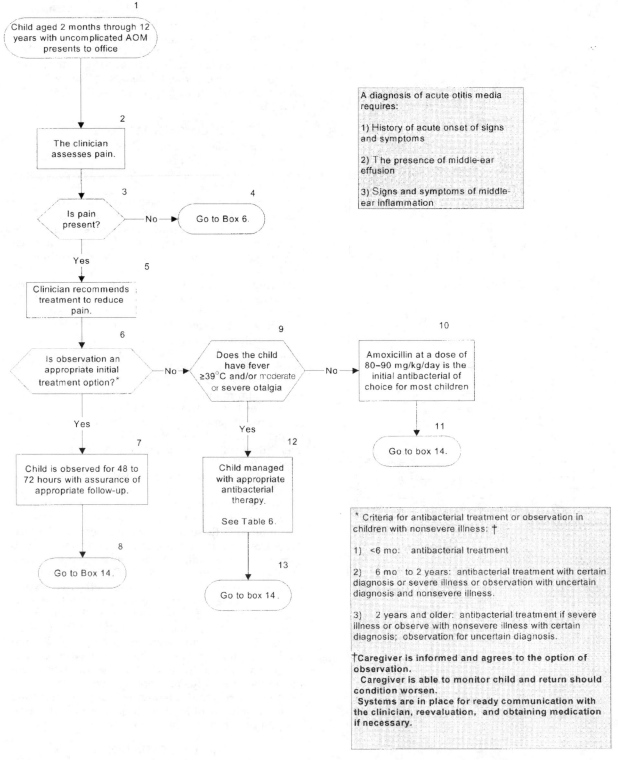

Fig 1. Management of AOM.

ments that have been used for AOM include homeopathy, acupuncture, herbal remedies, chiropractic treatments, and nutritional supplements.[130] Many physicians ask parents, caregivers, or older children if they are using medicines, supplements, or other means to maintain health or treat specific conditions;[131] however, parents/caregivers are often reluctant to tell their physicians that they are using

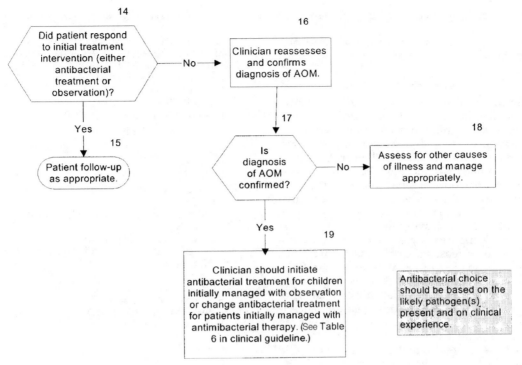

Fig 1. Continued.

complementary or alternative treatments.[132] Although most treatments are harmless, some are not. Some treatments can have a direct and dangerous effect, whereas others may interfere with the effects of conventional treatments.[30] Clinicians should become more informed about CAM, ask whether they are being used, and be ready to discuss potential benefits or risks.[133]

To date there are no studies that conclusively show a beneficial effect of alternative therapies used for AOM. Recent interest in the use of CAM has led to research efforts to investigate its efficacy.[134] It is difficult to design and conduct studies on certain forms of CAM because of the unique nature of the treatment.[135] Any study conducted will need to show proof of effectiveness of a specific therapy when compared with the natural history of AOM. Conclusions regarding CAM cannot be made until research evidence is available.

FUTURE RESEARCH

Despite the voluminous literature about AOM, there still are many opportunities for future research to continue to clarify the accurate diagnosis and most effective management of this common condition. Most important is that future studies address concerns regarding the quality and applicability of many studies in AOM.[21,69,78,100] Future studies should use standardized criteria for diagnosis, outcome, and severity of illness; increase sample size, which in general has been too limited to identify small but significant differences in clinical outcome; include children younger than 2 years and older than 12 years; use

doses of medication shown to achieve adequate levels in the middle ear to treat the target organisms successfully; and stratify outcomes by age and severity of illness. In addition, studies done in limited geographic areas must be replicated in other areas to ensure generalizability.

Some of the studies that should be considered include:

- Additional validation of standard definitions of AOM
- New or improved technologies for objective diagnosis of MEE
- Efficacy of education programs to improve clinician diagnostic skills
- Additional studies on pain management including topical agents, CAM, and role of tympanocentesis/myringotomy in pain management
- Large population-based studies on the benefits and risks of the "observation option" looking at antibacterial use; bacterial resistance; incidence of adverse events; long-term effects on hearing; persistence of MEE; and parent, patient, and clinician satisfaction
- Continued development of new antibacterial agents to address potential changes in resistance patterns of organisms responsible for AOM (studies on new agents must be appropriately designed and have adequate sample size to show clinical efficacy equal to or better than current agents)
- Randomized, controlled trials on duration of treatment in all age groups

- Vaccine research directed at more of the causative organisms of AOM
- Additional studies on potential measures to prevent AOM

SUMMARY

This clinical practice guideline provides evidence-based recommendations for the definition and management of AOM in children from 2 months through 12 years of age without signs or symptoms of systemic illness unrelated to the middle ear. It emphasizes accurate diagnosis and adherence to a consistent definition of AOM. Management of the pain associated with AOM is identified as an essential aspect of care. An option to observe a select group of children with AOM with symptomatic therapy for 48 to 72 hours is supported by evidence and may potentially lead to decreased use of antibacterial agents. If a decision is made to treat with an antibacterial agent, amoxicillin at a dose of 80 to 90 mg/kg per day is recommended as the initial antibacterial agent of choice for most children. Additional guidance is given for choosing an antibacterial agent when an alternative to amoxicillin is indicated. Also addressed is evidence related to the prevention of AOM and the role of CAM in the treatment of AOM. The recommendations are summarized in Fig. 1.

CONCLUSIONS

1. Recommendation: To diagnose AOM the clinician should confirm a history of acute onset, identify signs of MEE, and evaluate for the presence of signs and symptoms of middle-ear inflammation.
2. Strong recommendation: The management of AOM should include an assessment of pain. If pain is present, the clinician should recommend treatment to reduce pain.
3A. Option: Observation without use of antibacterial agents in a child with uncomplicated AOM is an option for selected children based on diagnostic certainty, age, illness severity, and assurance of follow-up.
3B. Recommendation: If a decision is made to treat with an antibacterial agent, the clinician should prescribe amoxicillin for most children.

   Option: When amoxicillin is used, the dose should be 80 to 90 mg/kg per day.

4. Recommendation: If the patient fails to respond to the initial management option within 48 to 72 hours, the clinician must reassess the patient to confirm AOM and exclude other causes of illness. If AOM is confirmed in the patient initially managed with observation, the clinician should begin antibacterial therapy. If the patient was initially managed with an antibacterial agent, the clinician should change the antibacterial agent.
5. Recommendation: Clinicians should encourage the prevention of AOM through reduction of risk factors.
6. No recommendation: There is insufficient evidence to make a recommendation regarding the use of CAM for AOM.

SUBCOMMITTEE ON MANAGEMENT OF ACUTE OTITIS MEDIA

Allan S. Lieberthal, MD, Cochairperson
Theodore G. Ganiats, MD, Cochairperson
Edward O. Cox, MD
Larry Culpepper, MD, MPH
Martin Mahoney, MD, PhD
Donald Miller, MD, MPH
Desmond K. Runyan, MD, DrPH
Nina Lisbeth Shapiro, MD
Ellen Wald, MD*

LIAISONS
Richard Besser, MD
　Centers for Disease Control and Prevention
Ellen Friedman, MD
　American Academy of Otolaryngology-Head and Neck Surgery
Norman Wendell Todd, MD
　American Academy of Otolaryngology-Head and Neck Surgery

CONSULTANTS
S. Michael Marcy, MD
Richard M. Rosenfeld, MD, MPH
Richard Shiffman, MD

STAFF
Maureen Hannley, PhD
Carla Herrerias, MPH
Bellinda Schoof, MHA, CPHQ

*Dr Ellen Wald withdrew from the Subcommittee on Management of Acute Otitis Media before publication of this guideline.

REFERENCES

1. Marcy M, Takata G, Chan LS, et al. Management of Acute Otitis Media. Evidence Report/Technology Assessment No. 15. AHRQ Publication No. 01-E010 Rockville, MD: Agency for Healthcare Research and Quality; 2001
2. Schappert SM. Office visits for otitis media: United States, 1975–90. Adv Data. 1992;214:1–18
3. Cherry DK, Woodwell DA. National ambulatory medical care survey: 2000 summary. Adv Data. 2002;328:1–32
4. McCaig LF, Besser RE, Hughes JM. Trends in antimicrobial prescribing rates for children and adolescents. JAMA. 2002;287:3096–3102
5. Niemela M, Uhari M, Jounio-Ervasti K, Luotonen J, Alho OP, Vierimaa E. Lack of specific symptomatology in children with acute otitis media. Pediatr Infect Dis J. 1994;13:765–768
6. Kontiokari T, Koivunen P, Niemela M, Pokka T, Uhari M. Symptoms of acute otitis media. Pediatr Infect Dis J. 1998;17:676–679
7. Pelton SI. Otoscopy for the diagnosis of otitis media. Pediatr Infect Dis J. 1998;17:540–543
8. Brookhouser PE. Use of tympanometry in office practice for diagnosis of otitis media. Pediatr Infect Dis J. 1998;17:544–551
9. Kimball S. Acoustic reflectometry: spectral gradient analysis for improved detection of middle ear effusion in children. Pediatr Infect Dis J. 1998;17:552–555
10. Barnett ED, Klein JO, Hawkins KA, Cabral HJ, Kenna M, Healy G. Comparison of spectral gradient acoustic reflectometry and other diagnostic techniques for detection of middle ear effusion in children with middle ear disease. Pediatr Infect Dis J. 1998;17:556–559
11. Block SL, Mandel E, McLinn S, et al. Spectral gradient acoustic reflectometry for detection of middle ear effusion by pediatricians and parents. Pediatr Infect Dis J. 1998;17:560–564
12. Block SL, Pichichero ME, McLinn S, Aronovitz G, Kimball S. Spectral gradient acoustic reflectometry: detection of middle ear effusion in suppurative acute otitis media. Pediatr Infect Dis J. 1999;18:741–744
13. Karma PH, Penttila MA, Sipila MM, Kataja MJ. Otoscopic diagnosis of middle ear effusion in acute and non-acute otitis media. I. The value of different otoscopic findings. Int J Pediatr Otorhinolaryngol. 1989;17:37–49
14. Karma PH, Sipila MM, Kataja MJ, Penttila MA. Pneumatic otoscopy and otitis media. II. Value of different tympanic membrane findings

and their combinations. In: Lim DJ, Bluestone CD, Klein JO, Nelson JD, Ogra PL, eds. *Recent Advances in Otitis Media: Proceedings of the Fifth International Symposium*. Burlington, ON, Canada: Decker Periodicals; 1993:41–45

15. Merifield DO, Miller GS. The etiology and clinical course of bullous myringitis. *Arch Otolaryngol*. 1966;84:487–489

16. Klein JO, McCracken GH Jr. Introduction: current assessments of diagnosis and management of otitis media. *Pediatr Infect Dis J*. 1998; 17:539

17. Pichichero ME, Poole MD. Assessing diagnostic accuracy and tympanocentesis skills in the management of otitis media. *Arch Pediatr Adolesc Med*. 2001;155:1137–1142

18. Pichichero ME. Diagnostic accuracy, tympanocentesis training performance, and antibiotic selection by pediatric residents in management of otitis media. *Pediatrics*. 2002;110:1064–1070

19. Chonmaitree T. Viral and bacterial interaction in acute otitis media. *Pediatr Infect Dis J*. 2000;19(suppl):S24–S30

20. Dowell SF, Marcy SM, Phillips WR, Gerber MA, Schwartz B. Otitis media—principles of judicious use of antimicrobial agents. *Pediatrics*. 1998;101:165–171

21. Wald ER. Acute otitis media: more trouble with the evidence. *Pediatr Infect Dis J*. 2003;22:103–104

22. Rosenfeld RM. Diagnostic certainty for acute otitis media. *Int J Pediatr Otorhinolaryngol*. 2002;64:89–95

23. Hayden GF, Schwartz RH. Characteristics of earache among children with acute otitis media. *Am J Dis Child*. 1985;139:721–723

24. Schechter NL. Management of pain associated with acute medical illness. In: Schechter NL, Berde CB, Yaster M, eds. *Pain in Infants, Children, and Adolescents*. Baltimore, MD: Williams & Wilkins; 1993: 537–538

25. American Academy of Pediatrics, Committee on Psychosocial Aspects of Child and Family Health; Task Force on Pain in Infants, Children, and Adolescents. The assessment and management of acute pain in infants, children, and adolescents. *Pediatrics*. 2001;108:793–797

26. Bertin L, Pons G, d'Athis P, et al. A randomized, double-blind, multicentre controlled trial of ibuprofen versus acetaminophen and placebo for symptoms of acute otitis media in children. *Fundam Clin Pharmacol*. 1996;10:387–392

27. Hoberman A, Paradise JL, Reynolds EA, Urkin J. Efficacy of Auralgan for treating ear pain in children with acute otitis media. *Arch Pediatr Adolesc Med*. 1997;151:675–678

28. Sarrell EM, Mandelberg A, Cohen HA. Efficacy of naturopathic extracts in the management of ear pain associated with acute otitis media. *Arch Pediatr Adolesc Med*. 2001;155:796–799

29. Barnett ED, Levatin JL, Chapman EH, et al. Challenges of evaluating homeopathic treatment of acute otitis media. *Pediatr Infect Dis J*. 2000; 19:273–275

30. Jacobs J, Springer DA, Crothers D. Homeopathic treatment of acute otitis media in children: a preliminary randomized placebo-controlled trial. *Pediatr Infect Dis J*. 2001;20:177–183

31. Rosenfeld RM, Bluestone CD. Clinical efficacy of surgical therapy. In: Rosenfeld RM, Bluestone CD, eds. *Evidence-Based Otitis Media*. 2nd ed. Hamilton, ON, Canada: BC Decker Inc; 2003:227–240

32. New York Region Otitis Project. *Observation Option Toolkit for Acute Otitis Media*. Publication No. 4894. New York, NY: State of New York, Department of Health; 2002

33. Rosenfeld RM. Observation option toolkit for acute otitis media. *Int J Pediatr Otorhinolaryngol*. 2001;58:1–8

34. Rosenfeld RM, Vertrees JE, Carr J, et al. Clinical efficacy of antimicrobial drugs for acute otitis media: metaanalysis of 5400 children from thirty-three randomized trials. *J Pediatr*. 1994;124:355–367

35. Del Mar C, Glasziou P, Hayem M. Are antibiotics indicated as initial treatment for children with acute otitis media? A meta-analysis. *BMJ*. 1997;314:1526–1529

36. Glasziou PP, Del Mar CB, Hayem M, Sanders SL. Antibiotics for acute otitis media in children. *Cochrane Database Syst Rev*. 2000;4:CD000219

37. Rosenfeld RM, Kay D. Natural history of untreated otitis media. In: Rosenfeld RM, Bluestone CD, eds. *Evidence-Based Otitis Media*. 2nd ed. Hamilton, ON, Canada: BC Decker Inc; 2003:180–198

38. Appelman CL, Van Balen FA, Van de Lisdonk EH, Van Weert HC, Eizenga WH. Otitis media acuta. NHG-standaard (eerste herziening) [in Dutch]. *Huisarts Wet*. 1999;42:362–366

39. van Buchem FL, Peeters MF, van't Hof MA. Acute otitis media: a new treatment strategy. *Br Med J (Clin Res Ed)*. 1985;290:1033–1037

40. Little P, Gould C, Williamson I, Moore M, Warner G, Dunleavey J. Pragmatic randomised controlled trial of two prescribing strategies for childhood acute otitis media. *BMJ*. 2001;322:336–342

41. Little P, Gould C, Moore M, Warner G, Dunleavey J, Williamson I. Predictors of poor outcome and benefits from antibiotics in children with acute otitis media: pragmatic randomised trial. *BMJ*. 2002;325:22

42. Kaleida PH, Casselbrant ML, Rockette HE, et al. Amoxicillin or myringotomy or both for acute otitis media: results of a randomized clinical trial. *Pediatrics*. 1991;87:466–474

43. Barry B, Gehanno P, Blumen M, Boucot I. Clinical outcome of acute otitis media caused by pneumococci with decreased susceptibility to penicillin. *Scand J Infect Dis*. 1994;26:446–452

44. Appelman CL, Claessen JQ, Touw-Otten FW, Hordijk GJ, de Melker RA. Co-amoxiclav in recurrent acute otitis media: placebo controlled study. *BMJ*. 1991;303:1450–1452

45. Froom J, Culpepper L, Grob P, et al. Diagnosis and antibiotic treatment of acute otitis media: report from International Primary Care Network. *BMJ*. 1990;300:582–586

46. Froom J, Culpepper L, Bridges-Webb C, et al. Effect of patient characteristics and disease manifestations on the outcome of acute otitis media at 2 months. *Arch Fam Med*. 1993;2:841–846

47. Shurin PA, Rehmus JM, Johnson CE, et al. Bacterial polysaccharide immune globulin for prophylaxis of acute otitis media in high-risk children. *J Pediatr*. 1993;123:801–810

48. Rudberg RD. Acute otitis media: comparative therapeutic results of sulfonamide and penicillin administered in various forms. *Acta Otolaryngol Suppl*. 1954;113:1–79

49. Palva T, Pulkkinen K. Mastoiditis. *J Laryngol Otol*. 1959;73:573–588

50. Hoppe JE, Koster S, Bootz F, Niethammer D. Acute mastoiditis—relevant once again. *Infection*. 1994;22:178–182

51. Bahadori RS, Schwartz RH, Ziai M. Acute mastoiditis in children: an increase in frequency in Northern Virginia. *Pediatr Infect Dis J*. 2000; 19:212–215

52. Faye-Lund H. Acute and latent mastoiditis. *J Laryngol Otol*. 1989;103: 1158–1160

53. Ghaffar FA, Wordemann M, McCracken GH Jr. Acute mastoiditis in children: a seventeen-year experience in Dallas, Texas. *Pediatr Infect Dis J*. 2001;20:376–380

54. Harley EH, Sdralis T, Berkowitz RG. Acute mastoiditis in children: a 12-year retrospective study. *Otolaryngol Head Neck Surg*. 1997;116: 26–30

55. Kaplan SL, Mason EO Jr, Wald ER, et al. Pneumococcal mastoiditis in children. *Pediatrics*. 2000;106:695–699

56. Kvestad E, Kvaerner KJ, Mair IW. Acute mastoiditis: predictors for surgery. *Int J Pediatr Otorhinolaryngol*. 2000;52:149–155

57. Linder TE, Briner HR, Bischoff T. Prevention of acute mastoiditis: fact or fiction? *Int J Pediatr Otorhinolaryngol*. 2000;56:129–134

58. Nadal D, Herrmann P, Baumann A, Fanconi A. Acute mastoiditis: clinical, microbiological, and therapeutic aspects. *Eur J Pediatr*. 1990; 149:560–564

59. Petersen CG, Ovesen T, Pedersen CB. Acute mastoidectomy in a Danish county from 1977 to 1996 with focus on the bacteriology. *Int J Pediatr Otorhinolaryngol*. 1998;45:21–29

60. Scott TA, Jackler RK. Acute mastoiditis in infancy: a sequela of unrecognized acute otitis media. *Otolaryngol Head Neck Surg*. 1989;101: 683–687

61. Dhooge IJ, Albers FW, Van Cauwenberge PB. Intratemporal and intracranial complications of acute suppurative otitis media in children: renewed interest. *Int J Pediatr Otorhinolaryngol*. 1999;49:S109–S114

62. Gliklich RE, Eavey RD, Iannuzzi RA, Camacho AE. A contemporary analysis of acute mastoiditis. *Arch Otolaryngol Head Neck Surg*. 1996; 122:135–139

63. Luntz M, Brodsky A, Nusem S, et al. Acute mastoiditis—the antibacterial agent era: a multicenter study. *Int J Pediatr Otorhinolaryngol*. 2001;57:1–9

64. Van Zuijlen DA, Schilder AG, Van Balen FA, Hoes AW. National differences in acute mastoiditis: relationship to prescribing patterns of antibiotics for acute otitis media? *Pediatr Infect Dis J*. 2001;20:140–144

65. Schutzman SA, Petrycki S, Fleisher GR. Bacteremia with otitis media. *Pediatrics*. 1991;87:48–53

66. Damoiseaux RA, van Balen FA, Hoes AW, Vaerheij TJ, de Melker RA. Primary care based randomised, double blind trial of amoxicillin versus placebo for acute otitis media in children aged under 2 years. *BMJ*. 2000;320:350–354

67. Kilpi T, Anttila M, Kallio MJ, Peltola H. Severity of childhood bacterial meningitis: duration of illness before diagnosis. *Lancet*. 1991;338: 406–409

68. Whitney CG, Farley MM, Hadler J, et al. Decline in invasive pneumococcal disease after the introduction of protein-polysaccharide conjugate vaccine. *N Engl J Med*. 2003;348:1737–1746

69. Dagan R, McCracken GH Jr. Flaws in design and conduct of clinical trials in acute otitis media. *Pediatr Infect Dis J.* 2002;21:894–902

70. Cates C. An evidence based approach to reducing antibiotic use in children with acute otitis media: controlled before and after study. *BMJ.* 1999;318:715–716

71. Siegel RM, Kiely M, Bien JP, et al. Treatment of otitis media with observation and a safety-net antibiotic prescription. *Pediatrics.* 2003; 112:527–531

72. Rosenfeld RM. Clinical efficacy of medical therapy. In: Rosenfeld RM, Bluestone CD, eds. *Evidence-Based Otitis Media.* 2nd ed. Hamilton, ON, Canada: BC Decker Inc; 2003:199–226

73. Burke P, Bain J, Robinson D, Dunleavey J. Acute red ear in children: controlled trial of non-antibiotic treatment in general practice. *BMJ.* 1991;303:558–562

74. Ruben RJ. Sequelae of antibiotic therapy. In: Rosenfeld RM, Bluestone CD, eds. *Evidence-Based Otitis Media.* Hamilton, ON, Canada: BC Decker Inc; 1999:303–314

75. Piglansky L, Leibovitz E, Raiz S, et al. Bacteriologic and clinical efficacy of high dose amoxicillin for therapy of acute otitis media in children. *Pediatr Infect Dis J.* 2003;22:405–413

76. Dagan R, Hoberman A, Johnson C, et al. Bacteriologic and clinical efficacy of high dose amoxicillin/clavulanate in children with acute otitis media. *Pediatr Infect Dis J.* 2001;20:829–837

77. Dagan R, Leibovitz E, Greenberg D, Yagupsky P, Fliss DM, Leiberman A. Early eradication of pathogens from middle ear fluid during antibiotic treatment of acute otitis media is associated with improved clinical outcome. *Pediatr Infect Dis J.* 1998;17:776–782

78. Marchant CD, Carlin SA, Johnson CE, Shurin PA. Measuring the comparative efficacy of antibacterial agents for acute otitis media: the "Pollyanna phenomenon." *J Pediatr.* 1992;120:72–77

79. Carlin SA, Marchant CD, Shurin PA, Johnson CE, Super DM, Rehmus JM. Host factors and early therapeutic response in acute otitis media. *J Pediatr.* 1991;118:178–183

80. Vogelman B, Gudmundsson S, Leggett J, Turnidge J, Ebert S, Craig WA. Correlation of antimicrobial pharmacokinetic parameters with therapeutic efficacy in an animal model. *J Infect Dis.* 1988;158:831–847

81. Craig W. Pharmacokinetic/pharmacodynamic parameters: rationale for antibacterial dosing of mice and men. *Clin Infect Dis.* 1998;26:1–10

82. Berman S. Otitis media in children. *N Engl J Med.* 1995;332:1560–1565

83. Klein JO. Otitis media. *Clin Infect Dis.* 1994;19:823–833

84. Block SL, Hedrick JA, Harrison CJ. Routine use of Prevnar in a pediatric practice profoundly alters the microbiology of acute otitis media. Paper presented at: Pediatric Academic Societies Annual Meeting; May 3–6, 2003; Seattle, WA

85. Pitkaranta A, Virolainen A, Jero J, Arruda E, Hayden FG. Detection of rhinovirus, respiratory syncytial virus, and coronavirus infections in acute otitis media by reverse transcriptase polymerase chain reaction. *Pediatrics.* 1998;102:291–295

86. Heikkinen T, Thint M, Chonmaitree T. Prevalence of various respiratory viruses in the middle ear during acute otitis media. *N Engl J Med.* 1999;340:260–264

87. Doern GV, Jones RN, Pfaller MA, Kugler K. *Haemophilus influenzae* and *Moraxella catarrhalis* from patients with community-acquired respiratory tract infections: antimicrobial susceptibility patterns from the SENTRY Antimicrobial Surveillance Program (United States and Canada, 1997). *Antimicrob Agents Chemother.* 1999;43:385–389

88. Sinus and Allergy Health Partnership. Antibacterial treatment guidelines for acute bacterial rhinosinusitis. *Otolaryngol Head Neck Surg.* 2000;123:S5–S31

89. Doern GV, Brueggemann AB, Pierce G, Holley HP Jr, Rauch A. Antibiotic resistance among clinical isolates of *Haemophilus influenzae* in the United States in 1994 and 1995 and detection of beta-lactamase-positive strains resistant to amoxicillin-clavulanate: results of a national multicenter surveillance study. *Antimicrob Agents Chemother.* 1997;41:292–297

90. Doern GV, Pfaller MA, Kugler K, Freeman J, Jones RN. Prevalence of antimicrobial resistance among respiratory tract isolates of *Streptococcus pneumoniae* in North America: 1997 results from the SENTRY Antimicrobial Surveillance Program. *Clin Infect Dis.* 1998;27:764–770

91. Jacobs MR, Felmingham D, Appelbaum PC, Gruneberg RN, Alexander Project Group. The Alexander Project 1998–2000: susceptibility of pathogens isolated from community-acquired respiratory tract infection to commonly used antimicrobial agents. *J Antimicrob Chemother.* 2003;52:229–246

92. Howie VM, Ploussard JH. Efficacy of fixed combination antibiotics versus separate components in otitis media. Effectiveness of erythromycin estolate, triple sulfonamide, ampicillin, erythromycin estolate-triple sulfonamide, and placebo in 280 patients with acute otitis media under two and one-half years of age. *Clin Pediatr (Phila).* 1972;11: 205–214

93. Klein JO. Microbiologic efficacy of antibacterial drugs for acute otitis media. *Pediatr Infect Dis J.* 1993;12:973–975

94. Barnett ED, Klein JO. The problem of resistant bacteria for the management of acute otitis media. *Pediatr Clin North Am.* 1995;42:509–517

95. Jacobs MR, Bajaksouzian S, Zilles A, Lin G, Pankuch GA, Appelbaum PC. Susceptibilities of *Streptococcus pneumoniae* and *Haemophilus influenzae* to 10 oral antimicrobial agents, based on pharmacodynamic parameters: 1997 U.S. Surveillance study. *Antimicrob Agents Chemother.* 1999;43:1901–1908

96. Wald ER, Mason EO Jr, Bradley JS, Barson WJ, Kaplan SL, US Pediatric Multicenter Pneumococcal Surveillance Group. Acute otitis media caused by *Streptococcus pneumoniae* in children's hospitals between 1994 and 1997. *Pediatr Infect Dis J.* 2001;20:34–39

97. Kellner JD, Ford-Jones EL. *Streptococcus pneumoniae* carriage in children attending 59 Canadian child care centers. Toronto Child Care Centre Study Group. *Arch Pediatr Adolesc Med.* 1999;153:495–502

98. Green SM, Rothrock SG. Single-dose intramuscular ceftriaxone for acute otitis media in children. *Pediatrics.* 1993;91:23–30

99. Leibovitz E, Piglansky L, Raiz S, Press J, Leiberman A, Dagan R. Bacteriologic and clinical efficacy of one day vs. three day intramuscular ceftriaxone for treatment of nonresponsive acute otitis media in children. *Pediatr Infect Dis J.* 2000;19:1040–1045

100. Paradise JL. Short-course antibacterial treatment for acute otitis media: not best for infants and young children. *JAMA.* 1997;278:1640–1642

101. Hoberman A, Paradise JL, Burch DJ, et al. Equivalent efficacy and reduced occurrence of diarrhea from a new formulation of amoxicillin/clavulanate potassium (Augmentin) for treatment of acute otitis media in children. *Pediatr Infect Dis J.* 1997;16:463–470

102. Cohen R, Levy C, Boucherat M, Langue J, de la Rocque F. A multicenter, randomized, double-blind trial of 5 versus 10 days of antibacterial agent therapy for acute otitis media in young children. *J Pediatr.* 1998;133:634–639

103. Cohen R, Levy C, Boucherat M, et al. Five vs. ten days of antibiotic therapy for acute otitis media in young children. *Pediatr Infect Dis J.* 2000;19:458–463

104. Pessey JJ, Gehanno P, Thoroddsen E, et al. Short course therapy with cefuroxime axetil for acute otitis media: results of a randomized multicenter comparison with amoxicillin/clavulanate. *Pediatr Infect Dis J.* 1999;18:854–859

105. Pichichero ME, Marsocci SM, Murphy ML, Hoeger W, Francis AB, Green JL. A prospective observational study of 5-, 7-, and 10-day antibiotic treatment for acute otitis media. *Otolaryngol Head Neck Surg.* 2001;124:381–387

106. Dowell SF, Butler JC, Giebink SG, et al. Acute otitis media: management and surveillance in an era of pneumococcal resistance—a report from the Drug-Resistant *Streptococcus pneumoniae* Therapeutic Working Group. *Pediatr Infect Dis J.* 1999;18:1–9

107. Leiberman A, Leibovitz E, Piglansky L, et al. Bacteriologic and clinical efficacy of trimethoprim-sulfamethoxazole for the treatment of acute otitis media. *Pediatr Infect Dis J.* 2001;20:260–264

108. Daly KA, Giebink GS. Clinical epidemiology of otitis media. *Pediatr Infect Dis J.* 2000;19(suppl 5):S31–S36

109. Paradise JL, Rockette HE, Colborn DK, et al. Otitis media in 2253 Pittsburgh-area infants: prevalence and risk factors during the first two years of life. *Pediatrics.* 1997;99:318–333

110. Kero P, Piekkala P. Factors affecting the occurrence of acute otitis media during the first year of life. *Acta Paediatr Scand.* 1987;76:618–623

111. Curns AT, Holman RC, Shay DK, et al. Outpatient and hospital visits associated with otitis media among American Indian and Alaska Native children younger than 5 years. *Pediatrics.* 2002;109(3). Available at: www.pediatrics.org/cgi/content/full/109/3/e41

112. Casselbrant ML, Mandel EM, Fall PA, et al. The hereditability of otitis media: a twin and triplet study. *JAMA.* 1999;282:2125–2130

113. Uhari M, Mantysaari K, Niemela M. A meta-analytic review of the risk factors for acute otitis media. *Clin Infect Dis.* 1996;22:1079–1083

114. Adderson EE. Preventing otitis media: medical approaches. *Pediatr Ann.* 1998;27:101–107

115. Brown CE, Magnuson B. On the physics of the infant feeding bottle and middle ear sequela: ear disease in infants can be associated with bottle feeding. *Int J Pediatr Otorhinolaryngol.* 2000;54:13–20

116. Niemela M, Pihakari O, Pokka T, Uhari M. Pacifier as a risk factor for acute otitis media: a randomized, controlled trial of parental counseling. *Pediatrics.* 2000;106:483–488

117. Etzel RA, Pattishall EN, Haley NJ, Fletcher RH, Henderson FW. Passive smoking and middle ear effusion among children in day care. *Pediatrics.* 1992;90:228–232

118. Ilicali OC, Keles N, Deger K, Savas I. Relationship of passive cigarette smoking to otitis media. *Arch Otolaryngol Head Neck Surg.* 1999;125: 758–762

119. Wellington M, Hall CB. Pacifier as a risk factor for acute otitis media [letter]. *Pediatrics.* 2002;109:351

120. Paradise JL, Ah-Tye C. Positional otitis media and otorrhea after tympanostomy-tube placement [letter]. *Pediatrics.* 2002;109:349–350

121. Clements DA, Langdon L, Bland C, Walter E. Influenza A vaccine decreases the incidence of otitis media in 6- to 30-month-old children in day care. *Arch Pediatr Adolesc Med.* 1995;149:1113–1117

122. Belshe RB, Gruber WC. Prevention of otitis media in children with live attenuated influenza vaccine given intranasally. *Pediatr Infect Dis J.* 2000;19(suppl 5):S66–S71

123. Hoberman A, Greenberg DP, Paradise JL, et al. Effectiveness of inactivated influenza vaccine in preventing acute otitis media in young children: a randomized controlled trial. *JAMA.* 2003;290:1608–1616

124. Eskola J, Kilpi T, Palmu A, et al. Efficacy of a pneumococcal conjugate vaccine against acute otitis media. *N Engl J Med.* 2001;344:403–409

125. Black S, Shinefield H, Fireman B, et al. Efficacy, safety and immunogenicity of heptavalent pneumococcal conjugate vaccine in children. *Pediatr Infect Dis J.* 2000;19:187–195

126. Jacobs MR. Prevention of otitis media: role of pneumococcal conjugate vaccines in reducing incidence and antibiotic resistance. *J Pediatr.* 2002;141:287–293

127. Fireman B, Black SB, Shinefield HR, Lee J, Lewis E, Ray P. Impact of the pneumococcal conjugate vaccine on otitis media. *Pediatr Infect Dis J.* 2003;22:10–16

128. Eisenberg DM, Kessler RC, Foster C, Norlock FE, Calkins DR, Delbanco TL. Unconventional medicine in the United States. *N Engl J Med.* 1993;328:246–252

129. Eisenberg DM, Davis R, Ettner S, et al. Trends in alternative medicine use in the United States, 1990–1997: results of a follow-up national survey. *JAMA.* 1998;280:1569–1575

130. Spigelblatt L, Laine-Ammara G, Pless IB, Guyver A. The use of alternative medicine by children. *Pediatrics.* 1994;94:811–814

131. Angell M, Kassirer JP. Alternative medicine—the risks of untested and unregulated remedies. *N Engl J Med.* 1998;339:839–841

132. Kemper KJ. *The Holistic Pediatrician: A Parent's Comprehensive Guide to Safe and Effective Therapies for the 25 Most Common Childhood Ailments.* New York, NY: Harper Perennial; 1996

133. American Academy of Pediatrics, Committee on Children With Disabilities. Counseling families who choose complementary and alternative medicine for their child with chronic illness or disability. *Pediatrics.* 2001;107:598–601

134. Grimm W, Muller HH. A randomized controlled trial of the effect of fluid extract of *Echinacea purpurea* on the incidence and severity of colds and respiratory infections. *Am J Med.* 1999;106:138–143

135. Barret B, Vohmann M, Calabrese C. Echinacea for upper respiratory infection. *J Fam Pract.* 1999;48:628–635

136. van Buchem FL, Dunk JH, van't Hof MA. Therapy of acute otitis media: myringotomy, antibiotics, or neither? A double-blind study in children. *Lancet.* 1981;2(8252):883–887

Otitis Media With Effusion

• *Clinical Practice Guideline*

AMERICAN ACADEMY OF PEDIATRICS

CLINICAL PRACTICE GUIDELINE

American Academy of Family Physicians, American Academy of Otolaryngology-Head and Neck Surgery, and American Academy of Pediatrics Subcommittee on Otitis Media With Effusion

Otitis Media With Effusion

ABSTRACT. The clinical practice guideline on otitis media with effusion (OME) provides evidence-based recommendations on diagnosing and managing OME in children. This is an update of the 1994 clinical practice guideline "Otitis Media With Effusion in Young Children," which was developed by the Agency for Healthcare Policy and Research (now the Agency for Healthcare Research and Quality). In contrast to the earlier guideline, which was limited to children 1 to 3 years old with no craniofacial or neurologic abnormalities or sensory deficits, the updated guideline applies to children aged 2 months through 12 years with or without developmental disabilities or underlying conditions that predispose to OME and its sequelae. The American Academy of Pediatrics, American Academy of Family Physicians, and American Academy of Otolaryngology-Head and Neck Surgery selected a subcommittee composed of experts in the fields of primary care, otolaryngology, infectious diseases, epidemiology, hearing, speech and language, and advanced-practice nursing to revise the OME guideline.

The subcommittee made a strong recommendation that clinicians use pneumatic otoscopy as the primary diagnostic method and distinguish OME from acute otitis media.

The subcommittee made recommendations that clinicians should 1) document the laterality, duration of effusion, and presence and severity of associated symptoms at each assessment of the child with OME, 2) distinguish the child with OME who is at risk for speech, language, or learning problems from other children with OME and more promptly evaluate hearing, speech, language, and need for intervention in children at risk, and 3) manage the child with OME who is not at risk with watchful waiting for 3 months from the date of effusion onset (if known) or diagnosis (if onset is unknown).

The subcommittee also made recommendations that 4) hearing testing be conducted when OME persists for 3 months or longer or at any time that language delay, learning problems, or a significant hearing loss is suspected in a child with OME, 5) children with persistent OME who are not at risk should be reexamined at 3- to 6-month intervals until the effusion is no longer present, significant hearing loss is identified, or structural abnormalities of the eardrum or middle ear are suspected, and 6) when a child becomes a surgical candidate (tympanostomy tube insertion is the preferred initial procedure). Adenoidectomy should not be performed unless a distinct indication exists (nasal obstruction, chronic adenoiditis); repeat surgery consists of adenoidectomy plus myringotomy with or without tubeinsertion. Tonsillectomy alone or myringotomy alone should not be used to treat OME.

The subcommittee made negative recommendations that 1) population-based screening programs for OME not be performed in healthy, asymptomatic children, and 2) because antihistamines and decongestants are ineffective for OME, they should not be used for treatment; antimicrobials and corticosteroids do not have long-term efficacy and should not be used for routine management.

The subcommittee gave as options that 1) tympanometry can be used to confirm the diagnosis of OME and 2) when children with OME are referred by the primary clinician for evaluation by an otolaryngologist, audiologist, or speech-language pathologist, the referring clinician should document the effusion duration and specific reason for referral (evaluation, surgery) and provide additional relevant information such as history of acute otitis media and developmental status of the child. The subcommittee made no recommendations for 1) complementary and alternative medicine as a treatment for OME, based on a lack of scientific evidence documenting efficacy, or 2) allergy management as a treatment for OME, based on insufficient evidence of therapeutic efficacy or a causal relationship between allergy and OME. Last, the panel compiled a list of research needs based on limitations of the evidence reviewed.

The purpose of this guideline is to inform clinicians of evidence-based methods to identify, monitor, and manage OME in children aged 2 months through 12 years. The guideline may not apply to children more than 12 years old, because OME is uncommon and the natural history is likely to differ from younger children who experience rapid developmental change. The target population includes children with or without developmental disabilities or underlying conditions that predispose to OME and its sequelae. The guideline is intended for use by providers of health care to children, including primary care and specialist physicians, nurses and nurse practitioners, physician assistants, audiologists, speech-language pathologists, and child-development specialists. The guideline is applicable to any setting in which children with OME would be identified, monitored, or managed.

This guideline is not intended as a sole source of guidance in evaluating children with OME. Rather, it is designed to assist primary care and other clinicians by providing an evidence-based framework for decision-making strategies. It is not intended to replace clinical judgment or establish a protocol for all children with this condition and may not provide the only appropriate approach to diagnosing and managing this problem. *Pediatrics* 2004;113:1412–1429; *acute otitis media, antibacterial, antibiotic.*

This document was approved by the American Academy of Otolaryngology–Head and Neck Surgery Foundation, Inc and the American Academy of Pediatrics, and is published in the May 2004 issue of *Otolaryngology-Head and Neck Surgery* and the May 2004 issue of *Pediatrics*.
PEDIATRICS (ISSN 0031 4005). Copyright © 2004 by the American Academy of Otolaryngology–Head and Neck Surgery Foundation, Inc and the American Academy of Pediatrics.

ABBREVIATIONS. OME, otitis media with effusion; AOM, acute otitis media; AAP, American Academy of Pediatrics; AHRQ, Agency for Healthcare Research and Quality; EPC, Southern California Evidence-Based Practice Center; CAM, complementary and alternative medicine; HL, hearing level.

Otitis media with effusion (OME) as discussed in this guideline is defined as the presence of fluid in the middle ear without signs or symptoms of acute ear infection.[1,2] OME is considered distinct from acute otitis media (AOM), which is defined as a history of acute onset of signs and symptoms, the presence of middle-ear effusion, and signs and symptoms of middle-ear inflammation. Persistent middle-ear fluid from OME results in decreased mobility of the tympanic membrane and serves as a barrier to sound conduction.[3] Approximately 2.2 million diagnosed episodes of OME occur annually in the United States, yielding a combined direct and indirect annual cost estimate of $4.0 billion.[2]

OME may occur spontaneously because of poor eustachian tube function or as an inflammatory response following AOM. Approximately 90% of children (80% of individual ears) have OME at some time before school age,[4] most often between ages 6 months and 4 years.[5] In the first year of life, >50% of children will experience OME, increasing to >60% by 2 years.[6] Many episodes resolve spontaneously within 3 months, but ~30% to 40% of children have recurrent OME, and 5% to 10% of episodes last 1 year or longer.[1,4,7]

The primary outcomes considered in the guideline include hearing loss; effects on speech, language, and learning; physiologic sequelae; health care utilization (medical, surgical); and quality of life.[1,2] The high prevalence of OME, difficulties in diagnosis and assessing duration, increased risk of conductive hearing loss, potential impact on language and cognition, and significant practice variations in management[8] make OME an important condition for the use of up-to-date evidence-based practice guidelines.

METHODS

General Methods and Literature Search

In developing an evidence-based clinical practice guideline on managing OME, the American Academy of Pediatrics (AAP), American Academy of Family Physicians, and American Academy of Otolaryngology-Head and Neck Surgery worked with the Agency for Healthcare Research and Quality (AHRQ) and other organizations. This effort included representatives from each partnering organization along with liaisons from audiology, speech-language pathology, informatics, and advanced-practice nursing. The most current literature on managing children with OME was reviewed, and research questions were developed to guide the evidence-review process.

The AHRQ report on OME from the Southern California Evidence-Based Practice Center (EPC) focused on key questions of natural history, diagnostic methods, and long-term speech, language, and hearing outcomes.[2] Searches were conducted through January 2000 in Medline, Embase, and the Cochrane Library. Additional articles were identified by review of reference listings in proceedings, reports, and other guidelines. The EPC accepted 970 articles for full review after screening 3200 abstracts. The EPC reviewed articles by using established quality criteria[9,10] and included randomized trials, prospective cohorts, and validations of diagnostic tests (validating cohort studies).

The AAP subcommittee on OME updated the AHRQ review with articles identified by an electronic Medline search through April 2003 and with additional material identified manually by subcommittee members. Copies of relevant articles were distributed to the subcommittee for consideration. A specific search for articles relevant to complementary and alternative medicine (CAM) was performed by using Medline and the Allied and Complementary Medicine Database through April 2003. Articles relevant to allergy and OME were identified by using Medline through April 2003. The subcommittee met 3 times over a 1-year period, ending in May 2003, with interval electronic review and feedback on each guideline draft to ensure accuracy of content and consistency with standardized criteria for reporting clinical practice guidelines.[11]

In May 2003, the Guidelines Review Group of the Yale Center for Medical Informatics used the Guideline Elements Model[12] to categorize content of the present draft guideline. Policy statements were parsed into component decision variables and actions and then assessed for decidability and executability. Quality appraisal using established criteria[13] was performed with Guideline Elements Model-Q Online.[14,15] Implementation issues were predicted by using the Implementability Rating Profile, an instrument under development by the Yale Guidelines Review Group (R. Shiffman, MD, written communication, May 2003). OME subcommittee members received summary results and modified an advanced draft of the guideline.

The final draft practice guideline underwent extensive peer review by numerous entities identified by the subcommittee. Comments were compiled and reviewed by the subcommittee cochairpersons. The recommendations contained in the practice guideline are based on the best available published data through April 2003. Where data are lacking, a combination of clinical experience and expert consensus was used. A scheduled review process will occur 5 years from publication or sooner if new compelling evidence warrants earlier consideration.

Classification of Evidence-Based Statements

Guidelines are intended to reduce inappropriate variations in clinical care, produce optimal health outcomes for patients, and minimize harm. The evidence-based approach to guideline development requires that the evidence supporting a policy be identified, appraised, and summarized and that an explicit link between evidence and statements be defined. Evidence-based statements reflect the quality of evidence and the balance of benefit and harm that is anticipated when the statement is followed. The AAP definitions for evidence-based statements[16] are listed in Tables 1 and 2.

Guidelines are never intended to overrule professional judgment; rather, they may be viewed as a relative constraint on individual clinician discretion in a particular clinical circumstance. Less frequent variation in practice is expected for a strong recommendation than might be expected with a recommendation. Options offer the most opportunity for practice variability.[17] All clinicians should always act and decide in a way that they believe will best serve their patients' interests and needs regardless of guideline recommendations. Guidelines represent the best judgment of a team of experienced clinicians and methodologists addressing the scientific evidence for a particular topic.[16]

Making recommendations about health practices involves value judgments on the desirability of various outcomes associated with management options. Value judgments applied by the OME subcommittee were made in an effort to minimize harm and diminish unnecessary therapy. Emphasis was placed on promptly identifying and managing children at risk for speech, language, or learning problems to maximize opportunities for beneficial outcomes. Direct costs also were considered in the statements concerning diagnosis and screening and to a lesser extent in other statements.

1A. PNEUMATIC OTOSCOPY: CLINICIANS SHOULD USE PNEUMATIC OTOSCOPY AS THE PRIMARY DIAGNOSTIC METHOD FOR OME, AND OME SHOULD BE DISTINGUISHED FROM AOM

This is a strong recommendation based on systematic review of cohort studies and the preponderance of benefit over harm.

TABLE 1.   Guideline Definitions for Evidence-Based Statements

Statement	Definition	Implication
Strong Recommendation	A strong recommendation means that the subcommittee believes that the benefits of the recommended approach clearly exceed the harms (or that the harms clearly exceed the benefits in the case of a strong negative recommendation) and that the quality of the supporting evidence is excellent (grade A or B).* In some clearly identified circumstances, strong recommendations may be made based on lesser evidence when high-quality evidence is impossible to obtain and the anticipated benefits strongly outweigh the harms.	Clinicians should follow a strong recommendation unless a clear and compelling rationale for an alternative approach is present.
Recommendation	A recommendation means that the subcommittee believes that the benefits exceed the harms (or that the harms exceed the benefits in the case of a negative recommendation), but the quality of evidence is not as strong (grade B or C).* In some clearly identified circumstances, recommendations may be made based on lesser evidence when high-quality evidence is impossible to obtain and the anticipated benefits outweigh the harms.	Clinicians also should generally follow a recommendation but should remain alert to new information and sensitive to patient preferences.
Option	An option means that either the quality of evidence that exists is suspect (grade D)* or that well-done studies (grade A, B, or C)* show little clear advantage to one approach versus another.	Clinicians should be flexible in their decision-making regarding appropriate practice, although they may set boundaries on alternatives; patient preference should have a substantial influencing role.
No Recommendation	No recommendation means that there is both a lack of pertinent evidence (grade D)* and an unclear balance between benefits and harms.	Clinicians should feel little constraint in their decision-making and be alert to new published evidence that clarifies the balance of benefit versus harm; patient preference should have a substantial influencing role.

* See Table 2 for the definitions of evidence grades.

TABLE 2.   Evidence Quality for Grades of Evidence

Grade	Evidence Quality
A	Well-designed, randomized, controlled trials or diagnostic studies performed on a population similar to the guideline's target population
B	Randomized, controlled trials or diagnostic studies with minor limitations; overwhelmingly consistent evidence from observational studies
C	Observational studies (case-control and cohort design)
D	Expert opinion, case reports, or reasoning from first principles (bench research or animal studies)

1B. TYMPANOMETRY: TYMPANOMETRY CAN BE USED TO CONFIRM THE DIAGNOSIS OF OME

This option is based on cohort studies and a balance of benefit and harm.

Diagnosing OME correctly is fundamental to proper management. Moreover, OME must be differentiated from AOM to avoid unnecessary antimicrobial use.[18,19]

OME is defined as fluid in the middle ear without signs or symptoms of acute ear infection.[2] The tympanic membrane is often cloudy with distinctly impaired mobility,[20] and an air-fluid level or bubble may be visible in the middle ear. Conversely, diagnosing AOM requires a history of acute onset of signs and symptoms, the presence of middle-ear effusion, and signs and symptoms of middle-ear inflammation. The critical distinguishing feature is that only AOM has acute signs and symptoms. Distinct redness of the tympanic membrane should not be a criterion for prescribing antibiotics, because it has poor predictive value for AOM and is present in ~5% of ears with OME.[20]

The AHRQ evidence report[2] systematically reviewed the sensitivity, specificity, and predictive values of 9 diagnostic methods for OME. Pneumatic otoscopy had the best balance of sensitivity and specificity, consistent with the 1994 guideline.[1] Meta-analysis revealed a pooled sensitivity of 94% (95% confidence interval: 91%–96%) and specificity of 80% (95% confidence interval: 75%–86%) for validated observers using pneumatic otoscopy versus myringotomy as the gold standard. Pneumatic otoscopy therefore should remain the primary method of OME diagnosis, because the instrument is readily available in practice settings, cost-effective, and accurate in experienced hands. Non–pneumatic otoscopy is not advised for primary diagnosis.

The accuracy of pneumatic otoscopy in routine clinical practice may be less than that shown in published results, because clinicians have varying training and experience.[21,22] When the diagnosis of OME is uncertain, tympanometry or acoustic reflectometry should be considered as an adjunct to pneumatic otoscopy. Tympanometry with a standard 226-Hz probe tone is reliable for infants 4 months old or older and has good interobserver agreement of curve patterns in routine clinical practice.[23,24] Younger infants require specialized equipment with a higher probe tone frequency. Tympanometry generates costs related to instrument purchase, annual calibration, and test administration. Acoustic reflectometry with spectral gradient analysis is a low-cost alternative to tympanometry that does not require an airtight seal in the ear canal; however, validation studies primarily have used children 2 years old or older with a high prevalence of OME.[25–27]

Although no research studies have examined whether pneumatic otoscopy causes discomfort, expert consensus suggests that the procedure does not have to be painful, especially when symptoms of acute infection (AOM) are absent. A nontraumatic examination is facilitated by using a gentle touch, restraining the child properly when necessary, and inserting the speculum only into the outer one third (cartilaginous portion) of the ear canal.[28] The pneumatic bulb should be compressed slightly before insertion, because OME often is associated with a negative middle-ear pressure, which can be assessed more accurately by releasing the already compressed bulb. The otoscope must be fully charged, the bulb (halogen or xenon) bright and luminescent,[29] and the insufflator bulb attached tightly to the head to avoid the loss of an air seal. The window must also be sealed.

Evidence Profile: Pneumatic Otoscopy

- Aggregate evidence quality: A, diagnostic studies in relevant populations.
- Benefit: improved diagnostic accuracy; inexpensive equipment.
- Harm: cost of training clinicians in pneumatic otoscopy.
- Benefits-harms assessment: preponderance of benefit over harm.
- Policy level: strong recommendation.

Evidence Profile: Tympanometry

- Aggregate evidence quality: B, diagnostic studies with minor limitations.
- Benefit: increased diagnostic accuracy beyond pneumatic otoscopy; documentation.
- Harm: acquisition cost, administrative burden, and recalibration.
- Benefits-harms assessment: balance of benefit and harm.
- Policy level: option.

1C. SCREENING: POPULATION-BASED SCREENING PROGRAMS FOR OME ARE NOT RECOMMENDED IN HEALTHY, ASYMPTOMATIC CHILDREN

This recommendation is based on randomized, controlled trials and cohort studies, with a preponderance of harm over benefit.

This recommendation concerns population-based screening programs of all children in a community or a school without regard to any preexisting symptoms or history of disease. This recommendation does not address hearing screening or monitoring of specific children with previous or recurrent OME.

OME is highly prevalent in young children. Screening surveys of healthy children ranging in age from infancy to 5 years old show a 15% to 40% point prevalence of middle-ear effusion.[5,7,30–36] Among children examined at regular intervals for a year, ~50% to 60% of child care center attendees[32] and 25% of school-aged children[37] were found to have a middle-ear effusion at some time during the examination period, with peak incidence during the winter months.

Population-based screening has not been found to influence short-term language outcomes,[33] and its long-term effects have not been evaluated in a randomized, clinical trial. Therefore, the recommendation against screening is based not only on the ability to identify OME but more importantly on a lack of demonstrable benefits from treating children so identified that exceed the favorable natural history of the disease. The New Zealand Health Technology Assessment[38] could not determine whether preschool screening for OME was effective. More recently, the Canadian Task Force on Preventive Health Care[39] reported that insufficient evidence was available to recommend including or excluding routine early screening for OME. Although screening for OME is not inherently harmful, potential risks include inaccurate diagnoses, overtreating self-limited disease, parental anxiety, and the costs of screening and unnecessary treatment.

Population-based screening is appropriate for conditions that are common, can be detected by a sensitive and specific test, and benefit from early detection and treatment.[40] The first 2 requirements are fulfilled by OME, which affects up to 80% of children by school entry[2,5,7] and can be screened easily with tympanometry (see recommendation 1B). Early detection and treatment of OME identified by screening, however, have not been shown to improve intelligence, receptive language, or expressive language.[2,39,41,42] Therefore, population-based screening for early detection of OME in asymptomatic children has not been shown to improve outcomes and is not recommended.

Evidence Profile: Screening

- Aggregate evidence quality: B, randomized, controlled trials with minor limitations and consistent evidence from observational studies.
- Benefit: potentially improved developmental outcomes, which have not been demonstrated in the best current evidence.

- Harm: inaccurate diagnosis (false-positive or false-negative), overtreating self-limited disease, parental anxiety, cost of screening, and/or unnecessary treatment.
- Benefits-harms assessment: preponderance of harm over benefit.
- Policy level: recommendation against.

2. DOCUMENTATION: CLINICIANS SHOULD DOCUMENT THE LATERALITY, DURATION OF EFFUSION, AND PRESENCE AND SEVERITY OF ASSOCIATED SYMPTOMS AT EACH ASSESSMENT OF THE CHILD WITH OME

This recommendation is based on observational studies and strong preponderance of benefit over harm.

Documentation in the medical record facilitates diagnosis and treatment and communicates pertinent information to other clinicians to ensure patient safety and reduce medical errors.[43] Management decisions in children with OME depend on effusion duration and laterality plus the nature and severity of associated symptoms. Therefore, these features should be documented at every medical encounter for OME. Although no studies have addressed documentation for OME specifically, there is room for improvement in documentation of ambulatory care medical records.[44]

Ideally, the time of onset and laterality of OME can be defined through diagnosis of an antecedent AOM, a history of acute onset of signs or symptoms directly referable to fluid in the middle ear, or the presence of an abnormal audiogram or tympanogram closely after a previously normal test. Unfortunately, these conditions are often lacking, and the clinician is forced to speculate on the onset and duration of fluid in the middle ear(s) in a child found to have OME at a routine office visit or school screening audiometry.

In ~40% to 50% of cases of OME, neither the affected children nor their parents or caregivers describe significant complaints referable to a middle-ear effusion.[45,46] In some children, however, OME may have associated signs and symptoms caused by inflammation or the presence of effusion (not acute infection) that should be documented, such as

- Mild intermittent ear pain, fullness, or "popping"
- Secondary manifestations of ear pain in infants, which may include ear rubbing, excessive irritability, and sleep disturbances
- Failure of infants to respond appropriately to voices or environmental sounds, such as not turning accurately toward the sound source
- Hearing loss, even when not specifically described by the child, suggested by seeming lack of attentiveness, behavioral changes, failure to respond to normal conversational-level speech, or the need for excessively high sound levels when using audio equipment or viewing television
- Recurrent episodes of AOM with persistent OME between episodes
- Problems with school performance
- Balance problems, unexplained clumsiness, or delayed gross motor development[47–50]
- Delayed speech or language development

The laterality (unilateral versus bilateral), duration of effusion, and presence and severity of associated symptoms should be documented in the medical record at each assessment of the child with OME. When OME duration is uncertain, the clinician must take whatever evidence is at hand and make a reasonable estimate.

Evidence Profile: Documentation

- Aggregate evidence quality: C, observational studies.
- Benefits: defines severity, duration has prognostic value, facilitates future communication with other clinicians, supports appropriate timing of intervention, and, if consistently unilateral, may identify a problem with specific ear other than OME (eg, retraction pocket or cholesteatoma).
- Harm: administrative burden.
- Benefits-harms assessment: preponderance of benefit over harm.
- Policy level: recommendation.

3. CHILD AT RISK: CLINICIANS SHOULD DISTINGUISH THE CHILD WITH OME WHO IS AT RISK FOR SPEECH, LANGUAGE, OR LEARNING PROBLEMS FROM OTHER CHILDREN WITH OME AND SHOULD EVALUATE HEARING, SPEECH, LANGUAGE, AND NEED FOR INTERVENTION MORE PROMPTLY

This recommendation is based on case series, the preponderance of benefit over harm, and ethical limitations in studying children with OME who are at risk.

The panel defines the child at risk as one who is at increased risk for developmental difficulties (delay or disorder) because of sensory, physical, cognitive, or behavioral factors listed in Table 3. These factors are not caused by OME but can make the child less tolerant of hearing loss or vestibular problems secondary to middle-ear effusion. In contrast the child with OME who is not at risk is otherwise healthy and does not have any of the factors shown in Table 3.

Earlier guidelines for managing OME have applied only to young children who are healthy and exhibit no developmental delays.[1] Studies of the relationship between OME and hearing loss or speech/language development typically exclude children with craniofacial anomalies, genetic syndromes, and other developmental disorders. Therefore, the available literature mainly applies to otherwise healthy children who meet inclusion criteria for randomized,

TABLE 3. Risk Factors for Developmental Difficulties*

Permanent hearing loss independent of OME
Suspected or diagnosed speech and language delay or disorder
Autism-spectrum disorder and other pervasive developmental disorders
Syndromes (eg, Down) or craniofacial disorders that include cognitive, speech, and language delays
Blindness or uncorrectable visual impairment
Cleft palate with or without associated syndrome
Developmental delay

* Sensory, physical, cognitive, or behavioral factors that place children who have OME at an increased risk for developmental difficulties (delay or disorder).

controlled trials. Few, if any, existing studies dealing with developmental sequelae caused by hearing loss from OME can be generalized to children who are at risk.

Children who are at risk for speech or language delay would likely be affected additionally by hearing problems from OME,[51] although definitive studies are lacking. For example, small comparative studies of children or adolescents with Down syndrome[52] or cerebral palsy[53] show poorer articulation and receptive language associated with a history of early otitis media. Large studies are unlikely to be forthcoming because of methodologic and ethical difficulties inherent in studying children who are delayed or at risk for further delays. Therefore, clinicians who manage children with OME should determine whether other conditions coexist that put a child at risk for developmental delay (Table 3) and then take these conditions into consideration when planning assessment and management.

Children with craniofacial anomalies (eg, cleft palate; Down syndrome; Robin sequence; coloboma, heart defect, choanal atresia, retarded growth and development, genital anomaly, and ear defect with deafness [CHARGE] association) have a higher prevalence of chronic OME, hearing loss (conductive and sensorineural), and speech or language delay than do children without these anomalies.[54–57] Other children may not be more prone to OME but are likely to have speech and language disorders, such as those children with permanent hearing loss independent of OME,[58,59] specific language impairment,[60] autism-spectrum disorders,[61] or syndromes that adversely affect cognitive and linguistic development. Some retrospective studies[52,62,63] have found that hearing loss caused by OME in children with cognitive delays, such as Down syndrome, has been associated with lower language levels. Children with language delays or disorders with OME histories perform more poorly on speech-perception tasks than do children with OME histories alone.[64,65]

Children with severe visual impairments may be more susceptible to the effects of OME, because they depend on hearing more than children with normal vision.[51] Any decrease in their most important remaining sensory input for language (hearing) may significantly compromise language development and their ability to interact and communicate with others. All children with severe visual impairments should be considered more vulnerable to OME sequelae, especially in the areas of balance, sound localization, and communication.

Management of the child with OME who is at increased risk for developmental delays should include hearing testing and speech and language evaluation and may include speech and language therapy concurrent with managing OME, hearing aids or other amplification devices for hearing loss independent of OME, tympanostomy tube insertion,[54,63,66,67] and hearing testing after OME resolves to document improvement, because OME can mask a permanent underlying hearing loss and delay detection.[59,68,69]

Evidence Profile: Child at Risk

- Aggregate evidence quality: C, observational studies of children at risk; D, expert opinion on the ability of prompt assessment and management to alter outcomes.
- Benefits: optimizing conditions for hearing, speech, and language; enabling children with special needs to reach their potential; avoiding limitations on the benefits of educational interventions because of hearing problems from OME.
- Harm: cost, time, and specific risks of medications or surgery.
- Benefits-harms assessment: exceptional preponderance of benefits over harm based on subcommittee consensus because of circumstances to date precluding randomized trials.
- Policy level: recommendation.

4. WATCHFUL WAITING: CLINICIANS SHOULD MANAGE THE CHILD WITH OME WHO IS NOT AT RISK WITH WATCHFUL WAITING FOR 3 MONTHS FROM THE DATE OF EFFUSION ONSET (IF KNOWN) OR DIAGNOSIS (IF ONSET IS UNKNOWN)

This recommendation is based on systematic review of cohort studies and the preponderance of benefit over harm.

This recommendation is based on the self-limited nature of most OME, which has been well documented in cohort studies and in control groups of randomized trials.[2,70]

The likelihood of spontaneous resolution of OME is determined by the cause and duration of effusion.[70] For example, ~75% to 90% of residual OME after an AOM episode resolves spontaneously by 3 months.[71–73] Similar outcomes of defined onset during a period of surveillance in a cohort study are observed for OME.[32,37] Another favorable situation involves improvement (not resolution) of newly detected OME defined as change in tympanogram from type B (flat curve) to non-B (anything other than a flat curve). Approximately 55% of children so defined improve by 3 months,[70] but one third will have OME relapse within the next 3 months.[4] Although a type B tympanogram is an imperfect measure of OME (81% sensitivity and 74% specificity versus myringotomy), it is the most widely reported measure suitable for deriving pooled resolution rates.[2,70]

Approximately 25% of newly detected OME of unknown prior duration in children 2 to 4 years old resolves by 3 months when resolution is defined as a change in tympanogram from type B to type A/C1 (peak pressure >200 daPa).[2,70,74–77] Resolution rates may be higher for infants and young children in whom the preexisting duration of effusion is generally shorter, and particularly for those observed prospectively in studies or in the course of well-child care. Documented bilateral OME of 3 months' duration or longer resolves spontaneously after 6 to 12 months in ~30% of children primarily 2 years old or older, with only marginal benefits if observed longer.[70]

Any intervention for OME (medical or surgical) other than observation carries some inherent harm. There is little harm associated with a specified period of observation in the child who is not at risk for speech, language, or learning problems. When observing children with OME, clinicians should inform the parent or caregiver that the child may experience reduced hearing until the effusion resolves, especially if it is bilateral. Clinicians may discuss strategies for optimizing the listening and learning environment until the effusion resolves. These strategies include speaking in close proximity to the child, facing the child and speaking clearly, repeating phrases when misunderstood, and providing preferential classroom seating.[78,79]

The recommendation for a 3-month period of observation is based on a clear preponderance of benefit over harm and is consistent with the original OME guideline intent of avoiding unnecessary surgery.[1] At the discretion of the clinician, this 3-month period of watchful waiting may include interval visits at which OME is monitored by using pneumatic otoscopy, tympanometry, or both. Factors to consider in determining the optimal interval(s) for follow-up include clinical judgment, parental comfort level, unique characteristics of the child and/or his environment, access to a health care system, and hearing levels (HLs) if known.

After documented resolution of OME in all affected ears, additional follow-up is unnecessary.

Evidence Profile: Watchful Waiting

- Aggregate evidence quality: B, systematic review of cohort studies.
- Benefit: avoid unnecessary interventions, take advantage of favorable natural history, and avoid unnecessary referrals and evaluations.
- Harm: delays in therapy for OME that will not resolve with observation; prolongation of hearing loss.
- Benefits-harms assessment: preponderance of benefit over harm.
- Policy level: recommendation.

5. MEDICATION: ANTIHISTAMINES AND DECONGESTANTS ARE INEFFECTIVE FOR OME AND ARE NOT RECOMMENDED FOR TREATMENT; ANTIMICROBIALS AND CORTICOSTEROIDS DO NOT HAVE LONG-TERM EFFICACY AND ARE NOT RECOMMENDED FOR ROUTINE MANAGEMENT

This recommendation is based on systematic review of randomized, controlled trials and the preponderance of harm over benefit.

Therapy for OME is appropriate only if persistent and clinically significant benefits can be achieved beyond spontaneous resolution. Although statistically significant benefits have been demonstrated for some medications, they are short-term and relatively small in magnitude. Moreover, significant adverse events may occur with all medical therapies.

The prior OME guideline[1] found no data supporting antihistamine-decongestant combinations in treating OME. Meta-analysis of 4 randomized trials showed no significant benefit for antihistamines or decongestants versus placebo. No additional studies have been published since 1994 to change this recommendation. Adverse effects of antihistamines and decongestants include insomnia, hyperactivity, drowsiness, behavioral change, and blood-pressure variability.

Long-term benefits of antimicrobial therapy for OME are unproved despite a modest short-term benefit for 2 to 8 weeks in randomized trials.[1,80,81] Initial benefits, however, can become nonsignificant within 2 weeks of stopping the medication.[82] Moreover, ~7 children would need to be treated with antimicrobials to achieve one short-term response.[1] Adverse effects of antimicrobials are significant and may include rashes, vomiting, diarrhea, allergic reactions, alteration of the child's nasopharyngeal flora, development of bacterial resistance,[83] and cost. Societal consequences include direct transmission of resistant bacterial pathogens in homes and child care centers.[84]

The prior OME guideline[1] did not recommend oral steroids for treating OME in children. A later meta-analysis[85] showed no benefit for oral steroid versus placebo within 2 weeks but did show a short-term benefit for oral steroid plus antimicrobial versus antimicrobial alone in 1 of 3 children treated. This benefit became nonsignificant after several weeks in a prior meta-analysis[1] and in a large, randomized trial.[86] Oral steroids can produce behavioral changes, increased appetite, and weight gain.[1] Additional adverse effects may include adrenal suppression, fatal varicella infection, and avascular necrosis of the femoral head.[3] Although intranasal steroids have fewer adverse effects, one randomized trial[87] showed statistically equivalent outcomes at 12 weeks for intranasal beclomethasone plus antimicrobials versus antimicrobials alone for OME.

Antimicrobial therapy with or without steroids has not been demonstrated to be effective in long-term resolution of OME, but in some cases this therapy can be considered an option because of short-term benefit in randomized trials, when the parent or caregiver expresses a strong aversion to impending surgery. In this circumstance, a single course of therapy for 10 to 14 days may be used. The likelihood that the OME will resolve long-term with these regimens is small, and prolonged or repetitive courses of antimicrobials or steroids are strongly not recommended.

Other nonsurgical therapies that are discussed in the OME literature include autoinflation of the eustachian tube, oral or intratympanic use of mucolytics, and systemic use of pharmacologic agents other than antimicrobials, steroids, and antihistamine-decongestants. Insufficient data exist for any of these therapies to be recommended in treating OME.[3]

Evidence Profile: Medication

- Aggregate evidence quality: A, systematic review of well-designed, randomized, controlled trials.

- Benefit: avoid side effects and reduce cost by not administering medications; avoid delays in definitive therapy caused by short-term improvement then relapse.
- Harm: adverse effects of specific medications as listed previously; societal impact of antimicrobial therapy on bacterial resistance and transmission of resistant pathogens.
- Benefits-harms assessment: preponderance of harm over benefit.
- Policy level: recommendation against.

6. HEARING AND LANGUAGE: HEARING TESTING IS RECOMMENDED WHEN OME PERSISTS FOR 3 MONTHS OR LONGER OR AT ANY TIME THAT LANGUAGE DELAY, LEARNING PROBLEMS, OR A SIGNIFICANT HEARING LOSS IS SUSPECTED IN A CHILD WITH OME; LANGUAGE TESTING SHOULD BE CONDUCTED FOR CHILDREN WITH HEARING LOSS

This recommendation is based on cohort studies and the preponderance of benefit over risk.

Hearing Testing

Hearing testing is recommended when OME persists for 3 months or longer or at any time that language delay, learning problems, or a significant hearing loss is suspected. Conductive hearing loss often accompanies OME[1,88] and may adversely affect binaural processing,[89] sound localization,[90] and speech perception in noise.[91–94] Hearing loss caused by OME may impair early language acquisition,[95–97] but the child's home environment has a greater impact on outcomes[98]; recent randomized trials[41,99,100] suggest no impact on children with OME who are not at risk as identified by screening or surveillance.

Studies examining hearing sensitivity in children with OME report that average pure-tone hearing loss at 4 frequencies (500, 1000, 2000, and 4000 Hz) ranges from normal hearing to moderate hearing loss (0–55 dB). The 50th percentile is an ~25-dB HL, and ~20% of ears exceed 35-dB HL.[101,102] Unilateral OME with hearing loss results in overall poorer binaural hearing than in infants with normal middle-ear function bilaterally.[103,104] However, based on limited research, there is evidence that children experiencing the greatest conductive hearing loss for the longest periods may be more likely to exhibit developmental and academic sequelae.[1,95,105]

Initial hearing testing for children 4 years old or older can be done in the primary care setting.[106] Testing should be performed in a quiet environment, preferably in a separate closed or sound-proofed area set aside specifically for that purpose. Conventional audiometry with earphones is performed with a fail criterion of more than 20-dB HL at 1 or more frequencies (500, 1000, 2000, and 4000 Hz) in either ear.[106,107] Methods not recommended as substitutes for primary care hearing testing include tympanometry and pneumatic otoscopy,[102] caregiver judgment regarding hearing loss,[108,109] speech audiometry, and tuning forks, acoustic reflectometry, and behavioral observation.[1]

Comprehensive audiologic evaluation is recommended for children who fail primary care testing, are less than 4 years old, or cannot be tested in the primary care setting. Audiologic assessment includes evaluating air-conduction and bone-conduction thresholds for pure tones, speech-detection or speech-recognition thresholds,[102] and measuring speech understanding if possible.[94] The method of assessment depends on the developmental age of the child and might include visual reinforcement or conditioned orienting-response audiometry for infants 6 to 24 months old, play audiometry for children 24 to 48 months old, or conventional screening audiometry for children 4 years old and older.[106] The auditory brainstem response and otoacoustic emission are tests of auditory pathway structural integrity, not hearing, and should not substitute for behavioral pure-tone audiometry.[106]

Language Testing

Language testing should be conducted for children with hearing loss (pure-tone average more than 20-dB HL on comprehensive audiometric evaluation). Testing for language delays is important, because communication is integral to all aspects of human functioning. Young children with speech and language delays during the preschool years are at risk for continued communication problems and later delays in reading and writing.[110–112] In one study, 6% to 8% of children 3 years old and 2% to 13% of kindergartners had language impairment.[113] Language intervention can improve communication and other functional outcomes for children with histories of OME.[114]

Children who experience repeated and persistent episodes of OME and associated hearing loss during early childhood may be at a disadvantage for learning speech and language.[79,115] Although Shekelle et al[2] concluded that there was no evidence to support the concern that OME during the first 3 years of life was related to later receptive or expressive language, this meta-analysis should be interpreted cautiously, because it did not examine specific language domains such as vocabulary and the independent variable was OME and not hearing loss. Other meta-analyses[79,115] have suggested at most a small negative association of OME and hearing loss on children's receptive and expressive language through the elementary school years. The clinical significance of these effects for language and learning is unclear for the child not at risk. For example, in one randomized trial,[100] prompt insertion of tympanostomy tubes for OME did not improve developmental outcomes at 3 years old regardless of baseline hearing. In another randomized trial,[116] however, prompt tube insertion achieved small benefits for children with bilateral OME and hearing loss.

Clinicians should ask the parent or caregiver about specific concerns regarding their child's language development. Children's speech and language can be tested at ages 6 to 36 months by direct engagement of a child and interviewing the parent using the Early Language Milestone Scale.[117] Other approaches require interviewing only the child's parent or caregiver, such as the MacArthur Communicative Development Inventory[118] and the Language Development Survey.[119] For older children, the Denver Developmental Screening Test II[120] can be used to screen general development including speech and language. Comprehensive speech and language evaluation is recommended for children who fail testing or whenever the child's parent or caregiver expresses concern.[121]

Evidence Profile: Hearing and Language

- Aggregate evidence quality: B, diagnostic studies with minor limitations; C, observational studies.
- Benefit: to detect hearing loss and language delay and identify strategies or interventions to improve developmental outcomes.
- Harm: parental anxiety, direct and indirect costs of assessment, and/or false-positive results.
- Balance of benefit and harm: preponderance of benefit over harm.
- Policy level: recommendation.

7. SURVEILLANCE: CHILDREN WITH PERSISTENT OME WHO ARE NOT AT RISK SHOULD BE REEXAMINED AT 3- TO 6-MONTH INTERVALS UNTIL THE EFFUSION IS NO LONGER PRESENT, SIGNIFICANT HEARING LOSS IS IDENTIFIED, OR STRUCTURAL ABNORMALITIES OF THE EARDRUM OR MIDDLE EAR ARE SUSPECTED

This recommendation is based on randomized, controlled trials and observational studies with a preponderance of benefit over harm.

If OME is asymptomatic and is likely to resolve spontaneously, intervention is unnecessary even if OME persists for more than 3 months. The clinician should determine whether risk factors exist that would predispose the child to undesirable sequelae or predict nonresolution of the effusion. As long as OME persists, the child is at risk for sequelae and must be reevaluated periodically for factors that would prompt intervention.

The 1994 OME guideline[1] recommended surgery for OME persisting 4 to 6 months with hearing loss but requires reconsideration because of later data on tubes and developmental sequelae.[122] For example, selecting surgical candidates using duration-based criteria (eg, OME >3 months or exceeding a cumulative threshold) does not improve developmental outcomes in infants and toddlers who are not at risk.[41,42,99,100] Additionally, the 1994 OME guideline did not specifically address managing effusion without significant hearing loss persisting more than 6 months.

Asymptomatic OME usually resolves spontaneously, but resolution rates decrease the longer the effusion has been present,[36,76,77] and relapse is common.[123] Risk factors that make spontaneous resolution less likely include[124,125]:

- Onset of OME in the summer or fall season
- Hearing loss more than 30-dB HL in the better-hearing ear

- History of prior tympanostomy tubes
- Not having had an adenoidectomy

Children with chronic OME are at risk for structural damage of the tympanic membrane[126] because the effusion contains leukotrienes, prostaglandins, and arachidonic acid metabolites that invoke a local inflammatory response.[127] Reactive changes may occur in the adjacent tympanic membrane and mucosal linings. A relative underventilation of the middle ear produces a negative pressure that predisposes to focal retraction pockets, generalized atelectasis of the tympanic membrane, and cholesteatoma.

Structural integrity is assessed by carefully examining the entire tympanic membrane, which, in many cases, can be accomplished by the primary care clinician using a handheld pneumatic otoscope. A search should be made for retraction pockets, ossicular erosion, and areas of atelectasis or atrophy. If there is any uncertainty that all observed structures are normal, the patient should be examined by using an otomicroscope. All children with these tympanic membrane conditions, regardless of OME duration, should have a comprehensive audiologic evaluation.

Conditions of the tympanic membrane that generally mandate inserting a tympanostomy tube are posterosuperior retraction pockets, ossicular erosion, adhesive atelectasis, and retraction pockets that accumulate keratin debris. Ongoing surveillance is mandatory, because the incidence of structural damage increases with effusion duration.[128]

As noted in recommendation 6, children with persistent OME for 3 months or longer should have their hearing tested. Based on these results, clinicians can identify 3 levels of action based on HLs obtained for the better-hearing ear using earphones or in sound field using speakers if the child is too young for ear-specific testing.

1. HLs of ≥40 dB (at least a moderate hearing loss): A comprehensive audiologic evaluation is indicated if not previously performed. If moderate hearing loss is documented and persists at this level, surgery is recommended, because persistent hearing loss of this magnitude that is permanent in nature has been shown to impact speech, language, and academic performance.[129–131]

2. HLs of 21 to 39 dB (mild hearing loss): A comprehensive audiologic evaluation is indicated if not previously performed. Mild sensorineural hearing loss has been associated with difficulties in speech, language, and academic performance in school,[129,132] and persistent mild conductive hearing loss from OME may have a similar impact. Further management should be individualized based on effusion duration, severity of hearing loss, and parent or caregiver preference and may include strategies to optimize the listening and learning environment (Table 4) or surgery. Repeat hearing testing should be performed in 3 to 6 months if OME persists at follow-up evaluation or tympanostomy tubes have not been placed.

3. HLs of ≤20 dB (normal hearing): A repeat hearing test should be performed in 3 to 6 months if OME persists at follow-up evaluation.

TABLE 4. Strategies for Optimizing the Listening-Learning Environment for Children With OME and Hearing Loss*

Get within 3 feet of the child before speaking.
Turn off competing audio signals such as unnecessary music and television in the background.
Face the child and speak clearly, using visual clues (hands, pictures) in addition to speech.
Slow the rate, raise the level, and enunciate speech directed at the child.
Read to or with the child, explaining pictures and asking questions.
Repeat words, phrases, and questions when misunderstood.
Assign preferential seating in the classroom near the teacher.
Use a frequency-modulated personal- or sound-field-amplification system in the classroom.

* Modified with permission from Roberts et al.[78,79]

In addition to hearing loss and speech or language delay, other factors may influence the decision to intervene for persistent OME. Roberts et al[98,133] showed that the caregiving environment is more strongly related to school outcome than was OME or hearing loss. Risk factors for delays in speech and language development caused by a poor caregiving environment included low maternal educational level, unfavorable child care environment, and low socioeconomic status. In such cases, these factors may be additive to the hearing loss in affecting lower school performance and classroom behavior problems.

Persistent OME may be associated with physical or behavioral symptoms including hyperactivity, poor attention, and behavioral problems in some studies[134–136] and reduced child quality of life.[46] Conversely, young children randomized to early versus late tube insertion for persistent OME showed no behavioral benefits from early surgery.[41,100] Children with chronic OME also have significantly poorer vestibular function and gross motor proficiency when compared with non-OME controls.[48–50] Moreover, vestibular function, behavior, and quality of life can improve after tympanostomy tube insertion.[47,137,138] Other physical symptoms of OME that, if present and persistent, may warrant surgery include otalgia, unexplained sleep disturbance, and coexisting recurrent AOM. Tubes reduce the absolute incidence of recurrent AOM by ~1 episode per child per year, but the relative risk reduction is 56%.[139]

The risks of continued observation of children with OME must be balanced against the risks of surgery. Children with persistent OME examined regularly at 3- to 6-month intervals, or sooner if OME-related symptoms develop, are most likely at low risk for physical, behavioral, or developmental sequelae of OME. Conversely, prolonged watchful waiting of OME is not appropriate when regular surveillance is impossible or when the child is at risk for developmental sequelae of OME because of comorbidities (Table 3). For these children, the risks of anesthesia and surgery (see recommendation 9) may be less than those of continued observation.

Evidence Profile: Surveillance

- Aggregate evidence quality: C, observational studies and some randomized trials.

- Benefit: avoiding interventions that do not improve outcomes.
- Harm: allowing structural abnormalities to develop in the tympanic membrane, underestimating the impact of hearing loss on a child, and/or failing to detect significant signs or symptoms that require intervention.
- Balance of benefit and harm: preponderance of benefit over harm.
- Policy level: recommendation.

8. REFERRAL: WHEN CHILDREN WITH OME ARE REFERRED BY THE PRIMARY CARE CLINICIAN FOR EVALUATION BY AN OTOLARYNGOLOGIST, AUDIOLOGIST, OR SPEECH-LANGUAGE PATHOLOGIST, THE REFERRING CLINICIAN SHOULD DOCUMENT THE EFFUSION DURATION AND SPECIFIC REASON FOR REFERRAL (EVALUATION, SURGERY) AND PROVIDE ADDITIONAL RELEVANT INFORMATION SUCH AS HISTORY OF AOM AND DEVELOPMENTAL STATUS OF THE CHILD

This option is based on panel consensus and a preponderance of benefit over harm.

This recommendation emphasizes the importance of communication between the referring primary care clinician and the otolaryngologist, audiologist, and speech-language pathologist. Parents and caregivers may be confused and frustrated when a recommendation for surgery is made for their child because of conflicting information about alternative management strategies. Choosing among management options is facilitated when primary care physicians and advanced-practice nurses who best know the patient's history of ear problems and general medical status provide the specialist with accurate information. Although there are no studies showing improved outcomes from better documentation of OME histories, there is a clear need for better mechanisms to convey information and expectations from primary care clinicians to consultants and subspecialists.[140–142]

When referring a child for evaluation to an otolaryngologist, the primary care physician should explain the following to the parent or caregiver of the patient:

- Reason for referral: Explain that the child is seeing an otolaryngologist for evaluation, which is likely to include ear examination and audiologic testing, and not necessarily simply to be scheduled for surgery.
- What to expect: Explain that surgery may be recommended, and let the parent know that the otolaryngologist will explain the options, benefits, and risks further.
- Decision-making process: Explain that there are many alternatives for management and that surgical decisions are elective; the parent or caregiver should be encouraged to express to the surgeon any concerns he or she may have about the recommendations made.

When referring a child to an otolaryngologist, audiologist, or speech-language pathologist, the minimum information that should be conveyed in writing includes:

- Duration of OME: State how long fluid has been present.
- Laterality of OME: State whether one or both ears have been affected.
- Results of prior hearing testing or tympanometry.
- Suspected speech or language problems: State whether there had been a delay in speech and language development or whether the parent or a caregiver has expressed concerns about the child's communication abilities, school achievement, or attentiveness.
- Conditions that might exacerbate the deleterious effects of OME: State whether the child has conditions such as permanent hearing loss, impaired cognition, developmental delays, cleft lip or palate, or an unstable or nonsupportive family or home environment.
- AOM history: State whether the child has a history of recurrent AOM.

Additional medical information that should be provided to the otolaryngologist by the primary care clinician includes:

- Parental attitude toward surgery: State whether the parents have expressed a strong preference for or against surgery as a management option.
- Related conditions that might require concomitant surgery: State whether there have been other conditions that might warrant surgery if the child is going to have general anesthesia (eg, nasal obstruction and snoring that might be an indication for adenoidectomy or obstructive breathing during sleep that might mean tonsillectomy is indicated).
- General health status: State whether there are any conditions that might present problems for surgery or administering general anesthesia, such as congenital heart abnormality, bleeding disorder, asthma or reactive airway disease, or family history of malignant hyperthermia.

After evaluating the child, the otolaryngologist, audiologist, or speech-language pathologist should inform the referring physician regarding his or her diagnostic impression, plans for additional assessment, and recommendations for ongoing monitoring and management.

Evidence Profile: Referral

- Aggregate evidence quality: C, observational studies.
- Benefit: better communication and improved decision-making.
- Harm: confidentiality concerns, administrative burden, and/or increased parent or caregiver anxiety.
- Benefits-harms assessment: balance of benefit and harm.
- Policy level: option.

9. SURGERY: WHEN A CHILD BECOMES A SURGICAL CANDIDATE, TYMPANOSTOMY TUBE INSERTION IS THE PREFERRED INITIAL PROCEDURE; ADENOIDECTOMY SHOULD NOT BE PERFORMED UNLESS A DISTINCT INDICATION EXISTS (NASAL OBSTRUCTION, CHRONIC ADENOIDITIS). REPEAT SURGERY CONSISTS OF ADENOIDECTOMY PLUS MYRINGOTOMY, WITH OR WITHOUT TUBE INSERTION. TONSILLECTOMY ALONE OR MYRINGOTOMY ALONE SHOULD NOT BE USED TO TREAT OME

This recommendation is based on randomized, controlled trials with a preponderance of benefit over harm.

Surgical candidacy for OME largely depends on hearing status, associated symptoms, the child's developmental risk (Table 3), and the anticipated chance of timely spontaneous resolution of the effusion. Candidates for surgery include children with OME lasting 4 months or longer with persistent hearing loss or other signs and symptoms, recurrent or persistent OME in children at risk regardless of hearing status, and OME and structural damage to the tympanic membrane or middle ear. Ultimately, the recommendation for surgery must be individualized based on consensus between the primary care physician, otolaryngologist, and parent or caregiver that a particular child would benefit from intervention. Children with OME of any duration who are at risk are candidates for earlier surgery.

Tympanostomy tubes are recommended for initial surgery because randomized trials show a mean 62% relative decrease in effusion prevalence and an absolute decrease of 128 effusion days per child during the next year.[139,143–145] HLs improve by a mean of 6 to 12 dB while the tubes remain patent.[146,147] Adenoidectomy plus myringotomy (without tube insertion) has comparable efficacy in children 4 years old or older[143] but is more invasive, with additional surgical and anesthetic risks. Similarly, the added risk of adenoidectomy outweighs the limited, short-term benefit for children 3 years old or older without prior tubes.[148] Consequently, adenoidectomy is not recommended for initial OME surgery unless a distinct indication exists, such as adenoiditis, postnasal obstruction, or chronic sinusitis.

Approximately 20% to 50% of children who have had tympanostomy tubes have OME relapse after tube extrusion that may require additional surgery.[144,145,149] When a child needs repeat surgery for OME, adenoidectomy is recommended (unless the child has an overt or submucous cleft palate), because it confers a 50% reduction in the need for future operations.[143,150,151] The benefit of adenoidectomy is apparent at 2 years old,[150] greatest for children 3 years old or older, and independent of adenoid size.[143,151,152] Myringotomy is performed concurrent with adenoidectomy. Myringotomy plus adenoidectomy is effective for children 4 years old or older,[143] but tube insertion is advised for younger children, when potential relapse of effusion must be minimized (eg, children at risk) or pronounced inflammation of the tympanic membrane and middle-ear mucosa is present.

Tonsillectomy or myringotomy alone (without adenoidectomy) is not recommended to treat OME. Although tonsillectomy is either ineffective[152] or of limited efficacy,[148,150] the risks of hemorrhage (~2%) and additional hospitalization outweigh any potential benefits unless a distinct indication for tonsillectomy exists. Myringotomy alone, without tube placement or adenoidectomy, is ineffective for chronic OME,[144,145] because the incision closes within several days. Laser-assisted myringotomy extends the ventilation period several weeks,[153] but randomized trials with concurrent controls have not been conducted to establish efficacy. In contrast, tympanostomy tubes ventilate the middle ear for an average of 12 to 14 months.[144,145]

Anesthesia mortality has been reported to be ~1: 50 000 for ambulatory surgery,[154] but the current fatality rate may be lower.[155] Laryngospasm and bronchospasm occur more often in children receiving anesthesia than adults. Tympanostomy tube sequelae are common[156] but are generally transient (otorrhea) or do not affect function (tympanosclerosis, focal atrophy, or shallow retraction pocket). Tympanic membrane perforations, which may require repair, are seen in 2% of children after placement of short-term (grommet-type) tubes and 17% after long-term tubes.[156] Adenoidectomy has a 0.2% to 0.5% incidence of hemorrhage[150,157] and 2% incidence of transient velopharyngeal insufficiency.[148] Other potential risks of adenoidectomy, such as nasopharyngeal stenosis and persistent velopharyngeal insufficiency, can be minimized with appropriate patient selection and surgical technique.

There is a clear preponderance of benefit over harm when considering the impact of surgery for OME on effusion prevalence, HLs, subsequent incidence of AOM, and the need for reoperation after adenoidectomy. Information about adenoidectomy in children less than 4 years old, however, remains limited. Although the cost of surgery and anesthesia is nontrivial, it is offset by reduced OME and AOM after tube placement and by reduced need for reoperation after adenoidectomy. Approximately 8 adenoidectomies are needed to avoid a single instance of tube reinsertion; however, each avoided surgery probably represents a larger reduction in the number of AOM and OME episodes, including those in children who did not require additional surgery.[150]

Evidence Profile: Surgery

- Aggregate evidence quality: B, randomized, controlled trials with minor limitations.
- Benefit: improved hearing, reduced prevalence of OME, reduced incidence of AOM, and less need for additional tube insertion (after adenoidectomy).
- Harm: risks of anesthesia and specific surgical procedures; sequelae of tympanostomy tubes.
- Benefits-harms assessment: preponderance of benefit over harm.
- Policy level: recommendation.

10. CAM: NO RECOMMENDATION IS MADE REGARDING CAM AS A TREATMENT FOR OME

There is no recommendation based on lack of scientific evidence documenting efficacy and an uncertain balance of harm and benefit.

The 1994 OME guideline[1] made no recommendation regarding CAM as a treatment for OME, and no subsequent controlled studies have been published to change this conclusion. The current statement of "no recommendation" is based on the lack of scientific evidence documenting efficacy plus the balance of benefit and harm.

Evidence concerning CAM is insufficient to determine whether the outcomes achieved for OME differ from those achieved by watchful waiting and spontaneous resolution. There are no randomized, controlled trials with adequate sample sizes on the efficacy of CAM for OME. Although many case reports and subjective reviews on CAM treatment of AOM were found, little is published on OME treatment or prevention. Homeopathy[158] and chiropractic treatments[159] were assessed in pilot studies with small numbers of patients that failed to show clinically or statistically significant benefits. Consequently, there is no research base on which to develop a recommendation concerning CAM for OME.

The natural history of OME in childhood (discussed previously) is such that almost any intervention can be "shown" to have helped in an anecdotal, uncontrolled report or case series. The efficacy of CAM or any other intervention for OME can only be shown with parallel-group, randomized, controlled trials with valid diagnostic methods and adequate sample sizes. Unproved modalities that have been claimed to provide benefit in middle-ear disease include osteopathic and chiropractic manipulation, dietary exclusions (such as dairy), herbal and other dietary supplements, acupuncture, traditional Chinese medicine, and homeopathy. None of these modalities, however, have been subjected yet to a published, peer-reviewed, clinical trial.

The absence of any published clinical trials also means that all reports of CAM adverse effects are anecdotal. A systematic review of recent evidence[160] found significant serious adverse effects of unconventional therapies for children, most of which were associated with inadequately regulated herbal medicines. One report on malpractice liability associated with CAM therapies[161] did not address childhood issues specifically. Allergic reactions to echinacea occur but seem to be rare in children.[162] A general concern about herbal products is the lack of any governmental oversight into product quality or purity.[160,163,164] Additionally, herbal products may alter blood levels of allopathic medications, including anticoagulants. A possible concern with homeopathy is the worsening of symptoms, which is viewed as a positive, early sign of homeopathic efficacy. The adverse effects of manipulative therapies (such as chiropractic treatments and osteopathy) in children are difficult to assess because of scant evidence, but a case series of 332 children treated for AOM or OME with chiropractic manipulation did not mention any side effects.[165] Quadriplegia has been reported, however, after spinal manipulation in an infant with torticollis.[166]

Evidence Profile: CAM

- Aggregate evidence quality: D, case series without controls.
- Benefit: not established.
- Harm: potentially significant depending on the intervention.
- Benefits-harms assessment: uncertain balance of benefit and harm.
- Policy level: no recommendation.

11. ALLERGY MANAGEMENT: NO RECOMMENDATION IS MADE REGARDING ALLERGY MANAGEMENT AS A TREATMENT FOR OME

There is no recommendation based on insufficient evidence of therapeutic efficacy or a causal relationship between allergy and OME.

The 1994 OME guideline[1] made no recommendation regarding allergy management as a treatment for OME, and no subsequent controlled studies have been published to change this conclusion. The current statement of "no recommendation" is based on insufficient evidence of therapeutic efficacy or a causal relationship between allergy and OME plus the balance of benefit and harm.

A linkage between allergy and OME has long been speculated but to date remains unquantified. The prevalence of allergy among OME patients has been reported to range from less than 10% to more than 80%.[167] Allergy has long been postulated to cause OME through its contribution to eustachian tube dysfunction.[168] The cellular response of respiratory mucosa to allergens has been well studied. Therefore, similar to other parts of respiratory mucosa, the mucosa lining the middle-ear cleft is capable of an allergic response.[169,170] Sensitivity to allergens varies among individuals, and atopy may involve neutrophils in type I allergic reactions that enhance the inflammatory response.[171]

The correlation between OME and allergy has been widely reported, but no prospective studies have examined the effects of immunotherapy compared with observation alone or other management options. Reports of OME cure after immunotherapy or food-elimination diets[172] are impossible to interpret without concurrent control groups because of the favorable natural history of most untreated OME. The documentation of allergy in published reports has been defined inconsistently (medical history, physical examination, skin-prick testing, nasal smears, serum immunoglobulin E and eosinophil counts, inflammatory mediators in effusions). Study groups have been drawn primarily from specialist offices, likely lack heterogeneity, and are not representative of general medical practice.

Evidence Profile: Allergy Management

- Aggregate evidence quality: D, case series without controls.

- Benefit: not established.
- Harm: adverse effects and cost of medication, physician evaluation, elimination diets, and desensitization.
- Benefits-harms assessment: balance of benefit and harm.
- Policy level: no recommendation.

RESEARCH NEEDS

Diagnosis

- Further standardize the definition of OME.
- Assess the performance characteristics of pneumatic otoscopy as a diagnostic test for OME when performed by primary care physicians and advanced-practice nurses in the routine office setting.
- Determine the optimal methods for teaching pneumatic otoscopy to residents and clinicians.
- Develop a brief, reliable, objective method for diagnosing OME.
- Develop a classification method for identifying the presence of OME for practical use by clinicians that is based on quantifiable tympanometric characteristics.
- Assess the usefulness of algorithms combining pneumatic otoscopy and tympanometry for detecting OME in clinical practice.
- Conduct additional validating cohort studies of acoustic reflectometry as a diagnostic method for OME, particularly in children less than 2 years old.

Child At Risk

- Better define the child with OME who is at risk for speech, language, and learning problems.
- Conduct large, multicenter, observational cohort studies to identify the child at risk who is most susceptible to potential adverse sequelae of OME.
- Conduct large, multicenter, observational cohort studies to analyze outcomes achieved with alternative management strategies for OME in children at risk.

Watchful Waiting

- Define the spontaneous resolution of OME in infants and young children (existing data are limited primarily to children 2 years old or older).
- Conduct large-scale, prospective cohort studies to obtain current data on the spontaneous resolution of newly diagnosed OME of unknown prior duration (existing data are primarily from the late 1970s and early 1980s).
- Develop prognostic indicators to identify the best candidates for watchful waiting.
- Determine whether the lack of impact from prompt insertion of tympanostomy tubes on speech and language outcomes seen in asymptomatic young children with OME identified by screening or intense surveillance can be generalized to older children with OME or to symptomatic children with OME referred for evaluation.

Medication

- Clarify which children, if any, should receive antimicrobials, steroids, or both for OME.
- Conduct a randomized, placebo-controlled trial on the efficacy of antimicrobial therapy, with or without concurrent oral steroid, in avoiding surgery in children with OME who are surgical candidates and have not received recent antimicrobials.
- Investigate the role of mucosal surface biofilms in refractory or recurrent OME and develop targeted interventions.

Hearing and Language

- Conduct longitudinal studies on the natural history of hearing loss accompanying OME.
- Develop improved methods for describing and quantifying the fluctuations in hearing of children with OME over time.
- Conduct prospective controlled studies on the relation of hearing loss associated with OME to later auditory, speech, language, behavioral, and academic sequelae.
- Develop reliable, brief, objective methods for estimating hearing loss associated with OME.
- Develop reliable, brief, objective methods for estimating speech or language delay associated with OME.
- Evaluate the benefits and administrative burden of language testing by primary care clinicians.
- Agree on the aspects of language that are vulnerable to or affected by hearing loss caused by OME, and reach a consensus on the best tools for measurement.
- Determine whether OME and associated hearing loss place children from special populations at greater risk for speech and language delays.

Surveillance

- Develop better tools for monitoring children with OME that are suitable for routine clinical care.
- Assess the value of new strategies for monitoring OME, such as acoustic reflectometry performed at home by the parent or caregiver, in optimizing surveillance.
- Improve our ability to identify children who would benefit from early surgery instead of prolonged surveillance.
- Promote early detection of structural abnormalities in the tympanic membrane associated with OME that may require surgery to prevent complications.
- Clarify and quantify the role of parent or caregiver education, socioeconomic status, and quality of the caregiving environment as modifiers of OME developmental outcomes.
- Develop methods for minimizing loss to follow-up during OME surveillance.

Surgery

- Define the role of adenoidectomy in children 3 years old or younger as a specific OME therapy.

- Conduct controlled trials on the efficacy of tympanostomy tubes for developmental outcomes in children with hearing loss, other symptoms, or speech and language delay.
- Conduct randomized, controlled trials of surgery versus no surgery that emphasize patient-based outcome measures (quality of life, functional health status) in addition to objective measures (effusion prevalence, HLs, AOM incidence, reoperation).
- Identify the optimal ways to incorporate parent or caregiver preference into surgical decision-making.

CAM

- Conduct randomized, controlled trials on the efficacy of CAM modalities for OME.
- Develop strategies to identify parents or caregivers who use CAM therapies for their child's OME, and encourage surveillance by the primary care clinician.

Allergy Management

- Evaluate the causal role of atopy in OME.
- Conduct randomized, controlled trials on the efficacy of allergy therapy for OME that are generalizable to the primary care setting.

CONCLUSIONS

This evidence-based practice guideline offers recommendations for identifying, monitoring, and managing the child with OME. The guideline emphasizes appropriate diagnosis and provides options for various management strategies including observation, medical intervention, and referral for surgical intervention. These recommendations should provide primary care physicians and other health care providers with assistance in managing children with OME.

SUBCOMMITTEE ON OTITIS MEDIA WITH EFFUSION
Richard M. Rosenfeld, MD, MPH, Cochairperson
    American Academy of Pediatrics
    American Academy of Otolaryngology-Head and Neck Surgery
Larry Culpepper, MD, MPH, Cochairperson
    American Academy of Family Physicians
Karen J. Doyle, MD, PhD
    American Academy of Otolaryngology-Head and Neck Surgery
Kenneth M. Grundfast, MD
    American Academy of Otolaryngology-Head and Neck Surgery
Alejandro Hoberman, MD
    American Academy of Pediatrics
Margaret A. Kenna, MD
    American Academy of Otolaryngology-Head and Neck Surgery
Allan S. Lieberthal, MD
    American Academy of Pediatrics
Martin Mahoney, MD, PhD
    American Academy of Family Physicians
Richard A. Wahl, MD
    American Academy of Pediatrics
Charles R. Woods, Jr, MD, MS
    American Academy of Pediatrics

Barbara Yawn, MD, MSc
American Academy of Family Physicians

CONSULTANTS
S. Michael Marcy, MD
Richard N. Shiffman, MD

LIAISONS
Linda Carlson, MS, CPNP
National Association of Pediatric Nurse
Practitioners
Judith Gravel, PhD
American Academy of Audiology
Joanne Roberts, PhD
American Speech-Language-Hearing Association
STAFF
Maureen Hannley, PhD
American Academy of Otolaryngology-Head and
Neck Surgery
Carla T. Herrerias, MPH
American Academy of Pediatrics
Bellinda K. Schoof, MHA, CPHQ
American Academy of Family Physicians

ACKNOWLEDGMENTS

Dr Marcy serves as a consultant to Abbott Laboratories Glaxo-SmithKline (vaccines).

REFERENCES

1. Stool SE, Berg AO, Berman S, et al. *Otitis Media With Effusion in Young Children. Clinical Practice Guideline, Number 12.* AHCPR Publication No. 94-0622. Rockville, MD: Agency for Health Care Policy and Research, Public Health Service, US Department of Health and Human Services; 1994

2. Shekelle P, Takata G, Chan LS, et al. *Diagnosis, Natural History, and Late Effects of Otitis Media With Effusion. Evidence Report/Technology Assessment No. 55.* AHRQ Publication No. 03-E023. Rockville, MD: Agency for Healthcare Research and Quality; 2003

3. Williamson I. Otitis media with effusion. *Clin Evid.* 2002;7:469–476

4. Tos M. Epidemiology and natural history of secretory otitis. *Am J Otol.* 1984;5:459–462

5. Paradise JL, Rockette HE, Colborn DK, et al. Otitis media in 2253 Pittsburgh area infants: prevalence and risk factors during the first two years of life. *Pediatrics.* 1997;99:318–333

6. Casselbrant ML, Mandel EM. Epidemiology. In: Rosenfeld RM, Bluestone CD, eds. *Evidence-Based Otitis Media.* 2nd ed. Hamilton, Ontario: BC Decker; 2003:147–162

7. Williamson IG, Dunleavy J, Baine J, Robinson D. The natural history of otitis media with effusion—a three-year study of the incidence and prevalence of abnormal tympanograms in four South West Hampshire infant and first schools. *J Laryngol Otol.* 1994;108:930–934

8. Coyte PC, Croxford R, Asche CV, To T, Feldman W, Friedberg J. Physician and population determinants of rates of middle-ear surgery in Ontario. *JAMA.* 2001;286:2128–2135

9. Tugwell P. How to read clinical journals: III. To learn the clinical course and prognosis of disease. *Can Med Assoc J.* 1981;124:869–872

10. Jaeschke R, Guyatt G, Sackett DL. Users' guides to the medical literature. III. How to use an article about a diagnostic test. A. Are the results of the study valid? Evidence-Based Medicine Working Group. *JAMA.* 1994;271:389–391

11. Shiffman RN, Shekelle P, Overhage JM, Slutsky J, Grimshaw J, Deshpande AM. Standardized reporting of clinical practice guidelines: a proposal from the Conference on Guideline Standardization. *Ann Intern Med.* 2003;139:493–498

12. Shiffman RN, Karras BT, Agrawal A, Chen R, Marenco L, Nath S. GEM: a proposal for a more comprehensive guideline document model using XML. *J Am Med Inform Assoc.* 2000;7:488–498

13. Shaneyfelt TM, Mayo-Smith MF, Rothwangl J. Are guidelines following guidelines? The methodological quality of clinical practice guidelines in the peer-reviewed medical literature. *JAMA.* 1999;281:1900–1905

14. Agrawal A, Shiffman RN. Evaluation of guideline quality using GEM-Q. *Medinfo.* 2001;10:1097–1101

15. Yale Center for Medical Informatics. GEM: The Guideline Elements Model. Available at: http://ycmi.med.yale.edu/GEM/. Accessed December 8, 2003

16. American Academy of Pediatrics, Steering Committee on Quality Improvement and Management. A taxonomy of recommendations for clinical practice guidelines. *Pediatrics.* 2004; In press

17. Eddy DM. *A Manual for Assessing Health Practices and Designing Practice Policies: The Explicit Approach.* Philadelphia, PA: American College of Physicians; 1992

18. Dowell SF, Marcy MS, Phillips WR, Gerber MA, Schwartz B. Otitis media—principles of judicious use of antimicrobial agents. *Pediatrics.* 1998;101:165–171

19. Dowell SF, Butler JC, Giebink GS, et al. Acute otitis media: management and surveillance in an era of pneumococcal resistance—a report from the Drug-Resistant *Streptococcus pneumoniae* Therapeutic Working Group. *Pediatr Infect Dis J.* 1999;18:1–9

20. Karma PH, Penttila MA, Sipila MM, Kataja MJ. Otoscopic diagnosis of middle ear effusion in acute and non-acute otitis media. I. The value of different otoscopic findings. *Int J Pediatr Otorhinolaryngol.* 1989;17:37–49

21. Pichichero ME, Poole MD. Assessing diagnostic accuracy and tympanocentesis skills in the management of otitis media. *Arch Pediatr Adolesc Med.* 2001;155:1137–1142

22. Steinbach WJ, Sectish TC. Pediatric resident training in the diagnosis and treatment of acute otitis media. *Pediatrics.* 2002;109:404–408

23. Palmu A, Puhakka H, Rahko T, Takala AK. Diagnostic value of tympanometry in infants in clinical practice. *Int J Pediatr Otorhinolaryngol.* 1999;49:207–213

24. van Balen FA, Aarts AM, De Melker RA. Tympanometry by general practitioners: reliable? *Int J Pediatr Otorhinolaryngol.* 1999;48:117–123

25. Block SL, Mandel E, McLinn S, et al. Spectral gradient acoustic reflectometry for the detection of middle ear effusion by pediatricians and parents. *Pediatr Infect Dis J.* 1998;17:560–564, 580

26. Barnett ED, Klein JO, Hawkins KA, Cabral HJ, Kenna M, Healy G. Comparison of spectral gradient acoustic reflectometry and other diagnostic techniques for detection of middle ear effusion in children with middle ear disease. *Pediatr Infect Dis J.* 1998;17:556–559, 580

27. Block SL, Pichichero ME, McLinn S, Aronovitz G, Kimball S. Spectral gradient acoustic reflectometry: detection of middle ear effusion by pediatricians in suppurative acute otitis media. *Pediatr Infect Dis J.* 1999;18:741–744

28. Schwartz RH. A practical approach to the otitis prone child. *Contemp Pediatr.* 1987;4:30–54

29. Barriga F, Schwartz RH, Hayden GF. Adequate illumination for otoscopy. Variations due to power source, bulb, and head and speculum design. *Am J Dis Child.* 1986;140:1237–1240

30. Sorenson CH, Jensen SH, Tos M. The post-winter prevalence of middle-ear effusion in four-year-old children, judged by tympanometry. *Int J Pediatr Otorhinolaryngol.* 1981;3:119–128

31. Fiellau-Nikolajsen M. Epidemiology of secretory otitis media. A descriptive cohort study. *Ann Otol Rhinol Laryngol.* 1983;92:172–177

32. Casselbrant ML, Brostoff LM, Cantekin EI, et al. Otitis media with effusion in preschool children. *Laryngoscope.* 1985;95:428–436

33. Zielhuis GA, Rach GH, van den Broek P. Screening for otitis media with effusion in preschool children. *Lancet.* 1989;1:311–314

34. Poulsen G, Tos M. Repetitive tympanometric screenings of two-year-old children. *Scand Audiol.* 1980;9:21–28

35. Tos M, Holm-Jensen S, Sorensen CH. Changes in prevalence of secretory otitis from summer to winter in four-year-old children. *Am J Otol.* 1981;2:324–327

36. Thomsen J, Tos M. Spontaneous improvement of secretory otitis. A long-term study. *Acta Otolaryngol.* 1981;92:493–499

37. Lous J, Fiellau-Nikolajsen M. Epidemiology of middle ear effusion and tubal dysfunction. A one-year prospective study comprising monthly tympanometry in 387 non-selected seven-year-old children. *Int J Pediatr Otorhinolaryngol.* 1981;3:303–317

38. New Zealand Health Technology Assessment. *Screening Programmes for the Detection of Otitis Media With Effusion and Conductive Hearing Loss in Pre-School and New Entrant School Children: A Critical Appraisal of the Literature.* Christchurch, New Zealand: New Zealand Health Technology Assessment; 1998:61

39. Canadian Task Force on Preventive Health Care. Screening for otitis media with effusion: recommendation statement from the Canadian Task Force on Preventive Health Care. *CMAJ.* 2001;165:1092–1093

40. US Preventive Services Task Force. *Guide to Clinical Preventive Services.* 2nd ed. Baltimore, MD: Williams & Wilkins; 1995

41. Paradise JL, Feldman HM, Campbell TF, et al. Effect of early or delayed insertion of tympanostomy tubes for persistent otitis media on

developmental outcomes at the age of three years. *N Engl J Med.* 2001;344:1179–1187

42. Rovers MM, Krabble PF, Straatman H, Ingels K, van der Wilt GJ, Zielhuis GA. Randomized controlled trial of the effect of ventilation tubes (grommets) on quality of life at age 1–2 years. *Arch Dis Child.* 2001;84:45–49

43. Wood DL. Documentation guidelines: evolution, future direction, and compliance. *Am J Med.* 2001;110:332–334

44. Soto CM, Kleinman KP, Simon SR. Quality and correlates of medical record documentation in the ambulatory care setting. *BMC Health Serv Res.* 2002;2:22–35

45. Marchant CD, Shurin PA, Turczyk VA, Wasikowski DE, Tutihasi MA, Kinney SE. Course and outcome of otitis media in early infancy: a prospective study. *J Pediatr.* 1984;104:826–831

46. Rosenfeld RM, Goldsmith AJ, Tetlus L, Balzano A. Quality of life for children with otitis media. *Arch Otolaryngol Head Neck Surg.* 1997;123:1049–1054

47. Casselbrant ML, Furman JM, Rubenstein E, Mandel EM. Effect of otitis media on the vestibular system in children. *Ann Otol Rhinol Laryngol.* 1995;104:620–624

48. Orlin MN, Effgen SK, Handler SD. Effect of otitis media with effusion on gross motor ability in preschool-aged children: preliminary findings. *Pediatrics.* 1997;99:334–337

49. Golz A, Angel-Yeger B, Parush S. Evaluation of balance disturbances in children with middle ear effusion. *Int J Pediatr Otorhinolaryngol.* 1998;43:21–26

50. Casselbrant ML, Redfern MS, Furman JM, Fall PA, Mandel EM. Visual-induced postural sway in children with and without otitis media. *Ann Otol Rhinol Laryngol.* 1998;107:401–405

51. Ruben R. Host susceptibility to otitis media sequelae. In: Rosenfeld RM, Bluestone CD, eds. *Evidence-Based Otitis Media.* 2nd ed. Hamilton, ON, Canada: BC Decker; 2003:505–514

52. Whiteman BC, Simpson GB, Compton WC. Relationship of otitis media and language impairment on adolescents with Down syndrome. *Ment Retard.* 1986;24:353–356

53. van der Vyver M, van der Merwe A, Tesner HE. The effects of otitis media on articulation in children with cerebral palsy. *Int J Rehabil Res.* 1988;11:386–389

54. Paradise JL, Bluestone CD. Early treatment of the universal otitis media of infants with cleft palate. *Pediatrics.* 1974;53:48–54

55. Schwartz DM, Schwartz RH. Acoustic impedance and otoscopic findings in young children with Down's syndrome. *Arch Otolaryngol.* 1978;104:652–656

56. Corey JP, Caldarelli DD, Gould HJ. Otopathology in cranial facial dysostosis. *Am J Otol.* 1987;8:14–17

57. Schonweiler R, Schonweiler B, Schmelzeisen R. Hearing capacity and speech production in 417 children with facial cleft abnormalities [in German]. *HNO.* 1994;42:691–696

58. Ruben RJ, Math R. Serous otitis media associated with sensorineural hearing loss in children. *Laryngoscope.* 1978;88:1139–1154

59. Brookhouser PE, Worthington DW, Kelly WJ. Middle ear disease in young children with sensorineural hearing loss. *Laryngoscope.* 1993;103:371–378

60. Rice ML. Specific language impairments: in search of diagnostic markers and genetic contributions. *Ment Retard Dev Disabil Res Rev.* 1997;3:350–357

61. Rosenhall U, Nordin V, Sandstrom M, Ahlsen G, Gillberg C. Autism and hearing loss. *J Autism Dev Disord.* 1999;29:349–357

62. Cunningham C, McArthur K. Hearing loss and treatment in young Down's syndrome children. *Child Care Health Dev.* 1981;7:357–374

63. Shott SR, Joseph A, Heithaus D. Hearing loss in children with Down syndrome. *Int J Pediatr Otorhinolaryngol.* 2001;61:199–205

64. Clarkson RL, Eimas PD, Marean GC. Speech perception in children with histories of recurrent otitis media. *J Acoust Soc Am.* 1989;85:926–933

65. Groenen P, Crul T, Maassen B, van Bon W. Perception of voicing cues by children with early otitis media with and without language impairment. *J Speech Hear Res.* 1996;39:43–54

66. Hubbard TW, Paradise JL, McWilliams BJ, Elster BA, Taylor FH. Consequences of unremitting middle-ear disease in early life. Otologic, audiologic, and developmental findings in children with cleft palate. *N Engl J Med.* 1985;312:1529–1534

67. Nunn DR, Derkay CS, Darrow DH, Magee W, Strasnick B. The effect of very early cleft palate closure on the need for ventilation tubes in the first years of life. *Laryngoscope.* 1995;105:905–908

68. Pappas DG, Flexer C, Shackelford L. Otological and habilitative management of children with Down syndrome. *Laryngoscope.* 1994;104:1065–1070

69. Vartiainen E. Otitis media with effusion in children with congenital or early-onset hearing impairment. *J Otolaryngol.* 2000;29:221–223

70. Rosenfeld RM, Kay D. Natural history of untreated otitis media. *Laryngoscope.* 2003;113:1645–1657

71. Teele DW, Klein JO, Rosner BA. Epidemiology of otitis media in children. *Ann Otol Rhinol Laryngol Suppl.* 1980;89:5–6

72. Mygind N, Meistrup-Larsen KI, Thomsen J, Thomsen VF, Josefsson K, Sorensen H. Penicillin in acute otitis media: a double-blind, placebo-controlled trial. *Clin Otolaryngol.* 1981;6:5–13

73. Burke P, Bain J, Robinson D, Dunleavey J. Acute red ear in children: controlled trial of nonantibiotic treatment in general practice. *BMJ.* 1991;303:558–562

74. Fiellau-Nikolajsen M, Lous J. Prospective tympanometry in 3-year-old children. A study of the spontaneous course of tympanometry types in a nonselected population. *Arch Otolaryngol.* 1979;105:461–466

75. Fiellau-Nikolajsen M. Tympanometry in 3-year-old children. Type of care as an epidemiological factor in secretory otitis media and tubal dysfunction in unselected populations of 3-year-old children. *ORL J Otorhinolaryngol Relat Spec.* 1979;41:193–205

76. Tos M. Spontaneous improvement of secretory otitis and impedance screening. *Arch Otolaryngol.* 1980;106:345–349

77. Tos M, Holm-Jensen S, Sorensen CH, Mogensen C. Spontaneous course and frequency of secretory otitis in 4-year-old children. *Arch Otolaryngol.* 1982;108:4–10

78. Roberts JE, Zeisel SA. *Ear Infections and Language Development.* Rockville, MD: American Speech-Language-Hearing Association and the National Center for Early Development and Learning; 2000

79. Roberts JE, Rosenfeld RM, Zeisel SA. Otitis media and speech and language: a meta-analysis of prospective studies. *Pediatrics.* 2004;113(3). Available at: www.pediatrics.org/cgi/content/full/113/3/e238

80. Williams RL, Chalmers TC, Stange KC, Chalmers FT, Bowlin SJ. Use of antibiotics in preventing recurrent otitis media and in treating otitis media with effusion. A meta-analytic attempt to resolve the brouhaha. *JAMA.* 1993;270:1344–1351

81. Rosenfeld RM, Post JC. Meta-analysis of antibiotics for the treatment of otitis media with effusion. *Otolaryngol Head Neck Surg.* 1992;106:378–386

82. Mandel EM, Rockette HE, Bluestone CD, Paradise JL, Nozza RJ. Efficacy of amoxicillin with and without decongestant-antihistamine for otitis media with effusion in children. Results of a double-blind, randomized trial. *N Engl J Med.* 1987;316:432–437

83. McCormick AW, Whitney CG, Farley MM, et al. Geographic diversity and temporal trends of antimicrobial resistance in *Streptococcus pneumoniae* in the United States. *Nat Med.* 2003;9:424–430

84. Levy SB. *The Antibiotic Paradox. How the Misuse of Antibiotic Destroys Their Curative Powers.* Cambridge, MA: Perseus Publishing; 2002

85. Butler CC, van der Voort JH. Oral or topical nasal steroids for hearing loss associated with otitis media with effusion in children. *Cochrane Database Syst Rev.* 2002;4:CD001935

86. Mandel EM, Casselbrant ML, Rockette HE, Fireman P, Kurs-Lasky M, Bluestone CD. Systemic steroid for chronic otitis media with effusion in children. *Pediatrics.* 2002;110:1071–1080

87. Tracy JM, Demain JG, Hoffman KM, Goetz DW. Intranasal beclomethasone as an adjunct to treatment of chronic middle ear effusion. *Ann Allergy Asthma Immunol.* 1998;80:198–206

88. Joint Committee on Infant Hearing. Year 2000 position statement: principles and guidelines for early hearing detection and intervention programs. *Am J Audiol.* 2000;9:9–29

89. Pillsbury HC, Grose JH, Hall JW III. Otitis media with effusion in children. Binaural hearing before and after corrective surgery. *Arch Otolaryngol Head Neck Surg.* 1991;117:718–723

90. Besing J, Koehnke J. A test of virtual auditory localization. *Ear Hear.* 1995;16:220–229

91. Jerger S, Jerger J, Alford BR, Abrams S. Development of speech intelligibility in children with recurrent otitis media. *Ear Hear.* 1983;4:138–145

92. Gravel JS, Wallace IF. Listening and language at 4 years of age: effects of early otitis media. *J Speech Hear Res.* 1992;35:588–595

93. Schilder AG, Snik AF, Straatman H, van den Broek P. The effect of otitis media with effusion at preschool age on some aspects of auditory perception at school age. *Ear Hear.* 1994;15:224–231

94. Rosenfeld RM, Madell JR, McMahon A. Auditory function in normal-hearing children with middle ear effusion. In: Lim DJ, Bluestone CD, Casselbrant M, Klein JO, Ogra PL, eds. *Recent Advances in Otitis Media: Proceedings of the 6th International Symposium.* Hamilton, ON, Canada: BC Decker; 1996:354–356

95. Friel-Patti S, Finitzo T. Language learning in a prospective study of otitis media with effusion in the first two years of life. *J Speech Hear Res.* 1990;33:188–194

96. Wallace IF, Gravel JS, McCarton CM, Stapells DR, Bernstein RS, Ruben RJ. Otitis media, auditory sensitivity, and language outcomes at one year. *Laryngoscope.* 1988;98:64–70

97. Roberts JE, Burchinal MR, Medley LP, et al. Otitis media, hearing sensitivity, and maternal responsiveness in relation to language during infancy. *J Pediatr.* 1995;126:481–489

98. Roberts JE, Burchinal MR, Zeisel SA. Otitis media in early childhood in relation to children's school-age language and academic skills. *Pediatrics.* 2002;110:696–706

99. Rovers MM, Straatman H, Ingels K, van der Wilt GJ, van den Broek P, Zielhuis GA. The effect of ventilation tubes on language development in infants with otitis media with effusion: a randomized trial. *Pediatrics.* 2000;106(3). Available at: www.pediatrics.org/cgi/content/full/106/3/e42

100. Paradise JL, Feldman HM, Campbell TF, et al. Early versus delayed insertion of tympanostomy tubes for persistent otitis media: developmental outcomes at the age of three years in relation to prerandomization illness patterns and hearing levels. *Pediatr Infect Dis J.* 2003;22:309–314

101. Kokko E. Chronic secretory otitis media in children. A clinical study. *Acta Otolaryngol Suppl.* 1974;327:1–44

102. Fria TJ, Cantekin EI, Eichler JA. Hearing acuity of children with otitis media with effusion. *Arch Otolaryngol.* 1985;111:10–16

103. Gravel JS, Wallace IF. Effects of otitis media with effusion on hearing in the first three years of life. *J Speech Lang Hear Res.* 2000;43:631–644

104. Roberts JE, Burchinal MR, Zeisel S, et al. Otitis media, the caregiving environment, and language and cognitive outcomes at 2 years. *Pediatrics.* 1998;102:346–354

105. Gravel JS, Wallace IF, Ruben RJ. Early otitis media and later educational risk. *Acta Otolaryngol.* 1995;115:279–281

106. Cunningham M, Cox EO; American Academy of Pediatrics, Committee on Practice and Ambulatory Medicine, Section on Otolaryngology and Bronchoesophagology. Hearing assessment in infants and children: recommendations beyond neonatal screening. *Pediatrics.* 2003;111:436–440

107. American Speech-Language-Hearing Association Panel on Audiologic Assessment. *Guidelines for Audiologic Screening.* Rockville, MD: American Speech-Language-Hearing Association; 1996

108. Rosenfeld RM, Goldsmith AJ, Madell JR. How accurate is parent rating of hearing for children with otitis media? *Arch Otolaryngol Head Neck Surg.* 1998;124:989–992

109. Brody R, Rosenfeld RM, Goldsmith AJ, Madell JR. Parents cannot detect mild hearing loss in children. *Otolaryngol Head Neck Surg.* 1999;121:681–686

110. Catts HW, Fey ME, Zhang X, Tomblin JB. Language basis of reading and reading disabilities: evidence from a longitudinal investigation. *Sci Stud Read.* 1999;3:331–362

111. Johnson CJ, Beitchman JH, Young A, et al. Fourteen-year follow-up of children with and without speech/language impairments: speech/language stability and outcomes. *J Speech Lang Hear Res.* 1999;42:744–760

112. Scarborough H, Dobrich W. Development of children with early language delay. *J Speech Hear Res.* 1990;33:70–83

113. Tomblin JB, Records NL, Buckwalter P, Zhang X, Smith E, O'Brien M. Prevalence of specific language impairment in kindergarten children. *J Speech Lang Hear Res.* 1997;40:1245–1260

114. Glade MJ. *Diagnostic and Therapeutic Technology Assessment: Speech Therapy in Patients With a Prior History of Recurrent Acute or Chronic Otitis Media With Effusion.* Chicago, IL: American Medical Association; 1996:1–14

115. Casby MW. Otitis media and language development: a meta-analysis. *Am J Speech Lang Pathol.* 2001;10:65–80

116. Maw R, Wilks J, Harvey I, Peters TJ, Golding J. Early surgery compared with watchful waiting for glue ear and effect on language development in preschool children: a randomised trial. *Lancet.* 1999;353:960–963

117. Coplan J. *Early Language Milestone Scale.* 2nd ed. Austin, TX: PRO-ED; 1983

118. Fenson L, Dale PS, Reznick JS, et al. *MacArthur Communicative Development Inventories. User's Guide and Technical Manual.* San Diego, CA: Singular Publishing Group; 1993

119. Rescoria L. The Language Development Survey: a screening tool for delayed language in toddlers. *J Speech Hear Dis.* 1989;54:587–599

120. Frankenburg WK, Dodds JA, Faucal A, et al. *Denver Developmental Screening Test II.* Denver, CO: University of Colorado Press; 1990

121. Klee T, Pearce K, Carson DK. Improving the positive predictive value of screening for developmental language disorder. *J Speech Lang Hear Res.* 2000;43:821–833

122. Shekelle PG, Ortiz E, Rhodes S, et al. Validity of the Agency for Healthcare Research and Quality clinical practice guidelines: how quickly do guidelines become outdated? *JAMA.* 2001;286:1461–1467

123. Zielhuis GA, Straatman H, Rach GH, van den Broek P. Analysis and presentation of data on the natural course of otitis media with effusion in children. *Int J Epidemiol.* 1990;19:1037–1044

124. MRC Multi-centre Otitis Media Study Group. Risk factors for persistence of bilateral otitis media with effusion. *Clin Otolaryngol.* 2001;26:147–156

125. van Balen FA, De Melker RA. Persistent otitis media with effusion: can it be predicted? A family practice follow-up study in children aged 6 months to 6 years. *J Fam Pract.* 2000;49:605–611

126. Sano S, Kamide Y, Schachern PA, Paparella MM. Micropathologic changes of pars tensa in children with otitis media with effusion. *Arch Otolaryngol Head Neck Surg.* 1994;120:815–819

127. Yellon RF, Doyle WJ, Whiteside TL, Diven WF, March AR, Fireman P. Cytokines, immunoglobulins, and bacterial pathogens in middle ear effusions. *Arch Otolaryngol Head Neck Surg.* 1995;121:865–869

128. Maw RA, Bawden R. Tympanic membrane atrophy, scarring, atelectasis and attic retraction in persistent, untreated otitis media with effusion and following ventilation tube insertion. *Int J Pediatr Otorhinolaryngol.* 1994;30:189–204

129. Davis JM, Elfenbein J, Schum R, Bentler RA. Effects of mild and moderate hearing impairment on language, educational, and psychosocial behavior of children. *J Speech Hear Disord.* 1986;51:53–62

130. Carney AE, Moeller MP. Treatment efficacy: hearing loss in children. *J Speech Lang Hear Res.* 1998;41:S61–S84

131. Karchmer MA, Allen TE. The functional assessment of deaf and hard of hearing students. *Am Ann Deaf.* 1999;144:68–77

132. Bess FH, Dodd-Murphy J, Parker RA. Children with minimal sensorineural hearing loss: prevalence, educational performance, and functional status. *Ear Hear.* 1998;19:339–354

133. Roberts JE, Burchinal MR, Jackson SC, et al. Otitis media in early childhood in relation to preschool language and school readiness skills among black children. *Pediatrics.* 2000;106:725–735

134. Haggard MP, Birkin JA, Browning GG, Gatehouse S, Lewis S. Behavior problems in otitis media. *Pediatr Infect Dis J.* 1994;13:S43–S50

135. Bennett KE, Haggard MP. Behaviour and cognitive outcomes from middle ear disease. *Arch Dis Child.* 1999;80:28–35

136. Bennett KE, Haggard MP, Silva PA, Stewart IA. Behaviour and developmental effects of otitis media with effusion into the teens. *Arch Dis Child.* 2001;85:91–95

137. Wilks J, Maw R, Peters TJ, Harvey I, Golding J. Randomised controlled trial of early surgery versus watchful waiting for glue ear: the effect on behavioural problems in pre-school children. *Clin Otolaryngol.* 2000;25:209–214

138. Rosenfeld RM, Bhaya MH, Bower CM, et al. Impact of tympanostomy tubes on child quality of life. *Arch Otolaryngol Head Neck Surg.* 2000;126:585–592

139. Rosenfeld RM, Bluestone CD. Clinical efficacy of surgical therapy. In: Rosenfeld RM, Bluestone CD, eds. *Evidence-Based Otitis Media.* 2nd ed. Hamilton, ON, Canada: BC Decker; 2003:227–240

140. Kuyvenhoven MM, De Melker RA. Referrals to specialists. An exploratory investigation of referrals by 13 general practitioners to medical and surgical departments. *Scand J Prim Health Care.* 1990;8:53–57

141. Haldis TA, Blankenship JC. Telephone reporting in the consultant-generalist relationship. *J Eval Clin Pract.* 2002;8:31–35

142. Reichman S. The generalist's patient and the subspecialist. *Am J Manag Care.* 2002;8:79–82

143. Gates GA, Avery CA, Prihoda TJ, Cooper JC Jr. Effectiveness of adenoidectomy and tympanostomy tubes in the treatment of chronic otitis media with effusion. *N Engl J Med.* 1987;317:1444–1451

144. Mandel EM, Rockette HE, Bluestone CD, Paradise JL, Nozza RJ. Myringotomy with and without tympanostomy tubes for chronic otitis media with effusion. *Arch Otolaryngol Head Neck Surg.* 1989;115:1217–1224

145. Mandel EM, Rockette HE, Bluestone CD, Paradise JL, Nozza RJ. Efficacy of myringotomy with and without tympanostomy tubes for chronic otitis media with effusion. *Pediatr Infect Dis J.* 1992;11:270–277

146. University of York Centre for Reviews and Dissemination. The treatment of persistent glue ear in children. *Eff Health Care.* 1992;4:1–16

147. Rovers MM, Straatman H, Ingels K, van der Wilt GJ, van den Broek P, Zielhuis GA. The effect of short-term ventilation tubes versus watchful waiting on hearing in young children with persistent otitis media with effusion: a randomized trial. *Ear Hear.* 2001;22:191–199

148. Paradise JL, Bluestone CD, Colborn DK, et al. Adenoidectomy and adenotonsillectomy for recurrent acute otitis media: parallel randomized clinical trials in children not previously treated with tympanostomy tubes. *JAMA*. 1999;282:945–953

149. Boston M, McCook J, Burke B, Derkay C. Incidence of and risk factors for additional tympanostomy tube insertion in children. *Arch Otolaryngol Head Neck Surg*. 2003;129:293–296

150. Coyte PC, Croxford R, McIsaac W, Feldman W, Friedberg J. The role of adjuvant adenoidectomy and tonsillectomy in the outcome of insertion of tympanostomy tubes. *N Engl J Med*. 2001;344:1188–1195

151. Paradise JL, Bluestone CD, Rogers KD, et al. Efficacy of adenoidectomy for recurrent otitis media in children previously treated with tympanostomy-tube placement. Results of parallel randomized and nonrandomized trials. *JAMA*. 1990;263:2066–2073

152. Maw AR. Chronic otitis media with effusion (glue ear) and adenotonsillectomy: prospective randomised controlled study. *Br Med J (Clin Res Ed)*. 1983;287:1586–1588

153. Cohen D, Schechter Y, Slatkine M, Gatt N, Perez R. Laser myringotomy in different age groups. *Arch Otolaryngol Head Neck Surg*. 2001;127:260–264

154. Holzman RS. Morbidity and mortality in pediatric anesthesia. *Pediatr Clin North Am*. 1994;41:239–256

155. Cottrell JE, Golden S. *Under the Mask: A Guide to Feeling Secure and Comfortable During Anesthesia and Surgery*. New Brunswick, NJ: Rutgers University Press; 2001

156. Kay DJ, Nelson M, Rosenfeld RM. Meta-analysis of tympanostomy tube sequelae. *Otolaryngol Head Neck Surg*. 2001;124:374–380

157. Crysdale WS, Russel D. Complications of tonsillectomy and adenoidectomy in 9409 children observed overnight. *CMAJ*. 1986;135:1139–1142

158. Harrison H, Fixsen A, Vickers A. A randomized comparison of homeopathic and standard care for the treatment of glue ear in children. *Complement Ther Med*. 1999;7:132–135

159. Sawyer CE, Evans RL, Boline PD, Branson R, Spicer A. A feasibility study of chiropractic spinal manipulation versus sham spinal manipulation for chronic otitis media with effusion in children. *J Manipulative Physiol Ther*. 1999;22:292–298

160. Ernst E. Serious adverse effects of unconventional therapies for children and adolescents: a systematic review of recent evidence. *Eur J Pediatr*. 2003;162:72–80

161. Cohen MH, Eisenberg DM. Potential physician malpractice liability associated with complementary and integrative medical therapies. *Ann Intern Med*. 2002;136:596–603

162. Mullins RJ, Heddle R. Adverse reactions associated with echinacea: the Australian experience. *Ann Allergy Asthma Immunol*. 2002;88:42–51

163. Miller LG, Hume A, Harris IM, et al. White paper on herbal products. American College of Clinical Pharmacy. *Pharmacotherapy*. 2000;20:877–891

164. Angell M, Kassirer JP. Alternative medicine—the risks of untested and unregulated remedies. *N Engl J Med*. 1998;339:839–841

165. Fallon JM. The role of chiropractic adjustment in the care and treatment of 332 children with otitis media. *J Clin Chiropractic Pediatr*. 1997;2:167–183

166. Shafrir Y, Kaufman BA. Quadriplegia after chiropractic manipulation in an infant with congenital torticollis caused by a spinal cord astrocytoma. *J Pediatr*. 1992;120:266–269

167. Corey JP, Adham RE, Abbass AH, Seligman I. The role of IgE-mediated hypersensitivity in otitis media with effusion. *Am J Otolaryngol*. 1994;15:138–144

168. Bernstein JM. Role of allergy in eustachian tube blockage and otitis media with effusion: a review. *Otolaryngol Head Neck Surg*. 1996;114:562–568

169. Ishii TM, Toriyama M, Suzuki JI. Histopathological study of otitis media with effusion. *Ann Otol Rhinol Laryngol*. 1980;89(suppl):83–86

170. Hurst DS, Venge P. Evidence of eosinophil, neutrophil, and mast-cell mediators in the effusion of OME patients with and without atopy. *Allergy*. 2000;55:435–441

171. Hurst DS, Venge P. The impact of atopy on neutrophil activity in middle ear effusion from children and adults with chronic otitis media. *Arch Otolaryngol Head Neck Surg*. 2002;128:561–566

172. Hurst DS. Allergy management of refractory serous otitis media. *Otolaryngol Head Neck Surg*. 1990;102:664–669

Management of Sinusitis

• •

- *Clinical Practice Guideline*
- *Technical Report Summary*

Readers of this clinical practice guideline are urged to review the technical report to enhance the evidence-based decision-making process. The full technical report is available on the enclosed CD-ROM.

AMERICAN ACADEMY OF PEDIATRICS

Subcommittee on Management of Sinusitis and Committee on Quality Improvement

Clinical Practice Guideline: Management of Sinusitis

ABSTRACT. This clinical practice guideline formulates recommendations for health care providers regarding the diagnosis, evaluation, and treatment of children, ages 1 to 21 years, with uncomplicated acute, subacute, and recurrent acute bacterial sinusitis. It was developed through a comprehensive search and analysis of the medical literature. Expert consensus opinion was used to enhance or formulate recommendations where data were insufficient.

A subcommittee, composed of pediatricians with expertise in infectious disease, allergy, epidemiology, family practice, and pediatric practice, supplemented with an otolaryngologist and radiologist, were selected to formulate the practice parameter. Several other groups (including members of the American College of Emergency Physicians, American Academy of Otolaryngology-Head and Neck Surgery, American Academy of Asthma, Allergy and Immunology, as well as numerous national committees and sections of the American Academy of Pediatrics) have reviewed and revised the guideline. Three specific issues were considered: 1) evidence for the efficacy of various antibiotics in children; 2) evidence for the efficacy of various ancillary, nonantibiotic regimens; and 3) the diagnostic accuracy and concordance of clinical symptoms, radiography (and other imaging methods), and sinus aspiration.

It is recommended that the diagnosis of acute bacterial sinusitis be based on clinical criteria in children ≤6 years of age who present with upper respiratory symptoms that are either persistent or severe. Although controversial, imaging studies may be necessary to confirm a diagnosis of acute bacterial sinusitis in children >6 years of age. Computed tomography scans of the paranasal sinuses should be reserved for children who present with complications of acute bacterial sinusitis or who have very persistent or recurrent infections and are not responsive to medical management.

There were only 5 controlled randomized trials and 8 case series on antimicrobial therapy for acute bacterial sinusitis in children. However, these data, plus data derived from the study of adults with acute bacterial sinusitis, support the recommendation that acute bacterial sinusitis be treated with antimicrobial therapy to achieve a more rapid clinical cure. Children with complications or suspected complications of acute bacterial sinusitis should be treated promptly and aggressively with antibiotics and, when appropriate, drainage. Based on controversial and limited data, no recommendations are made about the use of prophylactic antimicrobials, ancillary therapies, or complementary/alternative medicine for prevention and treatment of acute bacterial sinusitis.

This clinical practice guideline is not intended as a sole source of guidance in the diagnosis and management of acute bacterial sinusitis in children. It is designed to assist pediatricians by providing an analytic framework for evaluation and treatment. It is not intended to replace clinical judgment or establish a protocol for all patients with this condition.

ABBREVIATION. CT, computed tomography.

BACKGROUND

The ethmoid and the maxillary sinuses form in the third to fourth gestational month and, accordingly, are present at birth. The sphenoid sinuses are generally pneumatized by 5 years of age; the frontal sinuses appear at age 7 to 8 years but are not completely developed until late adolescence. The paranasal sinuses are a common site of infection in children and adolescents.[1] These infections are important as a cause of frequent morbidity and rarely may result in life-threatening complications. It may be difficult to distinguish children with uncomplicated viral upper respiratory infections or adenoiditis from those with an episode of acute bacterial sinusitis.[2] Most viral infections of the upper respiratory tract involve the nose and the paranasal sinuses (viral rhinosinusitis).[3] However, bacterial infections of the paranasal sinuses do not usually involve the nose. When the patient with bacterial infection of the paranasal sinuses has purulent (thick, colored, and opaque) nasal drainage, the site of infection is the paranasal sinuses; the nose is simply acting as a conduit for secretions produced in the sinuses.

The common predisposing events that set the stage for acute bacterial sinusitis are acute viral upper respiratory infections that result in a viral rhinosinusitis (a diffuse mucositis that predisposes to approximately 80% of bacterial sinus infections) and allergic inflammation (that predisposes to 20% of bacterial sinus infections).[4] Children have 6 to 8 viral upper respiratory infections each year; it is estimated that between 5% to 13% of these infections may be complicated by a secondary bacterial infection of the paranasal sinuses.[5–7] Acute bacterial otitis media and acute bacterial sinusitis are the most common complications of viral upper respiratory infections and are probably the most common indications for the prescription of antimicrobial agents.[8] The middle ear cavity connects to the nasopharynx via the eustachian tube. In a sense then, the middle ear cavity is also a paranasal sinus.[9] The pathogenesis and microbiology of acute otitis media and acute bacterial sinusitis are similar.[9] This similarity allows us to extrapolate information known about the treatment of acute otitis media and apply it to the treatment of acute bacterial sinusitis. This is especially helpful when considering antimicrobials and antibacterial resistance. Data on antimicrobial efficacy and antibacterial resistance also may be derived from the study of adult patients with acute sinusitis, in whom there have been more recent systematic inquiry.[10,11]

This practice guideline focuses on the diagnosis, evaluation, and treatment of children, ages 1 to 21 years, with uncomplicated acute, subacute, and recurrent acute bacterial sinusitis. Neonates and children younger than 1 year of age are not considered. Although bacterial sinusitis does occur rarely in children less than 1 year of age, their exclusion reflects, in part, the difficulty in conducting clinical investigation in this age group. This is a consequence of the small size of the paranasal sinuses and the difficulty in safely performing sinus aspiration.[12] This practice parameter does not apply to children with previously recognized anatomic abnormalities of their paranasal sinuses (facial dysmorphisms or trauma), immunodeficiencies, cystic fibrosis, or immotile cilia syndrome.

A discussion of chronic sinusitis (defined by the presence of symptoms for 90 days) and acute exacerbations of chronic sinusitis are not included in this guideline. The role of bacterial infection as a primary cause of chronic sinusitis is controversial.[11,13] Chronic inflammation of the paranasal sinuses may be a consequence of noninfectious conditions such as allergy, environmental pollutants, cystic fibrosis, or gastroesophageal reflux.

This guideline is intended for use by clinicians who treat children and adolescents in a variety of clinical settings including the office and emergency department. The purpose of the guideline is to encourage accurate diagnosis of bacterial sinusitis, appropriate use of imaging procedures, and judicious use of antibiotics.

DEFINITIONS

<u>Acute bacterial sinusitis:</u> Bacterial infection of the paranasal sinuses lasting less than 30 days in which symptoms resolve completely.

<u>Subacute bacterial sinusitis:</u> Bacterial infection of the paranasal sinuses lasting between 30 and 90 days in which symptoms resolve completely.

<u>Recurrent acute bacterial sinusitis:</u> Episodes of bacterial infection of the paranasal sinuses, each lasting less than 30 days and separated by intervals of at least 10 days during which the patient is asymptomatic.

<u>Chronic sinusitis:</u> Episodes of inflammation of the paranasal sinuses lasting more than 90 days. Patients have persistent residual respiratory symptoms such as cough, rhinorrhea, or nasal obstruction.

<u>Acute bacterial sinusitis superimposed on chronic sinusitis:</u> Patients with residual respiratory symptoms develop new respiratory symptoms. When treated with antimicrobials, these new symptoms resolve, but the underlying residual symptoms do not.[14]

METHODS

To develop the clinical practice guideline on the management of acute bacterial sinusitis, the American Academy of Pediatrics subcommittee partnered with the Agency for Healthcare Research and Quality and colleague organizations from family practice and otolaryngology. The Agency for Healthcare Research and Quality worked with the New England Medical Center Evidence-based Practice Center, as one of several centers that focus on conducting systematic reviews of the literature. A full report was produced by the New England Medical Center on the diagnosis and management of acute sinusitis.[15] However, because there were only 5 randomized studies in children, a supplemental analysis was conducted that included nonrandomized pediatric trials. The subcommittee used both reports to form the practice guideline recommendations but relied heavily on the pediatric supplement.[16]

For the pediatric supplement, the major research questions to be analyzed through the literature on acute bacterial sinusitis in childhood were 1) evidence for the efficacy of various antibiotics in children; 2) evidence for the efficacy of various ancillary, non-antibiotic regimens; and 3) the diagnostic accuracy and concordance of clinical symptoms, radiography (and other imaging methods), and sinus aspiration.

The literature was searched in Medline, complemented by Excerpta Medica, from 1966 through March 1999, using the word "sinusitis." Search criteria were limited to human studies and English language and appropriate pediatric terms. More than 1800 citations were reviewed. One hundred thirty-eight articles were fully examined, resulting in 21 qualifying studies. These studies included 5 controlled randomized trials and 8 case series on antimicrobial therapy, 3 controlled randomized trials on ancillary treatments, and 8 studies with information on diagnostic tests. The heterogeneity and paucity of the data did not allow for formal meta-analysis. When possible, rates were pooled across different studies and heterogeneity assessed.

The draft clinical practice guideline underwent extensive peer review by committees and sections within the American Academy of Pediatrics and by numerous outside organizations. Liaisons to the committee also distributed the draft within their organizations. Comments were compiled and reviewed by the subcommittee and relevant changes incorporated into the guideline.

The recommendations contained in this practice guideline are based on the best available data. Where data are lacking, a combination of evidence and expert opinion was used. Strong recommendations were based on high-quality scientific evidence or, when such was unavailable, strong expert consensus. Fair and weak recommendations are based on lesser-quality or limited data and expert consensus. Clinical options are identified as interventions for which the subcommittee could not find compelling positive or negative evidence. These clinical options are interventions that a reasonable health care professional may or may not wish to consider.

RECOMMENDATIONS

Methods of Diagnosis

Under normal circumstances the paranasal sinuses are assumed to be sterile.[17–19] However, the paranasal sinuses are in continuity with surface areas, such as the nasal mucosa and nasopharynx, which are heavily colonized with bacteria. Although it is reasonable to assume that the paranasal sinuses are frequently and transiently contaminated by bacteria from neighboring surfaces, these bacteria, which are present in low density, are probably removed by the normal function of the mucociliary apparatus. Accordingly, the gold standard for the diagnosis of acute bacterial sinusitis is the recovery of bacteria in high density ($\geq 10^4$ colony-forming units/mL) from the cavity of a paranasal sinus.[20] Although sinus aspiration is the gold standard for the diagnosis of acute bacterial sinusitis,[11] it is an invasive, time-consuming, and potentially painful procedure that should only be performed by a specialist (otolaryngologist). It is not a feasible method of diagnosis for the primary care practitioner and is not recommended for the routine diagnosis of bacterial sinus infections in children. However, the results of sinus aspiration have been correlated with clinical and radiographic findings in children with acute respiratory symptoms.[21,22]

Recommendation 1

The diagnosis of acute bacterial sinusitis is based on clinical criteria in children who present with upper respiratory symptoms that are either persistent or severe (strong recommendation based on limited scientific evidence and strong consensus of the panel).

Acute bacterial sinusitis is an infection of the paranasal sinuses lasting less than 30 days that presents with either persistent or severe symptoms.[4,23] Patients are asymptomatic after recovery from episodes of acute bacterial sinusitis.

Persistent symptoms are those that last longer than 10 to 14, but less than 30, days. Such symptoms include nasal or postnasal discharge (of any quality), daytime cough (which may be worse at night), or both.

Severe symptoms include a temperature of at least 102°F (39°C) and purulent nasal discharge present concurrently for at least 3 to 4 consecutive days in a child who seems ill. The child who seems toxic should be hospitalized and is not considered in this algorithm.

Uncomplicated viral upper respiratory infections generally last 5 to 7 days but may last longer.[24,25] Although the respiratory symptoms may not have completely resolved by the 10th day, almost always they have peaked in severity and begun to improve. Therefore, the persistence of respiratory symptoms without any evidence that they are beginning to resolve suggests the presence of a secondary bacterial infection. Significant fever or complaints of facial pain or headache are variable. It is important for the practitioner to attempt to differentiate between sequential episodes of uncomplicated viral upper respiratory tract infections (which may seem to coalesce in the mind of the patient or parent) from the onset of acute sinusitis with persistent symptoms. The objective of treatment of acute bacterial sinusitis is to foster rapid recovery, prevent suppurative complications, and minimize exacerbations of asthma (reactive airways diseases).[26]

Children with acute bacterial sinusitis who present with severe symptoms need to be distinguished from those with uncomplicated viral infections who are moderately ill. If fever is present at all in uncomplicated viral infections of the upper respiratory tract, it tends to be present early in the illness, usually accompanied by other constitutional symptoms such as headache and myalgias.[24] Generally, the constitutional symptoms resolve in the first 48 hours and then the respiratory symptoms become prominent. In most uncomplicated viral infections, purulent nasal discharge does not appear for several days. Accordingly, it is the concurrent presentation with high fever and purulent nasal discharge for at least 3 to 4

consecutive days that helps to define the severe presentation of acute bacterial sinusitis.[23] Children with severe onset of acute bacterial sinusitis may have an intense headache that is above or behind the eye; in general, they seem to be moderately ill.

Unfortunately, the physical examination does not generally contribute substantially to the diagnosis of acute bacterial sinusitis. This is explained by the similarity of physical findings in the patient with an uncomplicated viral rhinosinusitis and the patient with acute bacterial sinusitis.[2] In both instances, examination of the nasal mucosa may show mild erythema and swelling of the nasal turbinates with mucopurulent discharge. Facial pain is an unusual complaint in children. Facial tenderness is a rare finding in small children and may be unreliable as an indicator of acute bacterial sinusitis in older children and adolescents. Reproducible unilateral pain, present on percussion or direct pressure over the body of the frontal and maxillary sinuses, may indicate a diagnosis of acute bacterial sinusitis.[27] Likewise, observed or reported periorbital swelling is suggestive of ethmoid sinusitis. Examination of the tympanic membranes, pharynx, and cervical lymph nodes does not usually contribute to the diagnosis of acute bacterial sinusitis.

The value of the performance of transillumination of the sinuses to assess whether fluid is present in the maxillary and frontal paranasal sinuses is controversial. The technique is performed in a completely darkened room (after the examiner's eyes are adapted to the dark) by placing a transilluminator (high-intensity light beam) either in the mouth or against the cheek (for the maxillary sinuses) or under the medial aspect of the supraorbital ridge area (for the frontal sinuses) to assess the transmission of light through the sinus cavity.[27] Transillumination is difficult to perform correctly and has been shown to be unreliable in children younger than 10 years.[22,28] In the older child it may be helpful at the extremes of interpretation; if transillumination is normal, sinusitis is unlikely; if the transmission of light is absent, the maxillary or frontal sinus is likely to be filled with fluid.[18]

Subacute sinusitis is defined by the persistence of mild to moderate and often intermittent respiratory symptoms (nasal discharge, daytime cough, or both) for between 30 and 90 days. The nasal discharge may be of any quality, and cough is often worse at night. Low-grade fever may be periodic but is usually not prominent. The microbiology of subacute sinusitis is the same as that observed in patients with acute bacterial sinusitis.[29]

Patients with recurrent acute bacterial sinusitis are defined as having had 3 episodes of acute bacterial sinusitis in 6 months or 4 episodes in 12 months. The response to antibiotics is usually brisk and the patient is completely free of symptoms between episodes.

The most common cause of recurrent sinusitis is recurrent viral upper respiratory infection, often a consequence of attendance at day care or the presence of an older school-age sibling in the household. Other predisposing conditions include allergic and nonallergic rhinitis, cystic fibrosis, an immunodeficiency disorder (insufficient or dysfunctional immunoglobulins), ciliary dyskinesia, or an anatomic problem.[23]

Recommendation 2a

Imaging studies are not necessary to confirm a diagnosis of clinical sinusitis in children ≤6 years of age (strong recommendation based on limited scientific evidence and strong consensus of the panel).

In 1981, children between the ages of 2 and 16 years presenting with either persistent or severe symptoms were evaluated with sinus radiographs.[21,22] When children with persistent or severe symptoms were found to have abnormal sinus radiographs (complete opacification, mucosal thickening of at least 4 mm, or an air-fluid level), an aspiration of the maxillary sinus was performed. Bacteria in high density ($\geq 10^4$ colony-forming units/mL) were recovered in 70% to 75% of the children. This proportion of positive cultures (75%) is similar to the likelihood that a tympanocentesis will yield middle ear fluid with a positive culture for bacteria in children with otoscopic evidence of acute otitis media.[30]

In children with persistent symptoms, the history of protracted respiratory symptoms (>10 but <30 days without evidence of improvement) predicted significantly abnormal radiographs (complete opacification, mucosal thickening of at least 4 mm, or an air-fluid level) in 80% of children.[31] For children 6 years of age or younger, the history predicted abnormal sinus radiographs in 88% of children. For children older than 6 years, the history of persistent symptoms predicted abnormal sinus radiographs in 70%. The peak age for acute bacterial sinusitis is in children 6 years of age or younger. Accordingly, in this age group, because a positive history predicts the finding of abnormal sinus radiographs so frequently (and because history plus abnormal radiographs results in a positive sinus aspirate in 75% of cases), radiographs can be safely omitted and a diagnosis of acute bacterial sinusitis can be made on clinical criteria alone. Approximately 60% of children with symptoms of sinusitis (persistent or severe) will have bacteria recovered from an aspirate of the maxillary sinus.

In contrast to the general agreement that radiographs are not necessary in children 6 years of age or younger with persistent symptoms, the need for radiographs as a confirmatory test of acute sinusitis in children older than 6 years with persistent symptoms and for all children (regardless of age) with severe symptoms is controversial.[32,33] Some practitioners may elect to perform sinus radiographs with the expectation or suspicion that the study may be normal. A normal radiograph is powerful evidence that bacterial sinusitis is not the cause of the clinical syndrome.[34] However, the American College of Radiology has taken the position that the diagnosis of acute uncomplicated sinusitis should be made on clinical grounds alone.[35] They support this position by noting that plain radiographs of the paranasal sinuses are technically difficult to perform, particularly in very young children. Correct positioning may be difficult to achieve and therefore the radiographic images may overestimate and underestimate the presence of abnormalities within the paranasal sinuses.[36,37] The college would reserve the use of images for situations in which the patient does not recover or worsens during the course of appropriate antimicrobial therapy. Similarly, a recent set of guidelines generated by the Sinus and Allergy Health Partnership (representing numerous constituencies) does not recommend either radiographs or computed tomography (CT) or magnetic resonance imaging scans to diagnose uncomplicated cases of acute bacterial sinusitis in any age group.[1]

It is essential to recognize that abnormal images of the sinuses (either radiographs, CT, or magnetic resonance imaging) cannot stand alone as diagnostic evidence of acute bacterial sinusitis under any circumstances. Images can serve only as confirmatory measures of sinus disease in patients whose clinical histories are supportive of the diagnosis. Numerous investigations have demonstrated the high frequency of abnormal images in the paranasal sinuses of children undergoing imaging for indications other than suspected sinusitis.[38-40] In a study by Glasier et al,[39] almost 100% of young children who were undergoing CT examination for reasons other than sinus disease and who had an upper respiratory tract infection in the previous 2 weeks demonstrated soft tissue changes in their sinuses. A study by Gwaltney et al in 1994[3] found that abnormalities of the paranasal sinuses on CT scan are extremely common in young adults with acute (<72 hours) uncomplicated viral upper respiratory infections. This study and others serve to underscore that when abnormalities of the mucosa are present on images they indicate the presence of inflammation but do not disclose whether the inflammatory process is caused by viral infection, bacterial infection, allergy, or chemical irritation (eg, chlorine exposure in the swimmer).

Recommendation 2b

CT scans of the paranasal sinuses should be reserved for patients in whom surgery is being considered as a management strategy (strong recommendation based on good evidence and strong panel consensus).

Despite the limitations of CT scans,[3,38-40] they offer a detailed image of sinus anatomy and, when taken in conjunction with clinical findings, remain a useful adjunct to guide surgical treatment. Computed tomography scans are indicated in children who present with complications of acute bacterial sinus infection or those who have very persistent or recurrent infections that are not responsive to medical management.[33] In these instances, the image, preferably a complete CT scan of the paranasal sinuses, is essential to provide precise anatomic information to the clinician. These are instances in which the physician may be contemplating surgical intervention, including aspiration of the paranasal sinuses.

Recommendation 3

Antibiotics are recommended for the management of acute bacterial sinusitis to achieve a more rapid clinical cure (strong recommendation based on good evidence and strong panel consensus).

To promote the judicious use of antibiotics, it is essential that children diagnosed as having acute bacterial sinusitis meet the defining clinical presentations of "persistent" or "severe" disease as described previously.[41] This will minimize the number of children with uncomplicated viral upper respiratory tract infections who are treated with antimicrobials.

In a study comparing antimicrobial therapy with placebo in the treatment of children with the clinical and radiographic diagnosis of acute bacterial sinusitis, children receiving antimicrobial therapy recovered more quickly and more often than those receiving placebo.[31] On the third day of treatment, 83% of children receiving an antimicrobial were cured or improved compared with 51% of the children in the placebo group. (Forty-five percent of children receiving antimicrobial therapy were cured [complete resolution of respiratory symptoms] compared with 11% receiving placebo.) On the 10th day of treatment, 79% of children receiving an antimicrobial were cured or improved compared with 60% of children receiving placebo. Approximately 50% to 60% of children will improve gradually without the use of antimicrobials; however, the recovery of an additional 20% to 30% is delayed substantially compared with children who receive appropriate antibiotics.

A recent study by Garbutt et al[42] has challenged the notion that children identified as having acute sinusitis on clinical grounds alone (without the performance of images) will benefit from antimicrobial therapy. When children randomized to low-dose antibiotic therapy were compared with those receiving placebo there were no differences observed in outcome, either in the timing or frequency of recovery. The discrepancy in results between this investigation and the Wald[31] study may be attributable to the inclusion in this study of a larger cohort of older children (who may not have had sinusitis) and the exclusion of more seriously ill children with a temperature > 39°C or facial pain. Current recommendations for antibiotic management of uncomplicated sinusitis vary depending on a previous history of antibiotic exposure (in the previous 1–3 months), attendance at day care, and age. Some of the children in the Garbutt study might have qualified for high-dose amoxicillin-clavulanate to overcome antimicrobial resistant pathogens.

Comparative bacteriologic cure rates in studies of adults with acute sinusitis indicate the efficacy of antimicrobial treatment.[11,43] The findings of these studies indicate that antimicrobials in adequate doses with appropriate antibacterial spectra are highly effective in eradicating or substantially reducing bacteria in the sinus cavity, whereas those with inadequate spectrum or given in inadequate doses are not (Table 1).

TABLE 1. Comparative Bacteriologic Cure Rates (as Determined by Sinus Puncture) Among Adult Patients With Acute Community-Acquired Bacterial Sinusitis*

Comment Regarding Treatment	Number (%) of Bacteriologic Cures
Antibiotic concentration was ≥ MIC of causative bacteria	19/21 (90)
Antibiotic concentration was < MIC of causative bacteria	15/33 (45)
Appropriate antimicrobial and dose given	278/300 (93)
Suboptimal dose given	53/76 (70)

MIC indicates minimum inhibitory concentration.
* Adapted from Gwaltney.[11]

The microbiology of acute, subacute, and recurrent acute bacterial sinusitis has been outlined in several studies.[20–22] The principal bacterial pathogens are *Streptococcus pneumoniae*, nontypeable *Haemophilus influenzae*, and *Moraxella catarrhalis*. *S pneumoniae* is recovered from approximately 30% of children with acute bacterial sinusitis, whereas *H influenzae* and *M catarrhalis* are each recovered from about 20%.[23] In the remaining 30% of children, aspirates of the maxillary sinus are sterile. It is noteworthy that neither *Staphylococcus aureus* nor respiratory anaerobes are likely to be recovered from children with acute bacterial sinusitis.[22]

Currently, approximately 50% of *H influenzae* and 100% of *M catarrhalis* are likely to be β-lactamase positive nationwide.[44,45] Upper respiratory tract isolates of *S pneumoniae* are not susceptible to penicillin in 15% to 38% (average 25%) of children; approximately 50% are highly resistant to penicillin and the remaining half are intermediate in resistance.[1,46,47] The mechanism of penicillin resistance in *S pneumoniae* is an alteration of penicillin binding proteins. This phenomenon, which varies considerably according to geographic location, results in resistance to penicillin and cephalosporin. Table 2 shows the calculation for the likelihood that a child with acute bacterial sinusitis will harbor a resistant pathogen and not respond to treatment with amoxicillin. The following should be considered: the prevalence of each bacterial species as a cause of acute bacterial sinusitis, the prevalence of resistance among each bacterial species, and the rate of spontaneous improvement. Extrapolating from data derived from patients with acute otitis media, 15% of children with acute bacterial sinusitis caused by *S pneumoniae* will recover spontaneously, half of the children with acute bacterial sinusitis caused by *H influenzae* and half to three-quarters of the children infected with *M catarrhalis* also will recover spontaneously.[48] Furthermore, only *S pneumoniae* that are highly resistant to penicillin will not respond to conventional doses of amoxicillin. Accordingly, in the absence of any risk factors, approximately 80% of children with acute bacterial sinusitis will respond to treatment with amoxicillin. Risk factors for the presence of bacterial species that are likely to be resistant to amoxicillin include 1) attendance at day care, 2) recent receipt (< 90 days) of antimicrobial treatment, and 3) age less than 2 years.[49,50]

TABLE 2.   Calculation of the Likelihood that a Child With Acute Bacterial Sinusitis Will Fail Treatment With Standard Doses of Amoxicillin*†

Bacterial Species	Prevalence	Spontaneous Cure Rate (%)	Prevalence of Resistance (%)	Failure to Amoxicillin (%)
Streptococcus pneumoniae	30	15	25	3
Haemophilus influenzae	20	50	50	5
Moraxella catarrhalis	20	50–75	100	5–10

* This table is based on data obtained from treatment of acute otitis media.
† Consider that 50% of resistant strains are highly resistant to penicillin and only highly resistant isolates will fail to respond to standard doses of amoxicillin (45 mg/kg/day); Minimum inhibitory concentration (MIC) of susceptible *S pneumoniae* ≤0.1 μg/mL; MIC of moderately resistant *S pneumoniae* = 0.1–1.0 μg/mL; MIC of highly resistant *S pneumoniae* ≥2.0 μg/mL.

The desire to continue to use amoxicillin as first-line therapy in patients suspected of having acute bacterial sinusitis relates to its general effectiveness, safety, and tolerability; low cost; and narrow spectrum. For children younger than 2 years of age with uncomplicated acute bacterial sinusitis that is mild to moderate in degree of severity, who do not attend day care, and have not recently been treated with an antimicrobial, amoxicillin is recommended at either a usual dose of 45 mg/kg/d in 2 divided doses or a high dose of 90 mg/kg/d in 2 divided doses (Fig 1). If the patient is allergic to amoxicillin, either cefdinir (14 mg/kg/d in 1 or 2 doses), cefuroxime (30 mg/kg/d in 2 divided doses), or cefpodoxime (10 mg/kg/d once daily) can be used (only if the allergic reaction was not a type 1 hypersensitivity reaction). In cases of serious allergic reactions, clarithromycin (15 mg/kg/d in 2 divided doses) or azithromycin (10 mg/kg/d on day 1, 5 mg/kg/d × 4 days as a single daily dose) can be used in an effort to select an antimicrobial of an entirely different class. The Food and Drug Administration has not approved azithromycin for use in patients with sinusitis. Alternative therapy in the penicillin-allergic patient who is known to be infected with a penicillin-resistant *S pneumoniae* is clindamycin at 30 to 40 mg/kg/d in 3 divided doses.

Most patients with acute bacterial sinusitis who are treated with an appropriate antimicrobial agent respond promptly (within 48–72 hours) with a diminution of respiratory symptoms (reduction of nasal discharge and cough) and an improvement in general well-being.[11,23,31] If a patient fails to improve, either the antimicrobial is ineffective or the diagnosis of sinusitis is not correct.

If patients do not improve while receiving the usual dose of amoxicillin (45 mg/kg/d), have recently been treated with an antimicrobial, have an illness that is moderate or more severe, or attend day care, therapy should be initiated with high-dose amoxicillin-clavulanate (80–90 mg/kg/d of amoxicillin component, with 6.4 mg/kg/d of clavulanate in 2 divided doses). This dose of amoxicillin will yield sinus fluid levels that exceed the minimum inhibitory concentration of all *S pneumoniae* that are intermediate in resistance to penicillin and most, but not all, highly resistant *S pneumoniae*. There is sufficient potassium clavulanate to inhibit all β-lactamase producing *H influenzae* and *M catarrhalis*. Alternative therapies include cefdinir, cefuroxime, or cefpo-

doxime. A single dose of ceftriaxone (at 50 mg/kg/d), given either intravenously or intramuscularly, can be used in children with vomiting that precludes administration of oral antibiotics. Twenty-four hours later, when the child is clinically improved, an oral antibiotic is substituted to complete the therapy. Although trimethoprim-sulfamethoxazole and erythromycin-sulfisoxazole have traditionally been useful in the past as first- and second-line therapy for patients with acute bacterial sinusitis, recent pneumococcal surveillance studies indicate that resistance to these 2 combination agents is substantial.[51,52] Therefore, when patients fail to improve while receiving amoxicillin, neither trimethoprim-sulfamethoxazole nor erythromycin-sulfisoxazole are appropriate choices for antimicrobial therapy. For patients who do not improve with a second course of antibiotics or who are acutely ill, there are 2 options. It is appropriate to consult an otolaryngologist for consideration of maxillary sinus aspiration to obtain a sample of sinus secretions for culture and sensitivity so that therapy can be adjusted precisely. Alternatively, the physician may prescribe intravenous cefotaxime or ceftriaxone (either in hospital or at home) and refer to an otolaryngologist only if the patient does not improve on intravenous antibiotics. Some authorities recommend performing cultures of the middle meatus instead of aspiration of the maxillary sinus to determine the cause of acute bacterial sinusitis.[53] However, there are no data in children that have correlated cultures of the middle meatus with cultures of the maxillary sinus aspirate.[54]

The optimal duration of therapy for patients with acute bacterial sinusitis has not received systematic study. Often empiric recommendations are made for 10, 14, 21, or 28 days of therapy. An alternative suggestion has been made that antibiotic therapy be continued until the patient becomes free of symptoms and then for an additional 7 days.[23] This strategy, which individualizes treatment for each patient, results in a minimum course of 10 days and avoids prolonged courses of antibiotics in patients who are asymptomatic and thereby unlikely to be compliant.

Adjuvant Therapies

No recommendations are made based on controversial and limited data.

Adjuvant therapies used to supplement the effect of antimicrobials have received relatively little systematic investigation.[55] Available agents include sa-

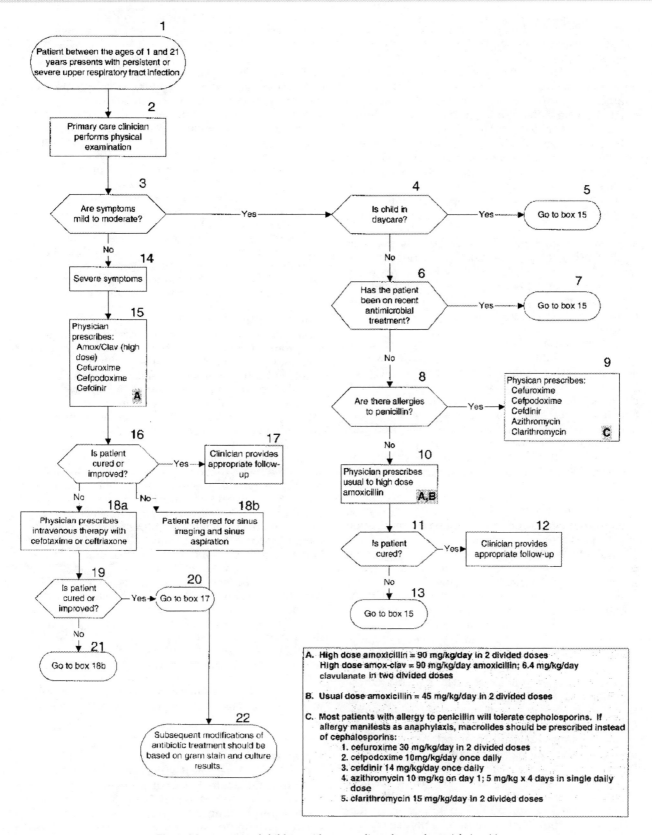

Fig 1. Management of children with uncomplicated acute bacterial sinusitis.

line nasal irrigation (hypertonic or normal saline), antihistamines, decongestants (topical or systemic), mucolytic agents, and topical intranasal steroids.

Currently there are no data to recommend the use of H1 antihistamines in nonallergic children with acute bacterial sinusitis. There is a single prospective study in which children with presumed acute bacterial sinusitis were randomized to receive either decongestant-antihistamine or placebo in addition to amoxicillin. The active treatment group received topical oxymetazoline and oral decongestant-antihistamine syrup (brompheniramine and phenylpropanolamine). No difference in clinical or radiographic resolution was noted between groups.[56]

There has been a single study of intranasal steroids as an adjunct to antibiotics in young children with presumed acute bacterial sinusitis. Intranasal budesonide spray had a modest effect on symptoms only during the second week of therapy.[57] A multicenter, double-blind, randomized, parallel trial evaluating flunisolide spray as an adjunct to oral antibiotic therapy was reported in patients at least 14 years of age.[58] The benefit of flunisolide was marginal and of minimal clinical importance. There is little reason to expect a substantial benefit from intranasal steroids in patients with acute bacterial sinusitis when antibiotics work effectively in the first 3 to 4 days of treatment.

No clinical trials of mucolytics have been reported in nonatopic children or adults with acute bacterial sinusitis.[59] Neither saline nose drops nor nasal spray have been studied in patients with acute bacterial sinusitis. However, by preventing crust formation and liquefying secretions, they may be helpful. In addition, saline also may act as a mild vasoconstrictor of nasal blood flow.[59] A method for performing a nasal saline flush was reported anecdotally by Schwartz.[60]

Antibiotic Prophylaxis

No recommendations are made based on limited and controversial data.

Antibiotic prophylaxis as a strategy to prevent infection in patients who experience recurrent episodes of acute bacterial sinusitis has not been systematically evaluated and is controversial.[59] Although previously successful in children who experience recurrent episodes of acute otitis media,[61,62] there is little enthusiasm for this approach in light of current concerns regarding the increasing prevalence of antibiotic-resistant organisms. Nonetheless, it may be used in a few highly selected patients whose infections have been defined meticulously (always fulfilling criteria for persistent or severe presentation) and are very frequent (at least 3 infections in 6 months or 4 infections in 12 months). Amoxicillin (20 mg/kg/d given at night) and sulfisoxazole (75 mg/kg/d in 2 divided doses) have been used successfully to prevent episodes of acute otitis media. Usually prophylaxis is maintained until the end of the respiratory season. It is appropriate to initiate an evaluation for factors that commonly predispose to episodes of recurrent acute bacterial sinusitis such as atopy, immunodeficiency, cystic fibrosis, and dysmotile cilia syndrome. Children with craniofacial abnormalities also are at risk to develop acute bacterial sinusitis.

Complementary/Alternative Medicine for Prevention and Treatment of Rhinosinusitis

No recommendations are made based on limited and controversial data.

A substantial number of children, adolescents, and their parents use nonprescription cold medicines or simple home-based remedies such as soups, fruit juices, or teas as alternatives or complements to conventional therapy for the treatment of upper respiratory infections including rhinosinusitis.[63,64] Others use herbal remedies and nutritional supplements or seek care from acupuncturists, chiropractors, homeopaths, naturopaths, aromatherapists, massage and therapeutic touch practitioners, and a variety of other healing modalities.[64–67]

Few of these therapies for upper respiratory tract infection or rhinosinusitis have been validated in randomized controlled trials. Claims that homeopathic medicines,[68–70] vitamin C preparations,[71] or zinc lozenges[72] prevent upper respiratory infections or hasten their resolution are controversial. A recently published study provides evidence that zinc nasal gel is effective in shortening the duration of symptoms of the common cold when taken within 24 hours of their onset.[73] Studies performed among adults indicating efficacy of *Echinacea* preparations in stimulating the immune system, thereby reducing the incidence, duration, or severity of respiratory infections, are debated[74,75]; however, a recent meta-analysis suggested a predominance of generally positive effects.[76]

Physicians treating children and young adults should be aware that many of their patients are using complementary therapies, often without informing them. Most of these remedies are harmless and, whether through pharmacologic or placebo effect, a perception of efficacy in providing relief from symptoms has stood the test of time. Nevertheless, many herbal medicines sold in the United States are of uncertain efficacy, content, and toxicity and carry a potential for serious adverse effects.[77] Of particular concern is the ability of the botanicals, either by direct interaction or by altering excretion mechanisms, to magnify or oppose the effect of conventional medicines that patients may be using concurrently.[78] Physicians should inquire about the use of complementary medicine for upper respiratory tract infections among their patients, particularly those on long-term medication for chronic conditions. Information on dietary supplements is available on a regularly updated Internet site.[79]

Recommendation 4

Children with complications or suspected complications of acute bacterial sinusitis should be treated promptly and aggressively. This should include referral to an otolaryngologist usually with the consultation of an infectious disease specialist, ophthalmologist, and neurosurgeon (strong recommendation based on strong consensus of the panel).

The complications of acute bacterial sinusitis usually involve either the orbit, the central nervous system, or both. Although rare, complications can result in permanent blindness or death if not treated promptly and appropriately.

Periorbital and intraorbital inflammation and infection are the most common complications of acute sinusitis and most often are caused by acute ethmoiditis. These disorders are commonly classified in relation to the orbital septum. The orbital septum is a sheet of connective tissue continuous with the periosteum of the orbital bones that separates tissues of the eyelid from those of the orbit. Preseptal inflammation involves only the eyelid, whereas postseptal inflammation involves structures of the orbit. Complications can be classified as 1) periorbital (or preseptal) cellulitis or sympathetic edema (periorbital cellulitis is not a true orbital complication. The periorbital swelling is attributable to passive venous congestion; infection is confined to the paranasal sinuses), 2) subperiosteal abscess, 3) orbital abscess, 4) orbital cellulitis, or 5) cavernous sinus thrombosis.

Mild cases of periorbital cellulitis (eyelid <50% closed) may be treated with appropriate oral antibiotic therapy as an outpatient with daily patient encounters. However, if the patient has not improved in 24 to 48 hours or if the infection is progressing rapidly, it is appropriate to admit the patient to the hospital for antimicrobial therapy consisting of intravenous ceftriaxone (100 mg/kg/d in 2 divided doses) or ampicillin-sulbactam (200 mg/kg/d in 4 divided doses). Vancomycin (60 mg/kg/d in 4 divided doses) may be added in children in whom infection is either known or likely to be caused by S pneumoniae that are highly resistant to penicillin.

If proptosis, impaired visual acuity, or impaired extraocular mobility are present on examination, a CT scan (preferably coronal thin cut with contrast) of the orbits/sinuses is essential to exclude a suppurative complication. In such cases, the patient should be evaluated by an otolaryngologist and an ophthalmologist. Suppurative complications generally require prompt surgical drainage. An exception to this is the patient with a small subperiosteal abscess and minimal ocular abnormalities for whom intravenous antibiotic treatment for 24 to 48 hours is recommended while performing frequent visual and mental status checks. Patients who have changes in visual acuity or mental status or who fail to improve within 24 to 48 hours require prompt surgical intervention and drainage of the abscess. Antibiotics can be altered, if inappropriate, when results of culture and sensitivity studies become available.

In patients with altered mental status, neurosurgical consultation is indicated. Signs of increased intracranial pressure (headache and vomiting) or nuchal rigidity require immediate CT scanning (with contrast) of the brain, orbits, and sinuses to exclude intracranial complications such as cavernous sinus thrombosis, osteomyelitis of the frontal bone (Pott's puffy tumor), meningitis, subdural empyema, epidural abscess, and brain abscess. Central nervous system complications, such as meningitis and empyemas, should be treated either with intravenous cefotaxime or ceftriaxone and vancomycin pending the results of culture and susceptibility testing.

AREAS FOR FUTURE RESEARCH

The extensive Medline searches to review the literature for the diagnosis and treatment of acute bacterial sinusitis in children uncovered the fact that there are scant data on which to base recommendations. Accordingly, areas for future research include the following:

1. Conduct more and larger studies correlating the clinical findings of acute bacterial sinusitis with findings of sinus aspiration, imaging, and treatment outcome.
2. Develop noninvasive strategies to accurately diagnose acute bacterial sinusitis in children.
   a. Correlate cultures obtained from the middle meatus of the maxillary sinus of infected individuals with cultures obtained from the maxillary sinus by puncture of the antrum.
   b. Develop imaging technology that differentiates bacterial infection from viral infection or allergic inflammation.
   c. Develop rapid diagnostic methods to image the sinuses without radiation.
3. Determine the optimal duration of antimicrobial therapy for children with acute bacterial sinusitis.
4. Determine the causes and treatment of subacute and recurrent acute bacterial sinusitis.
5. Determine the efficacy of prophylaxis with antimicrobials to prevent recurrent acute bacterial sinusitis.
6. Determine the impact of bacterial resistance among S pneumoniae, H influenzae, and M catarrhalis on outcome of treatment with antibiotics by the performance of randomized, double-blind, placebo-controlled studies in well-defined populations of patients.
7. Determine the role of adjuvant therapies (mucolytics, decongestants, antihistamines, etc) in patients with acute bacterial sinusitis by the performance of prospective, randomized, clinical trials.
8. Determine the role of complementary and alternative medicine strategies in patients with acute bacterial sinusitis by performing systematic, prospective, randomized clinical trials.
9. Assess the effect of the pneumococcal conjugate vaccine on the epidemiology of acute bacterial sinusitis.
10. Develop new bacterial and viral vaccines to reduce the incidence of acute bacterial sinusitis.

CONCLUSION

This clinical practice guideline provides evidence-based recommendations for the management of bacterial rhinosinusitis in children ages 1 to 21 years. The guideline emphasizes 1) appropriate diagnosis in children who present with persistent or severe upper respiratory symptoms; 2) the utility of imaging studies to confirm a diagnosis; 3) treatment therapies such as antibiotic use including prophylaxis, adjuvant treatment, and alternative interventions; and 4) management of complications. The guideline provides decision-making strategies for managing sinusitis to assist primary care providers in diagnosing and treating children with this common health problem.

ACKNOWLEDGMENTS

The subcommittee wishes to acknowledge the Agency for Healthcare Research and Quality and the New England Medical Center Evidence-based Practice Center for their work in developing the evidence report. We especially thank John P. A. Ioannidis, MD, and Joseph Lau, MD, for their work on the technical report.

SUBCOMMITTEE ON MANAGEMENT OF SINUSITIS
Ellen R. Wald, MD, Chairperson
W. Clayton Bordley, MD, MPH
David H. Darrow, MD, DDS
Katherine Teets Grimm, MD
Jack M. Gwaltney, Jr, MD
S. Michael Marcy, MD
Melvin O. Senac, Jr, MD
Paul V. Williams, MD

LIAISONS
Larry Culpepper, MD, MPH
    American Academy of Family Physicians
David L. Walner, MD
    American Academy of Otolaryngology-Head and Neck Surgery

STAFF
Carla Herrerias, MPH

COMMITTEE ON QUALITY IMPROVEMENT, 2000–2001
Charles J. Homer, MD, MPH, Chairperson
Richard D. Baltz, MD
Michael J. Goldberg, MD
Gerald B. Hickson, MD
Paul V. Miles, MD
Thomas B. Newman, MD, MPH
Joan E. Shook, MD
William M. Zurhellen, MD

LIAISONS
Charles H. Deitschel, Jr, MD
    Committee on Medical Liability
Denise Dougherty, PhD
    Agency for Healthcare Research and Quality Institutions
F. Lane France, MD
    Committee on Practice and Ambulatory Medicine
Kelly J. Kelleher, MD, MPH
    Section on Epidemiology
Betty A. Lowe, MD
    National Association of Children's Hospitals and Related Institutions
Ellen Schwalenstocker, MBA
    National Association of Children's Hospitals and Related Institutions
Richard N. Shiffman, MD
    Section on Computers and Other Technology

REFERENCES

1. Sinus and Allergy Health Partnership. Antimicrobial treatment guidelines for acute bacterial rhinosinusitis. *Otolaryngol Head Neck Surg.* 2000;123:5–31
2. Lusk RP, Stankiewicz JA. Pediatric rhinosinusitis. *Otolaryngol Head Neck Surg.* 1997;117:S53–S57
3. Gwaltney JM Jr, Phillips CD, Miller RD, Riker DK. Computed tomographic study of the common cold. *N Engl J Med.* 1994;330:25–30
4. Fireman P. Diagnosis of sinusitis in children: emphasis on the history and physical examination. *J Allergy Clin Immunol.* 1992;90:433–436
5. Aitken M, Taylor JA. Prevalence of clinical sinusitis in young children followed up by primary care pediatricians. *Arch Pediatr Adolesc Med.* 1998;152:244–248
6. Ueda D, Yoto Y. The ten-day mark as a practical diagnostic approach for acute paranasal sinusitis in children. *Pediatr Infect Dis J.* 1996;15:576–579
7. Wald ER, Guerra N, Byers C. Upper respiratory tract infections in young children: duration of and frequency of complications. *Pediatrics.* 1991;87:129–133
8. McCaig LF, Hughes JM. Trends in antimicrobial drug prescribing among office-based physicians in the United States [published erratum in *JAMA.* 1998;11:279]. *JAMA.* 1995;273:214–219
9. Parsons DS, Wald ER. Otitis media and sinusitis: similar diseases. *Otolaryngol Clin North Am.* 1996;29:11–25
10. Gwaltney JM Jr, Scheld WM, Sande MA, Sydnor A. The microbial etiology and antimicrobial therapy of adults with acute community-acquired sinusitis: a fifteen-year experience at the University of Virginia and review of other selected studies. *J Allergy Clin Immunol.* 1992;90:457–462
11. Gwaltney JM Jr. Acute community-acquired sinusitis. *Clin Infect Dis.* 1996;23:1209–1223
12. Wald ER. Purulent nasal discharge. *Pediatr Infect Dis J.* 1991;10:329–333
13. Wald ER. Chronic sinusitis in children. *J Pediatr.* 1995;127:339–347
14. International Rhinosinusitis Advisory Board. Infectious rhinosinusitis in adults: classification, etiology and management. *Ear Nose Throat J.* 1997;76(suppl):1–22
15. Lau J, Ioannidis JP, Wald ER. *Diagnosis and Treatment of Uncomplicated Acute Sinusitis in Children. Evidence Report/Technology Assessment: Number 9.* Rockville, MD: Agency for Healthcare Research and Quality, US Department of Health and Human Services; 2000. AHRQ Contract No. 290-97-0019. Available at: http://www.ahrq.gov/clinic/sinuschsum.htm. Accessed February 23, 2001
16. Lau J, Zucker D, Engels EA, et al. *Diagnosis and Treatment of Acute Bacterial Rhinosinusitis. Summary, Evidence Report/Technology Assessment: Number 9.* Rockville, MD: Agency for Healthcare Research and Quality, US Department of Health and Human Services; 1999. AHRQ Contract No. 290–97-0019. Available at: http://hstat.nlm.nih.gov/ftrs/tocview. Accessed February 23, 2001
17. Arruda LK, Mimica IM, Sole D, et al. Abnormal maxillary sinus radiographs in children: do they represent infection? *Pediatrics.* 1990;85:553–558
18. Evans FO, Sydnor JB, Moore WE, et al. Sinusitis of the maxillary antrum. *N Engl J Med.* 1975;293:735–739
19. Shapiro ED, Wald ER, Doyle WJ, Rohn D. Bacteriology of the maxillary sinus of rhesus monkeys. *Ann Otol Rhinol Laryngol.* 1982;91:150–151
20. Wald ER. Microbiology of acute and chronic sinusitis in children. *J Allergy Clin Immunol.* 1992;90:452–456
21. Wald ER, Milmoe GJ, Bowen A, Ledesma-Medina J, Salamon N, Bluestone CD. Acute maxillary sinusitis in children. *N Engl J Med.* 1981;304:749–754
22. Wald ER, Reilly JS, Casselbrant M, et al. Treatment of acute maxillary sinusitis in childhood: a comparative study of amoxicillin and cefaclor. *J Pediatr.* 1984;104:297–302
23. Wald ER. Sinusitis. *Pediatr Ann.* 1998;27:811–818
24. Gwaltney JM Jr, Hendley JO, Simon G, Jordan WS. Rhinovirus infection in an industrial population. II. Characteristics of illness and antibody response. *JAMA.* 1967;202:494–500
25. Gwaltney JM Jr, Buier RM, Rogers JL. The influence of signal variation, bias, noise, and effect size on statistical significance in treatment studies of the common cold. *Antiviral Res.* 1996;29:287–295
26. Slavin RG. Asthma and sinusitis. *J Allergy Clin Immunol.* 1992;90:534–537
27. Williams JW, Simel DL. Does this patient have sinusitis? Diagnosing acute sinusitis by history and physical examination. *JAMA.* 1993;270:1242–1246
28. Otten FW, Grote JJ. The diagnostic value of transillumination for maxillary sinusitis in children. *Int J Pediatr Otorhinolaryngol.* 1989;18:9–11
29. Wald ER, Byers C, Guerra N, Casselbrant M, Beste D. Subacute sinusitis in children. *J Pediatr.* 1989;115:28–32
30. Kline MW. Otitis media. In: McMillan JA, DeAngelis CD, Feigin RD, Warshaw JB, eds. *Oski's Pediatrics: Principles and Practice.* Philadelphia, PA: Lippincott Williams & Wilkins; 1999:1301–1304
31. Wald ER, Chiponis D, Ledesma-Medina J. Comparative effectiveness of amoxicillin and amoxicillin-clavulanate potassium in acute paranasal sinus infections in children: a double-blind, placebo-controlled trial. *Pediatrics.* 1986;77:795–800
32. Diament MJ. The diagnosis of sinusitis in infants and children: x-ray,

computed tomography and magnetic resonance imaging. *J Allergy Clin Immunol.* 1992;90:442–444

33. McAlister WH, Kronemer K. Imaging of sinusitis in children. *Pediatr Infect Dis J.* 1999;18:1019–1020

34. Kovatch AL, Wald ER, Ledesma-Medina J, Chiponis DM, Bedingfield B. Maxillary sinus radiographs in children with nonrespiratory complaints. *Pediatrics.* 1984;73:306–308

35. McAlister WH, Parker BR, Kushner DC, et al. Sinusitis in the pediatric population. In: *ACR Appropriateness Criteria.* Reston, VA: American College of Radiology; 2000. Available at: http://www.acr.org/departments/appropriateness_criteria/toc.html. Accessed February 23, 2001

36. Lazar RH, Younis RT, Parvey LS. Comparison of plain radiographs, coronal CT, and interoperative findings in children with chronic sinusitis. *Otolaryngol Head Neck Surg.* 1992;107:29–34

37. McAlister WH, Lusk R, Muntz HR. Comparison of plain radiographs and coronal CT scans in infants and children with recurrent sinusitis. *AJR Am J Roentgenol.* 1989;153:1259–1264

38. Kronemer KA, McAlister WH. Sinusitis and its imaging in the pediatric population. *Pediatr Radiol.* 1997;27:837–846

39. Glasier CM, Mallory GB, Steele RW. Significance of opacification of the maxillary and ethmoid sinuses in infants. *J Pediatr.* 1989;114:45–50

40. Diament MJ, Senac MO, Gilsanz V, Baker S, Gillespie T, Larsson S. Prevalence of incidental paranasal sinuses opacification in pediatric patients: a CT study. *J Comput Assist Tomogr.* 1987;11:426–431

41. Dowell SF, Marcy SM, Phillips WR, Gerber MA, Schwartz B. Principles of judicious use of antimicrobial agents for pediatric upper respiratory tract infections. *Pediatrics.* 1998;101(suppl):163–165

42. Garbutt JM, Goldstein M, Gellman E, Shannon W, Littenberg B. A randomized, placebo-controlled trial of antimicrobial treatment for children with clinically diagnosed acute sinusitis. *Pediatrics.* 2001;107:619–625

43. Gwaltney JM Jr. Acute community acquired bacterial sinusitis: to treat or not to treat. *Can Respir J.* 1999;6(suppl):46A–50A

44. Doern GV, Brueggemann AB, Pierce G, Holley HP, Rauch A. Antibiotic resistance among clinical isolates of *Haemophilus influenzae* in the United States in 1994 and 1995 and detection of beta-lactamase-positive strains resistant to amoxicillin-clavulanate; results of a national multicenter surveillance study. *Antimicrob Agents Chemother.* 1997;41:292–297

45. Doern GV, Jones RN, Pfaller MA, Kugler K. *Haemophilus influenzae* and *Moraxella catarrhalis* from patients with community-acquired respiratory tract infections: antimicrobial susceptibility patterns from the SENTRY antimicrobial Surveillance Program (United States and Canada, 1997). *Antimicrob Agents Chemother.* 1999;43:385–389

46. Centers for Disease Control and Prevention. Geographic variation in penicillin resistance in *Streptococcus pneumoniae*-selected sites, United States, 1997. *MMWR Morb Mortal Wkly Rep.* 1999;48:656–661

47. Dowell SF, Butler JC, Giebink GS, et al. Acute otitis media: management and surveillance in an era of pneumococcal resistance—a report from the Drug-resistant *Streptococcus pneumoniae* Therapeutic Working Group. *Pediatr Infect Dis J.* 1999;18:1–9

48. Howie VM, Ploussard JH. The "in vivo sensitivity test"—bacteriology of middle ear exudate during antimicrobial therapy in otitis media. *Pediatrics.* 1969;44:940–944

49. Block SL, Harrison CJ, Hedrick JA, et al. Penicillin-resistant *Streptococcus pneumoniae* in acute otitis media: risk factors, susceptibility patterns and antimicrobial management. *Pediatr Infect Dis J.* 1995;14:751–759

50. Levine OS, Farley M, Harrison LH, Lefkowitz L, McGeer A, Schwartz B. Risk factors for invasive pneumococcal disease in children: a population-based case-control study in North America. *Pediatrics.* 1999;103(3). Available at: http://www.pediatrics.org/cgi/content/full/103/3/e28. Accessed February 28, 2001

51. Jacobs MR, Bajaksouzian S, Zilles A, Lin G, Pankuch GA, Appelbaum PC. Susceptibilities of *Streptococcus pneumoniae* and *Haemophilus influenzae* to 10 oral antimicrobial agents based on pharmacodynamic parameters: 1997 US Surveillance study. *Antimicrob Agents Chemother.* 1999;43:1901–1908

52. Doern GV, Pfaller MA, Kugler K, Freeman J, Jones RN. Prevalence of antimicrobial resistance among respiratory tract isolates of *Streptococcus pneumoniae* in North American: 1997 results from the SENTRY antimicrobial surveillance program. *Clin Infect Dis.* 1998;27:764–770

53. Gold SM, Tami TA. Role of middle meatus aspiration culture in the diagnoses of chronic sinusitis. *Laryngoscope.* 1997;107:1586–1589

54. Gordts F, Abu Nasser I, Clement PA, Pierard D, Kaufman L. Bacteriology of the middle meatus in children. *Int J Pediatr Otorhinolaryngol.* 1999;48:163–167

55. Zeiger RS. Prospects for ancillary treatment of sinusitis in the 1990s. *J Allergy Clin Immunol.* 1992;90:478–495

56. McCormick DP, John SD, Swischuk LE, Uchida T. A double-blind, placebo-controlled trial of decongestant-antihistamine for the treatment of sinusitis in children. *Clin Pediatr (Phila).* 1996;35:457–460

57. Barlan IB, Erkan E, Bakir M, Berrak S, Basaran MM. Intranasal budesonide spray as an adjunct to oral antibiotic therapy for acute sinusitis in children. *Ann Allergy Asthma Immunol.* 1997;78:598–601

58. Meltzer EO, Orgel HA, Backhaus JW, et al. Intranasal flunisolide spray as an adjunct to oral antibiotic therapy for sinusitis. *J Allergy Clin Immunol.* 1993;92:812–823

59. Spector SL, Bernstein IL, Li JT, et al. Parameters for the diagnosis and management of sinusitis. *J Allergy Clin Immunol.* 1998;102:S107–S144

60. Schwartz RH. The nasal saline flush procedure. *Pediatr Infect Dis J.* 1997;16:725

61. Perrin JM, Charney E, MacWhinney JB, McInerny TK, Miller RL, Nazarian LF. Sulfisoxazole as chemoprophylaxis for recurrent otitis media: a double-blind crossover study in pediatric practice. *N Engl J Med.* 1974;291:664–667

62. Casselbrant ML, Kaleida PH, Rockette HE, et al. Efficacy of antimicrobial prophylaxis and of tympanostomy tube insertion for prevention of recurrent acute otitis media: results of a randomized clinical trial. *Pediatr Infect Dis J.* 1992;11:278–286

63. Krouse JH, Krouse HJ. Patient use of traditional and complementary therapies in treating rhinosinusitis before consulting an otolaryngologist. *Laryngoscope.* 1999;109:1223–1227

64. Pachter LM, Sumner T, Fontan A, Sneed M, Bernstein BA. Home-based therapies of the common cold among European American and ethnic minority families: the interface between alternative/complementary and folk medicine. *Arch Pediatr Adolesc Med.* 1998;152:1083–1088

65. Kemper KJ. *The Holistic Pediatrician: A Parent's Comprehensive Guide to Safe and Effective Therapies for the 25 Most Common Childhood Ailments.* New York, NY: Harper Perennial; 1996

66. Lee ACC, Kemper KJ. Homeopathy and naturopathy: practice characteristics and pediatric care. *Arch Pediatr Adolesc Med.* 2000;154:75–80

67. Spigelblatt L, Laine-Ammara G, Pless IB, Guyver A. The use of alternative medicine by children. *Pediatrics.* 1994;94:811–814

68. de Lange de Klerk ES, Blommers J, Kuik DJ, Bezemer PD, Feenstra L. Effect of homeopathic medicines on daily burden of symptoms in children with recurrent upper respiratory tract infections. *BMJ.* 1994;309:1329–1332

69. Langman MJ. Homeopathy trials: reason for good ones but are they warranted? *Lancet.* 1997;350:825

70. Vandenbroucke JP. Homeopathy trials: going nowhere. *Lancet.* 1997;350:824

71. Hemila H. Does vitamin C alleviate the symptoms of the common cold?—a review of current evidence. *Scand J Infect Dis.* 1994;26:1–6

72. Macknin ML, Piedmonte M, Calendine C, Janosky J, Wald E. Zinc gluconate lozenges for treating the common cold in children: a randomized controlled trial. *JAMA.* 1998;279:1962–1967

73. Hirt M, Novel S, Barron E. Zinc nasal gel for the treatment of common cold symptoms: a double-blind, placebo-controlled trial. *Ear Nose Throat J.* 2000;79:778–782

74. Grimm W, Muller HH. A randomized controlled trial of the effect of fluid extract of *Echinacea purpurea* on the incidence and severity of colds and respiratory infections. *Am J Med.* 1999;106:138–143

75. Turner RB, Riker DK, Gangemi JD. Ineffectiveness of echineacea for prevention of experimental rhinovirus colds. *Antimicrob Agents Chemother.* 2000;44:1708–1709

76. Barret B, Vohmann M, Calabrese C. Echinacea for upper respiratory infection. *J Fam Pract.* 1999;48:628–635

77. Angell M, Kassirer JP. Alternative medicine—the risks of untested and unregulated remedies. *N Engl J Med.* 1998;339:839–841

78. Fugh-Berman A. Herb-drug interactions. *Lancet.* 2000;355:134–138

79. Office of Dietary Supplements. International Bibliographic Information on Dietary Supplements (IBIDS) Database. Available at: http://ods.od.nih.gov/databases/ibids.html. Accessed February 23, 2001

ERRATUM

In the September 2001 issue of *Pediatrics* (2001;108:798–808) an error appeared on page 802 in the AAP statement entitled "Clinical Practice Guideline: Management of Sinusitis." In the paragraph under Table 1, *Streptococcus aureus* should read "*Staphylococcus aureus*".

ERRATUM

The following is the correct clinical algorithm that accompanies "Clinical Practice Guideline: Management of Sinusitis" (*Pediatrics.* 2001;108:798–808). Errors in the spelling and names of antimicrobial agents have been corrected.

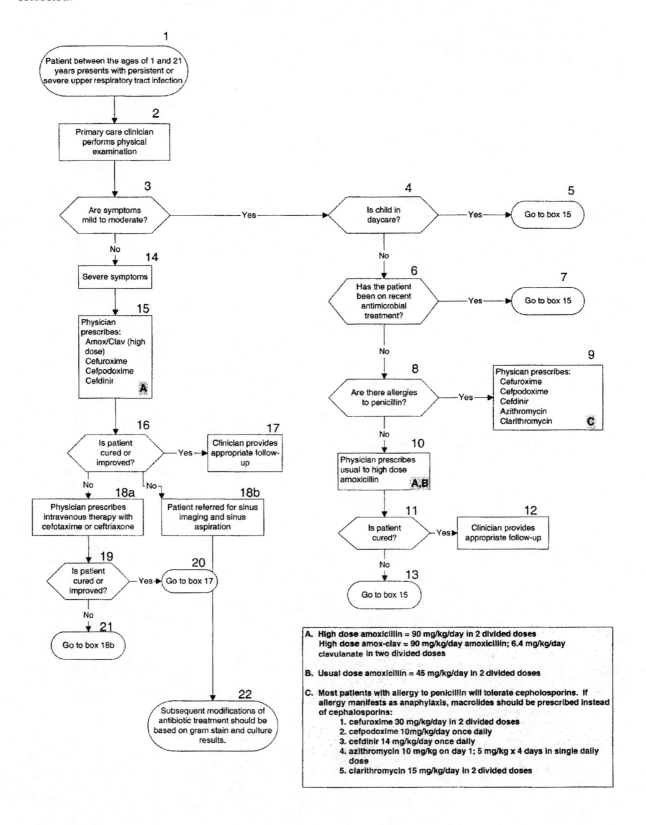

Technical Report Summary:
Evidence for the Diagnosis and Treatment of
Acute Uncomplicated Sinusitis in Children:
A Systematic Overview

Authors:

John P. A. Ioannidis, MD
Joseph Lau, MD

American Academy of Pediatrics
PO Box 927, 141 Northwest Point Blvd
Elk Grove Village, IL 60009-0927

For the complete technical report, including tables, figures, and references, please see the companion CD-ROM.

ABSTRACT. *Objective.* To evaluate and analyze the existing evidence for the diagnosis and treatment of acute uncomplicated sinusitis in children.

Design. A systematic overview and meta-analysis considered all pertinent studies with at least 10 children younger than 18 years with acute symptoms of <30 days and without serious complications.

Outcomes. Clinical improvement rates for intervention studies of antibiotics or ancillary measures; concordance of diagnostic tests (expressed as likelihood ratios).

Results. Of 1857 citations originally reviewed, we identified 21 qualifying studies, compared with 450 reports on complications of acute sinusitis and 233 nonsystematic reviews of the subject. The qualifying studies included 5 randomized, controlled trials and 8 case series on antibiotic therapy, 3 randomized, controlled trials on ancillary treatments, and 8 studies with information on diagnostic tests (including 3 therapeutic trials). Definitions and inclusion criteria were heterogeneous across studies. The pooled clinical improvement rate with antibiotics was 88% (177/202) in randomized, controlled trials and 92% (318/345) in nonrandomized studies; the improvement rates on no antibiotics were 60% and 80%, respectively. Improvement rates were significantly higher in nonrandomized studies (Mantel-Haenszel odds ratio: 1.79; 95% CI: 1.05–3.04, stratified for use of antibiotics). Data on ancillary measures were sparse and heterogeneous. In studies comparing clinical findings with plain film radiography, the pooled rate of abnormal radiographic findings against a clinical diagnosis of sinusitis was 73% (596/814; range: 55% to 96% between studies). There was poor concordance between clinical criteria, plain radiographs, ultrasonography, computed tomography, and fluid on aspiration in all available paired assessments (all positive likelihood ratios were <4 and all negative likelihood ratios were >0.2).

Conclusions. Good, high-quality evidence for acute uncomplicated sinusitis in children is limited. Diagnostic modalities show poor concordance, and treatment options are based on inadequate data. More evidence is needed for defining the optimal treatment and diagnostic methods for this common condition.

INTRODUCTION

Acute sinusitis is one of the most common community-acquired infections. One investigator estimated that there are as many as 1 billion episodes (viral, bacterial, or other) occurring each year in the US population. The condition is even more common in children than in adults. Given the frequency of this condition, the costs associated with its diagnosis and medical treatment (either antibiotics or ancillary measures) are large. However, evidence on the diagnosis and management of this common condition is limited and fragmented.

In 1997, the Agency for Healthcare Research and Quality contracted with the New England Medical Center Evidence-based Practice Center to produce an evidence report, titled "Diagnosis and Management of Acute Sinusitis." A supplemental analysis to include nonrandomized trials for the pediatrics population was added to this contract when only 2 relevant randomized studies

were found that studied exclusively pediatric populations. Although randomized studies are more likely to provide unbiased information, nonrandomized evidence may provide additional information and is needed when randomized data are sparse.

In this study, we systematically identified and analyzed all the accumulated evidence that pertains to the diagnosis and therapeutic management of acute uncomplicated sinusitis in children. The main questions addressed in this study are: 1) What is the evidence for the efficacy of various antibiotics in children with a diagnosis of acute sinusitis? 2) What is the evidence for the efficacy of various ancillary, nonantibiotic regimens in children with acute sinusitis? 3) What is the diagnostic accuracy and concordance of clinical symptoms, radiography, and other imaging methods and sinus aspiration for the diagnosis of acute sinusitis in children?

METHODS

Definitions

The definition of uncomplicated sinusitis excludes cases in which clinically evident neurologic, soft tissue, or other complications were present. Acute sinusitis is defined typically by a duration of symptoms of <30 days. We did not attempt to separate bacterial from nonbacterial cases in the considered reports. Cures and failures were recorded as defined by each individual study: "cure" generally meant resolution of all signs and symptoms, and "failure" generally signified no change or worsening of signs and symptoms. "Improvement" was typically used for intermediate changes, although some studies used the term without a distinction from "cure."

The reference standard for the diagnosis of acute uncomplicated bacterial sinusitis is sinus aspiration and culture; this is infrequently used because it is invasive, cumbersome to perform, and time-consuming. Other diagnostic parameters (clinical presentation, plain-film, and ultrasound) were compared to assess concordance rather than as proof of diagnostic accuracy.

Inclusion Criteria

Published reports on acute sinusitis qualified for inclusion regardless of study design if they studied at least 10 children younger than 18 years, or if subgroups of age younger than 18 years could be readily identified in the presented data. Studies of subacute and chronic sinusitis were excluded. Subgroup data on acute sinusitis (with at least 10 children) from reports in which chronic and acute sinusitis or other infections were considered, qualified for inclusion. Studies limited to complications (neurologic, local soft tissue, or other) of acute sinusitis were excluded.

Search Strategy

We searched Medline using a broad search strategy covering from January 1966 through March 1999. The word sinusitis was used in the search as a text word and as a medical subject heading. We then limited the search results to human studies and English language that included pediatric patients using the terms "infant, newborn," "infant," "child, preschool," "child," and "adolescence." The titles and abstracts of the citations produced by the search were screened for articles that may have data on treatment of acute sinusitis in the pediatric population.

As part of a previous project, we also had retrieved all published randomized, controlled trials on the management of acute uncomplicated sinusitis in all age groups. This collection of randomized, controlled trials had been generated based on Med-line searches complemented by Excerpta Medica searches, perusal of the Abstracts for the Interscience Conference on Antimicrobial Agents and Chemotherapy, review of bibliographies of retrieved studies, and communication with technical experts and colleagues in the field. Randomized, controlled trials were included in this collection with no foreign language restrictions. All identified randomized, controlled trials were screened for the presence of data in children.

Statistical Analysis

Given the paucity and heterogeneity of the data for specific questions, we did not attempt the application of formal meta-analytic techniques in most circumstances. When possible, rates were combined across different studies and heterogeneity was assessed with a χ^2 statistic. Odds ratios (ORs) for efficacy (clinical improvement) also were estimated by the Mantel-Haenszel formula stratified per antibiotic use.

For diagnostic modalities, we expressed concordance by using the positive likelihood ratio, which is calculated as

$$positive\ likelihood\ ratio = sensitivity / (1 - specificity)$$

and the negative likelihood ratio, which is calculated as

$$negative\ likelihood\ ratio = (1 - sensitivity) / specificity.$$

The positive likelihood ratio gives an estimate of how much more common a specific diagnostic finding in the positive group is versus the negative group, when positive and negative are defined by a different diagnostic standard. For example, a sensitivity of 50% with specificity of 90% corresponds to a positive likelihood ratio of 5. The higher the positive likelihood ratio, the better the concordance of the 2 diagnostic modalities. A positive likelihood ratio of 1 indicates that there is no concordance at all. There are no absolute cutoffs, but positive likelihood ratios between 1 and 5 are generally suggestive of poor concordance, while positive likelihood ratios >20 suggest strong concordance. The positive likelihood ratio can take values up to infinity. The inverse considerations hold true for the negative likelihood ratio, where good concordance is shown by diminishing values. A negative likelihood ratio of 1 also shows lack of concordance. Again, there are no absolute cutoffs, but negative likelihood ratios between 0.2 and 1 are generally suggestive of poor concordance, while negative likelihood ratios <0.05 suggest strong concordance.

All reported P values are 2-tailed.

RESULTS

Retrieved Reports

The Medline strategy produced 1857 articles. Of those, 1719 were rejected on the basis of their title and abstracts. Notably, these included 450 articles on complications of acute sinusitis and 233 non-systematic review articles without apparent primary original data. One hundred thirty-eight articles were retrieved in full and examined because the possibility that they might qualify could not be excluded from the title and/or abstract alone. A total of 21 studies qualified for inclusion.

Of 68 randomized, controlled trials on antibiotic treatment of acute sinusitis that we identified in the more extended search, only 5 dealt with exclusively a pediatric population. These 5 trials are among the 21 identified qualifying reports. For 30 additional randomized, controlled trials, the age range of the enrolled patients extended to younger than 18 years, but no separate data on children younger than 18 years were available, and the majority of the patients were presumably adults. For 23 of these 30 trials, the lower age limit was between 12 and 17 years, and for another 5 trials it was 10 or 11 years.

Of the 12 randomized, controlled trials on ancillary measures identified as part of the extended search, there were only 3 trials (with a total of 243 patients) that studied the efficacy of ancillary measures in the treatment of acute sinusitis in exclusively pediatric populations. The age range of the remaining 9 trials extended to as young as 9 to 20 years (younger than 12 years in 7 of them), but no separate data on the pediatric population were provided and the majority of the enrolled patients were presumably adults (upper age limit: 62 years to undefined).

Efficacy of Antibiotic Interventions

The efficacy of various antibiotic interventions was addressed in 5 randomized, controlled trials and 8 nonrandomized studies. These 13 qualifying studies were published between 1970 and 1997 and with 2 exceptions had been conducted at single centers by pediatricians or otolaryngologists. Nine of the 13 reports, including 6 of the 8 nonrandomized studies, originated outside the United States. Pharmaceutical sponsorship was clearly mentioned in 4 reports. The largest case series had 106 patients, and the largest randomized, controlled trial had 93 patients. Overall, 255 children had been studied in the 5 randomized, controlled trials, and 418 children had been studied in the 8 nonrandomized studies. Eight of the 13 reports did not specify the duration of symptoms. Puncture for aspiration/ irrigation was performed in 6 studies in selected children. Positive radiographic findings (typically combinations of air-fluid level, opacification, and/or mucosal thickening criteria) were required for the diagnosis of acute sinusitis in 9 of the 13 studies. Clinical symptoms and signs were typically the other mainstay of diagnosis, but there was large variability on how sinusitis was diagnosed as well as on the prevalence of various specific symptoms and signs as reported in the various studies.

An array of antibiotics were tested, while a placebo arm was present in 2 randomized, controlled trials and a "no antibiotic" treatment group was considered in 1 of the case series. The duration of treatment varied between 3 and 28 days. The 2 shorter courses (3 and 5 days) were with azithromycin, which retains high drug levels for several days after its discontinuation. All other studies used at least 7 days of therapy. Decongestants were either reported to be routinely prescribed or their use was not mentioned at all.

The response to treatment typically was assessed after 7 to 14 days, but it also was assessed at 21 days and 1 month in 2 early studies. Cure, improvement, and failure rates are shown. Overall, using the available data we estimated that the clinical improvement rate with antibiotics was 88% in randomized, controlled trials (177/202) and 92% (318/ 345) in nonrandomized studies. The rate of improvement on no antibiotics was 66% (33/50). It was 60% (21/35) in a randomized trial and 80% (12/15) in an observational study. The only randomized trial that compared antibiotics with placebo and provided cure rates found significantly better efficacy for antibiotics. There were no significant differences in the efficacy of various antibiotic regimens in direct randomized comparisons. Overall, there was a trend for higher improvement rates in the nonrandomized studies compared with the randomized studies (OR: 1.79; 95% CI: 1.05–3.04; $P = .03$ stratified for antibiotic use). Improvement rates were higher in nonrandomized studies versus randomized studies in the stratum of patients receiving antibiotics (OR: 1.66) and in the stratum of patients not receiving antibiotics (OR: 2.67). Improvement rates did not differ significantly between the various individual studies.

Data on outcome as documented by the performance of follow-up images were available from 5 studies; overall 81% (269/333) of images (plain film radiography or ultrasound) improved. Reporting of safety data were limited; the frequency of discontinuations of treatment attributable to side effects was mentioned per arm in only 5 studies. In all, there were 7 discontinuations attributable to side effects among 233 (3%) patients treated with antibiotics. In 1 placebo-controlled trial, the discontinuation rate attributable to side effects was 6 of 58 patients with antibiotics versus 2 of 35 patients with placebo (risk ratio: 1.8; 95% CI: 0.4–8.5).

Bacteriologic response with sinus aspirates obtained before and after treatment was assessed only in 2 studies. In the study by Ficnar et al, eradication was achieved with azithromycin in 3 of 3 patients who had isolated pathogens. Puhakka et al used sinus aspirates and exudates from sinus ostia for culture; information on the 2 sampling modes is not presented separately. In addition, the results on eradication are mixed with those of other infections and thus are not interpretable.

Efficacy of Ancillary Measures

Of the 3 trials qualifying for inclusion regarding the efficacy of ancillary measures, 1 trial enrolled children who had sinusitis on the basis of ultrasonography, in the absence of any symptoms, and addressed the value of lavage as adjunctive therapy to amoxicillin and a decongestant. The other 2 trials addressed, in a double-blind fashion, the efficacy of steroid or combination agents (nasal spray budenoside and a combination of nasal oxymetazoline in addition to oral liquid brompheniramine and phenylpropanolamine, respectively) against placebo.

None of the 3 studies used the categorization "cure-improvement-failure" for clinical outcomes. The study on lavage used strictly ultra-sonographic criteria. The other 2 studies used composite clinical and/or radiologic scores, and there was no statistically significant difference found at any of the addressed time points, except for a superiority of budenoside over placebo at the end of 2 weeks in terms of the clinical score. It should be noted that in this study, only 89 of the 151 enrolled patients were followed up adequately to be included in the analysis.

Concordance of Diagnostic Methods

We were able to identify only 5 studies that addressed the comparative diagnostic accuracy of at least 2 procedures used as diagnostic tools in children with acute sinusitis. In addition, 2 of the randomized, controlled trials on therapeutic measures provided data on percentage of abnormal radiographs among children with a clinical diagnosis of sinusitis; a third trial addressed the presence of aspiration fluid in the setting of abnormal ultrasonography without any symptoms being present. Thus, a total of 8 studies qualified for considerations pertaining to diagnostic concordance.

These diagnostic studies were very heterogeneous. Five of the 8 originated outside the United States. In several of them, radiology and/or otolaryngology specialists authored the reports, rather than general pediatricians. The study population was usually not adequately defined in terms of duration of symptoms, except in 2 randomized, controlled trials.

Of the 7 studies in which some or all patients had clinical symptoms or signs, plain film radiography was performed in 6, while plain films were considered to be worthless in a study of infants. In these 6 studies, the rate of abnormal plain film radiography findings (typically opacification, mucosal thickening, and/or air-fluid level) against a clinical diagnosis of sinusitis ranged from 55% to 96%. These rates were statistically significantly different across the various studies ($P = .001$). The pooled rate was 73% (596/814). The largest component of this variability is probably attributable to variability in the clinical definition of sinusitis. This could be discerned easily in the only study that used different thresholds for the clinical definition. When the subgroup of children who had only 1 of the 3 criteria of purulent secretion, history of upper respiratory secretion, and sinus pain or tenderness were considered, radiographic abnormalities were present only in 22/79 cases (28%). When 2 or 3 of these criteria were present, radiographic abnormalities were noted in 75/96 cases (78%).

Similar rates of abnormal radiographs also were seen in the 2 randomized, controlled trials that used strict clinical criteria for the diagnosis of acute sinusitis. Wald et al defined sinusitis by the presence of any nasal discharge and/or cough that were not improving for 10 to 30 days. Barlan et al defined sinusitis by the presence of at least 2 of 3 major criteria (purulent nasal discharge, pharyngeal discharge, cough) or 1 of them plus 2 of 9 minor ones with duration of at least 7 days. In these 2 randomized, controlled trials, abnormal radiographs were seen in 136/171 (80%) and 69/89 (78%) of children with a clinical diagnosis, respectively.

The other 3 studies that offer data on radiography and clinical diagnosis do not specify a priori explicit criteria for the clinical diagnosis of acute sinusitis. One study simply lists the percentage of various symptoms, while another does not give any clinical information on signs and symptoms. The third study states that the distinction between "sinusitis" and "rhinitis" was left to the impression of the clinician. Interestingly, the "rhinitis" group did not differ from the "sinusitis" group in the prevalence of fever, purulent secretion, sinus tenderness, or headache.

In a study of infants (newborn to 12 months of age), plain film radiographs were considered worthless and thus only computed tomography (CT) scans were evaluated. Excluding cases of sinus hypoplasia, evidence of CT involvement of the maxillary sinus(es) had an 87% (13/15) sensitivity, but only 41% (28/69) specificity against the clinical impression of upper respiratory infection symptoms. The positive predictive value is only 13/54 (24%), and the negative predictive value is 28/30 (93%). The respective figures for the ethmoid sinus(es) were sensitivity of 67% (10/15) and specificity of 61% (46/75), positive predictive value of 10/39 (26%) and negative predictive value of 46/51 (90%). Thus the concordance of CT scan and clinical impression in infants is very poor.

One study found good correlation between ultrasonographic findings and retrieval of fluid on aspiration: 68 of 72 sinuses with ultrasonographic abnormalities yielded fluid on aspiration, but aspiration was not attempted in any control group without ultrasonographic abnormalities. Cultures of the aspirate from 59 sinuses yielded microbial pathogens in less than half the cases (26/59). The only study to compare ultrasonography with plain film radiography and sinus fluid abnormalities among children with a clinical picture of sinusitis found very low concordance between these diagnostic techniques. Finally, abnormalities of plain film radiography had a poor concordance even with the simple presence of fluid in one study.

DISCUSSION

This study evaluated the available randomized and nonrandomized evidence on the diagnosis and management of acute sinusitis in children. Compared with the frequency of this common condition, the amount of high-quality evidence regarding diagnosis and treatment is remarkably limited. Most randomized data on adolescents may have been inextricably merged with data on adults in previous studies, and it is unclear whether adolescents should differ from adults in the diagnosis and management of acute sinusitis. However, for children younger than 12 years, evidence is sparse. Furthermore, it is hazardous to extrapolate evidence from adults to children given that children have a different and continuously changing anatomy and a higher incidence of viral upper respiratory tract infections.

There are few data on how to accurately diagnose acute sinusitis in childhood. Clinical criteria may not be very reliable. Plain film radiography shows only modest concordance with clinical diagnosis, and the concordance depends largely on how a clinical diagnosis is defined. Other imaging modalities have no clear role in the diagnosis of uncomplicated acute bacterial sinusitis. A decision analysis suggests that imaging studies may not be cost-effective for any level of previous suspicion of acute bacterial sinusitis.

Although 1 small trial has shown superiority of antibiotics over placebo, its applicability to settings where sinusitis is defined by different criteria is uncertain. The available evidence also suggests that the various antibiotics, among the several used for children with sinusitis, do not differ in their efficacy; nevertheless, given the sparse evidence and the high rate of spontaneous resolution, modest differences could have been missed. Furthermore, no studies have been reported in the era of increased resistance among isolates of *Streptococcus pneumoniae* and bacteriologic response data are almost nonexistent. There is no convincing evidence to support the use of ancillary treatment with decongestant-antihistamines and limited evidence on the use of steroids.

Therapy for children with acute uncomplicated sinusitis is controversial. The rates of spontaneous resolution are high. Antibiotics have been shown to be superior to placebo in a population defined by symptoms of nasal discharge or cough that were not improving for at least 10 days and positive radiographs. Perhaps obtaining a radiograph would not be necessary if these clinical criteria exist for >10 days because almost 80% of these children would have a positive radiograph. Empirical treatment with antibiotics may be warranted in such cases. However, there is no evidence to support the use of antibiotics in other groups of children, such as those without nasal discharge or cough, those with shorter duration of symptoms, or those with improving symptoms. Spontaneous recovery rates in these groups are likely to be too high for antibiotics to offer any meaningful benefit. Finally, if antibiotic treatment is prescribed in acute, uncomplicated cases of sinusitis, evidence supports the use of amoxicillin, unless there is a history of allergy to β-lactams. Currently, there is insufficient evidence to support the use of newer, broad-spectrum antibiotics, although increasing rates of antibiotic resistance should prompt the performance of properly designed studies.

Finally, the current evidence does not offer any clear indication for the use of ancillary measures. Although routinely used, there is no strong evidence from randomized, controlled trials to justify the use of antihistamines and decongestants in children. Evidence for the use of steroids comes from a single small trial. More data are needed to evaluate the usefulness of these agents.

The strongest message emanating from this report is the lack of standardized clinical criteria for defining acute bacterial sinusitis in children as well as the paucity of high-quality evidence for establishing the diagnosis and optimal management of this condition. Despite the presence of an extensive bibliography on sinusitis in children, actual evidence and primary data on the diagnosis and management of acute uncomplicated sinusitis are limited. We encountered 450 reports on complications of sinusitis, mostly case reports or case series. Although it is important to know about the rare complications of this disease, it is questionable whether all these case reports and small case series give us useful information when there is comparatively only a handful of studies that deal with the common uncomplicated forms of the infection. In addition, there were 233 nonsystematic review articles compared with approximately 20 primary studies with analyzable original data. The paucity of primary data may be attributable to the difficulties in applying the necessary rigorous diagnostic methodologies to generate high-quality information in children. Additional well-designed prospective studies are much needed to establish optimal diagnostic procedures and management of children suspected to have acute bacterial sinusitis.

Diagnosis and Management of Childhood Obstructive Sleep Apnea Syndrome

- *Clinical Practice Guideline*
- *Technical Report Summary*

Readers of this clinical practice guideline are urged to review the technical report to enhance the evidence-based decision-making process. The full technical report is available on the enclosed CD-ROM.

AMERICAN ACADEMY OF PEDIATRICS

Section on Pediatric Pulmonology, Subcommittee on Obstructive Sleep Apnea Syndrome

Clinical Practice Guideline: Diagnosis and Management of Childhood Obstructive Sleep Apnea Syndrome

ABSTRACT. This clinical practice guideline, intended for use by primary care clinicians, provides recommendations for the diagnosis and management of obstructive sleep apnea syndrome (OSAS).

The Section on Pediatric Pulmonology of the American Academy of Pediatrics selected a subcommittee composed of pediatricians and other experts in the fields of pulmonology and otolaryngology as well as experts from epidemiology and pediatric practice to develop an evidence base of literature on this topic. The resulting evidence report was used to formulate recommendations for the diagnosis and management of childhood OSAS.

The guideline contains the following recommendations for the diagnosis of OSAS: 1) all children should be screened for snoring; 2) complex high-risk patients should be referred to a specialist; 3) patients with cardiorespiratory failure cannot await elective evaluation; 4) diagnostic evaluation is useful in discriminating between primary snoring and OSAS, the gold standard being polysomnography; 5) adenotonsillectomy is the first line of treatment for most children, and continuous positive airway pressure is an option for those who are not candidates for surgery or do not respond to surgery; 6) high-risk patients should be monitored as inpatients postoperatively; 7) patients should be reevaluated postoperatively to determine whether additional treatment is required.

This clinical practice guideline is not intended as a sole source of guidance in the evaluation of children with OSAS. Rather, it is designed to assist primary care clinicians by providing a framework for diagnostic decision-making. It is not intended to replace clinical judgment or to establish a protocol for all children with this condition and may not provide the only appropriate approach to this problem. *Pediatrics* 2002;109:704–712; *obstructive sleep apnea, infant, child, adenoidectomy, tonsillectomy, meta-analysis, polysomnography, sleep disorders, snoring.*

ABBREVIATIONS. OSAS, obstructive sleep apnea syndrome; PS, primary snoring; REM, rapid eye movement; CPAP, continuous positive airway pressure; PPV, positive predictive value; NPV, negative predictive value.

INTRODUCTION

Obstructive sleep apnea syndrome (OSAS) is a common condition in childhood and can result in severe complications if left untreated. Nevertheless, there is no consensus on the best methods of evaluation and management of this syndrome in children. Therefore, the American Academy of

Pediatrics has supported the development of a practice guideline for the diagnosis and management of childhood OSAS.

The purpose of this clinical practice guideline is to 1) increase the recognition of OSAS by pediatricians to decrease diagnostic delay and avoid serious sequelae of OSAS; 2) evaluate diagnostic techniques; 3) describe treatment options; 4) provide guidelines for follow-up; and 5) discuss areas requiring additional research.

This practice guideline focuses on uncomplicated childhood OSAS, that is, the otherwise healthy child with OSAS associated with adenotonsillar hypertrophy and/or obesity who is being treated in the primary care setting. This guideline specifically excludes infants younger than 1 year, patients with central apnea or hypoventilation syndromes, and patients with OSAS associated with other medical disorders, including but not limited to Down syndrome, craniofacial anomalies, neuromuscular disease (including cerebral palsy), chronic lung disease, sickle cell disease, metabolic disease, or laryngomalacia. These important patient populations are too complex to discuss within the scope of this paper and require specialist consultation. In addition, patients with life-threatening OSAS who present in cardiorespiratory failure will not be covered here, because these patients require urgent treatment.

METHODS OF GUIDELINE DEVELOPMENT

Details of the methods of guideline development are included in the accompanying technical report published online.[1] Committee members signed forms confirming that they did not have a conflict of interest. The guidelines were based on data available from the medical literature. A computerized search of the National Library of Medicine's PubMed database (http://www.ncbi.nlm.nih.gov/entrez/query.fcgi?db=PubMed) from 1966–1999 (later updated to include 2000) was performed using the following keywords: sleep apnea syndrome, apnea, sleep disorders, snoring, polysomnography, airway obstruction, adenoidectomy, tonsillectomy (adverse effects, mortality), and sleep-disordered breathing. The search was limited to articles involving children. Studies involving infants, animal studies, and articles written in languages other than English were excluded. Reviews, case reports, letters to the editor, and abstracts were not included. A total of 2110 articles were found. Committee members then screened the articles, first by title and then by abstract, to obtain articles relevant to the guideline.

After screening, a total of 278 articles were reviewed in full by committee members. An additional 6 articles, primarily from foreign publications, could not be obtained from local libraries. None of these were considered particularly germane to the guideline. In addition to the literature search, committee members supplemented the articles with additional publications thought to be relevant and with those published after 1999. Details of the literature grading system are available in the accompanying technical report published online. Review of the literature revealed that there were very few randomized controlled studies. When the evidence was poor or lacking, there was extensive discussion among committee members to achieve consensus. The guideline notes whether a decision was based on objective evidence or on consensus decision.

DEFINITION

OSAS in children is a "disorder of breathing during sleep characterized by prolonged partial upper airway obstruction and/or intermittent complete obstruction (obstructive apnea) that disrupts normal ventilation during sleep and normal sleep patterns."[2] Symptoms include habitual (nightly) snoring (often with intermittent pauses, snorts, or gasps), disturbed sleep, and daytime neurobehavioral problems. Daytime sleepiness may occur but is uncommon in young children. Complications include neurocognitive impairment, behavioral problems, failure to thrive, and cor pulmonale, particularly in severe cases. Risk factors include adenotonsillar hypertrophy, obesity, craniofacial anomalies, and neuromuscular disorders. Only the first 2 risk factors are discussed in this guideline.

OSAS needs to be distinguished from primary snoring (PS), which is defined as snoring without obstructive apnea, frequent arousals from sleep, or gas exchange abnormalities.[3] Although PS is usually considered benign, this has not been well evaluated, because most studies of snoring children did not discriminate between PS and OSAS.

PREVALENCE

OSAS occurs in children of all ages, from neonates to adolescents. It is thought to be most common in preschool-aged children, which is the age when the tonsils and adenoids are the largest in relation to the underlying airway size.[4] Three studies have evaluated the prevalence of childhood OSAS. These studies did not use conventional polysomnography, used adult rather than pediatric polysomnographic criteria, or studied only a selected high-risk sample of the population; thus, a definitive epidemiologic study has not yet been performed. Despite these limitations, the 3 studies showed similar prevalence rates of approximately 2%.[5–7] In contrast, PS is more common; habitual snoring occurs in 3% to 12% of preschool-aged children.[5,6,8–10] Thus, the clinician needs a method to distinguish OSAS from PS. OSAS occurs equally among boys and girls.[7] One study indicated that the prevalence is higher among African American individuals than among white individuals.[7]

SEQUELAE OF OSAS

Untreated OSAS can result in serious morbidity. Early reports documented such complications as failure to thrive, cor pulmonale, and mental retardation.[11] These severe sequelae appear to be less common now, probably because of earlier diagnosis and treatment. Although failure to thrive is the exception these days, children with OSAS still tend to have a growth spurt after adenotonsillectomy.[12–14] In the past, cor pulmonale with heart failure was not an uncommon mode of presentation for OSAS in children, but it is now rare. Although overt right heart failure now occurs less often, asymptomatic degrees of pulmonary hypertension may be common.[15] Systemic hypertension can occur.[16–18] Many reports have suggested that children with OSAS are at risk of neurocognitive deficits, such as poor learning, behavioral problems, and attention-deficit/hyperactivity disorder.[19–22] However, many of these studies were case series based on histories obtained from parents of snoring children without objective evaluation, control groups, or sleep studies to distinguish PS from OSAS. One recent study showed that children with sleep-disordered breathing were more likely to do poorly at school, and many improved after adenotonsillectomy.[23] If untreated, OSAS may result in death. Early OSAS literature described children who presented with cardiorespiratory failure or coma, some of whom died.[24–26]

METHODS OF DIAGNOSIS

Diagnostic methods that have been scientifically evaluated include history and physical examination, audiotaping or videotaping, pulse oximetry, abbreviated polysomnography, and full polysomnography. The goals of diagnosis are to 1) identify patients who are at risk for adverse outcomes; 2) avoid unnecessary intervention in patients who are not at risk for adverse outcomes; and 3) evaluate which patients are at increased risk of complications resulting from adenotonsillectomy so that appropriate precautions can be taken.

History and Physical Examination

A sleep history screening for snoring should be part of routine health care visits. In children, OSAS is very unlikely in the absence of habitual snoring. If a history of nightly snoring is elicited, a more detailed history regarding labored breathing during sleep, observed apnea, restless sleep, diaphoresis, enuresis, cyanosis, excessive daytime sleepiness, and behavior or learning problems (including attention-deficit/hyperactivity disorder) should be obtained. Findings on physical examination during wakefulness are often normal. There may be nonspecific findings related to adenotonsillar hypertrophy, such as mouth breathing, nasal obstruction during wakefulness, adenoidal facies, and hyponasal speech. Evidence of complications of OSAS may be present. These include systemic hypertension, an increased pulmonic component of the second heart sound indicating pulmonary hypertension, and poor growth (although conversely, some children with OSAS are obese).

Although history and physical examination are useful to screen patients and determine which patients need additional investigation for OSAS, there is controversy about their roles in determining which patients require treatment. A number of studies have shown that there is no relation between the size of the tonsils and adenoids and presence of OSAS.[27-30] This is because OSAS is thought to be attributable to a combination of adenotonsillar hypertrophy and the neuromuscular tone of the upper airway during sleep rather than to structural abnormalities alone. Thus, the presence of large tonsils and adenoids does not necessarily indicate that the patient has OSAS.

An accurate diagnosis is required not only to ensure that appropriate treatment is provided and to avoid unnecessary treatment, but also to determine which children are at risk of complications resulting from treatment. Several studies have objectively evaluated the utility of a standardized history alone; history and physical examination; or history, physical examination, and audiotaping or videotaping to diagnose OSAS. In 1984, a study evaluated the efficacy of a questionnaire-derived OSAS score.[31] The questionnaire was administered first to patients with polysomnographically proven OSAS and controls without OSAS and then prospectively to snoring patients being evaluated for suspected OSAS. The score was able to distinguish between patients with known OSAS and controls. However, three quarters of subjects had an indeterminate score. A more recent study by the same authors with a much larger sample found that the score had a sensitivity of 35% and specificity of 39%.[32] A number of other studies have shown that this score has limited utility when applied to snoring children being evaluated for OSAS[33,34] or when applied to obese patients.[35,36] Thus, this questionnaire has minimal usefulness in the evaluation of OSAS.

Other studies have evaluated the utility of history and physical examination in distinguishing children with PS from those with OSAS.[33,34,37-41] None of these studies were able to reliably discriminate between OSAS and PS.

There are a number of reasons why the history can be misleading. The loudness of snoring does not necessarily correlate with the degree of obstructive apnea. Thus, children may have very noticeable snoring without apnea. Children with OSAS experience obstruction primarily during rapid eye movement (REM) sleep, which occurs predominantly in the early morning hours when their parents are not observing them,[42] thus leading to an underestimation of apnea. Some children have a pattern of persistent partial upper airway obstruction associated with gas exchange abnormalities, rather than discrete, cyclic apneas ("obstructive hypoventilation"[2]). These children will not manifest pauses and gasps in their snoring, and therefore, the condition may be misdiagnosed as PS.

Nocturnal Polysomnography

Nocturnal polysomnography (sleep study) is the only diagnostic technique shown to quantitate the ventilatory and sleep abnormalities associated with sleep-disordered breathing and is currently the gold standard. Polysomnography can be performed satisfactorily in children of any age, providing that appropriate equipment and trained staff are used. Furthermore, pediatric studies should be scored and interpreted using age-appropriate criteria as outlined in the American Thoracic Society consensus statement on pediatric polysomnography.[2] Polysomnography, by definition, can distinguish PS from OSAS. It can objectively determine the severity of OSAS and related gas exchange and sleep disturbances. As such, it can help determine the risk of postoperative complications (Table 1). However, although it is generally believed that children with severely abnormal results of sleep studies are at increased risk for complications of OSAS, formal studies have not been performed to evaluate the correlation between polysomnographic parameters and adverse outcomes in children with OSAS.[43] Thus, although we know which polysomnographic parameters are statistically abnormal,[44] studies have not definitively evaluated which polysomnographic criteria predict morbidity. In addition, there is currently a shortage of facilities that perform pediatric polysomnography. The availability of pediatric polysomnography is expected to improve, especially with the computerized equipment currently available.

Audiotaping or Videotaping

Two studies have examined the use of audiotaping,[33,41] and 1 study has examined the use of videotaping,[45] alone or combined with clinical findings, in establishing a diagnosis. In these studies, sensitivity ranged from 71% to 94%, and specificity ranged from 29% to 80%. Positive predictive values (PPVs) were 50%[41] and 75%[33] for audiotaping and 83% for videotaping.[45] Sounds of struggle on audiotapes were found to be more predictive of OSAS than were pauses.[33] The negative predictive value (NPV) ranged from 73% to 88%. Although these techniques may have promise, the discrepancies in results from different centers indicate that additional study is necessary.

Abbreviated Polysomnography

Several studies have evaluated abbreviated polysomnographic techniques. Overnight oximetry can be useful if it shows a pattern of cyclic desaturation. Brouillette et al[32] performed oximetry in a group of

---

TABLE 1. Risk Factors for Postoperative Respiratory Complications in Children With OSAS Undergoing Adenotonsillectomy

Age younger than 3 years
Severe OSAS on polysomnography
Cardiac complications of OSAS (eg, right ventricular hypertrophy)
Failure to thrive
Obesity
Prematurity
Recent respiratory infection
Craniofacial anomalies*
Neuromuscular disorders*

* Not discussed in these guidelines.

children with suspected OSAS and compared it with simultaneous full polysomnography. Patients with complex medical conditions were excluded. Compared with polysomnography, they found a PPV of 97% and an NPV of 47%, indicating that oximetry was useful when results were positive. However, patients with negative results of oximetry required full polysomnography for definitive diagnosis. False-positive results were found in patients with mild coexistent medical problems, such as obesity and asthma, suggesting that this technique is useful only in otherwise healthy children.

Nap polysomnography is appealing, because it can be performed in the daytime and is, therefore, more convenient for patients and laboratory staff. Studies have shown a PPV of 77% to 100% and an NPV of 17% to 49%.[46,47] In children with OSAS, overnight polysomnograms demonstrate more severe abnormalities than do nap studies. Thus, nap polysomnography may be useful if results are positive, although it may underestimate the severity of OSAS. An overnight study should be performed if the results of the nap study are negative. The difference in predictive value between nap and overnight studies is probably attributable to the decreased amount of REM sleep during nap studies as well as the decreased total sleep time.

Unattended home polysomnography in children has been evaluated by only 1 center.[48] Home polysomnography yielded similar results to laboratory studies. However, it should be noted that the equipment used in this study was relatively sophisticated and included respiratory inductive plethysmography (a method for determining ventilation without using oronasal sensors), oximeter pulse wave form, and videotaping. The utility of unattended home studies in children using commercially available 4- to 6-channel recording equipment has not been studied.

Summary of Diagnostic Techniques

In summary, history and physical examination are poor at predicting OSAS. Most studies have shown that abbreviated or screening techniques, such as videotaping, nocturnal pulse oximetry, and daytime nap polysomnography tend to be helpful if results are positive but have a poor predictive value if results are negative. Thus, children with negative study results should undergo a more comprehensive evaluation. The cost efficacy of these screening techniques is unclear and would depend, in part, on how many patients eventually required full polysomnography. In addition, the use of these techniques in evaluating the severity of OSAS (which is important in determining management, such as whether outpatient surgery should be performed) has not been evaluated.

TREATMENT OPTIONS

Tonsillectomy and Adenoidectomy

Adenotonsillectomy is the most common treatment for children with OSAS. Adenoidectomy alone may not be sufficient.[38,49] In otherwise healthy children with adenotonsillar hypertrophy, polysomnographic resolution occurs in 75% to 100%[37,49–51] after adenotonsillectomy; this is associated with symptom resolution.[37] Although obese children may have less satisfactory results, many will be adequately treated with adenotonsillectomy,[52] and it is generally the first-line therapy for these patients.

Potential complications of adenotonsillectomy include anesthetic complications; immediate postoperative problems, such as pain and poor oral intake; and hemorrhage. In addition, patients with OSAS may develop respiratory complications, such as worsening of OSAS or pulmonary edema, in the immediate postoperative period. Death attributable to respiratory complications in the immediate postoperative period has been reported in patients with severe OSAS. Identified risk factors are shown in Table 1.[53–58] High-risk patients should be hospitalized overnight after surgery and monitored continuously with pulse oximetry.

Continuous Positive Airway Pressure (CPAP)

For patients with specific surgical contraindications, minimal adenotonsillar tissue, or persistent OSAS after adenotonsillectomy or for those who prefer nonsurgical alternatives, CPAP therapy is an option.[59–61] However, unlike adenotonsillectomy, which is a 1-time procedure that is usually curative, CPAP will need to be used indefinitely. CPAP is delivered using an electronic device that delivers constant air pressure via a nasal mask, leading to mechanical stenting of the airway and improved functional residual capacity in the lungs. The pressure requirement varies among individuals; thus, CPAP must be titrated in the sleep laboratory before prescribing the device and periodically readjusted thereafter.[59] CPAP is a long-term therapy and requires frequent clinician assessment of adherence and efficacy. It is generally tolerated in older children.[59,60] Young children or older children with learning or behavioral problems may require behavioral or desensitization techniques to accept this form of therapy.[62] Attention to compliance with this therapy is crucial.

Other Treatment Modalities

Most adjunctive measures in the treatment of childhood OSAS have not been prospectively evaluated. Avoidance of environmental tobacco smoke and other indoor pollutants, avoidance of indoor allergens, and treatment of accompanying rhinitis may be helpful. In obese patients, weight loss strategies should be used. However, implementation of adjunctive therapies should not delay specific treatment of OSAS.

Oxygen therapy is sometimes prescribed in special cases to alleviate nocturnal hypoxemia in children with OSAS. However, there are few, if any, indications for its use in the otherwise healthy child with OSAS. Oxygen therapy does not prevent sleep-related upper airway obstruction and resultant problems, such as sleep fragmentation and increased work of breathing. Furthermore, it may worsen hy-

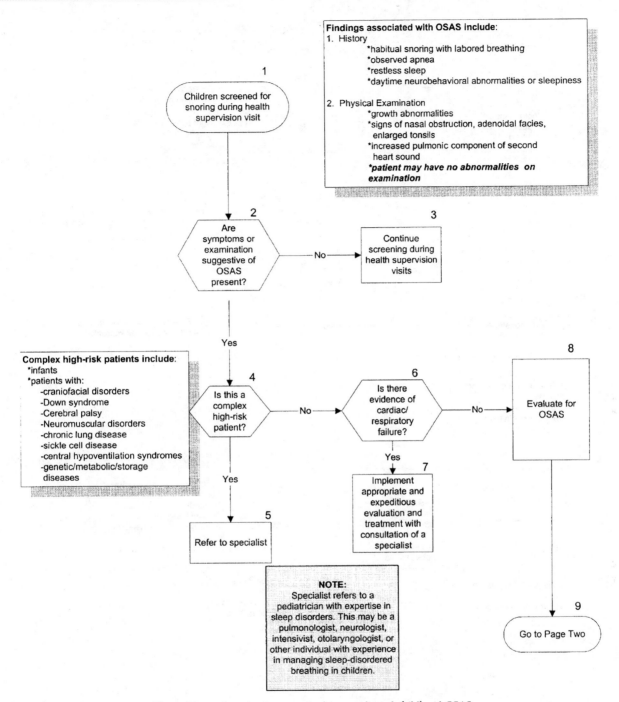

Fig 1. Diagnosis and management of uncomplicated childhood OSAS.

poventilation.[63] If oxygen therapy is to be used in children with OSAS, it should be evaluated during continuous Pco_2 monitoring to assess its effect on hypoventilation.

Other surgical options are available for patients not responding to usual treatment. These patients require care from pediatric surgical specialists. Surgical treatment options include uvulopharyngopalatoplasty, craniofacial surgery, and in severe cases, tracheostomy.

Follow-up of Patients Undergoing Surgical Treatment for OSAS

All patients should have clinical follow-up for reassessment of symptoms and signs associated with OSAS after initial treatment. Patients with mild to moderate OSAS who have complete resolution of symptoms and signs do not require objective testing to document resolution. Patients who have continued symptoms or signs, who have severe OSAS,[37] or

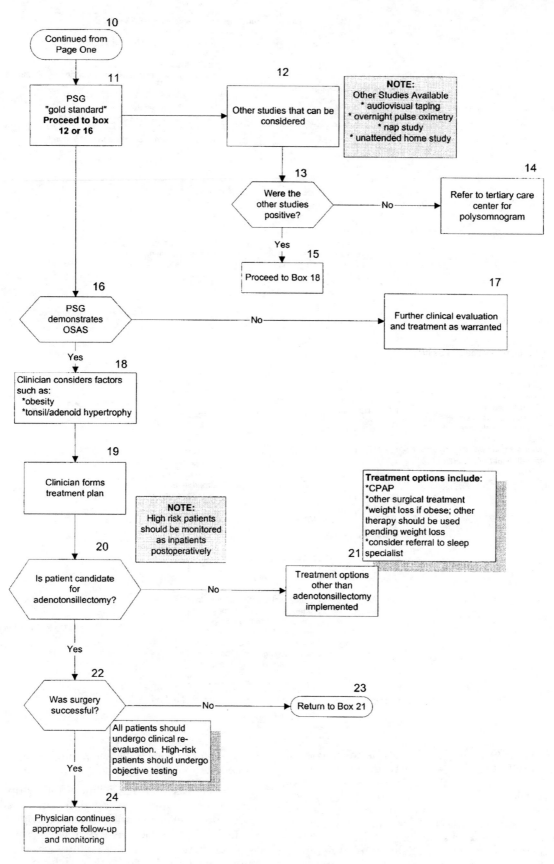

Fig 1. (continued)

who are obese require objective reevaluation to determine whether additional therapy, such as CPAP, is required. Objective data regarding timing of postoperative evaluation are not available. Most clinicians recommend waiting 6 to 8 weeks before reevaluation to ensure that upper airway, cardiac, and central nervous system remodeling is complete.

SUMMARY OF RECOMMENDATIONS FOR THE DIAGNOSIS AND MANAGEMENT OF UNCOMPLICATED CHILDHOOD OSAS

The following recommendations accompany an algorithm (Fig 1). As previously noted, these recommendations relate to otherwise healthy children older than 1 year with OSAS secondary to adenotonsillar hypertrophy and/or obesity and who are not in cardiorespiratory failure.

1. All children should be screened for snoring. As part of routine health care maintenance for all children, pediatricians should ask whether the patient snores. An affirmative answer should be followed by a more detailed evaluation. (Evidence for this recommendation is good, and the strength of the recommendation is strong.)
2. Complex, high-risk patients (Fig 1) should be referred to a specialist. (Evidence is good that these children are at increased surgical risk and require more complex management; the strength of the recommendation is strong.)
3. Patients with cardiorespiratory failure cannot await elective evaluation. It is expected that these patients will be in an intensive care setting and will be treated by a specialist; thus, these patients are not covered in this practice guideline.
4. Thorough diagnostic evaluation should be performed. History and physical examination have been shown to be poor at discriminating between PS and OSAS (evidence is strong). Polysomnography is the only method that quantifies ventilatory and sleep abnormalities and is recommended as the diagnostic test of choice. Other diagnostic techniques, such as videotaping, nocturnal pulse oximetry, and daytime nap studies, may be useful in discriminating between PS and OSAS if results of polysomnography are positive. However, they do not assess the severity of OSAS, which is useful for determining treatment and follow-up. In any case, because of their high rate of false-negative results, polysomnography should be performed in the event of negative results of the other diagnostic techniques. Additional study of audiotaping is necessary. (Evidence for and strength of the recommendation are strong.)
5. Adenotonsillectomy is the first line of treatment for most children. CPAP is an option for those who are not candidates for surgery or do not respond to surgery. (Evidence for and strength of the recommendation are strong.)
6. High-risk patients should be monitored as inpatients postoperatively. (Evidence that these patients are at high risk of postoperative complications is strong. Strength of the recommendation is strong.)
7. Patients should be reevaluated postoperatively to determine whether additional treatment is required. All patients should undergo clinical reevaluation. High-risk patients should undergo objective testing. (Evidence is good, strength of the recommendation is strong.)

RESEARCH RECOMMENDATIONS

Specific research questions have been delineated by an American Thoracic Society workshop.[43] Areas requiring additional investigation include:

1. Accurate prevalence data.
2. Identification of risk factors of complications resulting from OSAS, including the relationship of OSAS severity to specific outcomes.
3. Development and evaluation of low-cost, high-sensitivity, and high-specificity screening methods for OSAS.
4. Delineation of the natural history of treated and untreated PS and OSAS.
5. Assessment of long-term efficacy of adenotonsillectomy, CPAP, and other OSAS treatments.

SUBCOMMITTEE ON OBSTRUCTIVE SLEEP APNEA SYNDROME
Carole L. Marcus, MBBCh, Chairperson
Dale Chapman, MD
Sally Davidson Ward, MD
Susanna A. McColley, MD

LIAISONS
Lee J. Brooks, MD
    American College of Chest Physicians
Jacqueline Jones, MD
    Section on Otolaryngology and
    Bronchoesophagology
Michael S. Schechter, MD, MPH
    Epidemiologist

STAFF
Carla T. Herrerias, MPH

SECTION ON PEDIATRIC PULMONOLOGY, 2001–2002
Paul C. Stillwell, MD, Chairperson
Dale L. Chapman, MD
Sally L. Davidson Ward, MD
Michelle Howenstine, MD
Michael J. Light, MD
Susanna A. McColley, MD
David A. Schaeffer, MD
Jeffrey S. Wagener, MD

STAFF
Laura N. Laskosz, MPH

REFERENCES

1. Schechter MS, and the American Academy of Pediatrics, Section on Pediatric Pulmonology, Subcommittee on Obstructive Sleep Apnea Syndrome. Technical report: diagnosis and management of childhood obstructive sleep apnea syndrome. *Pediatrics*. 2002;109(4). Available at: http://www.pediatrics.org/cgi/content/full/109/4/e69
2. American Thoracic Society. Standards and indications for cardiopulmonary sleep studies in children. *Am J Respir Crit Care Med*. 1996;153: 866–878
3. American Sleep Disorders Association. *International Classification of Sleep Disorders, Revised: Diagnostic and Coding Manual*. Rochester, MN: American Sleep Disorders Association; 1997:195–197

4. Jeans WD, Fernando DC, Maw AR, Leighton BC. A longitudinal study of the growth of the nasopharynx and its contents in normal children. *Br J Radiol.* 1981;54:117–121

5. Ali NJ, Pitson DJ, Stradling JR. Snoring, sleep disturbance, and behaviour in 4–5 year olds. *Arch Dis Child.* 1993;68:360–366

6. Gislason T, Benediktsdottir B. Snoring, apneic episodes, and nocturnal hypoxemia among children 6 months to 6 years old. *Chest.* 1995;107:963–966

7. Redline S, Tishler PV, Schluchter M, Aylor J, Clark K, Graham G. Risk factors for sleep-disordered breathing in children. Associations with obesity, race, and respiratory problems. *Am J Respir Crit Care Med.* 1999;159:1527–1532

8. Teculescu DB, Caillier I, Perrin P, Rebstock E, Rauch A. Snoring in French preschool children. *Pediatr Pulmonol.* 1992;13:239–244

9. Hultcrantz E, Lofstrand-Tidestrom B, Ahlquist-Rastad J. The epidemiology of sleep related breathing disorder in children. *Int J Pediatr Otorhinolaryngol.* 1995;32(suppl):S63–S66

10. Owen GO, Canter RJ, Robinson A. Overnight pulse oximetry in snoring and non-snoring children. *Clin Otolaryngol.* 1995;20:402–406

11. Brouillette RT, Fernbach SK, Hunt CE. Obstructive sleep apnea in infants and children. *J Pediatr.* 1982;100:31–40

12. Marcus CL, Carroll JL, Koerner CB, Hamer A, Lutz J, Loughlin GM. Determinants of growth in children with the obstructive sleep apnea syndrome. *J Pediatr.* 1994;125:556–562

13. Lind M, Lundell B. Tonsillar hyperplasia in children: a cause of obstructive sleep apneas, CO_2 retention, and retarded growth. *Arch Otolaryngol Head Neck Surg.* 1982;108:650–654

14. Bar A, Tarasiuk A, Segev Y, Phillip M, Tal A. The effect of adenotonsillectomy on serum insulin-like growth factor-I and growth in children with obstructive sleep apnea syndrome. *J Pediatr.* 1999;135:76–80

15. Tal A, Leiberman A, Margulis G, Sofer S. Ventricular dysfunction in children with obstructive sleep apnea: radionuclide assessment. *Pediatr Pulmonol.* 1988;4:139–143

16. Guilleminault C, Eldridge FL, Simmons FB, Dement WC. Sleep apnea in eight children. *Pediatrics.* 1976;58:23–30

17. Serratto M, Harris VJ, Carr I. Upper airways obstruction. *Arch Dis Child.* 1981;56:153–155

18. Marcus CL, Greene MG, Carroll JL. Blood pressure in children with obstructive sleep apnea. *Am J Respir Crit Care Med.* 1998;157:1098–1103

19. Ali NJ, Pitson D, Stradling JR. Natural history of snoring and related behaviour problems between the ages of 4 and 7 years. *Arch Dis Child.* 1994;71:74–76

20. Weissbluth M, Davis AT, Poncher J, Reiff J. Signs of airway obstruction during sleep and behavioral, developmental, and academic problems. *J Dev Behav Pediatr.* 1983;4:119–121

21. Chervin RD, Dillon JE, Bassetti C, Ganoczy DA, Pituch KJ. Symptoms of sleep disorders, inattention, and hyperactivity in children. *Sleep.* 1997;20:1185–1192

22. Goldstein NA, Post C, Rosenfeld RM, Campbell TF. Impact of tonsillectomy and adenoidectomy on child behavior. *Arch Otolaryngol Head Neck Surg.* 2000;126:494–498

23. Gozal D. Sleep-disordered breathing and school performance in children. *Pediatrics.* 1998;102:616–620

24. Ross RD, Daniels SR, Loggie JM, Meyer RA, Ballard ET. Sleep apnea-associated hypertension and reversible left ventricular hypertrophy. *J Pediatr.* 1987;111:253–255

25. Kravath RE, Pollak CP, Borowiecki B, Weitzman ED. Obstructive sleep apnea and death associated with surgical correction of velopharyngeal incompetence. *J Pediatr.* 1980;96:645–648

26. Massumi RA, Sarin RK, Pooya M, et al. Tonsillar hypertrophy, airway obstruction, alveolar hypoventilation, and cor pulmonale in twin brothers. *Dis Chest.* 1969;55:110–114

27. Fernbach SK, Brouillette RT, Riggs TW, Hunt CE. Radiologic evaluation of adenoids and tonsils in children with obstructive apnea: plain films and fluoroscopy. *Pediatr Radiol.* 1983;13:258–265

28. Mahboubi S, Marsh RR, Potsic WP, Pasquariello PS. The lateral neck radiograph in adenotonsillar hyperplasia. *Int J Pediatr Otorhinolaryngol.* 1985;10:67–73

29. Laurikainen E, Erkinjuntti M, Alihanka J, Rikalainen H, Suonpaa J. Radiological parameters of the bony nasopharynx and the adenotonsillar size compared with sleep apnea episodes in children. *Int J Pediatr Otorhinolaryngol.* 1987;12:303–310

30. Brooks LJ, Stephens BM, Bacevice AM. Adenoid size is related to severity but not the number of episodes of obstructive apnea in children. *J Pediatr.* 1998;132:682–686

31. Brouillette RT, Hanson D, David R, et al. A diagnostic approach to suspected obstructive sleep apnea in children. *J Pediatr.* 1984;105:10–14

32. Brouillette RT, Morielli A, Leimanis A, Waters KA, Luciano R, Ducharme FM. Nocturnal pulse oximetry as an abbreviated testing modality for pediatric obstructive sleep apnea. *Pediatrics.* 2000;105:405–412

33. Lamm C, Mandeli J, Kattan M. Evaluation of home audiotapes as an abbreviated test for obstructive sleep apnea syndrome (OSAS) in children. *Pediatr Pulmonol.* 1999;27:267–272

34. Carroll JL, McColley SA, Marcus CL, Curtis S, Loughlin GM. Inability of clinical history to distinguish primary snoring from obstructive sleep apnea syndrome in children. *Chest.* 1995;108:610–618

35. Marcus CL, Curtis S, Koerner CB, Joffe A, Serwint JR, Loughlin GM. Evaluation of pulmonary function and polysomnography in obese children and adolescents. *Pediatr Pulmonol.* 1996;21:176–183

36. Mallory GB, Fiser DH, Jackson R. Sleep-associated breathing disorders in morbidly obese children and adolescents. *J Pediatr.* 1989;115:892–897

37. Suen JS, Arnold JE, Brooks LJ. Adenotonsillectomy for treatment of obstructive sleep apnea in children. *Arch Otolaryngol Head Neck Surg.* 1995;121:525–530

38. Nieminen P, Tolonen U, Lopponen H, Lopponen T, Luotonen J, Jokinen K. Snoring children: factors predicting sleep apnea. *Acta Otolaryngol Suppl.* 1997;529:190–194

39. Leach J, Olson J, Hermann J, Manning S. Polysomnographic and clinical findings in children with obstructive sleep apnea. *Arch Otolaryngol Head Neck Surg.* 1992;118:741–744

40. Wang RC, Elkins TP, Keech D, Wauquier A, Hubbard D. Accuracy of clinical evaluation in pediatric obstructive sleep apnea. *Otolaryngol Head Neck Surg.* 1998;118:69–73

41. Goldstein NA, Sculerati N, Walsleben JA, Bhatia N, Friedman DM, Rapoport DM. Clinical diagnosis of pediatric obstructive sleep apnea validated by polysomnography. *Otolaryngol Head Neck Surg.* 1994;111:611–617

42. Goh DY, Galster P, Marcus CL. Sleep architecture and respiratory disturbances in children with obstructive sleep apnea. *Am J Respir Crit Care Med.* 2000;162:682–686

43. American Thoracic Society. Cardiorespiratory sleep studies in children: establishment of normative data and polysomnographic predictors of morbidity. *Am J Respir Crit Care Med.* 1999;160:1381–1387

44. Marcus CL, Omlin KJ, Basinki DJ, et al. Normal polysomnographic values for children and adolescents. *Am Rev Respir Dis.* 1992;146:1235–1239

45. Sivan Y, Kornecki A, Schonfeld T. Screening obstructive sleep apnoea syndrome by home videotape recording in children. *Eur Respir J.* 1996;9:2127–2131

46. Saeed MM, Keens TG, Stabile MW, Bolokowicz J, Davidson WS. Should children with suspected obstructive sleep apnea syndrome and normal nap sleep studies have overnight sleep studies? *Chest.* 2000;118:360–365

47. Marcus CL, Keens TG, Ward SL. Comparison of nap and overnight polysomnography in children. *Pediatr Pulmonol.* 1992;13:16–21

48. Jacob SV, Morielli A, Mograss MA, Ducharme FM, Schloss MD, Brouillette RT. Home testing for pediatric obstructive sleep apnea syndrome secondary to adenotonsillar hypertrophy. *Pediatr Pulmonol.* 1995;20:241–252

49. Zucconi M, Strambi LF, Pestalozza G, Tessitore E, Smirne S. Habitual snoring and obstructive sleep apnea syndrome in children: effects of early tonsil surgery. *Int J Pediatr Otorhinolaryngol.* 1993;26:235–243

50. Nieminen P, Tolonen U, Lopponen H. Snoring and obstructive sleep apnea in children: a 6-month follow-up study. *Arch Otolaryngol Head Neck Surg.* 2000;126:481–486

51. Agren K, Nordlander B, Linder-Aronsson S, Zettergren-Wijk L, Svanborg E. Children with nocturnal upper airway obstruction: postoperative orthodontic and respiratory improvement. *Acta Otolaryngol.* 1998;118:581–587

52. Kudoh F, Sanai A. Effect of tonsillectomy and adenoidectomy on obese children with sleep-associated breathing disorders. *Acta Otolaryngol.* 1996;523(suppl):216–218

53. McColley SA, April MM, Carroll JL, Loughlin GM. Respiratory compromise after adenotonsillectomy in children with obstructive sleep apnea. *Arch Otolaryngol Head Neck Surg.* 1992;118:940–943

54. Rosen GM, Muckle RP, Mahowald MW, Goding GS, Ullevig C. Postoperative respiratory compromise in children with obstructive sleep apnea syndrome: can it be anticipated? *Pediatrics.* 1994;93:784–788

55. Ruboyianes JM, Cruz RM. Pediatric adenotonsillectomy for obstructive sleep apnea. *Ear Nose Throat J.* 1996;75:430–433

56. Rothschild MA, Catalano P, Biller HF. Ambulatory pediatric tonsillectomy and the identification of high-risk subgroups. *Otolaryngol Head Neck Surg.* 1994;110:203–210

57. Wiatrak BJ, Myer CM, Andrews TM. Complications of adenotonsillectomy in children under 3 years of age. *Am J Otolaryngol*. 1991;12:170–172

58. Biavati MJ, Manning SC, Phillips DC. Predictive factors for respiratory complications after tonsillectomy and adenoidectomy in children with OSA. *Arch Otolaryngol Head Neck Surg*. 1997;123:517–521

59. Marcus CL, Ward SL, Mallory GB, et al. Use of nasal continuous positive airway pressure as treatment of childhood obstructive sleep apnea. *J Pediatr*. 1995;127:88–94

60. Waters KA, Everett FM, Bruderer JW, Sullivan CE. Obstructive sleep apnea: the use of nasal CPAP in 80 children. *Am J Respir Crit Care Med*. 1995;152:780–785

61. Guilleminault C, Pelayo R, Clerk A, Leger D, Bocian RC. Home nasal continuous positive airway pressure in infants with sleep-disordered breathing. *J Pediatr*. 1995;127:905–912

62. Rains JC. Treatment of obstructive sleep apnea in pediatric patients. *Clin Pediatr (Phila)*. 1995;34:535–541

63. Marcus CL, Carroll JL, Bamford O, Pyzik P, Loughlin GM. Supplemental oxygen during sleep in children with sleep-disordered breathing. *Am J Respir Crit Care Med*. 1995;152:1297–1301

Technical Report Summary:
Diagnosis and Management of Childhood
Obstructive Sleep Apnea Syndrome

Authors:

Michael S. Schechter, MD, MPH,
and the Section on Pediatric Pulmonology,
Subcommittee on Obstructive Sleep Apnea Syndrome

American Academy of Pediatrics
PO Box 927, 141 Northwest Point Blvd
Elk Grove Village, IL 60009-0927

For the complete technical report, including tables, figures, and references, please see the companion CD-ROM.

ABSTRACT

Objective

This technical report describes the procedures involved in developing the recommendations of the Subcommittee on Obstructive Sleep Apnea Syndrome in children. The group of primary interest for this report was otherwise healthy children older than 1 year who might have adenotonsillar hypertrophy or obesity as underlying risk factors of obstructive sleep apnea syndrome (OSAS). The goals of the committee were to enhance the primary care clinician's ability to recognize OSAS, identify the most appropriate procedure for diagnosis of OSAS, identify risks associated with pediatric OSAS, and evaluate management options for OSAS.

Methods

A literature search was initially conducted for the years 1966–1999 and then updated to include 2000. The search was limited to English language literature concerning children older than 2 and younger than 18 years. Titles and abstracts were reviewed for relevance, and committee members reviewed in detail any possibly appropriate articles to determine eligibility for inclusion. Additional articles were obtained by a review of literature and committee members' files. Committee members compiled evidence tables and met to review and discuss the literature that was collected.

Results

A total of 2115 titles were reviewed, of which 113 provided relevant original data for analysis. These articles were mainly case series and cross-sectional studies; overall, very few methodologically strong cohort studies or randomized, controlled trials concerning OSAS have been published. In addition, a minority of studies satisfactorily differentiated primary snoring from true OSAS. Reports of the prevalence of habitual snoring in children ranged from 3.2% to 12.1%, and estimates of OSAS ranged from 0.7% to 10.3%; these studies were too heterogeneous for data pooling. Children with sleepdisordered breathing are at increased risk for hyperactivity and learning problems. The combined odds ratio for neurobehavioral abnormalities in snoring children compared with controls is 2.93 (95% confidence interval: 2.23 – 3.83). A number of case series have documented decreased somatic growth in children with OSAS; right ventricular dysfunction and systemic hypertension also have been reported in children with OSAS. However, the risk growth and cardiovascular problems cannot be quantified from the published literature. Overnight polysomnography (PSG) is recognized as the gold standard for diagnosis of OSAS, and there are currently no satisfactory alternatives. The diagnostic accuracy of symptom questionnaires and other purely clinical approaches is low. Pulse oximetry appears to be specific but insensitive. Other methods, including audiotaping or videotaping and nap or home overnight PSG, remain investigational. Adenotonsillectomy is curative in 75% to 100% of children with OSAS, including those who are obese. Up to 27% of children undergoing adenotonsillectomy for OSAS have postoperative respiratory complications, but estimates are varied. Risk factors for persistent OSAS after adenotonsillectomy include continued snoring and a high apnea-hypopnea index on the preoperative PSG.

Conclusions

OSAS is common in children and is associated with significant sequelae. Overnight PSG is currently the only reliable diagnostic modality that can differentiate OSAS from primary snoring. However, the PSG criteria for OSAS have not been definitively validated, and it is not clear that primary snoring without PSG-defined OSAS is benign. Adenotonsillectomy is the first-line treatment for OSAS but requires careful postoperative monitoring because of the high risk of respiratory complications. Adenotonsillectomy is usually curative, but children with persistent snoring (and perhaps with severely abnormal preoperative PSG results) should have PSG repeated postoperatively.

INTRODUCTION

This technical report describes in detail the procedures involved in developing recommendations as given in the accompanying practice guideline on obstructive sleep apnea syndrome (OSAS). A description of the process, methods of data compilation and analysis, and summaries of the conclusions of the committee will be given.

FORMULATION AND ARTICULATION OF THE QUESTION ADDRESSED BY THE COMMITTEE

Target Audience

The practice guideline is primarily aimed at office-based pediatricians and other primary care clinicians who treat children (family physicians, nurse practitioners, physician assistants). The secondary audience for the guideline includes pediatric pulmonologists, neurologists, otolaryngologists, and developmental/behavioral pediatricians.

Definitions

The primary focus of the committee was on OSAS in childhood. The committee agreed to use the definition provided in a statement from the American Thoracic Society with some additional elaboration of associated symptoms:

OSAS in children is a disorder of breathing during sleep characterized by prolonged partial upper airway obstruction and/or intermittent complete obstruction (obstructive apnea) that disrupts normal ventilation during sleep and normal sleep patterns. It is associated with symptoms including habitual (nightly) snoring, sleep difficulties, and/or daytime neurobehavioral problems. Complications may include growth abnormalities, neurologic disorders, and cor pulmonale, especially in severe cases. Various risk factors have been identified and are defined.

The committee sought to focus on otherwise healthy children who might have adenotonsillar hypertrophy or obesity as underlying risk factors and to specifically exclude infants younger than 1 year, children with central hypoventilation syndromes, and children at risk because of underlying abnormalities, such as craniofacial disorders; Down syndrome; cerebral palsy; neuromuscular disorders; chronic lung disease; sickle cell disease; genetic, metabolic, and storage diseases; and laryngomalacia.

Goals of the Committee

The committee sought to address several specific goals and questions:

1. *To enhance the primary care clinician's ability to recognize OSAS.* The committee believed that a certain amount of consciousness raising would be appropriate to alert the clinician to suspect the presence of OSAS. Thus, a catalog of associated signs and symptoms is provided in the accompanying practice guideline but will not be addressed in this technical report.
2. *To identify the most appropriate procedure for diagnosis of OSAS.* Approaches evaluated by the committee included history and physical examination, questionnaires, audiotaping or videotaping, nocturnal pulse oximetry, nap polysomnography (PSG), and ambulatory PSG, all of which would be compared with the gold standard, comprehensive overnight PSG, as defined by the American Thoracic Society. In view of the fact that overnight PSG is not readily available to children in all geographic areas, consideration was given to alternative diagnostic approaches even if their accuracy is suboptimal.
3. *To identify risks associated with pediatric OSAS.* In adults, OSAS is associated with excessive daytime sleepiness (leading to cognitive defects and increased mortality attributable to susceptibility to motor vehicle crashes), pulmonary hypertension, and systemic hypertension. The committee wished to evaluate the strength of pediatric data in this area.
4. *To evaluate management options for OSAS.* The committee sought to find data relating to adenotonsillectomy and alternative treatment modalities in the management of OSAS. The committee set out to evaluate the risk of complications after adenotonsillectomy in children with OSAS, especially given the fact that patients not suspected to have OSAS might undergo adenotonsillectomy for other indications. The postoperative complication of particular concern was respiratory compromise. Other complications of surgery, such as bleeding and pain, were not specifically addressed in relation to OSAS. In addition, data on postoperative recurrence and persistence of OSAS was sought.

METHODS

Literature Search

A literature search of the National Library of Medicine's PubMed database (http://www.ncbi.nlm.nih.gov/entrez/query. fcgi?db_PubMed) for the years 1966–1999 was conducted in August 1999 by staff at the American Academy of Pediatrics. The search was limited to English language literature concerning children older than 2 and younger than 18 years. The following search terms were used: sleep apnea syndrome; apnea; sleep disorders; snoring; polysomnography; airway obstruction; adenoidectomy; tonsillectomy (adverse effects, mortality); and sleep-disordered breathing.mp. This search was updated in November 2000 before preparation of this technical report.

Article Review

Titles and abstracts (when available) of articles found by the literature search were reviewed by committee members, and all those considered to be possibly relevant were marked for detailed review. Recent review articles were included to compare their bibliographies with the result of the automated literature search. Articles deemed possibly relevant were then printed and distributed to committee members for more detailed review. A literature review form was developed for this project to standardize this part of the process. Because there was a large number of articles requiring evaluation, some committee members recruited residents and fellows to assist in the performance of these reviews under their supervision. Although it became clear at this point that the number of articles that could be considered high quality by conventional epidemiologic standards was small, a low threshold was used to allow inclusion of any possibly relevant articles into the next level of review. At this point, articles were compiled and divided by the committee chair, additional articles were obtained by a review of literature, committee members' files were added, and committee members were assigned specific topics (as discussed previously in "Goals of the Committee") for detailed review and compilation of evidence tables. The findings of committee members were then presented at a follow-up meeting of the entire committee. A final review and compilation into evidence tables was performed by the lead author of this technical report (M.S.S.).

Calculation of prevalence, diagnostic test characteristics, and odds ratios were performed independently of the authors' reports, using data provided in the original articles. In 2 cases, authors were contacted for clarification of data. Where applicable, odds ratios from different studies were combined, using Mantel-Haenszel weights in stratified tables. Tests for heterogeneity are reported. All statistical calculations were performed using Stata 5.0 software (Stata Corporation, College Station, TX).

RESULTS

The literature search identified 2067 articles for initial review. Titles and abstracts (when available) of these articles were divided among the 7 committee members for perusal as an initial screening, and of those, 278 (16.2%) were retained for more detailed scrutiny. An additional 48 relevant publications were found outside this initial review. Articles were read in full if they appeared to have any relevance to childhood OSAS; included in this group were 70 general reviews and case reports or descriptive case series, which were used to allow committee members to gain a general sense of the literature and access their bibliographies. Among various committee members, the percentage of articles chosen for more detailed review ranged from 12.7% to 23.4%. This variability was statistically significant ($P = .007$ by Pearson χ^2). Excluding the methodologist, whose approach was the most permissive (23.4% acceptance rate), the range was 12.7% to 19.4%, and variability was not statistically significant ($P = .143$ by Pearson χ^2) among remaining committee members.

A total of 113 articles were found that contained original data relevant to the specific aims of this committee. Most of the publications that were reviewed in detail provided little quantitative data for analysis. In particular, most papers that were older than 5 years presented case series or poor-quality cohort studies or omitted important details. These lower-quality studies provide the background for current expert opinion but are otherwise of limited value and will not be listed in detail for this report. Studies that were of quantitative value are tabulated and were given quality ratings in the tables. Briefly, rating levels of studies on treatment efficacy were assigned as follows:

Level I—Randomized trials with low rates of false-positive (α) and/or false-negative (β) results (high power).

Level II—Randomized trials with high rates of false-positive (α) and/or false-negative (β) results (low power).

Level III—Nonrandomized concurrent cohort comparisons between contemporaneous patients who did and did not receive an intervention, or casecontrol or crosssectional studies with appropriate control group.

Level IV—Nonrandomized historical cohort comparisons between current patients who received an intervention and former patients (from the same institution or from the literature) who did not, or casecontrol or crosssectional studies for which control groups were suboptimally chosen.

Level V—Case series without controls.

Rating levels for diagnostic tests were assigned as follows:

Level 1—Independent blind comparison of patients from an appropriate spectrum of patients, all of whom have undergone both the diagnostic test and the reference standard.

Level 2—Independent blind or objective comparison performed in a set of nonconsecutive patients or confined to a narrow spectrum of study individuals (or both), all of whom have undergone both the diagnostic test and the reference standard.

Level 3—Independent blind or objective comparison of an appropriate spectrum of patients, but the reference standard was not applied to all.

Level 4—Reference standard was unobjective, unblinded, or not independent; positive and negative tests were verified using separate reference standards; or study was performed in an inappropriate spectrum of patients.

Prevalence of Snoring and OSAS
We found 7 studies that attempted to establish prevalence of snoring in childhood. These studies came from a variety of European countries, and all ascertained data via parent questionnaire. The prevalence of snoring in these studies ranged from 3.2% to 12.1%, which was significantly heterogeneous ($P < .0001$). The study by Gislason and Benediktsdottir seemed to be somewhat of an outlier, especially because the frequency of OSAS they reported was nearly the same as that of snoring, but with omission of that study, the heterogeneity remains significant ($P < .001$).

Three studies reported on prevalence of OSAS, and estimates ranged from 0.7% to 10.3%. All used very different criteria, including 1 that gave estimates based on 2 different criteria. The variability of these estimates was so great that no attempt was made to combine the data.

Sequelae of OSAS
Most published articles on complications of OSAS are reports of retrospective case series or prospectively collected, uncontrolled data comparing measures before and after surgical treatment. These articles are summarized in this report and in evidence tables.

Cognitive and Behavioral Abnormalities
The committee found 12 publications that evaluated the association of behavioral problems, especially hyperactivity or attention-deficit/hyperactivity disorder (ADHD), with sleep-disordered breathing. In an early case series of 50 children with OSAS documented by PSG, 84% had excessive daytime sleepiness, 76% had some behavior disturbance, 42% were hyperactive, and 16% had decreased school performance. A number of crosssectional studies have been done that compare the risk of behavioral problems in children who snore with that of a control population. None of these studies distinguish children with OSAS from those with primary snoring (PS). For the study of Weissbluth et al, parents of children attending a general pediatric practice were surveyed, and 71 children were reported to have behavioral or academic problems. Snoring, mouth breathing, and labored breathing when asleep were reported to be more than twice as common in these children as in the comparison group. The study of Chervin et al reported that 33% of children with ADHD were habitual snorers, compared with 11% of children attending a general psychiatric clinic and 9% attending a general pediatric clinic. A previously mentioned prevalence study by Ali et al found that children who were reported to snore during most nights were also reported to have more daytime sleepiness and hyperactivity than were children in a comparison group. Children were evaluated using Conners scales, and those with more severe sleep disturbance were also more likely to be at the 95th percentile on Conners subscales relating to hyperactive, inattentive, and aggressive behaviors. In a follow-up report, 29 of 60 children reported to snore 2 years previously no longer snored (weighted κ 0.52), although habitual snoring was again found to be associated with daytime sleepiness and hyperactivity. In another publication, the same authors identified 12 children with sleep-disordered breathing (by overnight pulse oximetry and videotaping), 11 snoring children without sleep-disordered breathing, and a control group not undergoing adenotonsillectomy and administered Conners scales, the Continuous Performance Test (a test of attention), and the Matching Familiar Figures Test (a test of vigilance). Significant improvement was found in Conners parent scale scores for aggressive, inattentive, and hyperactive behaviors; attention; and vigilance in the sleep-disordered breathing group after adenotonsillectomy, and similar

changes were found in the primary snorers postoperatively, but not in control groups. In a recent population-based cross-sectional study of 988 Portuguese children, Ferreira et al found that habitual snorers were twice as likely as nonsnorers to have an abnormal score on the Children's Behavioral Questionnaire. Finally, Blunden et al compared 16 children referred for adenotonsillectomy or snoring with a control group and found impaired selective and sustained attention scores only in the children who snored. They also reported that the snoring children had significantly lower average IQ scores. PSG was done in these children, but for purposes of analysis, the PS and OSAS groups were combined because preliminary analyses revealed no significant group differences on any neurocognitive or behavioral parameter (all $P > .05$). The authors pointed out that even patients with OSAS had very mild abnormalities (mean respiratory disturbance index [RDI] <1). Although it is possible that lack of power and selection bias may have contributed to their findings, the implication is that snoring without overt OSAS might be associated with neurocognitive abnormalities.

Although the 6 cross-sectional studies described previously all reported on slightly different behavioral and cognitive phenomena, their findings were pooled, and the results of this are shown. The Mantel-Haenszel test for heterogeneity was not significant ($P=.4577$). The combined odds ratio for neurobehavioral abnormalities in snoring children is 2.93 (95% confidence interval [CI], 2.23–3.83).

Several other papers are of interest but cannot be quantitatively combined. Goldstein et al had parents of 36 children who were referred for adenotonsillectomy because of clinically significant obstructive symptoms complete the Child Behavior Checklist and found that 10 (28%) had abnormal results. Postoperatively, 15 had a repeat evaluation, and only 2 (13%) still had abnormal results. This finding was not clinically significant, presumably because of lack of statistical power, but there was a clinically significant improvement in mean test scores postoperatively ($P < .001$).

Four studies used overnight PSG testing to establish a diagnosis of OSAS. Rosen reported on a series of 326 children referred for evaluation of snoring, of whom 59% met PSG criteria for OSAS. Daily tiredness was reported in 19%; excessive daytime sleepiness was reported in 10%; and behavior, school, or mood problems were reported in 9%, with no difference between the OSAS and non-OSAS groups. Gozal conducted an interesting study in which 297 first graders who were in the lowest 10th percentile academically were evaluated for sleepdisordered breathing by parent questionnaire combined with overnight (home) oximetry. Adenotonsillectomy was recommended in the 54 children (18.1%) with abnormal test results; 24 accepted surgery, and 30 did not. Mean grades increased from 2.43 ± 0.17 to 2.87 ± 0.19 in the children who had surgery, with no change in the untreated OSAS group or the non-OSAS group ($P < .001$).

The findings of an Australian study contrasted with the aforementioned papers. Thirty-nine children with PSG evidence of OSAS were followed 6 months after the initial PSG, and 24 had received adenotonsillectomy. These were compared with children who were waiting for intervention ($n = 5$; median apnea-hypopnea index [AHI]

= 5.5) or didn't require intervention ($n = 10$; median AHI = 3.1). Information on AHI was not given for the surgical group. At follow-up, children in the surgical and nonsurgical groups had improved sleep behavior. Intervention did not result in any statistically significant improvement in development or temperament, although the study was probably underpowered.

In summary, studies generally show a nearly threefold increase in behavior and neurocognitive abnormalities in children with sleep-disordered breathing. Most of these studies did not definitively differentiate children with PS from those with OSAS, so the true prevalence of behavior and learning problems in children with OSAS versus PS is not clear. It is possible, however, that PS, even in the absence of clear-cut OSAS, might place children at risk.

Growth

Four studies evaluating growth and OSAS were found. Marcus et al evaluated 14 prepubertal children with a mean age of 4 years ± 1 standard deviation who had OSAS documented by overnight PSG and measured caloric intake and sleeping energy expenditure as well as anthropomorphic measurements before and after adenotonsillectomy. Average sleeping energy expenditure decreased, and mean weight z score increased postoperatively without any change in caloric intake. Bar et al evaluated changes in growth and also measured insulin-like growth factor (IGF)-I and IGF-binding protein-3 levels before and 18 months after adenotonsillectomy. Both studies showed statistically significant increases in weight but not height; IGF-I levels increased and IGF-binding protein levels did not. An interesting report on the effect of adenotonsillectomy on growth included a group of obese and morbidly obese children and documented postoperative increases in weight and height, even in those children who were initially obese. The other 2 studies, which had poorer documentation of OSAS, reported similar results. None of these studies reported a comparison with a nonsurgical control group, comparison with children operated on for indications other than OSAS, or comparison with children who had PS.

Cardiovascular

Eight case reports or small series were found that documented cor pulmonale or hypertension, which reversed with adenotonsillectomy or other surgical correction in patients with clinically diagnosed OSAS. Two case series reported children with adenotonsillar hypertrophy with or without clinical airway obstruction who were found to have right ventricular dysfunction that reversed after adenotonsillectomy. One study described pulsus paradoxus and leftward shift of the interventricular septum secondary to snoring in 3 of 6 children with OSAS. This correlated with negative esophageal pressures but not with oxygen desaturation, and it reversed with nasal continuous positive airway pressure (CPAP). Tal et al used radionuclide ventriculography to evaluate ventricular function in 27 children referred for oropharyngeal obstruction who had abnormal Brouillette questionnaire scores for OSAS; PSG was not performed. They found decreased right ventricular ejection fraction in 37% of these children and abnormal wall motion in 67%. All of the 11 patients who had a repeat evaluation after adenotonsillectomy showed improvement. Systemic blood pressure was evaluated in a study of children referred for PSG. Higher diastolic pressures (adjusted for body mass index and age) were found in children with OSAS, compared with those with PS. The prevalence of blood pressure measurements >95th percentile was high in both groups (32% vs 19%, respectively), with a nonsignificant difference that may have been attributable to low power. The response after adenotonsillectomy was not reported. This was the only study that compared cardiovascular complications in children with OSAS versus those with PS.

Miscellaneous

One study reported on 115 enuretic children undergoing adenotonsillectomy for any indication. There was a 66% reduction in enuretic nights 1 month after surgery and a 77% decrease 6 months after surgery. In the group with secondary enuresis, 100% were dry 6 months after surgery.

Diagnosis of OSAS

Polysomnography

One of the problems in evaluating various methods of diagnosing OSAS in children is that the gold standard, overnight PSG, has not been well standardized in its performance or interpretation. Although recent consensus statements pertaining to standards and normative data should lessen this problem, the question of definition remains problematic. Pediatric sleep specialists use the adult model in describing a continuum of sleep-disordered breathing from PS to upper airway resistance syndrome to obstructive hypoventilation and OSAS. It is assumed that PS is a benign condition and OSAS is associated with undesirable complications. Normative standards for their polysomnographic determination have been chosen on the basis of statistical distribution of data, but it has not been established that those standards have any validity as predictors of the occurrence of complications. In other words:

"On the basis of normative data, an obstructive apnea index of 1 is often chosen as the cutoff for normality. However, while an apnea index of 1 is statistically significant (ie, at the 97.5th percentile for an asymptomatic, normative population), it is not known what level is clinically significant."

Of the few studies that compare children with polysomnographically defined OSAS with those with PS in regard to prevalence of complications, only 1 found a clear difference between the 2 groups. This is an important point, because with a poorly validated gold standard, statements regarding diagnostic accuracy of alternative methods of diagnosis become dubious. Finally, the test-retest reliability of overnight PSG, which in adults is no greater than 91% and possibly somewhat lower, has never been evaluated in children.

Having stated these points, additional analysis of the validity of alternative diagnostic approaches will be done assuming PSG as the gold standard. One additional benefit of overnight PSG is that in addition to establishing the diagnosis of OSAS, PSG also may be used to determine its severity. It has been suggested that the severity of OSAS is an important predictor of complications, particularly in the immediate postoperative period. None of the alternative diagnostic techniques discussed below have been evaluated for this purpose.

Questionnaires

In 1984, Brouillette et al reported high accuracy for a diagnostic questionnaire for OSAS in children with adenotonsillar hypertrophy. This questionnaire was initially tested on 23 children with OSAS and 46 controls. On the basis of this questionnaire, a 3-variable discriminant function was calculated as follows:

$$\text{OSAS score} = 1.42D + 1.41A + 0.71S - 3.83$$

where D is difficulty during sleep, A is apnea observed during sleep, and S is snoring. Values assigned to D and S were: 0 = never; 1 = occasionally; 2 = frequently; and 3 = always. Values assigned to A were: 0 = no; and 1 = yes. This system was then applied to a prospective group of 23 patients referred for evaluation of possible OSAS. The authors demonstrated that a score of >3.5 perfectly predicted the presence of OSAS by PSG; a score of <−1 perfectly predicted absence of OSAS; and a score in between was indeterminate. Unfortunately, there were 5 children who were believed to have a borderline PSG, confusing the issue somewhat. It appears that the choices of 3.5 and −1 as breakpoints in the score were made posthoc and were, thus, somewhat arbitrary. Since the initial publication of the questionnaire, 3 additional studies have been published detailing the results of its use. All of these studies prospectively evaluated similar groups of pediatric patients with a similar prevalence of OSAS; PSG with similar evaluation criteria was performed on all subjects, and all completed the same questionnaire applied in similar ways. This scoring system is sufficiently simple and straightforward, so its application can be expected to be fairly standard and replicable. Thus, data from these studies was combined, and conclusions were drawn accordingly.

The OSAS questionnaire by Brouillette et al performed much less well in subsequent applications. The 4 studies (including a later study by the same authors) included a total of 765 patients with an overall prevalence of OSAS confirmed by PSG of 60%. Applied to these patients, the score was indeterminate in 47%; in subjects who were categorized (ie, not indeterminate), its positive predictive value (PPV) was 65% and negative predictive value (NPV) was 46%. Using the pooled data for calculation, the likelihood ratio of positive questionnaire results is 1.24, and the likelihood ratio of negative questionnaire results is 0.78. Overall, the use of the questionnaire by Brouillette et al as a substitute for PSG would clearly be fraught with error, leading to numerous false-positive and falsenegative results in the diagnosis of OSAS.

Other publications reporting attempts at creating questionnaires or developing other purely clinical criteria to substitute for PSG are uninterpretable because of their failure to compare their criteria with PSG50–53 or unsuccessful in developing any reliable predictive criteria.

Audiotaping and Videotaping

Two studies have evaluated the use of home audiotaping, and 1 evaluated home videotaping, as a screening test for OSAS. The methods used to evaluate these techniques were different, so the data do not lend themselves to pooling. Sivan et al scored a 30-minute videotape in 58 children using 7 variables, including loudness and type of inspiratory noise, movements during sleep, number of waking episodes, number of apneas, chest retractions, and mouth breathing. The PSG results were abnormal in 62%. They reported a sensitivity of 94%, specificity of 68%, PPV of 83%, and NPV of 88%. Posthoc analysis (similar to what was done in the 1984 study by Brouillette et al) was performed in 2 ways, leading to the development of an indeterminate score and better test characteristics in the categorizable group. As might be expected, a scoring system that places a greater number of subjects into the indeterminate group leads to better NPV and PPV.

Goldstein et al developed a 7-item predictive score that considered the presence of snoring, respiratory pauses, gasping, sleeping with neck extended, daytime sleepiness, adenoid facies, and the presence of pauses in breathing of at least 5 seconds on an audiotape recorded by the parents. The criteria used to score each category were not precisely described, and there seemed to be significant variability in the evaluation of the audiotapes, which were reviewed for "at least 2 minutes…for each child, and an average of 10 minutes were generally reviewed. Various parts of the tape were sampled." Patients were categorized as definitely, possibly, or not likely having OSAS on the basis of these items, but no description was provided of how these items were scored and combined, and no measure of interobserver vari- ability was attempted, so reproducibility is unknown. A total of 30 children were studied prospectively, of whom 13 (43%) had OSAS confirmed by PSG. The authors reported a sensitivity of 92.3%, specificity of 29.4%, PPV of 50.0%, and NPV of 83.3%, which they calculated by combining the "definite" and "possible" groups into a positive screening category. If their possible group was eliminated from consideration (analogous to the way Brouillette et al treated indeterminate scores), a mild decrease in sensitivity (91%) and mild increases in specificity (38%) and PPV (56%) are seen.

Goldstein et al concluded that children whose results of evaluation for sleep apnea (as performed using their technique, including audiotaping) are negative do not need PSG, because the sensitivity of their clinical assessment is high. They recommended PSG for children who appear to have OSAS, because the specificity of clinical assessment is low. It is important to note that the percentage of positive results of PSG in their study (43%) was somewhat lower than the prevalence of approximately 60% reported in most studies of children referred for evaluation of possible OSAS. This is probably (at least in part) because they used more restrictive PSG criteria for diagnosing OSAS (AHI >15). If a population with a higher prevalence of OSAS were studied, it is likely that the PPV of the clinical evaluation by Goldstein et al would be higher and the NPV would be lower. In addition, the higher AHI as a diagnostic criterion might have biased the study toward the more severe end of the OSAS spectrum. The possibil-

ity of spectrum bias and the undocumented reproducibility of the tape evaluation raise the question of whether test characteristics will be as good if applied to a large, general population.

A second study of the use of home audiotaping as an abbreviated test for OSAS used 7 observers to analyze audiotapes of 29 children referred for evaluation; 48% were subsequently found to have positive PSG. Observers listened to 15 minutes of audiotape and specifically scored the presence of struggle sounds and respiratory pauses. A mean κ statistic of 0.70 (range, 0.50–0.93) was calculated, indicating moderately good interobserver agreement. The presence of a struggle sound on the audiotape gave the best posthoc test characteristics, with a sensitivity of 0.71, specificity of 80%, NPV of 73%, and PPV of 75%.

To summarize, the use of home audiotaping and videotaping has been inadequately investigated. Additional studies are necessary. It should be pointed out that there was no consensus of the committee regarding acceptable rates of false-negative and false-positive results for tests used as an alternative to PSG.

Pulse Oximetry

Seven studies were found that reported on pulse oximetry in children suspected of having OSAS. However, only 1 compared pulse oximetry to PSG. In this study involving 349 children, pulse oximetry was performed during PSG and was evaluated independently of the PSG interpretation, with well-defined criteria and excellent interobserver agreement. There were 89 PSGs (25.5%) performed in a sleep lab; the others were done at home, so the gold standard was not identical for all subjects. In this group, with a 60.2% prevalence of OSAS, the PPV was 97% (90 of 93). However, the NPV of the test (calculated by the authors by combining subjects with either inconclusive or negative tests) was only 53%. When the analysis was limited to subjects without any medical diagnoses other than adenotonsillar hypertrophy, the PPV was 100%, with an insubstantial change in NPV.

Given the test characteristic described, it appears that overnight pulse oximetry could provide an accurate screen for OSAS, insofar as a positive result may be a good predictor of an abnormal PSG result. However, the findings of the single study described in this report need to be replicated.

Nap Polysomnography

Two papers from the same institution have evaluated the utility of brief (1 hour) daytime nap studies in comparison with full overnight PSGs. The conclusions of both are generalizable to only a limited degree, however. Marcus et al studied 40 children referred for evaluation of possible OSAS, but this group was not representative of the type of patient addressed by this practice guideline, because only 35% had adenotonsillar hypertrophy as the underlying cause of their sleep disturbances. Other diagnoses included Down syndrome (40% of subjects), various upper airway abnormalities, and other neurologic and respiratory problems. Furthermore, 95% (38 of 40) of the patients studied had abnormal overnight PSG results, providing little opportunity to evaluate the test performance of nap studies in children with normal PSG results. The study by Saeed et al limited itself to children addressed by this practice guideline (age, 1–18 years; adenotonsillar hypertrophy; absence of other significant disease). They reported on the results of overnight PSG in children with normal and mildly abnormal nap study results. Patients with severely abnormal nap study results were excluded; they were assumed to have significant OSAS and, therefore, referred directly for tonsillectomy without overnight PSG (S.D. Ward, personal communication). In this group, for which prevalence of PSG-documented OSAS was 66%, the nap studies had a PPV of 77% and NPV of 49%. In fact, if children with more severely abnormal nap study results were included in the analysis and the investigators are correct in their assumption that these children all have abnormal overnight PSG results, then the sensitivity and PPV of nap studies is actually higher than that reported in this paper. Thus, it is possible that abnormal nap study results might provide a predictive value adequate to allow the recommendation for surgery without corroborative overnight PSG, but confirmation of this conclusion (asserted by the authors) is lacking. On the other hand, a nap study with negative results would still require a follow-up overnight PSG for confirmation.

Home Polysomnography

One group has published data comparing the results of PSG performed in children at home with those performed at the sleep laboratory. In a report of 21 children between the ages of 2 and 12 years who were studied in both environments, the sensitivity and specificity of home PSG varied depending on the severity of OSA. When an AHI >1 was used as the criterion for diagnosing OSAS, the sensitivity of home PSG was 100% and the specificity was 62%; for AHI >3, sensitivity was 88% and specificity was 77%; for AHI >5, sensitivity and specificity were both 100%. This group uses a sophisticated type of ambulatory PSG that is not commercially available and is not analogous to commercial systems. Also, their system did not allow for detection of obstructive hypoventilation. Furthermore, the subjects used in their report were not chosen sequentially or at random, and the authors describe a complex process for specifically selecting children for inclusion in the study. Nonetheless, the comparability of the results of home and sleep laboratory overnight PSG appears good; additional study using commercially available equipment in a more representative population would be helpful.

Treatment of OSAS

Tonsillectomy and/or Adenoidectomy

There are many published papers, primarily case reports and case series, that support the efficacy of tonsillectomy with or without adenoidectomy as treatment for OSAS. Most of these studies use relief of snoring and other clinical symptoms as their endpoint. Others cite improvement in growth, behavior, cardiovascular complications, or enuresis after surgery. Several papers suggest that adenotonsillectomy is effective treatment of OSAS even in children who are morbidly obese. Many of these studies are anecdotal and methodologically uninterpretable.

Frank et al were the first to use PSG to analyze the effect of surgery on OSAS in children. Of an initial group of 32 children referred for suspected OSAS, they reported on 7 who had PSG before and after adenotonsillectomy. These children had an average of 194 obstructive apneas per night preoperatively and 7 postoperatively (P < .025). They provide no breakdown of individual cure rate. Zucconi et al, using nocturnal or nap PSG, reported a 100% cure rate of OSAS in 29 children receiving adenotonsillectomy or adenoidectomy and monotonsillectomy and a 0% cure rate in 5 children receiving only adenoidectomy. Two more recent studies were methodologically superior regarding diagnosis of OSAS. Suen et al reported on 69 children referred for evaluation of possible OSAS; 35 (51%) had a RDI >5 and were referred for adenotonsillectomy, and 30 had the procedure. Follow-up PSG was performed in 26; all showed improvement, although 4 (15%) still had an RDI >5. All children with persistently high RDIs continued to snore, although 3 children with RDIs that had normalized continued to snore. Thus, adenotonsillectomy resulted in a cure rate of 85%, and the absence of postoperative snoring was associated with no treatment failures (NPV of postoperative snoring = 100%), whereas 57% of children who still snored continued to have abnormal PSG results (PPV = 57%). The authors of that paper emphasized that a high preoperative RDI was a strong predictor of abnormal postoperative RDI and suggested 19.1 as a cutoff. However, their data shows that the PPV of preoperative RDI ≥19.1 for a postoperative RDI >5 was 43% and the NPV was 95%, neither of which are as high as the predictive values afforded by the presence of persistent snoring postoperatively. The findings of Nieminen were similar, although their criteria for positive PSG results were slightly different (AHI >1). They reported a 95% cure rate for a group of 21 children after adenotonsillectomy or tonsillectomy; 1 of 5 children who continued to snore had postoperative PSG results that remained abnormal (PPV = 20%), and none of the children who stopped snoring had abnormal PSG results (NPV = 100%). The authors pointed out that 73% of this group had previously had their adenoids removed, implying confirmation of the lack of efficacy of adenoidectomy alone for relief of OSAS. This paper also mentioned in passing that 2 children with abnormal results of PSG did not have surgery; in 1, the follow-up PSG results were unchanged, and in the other, the results had normalized. Although no generalizations can be made on the basis of these data, it represents the only published report of follow-up PSG in children with OSAS who were not treated.

Several other papers reported PSG results in association with adenotonsillectomy, but these reports were somewhat less clearly written. Wiet et al reported a series of 48 patients in whom sleep studies were performed because of unclear history or physical findings, or complicated OSA. An AHI >5 was considered abnormal. Thirteen patients had no complicating medical factors, and of the 35 remaining, 20 were morbidly obese. All 13 uncomplicated patients had adenotonsillectomy. They had a significant decrease in mean AHI (from 23 to 6 [P < .01]); it was not stated whether any had residual abnormal postoperative PSG results. Of the obese patients, 12 of 20 had adenotonsillectomy alone, and the rest had uvulopharyngopalatoplasty in addition. It was not specified how the decision to perform uvulopharyngopalatoplasty was made, and the report of results for this group was not broken down by surgical procedure. Mean AHI in the obese group decreased from 33 to 4 ($P < .001$). Agren et al reported on a group of 20 children with "unequivocal anamnestic nocturnal obstructive breathing." The preoperative AHI was >5 in 10 children, and the apnea index (AI) was >1 in 17. Five of these patients had an adenoidectomy in the past. The terminology used in that paper was confusing, and it was not entirely clear whether AI meant apnea index or apnea-hypopnea index. Postoperatively, no AHI (or AI) was reported; it was stated that 5 patients still had some partial obstruction postoperatively, but all had a normal oxygen desaturation index (which had been abnormal in 13 preoperatively). Shintani et al described 134 children referred for snoring and clinical sleep apnea; 74 had a preoperative AHI >10, but for the rest of the group, the AHI was unspecified. Of this group, 114 had adenotonsillectomy, 13 had adenoidectomy, 4 had adenoidectomy with monotonsillectomy, and 3 had tonsillectomy alone, all presumably at the discretion of the surgeon. Using the authors' criterion for improvement of a postoperative decrease in AHI by 50%, 84.5% of children who had adenoidectomy and 75.4% of those who had adenotonsillectomy were improved postoperatively (difference between adenotonsillectomy and adenoidectomy, $P = .732$). In contrast to the findings of Suen et al, the preoperative AHI in this report did not predict the likelihood of treatment failure.

To summarize these studies, all of which were case series that were reported with variable rigor, it appears that adenotonsillectomy is curative in 75% to 100% of children, even if obese. The role of adenoidectomy alone is unclear. Postoperatively, children should be retested for OSAS if they continue to snore and possibly if the preoperative AHI was high.

Postoperative Complications and the
Need for Inpatient Monitoring
A number of publications have catalogued postoperative complications of adenotonsillectomy in large series of patients, but these will not be discussed further here. An additional large group of papers have described the risk of complications associated with outpatient adenotonsillectomy in the general population; these case series have generally excluded children with upper airway obstruction from consideration and also will not be discussed further. However, several papers provide data pertaining to complications of surgery in children undergoing adenotonsillectomy for upper airway obstruction, all specifically addressing the risk of postoperative respiratory obstruction. These authors define respiratory compromise in various ways but generally consider the need for supplemental oxygen as a minimum criterion. The papers report a wide range for the rate of postoperative respiratory complications (0%–27%), primarily because their populations include different proportions of children with neuromuscular, chromosomal, and craniofacial disorders. This variation makes the study groups too heterogeneous

for pooling of the data, and their inclusion of complex patients makes them less valid in estimating the risk of postoperative respiratory compromise in the population being addressed by this practice guideline. Young age (younger than 3 years) and associated medical problems were found in most papers to define the highest risk groups. High preoperative RDI also seems to be a risk factor for postoperative complications. Time to onset of respiratory compromise appears to be brief, although McColley et al reported that 1 patient took 14 hours to manifest respiratory symptoms.

All in all, children with OSAS clearly seem to be at high risk of postoperative respiratory compromise, and increased vigilance in postoperative monitoring is warranted.

Nasal CPAP
Several papers report on the successful use of CPAP in childhood. In children, CPAP is usually used when adenotonsillectomy is unsuccessful or contraindicated rather than as a primary treatment. Thus, most cases in the above reports describe children with complicated OSAS who are not the target group for this practice guideline. For example, of 80 children reported by Waters et al, 70 had previous adenotonsillar surgery; the 10 who did not were younger than 6 months or had other significant medical conditions. Of 94 patients reported by Marcus et al, only 2 of 18 patients whose OSAS was idiopathic (ie, not associated with another predisposing cause) had not had previous adenotonsillectomy; 1 of these patients had cystic fibrosis. All of the patients described by Guilleminault et al (1995) were younger than 1 year. All of the patients described by Rains et al and by Guilleminault et al (1986) had underlying predisposing abnormalities. All of the subjects described by Tirosh et al had previous adenotonsillectomy. These studies do confirm, however, that CPAP is efficacious in children.

CONCLUSIONS

Prevalence of Childhood OSAS
Snoring is a common occurrence in childhood, with reported prevalence between 3.2% and 12.1%. The prevalence of childhood OSAS is difficult to estimate, largely because published studies use different PSG criteria for its ascertainment. Reports range from 0.7% to 10.3%.

Sequelae of Childhood OSAS
Childhood OSAS is associated with several important sequelae and complications for which prevalence is unclear because of a lack of population-based cohort studies.

Neurobehavioral Complications
Cross-sectional studies suggest a nearly threefold increase in behavior problems and neurocognitive abnormalities in children with sleep-disordered breathing. Most of these studies did not definitively differentiate children with PS from those with OSAS, so the true prevalence of behavior and learning problems in children with OSAS versus PS is not clear.

Growth Inhibition

No systematic studies exist, but case series suggest that growth (especially weight gain) accelerates after surgery for OSAS, even in children with preexisting obesity, so it appears that OSAS has an inhibitory effect on growth. One study suggests that this effect is attributable to increased metabolic expenditures associated with OSAS.

Cardiovascular Complications

Cor pulmonale, right ventricular dysfunction, and pulmonary hypertension all have been reported in case reports and series, but their prevalence is unknown. These appear to be reversible after adenotonsillectomy. Systemic hypertension is a known complication of adult OSAS, and elevated diastolic blood pressure has been found in children with OSAS.

Diagnosis of OSAS

Overnight Polysomnography

The gold standard for diagnosis of OSAS is overnight PSG performed in a sleep lab. Methodologic standards and population-based normal ranges have recently been published, so although older published studies reflect a problem of variability in methods and interpretation, this has diminished in recent years. However, current normative standards for PSG determination of OSAS have been chosen on the basis of statistical distribution of data, and it has not been established that those standards have any validity as predictors of the occurrence of complications. Nonetheless, at the very least, it appears that the severity of PSG abnormality is an important predictor of complications in the immediate postoperative period after adenotonsillectomy.

Alternatives to PSG

Clinical evaluation, including the use of questionnaires such as the one published by Brouillette et al, has unacceptably low sensitivity and specificity for predicting OSAS. The use of home audiotaping and videotaping to supplement the clinical evaluation has been inadequately investigated. Additional studies are necessary before any statements about their validity can be made. Pulse oximetry and nap PSG appear to have high specificity and low sensitivity, meaning that positive test results are probably true, but negative test results would need to be confirmed using overnight PSG. The comparability of the results of home and sleep laboratory overnight PSG appears good, but additional study using commercially available equipment in a representative population is necessary for confirmation.

Treatment of OSAS

On the basis of case series that were reported with variable rigor, it appears that adenotonsillectomy is curative in 75% to 100% of children, even if the children are obese. The role of adenoidectomy alone is unclear. Postoperatively, children should be retested for OSAS if they continue to snore and possibly if the preoperative AHI was high. Children with OSAS clearly seem to be at high risk of postoperative respiratory compromise, and increased vigilance in postoperative monitoring is warranted, particularly in those with a high preoperative RDI. CPAP is effective in children, but it is usually used when adenotonsillectomy is delayed, contraindicated, or unsuccessful rather than as a primary treatment.

The Diagnosis, Treatment, and Evaluation of the Initial Urinary Tract Infection in Febrile Infants and Young Children

- *Clinical Practice Guideline*
- *Technical Report Summary*

Readers of this clinical practice guideline are urged to review the technical report to enhance the evidence-based decision-making process. The full technical report is available on the enclosed CD-ROM.

AMERICAN ACADEMY OF PEDIATRICS

Committee on Quality Improvement

Subcommittee on Urinary Tract Infection

Practice Parameter: The Diagnosis, Treatment, and Evaluation of the Initial Urinary Tract Infection in Febrile Infants and Young Children

ABSTRACT. *Objective.* To formulate recommendations for health care professionals about the diagnosis, treatment, and evaluation of an initial urinary tract infection (UTI) in febrile infants and young children (ages 2 months to 2 years).

Design. Comprehensive search and analysis of the medical literature, supplemented with consensus opinion of Subcommittee members.

Participants. The American Academy of Pediatrics (AAP) Committee on Quality Improvement selected a Subcommittee composed of pediatricians with expertise in the fields of epidemiology and informatics, infectious diseases, nephrology, pediatric practice, radiology, and urology to draft the parameter. The Subcommittee, the AAP Committee on Quality Improvement, a review panel of office-based practitioners, and other groups within and outside the AAP reviewed and revised the parameter.

Methods. The Subcommittee identified the population at highest risk of incurring renal damage from UTI—infants and young children with UTI and fever. A comprehensive bibliography on UTI in infants and young children was compiled. Literature was abstracted in a formal manner, and evidence tables were constructed. Decision analysis and cost-effectiveness analyses were performed to assess various strategies for diagnosis, treatment, and evaluation.

Technical Report. The overall problem of managing UTI in children between 2 months and 2 years of age was conceptualized as an evidence model. The model depicts the relationship between the steps in diagnosis and management of UTI. The steps are divided into the following four phases: 1) recognizing the child at risk for UTI, 2)

The recommendations in this statement do not indicate an exclusive course of treatment or serve as a standard of medical care. Variations, taking into account individual circumstances, may be appropriate.

"Practice Parameter: The Diagnosis, Treatment, and Evaluation of the Initial Urinary Tract Infection in Febrile Infants and Young Children" was reviewed by the appropriate committees and sections of the American Academy of Pediatrics (AAP), including the Committee on Infectious Diseases, the Committee on Medical Liability, and the Committee on Practice and Ambulatory Medicine; the Sections on Infectious Diseases, Nephrology, Radiology, and Urology; and the Chapter Review Group, a focus group of office-based pediatricians representing each AAP District: Gene R. Adams, MD; Charles S. Ball, MD; Robert M. Corwin, MD; Diane Fuquay, MD; Barbara M. Harley, MD; Michael J. Heimerl, MD; Thomas J. Herr, MD; Kenneth E. Matthews, MD; Robert D. Mines, MD; Lawrence C. Pakula, MD; Howard B. Weinblatt, MD; and Delosa A. Young, MD. The COQI and Subcommittee on UTI greatly appreciate the expertise of Richard N. Shiffman, MD, Center for Medical Informatics, Yale School of Medicine, for his input and analysis in the development of this practice guideline.

Comments also were solicited and received from the American Academy of Family Physicians, the American College of Emergency Physicians, and the American Urological Association.

PEDIATRICS (ISSN 0031 4005). Copyright © 1999 by the American Academy of Pediatrics.

making the diagnosis of UTI, 3) short-term treatment of UTI, and 4) evaluation of the child with UTI for possible urinary tract abnormality.

Phase 1 represents the recognition of the child at risk for UTI. Age and other clinical features define a prevalence or a prior probability of UTI, determining whether the diagnosis should be pursued.

Phase 2 depicts the diagnosis of UTI. Alternative diagnostic strategies may be characterized by their cost, sensitivity, and specificity. The result of testing is the division of patients into groups according to a relatively higher or lower probability of having a UTI. The probability of UTI in each of these groups depends not only on the sensitivity and specificity of the test, but also on the prior probability of the UTI among the children being tested. In this way, the usefulness of a diagnostic test depends on the prior probability of UTI established in Phase 1.

Phase 3 represents the short-term treatment of UTI. Alternatives for treatment of UTI may be compared, based on their likelihood of clearing the initial UTI.

Phase 4 depicts the imaging evaluation of infants with the diagnosis of UTI to identify those with urinary tract abnormalities such as vesicoureteral reflux (VUR). Children with VUR are believed to be at risk for ongoing renal damage with subsequent infections, resulting in hypertension and renal failure. Prophylactic antibiotic therapy or surgical procedures such as ureteral reimplantation may prevent progressive renal damage. Therefore, identifying urinary abnormalities may offer the benefit of preventing hypertension and renal failure.

Because the consequences of detection and early management of UTI are affected by subsequent evaluation and long-term management and, likewise, long-term management of patients with UTI depends on how they are detected at the outset, the Subcommittee elected to analyze the entire process from detection of UTI to the evaluation for, and consequences of, urinary tract abnormalities. The full analysis of these data can be found in the technical report. History of the literature review along with evidence-tables and a comprehensive bibliography also are available in the report. This report is published in *Pediatrics electronic pages* and can be accessed at the following URL: http://www.pediatrics.org/cgi/content/full/103/4/e54.

Results. Eleven recommendations are proposed for the diagnosis, management, and follow-up evaluation of infants and young children with unexplained fever who are later found to have a diagnosed UTI. Infants and young children are of particular concern because UTI in this age group (approximately 5%) may cause few recognizable signs or symptoms other than fever and has a higher potential for renal damage than in older children. Strategies for diagnosis and treatment depend on the clinician's assessment of the illness in the infant or young child. Diagnosis is based on the culture of a properly collected specimen of urine; urinalysis can only suggest the diagnosis. A sonogram should be performed on all infants and young children with fever and their first documented UTI; voiding cystourethrography or radionuclide cystography should be strongly considered.

ABBREVIATIONS. UTI, urinary tract infections; SPA, suprapubic aspiration; VUR, vesicoureteral reflux; WBC, white blood cell; TMP–SMX, trimethoprim–sulfamethoxazole; VCUG, voiding cystourethrography; RNC, radionuclide cystography.

The urinary tract is a relatively common site of infection in infants and young children. Urinary tract infections (UTIs) are important because they cause acute morbidity and may result in long-term medical problems, including hypertension and reduced renal function. Management of children with UTI involves repeated patient visits, use of antimicrobials, exposure to radiation, and cost. Accurate diagnosis is extremely important for two reasons: to permit identification, treatment, and evaluation of the children who are at risk for kidney damage and to avoid unnecessary treatment and evaluation of children who are not at risk, for whom interventions are costly and potentially harmful but provide no benefit. Infants and young children with UTI are of particular concern because the risk of renal damage is greatest in this age group and because the diagnosis is frequently challenging: the clinical presentation tends to be nonspecific and valid urine specimens cannot be obtained without invasive methods (suprapubic aspiration [SPA], transurethral catheterization).

Considerable variation in the methods of diagnosis, treatment, and evaluation of children with UTI was documented more than 2 decades ago.[1] Since then, various changes have been proposed to aid in diagnosis, treatment, and evaluation, but no data are available to suggest that such innovations have resulted in reduced variation in practice. This practice parameter focuses on the diagnosis, treatment, and evaluation of febrile infants and young children (2 months to 2 years of age). Excluded are those with obvious neurologic or anatomic abnormalities known to be associated with recurrent UTI and renal damage. Neonates and infants younger than 2 months have been excluded from consideration in this practice parameter. Children older than 2 years experiencing their first UTI also are excluded because they are more likely than younger children to have symptoms referable to the urinary tract, are less likely to have factors predisposing them to renal damage, and are at lower risk of developing renal damage.

This parameter is intended for use by clinicians who treat infants and young children in a variety of clinical settings (eg, office, emergency department, hospital).

METHODS

A comprehensive literature review was conducted to provide data for evidence tables that could be used to generate a decision tree. More than 2000 titles were identified from MEDLINE and bibliographies of current review articles from 1966 to 1996, and the authors' files. Of these, 402 articles contained relevant original data that were abstracted in a formal, standardized manner. An evidence-based model was developed using quantitative outcomes derived from the literature and cost data from the University of North Carolina. Decision analysis was used to perform risk analyses and cost-effectiveness analyses of alternative strategies for the diagnosis, management, and evaluation of UTI, using hypertension and end-stage renal disease as the undesirable outcomes. The calculated probability of undesirable outcome is the product of the probabilities of several steps (diagnosis, treatment, evaluation) and therefore is an estimate, influenced by approximations at each step. Cost-effectiveness of various strategies was assessed using the methods of Rice and associates[2] in which the break-even cost to prevent a chronic condition, such as hypertension or end-stage renal disease, is considered to be $700 000, an amount based on the estimated lifetime productivity of a healthy, young adult. Once this cost is assigned to the untoward clinical outcome (ie, hypertension or end-stage renal disease), it is possible to use the threshold method of decision-making.[3] The threshold approach to decision-making involves changing the value of a variable in the decision analysis to determine the value at which one strategy of diagnosis, treatment, and evaluation exceeds the break-even cost and an alternative strategy is preferred. Based on the results of these analyses and consensus, when necessary, an Algorithm was developed representing the strategies with the greatest benefit–risk characteristics. The strength of evidence on which recommendations were based was rated by the Subcommittee methodologist as strong, good, fair, or opinion/consensus. A detailed description of the methods by which the parameter was derived is available in a technical report from the American Academy of Pediatrics.

DIAGNOSIS

Recommendation 1

The presence of UTI should be considered in infants and young children 2 months to 2 years of age with unexplained fever (strength of evidence: strong).

The prevalence of UTI in infants and young children 2 months to 2 years of age who have no fever source evident from history or physical examination is high, ~5%.[4-8] The genders are not affected equally, however. The prevalence of UTI in febrile girls age 2 months to 2 years is more than twice that in boys (relative risk, 2.27). The prevalence of UTI in girls younger than 1 year of age is 6.5%; in boys, it is 3.3%. The prevalence of UTI in girls between 1 and 2 years of age is 8.1%; in boys it is 1.9%. The rate in circumcised boys is low, 0.2% to 0.4%.[9-13] The literature suggests that the rate in uncircumcised boys is 5 to 20 times higher than in circumcised boys.

Infants and young children are at higher risk than are older children for incurring acute renal injury with UTI. The incidence of vesicoureteral reflux (VUR) is higher in this age group than in older children (Fig 1), and the severity of VUR is greater, with the most severe form (with intrarenal reflux or pyelotubular backflow) virtually limited to infants.

Infants and young children with UTI warrant special attention because of the opportunity to prevent kidney damage. First, the UTI may bring to attention a child with an obstructive anomaly or severe VUR. Second, because infants and young children with UTI may have a febrile illness and no localizing findings, there may be a delay in diagnosis and treatment of the UTI. Clinical and experimental data support the concept that delay in instituting appro-

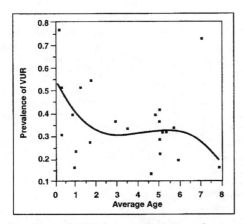

Fig 1. Prevalence of VUR by age. Plotted are the prevalences reported in 54 studies of urinary tract infections in children (references in Technical Report). The studies are weighted by sample size. The line is a third order polynomial fit to the data.

priate treatment of acute pyelonephritis increases the risk of kidney damage.[14,15] Third, the risk of renal damage increases as the number of recurrences increases[16] (Fig 2).

The presence of fever has long been considered a finding of special importance in infants and young children with UTI, because it has been accepted as a clinical marker of renal parenchymal involvement (pyelonephritis). The concept that otherwise unexplained fever in a child with UTI indicates that renal parenchymal involvement is based on comparison of children with high fever (39°C) and the clinical diagnosis of acute pyelonephritis with those with no fever (38°C) and a clinical diagnosis of cystitis.[17] Indirect tests for localization of the site of UTI, such as the presence of a reversible defect in renal concentrating ability and high levels of antibody titer to the infecting strains of *Escherichia coli*, and nonspecific tests of inflammation, such as elevated white blood cell (WBC) count, C-reactive protein, or sedimentation rate, are encountered more frequently in children with clinical pyelonephritis than in those with clinical cystitis. However, the indirect tests for localization of the site of infection and the nonspecific indicators of inflammation do not provide confirmatory evidence that the febrile infant or young child

with UTI has pyelonephritis. Cortical imaging studies using technetium 99 m Tc-dimercaptosuccinic acid (DMSA) or 99 m Tc-glucoheptonate may prove useful in determining whether the presence of high fever does identify children with pyelonephritis and distinguish them from those with cystitis; currently available studies with data that can be used to assess fever as a marker of pyelonephritis (defined by a positive scan) provide a wide range of sensitivity (53% to 84%) and specificity (44% to 92%).[18-20]

The likelihood that UTI is the cause of the fever may be increased if there is a history of crying on urination or of foul-smelling urine. An altered voiding pattern may be recognized as a symptom of UTI as early as the second year after birth in some children. Dysuria, urgency, frequency, or hesitancy may be present but are difficult to discern in this age group. Nonspecific signs and symptoms, such as irritability, vomiting, diarrhea, and failure to thrive, also may reflect the presence of UTI, but data are not available to assess the sensitivity, specificity, and predictive value of these clinical manifestations.

Decision analysis and cost-effectiveness analyses were performed, considering the different prevalences for age, gender, and circumcision status, and the prevalence of VUR by age. For girls and uncircumcised boys, it is cost-effective to pursue the diagnosis of UTI by invasive means and to perform imaging studies of the urinary tract. For circumcised boys younger than 1 year, the cost–benefit analysis is equivocal, but the Subcommittee supports the same diagnostic and evaluation measures as for girls and uncircumcised boys. Circumcised boys older than 1 year have a lower prevalence of UTI, and the prevalence of reflux is lower than that in those younger than 1 year. As a result, the cost-effectiveness analysis does not support invasive diagnostic procedures for all circumcised boys older than 1 year with unexplained fever. Analysis of a bag-collected specimen is a reasonable screening test in these boys, as long as they do not appear so ill as to warrant the initiation of antimicrobial therapy. Those who will be given antimicrobials on clinical grounds should have a specimen obtained for culture that is unlikely to be contaminated.

Recommendation 2

In infants and young children 2 months to 2 years of age with unexplained fever, the degree of toxicity, dehydration, and ability to retain oral intake must be carefully assessed (strength of evidence: strong).

In addition to seeking an explanation for fever, such as a source of infection, clinicians make a subjective assessment of the degree of illness or toxicity. Attempts have been made to objectify this assessment, using the prediction of bacteremia or serious bacterial infection as the outcome measure.[21] This clinical assessment, operationalized as whether antimicrobial therapy will be initiated, affects the diagnostic and therapeutic process regarding UTI as follows. If the clinician determines that the degree of illness warrants antimicrobial therapy, a valid urine

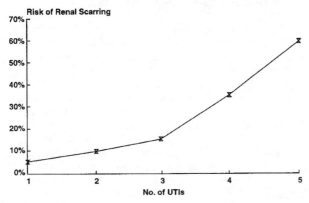

Fig 2. Relationship between renal scarring and number of urinary tract infections.[16]

specimen should be obtained before antimicrobials are administered, because the antimicrobials commonly prescribed in such situations will be effective against the usual urinary pathogens; invasive means are required to obtain such a specimen. If the clinician determines that the degree of illness does not require antimicrobial therapy, a urine culture is not essential immediately. In this situation, some clinicians may choose to obtain a specimen by noninvasive means (eg, in a collection bag attached to the perineum). The false-positive rate with such specimens dictates that before diagnosing UTI, all positive results be confirmed with culture of a urine specimen unlikely to be contaminated (see below).

Recommendation 3

If an infant or young child 2 months to 2 years of age with unexplained fever is assessed as being sufficiently ill to warrant immediate antimicrobial therapy, a urine specimen should be obtained by SPA or transurethral bladder catheterization; the diagnosis of UTI cannot be established by a culture of urine collected in a bag (strength of evidence: good).

Urine obtained by SPA or transurethral catheterization is unlikely to be contaminated and therefore is the preferred specimen for documenting UTI. In a clinical setting in which the physician has determined that immediate antimicrobial therapy is appropriate, the use of a bag-collected urine specimen is insufficient to document the presence of UTI.

Establishing a diagnosis of UTI requires a strategy that minimizes false-negative and false-positive results. Urine obtained by SPA is the least likely to be contaminated; urine obtained by transurethral bladder catheterization is next best. Either SPA or transurethral bladder catheterization should be used to establish the diagnosis of UTI. Cultures of urine specimens collected in a bag applied to the perineum have an unacceptably high false-positive rate; the combination of a 5% prevalence of UTI and a high rate of false-positive results (specificity, ~70%) results in a positive culture of urine collected in a bag to be a *false*-positive result 85% of the time. If antimicrobial therapy is initiated before obtaining a specimen of urine for culture that is unlikely to be contaminated, the opportunity may be lost to confirm the presence or establish the absence of UTI. Therefore, in the situation in which antimicrobial therapy will be initiated, SPA or catheterization is required to establish the diagnosis of UTI.

SPA has been considered the "gold standard" for obtaining urine for detecting bacteria in bladder urine accurately. The technique has limited risks. However, variable success rates for obtaining urine have been reported (23% to 90%),[16,22-24] technical expertise and experience are required, and many parents and physicians perceive the procedure as unacceptably invasive compared with catheterization. There may be no acceptable alternative in the boy with moderate or severe phimosis, however.

Urine obtained by transurethral catheterization of the urinary bladder for urine culture has a sensitivity of 95% and a specificity of 99% compared with that obtained by SPA.[23,25] Catheterization requires some skill and experience to obtain uncontaminated specimens, particularly in small infants, girls, and uncircumcised boys. Early studies in adults provided widely varying estimates of risk of introducing infection by a single, in–out catheterization. Turck and colleagues[26] demonstrated that the rate of bacteriuria secondary to transurethral catheterization in healthy young adults was considerably lower than that in hospitalized, older adults. Of the 200 healthy young adults studied, 100 men and 100 women, bacteriuria ultimately developed in only 1 woman—2 weeks after catheterization; bacteriuria was documented not to be present during the first 1 to 2 weeks after her catheterization. The risk of introducing infection in infants by transurethral catheterization has not been determined precisely, but it is the consensus of the Subcommittee that the risk is sufficiently low to recommend the procedure when UTI is suspected.

The techniques required for transurethral bladder catheterization and SPA are well described.[27] When SPA or transurethral catheterization is being attempted, the clinician should have a sterile container ready to collect a urine specimen voided because of the stimulus of the patient by manipulation in preparation for or during the procedure.

Recommendation 4

If an infant or young child 2 months to 2 years of age with unexplained fever is assessed as not being so ill as to require immediate antimicrobial therapy, there are two options (strength of evidence: good).

Option 1

Obtain and culture a urine specimen collected by SPA or transurethral bladder catheterization.

Option 2

Obtain a urine specimen by the most convenient means and perform a urinalysis. If the urinalysis suggests a UTI, obtain and culture a urine specimen collected by SPA or transurethral bladder catheterization; if urinalysis does not suggest a UTI, it is reasonable to follow the clinical course without initiating antimicrobial therapy, recognizing that a negative urinalysis does not rule out a UTI.

The option with the highest sensitivity is to obtain and culture a urine specimen collected by SPA or transurethral bladder catheterization; however, this approach may be resisted by some families and clinicians. In infants and young children assessed as *not* being so ill as to require immediate antimicrobial therapy, a urinalysis may help distinguish those with higher and lower likelihood of UTI. The urinalysis can be performed on any specimen, including one collected from a bag applied to the perineum, and has the advantage of convenience. The major disadvantage of collecting a specimen in a bag is that it is unsuitable for quantitative culture. In addition, there may be a delay of 1 hour or longer for the infant or young child to void; then, if the urinalysis suggests

UTI, a second specimen is required. The sensitivity of the bag method for detecting UTI is essentially 100%, but the false-positive rate of this method is also high, as demonstrated in several studies.[23,25,28] If the prevalence of UTI is 5%, 85% of positive cultures will be false-positive results; if the prevalence of UTI is 2% (febrile boys), the rate of false-positive results is 93%; if the prevalence of UTI is 0.2% (circumcised boys), the rate of false-positive results is 99%. The use of bag-collected urine specimens persists because collection of urine by this method is noninvasive and requires limited personnel time and expertise. Moreover, a negative (sterile) culture of a bag-collected urine specimen effectively eliminates the diagnosis of UTI, provided that the child is not receiving antimicrobials and that the urine is not contaminated with an antibacterial skin cleansing agent. Based on their experience, many clinicians believe that this collection technique has a low contamination rate under the following circumstances: the patient's perineum is properly cleansed and rinsed before application of the collection bag; the urine bag is removed promptly after urine is voided into the bag; and the specimen is refrigerated or processed immediately. Nevertheless, even if contamination from the perineal skin is minimized, there may be significant contamination from the vagina in girls or the prepuce in uncircumcised boys. Published results demonstrate that although a negative culture of a bag-collected specimen effectively rules out UTI, a positive culture does not document UTI. Confirmation requires culture of a specimen collected by transurethral bladder catheterization or SPA. Transurethral catheterization does not eliminate completely the possibility of contamination in girls and uncircumcised boys.

Of the components of urinalysis, the three most useful in the evaluation of possible UTI are leukocyte esterase test, nitrite test, and microscopy. A positive result on a leukocyte esterase test seems to be as sensitive as the identification of WBCs microscopically, but the sensitivity of either test is so low that the risk of missing UTI by either test alone is unacceptably high (Table 1). The nitrite test has a very high specificity and positive predictive value when urine specimens are processed promptly after collection. Using either a positive leukocyte esterase or nitrite test improves sensitivity at the expense of specificity; that is, there are many false-positive results. The wide range of reported test characteristics for microscopy indicates the difficulty in ensuring quality performance; the best results are achieved with skilled technicians processing fresh urine specimens.

The urinalysis cannot substitute for a urine culture to document the presence of UTI, but the urinalysis can be valuable in selecting individuals for prompt initiation of treatment while waiting for the results of the urine culture. Any of the following are suggestive (although not diagnostic) of UTI: positive result of a leukocyte esterase or nitrite test, more than 5 white blood cells per high-power field of a properly spun specimen, or bacteria present on an unspun Gram-stained specimen.

In circumcised boys, whose low a priori rate of UTI (0.2% to 0.4%) does not routinely justify an invasive, potentially traumatic procedure, a normal urinalysis reduces the likelihood of UTI as the cause of the fever still further, to the order of 0.1%.

Recommendation 5

Diagnosis of UTI requires a culture of the urine (strength of evidence: strong).

All urine specimens should be processed as expediently as possible. If the specimen is not processed promptly, it should be refrigerated to prevent the growth of organisms that can occur in urine at room temperature. For the same reason, specimens requiring transportation to another site for processing should be transported on ice.

The standard test for the diagnosis of UTI is a quantitative urine culture; no element of the urinalysis or combination of elements is as sensitive and specific. A properly collected urine specimen should be inoculated on culture media that will allow identification of urinary tract pathogens.

UTI is confirmed or excluded based on the number of colony-forming units that grow on the culture media. Defining significant colony counts with regard to the method of collection considers that the distal urethra is commonly colonized by the same bacteria that may cause UTI; thus, a low colony count may be present in a specimen obtained by voiding or by transurethral catheterization when bacteria are not present in bladder urine. As noted in Table 2, what constitutes a significant colony count depends on the collection method and the clinical status of the patient; definitions of positive and negative cultures are operational and not absolute. Significance also depends on the identification of the isolated organism as a pathogen. Organisms such as *Lactobacillus* species, coagulase-negative staphylococci, and *Corynebacterium* species are not considered clinically relevant urine isolates in the otherwise healthy 2-month to 2-year-old. Alternative culture methods such as the dipslide may have a place in the office setting; sensitivity is reported in the range of 87% to 100%, and specificity, 92% to 98%.

TREATMENT

Recommendation 6

If the infant or young child 2 months to 2 years of age with suspected UTI is assessed as toxic, dehydrated, or unable to retain oral intake, initial anti-

TABLE 1. Sensitivity and Specificity of Components of the Urinalysis, Alone and in Combination (References in Text)

Test	Sensitivity % (Range)	Specificity % (Range)
Leukocyte esterase	83 (67–94)	78 (64–92)
Nitrite	53 (15–82)	98 (90–100)
Leukocyte esterase *or* nitrite positive	93 (90–100)	72 (58–91)
Microscopy: WBCs	73 (32–100)	81 (45–98)
Microscopy: bacteria	81 (16–99)	83 (11–100)
Leukocyte esterase *or* nitrite *or* microscopy positive	99.8 (99–100)	70 (60–92)

TABLE 2.   Criteria for the Diagnosis of UTI[53]

Method of Collection	Colony Count (Pure Culture)	Probability of Infection (%)
SPA	Gram-negative bacilli: any number Gram-positive cocci: more than a few thousand	>99%
Transurethral catheterization	>10^5 10^4–10^5 10^3–10^4 <10^3	95%; Infection likely suspicious; repeat infection unlikely
Clean void		
Boy	>10^4	Infection likely
Girl	3 Specimens 10^5 2 Specimens 10^5 1 Specimen 10^5 5 × 10^4 – 10^5 10^4 – 5 × 10^4 <10^4	95% 90% 80% Suspicious, repeat Symptomatic: suspicious, repeat Asymptomatic: infection unlikely infection unlikely

microbial therapy should be administered parenterally and hospitalization should be considered (strength of evidence: opinion/consensus).

The goals of treatment of acute UTI are to eliminate the acute infection, to prevent urosepsis, and to reduce the likelihood of renal damage. Patients who are toxic-appearing, dehydrated, or unable to retain oral intake (including medications) should receive an antimicrobial parenterally (Table 3) until they are improved clinically and are able to retain oral fluids and medications. The parenteral route is recommended because it ensures optimal antimicrobial levels in these high-risk patients. Parenteral administration of an antimicrobial also should be considered when compliance with obtaining and/or administering an antimicrobial orally cannot be ensured. In patients with compromised renal function, the use of potentially nephrotoxic antimicrobials (eg, aminoglycosides) requires caution, and serum creatinine and peak and trough antimicrobial concentrations need to be monitored. The clinical conditions of most patients improve within 24 to 48 hours; the route of antimicrobial administration then can be changed to oral (Table 4) to complete a 7- to 14-day course of therapy.

Hospitalization is necessary if patients have clinical urosepsis or are considered likely to have bacteremia based on clinical or laboratory evaluation. These patients need careful monitoring and repeated clinical examinations.

For children who do not appear toxic but who are vomiting, or when noncompliance is a concern, options include beginning therapy in the hospital or administering an antimicrobial parenterally on an outpatient basis. The route of administration is changed to oral when the child is no longer vomiting, and compliance appears to be ensured.

Recommendation 7

In the infant or young child 2 months to 2 years of age who may not appear ill but who has a culture confirming the presence of UTI, antimicrobial therapy should be initiated, parenterally or orally (strength of evidence: good).

The usual choices for treatment of UTI orally include amoxicillin, a sulfonamide-containing antimicrobial (sulfisoxazole or trimethoprim–sulfamethoxazole [TMP–SMX]), or a cephalosporin (Table 4). Emerging resistance of *E coli* to ampicillin appears to have rendered ampicillin and amoxicillin less effective than alternative agents. Studies comparing amoxicillin with TMP–SMX have demonstrated consistently higher cure rates with TMP–SMX (4% to 42%), regardless of the duration of therapy (1 dose, 3 to 4 days, or 10 days).[29–45]

Agents that are excreted in the urine but do not achieve therapeutic concentrations in the bloodstream, such as nalidixic acid or nitrofurantoin, should not be used to treat UTI in febrile infants and young children in whom renal involvement is likely.

Recommendation 8

Infants and young children 2 months to 2 years of age with UTI who have not had the expected clinical response with 2 days of antimicrobial therapy

TABLE 3.   Some Antimicrobials for Parenteral Treatment of UTI

Antimicrobial	Daily Dosage
Ceftriaxone	75 mg/kg every 24 h
Cefotaxime	150 mg/kg/d divided every 6 h
Ceftazidime	150 mg/kg/d divided every 6 h
Cefazolin	50 mg/kg/d divided every 8 h
Gentamicin	7.5 mg/kg/d divided every 8 h
Tobramycin	5 mg/kg/d divided every 8 h
Ticarcillin	300 mg/kg/d divided every 6 h
Ampicillin	100 mg/kg/d divided every 6 h

TABLE 4.   Some Antimicrobials for Oral Treatment of UTI

Antimicrobial	Dosage
Amoxicillin	20–40 mg/kg/d in 3 doses
Sulfonamide	
TMP in combination with SMX	6–12 mg TMP, 30–60 mg SMX per kg per d in 2 doses
Sulfisoxazole	120–150 mg/kg/d in 4 doses
Cephalosporin	
Cefixime	8 mg/kg/d in 2 doses
Cefpodixime	10 mg/kg/d in 2 doses
Cefprozil	30 mg/kg/d in 2 doses
Cephalexin	50–100 mg/kg/d in 4 doses
Loracarbef	15–30 mg/kg/d in 2 doses

should be reevaluated and another urine specimen should be cultured (strength of evidence: good).

Routine reculturing of the urine after 2 days of antimicrobial therapy is generally not necessary if the infant or young child has had the expected clinical response and the uropathogen is determined to be sensitive to the antimicrobial being administered. Antimicrobial sensitivity testing is determined most commonly by the application of disks containing the usual serum concentration of the antimicrobial to the culture plate. Because many antimicrobial agents are excreted in the urine in extremely high concentrations, an intermediately sensitive organism may be fully eradicated. Studies of minimal inhibitory concentration may be required to clarify the appropriateness of a given antimicrobial. If the sensitivity of the organism to the chosen antimicrobial is determined to be intermediate or resistant, or if sensitivity testing is not performed, a "proof-of-bacteriologic cure" culture should be performed after 48 hours of treatment. Data are not available to determine that clinical response alone ensures bacteriologic cure.

Recommendation 9

Infants and young children 2 months to 2 years of age, including those whose treatment initially was administered parenterally, should complete a 7- to 14-day antimicrobial course orally (strength of evidence: strong).

In 8 of 10 comparisons of long treatment duration (7 to 10 days) and short duration (1 dose or up to 3 days), results were better with long duration, with an attributable improvement in outcome of 5% to 21%.[33,38,41,44–48] Most uncomplicated UTIs are eliminated with a 7- to 10-day antimicrobial course, but many experts prefer 14 days for ill-appearing children with clinical evidence of pyelonephritis. Data comparing 10 days and 14 days are not available.

Recommendation 10

After a 7- to 14-day course of antimicrobial therapy and sterilization of the urine, infants and young children 2 months to 2 years of age with UTI should receive antimicrobials in therapeutic or prophylactic dosages until the imaging studies are completed (strength of evidence: good).

Although this practice parameter deals with the acute UTI, it is important to recognize the significance of recurrent infections. The association between recurrent bouts of febrile UTI and renal scarring follows an exponential curve[16] (Fig 2). Because the risk of recurrence is highest during the first months after UTI, children treated for UTI should continue antimicrobial treatment or prophylaxis (Table 5) until the imaging studies are completed and assessed. Additional treatment is based on the imaging findings assuming sterilization of the urine.

EVALUATION: IMAGING

Recommendation 11

Infants and young children 2 months to 2 years of age with UTI who do not demonstrate the expected clinical response within 2 days of antimicrobial therapy should undergo ultrasonography promptly. Voiding cystourethrography (VCUG) or radionuclide cystography (RNC) is strongly encouraged to be performed at the earliest convenient time. Infants and young children who have the expected response to antimicrobials should have a sonogram performed at the earliest convenient time; a VCUG or RUC is strongly encouraged (strength of evidence: fair).

UTI in young children serve as a marker for abnormalities of the urinary tract. Imaging of the urinary tract is recommended in every febrile infant or young child with a first UTI to identify those with abnormalities that predispose to renal damage. Imaging should consist of urinary tract ultrasonography to detect dilatation secondary to obstruction and a study to detect VUR.

Ultrasonography

Urinary tract ultrasonography consists of examination of the kidneys to identify hydronephrosis and examination of the bladder to identify dilatation of the distal ureters, hypertrophy of the bladder wall, and the presence of ureteroceles. Previously, excretory urography (commonly called intravenous pyelography) was used to reveal these abnormalities, but now ultrasonography shows them more safely, less invasively, and often less expensively. Ultrasonography does have limitations, however. A normal ultrasound does not exclude VUR. Ultrasonography may show signs of acute renal inflammation and established renal scars, but it is not as sensitive as other renal imaging techniques.

Usually the timing of the ultrasound is not crucial, but when the rate of clinical improvement is slower than anticipated during treatment, ultrasonography should be performed promptly to look for a cause such as obstruction or abscess.

VUR

The most common abnormality detected in imaging studies is VUR (Fig 1). The rate of VUR among children younger than 1 year of age with UTI exceeds 50%. VUR is not an all-or-none phenomenon; grades of severity are recognized, designated I to V in the

TABLE 5.   Some Antimicrobials for Prophylaxis of UTI

Antimicrobial	Dosage
TMP in combination with SMX	2 mg of TMP, 10 mg of SMX per kg as single bedtime dose *or* 5 mg of TMP, 25 mg of SMX per kg twice per week
Nitrofurantoin	1–2 mg/kg as single daily dose
Sulfisoxazole	10–20 mg/kg divided every 12 h
Nalidixic acid	30 mg/kg divided every 12 h
Methenamine mandelate	75 mg/kg divided every 12 h

International Study Classification (International Reflux Study Committee, 1981), based on the extent of the reflux and associated dilatation of the ureter and pelvis. The grading of VUR is important because the natural history differs by grade, as does the risk of renal damage. Patients with high-grade VUR are 4 to 6 times more likely to have scarring than those with low-grade VUR and 8 to 10 times more likely than those without VUR.[16,49]

VCUG; RNC

Either traditional contrast VCUG or RNC is recommended for detecting reflux. Although children may have pyelonephritis without reflux, the child with reflux is at increased risk of pyelonephritis and of scarring from UTI. With VCUG and RNC, a voiding phase is important because some reflux occurs only during voiding. If the predicted bladder capacity is not reached, the study may underestimate the presence or degree of reflux.

VCUG with fluoroscopy characterizes reflux better than does RNC. In addition, RNC does not show urethral or bladder abnormalities; for this reason, boys, whose urethra must be examined for posterior urethral valves, or girls, who have symptoms of voiding dysfunction when not infected, should have a standard fluoroscopic contrast VCUG as part of their initial studies. RNC has a lower radiation dose and therefore may be preferred in follow-up examinations of children with reflux. However, the introduction of low-dose radiographic equipment has narrowed the gap in radiation between the VCUG and RNC.[50]

There is no benefit in delaying performance of these studies as long as the child is free of infection and bladder irritability is absent. While waiting for reflux study results, the child should be receiving an antimicrobial, either as part of the initial treatment or as posttreatment prophylaxis (Table 5).

Radionuclide Renal Scans

Renal cortical scintigraphy (with 99 m Tc-DMSA or 99 m Tc-glucoheptonate) and enhanced computed tomography are very sensitive means of identifying acute changes from pyelonephritis or renal scarring. However, the role of these imaging modalities in the clinical management of the child with UTI still is unclear.

CONCLUSIONS

Eleven recommendations are proposed for the diagnosis, management, and evaluation of infants and young children with UTI and unexplained fever. Infants and children younger than 2 years of age with unexplained fever are identified for particular concern because UTI has a high prevalence in this group (~5%), may cause few recognizable signs or symptoms other than fever, and has a greater potential for renal damage than in older children. Strategies of diagnosis and treatment depend on how ill the clinician assesses the infant or young child to be, ie, whether antimicrobial therapy is warranted immediately or can be delayed safely until the results of urine culture are avail-

able. Diagnosis is based on the culture of an appropriately collected specimen of urine; urinalysis can only suggest the diagnosis. Imaging studies should be performed on all infants and young children with a documented initial UTI.

AREAS FOR FUTURE RESEARCH

The relationship between UTI in infants and young children and reduced renal function in adults has been established but is not well characterized in quantitative terms. The ideal prospective cohort study from birth to age 40 to 50 years has not been conducted and is unlikely to be conducted. Thus, estimates of undesirable outcomes in adulthood, such as hypertension and end-stage renal disease, are based on the mathematical product of probabilities at several steps, each of which is subject to bias and error. Other attempts at decision analysis[51] and thoughtful literature review[52] have recognized the same limitations. Until recently, imaging tools available to assess the effect of UTI have been insensitive. With the imaging techniques available now, it may be possible to follow a cohort of infants and young children who present with fever and UTI to assess the development of scars and functional impairment. Research is underway in this area.

The development of noninvasive methods of obtaining a urine specimen or of techniques that obviate the need for invasive sampling would be valuable for general use. One component of the urinalysis that merits particular attention is the assessment of WBCs in the urine. Bacteriuria can occur without pyuria, but it is not clear whether pyuria is a specific marker for renal inflammation, obviating the need for culture if WBCs are not present in the urine. Research is underway in this area under conditions that optimize the detection of WBCs in the urine by microscopy. If studies continue to demonstrate usefulness of microscopy, the general applicability of the test will need to be studied, particularly in offices without on-site laboratories or trained laboratory staff. Special attention will need to be given to specimens from girls and from uncircumcised boys, particularly infants, because transurethral catheterization may be difficult and produce a contaminated specimen. An alternative to SPA, which is not commonly performed anymore, would be welcome in clinical practice and in research to clarify such issues as the true prevalence of UTI in young uncircumcised boys.

There is consensus about the antimicrobial treatment of infants and young children with acute UTI, but questions remain relating to the specific duration and route of therapy. Currently, the efficacy of orally administered treatment is being compared with parenterally administered treatment under controlled conditions. If orally administered therapy is as efficacious as that administered parenterally, concern about variable adherence to a prescribed regimen will remain and influence the decision of whether to hospitalize and whether to administer the antimicrobial(s) parenterally or orally.

As noted in the section "Evaluation: Imaging," ultrasonography is recommended to detect dilatation associated with obstruction and is preferred over other modalities because it is noninvasive and does not expose the child to radiation. Data defining the yield of positive findings were generated before the widespread use of fetal ultrasonography, and it is not clear that they are applicable today. The absence of extensive data from modern studies and variations in the frequency and quality of fetal ultrasonography do not permit a determination of whether ultrasonography can reasonably be omitted. Further complicating the assessment is the changing utilization of fetal ultrasonography under the financial pressures of managed care. Studies in this area will need to be defined carefully so that the generalizability and applicability to individual patients can be assessed.

A study to determine the presence and severity of VUR also is recommended. It is recognized, however, that pyelonephritis (defined by cortical scintigraphy) can occur in the absence of VUR (defined by VCUG or RNC) and that progressive renal scarring (defined by cortical scintigraphy) can occur in the absence of demonstrated VUR. Whether children with pyelonephritis (defined clinically or by cortical scintigraphy) who have normal results on VCUG or RNC benefit from antimicrobial prophylaxis is unknown but is being studied.

The role of cortical scintigraphy in the imaging examination of infants and young children with initial UTI is unclear and requires additional study. The demonstration by cortical scintigraphy of "cold" areas of decreased perfusion has led to the development of alternative imaging techniques, such as enhanced computed tomography and power Doppler ultrasonography. These modalities also can demonstrate hypoperfusion and have advantages, particularly power Doppler ultrasonography, which is noninvasive and does not expose the child to radiation. Studies are now in progress.

COMMITTEE ON QUALITY IMPROVEMENT, 1999
David A. Bergman, MD, Chairperson
Richard D. Baltz, MD
James R. Cooley, MD

LIAISON REPRESENTATIVES
Michael J. Goldberg, MD, Sections Liason
Gerald B. Hickson, MD

Algorithm

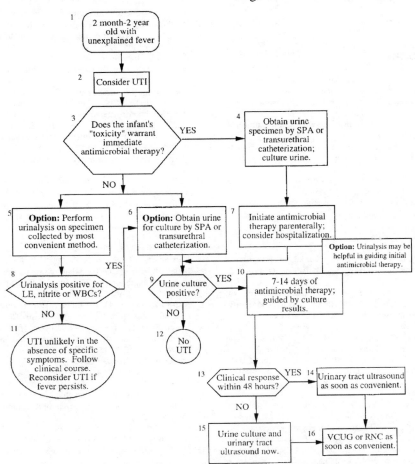

Charles J. Homer, MD, MPH, Section on
　Epidemiology Liaison
Paul V. Miles, MD
Joan E. Shook, MD
William M. Zurthellen, MD

LIAISON REPRESENTATIVE
Betty A. Lowe, MD, NACHRI Liaison

SUBCOMMITTEE ON URINARY TRACT
Kenneth B. Roberts, MD, Chairperson
Stephen M. Downs, MD, MS
Stanley Hellerstein, MD
Michael J. Holmes, MD, PhD
Robert L. Lebowitz, MD
Jacob A. Lohr, MD
Linda D. Shortliffe, MD
Russell W. Steele, MD

REFERENCES

1. Dolan TF Jr, Meyers A. A survey of office management of urinary tract infections in childhood. *Pediatrics*. 1973;52:21–24
2. Rice DP, Hodgeson TA, Kopstein AN. The economic costs of illness: a replication and update. *Health Care Financ Rev*. 1985;7:61–80
3. Pauker SG, Kassirer JP. The threshold approach to clinical decision making. *N Engl J Med*. 1980;302:1109–1117
4. Hoberman A, Chao HP, Keller DM, et al. Prevalence of urinary tract infection in febrile infants. *J Pediatr*. 1993;123:17–23
5. Roberts KB, Charney E, Sweren RJ, et al. Urinary tract infection in infants with unexplained fever: a collaborative study. *J Pediatr*. 1983;103:864–867
6. Bauchner H, Philipp B, Dahefsky G, Klein JO. Prevalence of bacteriuria in febrile children. *Pediatr Infect Dis J*. 1987;6:239–242
7. Bonadio WA. Urine culturing technique in febrile infants. *Pediatr Emerg Care*. 1987;3:75–78
8. North AF. Bacteriuria in children with acute febrile illnesses. *J Pediatr*. 1963;63:408–411
9. Ginsburg CM, McCracken GH Jr. Urinary tract infections in young infants. *Pediatrics*. 1982;69:409–412
10. Wiswell TE, Smith FR, Bass JW. Decreased incidence of urinary tract infections in circumcised male infants. *Pediatrics*. 1985;75:901–903
11. Wiswell TE, Roscelli JD. Corroborative evidence for the decreased incidence of urinary tract infections in circumcised male infants. *Pediatrics*. 1986;78:96–99
12. Wiswell TE, Hachey WE. Urinary tract infections and the uncircumcised state: an update. *Clin Pediatr*. 1993;32:130–134
13. Craig JC, Knight JF, Sureshjumar P, Mantz E, Roy LP. Effect of circumcision on incidence of urinary tract infection in preschool boys. *J Pediatr*. 1996;128:23–27
14. Winter AL, Hardy BE, Alton DJ, Arbus GS, Churchill BM. Acquired renal scars in children. *J Urol*. 1983;129:1190–1194
15. Smellie JM, Poulton A, Prescod NP. Retrospective study of children with renal scarring associated with reflux and urinary infection. *Br Med J*. 1994;308:1193–1196
16. Jodal U. The natural history of bacteriuria in childhood. *Infect Dis Clin North Am*. 1987;1:713–729
17. Winberg J, Andersen HJ, Bergstrom T, et al. Epidemiology of symptomatic urinary tract infection in childhood. *Acta Paediatr Scand*. 1974;252:1–20. Supplement
18. Tappin DM, Murphy AV, Mocan H, et al. A prospective study of children with first acute symptomatic E coli urinary tract infection: early 99 m technetium dimercaptosuccinic acid scan appearances. *Acta Paediatr Scand*. 1989;78:923–929
19. Verboven M, Ingels M, Delree M, Piepsz A. 99 mTc-DMSA scintigraphy in acute urinary tract infection in children. *Pediatr Radiol*. 1990;20:540–542
20. Rosenberg AR, Rossleigh MA, Brydon MP, Bass SJ, Leighton DM, Farnsworth RH. Evaluation of acute urinary tract infection in children by dimercaptosuccinic acid scintigraphy: a prospective study. *J Urol*. 1992;148:1746–1749. Part II
21. McCarthy PL, Sharpe MR, Spiesel SZ, et al. Observation scales to identify serious illness in febrile children. *Pediatrics*. 1982;70:802–809
22. Pryles CV, Atkin MD, Morse TS, Welch KJ. Comparative bacteriologic study of urine obtained from children by percutaneous suprapubic aspiration of the bladder and by catheter. *Pediatrics*. 1959;24:983–991
23. Leong YY, Tan KW. Bladder aspiration for diagnosis of urinary tract infection in infants and young children. *J Singapore Paediatr Soc*. 1976;18:43–47
24. Djojohadipringgo S, Abdul Hamid RH, Thahir S, Karim A, Darsono I. Bladder puncture in newborns—a bacteriological study. *Paediatr Indonesia*. 1976;16:527–534
25. Sorensen K, Lose G, Nathan E. Urinary tract infection and diurnal incontinence in girls. *Eur J Pediatr*. 1988;148:146–147
26. Turck M, Goffe B, Petersdorf RG. The urethral catheter and urinary tract infection. *J Urol*. 1962;88:834–837
27. Lohf J. *Pediatric Outpatient Procedures*. Philadelphia, PA: JB Lippincott Co; 1991:142–152
28. Shannon F, Sepp E, Rose G. The diagnosis of bacteriuria by bladder puncture in infancy and childhood. *Aust Paediatr J*. 1969;5:97–100
29. Cohen M. The first urinary tract infection in male children. *Am J Dis Child*. 1976;130:810–813
30. Ellerstein NS, Sullivan TD, Baliah T, Neter E. Trimethoprim/sulfamethoxazole and ampicillin in the treatment of acute urinary tract infections in children: a double-blind study. *Pediatrics*. 1977;60:245–247
31. Khan AJ, Ubriani RS, Bombach E, Agbayani MM, Ratner H, Evans HE. Initial urinary tract infection caused by *Proteus mirabilis* in infancy and childhood. *J Pediatr*. 1978;93:791–793
32. Howard JB, Howard JE. Trimethoprim–sulfamethoxazole vs sulfamethoxazole for acute urinary tract infections in children. *Am J Dis Child*. 1978;132:1085–1087
33. Wientzen RL, McCracken GH Jr, Petruska ML, Swinson SG, Kaijer B, Hanson LA. Localization and therapy of urinary tract infections of childhood. *Pediatrics*. 1979;63:467–474
34. Sullivan TD, Ellerstein NS, Neter E. The effects of ampicillin and trimethoprim/sulfamethoxazole on the periurethral flora of children with urinary tract infection. *Infection*. 1980;8:S339–S341. Supplement 3
35. Fennell RS, Luengnaruemitchai M, Iravani A, Garin EH, Walker RD, Richard GA. Urinary tract infections in children: effect of short course antibiotic therapy on recurrence rate in children with previous infections. *Clin Pediatr*. 1980;19:121–124
36. Shapiro ED, Wald ER. Single-dose amoxicillin treatment of urinary tract infections. *J Pediatr*. 1981;99:989–992
37. Helin I. Short-term treatment of lower urinary tract infections in children with trimethoprim/sulphadiazine. *Infection*. 1981;9:249–251
38. Pitt WR, Dyer SA, McNee JL, Burke JR. Single dose trimethoprim-sulphamethoxazole treatment of symptomatic urinary infection. *Arch Dis Child*. 1981;57:229–231
39. Avner ED, Ingelfinger JR, Herrin JT, et al. Single-dose amoxicillin therapy of uncomplicated pediatric urinary tract infections. *J Pediatr*. 1983;102:623–627
40. Aarbakke J, Opshaug O, Digranes A, Hoylandskjaer A, Fluge G, Fellner H. Clinical effect and pharmacokinetics of trimethoprim–sulphadiazine in children with urinary tract infections. *Eur J Clin Pharmacol*. 1983;24:267–271
41. Stahl G, Topf P, Fleisher GR, Normal ME, Rosenblum HW, Gruskin AB. Single-dose treatment of uncomplicated urinary tract infections in children. *Ann Emerg Med*. 1984;13:705–708
42. Hashemi G. Recurrent urinary tract infection. *Indian J Pediatr*. 1985;52:401–403
43. Rajkumar S, Saxena Y, Rajogopal V, Sierra MF. Trimethoprim in pediatric urinary tract infection. *Child Nephrol Urol*. 1988;9:77–81
44. Madrigal G, Odio CM, Mohs E, Guevara J, McCracken GH Jr. Single dose antibiotic therapy is not as effective as conventional regimens for management of acute urinary tract infections in children. *Pediatr Infect Dis J*. 1988;7:316–319
45. Nolan T, Lubitz L, Oberklaid F. Single dose trimethoprim for urinary tract infection. *Arch Dis Child*. 1989;64:581–586
46. Bailey RR, Abbott GD. Treatment of urinary tract infection with a single dose of trimethoprim–sulfamethoxazole. *Can Med Assoc J*. 1978;118:551–552
47. Bailey RR, Abbott GD. Treatment of urinary tract infection with a single dose of amoxycillin. *Nephron*. 1977;18:316–320
48. Copenhagen Study Group of Urinary Tract Infections in Children. Short-term treatment of acute urinary tract infection in girls. *Scand J Infect Dis*. 1991;23:213–220
49. McKerrow W, Davidson-Lamb N, Jones PF. Urinary tract infection in children. *Br Med J*. 1984;289:299–303
50. Kleinman PK, Diamond DA, Karellas A, Spevak MR, Nimkin K, Belanger P. Tailored low-dose fluoroscopic voiding cystourethrography for the reevaluation of vesicoureteral reflux in girls. *AJR Am J Roentgenol*. 1994;162:1151–1154
51. Kramer MS, Tange SM, Drummond KN, Mills EL. Urine testing in young febrile children: a risk–benefit analysis. *J Pediatr*. 1994;125:6–13
52. Dick PT, Feldman W. Routine diagnostic imaging for childhood urinary tract infections: a systematic overview. *J Pediatr*. 1996;128:15–22
53. Hellerstein S. Recurrent urinary tract infections in children. *Pediatr Infect Dis*. 1982;1:271–281

ERRATUM

For the practice guideline entitled, "Practice Parameter: The Diagnosis, Treatment, and Evaluation of the Initial Urinary Tract Infection in Febrile Infants and Young Children" (1999;103:843–852), the table below replaces the previously published Table 2 (1999;104:118) and should be used in conjunction with this practice guideline.

TABLE 2.   Criteria for the Diagnosis of Urinary Tract Infection[53]

Method of Collection	Colony Count (Pure Culture)	Probability of Infection (%)
Suprapubic aspiration	Gram-negative bacilli: any number Gram-positive cocci: more than a few thousand	>99%
Transurethral catheterization	>10^5	95%
	$10^4 - 10^5$	Infection likely
	$10^3 - 10^4$	Suspicious; repeat
	<10^3	Infection unlikely
Clean void		
Boy	>10^4	Infection likely
Girl	3 specimens $\geq 10^5$	95%
	2 specimens $\geq 10^5$	90%
	1 specimen $\geq 10^5$	80%
	$5 \times 10^4 - 10^5$	Suspicious; repeat
	$10^4 - 5 \times 10^4$	Symptomatic: suspicious; repeat
		Asymptomatic: infection unlikely
	<10^4	Infection unlikely

Technical Report Summary:
Urinary Tract Infections in Febrile Infants
and Young Children

Author:

Stephen M. Downs, MD, MS

American Academy of Pediatrics
PO Box 927, 141 Northwest Point Blvd
Elk Grove Village, IL 60009-0927

For the complete technical report, including tables, figures, and references, please see the companion CD-ROM.

ABSTRACT

Overview

The Urinary Tract Infection Subcommittee of the American Academy of Pediatrics' Committee on Quality Improvement has analyzed alternative strategies for the diagnosis and management of urinary tract infection (UTI) in children. The target population is limited to children between 2 months and 2 years of age who are examined because of fever without an obvious cause. Diagnosis and management of UTI in this group are especially challenging for these three reasons: 1) the manifestation of UTI tends to be nonspecific, and cases may be missed easily; 2) clean voided midstream urine specimens rarely can be obtained, leaving only urine collection methods that are invasive (transurethral catheterization or bladder tap) or result in nonspecific test results (bag urine); and 3) a substantial number of infants with UTI also may have structural or functional abnormalities of the urinary tract that put them at risk for ongoing renal damage, hypertension, and end-stage renal disease (ESRD).

Methods

To examine alternative management strategies for UTI in infants, a conceptual model of the steps in diagnosis and management of UTI was developed. The model was expanded into a decision tree. Probabilities for branch points in the decision tree were obtained by review of the literature on childhood UTI. Data were extracted on standardized forms. Cost data were obtained by literature review and from hospital billing data. The data were collated into evidence tables. Analysis of the decision tree was used to produce risk tables and incremental cost-effectiveness ratios for alternative strategies.

Results

Based on the results of this analysis and, when necessary, consensus opinion, the Committee developed recommendations for the management of UTI in this population. This document provides the evidence the Subcommittee used in the development of its recommendations.

Conclusions

The Subcommittee agreed that the objective of the practice guideline would be to minimize the risk of chronic renal damage within reasonable economic constraints. Steps involved in achieving these objectives are: 1) identifying UTI; 2) short-term treatment of UTI; and 3) evaluation for urinary tract abnormalities.

METHODS

Analysis of the data on UTI consisted of several steps. The Subcommittee met to define the target population, setting, and providers for whom the practice parameter is intended. Subcommittee members identified the outcomes of interest for the analysis. A conceptual evidence model of the diagnosis and management of UTI was developed. The evidence model was used to generate a decision tree.

A comprehensive review of the literature determined the probability estimates used in the tree. The tree was used to conduct risk analyses and cost-effectiveness analyses of alternative strategies for the diagnosis and management of UTI. Based on the results of these analyses and consensus when necessary, an algorithm representing the strategies with acceptable risk-benefit trade-offs was developed.

EVIDENCE MODEL

The overall problem of managing UTI in children between 2 months and 2 years of age was conceptualized as an evidence model. The model depicts the relationships between the steps in the diagnosis and management of UTI. The steps are divided into the following four phases: 1) recognizing the child at risk for UTI, 2) making the diagnosis of UTI, 3) short-term treatment of UTI, and 4) evaluation of the child with UTI for possible urinary tract abnormality.

Phase 1 represents the recognition of the child at risk for UTI. Age and other clinical features define a prevalence or *a priori* probability of UTI, determining whether the diagnosis should be pursued. If children at sufficiently high risk for UTI are not identified for diagnostic evaluation, the potential benefit of treatment will be lost. However, children with a sufficiently low likelihood of UTI should be saved the cost of diagnosis (and perhaps misdiagnosis) of UTI when the potential for benefit is minimal.

Phase 2 depicts the diagnosis of UTI. Alternative diagnostic strategies may be characterized by their cost, sensitivity, and specificity. The result of testing is the division of patients into groups according to a relatively higher or lower probability of having a UTI. The probability of UTI in each of these groups depends not only on the sensitivity and specificity of the test, but also on the prior probability of the UTI among the children being tested. In this way, the usefulness of a diagnostic test depends on the prior probability of UTI established in phase 1. Overdiagnosis of UTI may result in unnecessary treatment and unnecessary imaging evaluation for urinary tract abnormalities. Underdiagnosis will result in missing the opportunity to treat the acute infection and the consequences of possible underlying urinary tract abnormalities.

Phase 3 represents the short-term treatment of UTI. Alternatives for treatment of UTI may be compared, based on their likelihood of clearing the initial UTI (IUTI).

Phase 4 depicts the imaging evaluation of infants with the diagnosis of UTI to identify those with urinary tract abnormalities such as vesicoureteral reflux (VUR). Children with VUR are believed to be at risk for ongoing renal damage with subsequent infections, resulting in hypertension and renal failure. Prophylactic antibiotic therapy or surgical procedures such as ureteral reimplantation may prevent progressive renal damage. Therefore, identifying urinary abnormalities may offer the benefit of preventing hypertension and renal failure. Each alternative strategy for imaging evaluation can be characterized according to its cost, invasiveness, and test characteristics (sensitivity and specificity). The potential yield of an imaging evaluation will be affected by the accuracy of the initial diagnosis of UTI. If the probability of UTI is low because a nonspecific test was used to make the diagnosis, the cost of an imaging study will yield little benefit.

Therefore, the value of imaging strategies depends on the accuracy of the diagnosis of UTI in phase 2.

Because the consequences of detection and early management of UTI are affected by subsequent evaluation and long-term management and, likewise, long-term management of patients with UTI depends on how they are detected at the outset, the Subcommittee elected to analyze the entire process from detection of UTI to the evaluation for, and consequences of, urinary tract abnormalities.

Decision Tree

The conceptual model was used to develop a decision tree. The tree quantifies the relationship between alternative strategies for the diagnosis and treatment of UTI, the evaluation of children for abnormalities of the urinary tract, and the anticipated consequences of these alternative diagnostic and treatment strategies.

In the diagnosis and treatment of UTI, four alternatives are represented. As anchor points, the alternatives of treating all or treating none of the patients at risk are represented. Two alternative tests are represented in the other branches. The test characteristics and costs of these tests were adjusted to correspond with the tests the Subcommittee chose to evaluate. In this way, the Subcommittee compared alternative testing strategies.

In the decision tree, if a testing strategy is used, the result is positive or negative. A positive result was assumed to lead to a decision to treat and a negative result to a decision to observe without treatment. If treatment is chosen, presumptively or based on the results of a diagnostic test, a treatment complication may result. Rarely, as in the case of anaphylaxis, the complication may result in death.

For all other patients, there is a risk of urosepsis. This risk is the probability of UTI multiplied by the prevalence of urosepsis among infants with UTI. Assuming urosepsis behaves like bacteremia from other sources in infants, the infection may clear spontaneously in those who have urosepsis. The probability of clearing the infection is increased among those who receive antimicrobials. If urosepsis does not clear, hospitalization will result, and the child has a risk of dying.

Once the short-term outcome of the UTI has been resolved, the second decision is whether and how to image the urinary tract for structural and functional abnormalities. The three following options are modeled: 1) a full evaluation, including ultrasonography or an intravenous pyelogram and voiding cystourethrography (VCUG) or radionuclide cystourethrography (RCG); 2) ultrasonography alone; and 3) no evaluation.

The results of the evaluation are determined separately for each patient type. For patients who have no UTI (false-positive diagnosis of UTI), it is assumed that abnormalities are not present and the infant is not at increased risk of renal damage. Patients who have a true UTI may or may not have VUR. Among those with VUR, the reflux may be low grade (1 or 2) or high grade (3, 4, or 5).

The probability of having a positive result when imaging an abnormal urinary tract depends on the sensitivity of the imaging modality for the abnormality. For example,

ultrasonography is much more sensitive to high-grade VUR than to low-grade VUR. The analysis assumes that all imaging modalities have 100% specificity (ie, no false-positive diagnoses).

The result of the imaging evaluation would be used to select a treatment (surgical correction or antibiotic prophylaxis as appropriate) to prevent recurrent infections. An evaluation with normal results or no evaluation would lead to no therapy. Identifying the optimal therapy for a given urinary tract abnormality is beyond the scope of the present analysis.

Patients may or may not have recurrent UTI, defined as more than three infections in a 5-year period. Recurrent infections lead to progressive renal scarring. The risk of scarring is highest among those with high-grade VUR and lowest among those with no VUR. Therapeutic interventions reduce the risk of renal scarring by reducing VUR in the case of surgery or preventing infection in the case of antimicrobial prophylaxis.

Patients with progressive renal scarring are at increased risk of hypertension and ESRD. Those who do not experience these outcomes may have decreased renal function but will not have clinically important outcomes.

At the terminal nodes of each branch, the outcomes are tabulated as costs and clinical outcomes. Costs considered include the cost of diagnostic testing, treatment, complications of treatment, hospitalization for urosepsis, imaging studies, surgery or prophylaxis, management of hypertension, and ESRD. Clinical outcomes include chronic hypertension, renal failure, and death.

The decision tree was encoded and evaluated using the Decision Maker software Version 6.0 (Sonnenberg and Pauker, New England Medical Center, Boston, MA).

Literature Review

Articles for review were obtained from four sources in two rounds of searching. In the first round, the MEDLINE database was searched using four separate search strategies corresponding with the four phases of the diagnosis and treatment of UTI: recognition, diagnosis, short-term treatment, and imaging evaluation. The titles and abstracts resulting from these searches were distributed among the Subcommittee members who identified those that were definitely or potentially useful. These articles were reproduced in full.

In a second round of searching, articles were identified from three additional sources: the bibliographies of two recent reviews; a survey of the members of the Subcommittee, soliciting the articles they identified as most important and relevant to the analysis; and articles sought specifically to estimate costs for the management of chronic hypertension and ESRD. At each of the two rounds of searching, the articles were reviewed by the epidemiology consultant, and articles with no original data were removed.

The remaining articles were reviewed and data extracted using a data extraction form designed to identify estimates necessary to evaluate the decision model. In addition, the quality of each article was rated on a scale from 0 to 1 by using quality criteria adapted from Sackett and colleagues. Reviewers also provided a subjective rating of "good," "fair," or "poor" to each article. Data extracted were recorded in evidence tables, using an Excel (Microsoft Corporation, Redmond, WA) spreadsheet. A subset of 24 articles was reviewed twice by different reviewers to check interrater reliability. At the time of analysis of the decision models, the articles were reviewed again by the epidemiology consultant.

RESULTS

Literature Review

In the initial MEDLINE search, 1949 articles were identified. The title and abstract of each of these was reviewed by two members of the Subcommittee and identified as "useful," "potentially useful," or "not useful." After this review and elimination of duplicates, 430 articles were reproduced in full for data extraction. Of these, 105 were rejected because they contained no original data relevant to the analysis. In the second round, an additional 133 articles were identified. Twenty-six of these were rejected for lack of original data. A total of 432 articles were reviewed at least once.

The quality of the articles in this area is highly variable, but most articles met 50% or fewer of the quality criteria. Interrater reliability for quality scores was tested using a subset of the articles. Correlation of scores among reviewers was only fair ($r = 0.43$). Correlation among the readers' subjective ratings was less good ($r = 0.29$).

Age and Gender

The data indicate that the probability of finding UTI in febrile male infants is less than half that in females, and just greater than one third for males between 1 and 2 years of age. Findings from two studies report the prevalence of UTI by gender in an unbiased sample of febrile infants younger than 1 year. The studies show inconsistent results among males younger than 1 year. Among females, the prevalence was similar, 7.4% and 8.8%, respectively. Other studies also suggest a lower risk among males in older age groups.

Other studies used to estimate the effect of age and gender on the prevalence of UTI examined only children with confirmed UTI. Relative risk of UTI for a given gender was estimated from these studies using the odds ratio (OR), $P(\text{male} | \text{UTI}) / P(\text{female} | \text{UTI})$. Because this prevalence in males and females in the general population is ~50%, the OR is essentially the same as the ratio of the prevalence of UTI among males to the prevalence among females. The prevalence itself can be derived by assuming an overall prevalence of 5% for both genders and a 50% prevalence of males in the population, using the formula, $P(\text{UTI} | \text{male}) = P(\text{male} | \text{UTI}) \cdot P(\text{UTI}) / P(\text{male})$. The comparable formula was used for females.

Studies also were stratified by age. These data and the data for prevalence by gender were used to make crude estimates of the effect of age and gender on the prevalence of UTI in four subgroups: males younger than 1 year (3%), males older than 1 year (2%), females younger than 1 year (7%), and females older than 1 year (8%).

Circumcision

Several studies show a dramatic risk reduction among circumcised males. Most (but not all) of these data are retrospective, and the studies are plagued with missing data, but the findings are quite consistent. In all these studies, the probability of circumcision given UTI [$P(\text{circ} | \text{UTI})$] was reported. Relative risk was estimated by the OR, $P(\text{circ} | \text{UTI}) / P(\text{no circ} | \text{UTI})$. Estimates of prevalence of UTI given circumcision [$P(\text{UTI} | \text{circ})$] were calculated by assuming the previous probability of UTI regardless of circumcision status [$P(\text{UTI})$] is 5%, and the probability of circumcision (among males) is 70%. Prevalences are calculated using these estimates and Bayes' formula, $P(\text{UTI} | \text{circ}) = P(\text{circ} | \text{UTI}) \cdot P(\text{UTI}) / P(\text{circ})$. The results suggest that the prevalence of UTI among febrile male infants who are circumcised would be ~0.2%.

Most data come from studies of infants younger than 1 year, but the effect seems to persist even beyond infancy. Making the (reasonable) assumption that circumcision status is independent of age, circumcised males older than 1 year are at lowest risk.

Interestingly, circumcision could account for the gender differences in prevalence. If one assumes that febrile females and uncircumcised males have a UTI prevalence of 7%, that circumcised males have a prevalence of 0.2%, and that 70% of males are circumcised, then the prevalence of UTI among males would be $(0.3 \cdot 0.07) + (0.7 \cdot 0.002) = 0.022$ or 2%, a figure consistent with the data.

Tests for UTI

When an infant is considered to be at significant risk for UTI, the next step is to make the diagnosis. Choosing diagnostic criteria for UTI involves two competing considerations. A false-negative diagnosis will leave patients with UTI at risk for serious complications. A false-positive diagnosis may lead to unnecessary, invasive, and expensive testing. In evaluating alternative diagnostic tests for UTI, the Subcommittee defined as a "gold standard" any bacterial growth on a culture of urine obtained by suprapubic bladder aspiration (tap), ie, any bacterial growth on a culture of a urine specimen obtained by tap defines a UTI.

For the analysis, a culture of a urine specimen obtained by a tap was considered to have 100% sensitivity and specificity. However, this was not always used for comparisons in studies of other diagnostic strategies. Alternative diagnostic strategies fall into the three following areas: 1) urine analysis (UA) for immediate diagnostic information, 2) culture of a urine specimen obtained by urine bag or transurethral catheterization, and 3) culture of a urine specimen using the dipslide culture technique.

UA

The various components of the UA include the reagent slide tests, ie, LE, nitrite, blood, and protein, and microscopic examination for leukocytes or bacteria. The diagnostic characteristics of these tests have been evaluated individually and in combination. Tests can be combined serially, meaning all test results must be positive for the combination to be positive or, in parallel, meaning a positive result on any one of the tests defines a positive result for the combination. The serial strategy maximizes specificity at the expense of sensitivity, whereas parallel testing maximizes sensitivity at the expense of specificity.

Perhaps the most commonly used component of the UA used to evaluate a child who may have a UTI is the reagent strip (dipstick). Tests for UTI that are available on most reagent strips include the LE, nitrite, blood, and protein. The LE is the most sensitive single test. Its reported sensitivity ranges from 67% in a screening setting in which symptoms and, therefore, inflammation, would not be expected, to 94% in settings in which UTI is suspected. The specificity of LE generally is not as good. However, because the specificity describes the performance of the test on specimens from patients without a UTI, it is highly dependent on patient characteristics. The reported specificity varies from 63% to 92%.

The test for nitrite has a much higher specificity (90% to 100%) and lower sensitivity (16% to 82%). For this reason, nitrite may be useful for "ruling in" UTI when it is positive, but it has little value in ruling out UTI. Dipstick tests for blood and protein have poor sensitivity and specificity with respect to UTI. Therefore, the use of results for blood or protein from dipstick testing has a high likelihood of being misleading.

Carefully performed microscopic examination of the urine has high sensitivity and specificity in many studies. However, the wide range of reported test characteristics of microscopy for leukocytes or bacteria presumably reflects the difficulty of performing these tests well and the hazards of performing them poorly. In studies that have shown the best test characteristics, tests were performed by on-site laboratory technicians who often used counting chambers.

When examining the urine for bacteria, unstained and Gram-stained specimens seem to be effective. However, centrifugation of the specimen reduces the specificity of the test. The number of bacteria also is important. Using heavy bacterial counts as a diagnostic criterion results in low sensitivity and high specificity. The reverse applies when observation of any bacteria is considered a positive test.

Microscopy for leukocytes is variably sensitive (32% to 100%) and specific (45% to 97%). Studies with accurate results generally used mirrored counting chambers, on-site technicians, or both. Specimens also must be examined shortly after collection. A 3-hour delay results in a 35% drop in sensitivity. Finally, if the number of leukocytes considered abnormal is high, the test will be insensitive, if the number is low, it will be highly sensitive. The reverse is true for specificity.

A number of special tests have been evaluated for the diagnosis of UTI. The first is a modified nitrite test. This involves incubating a urine specimen for several hours with added nitrite before testing for nitrate. The reported sensitivity and specificity are 93% and 88%, respectively. However, comparable results have not been reported. Immunochemical studies for early detection of bacterial growth have not had impressive results.

Obtaining a Urine Specimen

The Subcommittee defined the gold standard definition of a UTI to be growth on a culture of a urine specimen obtained by tap. Often, however, performance of a bladder tap is resisted because it is invasive. Moreover, bladder taps may not yield urine specimens. Success rates for obtaining urine specimens vary between 23% and 90%. Although 100% success has been achieved when using ultrasonographic guidance, practitioners often use transurethral catheterization or urine bags to obtain urine specimens for culture.

Cultures of urine specimens obtained by catheterization have a specificity of 83% to 89% compared with cultures of urine specimens obtained by tap. However, if only cultures yielding >1000 CFU/mL are considered positive, catheterization cultures have a 95% sensitivity with a specificity of 99%.

Cultures of bag urine specimens are 100% sensitive, but they have a specificity between 14% and 84%. Therefore, because UTI is present in a small minority (5%) of patients tested, use of culture results from urine specimens obtained from the bag to rule in UTI is likely to result in large numbers of false-positive results. Specifically, with a prevalence of 5% and specificity of 70%, the positive predictive value of a positive culture of bag urine specimens would be 15%. That is, 85% of positive cultures of urine specimens obtained from a bag would be false-positive results.

Culturing Techniques

The standard culturing technique involves streaking on blood agar and MacConkey media. More recently, dipslide methods have been developed. The few studies of dipslide cultures that were reviewed reported sensitivities between 87% and 100% and specificities between 92% and 98%.

Consequences of a Missed Diagnosis of UTI

If the diagnosis of UTI is not made because it was not suspected or a test of insufficient sensitivity was used, three consequences may result. The first (see "Prevalence of Urinary Tract Abnormalities") is the lost opportunity to find a urinary tract abnormality that could result in renal damage. The second is the formation of new renal scars. Although repeated UTI lead to scarring (see "Progressive Renal Damage") and progressive scarring is associated with hypertension and ESRD, the role of scarring from a single UTI in long-term clinical consequences is unknown. Nevertheless, timely treatment of febrile UTI in children appears to be important in preventing scars.

The third consequence of missing the diagnosis of UTI results from the urosepsis that occurs in a small proportion of febrile infants with UTI. Among patients with febrile UTI, in the age group to which this analysis applies, the risk of concurrent bacteremia is between 2.2% and 9%. The natural history of bacteremia in infants with febrile UTI is not described. Common pediatric experience is that septic shock and death are rarely seen in this situation, suggesting that spontaneous resolution of bacteremia occurs in this situation as it does in others. However, evidence exists that among infants with bacteremia attributable to *Escherichia coli* in the presence of a UTI, fatality rates may be as high as 10% to 12%.

Short-term Treatment of UTI

In studying the short-term treatment of UTI, the two following issues were addressed: 1) What do the data suggest about the duration of outpatient antibiotic therapy? and 2) What is the best choice for presumptive oral antibiotic therapy for the infant with suspected UTI before culture results are available? From the data presented subsequently in this report, it may be reasonable to conclude the following. 1) Single-dose to 3-day therapy is not as effective as therapy of 7 days or longer (perhaps because of more rapid metabolism of antimicrobials in children), but that the minimal acceptable duration of therapy has not been demonstrated. 2) Cotrimoxazole appears to be superior to amoxicillin for presumptive antibiotic therapy of UTI, but local antibiotic susceptibility patterns should ultimately dictate the antibiotic choice.

Duration of Therapy

Several studies have compared treatment of pediatric UTI with varying durations of therapy. The data have been analyzed in two ways. First, studies that directly compared different durations of therapy were examined. Then, data were pooled by antibiotic and duration of therapy, and the pooled values were compared.

None of the studies of duration of therapy compared 7 days with 10 days. In seven studies with 10 comparisons between long duration (7 to 10 days) and short duration (one dose to 3 days), 8 of 10 comparisons showed better results with an attributable improvement in outcome of 5% to 21%.

When the data were pooled by agent and duration, no discernible differences were found in initial cure or relapse among one-dose, 3-day, and 10-day courses of amoxicillin. However, single-dose cotrimoxazole was 10% less effective than 1-, 3-, 7-, or 10-day therapy. Differences among the latter regimens were not discernible.

Agent

The data pooled by agent and duration of therapy were used to compare amoxicillin and cotrimoxazole. For therapies of one dose, 3 to 4 days, or 10 days, cotrimoxazole consistently shows better cure rates (4% to 42%).

Data comparing parenteral and oral therapy were not found. However, intramuscular ceftriaxone (one dose) or gentamicin (10 days) was 100% effective in resolving UTI in children in whom oral therapy had failed. No data are available that clarify the role of oral vs parenteral therapy for bacteremia in association with UTI. Drawing on analyses of unsuspected bacteremia in children without UTI, parenteral antibiotic therapy is 95% effective in clearing bacteremia.

Prevalence of Urinary Tract Abnormalities

UTI in young children is a marker for abnormalities of the urinary tract. By far, the most common abnormality is VUR, which may be present with different degrees of severity that are graded I to V according to whether the reflux reaches the kidney and the degree of dilation of the collecting system. The grade of VUR is important because it determines the likelihood of detecting VUR on radiologic evaluation and the probability of renal damage, hypertension, or renal failure.

VUR

The Subcommittee identified 77 studies that reported the prevalence of VUR among children with UTI. The range of reported values is wide which may be primarily attributed to small sample size. As the sample size grows, the prevalence reported converges at 30% to 40%. The prevalence appears to decrease with age.

Specific studies of the relationship between age and prevalence of VUR show similar results. For example, one study reported a 68% prevalence among boys younger than 1 year and 25% among boys 1 to 3 years. Another study of boys found some type of abnormality in 76% of boys younger than 10 years (~54% of these were VUR) and 15% in boys older than 10 years. A population-based study showed a peak prevalence of VUR among girls 1 to 3 years of age and a rapid drop-off (perhaps by half) by age 5. A much smaller study found VUR in 100% of 9 boys younger than 1 year of age with a UTI and in 74% of 34 boys 1 to 5 years of age.

This relationship was fitted to a third-degree polynomial and a spline. Although the data are insufficient to define a particular functional relationship, they suggest a decline in the prevalence of VUR with age that seems to be most rapid during the first year of life. It levels off somewhat between 1 and 5 years of age, then drops off again after age 5. When studies of children younger than 3 years were pooled, the prevalence was 50%.

For this analysis, grades of VUR were grouped into low grade (grades I and II) and high grade (grades III to V). This grouping reduces the precision of the analysis slightly because higher grade reflux is easier to detect with ultrasonography and poses a greater risk of subsequent renal damage than do the lower grades. However, these effects were represented in this model, making this a more detailed analysis than has been reported previously. Some studies grouped patients in a similar manner, but grade III VUR was variably grouped as high grade or low grade. For classification of results, the classification used in the articles was (by necessity) used in this analysis. Pooling the data gives a 51.1% prevalence of low-grade (grades I to II) VUR among patients with VUR.

Tests for VUR

The Subcommittee identified the gold standard test for detecting VUR as the VCUG or RCG. These studies have, by definition, 100% sensitivity and specificity. The Subcommittee also believed that renal ultrasonography or intravenous pyelography should be performed to identify obstructions or other structural renal abnormalities.

VCUG and RCG are expensive and invasive. Data were collected on the sensitivity and specificity of renal ultrasonography alone in the detection of VUR. Overall, renal ultrasonography has poor sensitivity (30% to 62%) and good specificity (85% to 100%) for VUR. The sensitivity is better, however, for high-grade VUR than for low-grade

VUR (82% to 100% vs 14% to 30%). The Subcommittee members believed that renal ultrasonography in young infants was less reliable than this. However, data supporting this point were not found.

Progressive Renal Damage

The evidence that links the presence of VUR to important clinical outcomes can only be assembled in a piecemeal way. The data link VUR to renal scarring in the presence of recurrent infection, and renal scarring is associated with subsequent hypertension and ESRD. The data support this model indirectly. However, there are no longitudinal data that link directly the presence of VUR in infants with febrile UTI and normal kidneys to the subsequent development of hypertension or ESRD. Therefore, it is difficult to quantify the strength of the relationship or the risk to such patients. The following discussion reviews evidence supporting each step in the hypothesized progression to renal damage.

Reflux and Scarring

The data demonstrate an association between VUR and subsequent renal scarring. More than 48 references reviewed reported renal scarring at rates between 1% and 40% in association with febrile UTI and VUR. Higher grades of VUR are associated with higher risk of scar progression. Patients with high-grade VUR are four to six times more likely to have scarring than those with low-grade VUR and eight to 10 times as likely as those without VUR. In one study of 84 consecutive children 2 to 70 months of age with their first recognized febrile UTI, the presence of VUR was 80% sensitive and 74% specific in predicting subsequent scarring in a follow-up period of 2 years or more. Of those with VUR, 30% had progressive renal scarring. Of those without VUR, only 4% did.

Recurrent Infections and Scarring

The association of VUR with renal scarring seems to be mediated through recurrent symptomatic infections. The association between recurrent bouts of febrile UTI and the risk of renal scarring in one study followed an exponential curve. Patients with no VUR or low-grade VUR and patients with no recurrences of UTI are at low risk for renal scarring. Thus, prophylactic antibiotic treatment of patients with VUR to prevent recurrences or surgical treatment to prevent VUR would be expected to prevent renal scarring.

ESRD and Hypertension

Retrospective examination of the causes of ESRD in registries of patients with renal failure shows that in 36% (of 9250 patients), the cause of ESRD is obstructive uropathy, renal hypoplasia or dysplasia, pyelonephritis, or a combination of these. Unfortunately, it is not possible to determine which patients originally had normal kidneys in whom disease progressed to ESRD because of VUR and recurrent infection. In the North American Renal Transplant Cooperative Study, the fraction of transplant recipients with reflux nephropathy is 102/2033, or 5%. Patients with pyelonephritis or interstitial nephritis make up another 2% of transplant recipients.

Most cohort studies to quantify the risk of ESRD and hypertension among patients with renal scarring and VUR are based on highly selected patients in whom extensive scarring already has occurred. Long-term studies show that ESRD develops in 3% to 10% of these patients. In addition, 10% may require nephrectomy, and 0.4% renal transplantation. One study followed women from their first UTI in childhood and found that abnormal renal function could be documented in 21% of those with severe scarring. However, this study also had a selected population and did not provide data on VUR.

The rate of hypertension in these and similar studies varies between 0% and 50%. It is apparently lowest in those with low-grade VUR and those with the least scarring. However, the quality of the studies relating VUR nephropathy with ESRD and hypertension was rated poor, and quantification of the relationship is weak. One study identified retrospectively a cohort of children 1 month to 16 years of age with VUR and measured blood pressure levels 5 months to 21 years (average, 9.6 years) after VUR was identified. There was an increase in the blood pressure level associated with increasing grades of VUR. However, none of the patients had hypertension.

Effectiveness of Prophylactic Antimicrobials and Surgical Correction

Ultimately the value of identifying VUR depends on the potential to prevent its long-term consequences. This depends on reducing recurrent infections with antibiotic prophylaxis or eliminating VUR surgically. The efficacy of these procedures is not well documented because controlled studies have not been performed. Studies in which patients receiving antibiotic prophylaxis are compared with those not taking antimicrobials suggest a 50% effectiveness whether comparing rates of reinfection or progression of scarring.

Cost Data

Cost data were derived from literature where available, the accounting department of the University of North Carolina (UNC) Hospital, and the physicians' fee schedule from the UNC Physicians and Associates. Estimates used in the decision model are given below.

UA and Culture

Based on the cost data from the UNC Hospital, the cost of a urine culture is $21.53 (charge, $26.00). The cost of a UA is $6.77 (charge, $15.00).

Treatment

The cost of short-term treatment of UTI varies substantially depending on the treatment chosen. Standard oral therapy, such as amoxicillin or trimethoprim-sulfamethoxazole, costs about $10 for a course. Newer, broad-spectrum oral therapy costs about $40 for a 10-day course. If parenteral therapy, such as intramuscular ceftriaxone, is given, the cost of the drug and the injection may be $125.

Complications of Therapy

For the analysis, only complications requiring a return visit to the physician were considered. This visit would cost a $50 clinic fee, plus a $50 professional fee, for a total of $100. Death attributable to anaphylaxis is rare. The additional cost of this complication was not added.

Cost of Urosepsis

It is assumed that sepsis that does not clear spontaneously or with antibiotic therapy will require hospital admission for intravenous antibiotic therapy at a cost of $10 000.

Imaging Evaluation

The two following imaging strategies were considered: 1) a full work-up, including renal ultrasonography and VCUG, and 2) renal ultrasonography alone. The cost of renal ultrasonography includes the hospital cost of $104 and the physician fee of $200, for a total of $304. The cost of the VCUG is the hospital cost of $123 plus the physician fee of $200, totaling $323. Thus, the full work-up costs $627.

Cost of Treatment of VUR

The estimated cost of antibiotic prophylaxis was based on low-dose nitrofurantoin. The weekly cost was $6 for an average of 3 years. The total is $1040. It was assumed that the cost of ureteral reimplantation surgery was similar.

Complications of VUR

Patients with VUR are at increased risk for recurrent UTI, at least until the VUR resolves. The period the child is at risk was assumed to be 3 years. The cost of these recurrences was based on the average cost of a clinic visit related to a diagnosis of UTI or pyelonephritis in infants at UNC, $134, plus the physician fee of $70. This was multiplied by three, the average number of infections expected over 3 years, for a total of $612.

The cost of ESRD was derived from data in previous analyses. Based on a 10-year period, including 10 years of dialysis or a year in which transplantation occurs followed by 8 years with a functioning graft, followed by 1 year of a failed graft, the cost of ESRD is ~$300 000. The cost of managing severe hypertension and its complications was estimated at $100 000 based on $2000 per year for 50 years.

Analysis of the Decision Model

Using data extracted from the literature as described in "Evidence Tables," probabilities and costs were inserted into the decision tree. Using baseline estimates, three types of analysis were conducted. First, a risk analysis was performed to determine the average cost and frequency of outcomes expected with each of four strategies. Next, a cost-effectiveness analysis was used to determine the incremental cost per major clinical outcome averted by the strategies. Finally, sensitivity and threshold analyses were performed to examine alternative strategies for evaluation and management of UTI.

Risk Analysis

Two risk analyses were performed. The first examined the costs and clinical outcomes expected with different strategies for making the diagnosis of UTI. The second compared alternative strategies for imaging the urinary tract of patients with UTI.

Diagnosis of UTI

The risk analysis of diagnostic strategies examines two anchor states. The first, "treat all," is presumptive antibiotic therapy for occult infection without testing. The second, "observe," is clinical observation without testing or treatment. Neither of these anchor strategies involves subsequent imaging of the urinary tract. Three testing strategies are evaluated. The first is the gold standard, culture of urine specimens obtained by suprapubic tap or transurethral catheter. The second is using a culture of the urine specimen obtained from the urine bag. Culture of bag urine specimens has 100% sensitivity and 70% specificity in the baseline analysis. The third strategy uses the cheaper but less reliable reagent strip as a test for UTI. A positive LE test result, a positive nitrite test result, or both, is considered a positive test result. The sensitivity and specificity of this strategy are 92% and 70%, respectively, based on median values. All three testing strategies include antibiotic therapy and imaging of the urinary tract of patients with positive test results.

The results of the risk analysis are presented as the number of outcomes expected per 100 000 infants treated by using each strategy. To observe patients without testing or treatment is the least expensive strategy. However, it results in inferior clinical outcomes, including death and hospitalization from urosepsis, hypertension, and ESRD. Presumptive treatment of all infants without testing costs slightly more than observing, but prevents hospitalization and death from urosepsis. Under the treat all strategy, it is impossible to select patients for imaging, and it is unreasonably expensive to image the urinary tracts of all patients (see "Cost-effectiveness Analysis"). Therefore, no patient in the treat all strategy undergoes imaging evaluation. As a result, there is no improvement in the rates of hypertension or ESRD.

Using culture of urine specimens obtained by catheterization or tap offers the lowest risk of death, because all children at risk for urosepsis are identified and there are no unnecessary treatments or treatment-related deaths. Moreover, because all children with UTI are identified for imaging evaluation, this strategy minimizes the risk of hypertension and ESRD.

Using a culture of bag urine specimens as a criterion for the diagnosis of UTI also identifies correctly all children with UTI. However, its poor specificity also results in many false-positive results. As a consequence, there are slightly more deaths (3 per million) attributable to unnecessary antibiotic treatment and many more imaging work-ups. This means an additional $47.2 million per 100 000 febrile infants with no improvement in clinical outcomes.

Using LE and nitrite as diagnostic criteria for UTI leaves a small number of UTIs undiagnosed and results in 2½ times as many imaging work-ups compared with a culture of urine specimens obtained by catheterization or tap. The result is poorer clinical outcomes at greater expense despite the lower cost of UA.

A fourth diagnostic strategy also was evaluated that used a full UA (reagent strip and microscopy) as an initial diagnostic test and treated any positive UA component as a positive result. A positive result would lead to presumptive treatment. However, positive results would be confirmed by a culture of urine specimens obtained by tap or catheterization before imaging was performed. This strategy has a sensitivity of virtually 100% and a specificity of 60% for making a treatment decision. Because positive results are confirmed with a culture of urine specimens obtained by catheterization or tap, the specificity is 100% for imaging. The cost of testing is higher for positive results because UA and culture are performed. Also, the false-positive results lead to more unnecessary treatment and the resulting costs and complications. However, there is a cost saving for patients with negative results of the UA because the UA costs less than the culture. Compared with a culture of specimens from all patients, there is a small net decrease in cost using UA followed by a culture of positive results. Moreover, this strategy has the advantage of allowing immediate treatment of patients at risk of UTI. The benefit of early treatment is difficult to quantify, but evidence suggests it reduces the risk of renal scarring. Although this strategy appears to be nearly as effective as (or perhaps more than) the culture of urine specimens obtained by catheterization or tap, its effectiveness depends on the accuracy of the urine microscopy. As noted above, the accuracy of urine microscopy is highly variable and apparently depends on the presence of an onsite technician. In many settings, this may be impossible or so expensive as to offset the benefits.

Imaging Strategies

Three imaging alternatives were evaluated by risk analysis. The first strategy was renal ultrasonography and VCUG. The second was renal ultrasonography alone, and the third was no imaging evaluation at all. The total cost associated with each strategy includes the cost of the imaging studies, the cost of treating abnormalities identified, and the cost of any complications incurred. Together, renal ultrasonography and VCUG will identify all cases of renal abnormalities. Renal ultrasonography alone detects ~42% of all abnormalities. However, most abnormalities (87%) missed by renal ultrasonography alone are low-grade VUR, which carries a lower risk of renal scarring. As a result, the differences in clinical outcomes (cases of hypertension and ESRD) are smaller between renal ultrasonography alone and the full evaluation.

Cost-effectiveness Analysis

Cost-effectiveness analysis was used to quantify the trade-offs between cost and clinical effect when moving from one clinical strategy to another. When one strategy offers a better clinical effect at a lower cost, it is said to be a dominant strategy. However, in most cases, the strategy with better clinical effect also has a higher cost. Cost-effectiveness analysis depicts the additional cost per unit

of improvement in clinical effect. For this analysis, the units of effect were defined as cases of death, ESRD, or hypertension prevented.

Strategies were compared using the incremental (or marginal) cost-effectiveness ratio, ie, the difference in cost among strategies divided by the difference in effect. The mathematical term is as follows:

$$\frac{\text{Cost}_b - \text{Cost}_a}{\text{Effect}_b - \text{Effect}_a}.$$

Diagnosis of UTI

The least expensive strategy for the diagnosis of UTI is to do nothing. This also is the least effective strategy. By comparison, treating all febrile 2-month to 2-year-olds for UTI without diagnostic testing or urinary tract imaging improves clinical effect at a cost of $61 000 per death prevented. However, it does not prevent ESRD or hypertension.

As an alternative, one could obtain a dipstick UA on all patients, culturing specimens from those for whom the results of UA were positive. Because UA costs less than culture, this strategy has the potential to save money. However, because UA does not have perfect sensitivity, a few cases will be missed. In addition, patients for whom the results of UA are positive will incur the costs of UA and culture. To evaluate this strategy, a new branch was added to the decision tree. The new branch is a dipstick UA. If results are positive, it is linked to the "test" branch; if results are negative, it is linked to the "observe" branch. Positive results involve the cost of the UA plus culture; negative results, only the cost of the UA. This strategy prevents an additional two cases of death or serious complication per 10 000 at a cost of $261 000 per case.

Culturing catheterization or tap urine specimens on all patients and then treating and imaging the urinary tracts of all patients with positive results is the most effective and most expensive strategy. It prevents an additional 2.5 cases of death or serious complication per 100 000 over culture-confirmed positive dipstick results at an additional cost of $434 000 per case prevented. Compared with the no testing strategy, culturing specimens from all patients prevents three cases of death or serious complication per 10 000 at a cost of $200 000 per case prevented.

The optimal strategy depends on the decision-maker's willingness to pay for each additional case prevented. For example, if that willingness to pay is between $261 000 and $434 000, then the positive results of the dipstick confirmed by culture is the best strategy. Culturing specimens from all patients will prevent a few additional cases, but the cost to prevent each of these additional cases exceeds the decision-maker's willingness to pay. If the decision-maker is willing to pay >$434 000 to prevent a case of death or serious complication, then culturing specimens from all patients is the right strategy.

Imaging Strategies

The cost-effectiveness of the alternative imaging strategies also was calculated. The least expensive alternative is to perform no evaluation. Renal ultrasonography alone will prevent almost three cases of ESRD or hypertension per

1000 studies done at a cost of $260 000 per case prevented. A VCUG prevents an additional one case of ESRD or hypertension per 1000 studies over renal ultrasonography at a cost of $353 000 per case.

Again, the optimal strategy depends on the decision-maker's willingness to pay for each additional case prevented. For example, if that willingness to pay is between $260 000 and $353 000, then renal ultrasonography alone is the best strategy. A VCUG will prevent a few additional cases, but the cost to prevent each of these additional cases exceeds the decision-maker's willingness to pay. If the decision maker is willing to pay >$353 000 to prevent a case, then renal ultrasonography and VCUG is the right strategy.

Sensitivity and Threshold Analysis

Choosing one alternative over another from the risk analyses involves striking a balance between the cost of an intervention and the improvement in clinical outcomes. When comparing alternatives, if one alternative provides better clinical outcomes at lower costs, it is the dominant alternative and is the obvious choice. However, in most circumstances, choosing an alternative requires a trade-off between costs and clinical benefit. For example, obtaining a urine specimen for culture by catheterization or tap on all febrile infants, treating those with positive cultures, and imaging their urinary tracts with VCUG and renal ultrasonography improve clinical outcome but at a substantially higher cost than doing none of these evaluations.

To select the optimal alternative and, moreover, to identify different clinical circumstances in which different alternatives may be better, it is first necessary to make explicit the trade-off between costs and clinical outcomes. This means identifying a "willingness to pay" for each untoward clinical outcome avoided. For the following analyses, a value of $700 000 was placed on each case of ESRD or hypertension prevented. This figure is based loosely on the life-time productivity of a healthy, young adult. Once this cost is assigned to each untoward clinical outcome, it is possible to use the threshold method of decision-making.

The threshold approach to decision-making involves changing the value of a variable in the decision analysis to determine the value at which one alternative becomes too expensive and another would be preferred. In the case of UTI, if the prior probability of UTI is sufficiently high, it costs <$700 000 to prevent a case of ESRD or hypertension by screening all febrile children. However, if the probability that a particular patient has a UTI is sufficiently low, the yield of a urine culture will be extremely low and a positive result of a UA will almost certainly be a false-positive. Under these circumstances, a strategy involving the evaluation of this child's urinary tract would cost >$700 000 per case of ESRD or hypertension prevented. Threshold analysis identifies the threshold probability of UTI above which evaluation would be cost-effective and below which it would not. A number of threshold analyses follow.

Prevalence of UTI and Prevalence of VUR

Because fever without an obvious cause is common in pediatric practice, culturing the urine of all febrile 2-month to 2-year-old children represents a substantial investment. The Subcommittee was interested in determining whether there were some clinical subpopulations in which the prevalence of UTI was low enough that culture was unnecessary. A threshold analysis was used to examine this question.

Cost of Culturing Urine Obtained by Urine Bag

Many practitioners prefer to culture urine specimens obtained by urine bag rather than by transurethral catheter or suprapubic tap because the urine bag is less invasive. However, culture of a urine specimen obtained by bag has low specificity. When the prevalence of UTI is low, as it is in febrile infants, the result is a large number of false-positive urine cultures. False-positive cultures lead to unnecessary antibiotic treatment and urinary tract evaluation. The result is additional costs with no clinical benefit. To examine these additional costs, the difference in costs between a strategy involving urine specimens obtained by catheterization or tap and a strategy involving specimens from bag urine was calculated at different levels of specificity for the urine bag. Results of the analysis imply that culturing urine specimens from bag urine in this setting can only be justified if one is willing to pay between $293 and $1340 per patient to use a urine bag rather than to obtain urine specimens by catheterization or tap.

Sensitivity and Specificity for UA

As an alternative to obtaining urine specimens for culture from all febrile children between 2 months and 2 years of age, one could use a UA to make the diagnosis of UTI. As noted previously, a carefully performed UA has high sensitivity and specificity. Two-way sensitivity analysis was used to determine the minimal sensitivity and specificity that would be necessary to justify the use of UA rather than culture. The results imply that a test must have a sensitivity >92% and a specificity >99% to be preferred over urine culture. This level of sensitivity and specificity is unlikely to be obtained in most clinical settings. Alternatively, several studies demonstrated that combinations of LE, nitrite, microscopy of fresh urine, in which any abnormality constituted a positive test result, yielded a sensitivity of >92%. If one of these tests were used to rule out UTI, and culture of urine specimens obtained by catheterization or tap were used to confirm UTI in positive results, the requisite sensitivity and specificity would be obtained.

Probability of UTI and Urinary Tract Imaging

The decision to image the urinary tracts of infants with documented UTI presumes that the diagnosis of UTI is certain. If an imperfect test (eg, using a bag urine specimen) is used to make the diagnosis of UTI, a substantial number of these patients in fact may not have had a UTI and, therefore, the yield of the imaging will be lower. Threshold analysis was used to determine the minimal probability of UTI that justified a full imaging evaluation. The analysis indicates that if the probability of UTI is <49%, imaging becomes too expensive. Bayes's theorem shows that among patients with a prevalence of UTI that is 5%, those who have a positive urine culture obtained by bag have a probability (positive predictive value) of UTI that is 15%, well below 49%. This implies that if the best evidence of the UTI available in a given patient is a positive culture of urine obtained by bag, additional imaging of the urinary tract is not justified.

Sensitivity of Renal Ultrasonography for VUR

Because VCUG is invasive and expensive, a threshold analysis was used to explore the possible use of renal ultrasonography alone in evaluating the urinary tracts of children with UTI. Renal ultrasonography has low sensitivity for low-grade VUR, but relatively higher sensitivity for high-grade VUR. Based on the professional opinion of the UTI Subcommittee, a sensitivity of 14% for low-grade VUR and 82% for high-grade VUR is a better reflection of the situation in children 2 months to 2 years of age. This implies that renal ultrasonography alone is an inadequate imaging evaluation for infants with UTI.

Risk of Renal Scarring With UTI

One area of relative uncertainty, in which quality data are lacking, is the risk of scarring in undetected or untreated VUR. This risk is higher for children with high-grade VUR than for those with low-grade VUR. Threshold analysis was used to explore how this risk of scarring affects the decision to culture urine specimens from all children 2 months to 2 years of age with fever and no obvious cause for the fever. Figure 14 plots the risk of scar progression given low-grade VUR on the x-axis and the risk of scar progression given high-grade VUR on the y-axis. For values that plot above and to the right of the threshold line, culture of urine specimens from all febrile infants is the preferred strategy. For values that plot below and to the left of the threshold line, no urine culture is the preferred strategy. The baseline estimates used in the analysis, 14% for low-grade VUR and 53% for high-grade VUR, are plotted on the graph. The risk of scarring because of untreated VUR seems to be high enough to justify culturing specimens from all febrile infants.

Risk of Hypertension and ESRD

The weakest probability estimates in the present analysis relate to the risk of ESRD and hypertension among patients who have progressive renal scarring attributable to VUR. Two-way sensitivity analysis was used to determine the effect of varying these estimates on the results of the analysis. Our best estimate of the risk of hypertension and ESRD justifies culturing urine specimens from febrile infants as a strategy to prevent these complications. However, the quality of evidence about the future risks of ESRD and hypertension among infants with UTI later found to have VUR is tenuous at best. This is an area that needs additional investigation.

RECOMMENDATIONS

Who Should Be Evaluated for UTI?

Under the assumptions of the analysis, all febrile children between the ages of 2 months and 24 months with no obvious cause of infection should be evaluated for UTI, with the exception of circumcised males older than 12 months.

Minimal Test Characteristics of Diagnosis of UTI

To be as cost-effective as a culture of a urine specimen obtained by transurethral catheter or suprapubic tap, a test must have a sensitivity of at least 92% and a specificity of at least 99%. With the possible exception of a complete UA performed within 1 hour of urine collection by an on-site laboratory technician, no other test meets these criteria.

Performing a dipstick UA and obtaining a urine specimen by catheterization or tap for culture from patients with a positive LE or nitrite test result is nearly as effective and slightly less costly than culturing specimens from all febrile children.

Treatment of UTI

The data suggest that short-term treatment of UTI should not be for <7 days. The data do not support treatment for >14 days if an appropriate clinical response is observed. There are no data comparing intravenous with oral administration of medications.

Evaluation of the Urinary Tract

Available data support the imaging evaluation of the urinary tracts of all 2- to 24-month-olds with their first documented UTI. Imaging should include VCUG and renal ultrasonography. The method for documenting the UTI must yield a positive predictive value of at least 49% to justify the evaluation. Culture of a urine specimen obtained by bag does not meet this criterion unless the previous probability of a UTI is >22%.

Endorsed Clinical Practice Guidelines

The American Academy of Pediatrics endorses and accepts as its policy the following guidelines from other organizations.

ALLERGEN IMMUNOTHERAPY

Allergen Immunotherapy: A Practice Parameter

American Academy of Allergy, Asthma, and Immunology and American College of Allergy, Asthma, and Immunology (1/03)

ASTHMA

Guidelines for the Diagnosis and Management of Asthma—Update on Selected Topics

National Asthma Education and Prevention Program (2002)

AUTISM

Screening and Diagnosis of Autism

Quality Standards Subcommittee of the American Academy of Neurology and the Child Neurology Society

ABSTRACT. Autism is a common disorder of childhood, affecting 1 in 500 children. Yet, it often remains unrecognized and undiagnosed until or after late preschool age because appropriate tools for routine developmental screening and screening specifically for autism have not been available. Early identification of children with autism and intensive, early intervention during the toddler and preschool years improves outcome for most young children with autism. This practice parameter reviews the available empirical evidence and gives specific recommendations for the identification of children with autism. This approach requires a dual process: 1) routine developmental surveillance and screening specifically for autism to be performed on all children to first identify those at risk for any type of atypical development, and to identify those specifically at risk for autism; and 2) to diagnose and evaluate autism, to differentiate autism from other developmental disorders. (8/00)

CEREBRAL PALSY

Diagnostic Assessment of the Child With Cerebral Palsy

Quality Standards Subcommittee of the American Academy of Neurology and the Practice Committee of the Child Neurology Society

ABSTRACT. *Objective*: The Quality Standards Subcommittee of the American Academy of Neurology and the Practice Committee of the Child Neurology Society develop practice parameters as strategies for patient management based on analysis of evidence. For this parameter the authors reviewed available evidence on the assessment of a child suspected of having cerebral palsy (CP), a nonprogressive disorder of posture or movement due to a lesion of the developing brain.

Methods: Relevant literature was reviewed, abstracted, and classified. Recommendations were based on a four-tiered scheme of evidence classification.

Results: CP is a common problem, occurring in about 2 to 2.5 per 1,000 live births. In order to establish that a brain abnormality exists in children with CP that may, in turn, suggest an etiology and prognosis, neuroimaging is recommended with MRI preferred to CT (Level A). Metabolic and genetic studies should not be routinely obtained in the evaluation of the child with CP (Level B). If the clinical history or findings on neuroimaging do not determine a specific structural abnormality or if there are additional and atypical features in the history or clinical examination, metabolic and genetic testing should be considered (Level C). Detection of a brain malformation in a child with CP warrants consideration of an underlying genetic or metabolic etiology. Because the incidence of cerebral infarction is high in children with hemiplegic CP, diagnostic testing for coagulation disorders should be considered (Level B). However, there is insufficient evidence at present to be precise as to what studies should be ordered. An EEG is not recommended unless there are features suggestive of epilepsy or a specific epileptic syndrome (Level A). Because children with CP may have associated deficits of mental retardation, ophthalmologic and hearing impairments, speech and language disorders, and oral-motor dysfunction, screening for these conditions should be part of the initial assessment (Level A).

Conclusions: Neuroimaging results in children with CP are commonly abnormal and may help determine the etiology. Screening for associated conditions is warranted as part of the initial evaluation. (3/04)

CONSTIPATION

Constipation in Infants and Children: Evaluation and Treatment

North American Society of Pediatric Gastroenterology, Hepatology, and Nutrition

ABSTRACT. **Background** Constipation, defined as a delay or difficulty in defecation, present for two or more weeks, is a common pediatric problem encountered by both primary and specialty medical providers.

Methods The Constipation Subcommittee of the Clinical Guidelines Committee of the North American Society for Pediatric Gastroenterology and Nutrition has formulated clinical practice guidelines for the management of pediatric constipation. The Constipation Subcommittee, consisting of two primary care pediatricians, a clinical epidemiologist and pediatric gastroenterologists, based its recommendations on an integration of a comprehensive and systematic review of the medical literature combined with expert opinion. Consensus was achieved through Nominal Group Technique, a structured quantitative method.

Results The Subcommittee developed two algorithms to assist with medical management, one for older infants and children and the second for infants less than one year of age. The guidelines provide recommendations for management by the primary care provider, including evaluation, initial treatment, follow-up management and indications for consultation by a specialist. The Constipation Subcommittee also provided recommendations for management by the pediatric gastroenterologist.

Conclusion This report, which has been endorsed by the Executive Council of the North American Society for Pediatric Gastroenterology and Nutrition, has been prepared as a general guideline to assist providers of medical care in the evaluation and treatment of constipation in children. It is not intended as a substitute for clinical judgment or as a protocol for the management of all patients with this problem. (3/00)

FLUORIDE
Recommendations for Using Fluoride to Prevent and Control Dental Caries in the United States

Centers for Disease Control and Prevention (8/01)

GASTROENTERITIS
Managing Acute Gastroenteritis Among Children: Oral Rehydration, Maintenance, and Nutritional Therapy

Centers for Disease Control and Prevention (11/03)

GASTROESOPHAGEAL REFLUX
Guidelines for Evaluation and Treatment of Gastroesophageal Reflux in Infants and Children

North American Society of Pediatric Gastroenterology, Hepatology, and Nutrition

ABSTRACT. Gastroesophageal reflux (GER), defined as passage of gastric contents into the esophagus, and GER disease (GERD), defined as symptoms or complications of GER, are common pediatric problems encountered by both primary and specialty medical providers. Clinical manifestations of GERD in children include vomiting, poor weight gain, dysphagia, abdominal or substernal pain, esophagitis and respiratory disorders. The GER Guideline Committee of the North American Society for Pediatric Gastroenterology and Nutrition has formulated a clinical practice guideline for the management of pediatric GER. The GER Guideline Committee, consisting of a primary care pediatrician, two clinical epidemiologists (who also practice primary care pediatrics) and five pediatric gastroenterologists, based its recommendations on an integration of a comprehensive and systematic review of the medical literature combined with expert opinion. Consensus was achieved through Nominal Group Technique, a structured quantitative method.

The Committee examined the value of diagnostic tests and treatment modalities commonly used for the management of GERD, and how those interventions can be applied to clinical situations in the infant and older child. The guideline provides recommendations for management by the primary care provider, including evaluation, initial treatment, follow-up management and indications for consultation by a specialist. The guideline also provides recommendations for management by the pediatric gastroenterologist.

This document represents the official recommendations of the North American Society for Pediatric Gastroenterology and Nutrition on the evaluation and treatment of gastroesophageal reflux in infants and children. The American Academy of Pediatrics has also endorsed these recommendations. The recommendations are summarized in a synopsis within the article. This review and recommendations are a general guideline and are not intended as a substitute for clinical judgment or as a protocol for the management of all patients with this problem. (2001)

GROUP B STREPTOCOCCAL DISEASE
Prevention of Perinatal Group B Streptococcal Disease

Centers for Disease Control and Prevention (8/02)

HELICOBACTER PYLORI INFECTION
Helicobacter pylori Infection in Children: Recommendations for Diagnosis and Treatment

North American Society of Pediatric Gastroenterology, Hepatology, and Nutrition (11/00)

HEMATOPOIETIC STEM CELL TRANSPLANT
Guidelines for Preventing Opportunistic Infections Among Hematopoietic Stem Cell Transplant Recipients

Centers for Disease Control and Prevention, Infectious Diseases Society of America, and the American Society of Blood and Marrow Transplantation (10/00)

INTRAVASCULAR CATHETER-RELATED INFECTIONS
Guidelines for the Prevention of Intravascular Catheter-Related Infections

Society of Critical Care Medicine, Infectious Diseases Society of America, Society for Healthcare Epidemiology of America, Surgical Infection Society, American College of Chest Physicians, American Thoracic Society, American Society of Critical Care Anesthesiologists, Association for Professionals in Infection Control and Epidemiology, Infusion Nurses Society, Oncology Nursing Society, Society of Cardiovascular and Interventional Radiology, American Academy of Pediatrics, and the Healthcare Infection Control Practices Advisory Committee of the Centers for Disease Control and Prevention

ABSTRACT. These guidelines have been developed for practitioners who insert catheters and for persons responsible for surveillance and control of infections in hospital, outpatient, and home health-care settings. This report was prepared by a working group comprising members from professional organizations representing the disciplines of critical care medicine, infectious diseases, health-care infection control, surgery, anesthesiology, interventional radiology, pulmonary medicine, pediatric medicine, and nursing. The working group was led by the Society of Critical Care Medicine (SCCM), in collaboration with the Infectious Disease Society of America (IDSA), Society for Healthcare Epidemiology of America (SHEA), Surgical Infection Society (SIS), American College of Chest Physicians (ACCP), American Thoracic Society (ATS), American Society of Critical Care Anesthesiologists (ASCCA), Association for Professionals in Infection Control and Epidemiology (APIC), Infusion Nurses Society (INS), Oncology Nursing Society (ONS), Society of Cardiovascular and Interventional Radiology (SCVIR), American Academy of Pediatrics (AAP), and the Healthcare Infection Control Practices Advisory Committee (HICPAC) of the Centers for Disease Control and Prevention (CDC) and is intended to replace the *Guideline for Prevention of Intravascular Device-Related Infections* published in 1996. These guidelines are intended to provide evidence-based recommendations for preventing catheter-related infections. Major areas of emphasis include 1) educating and training health-care providers who insert and maintain catheters; 2) using maximal sterile barrier precautions during central venous catheter insertion; 3) using a 2% chlorhexidine preparation for skin antisepsis; 4) avoiding routine replacement of central venous catheters as a strategy to prevent infection; and 5) using antiseptic/antibiotic impregnated short-term central venous catheters if the rate of infection is high despite adherence to other strategies (ie, education and training, maximal sterile barrier precautions, and 2% chlorhexidine for skin antisepsis). These guidelines also identify performance indicators that can be used locally by healthcare institutions or organizations to monitor their success in implementing these evidence-based recommendations. (2002)

LYME DISEASE

Practice Guidelines for the Treatment of Lyme Disease

Infectious Diseases Society of America (9/00)

MIGRAINE HEADACHE

Pharmacological Treatment of Migraine Headache in Children and Adolescents

Quality Standards Subcommittee of the American Academy of Neurology and the Practice Committee of the Child Neurology Society (12/04)

PALLIATIVE CARE

Clinical Practice Guidelines for Quality Palliative Care

National Consensus Project for Quality Palliative Care (5/04)

RADIOLOGY

Neuroimaging of the Neonate

Quality Standards Subcommittee of the American Academy of Neurology and the Practice Committee of the Child Neurology Society

ABSTRACT. *Objective:* The authors reviewed available evidence on neonatal neuroimaging strategies for evaluating both very low birth weight preterm infants and encephalopathic term neonates. *Imaging for the preterm neonate:* Routine screening cranial ultrasonography (US) should be performed on all infants of <30 weeks' gestation once between 7 and 14 days of age and should be optimally repeated between 36 and 40 weeks' postmenstrual age. This strategy detects lesions such as intraventricular hemorrhage, which influences clinical care, and those such as periventricular leukomalacia and low-pressure ventriculomegaly, which provide information about long-term neurodevelopmental outcome. There is insufficient evidence for routine MRI of all very low birth weight preterm infants with abnormal results of cranial US. *Imaging for the term infant:* Noncontrast CT should be performed to detect hemorrhagic lesions in the encephalopathic term infant with a history of birth trauma, low hematocrit, or coagulopathy. If CT findings are inconclusive, MRI should be performed between days 2 and 8 to assess the location and extent of injury. The pattern of injury identified with conventional MRI may provide diagnostic and prognostic information for term infants with evidence of encephalopathy. In particular, basal ganglia and thalamic lesions detected by conventional MRI are associated with poor neurodevelopmental outcome. Diffusion-weighted imaging may allow earlier detection of these cerebral injuries. *Recommendations:* US plays an established role in the management of preterm neonates of <30 weeks' gestation. US also provides valuable prognostic information when the infant reaches 40 weeks' postmenstrual age. For encephalopathic term infants, early CT should be used to exclude hemorrhage; MRI should be performed later in the first postnatal week to establish the pattern of injury and predict neurologic outcome. (6/02)

SEIZURE

Evaluating a First Nonfebrile Seizure in Children

Quality Standards Subcommittee of the American Academy of Neurology, the Child Neurology Society, and the American Epilepsy Society

ABSTRACT: Objective: The Quality Standards Subcommittee of the American Academy of Neurology develops practice parameters as strategies for patient management based on analysis of evidence. For this practice parameter, the authors reviewed available evidence on evaluation of the first nonfebrile seizure in children in order to make practice recommendations based on this available evidence. Methods: Multiple searches revealed relevant literature and each article was reviewed, abstracted, and classified. Recommendations were based on a three-tiered scheme of classification of the evidence. Results: Routine EEG as part of the diagnostic evaluation was recommended; other studies such as laboratory evaluations and neuroimaging studies were recommended as based on specific clinical circumstances. Conclusions: Further studies are needed using large, well-characterized samples and standardized data collection instruments. Collection of data regarding appropriate timing of evaluations would be important. (8/00)

Treatment of the Child With a First Unprovoked Seizure

Quality Standards Subcommittee of the American Academy of Neurology and the Practice Committee of the Child Neurology Society

ABSTRACT. The Quality Standards Subcommittee of the American Academy of Neurology and the Practice Committee of the Child Neurology Society develop practice parameters as strategies for patient management based on analysis of evidence regarding risks and benefits. This parameter reviews published literature relevant to the decision to begin treatment after a child or adolescent experiences a first unprovoked seizure and presents evidence-based practice recommendations. Reasons why treatment may be considered are discussed. Evidence is reviewed concerning risk of recurrence as well as effect of treatment on prevention of recurrence and development of chronic epilepsy. Studies of side effects of anticonvulsants commonly used to treat seizures in children are also reviewed. Relevant articles are classified according to the Quality Standards Subcommittee classification scheme. Treatment after a first unprovoked seizure appears to decrease the risk of a second seizure, but there are few data from studies involving only children. There appears to be no benefit of treatment with regard to the prognosis for long-term seizure remission. Antiepileptic drugs (AED) carry risks of side effects that are particularly important in children. The decision as to whether or not to treat children and adolescents who have experienced a first unprovoked seizure must be based on a risk–benefit assessment that weighs the risk of having another seizure against the risk of chronic AED therapy. The decision should be individualized and take into account both medical issues and patient and family preference. (1/03)

SPORTS MEDICINE
Prehospital Care of the Spine-Injured Athlete

Inter-Association Task Force for Appropriate Care of the Spine-Injured Athlete

ABSTRACT. *Objective:* The primary purpose of this paper is to provide guidelines for the prehospital management of a physically active person with a suspected spinal injury. A secondary purpose is to provide additional information that, although beyond the scope of prehospital care, may prove to be useful in understanding the need for a comprehensive approach when treating the spine and is valuable to the different types of clinicians for whom this document is intended.

Background: For many years, disagreements have occurred among various healthcare professionals as to the proper management of a spine-injured athlete, because each group of professionals had their own protocols. In 1998, the National Athletic Trainers' Association formed an inter-association task force to develop guidelines for the appropriate management of the catastrophically spine-injured athlete. Although not all catastrophic injuries are spine injuries and not all spine injuries are catastrophic, it is believed that the improper management of a suspected spinal injury can result in a secondary injury. Thus, it was important to develop standard guidelines to be used by all providers of prehospital care that ensured the safe management of the spine-injured athlete.

Recommendations: The Inter-Association Task Force for Appropriate Care of the Spine-Injured Athlete developed guidelines that were endorsed by the representatives of various healthcare specialties, including certified athletic trainers, physicians, and providers of emergency medical services. This paper provides more details and more thorough information on the guidelines that were developed and endorsed by the task force. (2001)

TOBACCO USE
Treating Tobacco Use and Dependence

US Department of Health and Human Services

ABSTRACT (excerpt). *Treating Tobacco Use and Dependence,* a Public Health Service-sponsored Clinical Practice Guideline, is a product of the Tobacco Use and Dependence Guideline Panel (ìthe panelî), consortium representatives, consultants, and staff. These 30 individuals were charged with the responsibility of identifying effective, experimentally validated tobacco dependence treatments and practices. The updated guideline was sponsored by a consortium of seven Federal Government and nonprofit organizations: the Agency for Healthcare Research and Quality (AHRQ); Centers for Disease Control and Prevention (CDC); National Cancer Institute (NCI); National Heart, Lung, and Blood Institute (NHLBI); National Institute on Drug Abuse (NIDA); Robert Wood Johnson Foundation (RWJF); and University of Wisconsin Medical School's Center for Tobacco Research and Intervention (CTRI). This guideline is an updated version of the 1996 *Smoking Cessation Clinical Practice Guideline No. 18* that was sponsored by the Agency for Health Care Policy and Research (now the AHRQ), U.S. Department of Health and Human Services. The original guideline reflected the extant scientific research literature published between 1975 and 1994.

The updated guideline was written because new, effective clinical treatments for tobacco dependence have been identified since 1994. The accelerating pace of tobacco research that prompted the update is reflected in the fact that 3,000 articles on tobacco were identified as published between 1975 and 1994, contributing to the original guideline. Another 3,000 were published between 1995 and 1999 and contributed to the updated guideline. These 6,000 articles were screened and reviewed to identify a much smaller group of articles that served as the basis for guideline data analyses and panel opinion.

This guideline contains strategies and recommendations designed to assist clinicians; tobacco dependence treatment specialists; and health care administrators, insurers, and purchasers in delivering and supporting effective treatments for tobacco use and dependence.... (6/00)

VESICOURETERAL REFLUX
Report on the Management of Primary Vesicoureteral Reflux in Children

American Urological Association (5/97)

SECTION 3

2004 Policies

From the American Academy of Pediatrics

• •

- ## *Policy Statements*
  ORGANIZATIONAL PRINCIPLES TO GUIDE AND DEFINE THE CHILD HEALTH CARE SYSTEM
  AND/OR IMPROVE THE HEALTH OF ALL CHILDREN

- ## *Clinical Reports*
  GUIDANCE FOR THE CLINICIAN IN RENDERING PEDIATRIC CARE

- ## *Technical Reports*
  BACKGROUND INFORMATION TO SUPPORT AMERICAN ACADEMY OF PEDIATRICS POLICY

INTRODUCTION

This section of the *Pediatric Clinical Practice Guidelines & Policies: A Compendium of Evidence-based Research for Pediatric Practice* manual is composed of policy statements, clinical reports, and technical reports issued by the American Academy of Pediatrics (AAP) and is designed as a quick reference tool for AAP members, staff, and other interested parties. Section 3 includes the full text of all AAP policies published in 2004. Section 4 is a compilation of all active AAP statements (through December 2004) arranged alphabetically, with abstracts where applicable. A committee index and subject index are also available. The enclosed CD-ROM contains the full text of all current policy statements, clinical reports, and technical reports (through December 2004). These materials should help answer questions that arise about the AAP position on child health care issues. **However, it should be remembered that AAP policy statements, clinical reports, and technical reports do not indicate an exclusive course of treatment or serve as a standard of medical care. Variations, taking into account individual circumstances, may be appropriate.**

The policy statements have been written by AAP committees, task forces, or sections and approved by the AAP Board of Directors. Most of these statements have appeared previously in *Pediatrics*, *AAP News*, or *News & Comments* (the forerunner of *AAP News*).

This section does not contain all AAP policies. It does not include

- Press releases.
- Motions and resolutions that were approved by the Board of Directors. These can be found in the Board of Directors' minutes.
- Policies in manuals, pamphlets, booklets, or other AAP publications. These items can be ordered through the AAP. Visit and order from our online Bookstore at www.aap.org/bookstore or call toll-free 888/227-1770.
- Testimony before Congress or government agencies.

Admission and Discharge Guidelines for the Pediatric Patient Requiring Intermediate Care

● ●

- *Clinical Report*

AMERICAN ACADEMY OF PEDIATRICS

CLINICAL REPORT
Guidance for the Clinician in Rendering Pediatric Care

David G. Jaimovich, MD, and the Committee on Hospital Care and Section on Critical Care

Admission and Discharge Guidelines for the Pediatric Patient Requiring Intermediate Care

ABSTRACT. During the past 3 decades, the specialty of pediatric critical care medicine has grown rapidly, leading to a number of pediatric intensive care units opening across the country. Many patients who are admitted to the hospital require a higher level of care than routine inpatient general pediatric care, yet not to the degree of intensity of pediatric critical care; therefore, an intermediate care level has been developed in institutions providing multidisciplinary subspecialty pediatric care. These patients may require frequent monitoring of vital signs and nursing interventions, but usually they do not require invasive monitoring. The admission of the pediatric intermediate care patient is guided by physiologic parameters depending on the respective organ system involved relative to an institution's resources and capacity to care for a patient in a general care environment. This report provides admission and discharge guidelines for intermediate pediatric care. Intermediate care promotes greater flexibility in patient triage and provides a cost-effective alternative to admission to a pediatric intensive care unit. This level of care may enhance the efficiency of care and make health care more affordable for patients receiving intermediate care. *Pediatrics* 2004; 113:1430–1433; *coordination of care, admission, discharge, multidisciplinary, intermediate care.*

The purpose of this statement is to provide lists of criteria that may be incorporated into multidisciplinary guidelines for the admission and discharge of children requiring intermediate care. Because of the continuous and rapidly changing developments in critical care pediatrics, these criteria may require periodic revision. Equally important, because of significant differences in personnel, facilities, and diagnostic and treatment capabilities from hospital to hospital, no single set of criteria will apply to every institution providing intermediate care.

Intermediate care is provided in acute care hospitals to a patient population with a severity of illness that does not require intensive care but does require greater services than those provided by routine inpatient general pediatric care. These patients may require frequent monitoring of vital signs and/or nursing interventions but usually will not require

invasive monitoring. The development of intermediate care services has been proposed as an appropriate means to enhance resource utilization for intermediately ill patients.[1–4] In light of the recent emphasis on cost containment, intermediate care promotes flexibility in patient triage, provides pediatric patients with monitoring and therapies tailored to their severity of illness, and may be a cost-effective alternative to admission to a pediatric intensive care unit. Patients with a low risk of, but potential for, significant deterioration and who are admitted for routine monitoring are excellent candidates for intermediate care.

Intermediate care is ideally provided in facilities that have a pediatric intensive care unit.[5] However, these resources may not be widely available, particularly in geographically remote regions, where tertiary pediatric centers may be several hours and hundreds of miles away. Therefore, this statement is also intended to provide guidance for the care of children requiring intermediate care in hospitals without a pediatric intensive care unit. These hospitals should ensure that the resources, facilities, and personnel needed to provide care beyond the level of a general pediatric medical-surgical unit are available; furthermore, they should have the ability to immediately stabilize a child who becomes critically ill. In addition, these hospitals should identify facilities with pediatric intensive care units to which patients can be transferred if their condition worsens.[6] Established transfer policies with these facilities can ensure timely and effective transition of care for these patients.

In a hospital that has a pediatric intensive care unit, these intermediate care admission and discharge guidelines should be compatible with the admission and discharge guidelines for the hospital's pediatric intensive care unit.[6] This statement provides a framework for individual hospitals to establish admission and discharge criteria for intermediate pediatric care. It is intended that these guidelines be modified by individual institutions, depending on the availability of resources, personnel, and equipment necessary to evaluate and treat a seriously ill child.

Physiologic parameters may be added to these guidelines according to individual patient care unit and institutional policies so that triage may be pro-

PEDIATRICS (ISSN 0031 4005). Copyright © 2004 by the American Academy of Pediatrics.

vided appropriately into and out of intermediate care. These criteria will need to be studied in relation to outcomes over the next several years, such as is done for pediatric intensive care units nationwide. Until that time these criteria, based on expert opinion, may assist hospitals and physicians in creating a safe environment for children with a higher intensity of service needs.

GUIDELINES FOR THE PATIENT REQUIRING INTERMEDIATE CARE

I. Respiratory Diseases

Patients with moderate pulmonary or airway disease requiring multidisciplinary intervention and frequent monitoring, including but not limited to the following, may be admitted:

A. Patients with the potential need for endotracheal intubation.
B. Patients requiring minimal support with mechanical ventilation delivered by mature and stable tracheostomy. This would apply primarily to children with chronic respiratory insufficiency.
C. Patients with progressive pulmonary (lower or upper airway) disease of moderate severity with risk of progression to respiratory failure or with obstruction potential.
D. Patients acutely requiring supplemental oxygen (fraction of inspired oxygen $\geq$0.5), regardless of cause.
E. Stable tracheotomy patients.
F. Patients requiring frequent (at intervals <2 hours), intermittent, or continuous nebulized medications (according to institutional guidelines).
G. Patients requiring apnea work-up and cardiorespiratory monitoring.

II. Cardiovascular Diseases

Patients with moderate cardiovascular disease requiring multidisciplinary intervention and frequent monitoring, including but not limited to the following, may be admitted:

A. Patients with non–life-threatening dysrhythmias with or without the need for cardioversion.
B. Patients with non–life-threatening cardiac disease requiring low-dose intravenous inotropic or vasodilator therapy.
C. Patients undergoing high-risk cardiac procedures who require close monitoring and who do not have hemodynamic or respiratory compromise.
D. Patients who have undergone closed-heart cardiovascular and intrathoracic surgical procedures, including patent ductus-arteriosis repair, vascular shunts, permanent pacemaker placement, and open thoracotomy who do not have hemodynamic or respiratory compromise.

III. Neurologic Diseases

Patients with non–life-threatening neurologic disease requiring multidisciplinary intervention, frequent monitoring, and neurologic assessment not more than every 2 hours, including but not limited to the following, may be admitted:

A. Patients with seizures who are responsive to therapy but require continuous cardiorespiratory monitoring and who do not have hemodynamic compromise but have the potential for respiratory compromise.
B. Patients with altered sensorium in whom neurologic deterioration or depression is unlikely and neurologic assessment is required.
C. Postoperative neurosurgical patients requiring cardiorespiratory monitoring.
D. Patients with acute inflammation or infections of the central nervous system without neurologic deficiency or other complications.
E. Patients with head trauma without progressive neurologic signs or symptoms.
F. Patients with progressive neuromuscular dysfunction without altered sensorium requiring cardiorespiratory monitoring.

IV. Hematologic/Oncologic Diseases

Patients with potentially unstable hematologic or oncologic disease or non–life-threatening bleeding requiring multidisciplinary intervention and frequent monitoring, including but not limited to the following, may be admitted:

A. Patients with severe anemia without hemodynamic or respiratory compromise.
B. Patients with moderate complications of sickle cell crisis, such as respiratory distress, without acute chest syndrome.
C. Patients with thrombocytopenia, anemia, neutropenia, or solid tumor who are at risk of cardiopulmonary compromise but who are currently stable and, as a result, require close cardiorespiratory monitoring.

V. Endocrine/Metabolic Diseases

Patients with potentially unstable endocrine or metabolic disease requiring multidisciplinary intervention and frequent monitoring, including but not limited to the following, may be admitted:

A. Patients with moderate diabetic ketoacidosis (blood glucose concentration <500 mg/dL or pH $\geq$7.2) requiring continuous insulin infusion therapy without altered sensorium.
B. Patients with other moderate electrolyte and/or metabolic abnormalities (requiring cardiac monitoring and therapeutic intervention), such as:
   1. Hypokalemia (blood potassium concentration <2.0 mEq) and hyperkalemia (blood potassium concentration >6.0 mEq)
   2. Hyponatremia and hypernatremia with alterations in clinical status (ie, seizures or altered mental status)
   3. Hypocalcemia or hypercalcemia.
   4. Hypoglycemia or hyperglycemia.
   5. Moderate metabolic acidosis requiring bicarbonate infusion.
C. Patients with inborn errors of metabolism requiring cardiorespiratory monitoring.

VI. Gastrointestinal Diseases

Patients with potentially unstable gastrointestinal disease requiring multidisciplinary intervention and frequent monitoring, including but not limited to the following, may be admitted:

A. Patients with acute gastrointestinal bleeding but who do not have hemodynamic or respiratory instability.
B. Patients with a gastrointestinal foreign body or other gastrointestinal problem requiring emergency endoscopy but who do not have cardiorespiratory compromise.
C. Patients who have chronic gastrointestinal or hepatobiliary insufficiency but do not have coma, hemodynamic, or respiratory instability.

VII. Surgery

All patients requiring multidisciplinary intervention and frequent monitoring who have undergone surgical procedures but who do not have hemodynamic or respiratory instability, including but not limited to the following, may be admitted:

A. Patients who have undergone cardiovascular surgery.
B. Patients who have undergone thoracic surgery.
C. Patients who have undergone neurosurgical procedures.
D. Patients who have undergone upper or lower airway surgery.
E. Patients who have undergone craniofacial surgery.
F. Patients who have had thoracic or abdominal trauma.
G. Patients being treated for multiple traumatic injuries.

VIII. Renal Diseases

Patients with potentially unstable renal disease requiring multidisciplinary intervention and frequent monitoring, including but not limited to the following, may be admitted:

A. Patients with hypertension without seizures, encephalopathy, or other symptoms, but who require frequent intermittent therapeutic intravenous or orally administered medication.
B. Patients with noncomplicated nephrotic syndrome (regardless of cause) with chronic hypertension requiring frequent blood pressure monitoring.
C. Patients with renal failure, regardless of cause.
D. Patients requiring chronic hemodialysis or peritoneal dialysis.

IX. Multisystem and Other Diseases

Patients with potentially unstable multisystem disease requiring multidisciplinary intervention and frequent monitoring, including but not limited to the following, may be admitted:

A. Patients requiring the application of special technologic needs, including:
   1. Use of respiratory assistance, such as continuous positive airway pressure, bilevel positive airway pressure, or chronic home ventilation.
   2. Tracheostomy care requiring frequent pulmonary hygiene and suctioning.
   3. Pleural or pericardial drains after initial stabilization (for patients who do not have respiratory or hemodynamic compromise).
   4. Medications or resource needs in excess of those provided in the general patient care unit.
B. Patients who are direct admissions from another health care facility outside the hospital (may be directly admitted for intermediate care).
C. Patients with uncomplicated toxic ingestion who do not have cardiovascular or respiratory compromise and who require cardiorespiratory monitoring.

DISCHARGE AND TRANSFER GUIDELINES FOR THE INTERMEDIATE CARE PATIENT

Patients will be evaluated and considered for transfer to general care or special care units when the disease process has reversed or the physiologic condition that prompted admission has resolved and the need for multidisciplinary intervention and treatment is no longer present.

The decision to transfer or discharge to home will be made on the basis of the following criteria:

A. If patient's condition deteriorates and he or she requires care beyond the capabilities of the unit providing intermediate care, he or she should be admitted or readmitted to a pediatric intensive care unit.
B. Patient should be transferred to a floor or specialty care unit or discharged from the hospital, as appropriate, if the following criteria apply:
   1. Patient has stable hemodynamic parameters for at least 6 to 12 hours.
   2. Patient has stable respiratory status and has been extubated with evidence of acceptable gas exchange for more than 4 hours.
   3. Patient has minimal oxygen requirements as evidenced by a fraction of inspired oxygen of 0.4 or less.
   4. Intravenous inotropic support, vasodilators, and antiarrhythmic drugs are no longer required, or, when applicable, low doses of these medications may be administered to otherwise stable patients in a designated patient care unit.
   5. Cardiac arrhythmias are controlled for a reasonable period of time but not less than 24 hours.
   6. Patient has neurologic stability with control of seizures for a reasonable period of time.
   7. All invasive hemodynamic monitoring devices have been removed (eg, arterial lines).
   8. Patient who had required chronic mechanical ventilation and has experienced resolution of the acute illness that required intermediate or

intensive care has now returned to baseline clinical status.

9. Patient will require peritoneal dialysis or hemodialysis on a routine basis and therefore may receive these treatments as an outpatient or in a designated patient care unit.

10. The need for multidisciplinary intervention is predictable and compatible with policies of the receiving patient care unit.

11. The health care team, after careful multidisciplinary assessment and together with the patient's family, decides that there would be no benefit to keeping the child hospitalized or that the course of treatment is medically futile.

COMMITTEE ON HOSPITAL CARE, 2001-2002
John M. Neff, MD, Chairperson
Jerrold M. Eichner, MD
David R. Hardy, MD
Jack M. Percelay, MD, MPH
Ted Sigrest, MD
Erin R. Stucky, MD

LIAISONS
Susan Dull, RN, MSN, MBA
  National Association of Children's Hospitals and Related Institutions
Mary T. Perkins, RN, DNSc
  American Hospital Association
Jerriann M. Wilson, CCLS, MEd
  Child Life Council

CONSULTANTS
Timothy E. Corden, MD
Michael D. Klein, MD
Mary O'Connor, MD, MPH
Theodore Striker, MD

STAFF
Stephanie Mucha, MPH

SECTION ON CRITICAL CARE, 2001-2002
M. Michele Moss, MD, Chairperson
Alice Ackerman, MD
Thomas Bojko, MD
Brahm Goldstein, MD
Stephanie A. Storgion, MD
Otwell Timmons, MD

LIAISON
Richard J. Brilli, MD
  Society of Critical Care Medicine

CONSULTANTS
Lynda J. Means, MD
Anthony L. Pearson-Shaver, MD
Timothy S. Yeh, MD, Immediate Past Chairperson

STAFF
Sue Tellez

SOCIETY OF CRITICAL CARE MEDICINE
  PEDIATRIC SECTION, ADMISSION CRITERIA TASK FORCE
David G. Jaimovich, MD, Chairperson
Lucian K. DeNicola, MD
Gabriel "Gabby" Hauser, MD
Jan Kronick, MD
Kristan Outwater, MD
Tom Rice, MD
Kathy Rosenthal, RN, MN, CCRN
Sara White, MD
Madolin Witte, MD

REFERENCES

1. Zimmerman JE, Wagner DP, Knaus WA, Williams JF, Kolakowski D, Draper EA. The use of risk predictions to identify candidates for intermediate care units: implications for intensive care utilization and cost. *Chest.* 1995;108:490–499

2. Teres D, Steingrub J. Can intermediate care substitute for intensive care? *Crit Care Med.* 1987;15:280

3. Popovich J Jr. Intermediate care units: graded care options. *Chest.* 1991; 99:4–5

4. Kalb PE, Miller DH. Utilization strategies for intensive care units. JAMA. 1989;261:2389–2395

5. American Academy of Pediatrics, Committee on Hospital Care; and Society of Critical Care Medicine, Pediatric Section. Guidelines and levels of care for pediatric intensive care units. *Pediatrics.* 1993;92:166–175

6. American Academy of Pediatrics, Committee on Hospital Care and Section on Critical Care; and Society of Critical Care Medicine, Pediatric Section, Admission Criteria Task Force. Guidelines for developing admission and discharge policies for the pediatric intensive care unit. *Pediatrics.* 1999;103:840–842

All clinical reports from the American Academy of Pediatrics automatically expire 5 years after publication unless reaffirmed, revised, or retired at or before that time.

Age Terminology During the Perinatal Period

- *Policy Statement*

AMERICAN ACADEMY OF PEDIATRICS

Policy Statement
Organizational Principles to Guide and Define the Child Health Care System and/or Improve the Health of All Children

Committee on Fetus and Newborn

Age Terminology During the Perinatal Period

ABSTRACT. Consistent definitions to describe the length of gestation and age in neonates are needed to compare neurodevelopmental, medical, and growth outcomes. The purposes of this policy statement are to review conventional definitions of age during the perinatal period and to recommend use of standard terminology including gestational age, postmenstrual age, chronological age, corrected age, adjusted age, and estimated date of delivery. *Pediatrics* 2004;114:1362–1364; *gestational age, postmenstrual age, chronological age, menstrual age, conceptional age, postconceptual age, corrected age, adjusted age, estimated date of delivery, estimated date of confinement.*

INTRODUCTION

Consistent definitions to describe the length of gestation and age in neonates are needed to compare neurodevelopmental, medical, and growth outcomes. The terms "gestational age," "postmenstrual age," "corrected age," and "postconceptional age" have frequently been defined unconventionally,[1,2] misapplied,[3–5] or left undefined.[6,7] Inconsistent use of terminology limits the accurate interpretation of data on health outcomes for newborn infants, especially for those born preterm or conceived using assisted reproductive technology. The purposes of this statement are to review conventional definitions of age during the perinatal period and to recommend standard terminology.

"Gestational age" (or "menstrual age") is the time elapsed between the first day of the last normal menstrual period and the day of delivery (Fig 1).[8–10] The first day of the last menstrual period occurs approximately 2 weeks before ovulation and approximately 3 weeks before implantation of the blastocyst. Because most women know when their last period began but not when ovulation occurred, this definition traditionally has been used when estimating the expected date of delivery. As long as menstrual dates are remembered accurately, this method of estimating the date of delivery is reliable.[11] Minor inaccuracy (4–6 days) in the expected date of delivery determined from menstrual dates is attributable to inherent biological variability in the relative timing of onset of the last menstrual period, fertilization of the egg, and implantation of the blastocyst.[12] Additional inaccuracy (weeks) may occur in women

who have menstrual cycles that are irregular or variable in duration or if breakthrough bleeding occurs around the time of conception. Gestational age is conventionally expressed as completed weeks. Therefore, a 25-week, 5-day fetus is considered a 25-week fetus. To round the gestational age of such a fetus to 26 weeks is inconsistent with national and international norms.[2] The term "gestational age" should be used instead of "menstrual age" to describe the age of the fetus or newborn infant.

"Chronological age" (or "postnatal" age) is the time elapsed after birth (Fig 1). It is usually described in days, weeks, months, and/or years. This is different from the term "postmenstrual age." Postmenstrual age is the time elapsed between the first day of the last menstrual period and birth (gestational age) plus the time elapsed after birth (chronological age). Postmenstrual age is usually described in number of weeks and is most frequently applied during the perinatal period beginning after the day of birth. Therefore, a preterm infant born at a gestational age of 33 weeks who is currently 10 weeks old (chronological age) would have a postmenstrual age of 43 weeks. When postmenstrual age is quantitated in weeks and days for postnatal management reasons, a 33-week, 1-day gestational age infant who is 10 weeks, 5 days chronological age would have a postmenstrual age of 43 weeks, 6 days.

"Corrected age" (or "adjusted age") is a term most appropriately used to describe children up to 3 years of age who were born preterm (Fig 1). This term is preferred to "corrected gestational age" or "gestational age" and represents the age of the child from the expected date of delivery.[13,14] Corrected age is calculated by subtracting the number of weeks born before 40 weeks of gestation from the chronological age. Therefore, a 24-month-old, former 28-week gestational age infant has a corrected age of 21 months according to the following equation:

$$24 \text{ months} - [(40 \text{ weeks} - 28 \text{ weeks})$$
$$\times 1 \text{ month}/4 \text{ weeks}]$$

Corrected age and chronological age are not synonymous in preterm infants. Additionally, the term "corrected age" should be used instead of "adjusted age."

"Conceptional age" is the time elapsed between the day of conception and the day of delivery. (The term "conceptual age" is incorrect and should not be

doi:10.1542/peds.2004-1915
PEDIATRICS (ISSN 0031 4005). Copyright © 2004 by the American Academy of Pediatrics.

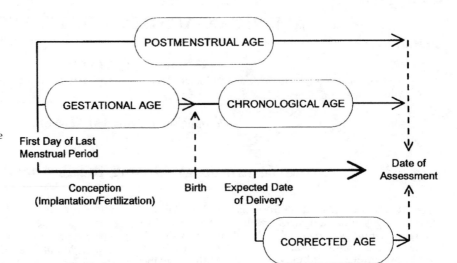

Fig 1. Age terminology during the perinatal period.

used.) Because assisted reproductive technologies accurately define the date of fertilization or implantation, a precise conceptional age can be determined in pregnancies resulting from such technologies. Much of the variability inherent in other methods of gestational age determination,[11–13] except for that attributed to timing of implantation, is eliminated when the date of conception is determined during assisted reproductive procedures. The convention for calculating gestational age when the date of conception is known is to add 2 weeks to the conceptional age.[10] Therefore, gestational age is 2 weeks longer than conceptional age; they are not synonymous terms. When describing the age of a fetus or neonate, "gestational age" is the term conventionally applied. This is particularly important for interpreting outcome studies of preterm infants. As an example, a preterm infant conceived using assisted reproductive technology who has a conceptional age of 25 weeks has a gestational age of 27 weeks. Outcomes for this infant should be compared with those of 27-week gestational age infants, not 25-week gestational age infants. To avoid confusion, the term "gestational age" should be used. The terms "conceptional age" and "postconceptional age," reflecting the time elapsed after conception, should not be used.

Gestational age is often determined by the "best obstetric estimate," which is based on a combination of the first day of last menstrual period, physical examination of the mother, prenatal ultrasonography, and history of assisted reproduction. The best obstetric estimate is necessary because of gaps in obstetric information and the inherent variability (as great as 2 weeks) in methods of gestational age estimation.[8,10,14–19] Postnatal physical examination of the infant is sometimes used as a method to determine gestational age if the best obstetric estimate seems inaccurate. Therefore, methods of determining gestational age should be clearly stated so that the variability inherent in these estimations can be considered when outcomes are interpreted.[8,10,14–19]

RECOMMENDATIONS

1. Standardized terminology should be used when defining ages and comparing outcomes of fetuses and newborns. The recommended terms (Table 1) are:

   - Gestational age (completed weeks): time elapsed between the first day of the last menstrual period and the day of delivery. If pregnancy was achieved using assisted reproductive technology, gestational age is calculated by adding 2 weeks to the conceptional age.
   - Chronological age (days, weeks, months, or years): time elapsed from birth.
   - Postmenstrual age (weeks): gestational age plus chronological age.
   - Corrected age (weeks or months): chronological age reduced by the number of weeks born before 40 weeks of gestation; the term should be used only for children up to 3 years of age who were born preterm.

2. During the perinatal period neonatal hospital stay, "postmenstrual age" is preferred to describe

TABLE 1. Age Terminology During the Perinatal Period

Term	Definition	Units of Time
Gestational age	Time elapsed between the first day of the last menstrual period and the day of delivery	Completed weeks
Chronological age	Time elapsed since birth	Days, weeks, months, years
Postmenstrual age	Gestational age + chronological age	Weeks
Corrected age	Chronological age reduced by the number of weeks born before 40 weeks of gestation	Weeks, months

the age of preterm infants. After the perinatal period, "corrected age" is the preferred term.

3. "Conceptional age," "postconceptional age," "conceptual age," and "postconceptual age" should not be used in clinical pediatrics.

4. Publications reporting fetal and neonatal outcomes should clearly describe methods used to determine gestational age.

COMMITTEE ON FETUS AND NEWBORN, 2003–2004
Lillian R. Blackmon, MD, Chairperson
Daniel G. Batton, MD
Edward F. Bell, MD
Susan E. Denson, MD
*William A. Engle, MD
William P. Kanto, Jr, MD
Gilbert I. Martin, MD
Ann Stark, MD

LIAISONS
Keith J. Barrington, MD
   Canadian Paediatric Society
Tonse N. K. Raju, MD, DCH
   National Institutes of Health
Laura E. Riley, MD
   American College of Obstetricians and
   Gynecologists
Kay M. Tomashek, MD, MPH
   Centers for Disease Control and Prevention
Carol Wallman, MSN, RNC, NNP
   National Association of Neonatal Nurses

STAFF
Jim Couto, MA

*Lead author

REFERENCES

1. Malloy MH, Hoffman HJ. Prematurity, sudden infant death syndrome, and age of death. *Pediatrics*. 1995;96:464–471
2. Bernstein IM, Horbar JD, Badger GJ, Ohlsson A, Golan A. Morbidity and mortality among very-low-birth-weight neonates with intrauterine growth restriction. The Vermont Oxford Network. *Am J Obstet Gynecol*. 2000;182:198–206
3. Ellenhorn MJ, ed. Toxicokinetics. In: *Ellenhorn's Medical Toxicology: Diagnosis and Treatment of Human Poisoning*. 2nd ed. Philadelphia, PA: Williams and Wilkins; 1997:128–148
4. DeVivo DC, Koenigsberger MR. Intracranial hemorrhage. In: Rudolph AM, ed. *Rudolph's Pediatrics*. 20th ed. Stamford, CT: Appleton & Lange; 1996:1877
5. Moriette G, Paris-Llado S, Walti H, et al. Prospective randomized multicenter comparison of high-frequency oscillatory ventilation and conventional ventilation in preterm infants of less than 30 weeks with respiratory distress syndrome. *Pediatrics*. 2001;107:363–372
6. Ramanathan R, Corwin MJ, Hunt CE, et al. Cardiorespiratory events recorded on home monitors: comparison of healthy infants with those at increased risk for SIDS. *JAMA*. 2001;285:2199–2207
7. Pierrat V, Duquennoy C, van Haastert IC, Ernst M, Guilley N, deVries LS. Ultrasound diagnosis and neurodevelopmental outcome of localized and extensive cystic periventricular leucomalacia. *Arch Dis Child Fetal Neonatal Ed*. 2001;84:F151–F156
8. American Academy of Pediatrics, American College of Obstetricians and Gynecologists. *Guidelines for Perinatal Care*. 5th ed. Washington, DC: American College of Obstetricians and Gynecologists; 2002:378–379
9. Cunningham FG, Gant NF, Gilstrap LC III, Hauth JC, Wenstrom KD, Leveno KJ, eds. *Williams Obstetrics*. 21st ed. New York, NY: McGraw-Hill; 2001:129–165
10. Craven C, Ward K. Embryology, fetus and placenta: normal and abnormal. In: Scott JR, DiSaia PJ, Hammond CB, Spellacy WN, eds. *Danforth's Obstetrics and Gynecology*. 8th ed. Philadelphia, PA: Lippincott Williams & Wilkins; 1999:29–46
11. Rossavik IK, Fishburne JI. Conceptional age, menstrual age, and ultrasound age: a second-trimester comparison of pregnancies dated of known conception date with pregnancies dated from last menstrual period. *Obstet Gynecol*. 1989;73:243–249
12. Shepherd TH. Developmental pathology of the embryonic and previable fetal periods. In: Avery GB, Fletcher MA, MacDonald MG, eds. *Neonatology: Pathophysiology and Management of the Newborn*. 4th ed. Philadelphia, PA: JB Lippincott Co; 1994:109–125
13. Bennett FC. Developmental outcome. In: Avery GB, Fletcher MA, MacDonald MG, eds. *Neonatology: Pathophysiology and Management of the Newborn*. 4th ed. Philadelphia, PA: JB Lippincott Co; 1994:1367–1386
14. DiPietro JA, Allen MC. Estimation of gestational age: implications for developmental research. *Child Dev*. 1991;62:1184–1199
15. Sohaey R, Branch DW. Ultrasound in obstetrics. In: Scott JR, DiSaia PJ, Hammond CB, Spellacy WN, eds. *Danforth's Obstetrics and Gynecology*. 8th ed. Philadelphia, PA: Lippincott Williams & Wilkins; 1999:213–242
16. American Academy of Pediatrics, American College of Obstetrics and Gynecology. *Guidelines for Perinatal Care*. 5th ed. Washington, DC: American College of Obstetrics and Gynecology; 2002:199–202
17. Goldenberg RL, Davis RO, Cutter GR, Hoffman HJ, Brumfield CG, Foster JM. Prematurity, postdates, and growth retardation: the influence of use of ultrasonography on reported gestational age. *Am J Obstet Gynecol*. 1989;160:462–470
18. Berg AT. Menstrual cycle length and calculation of gestational age. *Am J Epidemiol*. 1991;133:585–589
19. Mustafa G, David RJ. Comparative accuracy of clinical estimate versus menstrual gestational age in computerized birth certificates. *Public Health Rep*. 2001;116:15–21

Ambient Air Pollution: Health Hazards to Children

● ●

- *Policy Statement*

AMERICAN ACADEMY OF PEDIATRICS

POLICY STATEMENT
Organizational Principles to Guide and Define the Child Health Care System and/or Improve the Health of All Children

Committee on Environmental Health

Ambient Air Pollution: Health Hazards to Children

ABSTRACT. Ambient (outdoor) air pollution is now recognized as an important problem, both nationally and worldwide. Our scientific understanding of the spectrum of health effects of air pollution has increased, and numerous studies are finding important health effects from air pollution at levels once considered safe. Children and infants are among the most susceptible to many of the air pollutants. In addition to associations between air pollution and respiratory symptoms, asthma exacerbations, and asthma hospitalizations, recent studies have found links between air pollution and preterm birth, infant mortality, deficits in lung growth, and possibly, development of asthma. This policy statement summarizes the recent literature linking ambient air pollution to adverse health outcomes in children and includes a perspective on the current regulatory process. The statement provides advice to pediatricians on how to integrate issues regarding air quality and health into patient education and children's environmental health advocacy and concludes with recommendations to the government on promotion of effective air-pollution policies to ensure protection of children's health. *Pediatrics* 2004;114:1699–1707; *air pollution, adverse effects, children, asthma, environmental health.*

ABBREVIATIONS. $PM_{2.5}$, particulate matter with a median aerodynamic diameter less than 2.5 μm; PM_{10}, particulate matter with a median aerodynamic diameter less than 10 μm; EPA, Environmental Protection Agency; HAP, hazardous air pollutant; AQI, air quality index.

INTRODUCTION

Although it has been 3 decades since passage of the Clean Air Act in 1970 (Pub L No. 91–604), the air in many parts of the United States is far from clean. Air quality has improved in some areas but decreased in others.[1] In addition, there are important health effects from air pollutants at levels once considered safe. Children and infants are among the most susceptible to many of the air pollutants.

In 2002, approximately 146 million Americans were living in areas where monitored air failed to meet the 1997 National Ambient Air Quality Standards for at least 1 of the 6 "criteria air pollutants": ozone, particulate matter, sulfur dioxide, nitrogen dioxide, carbon monoxide, and lead (Table 1).[1] Although the standards for ozone and particulate matter were revised in 1997, legal barriers have delayed

doi:10.1542/peds.2004-2166
PEDIATRICS (ISSN 0031 4005). Copyright © 2004 by the American Academy of Pediatrics.

timely implementation.[2] Recent reports have identified adverse health effects at levels near or below the current standards for ozone, particulate matter, and nitrogen dioxide. Thus, the 1997 federal standards may not adequately protect children. Additionally, numerous other toxic air pollutants are of public health concern.[3]

Outdoor air pollution is also a major problem in developing countries. The World Health Organization found that the air quality in large cities in many developing countries is remarkably poor and that very large numbers of people in those countries are exposed to ambient concentrations of air pollutants well above the World Health Organization guidelines for air quality (www.who.int/ceh/publications/en/11airpollution.pdf).

Scientific understanding of the health effects of air pollution, including effects on children, has increased in the last decade. This statement updates a 1993 American Academy of Pediatrics (AAP) statement titled "Ambient Air Pollution: Respiratory Hazards to Children."[4]

EFFECTS OF AIR POLLUTION ON CHILDREN

Children are more vulnerable to the adverse effects of air pollution than are adults. Eighty percent of alveoli are formed postnatally, and changes in the lung continue through adolescence.[5] During the early postneonatal period, the developing lung is highly susceptible to damage after exposure to environmental toxicants.[5–7]

Children have increased exposure to many air pollutants compared with adults because of higher minute ventilation and higher levels of physical activity.[8] Because children spend more time outdoors than do adults, they have increased exposure to outdoor air pollution.[9,10]

Infants, children, the elderly, and those with cardiopulmonary disease are among the most susceptible to adverse health effects from criteria pollutants.[11–15] Lead is neurotoxic, especially during early childhood. Carbon monoxide interferes with oxygen transport through the formation of carboxyhemoglobin. Other criteria pollutants (ozone, sulfur dioxide, particulate matter, nitrogen dioxide) have respiratory effects in children and adults, including increased respiratory tract illness, asthma exacerbations, and decreased lung function (eg, changes in peak flow).[11–12] In adults, particulate air pollution is associated with respiratory and cardiovascular hos-

TABLE 1.　National Ambient Air Quality Standards for Criteria Air Pollutants, 1997

Pollutant	Primary Standards*
Ozone	
1-h average	0.12 ppm (235 μg/m^3)
8-h average	0.08 ppm (157 μg/m^3)
PM$_{10}$	
Annual arithmetic mean	50 μg/m^3
24-h average	150 μg/m^3
PM$_{2.5}$	
Annual arithmetic mean	15 μg/m^3
24-h average	65 μg/m^3
Sulfur dioxide	
Annual arithmetic mean	0.03 ppm (80 μg/m^3)
24-h average	0.14 ppm (365 μg/m^3)
Nitrogen dioxide	
Annual arithmetic mean	0.053 ppm (100 μg/m^3)
Carbon monoxide	
8-h average	9 ppm (10 mg/m^3)
1-h average	35 ppm (40 mg/m^3)
Lead	
Quarterly average	1.5 μg/m^3

Additional information on air quality standards are available at www.epa.gov/air/criteria.html.

* People residing in regions with pollutant concentrations above the primary standard may experience adverse health effects from poor air quality.

pitalizations, cardiovascular mortality,[16] and lung cancer.[17] Air pollution also has effects on indirect health indicators such as health care utilization and school absences.[11–13]

Although numerous studies have shown that outdoor air pollution exacerbates asthma, the effect of outdoor air pollution on the development of asthma has been less clear. Recently, a prospective study found that the risk of developing asthma was not greater, overall, in children living in communities with high levels of ozone or particulate air pollution. However, in communities with high levels of ozone, there was an increased risk of developing asthma in a small subset of children involved in heavy exercise (participation in 3 or more team sports per year [relative risk: 3.3; 95% confidence interval: 1.9–5.8]). This increased risk with heavy exercise was not seen in low-ozone communities. Time spent outside was also associated with new cases of asthma in high-ozone communities (relative risk: 1.4; 95% confidence interval: 1.0–2.1) but not in low-ozone communities.[18] Additional studies are needed to define the role of outdoor air pollution in the development of asthma.

Children in communities with higher levels of urban air pollution (acid vapor, nitrogen dioxide, particulate matter with a median aerodynamic diameter less than 2.5 μm [PM$_{2.5}$], and elemental carbon [a component of diesel exhaust]) had decreased lung function growth, and children who spent more time outdoors had larger deficits in the growth rate of lung function.[19,20] Ambient air pollution (especially particulate matter with a median aerodynamic diameter less than 10 μm [PM$_{10}$]) has also been associated with several adverse birth outcomes, as discussed in the next section.

Levels of ozone and particulate matter are high enough in many parts of the United States to present health hazards to children.[1] Additionally, National Ambient Air Quality Standards for nitrogen dioxide may not be protective. Findings on these pollutants are summarized here.

Ozone

Ambient ozone is formed by the action of sunlight on nitrogen oxides and reactive hydrocarbons, both of which are emitted by motor vehicles and industrial sources. The levels tend to be highest on warm, sunny, windless days and often peak in midafternoon, when children are most likely to be playing outside.

Ozone is a powerful oxidant and respiratory tract irritant in adults and children, causing shortness of breath, chest pain when inhaling deeply, wheezing, and cough.[11] Children have decreases in lung function, increased respiratory tract symptoms, and asthma exacerbations on days with higher levels of ambient ozone.[11,21–23] Increases in ambient ozone have been associated with respiratory or asthma hospitalizations,[24,25] emergency department visits for asthma,[26] and school absences for respiratory tract illness.[27] In Atlanta, Georgia, summertime children's emergency department visits for asthma increased 37% after 6 days when ozone levels exceeded 0.11 ppm.[25] In southern California, school absences for respiratory tract illness increased 63% in association with a 0.02-ppm increase in ozone.[27]

In healthy adults, ozone causes airway inflammation and hyperreactivity, decrements in pulmonary function, and increased respiratory tract symptoms.[11] Ozone exposures at concentrations of 0.12 ppm or higher can result in decrements in lung function after subsequent challenge with aeroallergen.[28] Although most of the controlled studies of ozone exposure have been performed with adults, it is reasonable to believe that the results of these findings could be extended to children.

Ozone may be toxic at concentrations lower than 0.08 ppm, the current federal regulatory standard. Field studies suggest potential thresholds of between 0.04 and 0.08 ppm (1-hour average) for effects on lung function.[29–31] Recent studies of hospitalizations for respiratory tract illness in young children and emergency department visits for asthma suggest that the effects of ozone may occur at ambient concentrations below 0.09 ppm.[32,33] Another study found associations of ozone and respiratory symptoms in children with asthma at levels below the current US Environmental Protection Agency (EPA) standards.[34] If these findings are confirmed, the ozone standards may need additional revision.

In addition to studies on short-term effects, 2 recent studies of college freshmen suggest that increasing cumulative childhood exposure to ozone may affect lung function when exposed children reach young adulthood, particularly in measures of flow in small airways.[35,36] Early childhood exposures may, therefore, be particularly important.[35]

Particulate Matter

PM$_{10}$ is small enough to reach the lower respiratory tract and has been associated with a wide range of serious health effects. PM$_{10}$ is a heterogeneous mixture of small solid or liquid particles of varying composition found in the atmosphere. Fine particles ($PM_{2.5}$) are emitted from combustion processes (especially diesel-powered engines, power generation, and wood burning) and from some industrial activities. Coarse particles (diameter between 2.5 and 10 μm) include windblown dust from dirt roads or soil and dust particles created by crushing and grinding operations. Toxicity of particles may vary with composition.[37,38]

Particle pollution contributes to excess mortality and hospitalizations for cardiac and respiratory tract disease.[14,39–41] The mechanism for particulate matter–associated cardiac effects may be related to disturbances in the cardiac autonomic nervous system, cardiac arrhythmias, or increased blood concentrations of markers of cardiovascular risk (eg, fibrinogen).[16,42]

Daily changes in mortality rates and numbers of people hospitalized are linked to changes in particulate air pollution.[14,39–41] These studies and others have estimated that for every 10 μg/m^3 increase in PM_{10}, there is an increase in the daily mortality rate between 0.5% and 1.6%. Effects were seen even in cities with mean annual PM_{10} concentrations between 25 and 35 μg/m^3. These recent studies suggest that even the current federal standards for $PM_{2.5}$ (24-hour standard = 65 μg/m^3; annual standard = 15 μg/m^3) and PM_{10} (24-hour standard = 150 μg/m^3; annual standard = 50 μg/m^3) should be lowered to protect public health. In 2002, California adopted more stringent standards for particulate matter: the annual average standard for $PM_{2.5}$ is 12 μg/m^3 and for PM_{10} is 20 μg/m^3.[43]

In children, particulate pollution affects lung function[44–46] and lung growth.[19] In a prospective cohort of children living in southern California, children with asthma living in communities with increased levels of air pollution (especially particulates, nitrogen dioxide, and acid vapor) were more likely to have bronchitis symptoms. In this study, bronchitis symptoms refers to a parental report of "one or more episodes of 'bronchitis' in the past 12 months" or report that, "apart from colds, the child usually seems to be congested in the chest or able to bring up phlegm").[47] The same mix of air pollutants was also associated with deficits in lung growth (as measured by lung function tests).[19] Recent studies in different countries have also found associations between ambient air pollution (especially particulates and/or carbon monoxide) and postneonatal infant mortality (attributable to respiratory causes and possibly sudden infant death syndrome),[48,49] low birth weight,[50–53] and preterm birth.[51,54–56]

The relative contribution of fine versus coarse particles to adverse health effects is being investigated. In studies of cities on the East Coast, fine particles seem to be important.[57] In other areas, coarse particles have a stronger or similar effect.[58] Several studies have found that fine particles from power plants and motor vehicles[59] or industrial sources[60] may be more closely associated with mortality.

Nitrogen Dioxide

Nitrogen dioxide is a gaseous pollutant produced by high-temperature combustion. The main outdoor sources of nitrogen dioxide include diesel and gasoline-powered engines and power plants. Levels of nitrogen dioxide around urban monitors have decreased over the past 20 years. Currently, all areas of the country meet the national air quality standard for nitrogen dioxide of 0.053 ppm (100 μg/m^3), measured as an annual arithmetic mean. However, national emissions (overall production) of nitrogen oxides have actually increased in the past 20 years because of an increase in nitrogen oxide emissions from diesel vehicles.[1] This increase is of concern, because nitrogen oxide emissions contribute to ground-level ozone (smog) and other environmental problems such as acid rain.[1]

Controlled-exposure studies of people with asthma have found that short-term exposures (30 minutes) to nitrogen dioxide at concentrations as low as 0.26 ppm can enhance the allergic response after subsequent challenge with allergens.[61,62] These findings are of concern, because some urban communities that are in compliance with the federal standards for nitrogen dioxide (annual average) may experience substantial short-term peak concentrations (1-hour average) that exceed 0.25 ppm. Confirmation of these studies is needed.

Epidemiologic studies have reported relationships between increased ambient nitrogen dioxide and risks of respiratory tract symptoms[63,64] and asthma exacerbations.[65] As noted previously, children with asthma living in communities with increased levels of air pollution (especially nitrogen dioxide, acid vapor, and particulates) were more likely to have bronchitis symptoms.[47] The same mix of air pollutants was also associated with deficits in lung growth (as measured by lung function tests).[19] These effects were increased in children who spent more time outdoors.

The epidemiologic studies of health effects associated with nitrogen dioxide should be interpreted with caution. Increased levels of ambient nitrogen dioxide may be a marker for exposure to traffic emissions or other combustion-related pollution. An independent role of nitrogen dioxide cannot be clearly established because of the high covariation between ambient nitrogen dioxide and other pollutants. Nonetheless, these studies illustrate that adverse respiratory tract effects are seen in urban areas where traffic is a dominant source of air pollution.

Traffic-Related Pollution

Motor vehicles pollute the air through tailpipe exhaust emissions and fuel evaporation, contributing to carbon monoxide, $PM_{2.5}$, nitrogen oxides, hydrocarbons, other hazardous air pollutants (HAPs), and ozone formation. Motor vehicles represent the principal source of air pollution in many communities, and concentrations of traffic pollutants are greater near major roads.[66] Recently, investigators (primarily in Europe and Japan) have found increased adverse health effects among those living near busy roads.

Studies examining associations between adverse respiratory tract health and traffic have been reviewed.[67] Increased respiratory tract complications in children (eg, wheezing, chronic productive cough, and asthma hospitalizations) have been associated with residence near areas of high traffic density (particularly truck traffic).[68–71] Other investigators have linked various childhood cancers to proximity to traffic.[72–74]

Diesel exhaust, a major source of fine particulates in urban areas, is carcinogenic. Numerous studies have found an association between occupational exposure to diesel exhaust and lung cancer.[75] On the basis of extensive toxicologic and epidemiologic evidence, national and international health authorities, including the EPA and the International Agency for Research on Cancer, have concluded that there is considerable evidence of an association between exposure to diesel exhaust and an increased risk of lung cancer.[76,77] Additionally, fine particles in diesel exhaust may enhance allergic and inflammatory responses to antigen challenge and may facilitate development of new allergies.[78,79] Thus, diesel exhaust exposure may worsen symptoms in those with allergic rhinitis or asthma.

School buses operate in proximity to children, and most of the nation's school bus fleets run on diesel fuel. The EPA and some state agencies are establishing programs to eliminate unnecessary school bus idling and to promote use of cleaner buses to decrease children's exposures to diesel exhaust and the amount of air pollution created by diesel school buses (www.epa.gov/cleanschoolbus). A recent pilot study found that a child riding inside a school bus may be exposed to as much as 4 times the level of diesel exhaust as someone riding in a car.[80] These findings underscore the importance of advocating for school districts to replace diesel buses or retrofit them with pollution-reducing devices and limit school bus idling where children congregate as soon as possible.

Other Air Pollutants

Airborne levels of lead, sulfur dioxide, and carbon monoxide have decreased dramatically because of the implementation of control measures. However, levels of these pollutants may still be high near major sources. For example, high lead levels may be found near metals-processing industries, high sulfur dioxide levels may occur near large industrial facilities (especially coal-fired power plants), and high levels of carbon monoxide may occur in areas with heavy traffic congestion.[1]

In addition to criteria air pollutants, there are numerous other air pollutants produced by motor vehicles, industrial facilities, residential wood combustion, agricultural burning, and other sources that are hazardous to children. More than 50000 chemicals are used commercially, and many are released into the air. For most of these chemicals, data on toxicity are sparse.[81] Some pollutants remain airborne or react in the atmosphere to produce other harmful substances. Other air pollutants deposit into and contaminate land and water. Some toxic air pollutants such as lead, mercury, and dioxins degrade slowly or not at all. These pollutants may bioaccumulate in animals at the top of the food chain, including humans. Children can be exposed to toxic air pollutants through contaminated air, water, soil, and food.[3] One example of a persistent pollutant emitted into ambient air that leads to exposure through another route is mercury, a developmental neurotoxicant.[82] Industrial emissions, especially from coal-fired power plants, are the leading source of environmental mercury. Although the levels of airborne mercury may not be hazardous, mercury deposits into soil and surface waters and ultimately accumulates in fish.[82]

The HAPs, often referred to as "toxic air contaminants" or "air toxics," refer to 188 pollutants and chemical groups known or suspected to cause serious health effects including cancer, birth defects, and respiratory tract and neurologic illness.[3,83] The Clean Air Act directs the EPA to regulate HAPs, which include compounds such as polycyclic aromatic hydrocarbons, acrolein, and benzene from fuel or fuel combustion; solvents such as hexane and toluene; hexavalent chromium from chrome-plating facilities; perchloroethylene from dry-cleaning plants; asbestos; metals (eg, mercury and cadmium); and persistent organic pollutants such as polychlorinated biphenyls. In 2001, diesel exhaust was listed as a mobile-source HAP. Many of these compounds are included in a priority list of 33 HAPs that are of special concern because of their widespread use and potential carcinogenicity and teratogenicity.[81] The priority list and general sources of these compounds are available on the EPA Web site (www.epa.gov/ttn/atw/nata).

Limited monitoring data suggest that concentrations of some HAPs may exceed the goals of the Clean Air Act in many cities.[84] Mobile sources (on- and off-road vehicles) account for approximately half of the emissions[3] but may contribute to 90% of the cancer risk (www.scorecard.org/env-releases/hap/us.tcl). A number of studies assessing health risks have found that estimated levels of some of the HAPs are a potential public health problem in many parts of the United States.[3,84–86] For example, estimated concentrations of benzene, formaldehyde, and 1,3-butadiene may contribute to extra cases of cancer (at least 1 extra case per million population exposed) in more than 90% of the census tracts in the contiguous United States. Additionally, the most recent national cancer-risk assessment for HAPs (1996 data) did not include diesel exhaust in the risk estimates.[3] The health risks may also be underestimated, because there is limited information on toxicity values for many of the HAPs,[87] and the risk models did not consider the potential for increased risk in children. These findings underscore the need for better ways to decrease toxic air emissions and assess exposures and risks.

Air-pollution episodes created by disasters (eg, accidents, volcanoes, forest fires, and acts of terrorism) can also create hazards for children. A discussion of these events and of bioaerosols in ambient air (eg, fungal spores and pollen) is beyond the scope of this policy statement. Additionally, this statement does not address the hazards of indoor air pollution.

PREVENTION

Public health interventions to improve air quality can improve health at the population level. A decrease in levels of air pollution in former East Germany after reunification was associated with a decrease in parent-reported bronchitis[88] and improved lung function.[89] During the 1996 Summer Olympics in Atlanta, Georgia, extensive programs were implemented to improve mass transportation and decrease anticipated downtown traffic congestion. These programs were successful and were associated with a prolonged decrease in ozone pollution and significantly lower rates of childhood asthma visits during this period.[90] Closure of a steel mill in Utah Valley and resultant reductions in particulate matter were associated with a twofold decrease in hospitalizations for asthma in preschool children.[91,92] Finally, lung function improved in children who moved away from communities with high particulate air pollution, compared with those who remained or moved to communities with comparable particulate air pollution.[93] These studies provide support for continued efforts to decrease air pollution and improve health via decreases in motor vehicle traffic and industrial emissions. Dietary factors may play a role in modulating the effects of air pollution in children. A recent study in Mexico City, Mexico, found that children with asthma given antioxidant supplements were less affected by ozone compared with a control group that did not receive supplementation.[94] Additional studies are needed to explore this issue further.

Air Pollution and the Regulatory Process

The Clean Air Act of 1970 mandated the EPA to establish the National Ambient Air Quality Standards (Table 1). Standards were set for criteria air pollutants because they are common, widespread, and known to be harmful to public health and the environment.[11,12,83,95] The standards are reviewed every 5 years and set to protect public health, including the health of "sensitive" populations such as people with asthma, children, and the elderly. These standards are set without considering the costs of attaining these levels.

The standards for ozone and particulate matter were revised in 1997 on the basis of numerous scientific studies showing that the previous standards were not adequate to ensure health protection. Legal challenges were made by the American Trucking Associations, the US Chamber of Commerce, and other state and local business groups. However, the Supreme Court ultimately supported the EPA and ordered implementation of the standards.[2] Establishing implementation plans will be a lengthy process that will require the coordinated efforts of the EPA, state and local governments, and industry and environmental organizations.

Population exposures to toxic air contaminants may be of substantial public health concern.[84,86] In contrast to criteria pollutants, monitoring of toxic air contaminants is more limited. Exposures are estimated on the basis of reported emissions and may underestimate actual exposures.[87] The EPA is mandated to develop regulations through a lengthy process that first sets standards to control emissions on the basis of best-available technology. After maximum available control technology emission standards are established, the EPA must assess the risk remaining after emission decreases for the source take effect (residual risk).

To date, the EPA has focused primarily on establishing technology-based emission standards,[3] and this has been a slow process for some sources (eg, mobile toxic air contaminants and mercury emissions). Nationwide, emissions of toxic air contaminants have dropped approximately 24% from baseline (1990–1993) because of regulation and voluntary decreases by industry. With the current plans for gradual fleet turnover and implementation of controls for motor vehicles and fuels, the EPA projects that toxic air-contaminant emissions from gasoline-powered and diesel mobile sources will not be decreased to 75% and 90% of baseline (1990–1993) levels, respectively, until the year 2020.[3] However, major decreases could be more rapidly achieved simply from a prompt, wider application of existing technology.

Protecting populations from exposure to the harmful effects of air pollutants will require effective control measures. Industry (eg, coal-burning power plants, refineries, and chemical plants) and motor vehicles (both gasoline- and diesel-powered) are major sources of criteria pollutants and HAPs.[11,12] For example, coal-fired power plants are important sources of nitrogen oxides (precursors of ozone), particulates, and sulfur dioxide and are the largest sources of mercury emission in the United States. Smaller sources such as dry cleaners, auto body shops, and wood-burning fireplaces can also affect air quality locally. Municipal and hospital waste incinerators release toxic air pollutants including mercury, lead, cadmium, and dioxin emissions. Depending on weather conditions and individual physicochemical properties, some pollutants can be carried by air currents to areas many miles from the source.

In numerous cities in the United States, the personal automobile is the single greatest polluter, because emissions from millions of vehicles on the road add up. Despite significant technologic advances that have led to tighter pollution control from vehicles, emissions vary substantially between vehicles, particularly between classes of vehicles, because of differences in fuel-economy standards set by regulatory agencies. For instance, the corporate average fuel-economy standards have less stringent fuel-economy requirements (average: 20.7 miles per gallon) for light-duty trucks, sport utility vehicles, and minivans, compared with passenger cars (average: 27.5 miles per gallon). The former group of vehicles tends to have higher emissions of air pollutants, higher fuel consumption, and higher emissions of greenhouse gases.[96,97] Information on emissions and fuel-economy ratings for recent models and a guide for choosing clean, fuel-efficient vehicles are available from the EPA Web site (www.epa.gov/greenvehicles/index.htm). The high levels of particulate emissions from diesel-powered buses and trucks must also be addressed. More than 70% of fine particle emissions from traffic are attributable to diesel-powered buses and trucks.

Driving a private car is probably a typical citizen's most "polluting" daily activity, yet in many cases, individuals have few alternative forms of transportation. Thus, urban planning and smart growth are imperative. Urban sprawl affects land use, transportation, and social and economic development and ultimately has important implications for public health.[98] Ways in which individuals can help to decrease air pollution are available at www.epa.gov/air/actions and www.arb.ca.gov/html/brochure/50things.htm.

Air Quality Index

The air quality index (AQI) provides local information on air quality and potential health concerns at the observed (or forecasted) levels of air pollution and can be a useful tool for educating families about local air quality and health.[99] The AQI is reported daily in metropolitan areas, often as part of local weather forecasts on television or radio or in newspapers. The AQI divides air-pollution levels into 6 categories of risk for 5 common pollutants (ozone, PM_{10}, nitrogen dioxide, carbon monoxide, and sulfur dioxide). Each category has a descriptive name reflecting levels of health concern (ranging from good through very hazardous), an associated color, and an advisory statement. Information about air quality in a specific area can be obtained from www.epa.gov/air/urbanair/index.html, www.scorecard.org, or www.weather.com. Although many states and local air districts actively forecast and disseminate health warnings, the challenge is to have people take actions to protect themselves and decrease activities that cause air pollution.

Pediatric Environmental Health[100] from the AAP provides additional information about the outdoor air pollutants and the use of the AQI.

CONCLUSIONS

Ambient air pollution has important and diverse health effects, and infants and children are among the most susceptible. Currently, levels of ozone and particulates remain unhealthful in many parts of the United States, and the current National Ambient Air Quality Standards may not protect the public adequately. There is a compelling need to move forward on efforts to ensure clean air for all.

The assurance of healthy air for children to breathe is beyond the control of an individual pediatrician, and there are no easy solutions. State chapters of the AAP, as well as individual members, can play an important role as advocates for children's environmental health. Areas of involvement might include working with community coalitions in support of strong pollution-control measures and informing local and national representatives and policy makers about the harmful effects of the environment on children's health. Advocates for children's health are needed in discussions about land use and transportation issues. Pediatricians can also advocate for energy-saving (and pollution-minimizing) lifestyles to their patients' families, especially regarding vehicles driven.

In communities with poor air quality, pediatricians can play a role in educating children with asthma or other chronic respiratory tract disease and their families about the harmful effects of air pollution. Patients and families can be counseled on following the AQI to determine when local air-pollution levels pose a health concern. Ozone levels tend to be highest in the afternoon, and it may be possible to decrease children's exposure by scheduling strenuous outdoor activity earlier in the day.

As pediatricians become better informed about local air quality issues in their communities (eg, ozone, nearby industrial facilities, traffic, diesel buses, wood burning, etc), these local concerns can provide a starting point for discussion and education.

Pediatricians who serve as physicians for schools or for team sports should be aware of the health implications of pollution alerts to provide appropriate guidance to school and sports officials, particularly in communities with high levels of ozone.

RECOMMENDATIONS

1. The National Ambient Air Quality Standards are designed to protect the public. To achieve this, the following points should be addressed:

    - The revised standards for ozone and particulate matter adopted by the EPA in 1997 should be promptly implemented.
    - During implementation, the standards should not be weakened in any way that decreases the protection of children's health.
    - Because recent studies suggest that current standards for PM_{10}, $PM_{2.5}$, ozone, and nitrogen dioxide may not be protecting children, the standards should be promptly reviewed and revised.
    - Because the law requires that the most vulnerable groups be protected when setting or revising the air quality standards, the potential effects of air pollution on the fetus, infant, and child should be evaluated, and all standards should include a margin of safety for protection of children.

2. The current measures to protect children from exposures to HAPs are not effective and should be critically reevaluated. The EPA should focus on prompt implementation of the Clean Air Act Amendments of 1990 (Pub L No. 101–549) to decrease HAPs. Additional monitoring for HAPs should be undertaken to allow more accurate characterization of children's exposures to these compounds. Risk assessments for HAPs should be reviewed to ensure that goals are protective of children. Control measures that specifically protect children's health should be implemented.

3. States and local air districts with air quality concerns should actively implement forecasting and

dissemination of health warnings in ways that help people take actions to protect themselves and decrease activities that cause air pollution.

4. Children's exposure to diesel exhaust particles should be decreased. Idling of diesel vehicles in places where children live and congregate should be minimized. Ongoing programs to fund conversion of diesel school bus fleets to cleaner alternative fuels and technologies should be pursued.

5. Industrial emissions of mercury should be decreased.

6. Federal and state governments' policies should encourage reductions in mobile and stationary sources of air pollution, including increased support for mass transit, carpooling, retiring or retrofitting old power plants that do not meet current pollution-control standards, and programs that support marked improvements in fuel emissions of gasoline- and diesel-powered vehicles. Additionally, the development of alternative fuel fleets, low-sulfur diesel, and other "low-emission" strategies (eg, retrofit of existing diesel engines) should be promoted. Before promoting new alternative fuels, these alternative fuel sources should be critically evaluated and determined by governmental authorities to have a good safety profile.

7. The same overall fuel-economy standard should apply to all passenger vehicles. Programs that allow certain passenger vehicles to be exempt from the usual fuel-economy standards should be abolished.

8. City and land-use planning should encourage the design and redevelopment of communities to promote mass transit, carpooling, pedestrian walkways, and bicycle use.

9. Siting of school and child care facilities should include consideration of proximity to roads with heavy traffic and other sources of air pollution. New schools should be located to avoid "hot spots" of localized pollution.

COMMITTEE ON ENVIRONMENTAL HEALTH, 2003–2004
Michael W. Shannon, MD, MPH, Chairperson
Dana Best, MD, MPH
Helen J. Binns, MD, MPH
Christine L. Johnson, MD
*Janice J. Kim, MD, PhD, MPH
Lynnette J. Mazur, MD, MPH
David W. Reynolds, MD
James R. Roberts, MD, MPH
William B. Weil, Jr, MD

Sophie J. Balk, MD
  Past Committee Chairperson
Mark Miller, MD, MPH
  Past Committee Member
Katherine M. Shea, MD, MPH
  Past Committee Member

CONSULTANT
Michael Lipsett, MD
  California Department of Health Services

LIAISONS
Robert H. Johnson, MD
  Centers for Disease Control and Prevention/Agency
  for Toxic Substances and Disease Registry

Martha Linet, MD
  National Cancer Institute
Walter Rogan, MD
  National Institute of Environmental Health Sciences

STAFF
Paul Spire

*Lead author

REFERENCES

1. US Environmental Protection Agency. Latest findings on national air quality: 2000 status and trends. Research Triangle Park, NC: Environmental Protection Agency; 2001. Publication No. EPA 454/K-01-002. Available at: www.epa.gov/airtrends/reports.html. Accessed August 8, 2003

2. US Environmental Protection Agency. Supreme Court upholds EPA position on smog, particulate rules [press release]. Available at: www.epa.gov/airlinks/rehear.htm. Accessed October 29, 2004

3. US Environmental Protection Agency. About air toxics, health and ecologic effects. Available at: www.epa.gov/air/toxicair/newtoxics.html. Accessed August 8, 2003

4. American Academy of Pediatrics, Committee on Environmental Health. Ambient air pollution: respiratory hazards to children. *Pediatrics*. 1993;91:1210–1213

5. Dietert RR, Etzel RA, Chen D, et al. Workshop to identify critical windows of exposure for children's health: immune and respiratory systems work group summary. *Environ Health Perspect*. 2000;108(suppl 3):483–490

6. Plopper CG, Fanucchi MV. Do urban environmental pollutants exacerbate childhood lung diseases? *Environ Health Perspect*. 2000;108: A252–A253

7. Pinkerton KE, Joad JP. The mammalian respiratory system and critical windows of exposure for children's health. *Environ Health Perspect*. 2000;108(suppl 3):457–462

8. Plunkett LM, Turnbull D, Rodricks JV. Differences between adults and children affecting exposure assessment. In: Guzelian PS, Henry CJ, Olin SS, eds. *Similarities and Differences Between Children and Adults: Implications for Risk Assessment*. Washington, DC: ILSI Press; 1992: 79–96

9. Wiley JA, Robinson JP, Piazza T, et al. *Activity Patterns of California Residents: Final Report*. Sacramento, CA: California Air Resources Board; 1991. Publication No. A6-177-33

10. Wiley JA, Robinson JP, Cheng YT, Piazza T, Stork L, Pladsen K. *Study of Children's Activity Patterns: Final Report*. Sacramento, CA: California Air Resources Board; 1991. Publication No. A733-149

11. American Thoracic Society, Committee of the Environmental and Occupational Health Assembly. Health effects of outdoor air pollution. Part 1. *Am J Respir Crit Care Med*. 1996;153:3–50

12. American Thoracic Society, Committee of the Environmental and Occupational Health Assembly. Health effects of outdoor air pollution. Part 2. *Am J Respir Crit Care Med*. 1996;153:477–498

13. Bates DV. The effects of air pollution on children. *Environ Health Perspect*. 1995;103(suppl 6):49–53

14. US Environmental Protection Agency. *Air Quality Criteria for Particulate Matter*, Vol. II. Research Triangle Park, NC: Environmental Protection Agency; 2001. Publication No. EPA/600/P-99/002bB

15. US Environmental Protection Agency. *Air Quality Criteria for Ozone and Related Photochemical Oxidants*, Vol. III. Research Triangle Park, NC: Environmental Protection Agency; 1996. Publication No. EPA/600/P-93/004a-cF

16. Dockery DW. Epidemiologic evidence of cardiovascular effects of particulate air pollution. *Environ Health Perspect*. 2001;109(suppl 4): 483–486

17. Pope CA III, Burnett RT, Thun MJ, et al. Lung cancer, cardiopulmonary mortality, and long-term exposure to fine particulate air pollution. *JAMA*. 2002;287:1132–114118.

18. McConnell R, Berhane K, Gilliland F, et al. Asthma in exercising children exposed to ozone: a cohort study [published correction appears in: *Lancet*. 2002;359:896]. *Lancet*. 2002;359:386–391

19. Gauderman WJ, McConnell R, Gilliland F, et al. Association between air pollution and lung function growth in southern California children. *Am J Respir Crit Care Med*. 2000;162:1383–1390

20. Gauderman WJ, Gilliland GF, Vora H, et al. Association between air pollution and lung function growth in southern California children: results from a second cohort. *Am J Respir Crit Care Med*. 2002;166:76–84

21. Kinney PL, Thurston GD, Raizenne M. The effects of ambient ozone on lung function in children: a reanalysis of six summer camp studies. *Environ Health Perspect.* 1996;104:170–174

22. Thurston GD, Lippmann M, Scott MB, Fine JM. Summertime haze air pollution and children with asthma. *Am J Respir Crit Care Med.* 1997; 155:654–660

23. Ostro BD, Lipsett MJ, Mann JK, Braxton-Owens H, White MC. Air pollution and asthma exacerbations among African-American children in Los Angeles. *Inhal Toxicol.* 1995;7:711–722

24. Thurston GD, Ito K, Hayes CG, Bates DV, Lippmann M. Respiratory hospital admissions and summertime haze air pollution in Toronto, Ontario: consideration of the role of acid aerosols. *Environ Res.* 1994; 65:271–290

25. White MC, Etzel RA, Wilcox WD, Lloyd C. Exacerbations of childhood asthma and ozone pollution in Atlanta. *Environ Res.* 1994;65:56–68

26. Tolbert PE, Mulholland JA, MacIntosh DL, et al. Air quality and pediatric emergency room visits for asthma in Atlanta, Georgia, USA. *Am J Epidemiol.* 2000;151:798–810

27. Gilliland FD, Berhane K, Rappaport EB, et al. The effects of ambient air pollution on school absenteeism due to respiratory illnesses. *Epidemiology.* 2001;12:43–54

28. Molfino NA, Wright SC, Katz I, et al. Effect of low concentration of ozone on inhaled allergen responses in asthmatic subjects. *Lancet.* 1991;338:199–203

29. Castillejos M, Gold DR, Damokosh AI, et al. Acute effects of ozone on the pulmonary function of exercising schoolchildren from Mexico City. *Am J Respir Crit Care Med.* 1995;152:1501–1507

30. Chen PC, Lai YM, Chan CC, Hwang JS, Yang CY, Wang JD. Short-term effect of ozone on the pulmonary function of children in primary school. *Environ Health Perspect.* 1999;107:921–925

31. Korrick SA, Neas LM, Dockery DW, et al. Effects of ozone and other pollutants on the pulmonary function of adult hikers. *Environ Health Perspect.* 1998;106:93–99

32. Burnett RT, Smith-Doiron M, Stieb D, et al. Association between ozone and hospitalization for acute respiratory diseases in children less than 2 years of age. *Am J Epidemiol.* 2001;153:444–452

33. Stieb DM, Burnett RT, Beveridge RC, Brook JR. Association between ozone and asthma emergency department visits in Saint John, New Brunswick, Canada. *Environ Health Perspect.* 1996;104:1354–1360

34. Gent JF, Tiche EW, Holford TR, et al. Association of low-level ozone and fine particles with respiratory symptoms in children with asthma. *JAMA.* 2003;290:1859–1867

35. Kunzli N, Lurmann F, Segal M, Ngo L, Balmes J, Tager IB. Association between lifetime ambient ozone exposure and pulmonary function in college freshmen—results of a pilot study. *Environ Res.* 1997;72:8–23

36. Galizia A, Kinney PL. Long-term residence in areas of high ozone: associations with respiratory health in a nationwide sample of non-smoking young adults. *Environ Health Perspect.* 1999;107:675–679

37. Ghio AJ, Silbajoris R, Carson JL, Samet JM. Biologic effects of oil fly ash. *Environ Health Perspect.* 2002;110(suppl 1):89–94

38. Pandya RJ, Solomon G, Kinner A, Balmes JR. Diesel exhaust and asthma: hypotheses and molecular mechanisms of action. *Environ Health Perspect.* 2002;110(suppl 1):103–112

39. Dockery DW, Pope CA III. Acute respiratory effects of particulate air pollution. *Annu Rev Public Health.* 1994;15:107–132

40. Schwartz J. Air pollution and daily mortality: a review and meta analysis. *Environ Res.* 1994;64:36–52

41. Samet JM, Dominici F, Curriero FC, Coursac I, Zeger SL. Fine particulate air pollution and mortality in 20 U.S. cities, 1987–1994. *N Engl J Med.* 2000;343:1742–1749

42. Schwartz J. Air pollution and blood markers of cardiovascular risk. *Environ Health Perspect.* 2001;109(suppl 3):405–409

43. California Air Resources Board. June 20, 2002 board meeting summary. Sacramento, CA: California Air Resources Board; 2002. Available at: www.arb.ca.gov/research/aaqs/std-rs/bdsum620/bdsum620.htm. Accessed August 8, 2003

44. Hoek G, Dockery DW, Pope A, Neas L, Roemer W, Brunekreef B. Association between PM10 and decrements in peak expiratory flow rates in children: reanalysis of data from five panel studies. *Eur Respir J.* 1998;11:1307–1311

45. Ostro B, Lipsett M, Mann J, Braxton-Owens H, White M. Air pollution and exacerbation of asthma in African-American children in Los Angeles. *Epidemiology.* 2001;12:200–208

46. Yu O, Sheppard L, Lumley T, Koenig JQ, Shapiro GG. Effects of ambient air pollution on symptoms of asthma in Seattle-area children enrolled in the CAMP study. *Environ Health Perspect.* 2000;108: 1209–1214

47. McConnell R, Berhane K, Gilliland F, et al. Air pollution and bronchitic symptoms in Southern California children with asthma. *Environ Health Perspect.* 1999;107:757–760

48. Woodruff TJ, Grillo J, Schoendorf KC. The relationship between selected causes of postneonatal infant mortality and particulate air pollution in the United States. *Environ Health Perspect.* 1997;105:608–612

49. Bobak M, Leon DA. The effect of air pollution on infant mortality appears specific for respiratory causes in the postneonatal period. *Epidemiology.* 1999;10:666–670

50. Ritz B, Yu F. The effect of ambient carbon monoxide on low birth weight among children born in southern California between 1989 and 1993. *Environ Health Perspect.* 1999;107:17–25

51. Bobak M. Outdoor air pollution, low birth weight, and prematurity. *Environ Health Perspect.* 2000;108:173–176

52. Dejmek J, Solansky I, Benes I, Lenicek J, Sram RJ. The impact of polycyclic aromatic hydrocarbons and fine particles on pregnancy outcome. *Environ Health Perspect.* 2000;108:1159–1164

53. Wang X, Ding H, Ryan L, Xu X. Association between air pollution and low birth weight: a community-based study. *Environ Health Perspect.* 1997;105:514–520

54. Ritz B, Yu F, Chapa G, Fruin S. Effect of air pollution on preterm birth among children born in Southern California between 1989 and 1993. *Epidemiology.* 2000;11:502–511

55. Ha EH, Hong YC, Lee BE, Woo BH, Schwartz J, Christiani DC. Is air pollution a risk factor for low birth weight in Seoul? *Epidemiology.* 2001;12:643–648

56. Xu X, Ding H, Wang X. Acute effects of total suspended particles and sulfur dioxides on preterm delivery: a community-based cohort study. *Arch Environ Health.* 1995;50:407–415

57. Schwartz J. Air pollution and hospital admissions for respiratory disease. *Epidemiology.* 1996;7:20–28

58. Ostro BD, Broadwin R, Lipsett MJ. Coarse and fine particles and daily mortality in the Coachella Valley, California: a follow-up study. *J Expo Anal Environ Epidemiol.* 2000;10:412–419

59. Laden F, Neas LM, Dockery DW, Schwartz J. Association of fine particulate matter from different sources with daily mortality in six US cities. *Environ Health Perspect.* 2000;108:941–947

60. Ozkaynak H, Thurston GD. Associations between 1980 U.S. mortality rates and alternative measures of airborne particle concentration. *Risk Anal.* 1987;7:449–461

61. Strand V, Svartengren M, Rak S, Barck C, Bylin G. Repeated exposure to an ambient level of NO₂ enhances asthmatic response to a nonsymptomatic allergen dose. *Eur Respir J.* 1998;12:6–12

62. Tunnicliffe WS, Burge PS, Ayres JG. Effect of domestic concentrations of nitrogen dioxide on airway responses to inhaled allergen in asthmatic patients. *Lancet.* 1994;344:1733–1736

63. Hajat S, Haines A, Goubet SA, Atkinson RW, Anderson HR. Association of air pollution with daily GP consultations for asthma and other lower respiratory conditions in London. *Thorax.* 1999;54:597–605

64. Shima M, Adachi M. Effect of outdoor and indoor nitrogen dioxide on respiratory symptoms in schoolchildren. *Int J Epidemiol.* 2000;29: 862–870

65. Lipsett M, Hurley S, Ostro B. Air pollution and emergency room visits for asthma in Santa Clara County, California. *Environ Health Perspect.* 1997;105:216–222

66. Zhu Y, Hinds WC, Kim S, Sioutas C. Concentration and size distribution of ultrafine particles near a major highway. *J Air Waste Manag Assoc.* 2002;52:1032–1042

67. Delfino RJ. Epidemiologic evidence for asthma and exposure to air toxics: linkages between occupational, indoor, and community air pollution research. *Environ Health Perspect.* 2002;110(suppl 4):573–589

68. Edwards J, Walters S, Griffiths RK. Hospital admissions for asthma in preschool children: relationship to major roads in Birmingham, United Kingdom. *Arch Environ Health.* 1994;49:223–227

69. van Vliet P, Knape M, de Hartog J, Janssen N, Harssema H, Brunekreef B. Motor vehicle exhaust and chronic respiratory symptoms in children living near freeways. *Environ Res.* 1997;74:122–132

70. Brunekreef B, Janssen NA, de Hartog J, Harssema H, Knape M, van Vliet P. Air pollution from truck traffic and lung function in children living near motorways. *Epidemiology.* 1997;8:298–303

71. Ciccone G, Forastiere F, Agabiti N, et al. Road traffic and adverse respiratory effects in children. SIDRIA Collaborative Group. *Occup Environ Med.* 1998;55:771–778

72. Feychting M, Svensson D, Ahlbom A. Exposure to motor vehicle exhaust and childhood cancer. *Scand J Work Environ Health.* 1998;24: 8–11

73. Pearson RL, Wachtel H, Ebi KL. Distance-weighted traffic density in proximity to a home is a risk factor for leukemia and other childhood cancers. *J Air Waste Manag Assoc.* 2000;50:175–180

74. Raaschou-Nielsen O, Hertel O, Thomsen BL, Olsen JH. Air pollution from traffic at the residence of children with cancer. *Am J Epidemiol.* 2001;153:433–443

75. Lipsett M, Campleman S. Occupational exposure to diesel exhaust and lung cancer: a meta-analysis. *Am J Public Health.* 1999;89:1009–1017

76. US Environmental Protection Agency. *Health Assessment Document for Diesel Engine Exhaust.* Washington, DC: Office of Research and Development NCfEA; 2002. EPA/600/8–909/057F

77. International Agency for Research on Cancer. *IARC Monographs on the Evaluation of Carcinogenic Risks to Humans: Diesel and Gasoline Engine Exhausts and Some Nitroarenes.* Vol 46. Lyon, France: International Agency for Research on Cancer; 1989:458

78. Diaz-Sanchez D, Garcia MP, Wang M, Jyrala M, Saxon A. Nasal challenge with diesel exhaust particles can induce sensitization to a neoallergen in the human mucosa. *J Allergy Clin Immunol.* 1999;104:1183–1188

79. Nel AE, Diaz-Sanchez D, Ng D, Hiura T, Saxon A. Enhancement of allergic inflammation by the interaction between diesel exhaust particles and the immune system. *J Allergy Clin Immunol.* 1998;102:539–554

80. Solomon GM, Campbell T, Feuer GR, Masters J, Samkian A, Paul KA. *No Breathing in the Aisles: Diesel Exhaust Inside School Buses.* New York, NY: Natural Resources Defense Council; 2001. Available at: www.nrdc.org/air/transportation/schoolbus/sbusinx.asp. Accessed August 8, 2003

81. Leikauf GD. Hazardous air pollutants and asthma. *Environ Health Perspect.* 2002;110(suppl 4):505–526

82. American Academy of Pediatrics, Goldman LR, Shannon MW, Committee on Environmental Health. Technical report: mercury in the environment: implications for pediatricians. *Pediatrics.* 2001;108:197–205

83. Suh HH, Bahadori T, Vallarino J, Spengler JD. Criteria air pollutants and toxic air pollutants. *Environ Health Perspect.* 2000;108(suppl 4):625–633

84. Woodruff TJ, Axelrad DA, Caldwell J, Morello-Frosch R, Rosenbaum A. Public health implications of 1990 air toxics concentrations across the United States. *Environ Health Perspect.* 1998;106:245–251

85. Nazemi MA. *Multiple Air Toxics Exposure Study (MATES-II) in the South Coast Air Basin.* Diamond Bar, CA: South Coast Air Quality Management District; 2000

86. Morello-Frosch RA, Woodruff TJ, Axelrad DA, Caldwell JC. Air toxics and health risks in California: the public health implications of outdoor concentrations. *Risk Anal.* 2000;20:273–291

87. Kyle AD, Wright CC, Caldwell JC, Buffler PA, Woodruff TJ. Evaluating the health significance of hazardous air pollutants using monitoring data. *Public Health Rep.* 2001;116:32–44

88. Heinrich J, Hoelscher B, Wichmann HE. Decline of ambient air pollution and respiratory symptoms in children. *Am J Respir Crit Care Med.* 2000;161:1930–1936

89. Frye C, Hoelscher B, Cyrys J, Wjst M, Wichmann HE, Heinrich J. Association of lung function with declining ambient air pollution. *Environ Health Perspect.* 2003;111:383–387

90. Friedman MS, Powell KE, Hutwagner L, Graham LM, Teague WG. Impact of changes in transportation and commuting behaviors during the 1996 Summer Olympic Games in Atlanta on air quality and childhood asthma. *JAMA.* 2001;285:897–905

91. Pope CA III. Respiratory hospital admissions associated with PM10 pollution in Utah, Salt Lake, and Cache Valleys. *Arch Environ Health.* 1991;46:90–97

92. Pope CA III. Particulate pollution and health: a review of the Utah valley experience. *J Expo Anal Environ Epidemiol.* 1996;6:23–34

93. Avol EL, Gauderman WJ, Tan SM, London SJ, Peters JM. Respiratory effects of relocating to areas of differing air pollution levels. *Am J Respir Crit Care Med.* 2001;164:2067–2072

94. Romieu I, Sienra-Monge JJ, Ramirez-Aguilar M, et al. Antioxidant supplementation and lung functions among children with asthma exposed to high levels of air pollutants. *Am J Respir Crit Care Med.* 2002;166:703–709

95. US Environmental Protection Agency. *The Plain English Guide To The Clean Air Act.* 1993. EPA-400-K-93-001. Available at: www.epa.gov/oar/oaqps/peg_caa/pegcaain.html. Accessed October 26, 2004

96. National Research Council. *Effectiveness and Impact of Corporate Average Fuel Economy (CAFE) Standards.* Washington, DC: National Academies Press; 2002. Available at: www.nap.edu/books/0309076013/html. Accessed August 8, 2003

97. Hwang R, Millis B, Spencer T. *Clean Getaway: Toward Safe and Efficient Vehicles.* New York, NY: Natural Resources Defense Council; 2001. Available at: www.nrdc.org/air/transportation/cafe/cafeinx.asp. Accessed August 8, 2003

98. Jackson RJ, Kochtitzky C. *Creating a Health Environment: The Impact of the Built Environment on Public Health.* Washington, DC: Sprawl Watch Clearinghouse. Available at: www.sprawlwatch.org/health.pdf. Accessed August 8, 2003

99. US Environmental Protection Agency, Office of Air and Radiation. *Air Quality Index: A Guide to Air Quality and Your Health.* Research Triangle Park, NC: Environmental Protection Agency; 2000. Publication No. EPA-454/R-00-005. Available at: www.epa.gov/airnow/aqibroch. Accessed August 8, 2003

100. American Academy of Pediatrics, Committee on Environmental Health. Outdoor air pollutants. In: Etzel RA, Balk SJ, eds. *Pediatric Environmental Health.* 2nd ed. Elk Grove Village, IL: American Academy of Pediatrics; 2003;:69–86

All policy statements from the American Academy of Pediatrics automatically expire 5 years after publication unless reaffirmed, revised, or retired at or before that time.

Application of the Resource-Based Relative Value Scale System to Pediatrics

- *Policy Statement*

AMERICAN ACADEMY OF PEDIATRICS

POLICY STATEMENT
Organizational Principles to Guide and Define the Child Health Care System and/or Improve the Health of All Children

Committee on Coding and Nomenclature

Application of the Resource-Based Relative Value Scale System to Pediatrics

ABSTRACT. In today's rapidly changing health care environment, it is crucial to understand the genesis and principles behind the Medicare Resource-Based Relative Value Scale (RBRVS) physician fee schedule. Many third-party payers, including state Medicaid programs, BlueCross BlueShield, and managed care organizations, use variations of the Medicare RBRVS to determine physician reimbursement and capitation rates. Because the RBRVS fee schedule was created originally for Medicare only, pediatric-specific Current Procedural Terminology (CPT) codes and pediatric practice expense calculations were not included. The American Academy of Pediatrics supports the use of CPT codes and the RBRVS physician fee schedule and continues to work to rectify certain inequities of the RBRVS system as they pertain to pediatrics. *Pediatrics* 2004;113:1437–1440; *reimbursement, coding, RBRVS.*

ABBREVIATIONS. RBRVS, Resource-Based Relative Value Scale; CF, conversion factor; RVU, relative value unit; AAP, American Academy of Pediatrics; CPT, Current Procedural Terminology; AMA, American Medical Association; CMS, Centers for Medicare and Medicaid Services.

BACKGROUND

The Medicare Resource-Based Relative Value Scale (RBRVS) physician fee schedule was developed to recognize objective measures of physician work while creating equity in physician reimbursement based on physician work for services across all specialties. The RBRVS system, which is based on uniform definitions of physician work, has eliminated many of the more dramatic reimbursement irregularities within the Medicare physician fee schedule. Each year, Congress establishes a budget for Medicare by setting a single conversion factor (CF). This CF (dollars per relative value unit [RVU]) is a national dollar value that converts the anticipated total RVUs into legislatively set payment amounts (RVU × CF = payment) for the purposes of reimbursing physicians for Medicare services provided. The annual assignment by the Centers for Medicare and Medicaid Services (CMS) of the CF is based on variations primarily in adult Medicare utilization and the requirement for CMS to operate within a legislatively determined budget. Changes in the CF should not be assumed to reflect pediatrics

PEDIATRICS (ISSN 0031 4005). Copyright © 2004 by the American Academy of Pediatrics.

utilization rates or effect a decrease in reimbursement for children's services.

In an effort to deal with the limitations of the RBRVS system as it was designed originally and recognizing that there were only limited pediatric-specific procedures in the Medicare database, the American Academy of Pediatrics (AAP) has continued to propose new Current Procedural Terminology (CPT) codes relevant to pediatrics to the CPT Editorial Panel of the American Medical Association (AMA) over the past years. Some of these CPT codes have been accepted and incorporated into the CPT nomenclature. The AAP Committee on Coding and Nomenclature (previously the Committee on Coding and Reimbursement and the RBRVS Project Advisory Committee) actively works within the CPT Editorial Panel process by submitting CPT codes relevant to pediatrics as well as within the AMA/Specialty Society Relative Value Scale Update Committee process to provide CMS with RVU recommendations that accurately reflect the work involved in providing services to children. Although CMS has assigned physician work values to most CPT codes within the Medicare RBRVS physician fee schedule, the current fee schedule has yet to assign specific reimbursement for several services commonly or uniquely associated with pediatric care (eg, vision screening, case management services, and child abuse services). The present Medicare-based system also has not uniformly recognized many of the aspects of providing care to infants and children, particularly those services for children that require increased physician work compared with similar services for adults.

The RBRVS physician fee schedule was implemented initially by CMS (the Health Care Financing Administration at the time) as a mechanism for the reimbursement of physician services provided to Medicare recipients. CMS neither designed nor planned its system to be a universal reimbursement system for services to all patient populations, such as those commonly covered by state Medicaid programs or commercial insurers. Despite this design limitation, most commercial and public payers have moved rapidly to adopt this method of reimbursement. A recent report by the AMA revealed that 74% of the private plans surveyed in 2002 reported some use of an RBRVS payment system, compared with

63% in 1998.[1] The work estimates driving the RBRVS Medicare physician fee schedule were developed primarily to reflect the services rendered to the typical Medicare patient and, as such, do not always accurately reflect the breadth and scope of work expended in providing care for newborns, infants, and children. A few Medicaid programs that adopted the Medicare RBRVS physician fee schedule to reimburse physicians instituted a separate and higher CF for some pediatric services. Some of these Medicaid programs have maintained a higher pediatric CF or established auxiliary fee schedules or case management fees to augment physician reimbursement for children's care.

Despite these limitations, the AAP advocates the use of the RBRVS physician fee schedule, expanded for pediatric patients, as an appropriate and fundamentally fair system for reimbursing pediatric services. The AAP believes that an RBRVS-based fee schedule, supported by objective assessments of physician work, is more consistent and equitable than the "customary, prevailing, and reasonable" reimbursement system under which physicians historically have been paid for their services. However, if appropriate access to health care is to be ensured for all children, Medicaid programs and other payers must recognize the inequities in reimbursement for some pediatric services within the RBRVS system and work with the AAP, AMA, and CMS to correct these deficiencies. Additionally, all payers (most importantly Medicaid) must recognize the importance of incorporating and reimbursing for all services listed under RBRVS while refining their payment schedules to correspond to the annual updates and revisions of the CMS. State-specific non-RBRVS payment methodologies cannot be endorsed, because they are often arbitrary and do not recognize objective differences in physician work. Payers also must acknowledge and embrace the CMS 5-year review of relative work values and its recent efforts to implement an accurate, resource-based approach to the practice expense portion of total RVUs. The AAP recognizes that the CMS annual budget neutrality adjustments to the RVUs may be necessary to comply with congressional requirements placed on the Medicare budget and fee schedule; however, private payers and state Medicaid programs must recognize that these adjustments are merely attributable to budgetary constraints imposed by Congress (budget neutrality) and do not reflect changes in the provision of care or the amount of work expended in providing a specific physician service.

The CMS has recognized that a Medicare-driven reimbursement tool may underrepresent or undervalue pediatric work. To account for this, Congress mandated that the CMS revisit this pediatric work issue as part of a normal 5-year review process specifically to evaluate whether codes for pediatric services are valued correctly. Although the AAP appreciates the attempts by the CMS to account for pediatric work more equitably, it is still important to remember that pediatricians were severely underrepresented in the original Hsiao et al study[2] that led to the creation of the original RVUs for physician work. Despite this deficiency, the overall fairness of the system that was created rapidly led to its incorporation into reimbursement formulas for children's health care services by many third-party payers as well as by state Medicaid programs. The assumption that there is equivalency of work between pediatricians and pediatric subspecialists to that of internists and adult subspecialists has not been rigorously studied. In some pediatric subspecialties (eg, pediatric cardiology and pediatric nephrology), in which valid survey data have been collected, there is quantifiable proof of underestimation of total physician work, particularly in situations in which major physiologic and developmental differences exist.[3,4]

The AAP believes that the unique characteristics of children's health care services have not yet been incorporated sufficiently into the corpus of medical and surgical procedural codes for services provided to children despite Congress' admonition to the CMS. The AAP supports the continued efforts of CPT and the CMS through the CPT and AMA/Specialty Society Relative Value Scale Update Committee processes to address this problem. The AAP also appreciates their commitment, through the CPT process, to represent more effectively the diversity of CPT codes specific to children and to assign appropriate work values to these procedures and services.

It is essential that the RBRVS survey process include an adequate pediatric sample size and valid survey questions. To that end, the AAP must ensure accurate survey completion by physicians who deliver health care services to children and are knowledgeable about the RBRVS system and the survey process. It is inappropriate and not in the best interest of pediatricians to simply extrapolate work values assigned for services to children from those values determined by surveying physicians who primarily provide adult services. The RBRVS system assigns value to each procedure based on physician work (including preservice, intraservice, and postservice time and effort), office practice expense, and procedure-based malpractice expense. Differences between adult and pediatric services can be demonstrated in each of those RBRVS system components.

Physician Work: Preservice, Intraservice, and Postservice Time

Children typically exhibit anxiety and fear when examined or during procedures resulting in the need for additional time and effort by the physician to respond to and prepare the child for the examination or procedures. This uniformly adds more time and stress to the preservice and intraservice periods compared with that required by the average adult patient. Children require constant adaptations to the physical examination, applied technology, or procedures in response to their constantly changing behavior and level of cooperation. Small physical size and limited ability to cooperate may also extend intraservice time. Follow-up communication with child care facilities, schools, absent parents, or extended family (eg, grandparents) requires increased postservice times.

Practice Expense

The practice expense component of the RBRVS includes clinical staff time, medical supplies, and medical equipment, accounting for, on average, 42% of the total RVU for a code. The costs of supplies and equipment are not proportional to a child's size. Therefore, arbitrary reductions of medical supplies and equipment based on patient size are inappropriate. Major factors affecting pediatric practice expense as compared with many other specialties are the high volume of lower-intensity office visits, the large volume of telephone management services, and the case management and administrative work required. As an example, high patient turnover requires more examination rooms per provider to maintain physician efficiency, as compared with specialties that see 1 to 3 patients per hour. High volume requires more clerical staff to deal with larger patient-flow volume and resulting phone calls; recognizing that 40% to 50% of most pediatric office volume is booked within 24 hours of the encounter, staff members are forced to do insurance verification at the time of patient arrival, which affects their ability to process patients efficiently. Providing care to young children also requires more direct hands-on staff time, results in less efficient room use because of difficulties dressing and undressing patients, and is marked by increased complexity and time in collecting laboratory specimens. These factors need to be accounted for in any resource-based practice expense study and in the resulting practice expense calculations for services for children.

Professional Liability RVUs

The RBRVS system assigns RVUs to cover the malpractice expenses incurred by physicians. These malpractice RVUs, originally calculated for office-based pediatricians, may systematically undervalue the practice liability costs for some pediatric specialties. The prolonged statutes of limitation on child-related legal actions, as compared with adult care, result in increased malpractice risk exposure for physicians providing services for children, compared with adults. In many states, that risk is measured in decades rather than years. As such, physicians treating minors are required to purchase an "extended reporting endorsement" to cover the risk until the patient achieves the age of majority, which imposes additional practice expenses in retaining medical records and the attendant security protections for that protracted period. This difference in exposure is not calculated into the RBRVS system and was not included in the initial Hsiao et al study.[2] Pediatric-specific survey data for malpractice expense should be used for this component when assigning final RVU valuations. Without pediatric-specific CPT codes, however, there is no way to do this without having different CFs for pediatric patients.

OTHER REIMBURSEMENT FACTORS

CPT Code Set

The AAP recognizes that the CPT code set is the accepted standard for coding physician services and communicating with third-party payers and is required for electronic data exchange under the Health Insurance Portability and Accountability Act of 1996 (HIPAA) regulations. Third-party payers, however, do not necessarily recognize nor reimburse for the full spectrum of health care services represented by the complete CPT code set, nor does HIPAA require insurers to reimburse for all CPT codes, merely to accept transactions electronically that include CPT procedure codes. The AAP strongly advocates for the acceptance and reimbursement for the complete CPT code set by all payers and encourages members to work to that end in negotiating contracts with individual payers.

National Pediatric Database

To better understand the spectrum, frequency, and regional variations in health care services for children, the AAP urges the creation of a national database for services to children analogous to Medicare's Part B Medicare Data Files, which contain Part B Medicare claims information. A national database for health care services for children is critical for making the Office of the Inspector General (OIG) Medicare and Medicaid compliance program applicable to pediatricians. The current use of Medicare-based utilization patterns inappropriately labels pediatricians as "outliers" and potential targets for health care fraud investigations. Finally, only by understanding the frequency with which codes for pediatric services are reported will the AAP be able to analyze utilization patterns and the effects of new codes on total health care costs. A pediatric database analogous to the Part B Medicare Data Files database should be encouraged or legislated and published annually.

RECOMMENDATIONS

1. The principles of the Medicare RBRVS system should be supported as an intrinsically more reasoned and equitable reimbursement methodology than alternative systems.
2. Work should continue within the RBRVS system to remove implementation inequities and ensure that the RBRVS system appropriately accounts for the work and expense in caring for neonates, infants, and children.
3. All payers should recognize the full spectrum of CPT codes and their guidelines.
4. Movement to an alternative to RBRVS should be supported only if the alternative system represents a significant enhancement and is responsive to the needs of children.

Committee on Coding and Nomenclature, 2003–2004
Richard J. Haynes, MD, Chairperson
Joel F. Bradley, Jr, MD
Robert S. Gerstle, MD*
Steven E. Krug, MD
Jeffrey F. Linzer, Sr, MD
Julia M. Pillsbury, DO
Richard H. Tuck, MD
Patience H. White, MD

CONSULTANTS
Diller B. Groff, MD
Richard A. Molteni, MD

LIAISON
Eugene S. Wiener, MD
    American Pediatric Surgical Association

STAFF
Linda J. Walsh, MAB

*Lead Author

REFERENCES

1. Gallagher PE, Klemp T, Smith SL, eds. *CPA Medicare RBRVS: The Physicians' Guide*. 5th ed. Chicago, IL: Coding and Medical Information Systems Group, American Medical Association; 2002
2. Hsiao WC, Braun P, Dunn D, Becker ER. Resource-based relative values: an overview. *JAMA*. 1998;260:2347–2353
3. Arnold W, Alexander S. Cost, work, reimbursement, and the pediatric nephrologist in the United States Medicare/End-Stage Renal Disease Program. *Pediatr Nephrol*. 1997;11:250–257
4. Garson A Jr, Wolk MJ, Morrin SB, Gold W, Dickstein M, Dobson A. Resource-based relative value scale for children—comparison of pediatric and adult cardiology work values. *Cardiol Young*. 1995;5:210–216

Classifying Recommendations for Clinical Practice Guidelines

• *Policy Statement*

AMERICAN ACADEMY OF PEDIATRICS

POLICY STATEMENT
Organizational Principles to Guide and Define the Child Health Care System and/or Improve the Health of All Children

Steering Committee on Quality Improvement and Management

Classifying Recommendations for Clinical Practice Guidelines

ABSTRACT. Clinical practice guidelines are intended to improve the quality of clinical care by reducing inappropriate variations, producing optimal outcomes for patients, minimizing harm, and promoting cost-effective practices. This statement proposes an explicit classification of recommendations for clinical practice guidelines of the American Academy of Pediatrics (AAP) to promote communication among guideline developers, implementers, and other users of guideline knowledge, to improve consistency, and to facilitate user understanding. The statement describes 3 sequential activities in developing evidence-based clinical practice guidelines and related policies: 1) determination of the aggregate evidence quality in support of a proposed recommendation; 2) evaluation of the anticipated balance between benefits and harms when the recommendation is carried out; and 3) designation of recommendation strength. An individual policy can be reported as a "strong recommendation," "recommendation," "option," or "no recommendation." Use of this classification is intended to improve consistency and increase the transparency of the guideline-development process, facilitate understanding of AAP clinical practice guidelines, and enhance both the utility and credibility of AAP clinical practice guidelines. *Pediatrics* 2004;114:874–877; *practice guidelines, evidence-based, recommendation, classification system.*

ABBREVIATION. AAP, American Academy of Pediatrics.

INTRODUCTION

Clinical practice guidelines are intended to reduce inappropriate variations in clinical care, minimize harm, promote cost-effective practice, and produce optimal health outcomes for patients. Evidence-based guidelines use a systematic process to select and review scientific evidence to develop policy. In a clinical practice guideline, policy is stated in terms of recommendations. Recommendations are the guideline components that are intended to influence practitioner and patient behavior.

The contemporary, evidence-based approach to guideline development differs from other methods of creating policy in several ways, including:

1. The high level of rigor with which the evidence in support of a policy is identified, appraised, and summarized, and

2. The explicit linkage between recommendations and the evidence that supports them.

Like all scientists, evidence-based guideline developers define their methods first and then allow their methods to lead to the results rather than deciding first on the outcome.

A variety of systems have been used to convey information to guideline readers regarding the quality of evidence that supports a given recommendation and the strength assigned to the recommendation by guideline developers. A large number of numeric and alphabetic codes contribute to general confusion about the meaning of these scales. A recent evidence report prepared by the Agency for Healthcare Research and Quality found 121 scales, checklists, or other types of instruments for rating evidence quality.[1]

The American Academy of Pediatrics (AAP) develops clinical practice guidelines internally through various entities and in collaboration with other organizations and also considers for endorsement guidelines developed by external organizations. Clearly, the method used to classify recommendations in clinical practice guidelines should be consistent and explicit. A unified approach will facilitate communication between guideline developers and users and promote appropriate interpretation and application of guidelines by clinicians.

The objective of this statement is to describe a system for defining recommendation strength for AAP evidence-based practice guidelines that is clear, informative, and helpful to users. A common current approach to indicate the strength of a recommendation is to append a term to describe the "level of consensus" or, in some instances, fervor achieved. Because this judgment may not reflect unanimity of the development team and can be influenced disproportionately by vociferous or persuasive team members, it represents a lapse in an otherwise explicit system to link guideline statements to the strength of evidence and recommendation.

The proposed system was derived from existing systems that support the principle of using explicit criteria for guideline development. This system is intended for use by the AAP in the process of developing evidence-based clinical practice guidelines. This statement describes 3 sequential processes in evidence-based policy setting: 1) determination of evidence quality in support of a proposed recom-

DOI: 10.1542/peds.2004-1260
PEDIATRICS (ISSN 0031 4005). Copyright © 2004 by the American Academy of Pediatrics.

mendation; 2) evaluation of the balance between anticipated benefits and harms when the recommendation is carried out; and 3) designation of recommendation strength.

CLASSIFICATION PROCEDURE

1. Assess Evidence Quality: Individual and Aggregate

Quality appraisal of individual studies examines both the type of study and the rigor of the investigator's adherence to methodologic principles. Evidence quality refers to "the extent to which all aspects of a study's design and conduct can be shown to protect against systematic bias, nonsystematic bias, and inferential error."[2] Systematic errors include selection bias and confounding, in which values tend to be inaccurate in a particular direction. Nonsystematic errors are attributable to chance. Inferential errors result from problems in data analysis and interpretation, such as choice of the wrong statistical measure or wrongly rejecting the null hypothesis.

Highest-quality evidence for therapeutic interventions comes from well-designed and well-conducted randomized, controlled trials performed on a population similar to the guideline's target population. The lowest-quality evidence is derived from case reports, reasoning from first principles of pathophysiology, and expert opinion based on ill-defined "clinical experience." Intermediate-quality evidence is associated with a randomized, controlled trial with "nonfatal flaws" or methodologic limitations (for example, one performed on a group from a population different from the target population, therefore requiring that findings be extrapolated) or with an observational design such as a case-control or cohort study. For studies of diagnostic tests, the representativeness of the population studied, the adequacy of the description of the test, the appropriateness of the reference standard against which the test is compared, and the methods used to avoid bias in interpretation of results (such as blinded comparison with the reference standard) are criteria for judging quality.[3]

After systematically reviewing the literature for studies that bear on a policy decision, evidence-based guideline developers must carefully review each study, extract the findings, and appraise both the quality of the study design and its execution. The specific quality criteria applied depend on the design and type of study. For example, appraisal of controlled trials requires consideration of the adequacy of randomization and blinding and loss to follow-up; assessing case-control studies requires consideration of the appropriateness of matching cases and controls.

Next, guideline developers must consider the quality of the aggregate of studies that bear on the issue. Judging the strength of a body of evidence requires careful consideration of the consistency of the results of individual studies, the magnitude of the effect that the studies detect, and the individual and aggregate sample sizes of these studies.[1]

2. Assess Anticipated Balance Between Benefits and Harms

The anticipated benefit, harm, risk, and cost of adherence to a guideline recommendation constitute the second factor that influences the strength of a recommendation. Guyatt et al[4] suggest looking at the clarity of the balance between benefits and harms. When the evidence indicates a clear benefit not offset by important harms or costs or a clear harm not mitigated by important benefit, stronger recommendations are possible. On the other hand, when the magnitude of the benefit is small or benefits are present but offset by important adverse consequences, the equilibrium between benefits and harms prevents a strong recommendation. A clear preponderance of benefit or harm supports stronger statements for or against a course of action. When the benefit-harm assessment is balanced, no matter how good the studies, practitioners should be offered options rather than recommendations. Such cases mirror the situation described by Bass,[5] in which "there is adequate evidence at hand to support those who wish to treat...yet the evidence is not so overwhelming as to suggest that those who do not choose to use this form of therapy are in error."

3. Assign Recommendation Strength

Recommendation strength communicates the guideline developers' (and the sponsoring organizations') assessment of the importance of adherence to a particular recommendation and is based on both the quality of the supporting evidence and the magnitude of the potential benefit or harm. The proposed classification defines 4 levels of policy (strong recommendation, recommendation, option, and no recommendation) based on:

- Four levels of aggregate evidence quality: A, B, C, and D (see Fig 1);
- Two benefit-harm assessments: clear (ie, substantial) preponderance of benefit or harm versus a relative balance of benefits and harms; and
- A category for recommendation under exceptional situations in which evidence cannot be obtained but clear benefits or harm are evident.

Because guideline recommendations are prescriptive or proscriptive (constraining variation in practice), guideline developers must follow an approach that has a high likelihood of doing more good than harm. The more restrictive the guidance (strong recommendation), the more certain the guideline developers and endorsers must be of its correctness. The AAP believes that its policy makers should be cautious about classifying a recommendation as strong, lest they jeopardize their credibility by making statements that do not stand up to scientific scrutiny. Most recommendations are likely to be just that: recommendations.

When the evidence is of low quality and the benefit-harm equilibrium is balanced, guideline developers generally should not constrain the clinician's discretion by making a recommendation but instead should designate acceptable alternatives as options.

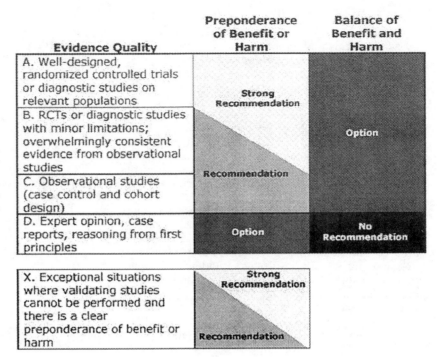

Fig 1. Integrating evidence quality appraisal with an assessment of the anticipated balance between benefits and harms if a policy is carried out leads to designation of a policy as a strong recommendation, recommendation, option, or no recommendation.

Although options do not direct clinicians' actions toward one activity or another, they may place boundaries by delineating appropriate alternative practices.

When the evidence is scant and the balance of benefit and harm is unknown, as for example with some complementary and alternative medicine practices, no recommendation regarding therapy may be possible. Stating that no recommendation is possible provides information but little direction to the clinician. No-recommendation statements are therefore of limited utility and should be discouraged. In some cases, guideline developers still may be able to make policy or offer options based on evidence. For example, although there may be no evidence of effectiveness of a complementary and alternative medicine practice, developers may be able to recommend that clinicians should inquire about use of complementary and alternative medicine and counsel about potential interactions. In other circumstances, guideline developers might suggest individualization on the basis of risk and values.

In some cases, a recommendation or strong recommendation may be made when analysis of the balance of benefits and harms demonstrates an exceptional preponderance of benefit or harm and it would be unethical to perform clinical trials to "prove" the point. These are almost exclusively situations of a medical (not social or political) nature. For example, the anticipated benefit of a recommendation for prescribing anthrax prophylaxis to exposed patients clearly outweighs the expected harms and calls for a strong recommendation, although studies do not exist to support the practice. Such situations with poor evidence but a highly unbalanced benefit-harm equation must be unmistakably differentiated from other circumstances in which

high-quality evidence supports strong recommendations. Requiring the authors to explicitly state the benefit-harm proposition opens it up for constructive debate.

INTERPRETING GUIDELINE RECOMMENDATIONS

How should a clinician interpret recommendations from the AAP in light of the proposed criteria for guideline recommendations? Guidelines are never intended to overrule professional judgment; rather, they may be viewed as a relative constraint on individual clinician discretion in a particular clinical circumstance. Less frequent variation in practice is expected for a strong recommendation than might be expected with a recommendation. Options offer the most opportunity for practice variability.[6] Clinicians should always act and make decisions on behalf of their patients' best interests and needs regardless of guideline recommendations. Guidelines represent the best judgment of a team of experienced clinicians and methodologists addressing the scientific evidence for a particular clinical topic.

A strong recommendation means that the committee believes that the benefits of the recommended approach clearly exceed the harms of that approach (or, in the case of a strong negative recommendation, that the harms clearly exceed the benefits) and that the quality of the evidence supporting this approach is either excellent or impossible to obtain. Clinicians should follow such guidance unless a clear and compelling rationale for acting in a contrary manner is present.

A recommendation means that the committee believes that the benefits exceed the harms (or, in the case of a negative recommendation, that the harms exceed the benefits), but the quality of the evidence on which this recommendation is based is not as strong. Clinicians also generally should follow such guidance but also should be alert to new information and sensitive to patient preferences.

An option means either that the evidence quality that exists is suspect or that well-designed, well-conducted studies have demonstrated little clear advantage to one approach versus another. Options offer clinicians flexibility in their decision-making regarding appropriate practice, although they may set boundaries on alternatives. Patient preference should have a substantial role in influencing clinical decision-making, particularly when policies are expressed as options.

No recommendation is made when there is both a lack of pertinent evidence and an unclear balance between benefits and harms. Clinicians should feel little constraint in their decision-making when addressing areas with insufficient evidence. Patient preference should have a substantial role in influencing clinical decision-making.

The AAP believes that adoption of an explicit, consistent classification of recommendations will facilitate communication between the AAP entities that develop guidelines (committees, sections, and task forces and the board of directors) and pediatricians who apply them to clinical practice. We recognize that any classification system may be considered by payors in making reimbursement decisions. This classification is intended only to increase transparency and to enhance the utility and credibility of AAP clinical practice guidelines. Direct linkage of this classification to reimbursement decisions would be overly simplistic, because recommendation strength is one of many factors that should be considered in developing reimbursement policy. Experience and new knowledge will likely require periodic revision of the proposed classification system.

STEERING COMMITTEE ON QUALITY IMPROVEMENT AND
  MANAGEMENT, 2003–2004
Charles J. Homer, MD, MPH, Chairperson
Carole M. Lannon, MD, MPH, Director

Norman Harbaugh, MD
Elizabeth Susan Hodgson, MD
*Edgar K. Marcuse, MD, MPH
*Richard N. Shiffman, MD
Lisa Simpson, MB, BCh

LIAISONS
Jay Berkelhamer, MD
Paul Darden, MD
  Section on Epidemiology
Denise Dougherty, PhD
  Agency for Healthcare Research and Quality
Ellen Schwalenstocker, MBA
  National Association of Children's Hospitals and
  Related Institutions

STAFF
Junelle P. Speller

*Lead authors

REFERENCES

1. West S, King V, Carey TS, et al. *Systems to Rate the Strength of Scientific Evidence. Evidence Report/Technology Assessment no. 47.* Research Triangle Park, NC: Research Triangle Institute-University of North Carolina Evidence-Based Practice Center; 2002. AHRQ Publication no. 02-E016
2. Lohr KN, Carey TS. Assessing "best evidence": issues in grading the quality of studies for systematic reviews. *Jt Comm J Qual Improv.* 1999; 25:470–479
3. Bossuyt PM, Reitsma JB, Bruns DE, et al. Towards complete and accurate reporting of studies of diagnostic accuracy: the STARD initiative. *Ann Intern Med.* 2003;138:40–44
4. Guyatt G, Sinclair J, Cook D, Jaeschke R, Schuenemann H, Pauker S. Moving from evidence to action: grading recommendations—a qualitative approach. In: Guyatt G, Rennie D, eds. *Users' Guides to the Medical Literature: A Manual for Evidence-Based Clinical Practice.* Chicago, IL: American Medical Association Press; 2002:599–608
5. Bass JW. Corticosteroids in croup [letter]. *JAMA.* 1972;221:1164
6. Eddy DM. *A Manual for Assessing Health Practices and Designing Practice Policies: The Explicit Approach.* Philadelphia, PA: American College of Physicians; 1992

Dealing With the Parent Whose Judgment Is Impaired by Alcohol or Drugs: Legal and Ethical Considerations

- *Clinical Report*

AMERICAN ACADEMY OF PEDIATRICS

CLINICAL REPORT
Guidance for the Clinician in Rendering Pediatric Care

John J. Fraser, Jr, MD, JD; Gary N. McAbee, DO, JD; and the Committee on Medical Liability

Dealing With the Parent Whose Judgment Is Impaired by Alcohol or Drugs: Legal and Ethical Considerations

ABSTRACT. An estimated 11 to 17.5 million children are being raised by a substance-abusing parent or guardian. The importance of this statistic is undeniable, particularly when a patient is brought to a pediatric office by a parent or guardian exhibiting symptoms of judgment impairment. Although the physician-patient relationship exists between the pediatrician and the minor patient, other obligations (some perceived and some real) should be considered as well. In managing encounters with impaired parents who may become disruptive or dangerous, pediatricians should be aware of their responsibilities before acting. In addition to fulfilling the duty involved with an established physician-patient relationship, the pediatrician should take reasonable care to safeguard patient confidentiality; protect the safety of the patient and other patients, visitors, and employees; and comply with reporting mandates. This clinical report identifies and discusses the legal and ethical concepts related to these circumstances. The report offers implementation suggestions when establishing anticipatory office procedures and training programs for staff on what to do (and not do) in such situations to maximize the patient's well-being and safety and minimize the liability of the pediatrician. *Pediatrics* 2004;114:869–873; *judgment impaired, alcohol, substance abuse, disruptive parent, informed permission, informed consent.*

ABBREVIATIONS. AAP, American Academy of Pediatrics; HHS, US Department of Health and Human Services; OSHA, Occupational Safety and Health Administration.

INTRODUCTION

In the course of providing health care services to children, pediatricians may encounter situations in which a patient arrives at the office accompanied by a parent, guardian, or caregiver who displays signs of judgment impairment. In these circumstances, pediatricians are challenged by an array of professional, ethical, and legal obligations, some of which may conflict. Pediatricians have sought guidance from the American Academy of Pediatrics (AAP) on how to respond to these potentially volatile and risk-laden scenarios. The purpose of this clinical report is to analyze the physician's poten-

The guidance in this report does not indicate an exclusive course of treatment or serve as a standard of medical care. Variations, taking into account individual circumstances, may be appropriate.
DOI: 10.1542/peds.2004-1234
PEDIATRICS (ISSN 0031 4005). Copyright © 2004 by the American Academy of Pediatrics.

tially conflicting duties and suggest ways that he or she can help both the child and the judgment-impaired adult in a situation fraught with legal complexity. This clinical report primarily addresses the situation in which the judgment of the parent, guardian, or caregiver is impaired by use of alcohol or drugs. However, the principles should be applicable to judgment impairment attributable to any cause (eg, prescription medication use, unstable medical condition such as diabetes, suspected dementia).

SCOPE OF THE PROBLEM

The Children of Alcoholics Foundation estimates that there are between 11 and 17.5 million children in the United States younger than 18 years currently living with a parent with alcoholism.[1] The number of children living in homes with an adult who abuses drugs is unknown. Clearly, this represents a substantial public health problem that most pediatricians will encounter at some point in their careers. Encounters with children accompanied by an impaired parent may take place wherever pediatric services are delivered. This report focuses on the legal and ethical issues pediatricians and their staff should consider when a patient's parent or guardian arrives at a pediatric office in a judgment-impaired state.

The profound effects of parental substance abuse on children have been described throughout the pediatric literature and summarized comprehensively in various AAP policy statements[2–4] and the manual on substance abuse.[5] A multidisciplinary working group developed a consensus paper titled "Core Competencies for Involvement of Health Care Providers in the Care of Children and Adolescents in Families Affected by Substance Abuse"[6] to identify the pivotal role of the primary health care professional in addressing the health needs of children in substance-abusing environments. It also suggests levels of responsibility and competencies for health care professionals in protecting the health and safety of these children. By virtue of their training and experience, pediatricians are well aware of the long-term risks to the child's physical, mental, and developmental health and safety associated with parental substance abuse. Therefore, it is not necessary for this clinical report to address the effects of parental substance abuse on the child. Instead, the report outlines the immediate risks and legal considerations associated with managing a parent or guardian whose judgment is impaired from alcohol or drugs during a pediatric office visit.

LEGAL CONSIDERATIONS

Pediatricians should consider the following legal principles when dealing with the parent whose judgment is temporarily impaired by alcohol or drugs:

- the physician-patient relationship;
- the duty to act in the best interest and for the safety of the patient;
- the need to obtain informed consent;
- the importance of safeguarding patient confidentiality;
- the mandated reporting of suspected child abuse and neglect; and
- the duty as an employer and business owner to protect the safety of employees and visitors in the office.

At times, there may be apparent conflict in these obligations. Every case is unique. The general considerations in this report are provided to enable pediatricians to develop office policies responsive to these situations. In translating this guidance into office policy, pediatricians should seek advice from competent legal counsel to ensure that the office policy is appropriate for a specific health care facility in a given state. The report's implementation suggestions serve as general guidance and, as such, should not be considered a specific course of action for a specific situation.

PHYSICIAN-PATIENT RELATIONSHIP

The parents, guardians, or caregivers who accompany infants, children, adolescents, and young adults play an important role in pediatric encounters. Depending on the age and circumstances of the patient, the adult often provides consent to treatment, furnishes pertinent historical information on the family and the child, and is financially responsible for medical care. Nevertheless, the pediatrician needs to remember that the physician-patient relationship exists between the pediatrician and the child. Thus, the pediatrician's first duty is to the patient.

The physician-patient relationship conveys many duties; one is to prevent harm. If there is reason to believe that the parent's impaired judgment substantially risks harming the patient or others, the pediatrician should attempt to decrease that risk by the least restrictive means. For instance, an impaired parent should not be allowed to drive. Not only would the patient be in considerable danger if allowed to ride in a motor vehicle being driven by someone under the influence of chemical substances, but the parent and the public also would be endangered. Depending on the circumstances, taking appropriate action could involve securing alternate transportation (eg, calling a taxi, contacting another family member to intervene). It may necessitate reporting the situation to the appropriate authorities including police or child protective services if discussion with the parent fails to result in a safe and satisfactory resolution. Local laws regarding public drunkenness or impairment may specify the appropriate course of action. Failing to fulfill the duty owed to a patient may constitute medical negligence and may even subject the pediatrician to liability from third parties.

BEST INTEREST OF THE PATIENT

Parents are presumed to have the best interests of their children at heart. Parents exhibiting signs of alcohol or drug impairment may be incapable of caring for a child properly. Therefore, the pediatrician's actions should be guided by the child's best interest, especially when the parent's condition compromises his or her ability to share that interest.

CONSENT TO CARE

Consent to care is a complicated concept in pediatrics. The ethical and legal considerations have been articulated in a number of AAP policy statements.[7–9] Pediatricians should be aware that it is likely that judgment-impaired parents are incapable of giving informed consent for their children's medical treatment. Pediatricians may have to use their judgment in determining whether a parent is incapable of consenting for a child. In some situations, it may be apparent that the parent has recently used alcohol or drugs but may not necessarily be impaired. In these circumstances, the pediatrician should be very careful about providing nonemergent care because of liability concerns brought forth later about insufficient informed consent. Therefore, if the child, by virtue of age or legal status, cannot consent to his or her own medical treatment and the parent's competency to do so is uncertain because of the chemical impairment, it would be advisable to postpone routine nonurgent medical care until consent can be obtained. To provide nonurgent care without consent would risk allegations of unauthorized treatment and even battery.[10,11]

However, in hospital emergency departments, the Emergency Medical Treatment and Active Labor Act[12] (EMTALA) plays a role. Under this act, a physician in certain situations may be mandated to screen for an emergency medical condition regardless of consent. Additional care may need to be given in the absence of consent if a delay would result in a threat of harm to the child's life or health. The EMTALA requirement for a medical screening examination does not apply to physician offices.

CONFIDENTIALITY AND PRIVACY

Parents have a reasonable expectation that information provided to the child's physician during a medical encounter will be considered confidential and protected by applicable laws. Thus, physicians should take reasonable care to safeguard health information obtained from the parent or guardian concerning the family (health and social history). Additional safeguards may be needed for sensitive topics such as substance abuse. These efforts should be reflected in the medical office's security policies for protecting patient records and other forms of identifiable health data according to any state and federal

(Health Insurance Portability and Accountability Act of 1996 [HIPAA]) laws.[13,14]

Due care should be taken to ensure that discussions with parents, patients, and appropriate government agencies concerning the substance-abuse problem and the family are conducted in a manner that protects confidentiality. For example, if the receptionist notices that an adult appears to be intoxicated when checking in for an appointment, it might be prudent to isolate the impaired person from others so that he or she can be spoken to privately. That would be preferable to confronting the impaired parent in the reception area in the presence of his or her child and others. The office could have a policy in place to summon the impaired parent as though it were time for the child's appointment and usher him or her into a more private location (eg, an office, conference room, or examining room) and take the child ostensibly to be weighed or measured in another room. This not only would minimize the risk of the conversation being overheard by others but also could afford an opportunity to discuss the problem without the child being present. However, if the impaired parent is disruptive in the office reception area, quick action may be needed to contain the situation, and in such instances, keeping the impaired person from harming others would take precedence over preserving the confidentiality of his or her chemical impairment.

MANDATED REPORTING

Every state has enacted laws to mandate reporting of child abuse and neglect. This is a legal obligation that is extended to children outside the physician-patient relationship. The physician must put the child's best interest before the parent's expectation of privacy and comply with mandated reporting to child protective services.[15–17]

An issue paper from the US Department of Health and Human Services (HHS) titled "Current Trends in Child Maltreatment Reporting Laws" summarizes how the standards used to determine when a mandatory reporter is required to notify authorities of abuse or neglect vary slightly from state to state.[18] These variances include who is a mandated reporter, the level of knowledge or suspicion of abuse necessary to report, and what constitutes abuse. The HHS issue paper provides a summary of common themes and general information on this complex topic. State Web sites may offer additional guidance to health care providers on mandated reporting of child abuse. However, specific legal advice interpreting the applicable laws and regulations is necessary when developing office policies for these situations.

It is important that mandated reporters understand these nuances in their state law. The patient should be carefully assessed for other signs of neglect or abuse. To do otherwise puts the pediatrician at risk of prosecution for failure to report suspected abuse or neglect of the patient. Should the patient subsequently be harmed as a consequence of the physician failing to act, the physician could be sued for medical negligence or face possible sanctions from a state licensing board. Anyone who is mandated to report suspected child abuse or maltreatment and fails to do so could be subject to criminal charges and could be sued in a civil court for monetary damages for any harm caused by their failure to report.

Two states impose penalties on mandatory reporters who intentionally, negligently, or purposefully fail to report suspected abuse. A few states impose penalties without imposing a standard. Failure to report is classified as a misdemeanor in approximately 35 states. Typically, sanctions are in the form of a fine and/or imprisonment.

Of greater impact on mandatory reporters themselves are the provisions exposing them to civil lawsuits for failure to report. The potential financial liability for additional injury of a child whose maltreatment should have been detected and prevented by a timely report can be considerable.

If a mandated reporter makes a report in earnest concern for the welfare of the child, that reporter is immune from any criminal or civil liability that may result. However, this good-faith immunity may not be available when the liability results from willful misconduct or gross negligence by the mandated reporter. Approximately 30 states impose penalties for false reporting of abuse. The most common standards used are knowingly and/or willfully filing an unproven report of abuse or neglect. A few jurisdictions impose penalties for intentionally making an unproven notification of abuse or neglect.[18]

GENERAL DUTY

In recent years, health care facilities have become targets of violence. Thus, the Occupational Safety and Health Administration (OSHA) has imposed regulations requiring health care employers to establish policies and procedures to safeguard employees from violent actions. Specific recommendations are enumerated in the OSHA regulations under the general duty heading.[19] Several documents are available on the OSHA Web site (www.osha.gov) that can be helpful in establishing practical step-by-step safety policies to protect employees in health care settings from potentially violent visitors.

IMPLEMENTATION SUGGESTIONS

The following suggestions are intended to help pediatricians implement office policies and procedures that may minimize legal risks should a patient arrive at the medical office in the care of an adult whose judgment is impaired.

Safety

Conduct a safety audit of your facility, including procedures for management of judgment-impaired visitors. Establish an office policy and train staff to respond appropriately. Incorporate this policy into your OSHA compliance program. Review and update the policy periodically. If the procedure is implemented, document the incident, how it was handled, and any injuries that occurred and evaluate whether the safety policy needs to be revised as a result of this occurrence. Maintain these records in a secure area of the office. Contact your professional liability insurance company to determine whether consulting services for developing such a loss-prevention program are available.

Confidentiality

Verify the confidentiality laws applicable in these situations and align your office confidentiality policies with these laws. Unless state laws indicate otherwise, the physician's duty to the patient should take precedence over the parent's expectation of confidentiality. Discuss with the parent your concerns regarding the risk to the child caused by his or her impairment in a compassionate, nonjudgmental fashion. Use the benefit of your previous rapport and professional relationship to show that the concern is for both the child's and the parent's welfare. Both the child and the parent should know what is happening and why it is necessary. Provide a referral for counseling to address the parent's substance abuse and its effect on the child. The Substance Abuse and Mental Health Services Administration of the HHS maintains a searchable directory of 12 000 facilities with treatment programs for drug and alcohol abuse throughout the United States (http://findtreatment. samhsa.gov).

Consent

Remember that an impaired parent cannot consent to medical treatment for the child. Therefore, it would be prudent to postpone nonurgent pediatric care until a time at which consent can be obtained. If no care is delivered, it is suggested that the physician document in the medical record that "valid and sufficient consent was not given by the parent for treatment today."

Mandated Reporting

It would be difficult to imagine how children under the care of an adult whose judgment is sporadically or habitually impaired by alcohol or drugs would not be at risk of harm. Use your best clinical judgment to determine the specific risks that the parent's condition poses to the child, and take action accordingly. Be knowledgeable of your state's laws governing reporting child abuse, standards of abuse, and consequences of failing to report for mandated reporters. Contacting child protective service agencies may be the only way to get treatment for the parent and protection for the child. If you believe that the judgment-impaired person may harm himself or herself or others, take action in accordance with applicable laws. Summoning for police escort or emergency personnel to transport the impaired adult to the emergency department for evaluation and treatment may be necessary. Should the child's custodial parent or guardian agree to it, it may be preferable to release the child to the care of a relative rather than have the child accompany the parent to the emergency department or police station. However, child protective services may be in the best situation to make such determinations.

The greatest risk is to do nothing.

REFERENCES

1. Johnson JL, Leff M. Children of substance abusers: overview of research findings. *Pediatrics.* 1999;103:1085–1099
2. American Academy of Pediatrics, Committee on Substance Abuse. Alcohol use and abuse: a pediatric concern. *Pediatrics.* 1995;95:439–442
3. American Academy of Pediatrics, Committee on Substance Abuse. Indications for management and referral of patients involved in substance abuse. *Pediatrics.* 2000;106:143–148
4. American Academy of Pediatrics, Committee on Early Childhood, Adoption, and Dependent Care. The pediatrician's role in family support programs. *Pediatrics.* 2001;107:195–197
5. American Academy of Pediatrics, Committee on Substance Abuse. *Substance Abuse: A Guide for Health Professionals.* 2nd ed. Schydlower M, ed. Elk Grove Village, IL: American Academy of Pediatrics; 2002
6. Adger H Jr, Macdonald DI, Wenger S. Core competencies for involvement of health care providers in the care of children and adolescents in families affected by substance abuse. *Pediatrics.* 1999;103:1083–1084
7. American Academy of Pediatrics, Committee on Bioethics. Informed consent, parental permission, and assent in pediatric practice. *Pediatrics.* 1995;95:314–317
8. American Academy of Pediatrics, Committee on Pediatric Emergency Medicine. Consent for medical services for children and adolescents. *Pediatrics.* 1993;92:290–291
9. American Academy of Pediatrics, Committee on Bioethics. Religious objections to medical care. *Pediatrics.* 1997;99:279–281
10. *Hodge v Lafayette General Hospital,* 399 So 2d 744 (La App 3rd Cir 1981)
11. *Buie v Reynolds,* 571 P2d 1230 (Okla Ct App 1977)
12. Emergency Medical Treatment and Active Labor Act. 42 USC §1395dd (1986)
13. American Academy of Pediatrics, Pediatric Practice Action Group and Task Force on Medical Informatics. Privacy protection and health information: patient rights and pediatrician responsibilities. *Pediatrics.* 1999;104:973–977
14. Security and electronic signature standards–HCFA. Proposed rule. *Fed Regist.* 1998;63:43242–43280
15. American Academy of Pediatrics, Committee on Child Abuse and Neglect. Public disclosure of private information about victims of abuse. *Pediatrics.* 1991;87:261
16. American Academy of Pediatrics, Committee on Hospital Care and Committee on Child Abuse and Neglect. Medical necessity for the hospitalization of the abused and neglected child. *Pediatrics.* 1998;101:715–716

17. American Academy of Pediatrics, Task Force on Violence. The role of the pediatrician in youth violence prevention in clinical practice and at the community level. *Pediatrics.* 1999;103:173–181

18. US Department of Health and Human Services. Current Trends in Child Maltreatment Reporting Laws. Child Abuse and Neglect State Statutes Series. Issue Paper. Washington, DC: National Clearinghouse on Child Abuse and Neglect Information; 2002. Available at: http://nccanch. acf.hhs.gov/general/legal/statutes/issue/report.cfm. Accessed November 7, 2003

19. US Occupational Safety and Health Administration. *Guidelines for Preventing Workplace Violence for Health Care and Social Service Workers.* Washington, DC: US Department of Labor; 2003. Publication No. 3148. Available at: www.osha.gov/SLTC/workplaceviolence/healthcare/ index.html. Accessed November 7, 2003

All clinical reports from the American Academy of Pediatrics automatically expire 5 years after publication unless reaffirmed, revised, or retired at or before that time.

Do-Not-Resuscitate Orders for Pediatric Patients Who Require Anesthesia and Surgery

● ●

- *Clinical Report*

AMERICAN ACADEMY OF PEDIATRICS

CLINICAL REPORT
Guidance for the Clinician in Rendering Pediatric Care

Mary E. Fallat, MD; Jayant K. Deshpande, MD; and the Section on Surgery, Section on Anesthesia and Pain Medicine, and Committee on Bioethics

Do-Not-Resuscitate Orders for Pediatric Patients Who Require Anesthesia and Surgery

ABSTRACT. This clinical report addresses the topic of preexisting do-not-resuscitate (DNR) orders for children undergoing anesthesia and surgery. Pertinent issues addressed include the rights of children, surrogate decision-making, the process of informed consent, and the roles of surgeons and anesthesiologists. The reevaluation process of DNR orders called "required reconsideration" can be incorporated into the process of informed consent for surgery and anesthesia. Care should be taken to distinguish between goal-directed and procedure-directed approaches to DNR orders. By giving parents or other surrogates and clinicians the option of deciding from among full resuscitation, limitations based on procedures, or limitations based on goals, the child's needs are individualized and better served. *Pediatrics* 2004;114: 1686–1692; *anesthesia, pediatric surgery, pediatrics, children, resuscitation, cardiac arrest, respiratory arrest.*

ABBREVIATIONS. DNR, do-not-resuscitate; CPR, cardiopulmonary resuscitation; ASA, American Society of Anesthesiologists; ACS, American College of Surgeons.

CONSIDERATIONS FOR CHILDREN WITH DO-NOT-RESUSCITATE ORDERS WHO REQUIRE ANESTHESIA AND SURGERY

In the 1970s, the Critical Care Committee at the Massachusetts General Hospital developed the original do-not-resuscitate (DNR) guidelines in response to nursing requests for clarification of what should be done when cardiopulmonary resuscitation (CPR) was unwanted or believed to be unwarranted by a patient or surrogate.[1] DNR orders are clinically and ethically appropriate when the burdens of resuscitation exceed the expected benefit. Currently, all hospitals seeking accreditation from the Joint Commission on Accreditation of Healthcare Organizations are required to have a DNR policy in place.[2–6] This policy should define a DNR order and describe the guidelines for its inclusion on a patient's medical record. A DNR order is a written order by an attending physician and precludes resuscitative efforts being undertaken in the event of cardiopulmonary ar-

rest. DNR orders should not have implications regarding the use of other therapeutic interventions that may be appropriate for the patient, including surgery and anesthesia.[7,8]

The controversial topic of DNR orders for patients undergoing surgery and anesthesia has received growing attention in the medical literature since the early 1990s. However, the literature does not specifically address the pediatric age group. For children, DNR orders are written when (1) in the judgment of the treating physician, an attempt to resuscitate the child would not benefit the child and (2) the parent or surrogate decision-maker (with the assent of an age-appropriate child) expresses his or her preference that CPR be withheld in the event that the child suffers a cardiopulmonary arrest, as long as this is in accordance with the child's best interests.[7,9] DNR orders are written on the assumption that cardiopulmonary arrest will be a spontaneous event that is the culmination of the dying process of a child who has a terminal illness or a poor quality of life. The dilemma surgeons and anesthesiologists are confronted with regarding children with DNR orders undergoing an operative procedure is twofold: (1) anesthesia promotes some degree of hemodynamic abnormality that may result in cardiopulmonary arrest, and (2) many routine anesthetic manipulations can be classified as resuscitative measures.

A number of hospitals across the nation still do not have a policy that specifically addresses the extent to which DNR orders apply in the operating room[2,5,10,11] or have a policy that mandates suspension of DNR orders.[9] According to 1 study, surgical procedures are performed in ~15% of patients with DNR orders.[12] The American Academy of Pediatrics and the American Society of Anesthesiologists (ASA) have issued guidelines on forgoing life-sustaining medical treatment, issues of informed consent,[13,14] and evaluation and preparation of pediatric patients undergoing anesthesia.[15] None of these policies address in detail the approach to be taken when an operative procedure is considered for a child with an existing DNR order. This encounter includes the dilemmas of who should assume responsibility (ie, the primary care physician, the surgeon, or the anesthesiologist) for discussing with the parent or surrogate decision-maker the potential risks of cardiopulmo-

The guidance in this report does not indicate an exclusive course of treatment or serve as a standard of medical care. Variations, taking into account individual circumstances, may be appropriate.

doi:10.1542/peds.2004-2119

PEDIATRICS (ISSN 0031 4005). Copyright © 2004 by the American Academy of Pediatrics.

nary arrest during surgery and anesthesia, whether the DNR order should be temporarily suspended during the procedure, and how long a temporary suspension should last if this option is chosen.

SURVEY OF SECTIONS ON SURGERY AND ANESTHESIA

The relevance of this topic was assessed by distributing a survey to the 570 members of the Section on Surgery and 293 members of the Section on Anesthesiology of the American Academy of Pediatrics in 1995. The survey was returned by 242 surgeons (42.5%) and 107 anesthesiologists (36.5%). Demographic data on the respondents are shown in Table 1.

For each group, surgeons and anesthesiologists, finite sample confidence intervals for proportions were computed.[16] The finite population correction factor was used for hypotheses testing as needed.[16] Statistical software used included SPSS version 10 (SPSS Inc, Chicago, IL [2000]) and StatXact version 4 (Cytel Software Inc, Cambridge, MA [2000]).

The majority of surgeons (88.8%) and anesthesiologists (86%) had been asked to operate on or provide anesthesia to a child with a DNR order in place at the time of surgery, and most indicated that they would not refuse to provide these services. Most surgeons (75.3%) and anesthesiologists (69.2%) would agree to honor a DNR order during a palliative operative procedure, but smaller percentages of surgeons (49.6%) and anesthesiologists (46.7%) were willing to honor a DNR order during an elective operative procedure. More than 95% of surgeons and anesthesiologists discuss resuscitation issues before surgery with parents of children who have standing DNR orders, and a majority of each group felt that there should be a hospital policy for children with DNR orders in the operating room. Only 50.5% of anesthesiologists and 27.5% of surgeons stated that their hospital has such a policy in place.

Surgeons and anesthesiologists then were asked which resuscitation maneuvers should be withheld during intraoperative arrest in a child with a DNR order. Results are summarized in Table 2.

The majority of anesthesiologists (86%) and surgeons (94.7%) were willing to withdraw life support at the request of the family a few days after surgery if a child suffered an arrest in the operating room, was resuscitated, and had an adverse change in quality of life. The majority of anesthesiologists (55.1%) felt that the perioperative period ended when the child left the recovery room, with only 38.2% of surgeons agreeing ($P = .0037$). Many anesthesiologists (22.4%) and surgeons (39.5%) felt that the perioperative period should be extended until 24 hours after surgery.

DISCUSSION

The medical literature contains some ambiguities on the scope of a DNR order and the resuscitative interventions it prevents during surgery and anesthesia. Resuscitative interventions may be broadly defined as any maneuvers and techniques used to prevent or reverse cardiopulmonary arrest.[17] However, this definition is inappropriate in an operative setting, because anesthetic agents routinely promote cardiovascular instability.[2,5,11,18] Perioperatively, resuscitative measures should only refer to the measures undertaken to restore life once a cardiopulmonary arrest has occurred.[8,19] Surveys of physicians and patients with DNR orders confirm that clarification is needed on the interpretation of a DNR order, especially its applicability in the operating room.[12,20–22]

Physicians caring for children have a duty to respect the wishes of the child and family, to do good (beneficence), and to avoid harm (nonmaleficence), which may lead to conflicting considerations for a child with a DNR order. Some physicians believe that honoring a DNR request harms a child by allowing a potentially reversible death to occur. On the other hand, the child's welfare is best served by not having a poor quality of life unnecessarily prolonged and not having to endure ineffective therapy.[23] Older children and adolescents should be included in the decision-making process (patient assent) when their neurologic status, development, and level of maturity allow. However, legally they require a surrogate decision-maker to act on their behalf (surrogate or parental permission).[14] A child's surrogate, usually a parent, should be the person presumed to be the most appropriate and capable to determine what actions would be in the best interest of the child. Conflicts arise when the parent or other surrogate and/or child and the physician fail to agree on what would be optimal care under a given set of circumstances.

Informed Consent

To respect the child's and family's wishes, physicians must obtain informed permission from a parent or surrogate before a child can undergo any medical intervention including surgery and resuscitation. Ordinarily, resuscitation efforts do not require informed consent, because they are deemed emergency interventions and consent is implied. However, terminally ill or severely disabled children and their parents are often confronted with the decision of whether resuscitation should be attempted in the

TABLE 1. Demographics of Respondents to Survey Regarding DNR Orders

	Pediatric Surgeons	Pediatric Anesthesiologists
Demographics		
Median age, y	50 (35–81)	44 (32–63)
Median years in practice, y	18 (3–45)	11 (2–41)
Practice characteristics,* n (%)		
Full-time university	132 (54.8)	55 (51.4)
University clinical affiliate	57 (23.4)	30 (28.0)
Private practice	68 (28.2)	26 (24.3)
Military	3 (1.2)	0 (0)
Hospital type,* n (%)		
Children's hospital	116 (49.2)	55 (51.4)
University hospital	95 (40.3)	36 (3.6)
Community hospital	53 (22.5)	17 (15.9)
Military hospital	2 (0.8)	0 (0)

* A small number of surgeons and anesthesiologists reported multiple affiliations.

TABLE 2.   Responses When Asked Whether Resuscitation Maneuvers Should Be Withheld During Intraoperative Arrest in a Child With a DNR Order

	Pediatric Surgeons*		Pediatric Anesthesiologists		P Value
	Yes, %	No	Yes, %	No	
Maneuver					
Positive-pressure ventilation	60 (26.7)	165	23 (21.5)	84	NS
Vasoactive drugs	93 (41.5)	131	34 (31.8)	73	.0005
Endotracheal intubation	63 (28.1)	161	22 (20.6)	85	NS
Defibrillation	166 (73.8)	56	65 (60.7)	42	.0092
Closed cardiac massage	175 (77.4)	51	36 (33.6)	71	<.00005

NS indicates not significant.
* Some respondents did not answer every question

event the child's underlying disease results in cardiopulmonary arrest.

Customarily, physicians will approach the parent or surrogate about instituting a DNR order when it is felt that resuscitation of the child would not be beneficial and would only prolong the time to death.[22] When a parent or surrogate consents to a DNR order, it is under the assumption that cardiopulmonary arrest will be a direct consequence of the child's underlying disease. Surgery and anesthesia constitute a change in the child's medical status, because they introduce additional risks to the patient. Because surgeons and anesthesiologists are rarely involved in the original DNR decision, they cannot be certain that the implications of the DNR status in the perioperative setting were discussed with the patient's parent (or other surrogate).[3] Therefore, the parent or surrogate, the surgeon, and the anesthesiologist should reevaluate the DNR order for a child who requires an operative procedure. This reevaluation process has been called "required reconsideration"[3] and should be incorporated into the process of informed consent for surgery and anesthesia. Discussions regarding consent under these circumstances should be initiated by attending staff, particularly in hospitals with residency teaching programs in which residents may be routinely involved in the consent process.

The surgeon and anesthesiologist must approach the parents and child with compassion. There is often no previous relationship established between the patient, parents, and surgical team, precluding a brief preoperative assessment. "Active listening" is essential. The parent or surrogate should be asked about specific interventions and their understanding of the relative merits of each of these interventions during resuscitation (Table 3).[15] Airway management should be determined by what is mandated by the child's condition and the surgical procedure. Specific prohibition of tracheal intubation is problematic, and beliefs and concerns must be carefully elicited and discussed. Exceptions to the injunctions against intervention should be specifically noted in the patient's medical record. The parent may agree to a temporary suspension of the DNR order during the perioperative period. If so, the temporal end point to the DNR suspension needs to be recorded as well. If an agreement cannot be obtained after thorough discussion, the wishes of the informed parent or surro-

TABLE 3.   Potential Interventions During Resuscitation

Airway management
  Supplemental oxygen
  Oral airway
  Bag and mask ventilation
  Intubation
Arterial puncture
Needle thoracentesis
Chest tube insertion
Blood product transfusion
Invasive monitoring
Chest compressions
Defibrillation
Cardiac pacing
Arrest medications (epinephrine, atropine, sodium bicarbonate, calcium, other vasoactive drugs)
Postoperative ventilatory support

gate must prevail. In some cases, the parents may feel that the burden of a therapy is not worth the potential benefits and decline the procedure. When an individual physician feels that the parent's wishes are inconsistent with his or her medical, ethical, or moral views, the physician should withdraw from the case after ensuring continuity of care[13] and could consider consulting the institutional ethics committee.

Role of the Surgeon

The following are operative interventions that might be considered for a pediatric patient with a DNR order:

1. Provision of a support device that will enable the child to be discharged from the hospital (eg, gastrostomy tube or tracheostomy).
2. Urgent surgery for a condition unrelated to the underlying chronic problem (eg, acute appendicitis in a terminal cancer patient).
3. Urgent surgery for a condition related to the underlying chronic problem but not believed to be a terminal event (eg, a pathologic fracture or bowel obstruction).
4. A procedure to decrease pain.
5. A procedure to provide vascular access.

It is the duty of the operating surgeon to discuss risks of a procedure with the parent or other surrogate of any pediatric patient, including how the patient's condition might influence the risk of anesthesia. The American College of Surgeons (ACS) issued a statement to guide surgeons in operating on patients with an active DNR order.[24] The ACS statement does not make specific reference to patient surrogates, although it is implied.[24] It is expected that the surgeon will advise parents or other surrogates and the child (if developmentally appropriate) regarding operative risks and benefits and advocate a policy of required reconsideration of previous DNR orders. The results of all discussions should be documented in the patient's medical record. The surgeon should also ultimately convey the patient's wishes to the members of the entire operating room team, help operating team members understand the patient's or surrogate's wishes, and find alternate team members to replace individuals who disagree with the patient's or surrogate's wishes. With children, the difficulty arises when there is no one who is willing to honor a family's wish to continue the DNR status during the anesthesia and surgery. Stalemates such as this should be referred to the ethics committee of the institution.

Role of the Anesthesiologist

In 1994 and 1999, the ASA released recommendations on caring for surgical patients with active DNR orders.[15] These guidelines explicitly reject the practice of automatically rescinding the DNR order before procedures involving the use of anesthesia, because this practice "may not sufficiently address a patient's rights to self-determination in a responsible and ethical manner."[15] The purpose of required reconsideration of DNR orders is to determine what is best for the patient under the circumstances, not to convince the patient and family to have the DNR order suspended. The guidelines proposed by the ASA clearly recommend that all physicians involved in the case (primary physician, surgeon, and anesthesiologist) discuss together with the patient (or other surrogate) the appropriateness of maintaining the DNR order during the operation. The 1999 guidelines distinguish between goal-directed and procedure-directed DNR orders.[15] Model procedure-specific DNR documentation forms are published and may be modified for individual hospital use.[9]

A goal-directed approach focuses on the patient's goals, values, and preferences rather than on individual procedures. The primary goal is to do everything to prevent the need for resuscitation, but if it occurs, this approach recognizes that patients are often less concerned with technical details of the resuscitation than with more subjective and personal issues regarding quality of life before and after resuscitation. This model promulgates an approach that honors the family's treatment goals while reflecting the reality and unique aspects of the perioperative environment. However, some anesthesiologists are uncomfortable with the indeterminate nature of a goal-directed DNR order and have ethical or legal concerns about having such crucial decisions rest solely on their best judgment at the time of arrest.

Goal-directed DNR orders may be less feasible if the anesthesiologist and surgeon caring for the child have not established a relationship with the family before surgery. A procedure-directed approach may be more appropriate in these circumstances, which involves careful consideration of a series of specific interventions that are likely to be used (Table 3). Each must be placed in the context of the child's usual quality of life and likelihood of the ability of the procedure to produce the desired effect, given his or her unique physiology. This approach has limited flexibility when an unexpected situation occurs.[9]

Perioperative suspension of the DNR order is considered by some anesthesiologists to be the ideal compromise, because it enables the physician to act without restraint while providing the patient with a realistic chance of achieving the operative goals.[10,25] Anesthetic agents and techniques may promote some degree of hemodynamic and respiratory abnormality, especially in patients with a deteriorated health condition.[2] The deliberate depression of vital functions by the anesthetic may require resuscitative measures to stabilize the patient.[11] Consequently, controversy about the use of these interventions arises when the patient has a written DNR order. Many of the routine anesthetic interventions performed as part of operative maintenance are considered resuscitative measures under different circumstances. These interventions include the use of paralytic agents, vasoactive drugs, blood products, and positive-pressure ventilation. This overlap in terminology promotes confusion and inconsistencies among physicians on the interpretation of a patient's DNR order and what it implies in an operative setting. Keffer and Keffer[8,19] proposed that resuscitation in the operating room be defined as "those measures undertaken to reestablish cardiac rhythm once a cardiac arrest has occurred."[8(p644)] This definition establishes a simple end point beyond which a patient's wish not to be resuscitated would come into play.

The anesthesiologists' concern for patient comfort during the procedure may support perioperative suspension of DNR orders. An active DNR order restricts the physicians' ability to treat any complications of their own procedure during anesthesia. Faced with this dilemma, anesthesiologists are forced to decrease the risk of cardiopulmonary arrest by increasing hemodynamic stability through the use of less anesthetic.[2,11,26] For the patient, this may potentially result in more discomfort and suffering.

One reason to distinguish DNR in the operating room from DNR in other settings is the difference in the success rate of CPR administered for a spontaneous cardiopulmonary arrest versus one that results from anesthesia. Anesthetic-related arrests are believed to be more easily reversible because of the immediate ability to respond and the controlled nature of the event.[3,19,26,27] One study of surgical patients suggested that when a cardiac arrest was ascribed to anesthesia, 92% of the patients were resuscitated successfully.[3,28] However, it is difficult to determine how these statistics apply to terminally ill patients with a DNR designation, because the survey was very broad and inclusive. A more relevant survey was conducted on 4301 seriously ill adult patients, and a few underwent an operative procedure and had previously written DNR orders in their medical records. Only 3 of the 57 patients with DNR orders (5%) experienced an intraoperative cardiopulmonary arrest, but all died within 5 days of operation.[29]

Traditionally, CPR has been considered a success if the patient survives the initial resuscitation effort. For patients with DNR orders, the success of CPR may be better gauged on the length of patient survival[7] and expected quality of life after resuscitation. Using this definition, CPR may be inappropriate from the parent's or surrogate's viewpoint if resuscitation has the overwhelming probability of resulting in patient suffering and only prolonging the time to death.[7] Anesthesiologists have the duty to inform the parent or other surrogate of the risks and potential benefits of intraoperative resuscitation. Required reconsideration as part of the process of informed consent for anesthesia eliminates ambiguities and misunderstandings associated with patients who have DNR orders by providing anesthesiologists with the opportunity to educate the parent (or other surrogate) to become familiar with their values and perceptions of the child's quality of life and together clarify how the child's DNR order should be interpreted perioperatively. By giving parents or surrogates and clinicians the option of deciding from among full resuscitation, limitations based on procedures, or limitations based on goals, the child's needs are individualized and better served. Regardless of the decision made by the parent or other surrogate, the individual acting on behalf of the child must be readily available for consultation during the procedure. The ASA, like the ACS, advocates that physicians withdraw from a case when they are unwilling or unable to respect and implement a patient's (or other surrogate's) decision to limit the use of resuscitation.[15,24]

If DNR Orders Are Suspended: Qualification of Perioperative Interval

If the family or medical personnel involved in a child's care choose to suspend DNR orders during anesthesia and surgery, it is necessary to define the duration of suspension.[30] The physiologic effects of anesthesia and surgery rarely terminate at the end of the procedure, but the duration thereafter depends on the anesthetic technique used and the type of surgical procedure performed. The acute effects of most anesthetic medications generally resolve within several hours or 1 day after surgery, and most anesthesiologists visit the patient the day after a surgical procedure and document recovery status in the patient record. Recovery of respiratory function after surgery depends on preoperative pulmonary function, chronicity of illness, and length of the procedure. Some patients will experience cardiopulmonary arrest during or immediately after surgery, which may be the result of an acute and reversible complication. It is appropriate to use mechanical ventilation after surgery as long as the patient continues to show significant and sustained improvement in pulmonary function. Once the patient ceases to recover or deteriorates, withdrawal of ventilatory

support should be considered. Generally speaking, the suspension of DNR orders should continue until the postanesthetic visit, until the patient has been weaned from mechanical ventilation, or until the primary physician involved in the patient's care and the family agree to reinstate the DNR order.

The surgeon and anesthesiologist should feel comfortable, and should be allowed, to reinstate a DNR order intraoperatively through consultation with the family under certain conditions. For example, if cardiac arrest occurs during surgery and it is apparent that the arrest is the result of an irreversible underlying disease or complication and that CPR would only allow continued deterioration, the DNR order should be reinstated. If resuscitation measures are withheld and intraoperative arrest occurs, such a death should be classified as "expected" for quality-assurance purposes rather than "unexpected." Expected deaths do not require mandatory quality-assurance review.[18,31]

IMPLEMENTING "REQUIRED RECONSIDERATION"

Hospitals are encouraged to develop and maintain written policies permitting the forgoing of life-sustaining treatment of patients, including children, in appropriate circumstances.[13] Once a DNR order is in place according to accepted standards, it is important that it be reviewed before surgery to determine applicability in the operating room and the postoperative recovery period. Hospitals wishing to develop a "required reconsideration" policy (Table 4) may want to address the following elements:

- Include in the discussion with a child's parent or other surrogate information about the likelihood of requiring resuscitative measures, a description of these measures and their reversibility, the chance of success, and possible outcomes with and without resuscitation. Establish an agreement about what, if any, resuscitative measures will be instituted during the procedure.
- Make the decision to uphold or suspend a DNR order on the basis of the planned procedure, the anticipated benefit for the child, and the likelihood of patient compromise as a result of the procedure.
- Document the salient features of the physician-family discussion in the medical record.
- Communicate plans to honor an intraoperative DNR order among relevant staff.
- Require any physician or other health care professional who is unwilling to honor a family's refusal

---

TABLE 4. Required Reconsideration Options for Pediatric Patients With DNR Orders Who Require Anesthesia and Surgery

Full resuscitation
  Perioperative suspension of DNR orders with qualification of perioperative interval
Goal-directed approach
  Focuses on patient goals, values, and preferences
  Implies personal relationship between physician and patient/family with understanding of quality-of-life concerns
  Most subjective approach
Procedure-directed approach
  Specific interventions (see Table 3) placed in context of child's quality of life are each reviewed prior to procedure

of resuscitation to withdraw from the case and allow others to assume care. The withdrawing physician or health care professional should make a conscientious effort to identify another physician who is willing to honor the DNR request.[13]

- Recognize that a patient's or surrogate's decision to refuse intraoperative resuscitation can be compatible with the provision of therapeutic measures to treat conditions other than arrest. This decision does not necessarily imply limits on other forms of care such as intensive care.
- If the family chooses to rescind the DNR order in the operating room and arrest occurs with resuscitation, but the patient's process of dying has only been prolonged, make a provision to discuss withdrawal of life support after a determined amount of time.[3,5,19]

SECTION ON SURGERY, 2004–2005
Donna A. Caniano, MD, Chairperson
Richard R. Ricketts, MD
Brad W. Warner, MD
Kurt D. Newman, MD
Michael D. Klein, MD

Ann M. Kosloske, MD
  Past Section Chairperson
Richard Andrassy, MD
  Past Section Chairperson
Richard Azizkhan, MD
  Past Section Chairperson
Thomas R. Weber, MD
  Past Section Chairperson

CONSULTANTS
Jane Goldsmith, PhD
Katia G. Santos, MD

STAFF
Chelsea Kirk

SECTION ON ANESTHESIOLOGY AND PAIN MEDICINE,
  2004–2005
Thomas Mancuso, MD, Chairperson
Joseph Cravero, MD
Constance Houck, MD
Zeev Kain, MD
Lynne Maxwell, MD
Robert Valley, MD
Rita Agarwal, MD

Lynne Ferrari, MD
  Past Section Chairperson
Patty Davidson, MD
  Past Section Executive Committee Member
Jayant K. Deshpande, MD
  Past Section Executive Committee Member

STAFF
Kathleen Kuk Ozmeral

COMMITTEE ON BIOETHICS, 2004–2005
Jeffrey R. Botkin, MD, MPH
Douglas S. Diekema, MD, MPH
Mary E. Fallat, MD
Eric D. Kodish, MD
Steven R. Leuthner, MD

Lainie Friedman Ross, MD, PhD
G. Kevin Donovan, MD, MLA

John T. Truman, MD, MPH
  Past Committee Member
Benjamin S. Wilfond, MD
  Past Committee Member

LIAISONS
Christine E. Harrison, MD
  Canadian Paediatric Society
Neil W. Boris, MD
  American Academy of Child and Adolescent
  Psychiatry
Marcia Levetown, MD
  American Board of Pediatrics
Arlene J. Morales, MD
  American College of Obstetricians and
  Gynecologists

Alessandra (Sandi) Kazura, MD
  Past Committee Liaison
Ernest F. Krug, III, MDiv, MD
  Past Committee Liaison
Michael K. Lindsay, MD
  Past Committee Liaison

CONSULTANT
Dena S. Davis, JD, PhD

STAFF
Alison Baker, MS

REFERENCES

1. Critical Care Committee of the Massachusetts General Hospital. Optimum care for hopelessly ill patients. *N Engl J Med.* 1976,295:362–364
2. Anderson EF, Freeman JW. Management of the do-not-resuscitate patient undergoing anesthesia and surgery. *S D J Med.* 1992,45:315–317
3. Cohen B, Cohen PJ. Sounding board: do-not-resuscitate order in the operating room. *N Engl J Med.* 1991,325:1879–1882
4. Jacobson BS. Ethical dilemmas of do-not-resuscitate orders in surgery. *AORN J.* 1994,60:449–452
5. Reeder JM. Do-not-resuscitate orders in the operating room. *AORN J.* 1993,57:947–951
6. Stevens WC. "Do-not-resuscitate" orders in operating rooms. *West J Med.* 1992,157:563–564
7. American Medical Association, Council on Ethical and Judicial Affairs. Guidelines for the appropriate use of do-not-resuscitate orders. *JAMA.* 1991,265:1868–1871
8. Keffer MJ, Keffer HL. The do-not-resuscitate order. Moral responsibilities of the perioperative nurse. *AORN J.* 1994,59:641–645, 648–650
9. Truog RD, Waisel DB, Burns JP. DNR in the OR: a goal-directed approach. *Anesthesiology.* 1999,90:289–295
10. Cohen NH. Do not resuscitate orders in the operating room: the birth of a policy. *Camb Q Healthc Ethics.* 1995,4:103–110
11. Truog RD. "Do-not-resuscitate" orders during anesthesia and surgery. *Anesthesiology.* 1991,74:606–608
12. La Puma J, Silverstein MD, Stocking CB, Roland D, Siegler M. Life-sustaining treatment. A prospective study of patients with DNR orders in a teaching hospital. *Arch Intern Med.* 1988,148:2193–2198
13. American Academy of Pediatrics, Committee on Bioethics. Guidelines on foregoing life-sustaining medical treatment. *Pediatrics.* 1994,93:532–536
14. American Academy of Pediatrics, Committee on Bioethics. Informed consent, parental permission, and assent in pediatric practice. *Pediatrics.* 1995,95:314–317
15. American Society of Anesthesiologists, Committee on Ethics. Ethical guidelines for the anesthesia care of patients with do not resuscitate orders or other directives that limit treatment. Available at: www.asahq.org/publicationsAndServices/standards/09.html. Accessed October 17, 2004
16. Cochran WG, ed. *Sampling Techniques.* 3rd ed. New York, NY: John Wiley & Sons; 1977:58–60

17. Walker RM. DNR in the OR: resuscitation as an operative risk. *JAMA.* 1991,266:2407–2412

18. Igoe S, Cascella S, Stockdale K. Ethics in the OR: DNR and patient autonomy. *Nurs Manage.* 1993,24:112A, 112D, 112H

19. Keffer MJ, Keffer HL. Do-not-resuscitate in the operating room: moral obligations of anesthesiologists. *Anesth Analg.* 1992,74:901–905

20. Clemency MV, Thompson NJ. "Do-not-resuscitate" (DNR) orders and the anesthesiologist: a survey. *Anesth Analg.* 1993,76:394–401

21. Clemency MV, Thompson NJ. "Do-not-resuscitate" (DNR) orders in the perioperative period—a comparison of the perspectives of anesthesiologists, internists, and surgeons. *Anesth Analg.* 1994,78:651–658

22. Murphy EK. Do-not-resuscitate orders in the OR. *AORN J.* 1993,58:399–401

23. American Academy of Pediatrics, Committee on Bioethics and Committee on Hospital Care. Palliative care for children. *Pediatrics.* 2000,106:351–357

24. American College of Surgeons. Statement of the American College of Surgeons on advance directives by patients. "Do not resuscitate" in the operating room. *Bull Am Coll Surg.* 1994,79(9):29

25. Fine PG, Jackson SH. Do not resuscitate in the operating room: more than rights and wrongs. *Am J Anesthesiol.* 1995,22:46–51

26. Bernat JL, Grabowski EW. Suspending do-not-resuscitate orders during anesthesia and surgery. *Surg Neurol.* 1993,40:7–9

27. Martin RL, Soifer BE, Stevens WC. Ethical issues in anesthesia: management of the do-not-resuscitate patient. *Anesth Analg.* 1991,73:221–225

28. Olsson GL, Hallen B. Cardiac arrest during anaesthesia: a computer-aided study in 250,543 anaesthetics. *Acta Anaesthesiol Scand.* 1988,32:653–664

29. Wenger NS, Greengold NL, Oye RK, et al. Patients with DNR orders in the operating room: surgery, resuscitation, and outcomes. *J Clin Ethics.* 1977,8:250–257

30. Clemency MV, Thompson NJ. Do not resuscitate orders in the perioperative period: patient perspectives. *Anesth Analg.* 1997,84:859–864

31. Youngner SJ, Cascorbi HF, Shuck JM. DNR in the operating room: not really a paradox. *JAMA.* 1991,266:2433–2434

All clinical reports from the American Academy of Pediatrics automatically expire 5 years after publication unless reaffirmed, revised, or retired at or before that time.

E-mail Communication Between Pediatricians and Their Patients

• *Clinical Report*

AMERICAN ACADEMY OF PEDIATRICS

CLINICAL REPORT
Guidance for the Clinician in Rendering Pediatric Care

Robert S. Gerstle, MD, and the Task Force on Medical Informatics

E-mail Communication Between Pediatricians and Their Patients

ABSTRACT. This report addresses specific e-mail patient communication issues relevant to pediatricians and their appropriate use of e-mail in the office setting. The report briefly reviews: 1) e-mail privacy and security concerns; 2) e-mail in the office environment; 3) the legal status of e-mail; and 4) available e-mail technologic solutions. *Pediatrics* 2004;114:317–321; *electronic communications, health care delivery, medical liability, e-mail, pediatrics.*

ABBREVIATIONS. HIPAA, Health Insurance Portability and Accountability Act; PHI, protected health information.

The American Academy of Pediatrics Periodic Survey of Fellows No. 51 documented that of the 1616 active US members reporting from October 2001 to February 2002, 14% already use e-mail to communicate with patients. Reasons cited for using e-mail included managing requests for prescription refills (54%), communicating test results (41%), and scheduling appointments (37%). Reasons for not using e-mail to communicate with patients included lack of physician time (52%), lack of office staff time (42%), concerns about privacy or confidentiality (45%), lack of interest in communicating via e-mail (38%), and too few patients with e-mail (34%).[1] The volume of e-mail sent daily in the United States was expected to exceed 9 billion messages in 2003.[2] A Harris Interactive survey reported in April 2002 that "about 90% of US adults who use the Internet say they would like to communicate with their physicians online . . . ."[3] The study went on to report, "56% said that ability to communicate with their physician online would help influence their choice of physician."

The popularity of e-mail is attributable to some of its unique characteristics, namely its ability to allow asynchronous communication and rapid message transfer, making it a hybrid of the telephone and the written letter.[4] As it is used, e-mail is a more informal means of communication than the letter, but more rapidly transmitted. Like a letter, it can be sent or read by the recipient at convenient times, avoiding "telephone tag." In addition, it is "self-document-ing," providing a lasting copy for future reference. Thus, it is no surprise that pediatric patients and their families share the desire to use e-mail to communicate with their pediatricians.[3–5] E-mail would seem to offer physicians and patients obvious benefits for facilitating communication. Therefore, it may seem somewhat surprising that there has been relatively slow adoption of e-mail as a patient communication tool by pediatricians and other physicians.[4] There are many reasons for this, including but not limited to concerns about maintaining the confidentiality of e-mail, physician concerns about the potential volume of e-mail correspondence, and potential legal issues.[1,5]

BACKGROUND: E-MAIL TECHNOLOGY

The transmission of e-mail messages requires: 1) access to a global network of linked computers, called the Internet; 2) the existence of an addressing system that enables messages to be routed through that network of computers to their correct destinations; and 3) programs that split messages into standard-sized "pieces," pack them into electronic "envelopes" or packets that have address information for routing each packet, and reassemble the message at the intended destination.

By design, the Internet is a very robust communication system with an architecture that was structured to maintain communication in case of national disasters that might result in the destruction of significant amounts of the national communications network (such as in the case of nuclear war). Messages transmitted across the Internet are not normally encrypted; nor is there typically authentication of author identity. Lack of encryption allows those with access to the Internet network to intercept, read, or potentially alter messages as they pass to their final destinations. These risks are not unique to e-mail. Telephones can be tapped (legally or illegally); scanners can monitor portable telephone communications; traditional mail can be intercepted, read, or altered, and letters can be forged. Despite potential confidentiality and security risks, it seems on the basis of volume alone that most people are comfortable using e-mail, particularly for relatively trivial or mundane communication needs. The perceived benefits of this fast, asynchronous, and relatively inexpensive form of communication appear to outweigh the risks to most users.

PRIVACY AND SECURITY RISKS

Physicians have special ethical and legal obligations to maintain the privacy and confidentiality of their communications with and regarding patients. Additionally, pediatricians and others who provide medical services to children and adolescents have special burdens and responsibilities by the nature of their patient population.[6,7] E-mail communication with patients adds complexity and responsibilities for the pediatrician, the office staff, and the patient and patient's family.

Pediatricians have the legal responsibility, whenever health information is requested by or communicated to an individual, to ensure that: 1) the individual has a legitimate right to release or gain access to that information before releasing or communicating that information by letter, by phone, in person, or by e-mail; 2) the information is directed only to those having a right to receive it; and 3) the information is accurately transmitted and received. These are the requirements to ensure the authenticity, confidentiality, and integrity of information exchange.[8,9]

Authenticity refers to a recipient's ability to positively know the identity of an individual sending a communication.[10] Anyone can send e-mail with virtually anyone's name attached to it. The inability of e-mail to provide methods of authentication presents a significant risk to patients and physicians. E-mail authentication has been one of the more difficult issues to address when using e-mail for medical communication. Two general solutions to the authentication problem, digital certificates and secure networks, will be discussed briefly later in this report.

Confidentiality refers to the need to protect information from those who have no legitimate right to the information presented.[11] Risks to patient confidentiality occur when multiple individuals (eg, family members) share the same e-mail address, when access passwords are not used or are not kept secured, when computers are left on and unattended without logging out of e-mail, or when e-mail at work or at school is used for personal communication. Using e-mail on systems that belong to employers, other organizations, or schools presents particular problems. Many e-mail users do not know that most organizations and companies, as policy, consider organizational e-mail to be their property and reserve the right to read e-mail on their systems. Another threat to confidentiality results from the ease with which e-mail messages can be misaddressed and erroneously sent to unintended recipients, instantaneously broadcast to multiple recipients, or forwarded by others to unintended recipients.

Integrity of message transmission refers to having absolute knowledge that the message received was unaltered and identical to the one transmitted and that the message was sent and received by the appropriate person.[11] Because e-mail messages can be intercepted, especially by hackers who break into an e-mail server but also by individuals who might gain access to another's personal electronic mailbox, there may be justifiable concern about integrity of messages. Of more concern is that a message sent to one individual might be altered by the recipient. The altered message, its intent perhaps drastically changed, might then be forwarded to another person.

E-MAIL IN THE PHYSICIAN OFFICE ENVIRONMENT

Office e-mail and confidentiality policies, procedures, and processes need to be in place before e-mail with patients can successfully, safely, and effectively be used in the office. Merely distributing or advertising a practice's e-mail address to patients may have unintended consequences. This address will rapidly become quite public, resulting in the office receiving a variety of unsolicited e-mail. A major concern is that individuals who are not current office patients may e-mail the office with medical questions. Office processes may get mired with the volume of e-mail received. The practice needs a way to determine which messages are from "legitimate" or established patients or families and needs to decide whether it will respond to queries from nonpatients. Distinguishing which messages are from current patients from those that are not can be difficult. E-mail address names may be aliases (eg, Superstud2) or common or nonunique names (eg, David Miller or Jose Rivera). Pediatric offices typically identify patients by the child's name but may have problems identifying e-mail from a parent, particularly if the message does not reference the child's name and birth date. Incorporating structured e-mail forms that require specific patient identifying information (eg, first and last name, date of birth, and practice identification or Social Security number) to be completed as part of the message helps simplify patient identification. In addition, the use of passwords as a means of identification and access can diminish the risk of outside or inappropriate access to communications.

Another concern beyond identification is that of e-mail attachments. E-mail attachments can cause a variety of problems, including the transmission of computer viruses (potentially paralyzing the computer system), the use of excessive memory, the need to read and print messages and attached documents for inclusion in patient records (using staff resources), or the need for versions of software that are not available on the office system. To rectify this issue, pediatric offices can consider restricting the use of attachments as part of patient messages. Attachments might be restricted to reports or attachments from professional sources, such as other physician offices, emergency departments, and hospital medical records departments. Having the ability to control which users may append attachments can lend a lot of flexibility to an e-mail system.

Occasionally, situations occur in which an office may want to have the ability to block the receipt of e-mail from certain individuals. E-mail systems that allow the office the ability to inactivate passwords or block e-mail from specific individuals can effectively restrict e-mail system access for selected patients by the office when necessary.

It is very important for practices to set realistic expectations for e-mail and communicate those expectations to families. Patients must understand what the office considers a reasonable response time for nonurgent messages and must understand that emergency communication is appropriately handled by telephone, not by e-mail. Communications that are usually appropriate for e-mail include routine appointment requests, billing questions, routine prescription refill requests, provision of follow-up information, and chronic disease management questions. By providing patients with office e-mail policies in written form before they receive an e-mail password, posting the policies on the practice Web site, and verbally reinforcing these policies, pediatricians and their staffs can help patients to understand and adhere to the appropriate use of e-mail.

There are other considerations the pediatrician needs to address before providing pediatric patients with e-mail access to the office. Policies can address the age at which pediatric patients can begin to send e-mail to the office themselves. Will children and parents receive the same brochures and sign the same consents (or assents)? Will parental permission be required before a child can receive a password to access office e-mail? Although there are not necessarily any right or wrong strategies, patients and their parents must know and understand office practices and policies.

Patients typically desire to communicate by e-mail with their physician's office to schedule appointments, refill prescriptions, resolve billing questions, request referrals, obtain test results, get forms or immunization records completed, ask nonurgent medical questions, or provide medical follow-up. Most of these tasks can be delegated to an appropriate office staff member. Patients must understand who in the office will read and triage e-mail as well as the limits to privacy that messages will have in the office. Patients must know when, for example, messages addressed to a particular individual in the office, even about personal matters, may be first subjected to clerical or nurse review. E-mail systems that can automatically triage messages to the appropriate office staff member, depending on the type of message, can improve efficiency and patient confidentiality. Patients can be informed that by restricting e-mail messages to one issue per message, message triage efficiency and patient confidentiality might be enhanced. The office also needs to have policies and processes to address messages that arrive when a pediatrician or designated office staff person is unavailable or has elected not to have the messages forwarded to them, and to address e-mail received on weekends, holidays, or whenever the office is closed. Routine policies can be incorporated into a patient e-mail brochure, and the policy can be reinforced using the "auto reply" feature included in most e-mail software, stating when action will be taken on messages and telling the patient to call the office for more urgent matters. Copies of e-mail messages with responses can be incorporated into patient charts. Patients can be advised to retain copies of e-mail sent by the office to avoid their forgetting or misunderstanding the intent of messages.

A well-constructed patient brochure outlining office e-mail policies and the appropriate use of e-mail will help control patient expectations and prevent misuse of e-mail by patients. Although some offices may require patients to sign a consent form allowing e-mail communication, it is more important that patients and parents clearly understand the differences among, and appropriate use of, each available form of communication. It is a good practice to document that each patient has been provided with written information that addresses the appropriate use of e-mail and office policies and procedures that support e-mail. This information can be provided before office e-mail addresses or access passwords are given to patients.

Drawing an analogy to telephone communications, e-mail communication is another way to enhance patient communication and satisfaction and to build goodwill. Just as there are no regulations that preclude charging patients for telephone advice, except as may be contained in insurance contracts, there are no restrictions on charging patients for advice rendered by e-mail. Some insurers have begun to consider e-mail an important part of chronic disease management and have started to selectively reimburse physicians for e-mail communication related to disease management.[12,13] More plans are expected to begin reimbursing clinicians for online consultation for both acute and chronic conditions. Because e-mail self-documents, it can provide the evidence of medical work that telephonic communication does not offer. Thus, insurers have been more willing to consider reimbursement for e-mail interactions. *Current Procedural Terminology*[14] codes for care plan oversight (99374-99380) already exist and are reimbursable under some insurance plans.[15] Case management services telephone calls (99371-99373) presently are restricted to telephone use but might be broadened in the future to include e-mail services.

LEGAL STATUS OF E-MAIL IN HEALTH CARE

The Health Insurance Portability and Accountability Act (HIPAA)[8,9] privacy and security regulations apply to e-mail communications that contain a patient's protected health information (PHI), as defined in HIPAA privacy regulations.[16] HIPAA requires encryption of messages when sending PHI over the Internet. If the pediatrician is using a third party to manage the e-mail system, HIPAA privacy regulations require a written business associate agreement with the service provider. HIPAA privacy regulations require that physician offices provide each of their patients or patient's families with an outline of the office's privacy practices. Final HIPAA security regulations[9] released on February 20, 2003, require physician office networks to have appropriate protection (firewalls and physical security) to prevent unauthorized individuals from gaining access to clinical e-mail or medical records, and to have appropriate safeguards to prevent the loss or unauthorized access to or distribution of PHI. Privacy regulations under HIPAA also require the ability to provide for author and user authentication for e-mail transmissions.

Just as for telemedicine, issues related to medical licensing and jurisdiction can be raised when communicating with patients and providing patient care or advice across state lines by e-mail. Although it is unlikely the pediatrician would be in jeopardy of prosecution for practicing medicine without a license by giving medical advice to an established patient via e-mail, it is important that pediatricians check their state's law on this issue. Some states have begun to address this issue in their state medical practice legislation, with the possibility of requiring a state medical license for such transactions.

There can also be medical liability risks related to providing "medical care" by e-mail or Internet communication. Before medical liability can exist, one must demonstrate that a patient-physician relationship has been formed. The establishment of the patient-physician relationship, or "duty," has not been well clarified when using e-mail or the Internet exclusively to provide advice in the absence of any physical contact. Arguably, an analogy can be drawn to the situation in which a physician provides general information on a local radio or television broadcast. In such cases, in which information is general in nature and not meant to diagnose or treat a specific individual, there is no relationship or duty established. Although case law has not been well established, there have been concerns raised as to whether a patient-provider relationship would be initiated when advice is given in an online forum ("bulletin board" or "chat room"). However, in cases in which there is a previous patient-physician relationship or in which a Web site is created to solicit patient queries, the risk of medical liability is greater.

Failure to meet patients' service expectations or follow one's own office policies and procedures can result in liability. The situation in which a physician fails to respond in an appropriate time frame to a patient e-mail, resulting in an adverse outcome, for example, might present a liability risk, emphasizing the need to educate patients about the appropriate use of e-mail and about appropriate response time expectations. Patients must be instructed and must understand when it is appropriate to escalate queries by telephoning the office directly. Although e-mail is widely used, neither the legal nor medical liability communities have significant precedents for dealing with potential e-mail communication risks. Pediatricians should monitor for the development of such precedents in the future.

E-MAIL TECHNOLOGIC SOLUTIONS

There are two commercially available solutions to the problem of providing authenticated, confidential, secure e-mail: secure servers or digital signatures.[17] Each of these approaches affords remedies for authentication of identities and facilitates secure communication with patients. No system, however, is perfect. Any system depends on patients and providers recognizing their responsibilities to keep passwords private and secure and to log off of systems properly when leaving computers unattended.

The secure server solution is analogous to doing banking online. The pediatrician's office must initially authenticate the identity of the patient, such as at the time of an office visit, and provide a sign-on code and temporary password specific to that individual. When the patient logs on to the system for the first time, he or she then changes the temporary password to a new and confidential one known only to the user. When a message is sent to that patient's system mailbox by the office, a secondary nonsecured notice is sent to the patient's identified home e-mail account alerting the patient to log on to his or her secure mailbox on the system. Logging on is accomplished securely using the patient's confidential password and via the Web browser's secure socket layer. Secure socket layer transmission across the Internet is encrypted between the mail server and the patient. Only the individual with the password to that account has access to it. From the secure mailbox, patients can also securely send messages back to the pediatric office. Such messages reside on the server, and the office logs on to the mail system securely, as does the patient. In this type of system, unencrypted messages containing medical information never travel on the Internet.

Digital signatures rely on the use of "keys" to encode (encrypt) messages sent across the Internet. The sender of a message has a private key that is used for coding the message. The receiver has a complementary public key to decode the message, thus making it readable.[18] These keys are not physical devices but rather strings of random characters that are used in the mathematical encrypting algorithm. Authentication of identity occurs before a key is released to a user, and a certification authority handles management of public and private keys. Authentication can still be an issue depending on the identity control mechanisms used.[17,18] Presently, these systems are complex to administer and cumbersome to use. However, in the future, perhaps by using smart cards or biometric forms of authentication (eg, fingerprint readers), these systems may grow in popularity.

Commercially available e-mail systems can provide added value beyond simply the ability to transmit and receive e-mail. They can provide e-mail encryption, authentication, and password management; can facilitate automatic triaging of messages on the basis of message type; and can provide the ability to "auto-fax" prescriptions to pharmacies. Some systems can assign "rights" to certain users (such as to append attachments) or allow for associated business transactions (charges for communications) to be handled online. Costs of these systems can vary widely, but for a very modest cost, most offices can implement basic secured messaging.

CONCLUSION

Successful communication between patients and pediatricians is an essential element to providing quality care and maintaining patient satisfaction. Although under certain circumstances, only face-to-face communication is appropriate, there are other times when other forms of communication, including direct telephone contact, facsimile transmission, traditional mail, and now, e-mail would be appropriate—although they should not be considered interchangeable. Pediatricians and their patients must be aware of the risks, benefits, and limitations of any form of communication. E-mail is still an emerging vehicle for communication. Its ability to allow for the rapid asynchronous transmittal of messages and to "self-document" makes it particularly popular despite the potential confidentiality risks. These risks can be acceptably minimized with appropriate forethought and planning.

TASK FORCE ON MEDICAL INFORMATICS, 2001–2002
Edward M. Gotlieb, MD, Chairperson
Robert S. Gerstle, MD
Allan S. Lieberthal, MD
Richard N. Shiffman, MD
S. Andrew Spooner, MD, MS
Melvin S. Stern, MD

STAFF
Aiysha Johnson, MA

REFERENCES

1. American Academy of Pediatrics, Division of Health Policy Research. *Periodic Survey of Fellows 51: Use of Computers and Other Technology, Executive Summary.* Elk Grove Village, IL: American Academy of Pediatrics; 2003

2. Walker J. The electronic records committee and state standards [slide presentation]. Columbus, OH: Ohio Historical Society; 2001. Available at: http://www.ohiohistory.org/resource/lgr/DeptofEd.ppt. Accessed August 9, 2003

3. Harris Interactive. Many patients willing to pay for online communication with their physicians [press release]. Rochester, NY: Harris Interactive; April 11, 2002. Available at: http://www.harrisinteractive.com/news/allnewsbydate.asp?NewsID=446. Accessed August 9, 2003

4. Bauchner H, Adams W, Burstin H. You've got mail: issues in communicating with patients and their families by e-mail. *Pediatrics.* 2002;109:954–956

5. Kleiner KD, Akers R, Burke BL, Werner EJ. Parent and physician attitudes regarding electronic communication in pediatric practices. *Pediatrics.* 2002;109:740–744

6. American Academy of Pediatrics, Pediatric Practice Action Group and Task Force on Medical Informatics. Privacy protection of health information: patient rights and pediatrician responsibilities. *Pediatrics.* 1999;104:973–977

7. American Academy of Pediatrics. Confidentiality in adolescent health care. *AAP News. April* 1989:9.Available at: http://www.aap.org/policy/104.html. Accessed August 9, 2003

8. Department of Health and Human Services, Office for Civil Rights. Medical privacy—national standards to protect the privacy of personal health information. 45 CFR §160, 164 (2000). Available at: http://www.hhs.gov/ocr/hipaa/finalreg.html. Accessed August 9, 2003

9. Department of Health and Human Services. Health insurance reform: security standards: final rule. *Federal Register.* February 20, 2003. Available at: http://a257.g.akamaitech.net/7/257/2422/14mar20010800/edocket.access.gpo.gov/2003/pdf/03-3877.pdf. Accessed August 9, 2003

10. Brooks P, Leyland P. Security: privacy, authenticity, and integrity. Available at: http://www.ac.uk.pgp.net/pgpnet/secemail/q4/node4.html. Accessed November 7, 2003

11. US Dept of Homeland Security. Critical infrastructure glossary of terms and acronyms. Available at: http://www.ciao.gov/ciao_document_library/glossary/C.htm. Accessed November 7, 2003

12. University of Illinois at Chicago, Division of Specialized Care for Children. Fee schedule for medical home services. Available at: http://internet.dscc.uic.edu/forms/medicalhome/0302.pdf. Accessed August 9, 2003

13. Bottom Line Medical Administrative Consultants, Inc. *Telephone Management: How Much Is Your Practice Losing?* Lake Wales, FL: Bottom Line Medical Administrative Consultants Inc; Available at: http://bottomlinemedicalconsultants.com/telephonemngmnt.html. Accessed August 9, 2003

14. American Medical Association. *CPT 2003: Standard Edition. Current Procedural Terminology.* Chicago, IL: American Medical Association; 2002

15. Appleby J. Insurers, doctors ponder implications of e-consultations. *USA Today. March* 26, 2001:1B, 5B

16. Health Insurance Portability and Accountability Act. Pub L No. 104-191 (1996)

17. Beer K. Secure messaging strategies for healthcare IT professionals. Available at: http://www.privacysecuritynetwork.com/healthnews/symposia/emailstrat.htm. Accessed November 7, 2003

18. VeriSign. What is a digital ID? Available at: shttps://digitalid.verisign.com/client/help/id_intro.htm#what_is_id. Accessed August 9, 2003

GENERAL SOURCES

Kane B, Sands DZ. American Medical Informatics Association white paper: guidelines for the clinical use of electronic mail with patients. *J Am Med Inform Assoc.* 1998;5:104–111

Burrington-Brown J, Hughes G. *AHIMA Practice Brief: Provider-Patient E-mail Security.* Chicago, IL: American Health Information Management Association; 2003. Available at: http://library.ahima.org/xpedio/groups/public/documents/ahima/pub_bok1_019873.html. Accessed August 9, 2003

American Medical Association. *Guidelines for Physician-Patient Electronic Communications.* Chicago, IL: American Medical Association; 2001. Available at: http://www.ama-assn.org/ama/pub/category/2386.html. Accessed August 9, 2003

Bisker S, Tracy M, Jansen W. *Guidelines on Electronic Mail Security: Recommendations of the National Institute of Standards and Technology.* Special Publication 800-45 6. US Department of Commerce, National Institute of Standards and Technology; 2002

Gerberick, Dahl A. Encryption and secure e-mail, an overview. Available at: http://64.78.52.225/initiatives/e-mail/background/Encryptn+SecureEmailOverview.doc. Accessed August 9, 2003

All clinical reports from the American Academy of Pediatrics automatically expire 5 years after publication unless reaffirmed, revised, or retired at or before that time.

Ensuring Culturally Effective Pediatric Care: Implications for Education and Health Policy

- *Policy Statement*

AMERICAN ACADEMY OF PEDIATRICS

POLICY STATEMENT
Organizational Principles to Guide and Define the Child Health Care System and/or Improve the Health of All Children

Committee on Pediatric Workforce

Ensuring Culturally Effective Pediatric Care: Implications for Education and Health Policy

ABSTRACT. This policy statement defines culturally effective health care and describes its importance for pediatrics and the health of children. The statement also defines cultural effectiveness, cultural sensitivity, and cultural competence and describes the importance of these concepts for training in medical school, residency, and continuing medical education. The statement is based on the conviction that culturally effective health care is vital and a critical social value and that the knowledge and skills necessary for providing culturally effective health care can be taught and acquired through focused curricula throughout the spectrum of lifelong learning, from premedical education and medical school through residency and continuing medical education. The American Academy of Pediatrics also believes that these educational efforts must be supported through health policy and advocacy activities that promote the delivery of culturally effective pediatric care. *Pediatrics* 2004;114:1677–1685; *culture, cultural competence, cultural sensitivity, culturally effective care, diversity, ethnicity, health literacy, minorities, pediatric, racial.*

ABBREVIATIONS. AAP, American Academy of Pediatrics; AMA, American Medical Association; CME, continuing medical education; APA, Ambulatory Pediatric Association.

INTRODUCTION

The mission of the American Academy of Pediatrics (AAP) is to attain optimal physical, mental, and social health and well-being for all infants, children, adolescents, and young adults. To this end, the AAP recognizes that the increasing cultural diversity of the patient population has implications for the provision of pediatric health services and for conducting child advocacy, health policy, and health services research.

Over time, the cultural attributes of children and families, including but not limited to race, ethnicity, language, religion, sexual orientation, gender, disability, and socioeconomic status, will likely continue to be different from those of the individual pediatrician or child health professional. Indeed, the most recent data from the US Census Bureau project that by the year 2020, 44.5% of American children 0 to 19 years of age will belong to a racial or ethnic minority group.[1] Consideration of cultural attributes

in addition to race and ethnicity would greatly increase this projection of diversity. As the Future of Pediatric Education II Task Force noted, "These changing demographics are likely to have implications for the utilization of medical services, as well as for the acceptance of interventions by caregivers. In addition, other special populations—including homeless children, children in migrant families, and children in foster care—will reflect even more cultural and ethnic diversity and will require sensitive attention from the pediatricians and other child health professionals who provide care for them."[2(p173)]

The disparity in cultural attributes between health care professionals and their patients and patients' families or guardians will require educational interventions to ensure that pediatricians and other health care professionals are able to provide culturally effective care to a diverse patient population.[3] The AAP, therefore, reaffirms the importance of establishing and promoting an organizational policy on the provision of culturally effective pediatric health care, which it regards as vital and a critical social value.

Throughout this statement, the term "pediatricians" refers not only to general pediatricians but also to pediatric subspecialists and pediatric surgical specialists. The AAP continues to embrace the concept of the pediatric health care team and recognizes the need for all health care professionals to deliver culturally effective care. However, the scope of this statement is limited to addressing this issue from a pediatrician perspective, providing a key reference point for this discourse. The AAP encourages child health care professionals other than pediatricians to embrace the concepts presented here and implement them accordingly, because this topic concerns the health and well-being of children, regardless of the individual providing health care services.

Culturally effective pediatric health care can be defined as the delivery of care within the context of appropriate physician knowledge, understanding, and appreciation of all cultural distinctions leading to optimal health outcomes. For the purposes of this policy statement, the term "culture" is used to signify the full spectrum of values, behaviors, customs, language, race, ethnicity, gender, sexual orientation, religious beliefs, socioeconomic status, and other distinct attributes of population groups. Given the com-

doi:10.1542/peds.2004-2091
PEDIATRICS (ISSN 0031 4005). Copyright © 2004 by the American Academy of Pediatrics.

plexities of the term "culture," a complete analysis of the specific effect of each aspect is beyond the scope of this statement. Rather, the focus remains on strategies, whether universally applicable or specifically targeted, that can be applied to one or all of the components of culture to improve the delivery of culturally effective care. Additionally, significant emphasis is placed on barriers to access to care that can be related to a low level of health literacy or unique health care needs, along with considerations of the traditional aspects of culture.

Because several terms have been used in the medical community to denote the concepts embodied by "culturally effective health care," some initial clarification of terminology is required. The American Medical Association (AMA) considers "cultural competence" and "culturally effective health care" synonymous terms but has retained use of the term "cultural competence" because of its widespread use and acceptance in the literature.[4] Over time, the scope of cultural competence has been expanded beyond the traditional realms of race and ethnicity to incorporate a wider range of personal attributes, health care services, and definitions of health, well-being, and illness. The literature and recent national mandates, for instance, demonstrate that there is great interest in expanding the concept of cultural competence to include access to interpreter services in health care settings and consideration of individual health and illness experiences as well as mechanisms to ensure the right to respectful and nondiscriminatory care.[5–7] The AAP believes, however, that "culturally effective pediatric care" is a more inclusive term than "cultural competence," because it encompasses the values of competence but more importantly focuses on the outcomes of the physician-patient or physician-family interaction.

At the level of the individual pediatrician, culturally effective health care requires acquisition of knowledge, development of skills, and demonstration of behaviors and attitudes that are appropriate to care for patients and families with a wide variety of cultural attributes. In addition, physician self-reflection, self-knowledge, and self-critique have been identified as critical components of competence.[8] Along with requiring these knowledge bases, skills, behaviors, and attitudes, commonly referred to as cultural competence and cultural sensitivity, culturally effective health care emphasizes the need for continued monitoring and documentation of measurable outcomes.

To promote the provision of culturally effective health care to pediatric patients, the AAP reaffirms its commitment to participate in the development and implementation of educational materials and courses. As such, the AAP maintains that culturally effective health care should be promoted through health policy and education at all levels, from premedical education and medical school through residency education and continuing medical education (CME). At every level of education, child health professionals must be able to interact effectively and respectfully with patients and their families regardless of the cultural differences that may exist between

them. These educational efforts should enhance the knowledge and understanding of pediatricians and child health care professionals other than pediatricians about the cultures of their patients and their families and increase their ability to provide care in a manner that is responsive to the individual needs of each patient. Educational programs must focus also on the enhancement of interpersonal and communication skills, which are essential to nurturing the pediatrician-patient or pediatrician-family relationship and optimizing the health status of patients.

The focus of this policy statement remains on strategies that can significantly improve patient outcomes for all infants, children, adolescents, and young adults in a diverse nation. Having defined the key terms to be used throughout the statement, some background information is provided on the scope of cultural distinctions and describes the current educational landscape regarding cultural education. After this, the statement outlines educational imperatives to expand on the current system and provides specific AAP recommendations for improving culturally effective care through educational and health policy reform.

BACKGROUND

Innate Cultural Attributes

In its 1994 report, the AAP Task Force on Minority Children's Access to Pediatric Care[9] expressed concern that the health services provided by many institutions in the United States reflect the values of the racial and ethnic majority culture (ie, white European). Patients and families that have different cultural attributes may experience difficulties in their interactions with health care professionals, and these difficulties may have an adverse effect on the delivery of health care. This is a concern for racial and ethnic minority children, for example, because according to standard indicators of child health status (including low birth weight, infant mortality, and immunization rates), these children are, in general, less healthy than are white children. The task force's report identified potential barriers to quality health care services for racial and ethnic minority children, including poverty, geographic factors, lack of provider cultural sensitivity, racism, and other forms of prejudice.

In the years since the 1994 report, discussions of health disparities among other minority patient populations and their families have emerged and expanded the discussion of culturally effective health care. In particular, sexual orientation,[10] socioeconomic status, religion, and gender have been identified as cultural factors that affect the delivery of health care. Although a comprehensive overview of how each aspect affects individuals cannot be provided here, there has been increasing recognition of the unique health and wellness concerns and potential barriers to access to quality health care for certain groups of individuals. For example, gay, lesbian, and transgendered youth are disproportionately affected by human immunodeficiency virus infection, suicide, substance use, and violence.[11] Varying socioeconomic circumstances present their own concerns that have been proven to have detrimental effects on the well-being of adolescents and children well into adulthood.[12] Similarly, religious issues challenge the pediatrician, as illustrated by 1 study[13] that describes the practical implications of Islamic ethical and moral norms in pediatric clinical practice. Another attribute that has proven to affect health care is gender, as 1 study[14] recounts the influence it has on patient-physician communication and consequently on health care.

Regardless of their background, all patients and their families have culturally based concepts about health, disease, and illness. At the same time, the cultural attributes of the pediatrician may differ from that of the patient or family or the pediatrician's colleagues. Given this variation, and because miscommunication between health care professionals as attributable to cultural differences may also lead to poorer health outcomes, the AAP previously addressed the need to enhance the diversity of the pediatric workforce as a strategy to improve patient care outcomes.[15] These differing cultural attributes are especially significant when they affect patients' and their families' beliefs about health, illness, and treatments and conflict with the pediatrician's diagnosis or management plan. In this scenario, cultural differences may become barriers to access to care or the provision of optimal pediatric health care services.

Communication and Language

In addition to innate cultural distinctions, there is an inherent imbalance of power in all physician-patient relationships as the patient and/or the patient's family seeks advice or care from a pediatrician in his or her role as an expert or consultant. This imbalance may be even more pronounced when patients and their families are from minority groups, because they may experience "communication anxiety" when dealing with people in expert roles.[16] Failure to appreciate this imbalance may lead to miscommunication, posing an even greater barrier to health care services.

Cultural variations in verbal and nonverbal communication can be a major barrier to effective pediatric care. Although the role of culturally linked behaviors that may influence the physician-patient interaction, including eye contact, body language, and communication styles, has not been fully explored,[17] language barriers have been shown to have a major effect on health care. Parents and their children in the United States increasingly speak a language other than English at home and/or have limited English proficiency. In addition, communication with families dependent on the use of American Sign Language and/or lip reading may pose significant challenges. When the pediatrician and his or her patient and patient's family do not speak the same language with fluency, there is a potential for misunderstandings such as an inaccurate history, misunderstanding of therapies, and deferred medical visits.[18,19] This barrier could be addressed through the use of medical interpreters or bilingual pediatricians and other pediatric health care professionals to meet the needs of children whose parents are not proficient enough to interact with members of the health care system in English.[20] Some pediatricians, medical educators, and policy makers have identified concerns with the use of medical interpreters, including concerns about the lack of required or standardized training. Translation errors, ranging from omission to substitution to editorialization, have implications for patient safety as well as potential clinical consequences.[18,19] An alternative to this personnel-intensive effort is the burgeoning use of technology in the medical sector. Because many times an interpreter is not available, technology can enable use of an off-site translator who interprets and relays through headphones to both the physician and the patient. Video and telecommunication may become prominent in the future as alternatives to on-site interpreters.

The US Department of Health and Human Services, in its March 2001 *National Standards for Culturally and Linguistically Appropriate Services in Health Care: Final Report,*[7] established 14 national standards, several of which concern services for individuals with limited English proficiency. Standard 4 states that "health care organizations must offer and provide language assistance services, including bilingual staff and interpreter services, at no cost to each patient/consumer with limited English proficiency at all points of contact, in a timely manner during all hours of operation." Although the AAP supports this and other efforts to provide culturally effective pediatric health care, the AAP is opposed to unfunded mandates such as those pertaining to interpreter and/or translation services that will further erode the beleaguered health care delivery system and lead to access problems for Medicaid patients, most of whom are children.[21] Government mandates to improve the provision of culturally effective health care must be accompanied by the funding and infrastructure necessary to implement these programs and achieve the identified outcomes. The AAP opposes the use of children and adolescents as medical interpreters for their parents and family members and calls for adequate funding to defray the cost of using professionally trained medical interpreters and/or translation services.

Health Literacy

Another facet of the relationship between language and culturally effective pediatric care is health literacy. Healthy People 2010 defines health literacy as "the degree to which individuals have the capacity to obtain, process, and understand basic health information and services needed to make appropriate health decisions."[22] Although this is a particular problem for individuals with low or marginal literacy skills, health literacy can also affect patients and families with adequate language literacy. Many individuals find the complex wording of insurance statements, benefits coverage, hospital admissions forms, prescription drug information sheets, and similar documents to be confusing. Low health literacy for pediatric patients and their families, similar to limited English proficiency, is a barrier to the provision of optimal pediatric health care. A number of AAP policies ranging from hearing detection[23] to Medicaid[24] have addressed these issues and call for materials to be produced in languages other than English for patients and families of diverse cultures and for consumers with low literacy. There is, however, no current AAP policy that specifically addresses low health literacy for patients and their families in all cultures. The AAP is currently and will continue addressing this topic through research, education, and other appropriate venues.

Although health literacy may not be a distinct cultural attribute, language and health literacy are greatly affected by cultural distinctions and, if low, directly contribute to unfavorable patient outcomes among minority groups. Background on these issues was provided to demonstrate how addressing these topics will improve cultural effectiveness of health care.

CURRENT STATUS OF EDUCATIONAL EFFORTS

To provide culturally effective health care for pediatric patients, education and training are needed for pediatricians and child health professionals at all levels and stages of careers and in all practice settings. The AAP recognizes the value of educational tools and programs and calls for their development and incorporation at all levels of pediatric education and child advocacy: medical school, residency training, and CME. A variety of programs, seminars, workshops, and residency curricula already exist across the country with great variation in educational content, focus, priorities, faculty support, and availability and with limited and/or variable descriptions of outcome measures.

Medical Student Education

The literature pertaining to teaching multicultural issues to medical students is robust, although many medical educators believe that training physicians to provide culturally effective care should begin earlier as part of undergraduate premedical curricula. Some medical educators have suggested that these educational endeavors should focus less on individual attitudes and the characteristics of minority groups and more on discussions pertaining to social barriers and inequities at the institutional or systems level.[25,26] Others have raised concerns about the model of addressing multiculturalism and cultural competence through lectures and occasional workshops and have argued for the incorporation of these topics as a continuum throughout medical school. The most prominent options for the latter approach include finding space in existing courses on patient-physician relationships and medical interviewing, for example, and developing "thoughtfully prepared instructional material throughout the four-year curriculum."[26,27] Drouin and Rivet support the premise that "communication in health care delivery is usually enhanced when the professional speaks in the patient's mother tongue and is familiar with the patient's culture and context."[28(p599)] The development of a communications skills laboratory within the medical school is one strategy to allow acquisition of language skills in a controlled environment, using simulated patients who provide feedback to students regarding their perceptions of the quality of the communication during the encounter.[28] The need for practical experience, mentoring, role models, and, in particular, evaluation tools has been stressed.[29,30]

Several specialties, including internal medicine and family medicine, have developed cross-cultural or multicultural curricula.[31–33] As a joint effort, the Council on Medical Student Education in Pediatrics and the Ambulatory Pediatric Association (APA) developed in 1995 the "General Pediatric Clerkship Curriculum and Resource Manual" for clerkship directors to encourage the use of formal curricular goals and objectives. The manual, which was revised in February 2002, cites cultural sensitivity and tolerance of difference among the important personal characteristics that are essential foundations for the medical student. This manual also outlines learning objectives and competencies for medical students that relate to the provision of culturally effective health care, with reference to cultural, ethnic, and socioeconomic factors.[34]

Residency Education

The program requirements for residency education in pediatrics developed by the Pediatric Residency Review Committee call for structured educational experiences that prepare residents for the role of child health advocate within the community and inclusion of the multicultural dimensions of health care in the curriculum.[35] To prepare residents to fulfill the needs of all their patients, the Future of Pediatric Education II Task Force recommended that all pediatric residents design and implement an individualized professional education (CME) plan by the third year of residency training that incorporates anticipated needs for their future practice.[2]

In 1995, the APA published its "Educational Guidelines for Residency Training in General Pediatrics,"[36] which soon became an essential tool for educators of pediatric residents. The APA began the revision of this important document in 2002, with a particular emphasis on tailoring the guidelines to support and mirror the 6 core competencies for residency education in all specialties established by the Accreditation Council for Graduate Medical Education. The APA adopted these 6 competencies of patient care: medical knowledge; practice-based learning and improvement; interpersonal and communication skills; professionalism; and systems-based practice. Under these competencies, the APA included considerable language related to the provision of culturally effective pediatric care. For example, the guidelines define professionalism as "demonstrat[ing] a commitment to carrying out professional responsibilities, adherence to ethical principles, and sensitivity to diversity," which includes "demonstrat[ing] sensitivity and responsiveness to patients' and colleagues' gender, age, culture, disabilities, ethnicity, and sexual orientation."[36] Language on culturally effective care also appears in the sections on patient care and interpersonal communication skills.

CME

Beyond residency training, pediatricians and other child health professionals can benefit from CME to enhance the provision of culturally effective health care. The AAP incorporates culturally effective pediatric care into its CME programming primarily, at this point, through the SuperCME, an activity serving more than 700 practicing general pediatricians. SuperCME will serve as a culturally effective care model for future AAP CME activities, demonstrating how the topic of culturally effective pediatric care can be infused into overall programming and specifically how to incorporate dimensions of culturally effective pediatric care into clinical presentations. In support of the latter component, the AAP Committee on Continuing Medical Education is engaged in the creation of CME guidelines that will assist physician volunteer CME program planners in including culturally effective pediatric care within the program design and CME faculty in preparing their materials and learning how they, too, might incorporate this topic through individual presentations. The goal is to raise awareness of the multifaceted dimensions of culturally effective pediatric care by ensuring that this topic is incorporated into CME activities appropriately.

Pediatricians, moreover, should become knowledgeable about the resources available to their patients and families within their institutions (offices, hospitals), health maintenance organizations, and communities. Pediatricians therefore should find opportunities to partner with institutions such as third-party payers, hospitals, health departments, and education departments to advocate for the culturally specific needs of their patients and, thereby, increase patient satisfaction and quality of health care. Although Medicaid and other public insurers are placing increased emphasis on "cultural competence" and quality care,[37] few tools exist for health care payers to measure the outcomes of processes implemented to ensure culturally effective care. The use of patient-satisfaction scoring systems that assess shared decision-making, mutual respect, trust, and other culturally sensitive parameters should be encouraged. Survey instruments should use quality measures that are within the scope of responsibility of the health care professional, and the results of these surveys should be used to identify priorities for continuing education. When carefully designed to reflect the health and wellness values of the specific community being surveyed, such outcomes-driven efforts will allow greater focus on the effectiveness of interventions designed to monitor and ensure quality care.

EDUCATIONAL STRATEGIES AND RESOURCES

The medical literature on cultural competence and sensitivity provides guidance for enhancing cultural effectiveness in pediatrics. In addition, other resources exist that may be helpful in identifying important components for educational activities. For example, *Delivering Culturally Competent Health Care for Adolescents: A Guide for Primary Health Care Providers*[38] discusses how to assess cultural factors within a health history and also how to modify patient management plans to accommodate cultural influences.

Educational programs may include a component that allows the individual participant to analyze personal beliefs and values. Programs may focus on the communication aspects of providing culturally effective health care by exploring how assumptions and stereotypes influence interactions between health care professionals and patients or their families as well as between health care professionals. Programs need not be all-inclusive or completely group-specific to discuss variations in the values and communication styles of various cultural groups. Indeed, training in the provision of culturally effective care may include teaching physician skills that are applicable to interacting with many cultural groups as well as those that are targeted at providing care to a specific cultural group. Because individuals are influenced by their own personal experiences and may or may not subscribe to group assumed norms, individuals who share the same cultural background may think and act quite differently. For this reason, it is important that programs intended to address the cultural values and practices of specific groups not perpetuate stereotypes. Also, culture is not static; changes occur over time. An appreciation of cultural change and the significance of intracultural diversity (variation among individuals within the same culture) helps to prevent cultural stereotyping.[39] Programs aimed at enhancing the provision of culturally effective health care should be tailored to the demographics of the pediatric population or community the pediatrician serves.

Many patient populations and communities suffer from poorer health compared with other populations. Reliable data have shown that patients who belong to racial, ethnic, linguistic, or other minority groups tend to have greater morbidity than do white, English-speaking patients.[40–46] The reasons for these health disparities are numerous, including cultural beliefs about health care and healing, dietary deficiency, insufficient exercise, barriers to access to health care resources, financial indigence, inadequate insurance coverage, and inability to communicate with English-speaking health care professionals. None of these reasons is exclusive; health outcomes can be more greatly affected by the additive effects of more than one of these factors. In particular, varying levels of health literacy may present considerable barriers to improving one's health. Strategies to overcome these barriers to eliminating health disparities are complex and often costly. However, the education of pediatricians has the potential to improve the provision of culturally effective care. At the medical school and residency levels, for example, institutions and programs are encouraged to set an example by supporting and, if possible, offering incentives for students and residents to demonstrate medical proficiency in a second language before graduation, possibly corresponding to a substantial underserved patient population that they anticipate serving.[28] It is recognized that such a suggestion, although popular in some venues, is also problematic and therefore requires additional monitoring and discussion before achieving the status of a recommendation or mandate. Another educational endeavor that merits institutional and program support is teaching students and residents how to use to their best advantage (and how to evaluate) professional medical interpreters and translation services. At a minimum, medical school curricula and pediatric residency education programs should include educational components that identify the implications of low English proficiency, low literacy, and low health literacy on pediatric health care and offer strategies for remediating these problems.

At the CME level, new programs emphasizing skills needed to care for an increasingly diverse patient population and address health disparities are already being offered. The AAP has established a diversity track at its SuperCME, and the APA offers special-interest group workshops on serving the underserved; culture, ethnicity, and health care; and race and medicine, which seek to teach pediatricians how to meet the unique health care needs of patients of ethnic minority groups. In addition, the Henry J. Kaiser Family Foundation and the Robert Wood Johnson Foundation, in collaboration with other key groups, have launched the Initiative to Engage Physicians in Dialogue About Racial/Ethnic Disparities in Medical Care to raise awareness among physicians about health disparities, starting with cardiac conditions among African American individuals, and to teach them to take a leadership role in addressing health disparities among patient populations at greater risk.[47] The Objectives for Improving Health in Healthy People 2010 identify strategies for addressing language barriers, including health literacy, and call for the development of materials for individuals with low literacy. The report also calls on organizations, community groups, schools, and others to offer programs that target skill improvement for individuals with low literacy and limited English proficiency.[22] Programs that provide multilingual prescription or drug information are needed. The AMA Foundation has been working to raise awareness of health literacy within the health care community and has awarded funds to state and county medical societies, along with several medical specialty societies, including the AAP. The AMA has also developed a Health Literacy Educational Kit and train-the-trainers sessions, in which AAP members have participated.[48,49]

Education and training to enhance the provision of culturally effective health care must be integrated into lifelong learning for pediatricians and other child health professionals and include didactic and experiential components. Toolboxes, such as the one developed by the University of California, San Francisco Center for the Health Professions,[50] provide a concrete curriculum with defined objectives for learning and application in clinical care and other professional activities. The AAP has also developed a Web page devoted to the provision of culturally effective pediatric care that provides a variety of educational resources, policy, and data on this issue.[51] Using such modalities, current and future pediatricians and other child health professionals can become better prepared to meet the needs of children from culturally diverse backgrounds, including racial and ethnic minority groups.

HEALTH POLICY IMPLICATIONS

Full participation by the pediatric community is critical to the delivery of culturally effective pediatric care. However, pediatricians will not be able to provide this care without the financial and infrastructure support of the health care system. Recent years have seen a noteworthy increase in the number of federal, state, national, and community organizations/agencies that are generating reports, guidelines, and strategies to address various facets of culturally effective health care delivery.[2,7,16,22,38,41,43,45,47–50,52]

Although mandates from government agencies and regulatory bodies have served as important policy leverage or motivation to promote the provision of culturally effective care, these mandates have been largely unfunded, implying that academic institutions, hospitals, pediatricians, and other physicians must defray the costs of their implementation.[6,7,53,54] Decreasing reimbursement to physician practices for clinical care and decreasing hospital operating margins have rendered these mandates largely impracticable. Additionally, financial and other incentives from insurers, government agencies, and other payers to reward physicians and hospitals for delivering culturally effective care have been meager and have not supplied the impetus and support to encourage fundamental systemic changes, which are often costly.

In an era when cost containment is an urgent priority for the health care community, research has a pivotal role in changing the societal value of culturally effective health care. The AAP regards culturally effective pediatric care as vital and a critical social value. However, many health care payers, employers, institutions, and others fear exacerbating current financial pressures and hardship when trying to provide such care. Reliable and timely data to demonstrate long-term decreases in health care costs, appropriate use of health care services, and improved patient health outcome measures would provide a solid foundation for addressing valid concerns about the financial implications of providing culturally effective care. To this end, culturally effective knowledge and skills need to be applied to research development and implementation. From a quality-of-care perspective, moreover, this research would allow policy makers to identify patient populations at risk and to develop strategies to address health disparities at national, regional, state, and local levels.

Indeed, because the delivery of health care services in the United States is regulated and directed by many entities at many levels, the provision of culturally effective pediatric care will depend on a coordinated effort by all stakeholders in child health. The development of sound and responsible health policy will have to address the aforementioned issues and others that act as barriers to optimal pediatric care.

Pediatricians are not alone in seeking solutions to improve the delivery of pediatric health care. Pediatricians, other health care professionals, community groups, health care payers and insurers, regulatory and accrediting bodies, legislators, and others have significant roles to play in ensuring culturally effective pediatric care and will have to participate in health policy deliberations on this topic. Broad-based participation will ensure that a pediatric focus and perspective are brought to bear on decisions that have a direct effect on the quality of care that is delivered to children. In particular, stakeholders will have to advocate for the necessary financial, regulatory, and other support among decision-makers to implement necessary changes to the US health care delivery system. Of prime importance will be advocacy for patient access to care using key parameters such as scope of services and benefits available; convenience of service organization; patient satisfaction; geographic, temporal, cultural, and language accessibility; and out-of-pocket costs.[54,55] It is critical that the needs and perspectives of the pediatric population and their parents, families, and caregivers be represented in all such policy development and regulatory action. The AAP, on behalf of the pediatric community, must actively participate at the national and chapter levels in these wider health policy deliberations and initiatives that seek to address issues pertinent to the provision of culturally effective care.

CONCLUSIONS

Since adoption of the *Report of the AAP Task Force on Minority Children's Access to Pediatric Care*,[9] the AAP has strengthened its commitment to ensure that all infants, children, adolescents, and young adults have access to optimal and culturally effective pediatric care, ideally through a medical home.[56] Additionally, the AAP acknowledges that culturally effective pediatric care is multifaceted, complex, and often costly. The AAP believes that the education of pediatricians about cultural attributes and about the importance of implementing culturally effective practices and policies is essential. Because pediatricians are committed to lifelong learning, education that will enhance the provision of such care must be available at all levels, from premedical education and medical school through residency education and CME. This policy statement describes some of the approaches that are available. One approach is not endorsed in lieu of another. It is noteworthy that new ideas and tools are being generated at a rapid rate. The AAP hopes that this policy statement will serve as a springboard to foster ongoing discussion, in many forums, about the application and efficacy of existing and new educational methods.

The individual pediatrician needs educational tools; the pediatric community needs the results of outcomes research to bolster, validate, and sustain their effort; institutions need support and encouragement to provide appropriate and effective education and training; foundations and other organizations need to have a pediatric perspective in all health care

and policy development considerations; and the legislative arena, including federal and state agencies, needs to provide the funding and infrastructure necessary to implement and evaluate mandates. The AAP has played and must continue to play a pivotal role in all these important health policy deliberations.

The AAP is committed to advocating for pediatric patients and families by participating in public policy deliberations pertaining to the delivery of culturally effective health care. To promote the provision of culturally effective health care to pediatric patients, the AAP recommends the following:

1. The AAP, along with health care organizations at all levels, should continue to participate in the development and evaluation of curricular programs, such as toolboxes, that teach health care professionals to be supportive of cultural diversity and sensitive to cultural differences and behavior. These curricular programs also should teach health care professionals to understand their own cultural norms and how they relate to patient care activities. Programs should be tailored to the unique needs of the learner at each stage within the spectrum of lifelong learning from premedical education and medical school through residency and CME. The curricula should address issues including but not limited to cultural beliefs, values, behaviors, customs, language (including health literacy), sexual orientation, religious beliefs, disability, socioeconomic status, and other distinct attributes.

2. Recognizing that institutional commitment is necessary to ensure the provision of culturally effective care, pediatricians must work with hospitals, offices, managed care organizations, and commercial and government insurance payers to develop policies and plans that address identified community needs and support community health efforts. Such policies and processes should include considerations of disparities between the diversity profiles of physicians and other caregivers and that of patients and families being served.

3. Government mandates to improve the provision of culturally effective health care must be accompanied by the funding and infrastructure necessary to implement these programs and achieve the identified outcomes. Health care payers and health care professionals should not be mandated to defray the costs of these programs out of their own pockets at a time when reimbursement for health care services is declining and weakening the financial viability of health care systems.

4. Federal and state incentive programs should be established to encourage the implementation of national and community-based programs to improve the delivery of culturally effective health care. These programs should contain an evaluative component to measure improved health care access and outcomes through the generation and dissemination of reliable data. Third-party payers, health care organizations, industry, and charitable foundations should be encouraged to establish

incentive programs that reward physicians for demonstrating improved outcomes in providing culturally effective health care. Public and private incentive programs should be considered as a strategy for encouraging physicians to practice in medically underserved areas, in which are large numbers of patients from minority (eg, racial, ethnic, cultural, linguistic) groups.

5. Medical students and residents should be encouraged to demonstrate proficiency in a second language in clinical settings corresponding to that of a substantial percentage of the patient population being served before graduation and should be rewarded for doing so as a strategy to improve the provision of culturally effective health care.

6. Pediatricians should assume a leadership role in advocating for culturally effective health care for all infants, children, adolescents, and young adults by ensuring that all public policy on these issues is in consonance with the best interests of pediatric patients and their families.

COMMITTEE ON PEDIATRIC WORKFORCE, 2004–2005
Michael R. Anderson, MD, Chairperson
Aaron L. Friedman, MD
Gerald S. Gilchrist, MD
David C. Goodman, MD, MS
Beth A. Pletcher, MD
Scott A. Shipman, MD, MPH
Richard P. Shugerman, MD
Rachel E. Wallace, MD, MS

Carol D. Berkowitz, MD
    Past Committee Member
*Carmelita V. Britton, MD
    Past Committee Chairperson
Kristan Outwater, MD
    Past Committee Member
Richard J. Pan, MD, MPH
    Past Committee Member
Debra R. Sowell, MD, MPH
    Past Committee Member

LIAISON
Gail A. McGuinness, MD
    American Board of Pediatrics

STAFF
Holly J. Mulvey, MA

*Lead author

ACKNOWLEDGMENT

We acknowledge the contributions of Sanjum S. Sethi, an intern in the American Academy of Pediatrics Division of Graduate Medical Education and Pediatric Workforce, to the development of this policy statement.

REFERENCES

1. US Census Bureau. *Projections of the Total Resident Population by 5-Year Age Groups, Race, and Hispanic Origin With Special Age Categories*. Middle Series, 2016–2020. Washington, DC: Population Projections Program, Population Division, US Census Bureau; 2000. Available at: www.census.gov/population/projections/nation/summary/np-t4-e.txt. Accessed December 15, 2003

2. Future of Pediatric Education II Task Force. The Future of Pediatric Education II: organizing pediatric education to meet the needs of infants, children, adolescents, and young adults in the 21st century. *Pediatrics*. 2000;105(1 pt 2):163–212

3. Stoddard JJ, Back MR, Brotherton, SE. The respective racial and ethnic diversity of US pediatricians and American children. *Pediatrics*. 2000; 105:27–31

4. American Medical Association, Council on Medical Education. Report of the Council on Medical Education: Enhancing the Cultural Competence of Physicians. Chicago, IL: American Medical Association; 1998. CME Report 5-A-98

5. Brach C, Fraser I. Can cultural competency reduce racial and ethnic health disparities? A review and conceptual model. *Med Care Res Rev*. 2000;57(suppl 1):181–217

6. Roberts CM. Meeting the needs of patients with limited English proficiency. *J Med Pract Manage*. 2001;17:71–75

7. US Department of Health and Human Services, Office of Minority Health. *Final National Standards on Culturally and Linguistically Appropriate Services (CLAS) in Health Care Published*. Rockville, MD: US Department of Health and Human Services; 2001. Available at: www.omhrc.gov/inetpub/wwwroot/cultural/cultural4.htm. Accessed December 15, 2003

8. Tervalon M, Murray-Garcia J. Cultural humility versus cultural competence: a critical distinction in defining physician training outcomes in multicultural education. *J Health Care Poor Underserved*. 1998; 9:117–125

9. American Academy of Pediatrics, Task Force on Minority Children's Access to Pediatric Care. *Report of the AAP Task Force on Minority Children's Access to Care*. Elk Grove Village, IL: American Academy of Pediatrics; 1994

10. American Academy of Pediatrics, Frankowski BL, Committee on Adolescence. Sexual orientation and adolescents. *Pediatrics*. 2004;113: 1827–1832

11. Garofalo R, Katz E. Health care issues of gay and lesbian youth. *Curr Opin Pediatr*. 2001;13:298–302

12. Huurre T, Aro H, Rahkonen O. Well-being and health behaviour by parental socioeconomic status: a follow-up study of adolescents aged 16 until age 32 years. *Soc Psychiatry Psychiatr Epidemiol*. 2003;38:249–255

13. Hedayat KM, Pirzadeh R. Issues in Islamic biomedical ethics: a primer for the pediatrician. *Pediatrics*. 2001;108:965–971

14. Street RL Jr. Gender differences in health care provider-patient communication: are they due to style, stereotypes, or accommodation? *Patient Educ Couns*. 2002;48:201–206

15. American Academy of Pediatrics, Committee on Pediatric Workforce. Enhancing the racial and ethnic diversity of the pediatric workforce. *Pediatrics*. 2000;105:129–131

16. Boyd CB. Cultures in contrast: developing empowering cross cultural partnerships. Workshop presented at: University of Illinois; March 9, 1996; Chicago, IL

17. Cooper-Patrick L, Gallo JJ, Gonzales JJ, et al. Race, gender, and partnership in the patient-physician relationship. *JAMA*. 1999 11;282:583–589

18. Flores G, Laws MB, Mayo SJ, et al. Errors in medical interpretation and their potential clinical consequences in pediatric encounters. *Pediatrics*. 2003;111:6–14

19. Flores G, Abreu M, Olivar MA, Kastner B. Access barriers to health care for Latino children. *Arch Pediatr Adolesc Med*. 1998;152:1119–1125

20. Weinick RM, Krauss NA. Racial/ethnic differences in children's access to care. *Am J Public Health*. 2000;90:1771–1774

21. Cooper LZ, American Academy of Pediatrics. Letter to Deeana Jang, US Department of Health and Human Services, Office of Civil Rights. Elk Grove Village, IL: American Academy of Pediatrics; April 2, 2002

22. US Department of Health and Human Services, Office of Disease Prevention and Health Promotion. Healthy People 2010. Available at: www.healthypeople.gov/Document/HTML/Volume1/11HealthCom. htm#_Toc490471359. Accessed December 15, 2003

23. Joint Committee on Infant Hearing, American Academy of Audiology, American Academy of Pediatrics, American Speech-Language-Hearing Association, Directors of Speech and Hearing Programs in State Health and Welfare Agencies. Year 2000 position statement: principles and guidelines for early hearing detection and intervention programs. *Pediatrics*. 2000;106:798–817

24. American Academy of Pediatrics, Committee on Child Health Financing. Medicaid policy statement. *Pediatrics*. 1999;104:344–347

25. Green AR, Betancourt JR, Carrillo JE. Integrating social factors into cross-cultural medical education. *Acad Med*. 2002;77:193–197

26. Wear D. Insurgent multiculturalism: rethinking how and why we teach culture in medical education. *Acad Med*. 2003;78:549–554

27. Taylor JS. Confronting "culture" in medicine's "culture of no culture." *Acad Med*. 2003;78:555–559

28. Drouin J, Rivet C. Training medical students to communicate with a linguistic minority group. *Acad Med*. 2003;78:599–604

29. Wright SM, Carrese JA. Serving as a physician role model for a diverse population of medical learners. *Acad Med.* 2003;78:623–628

30. Dolhun EP, Munoz C, Grumbach K. Cross-cultural education in U.S. medical schools: development of an assessment tool. *Acad Med.* 2003; 78:615–622

31. Carrillo JE, Green AR, Betancourt JR. Cross-cultural primary care: a patient-based approach. *Ann Intern Med.* 1999;18:130:829–834

32. Like RC, Steiner RP, Rubel AJ. STFM core curriculum guidelines. Recommended core curriculum guidelines on culturally sensitive and competent health care. *Fam Med.* 1996;28:291–297

33. Culhane-Pera KA, Reif C, Egli E, Baker NJ, Kassekert R. A curriculum for multicultural education in family medicine. *Fam Med.* 1997;29: 719–723

34. Council on Medical Student Education in Pediatrics and the Ambulatory Pediatric Association. General pediatric clerkship curriculum and resource manual. Revised June 2002. Available at: www.comsep.org/Curriculum/CurriculumCompetencies/index.htm. Accessed December 15, 2003

35. Mulvey HJ, Ogle-Jewett EAB, Cheng TL, Johnson RL. Pediatric residency education. *Pediatrics.* 2000;106:323–329

36. Ambulatory Pediatric Association. Competencies and elements with goals/objectives from the educational guidelines. Available at: www.ambpeds.org/egtest/pedicompxref.htm. Accessed December 15, 2003

37. Medicaid Program, Managed care, Proposed rule. 63 *Federal Register* 52021–52092 (1998). Provision of services (codified at 42 CFR §438.306 [e][4])

38. Fleming M, Towey K. *Delivering Culturally Competent Health Care for Adolescents: A Guide for Primary Health Care Providers.* Chicago, IL: American Medical Association; 2003

39. Pachter LM, Harwood RL. Culture and child behavior and psychosocial development. *J Dev Behav Pediatr.* 1996;17:191–198

40. Betancourt JR, Green AR, Carrillo JE. *Cultural Competence in Health Care: Emerging Frameworks and Practical Approaches.* New York, NY: The Commonwealth Fund; 2002

41. Collins KS, Hughes DL, Doty MM, Ives BL, Edwards JN, Tenney K. *Diverse Communities, Common Concerns: Assessing Health Care Quality For Minority Americans. Findings From The Commonwealth Fund 2001 Health Care Quality Survey.* New York, NY: The Commonwealth Fund; 2002

42. Collins KS, Tenney K, Hughes DL. *Quality of Health Care for African Americans.* New York, NY: The Commonwealth Fund; 2002

43. Doty MM. *Hispanic Patients' Double Burden: Lack of Health Insurance and Limited English.* New York, NY: The Commonwealth Fund; 2003

44. Doty MM, Ives BL. *Quality of Health Care for Hispanic Populations.* New York, NY: The Commonwealth Fund; 2002

45. Hughes DL. *Quality of Health Care for Asian Americans.* New York, NY: The Commonwealth Fund; 2002

46. Perot RT, Youdelman M. *Racial, Ethnic, and Primary Language Data Collection in the Health Care System: An Assessment of Federal Policies and Practices.* New York, NY: The Commonwealth Fund; 2001

47. Henry J Kaiser Family Foundation, Robert Wood Johnson Foundation. Help understand why. Available at: www.kff.org/whythedifference. Accessed December 15, 2003

48. A Cure for Confusion: AMA Foundation and Pfizer Working Together in Health Literacy Campaign [press release]. Chicago, IL: American Medical Association Foundation; September 19, 2002. Available at: www.ama-assn.org/ama/pub/category/9059.html. Accessed December 15, 2003

49. American Medical Association Foundation. 2003 Health literacy educational kit. Chicago, IL: American Medical Association; 2003. Available at: www.ama-assn.org/ama/pub/category/9913.html. Accessed December 15, 2003

50. Mutha S, Allen C, Welch M. *Toward Culturally Competent Care: A Toolbox for Teaching Communication Strategies.* San Francisco, CA: University of California; 2002

51. American Academy of Pediatrics, Department of Community Pediatrics. Culturally effective pediatric care. Available at: www.aap.org/commpeds/cepc. Accessed December 15, 2003

52. Accreditation Council for Graduate Medical Education. ACGME Outcome Project competencies. Available at: www.acgme.org/outcome/comp/compHome.asp. Accessed December 15, 2003

53. Liaison Committee on Medical Education. Educational program for the M.D. degree: educational objectives. Available at: www.lcme.org/functionslist.htm#educational%20objectives. Accessed December 15, 2003

54. Penchansky R, Thomas JW. The concept of access: definition and relationship to consumer satisfaction. *Med Care.* 1981;19:127–140

55. Zweifler J, Gonzalez AM. Teaching residents to care for culturally diverse populations. *Acad Med.* 1998;73:1056–1061

56. American Academy of Pediatrics, Medical Home Initiatives for Children With Special Needs Project Advisory Committee. The medical home. *Pediatrics.* 2002;110:184–186

All policy statements from the American Academy of Pediatrics automatically expire 5 years after publication unless reaffirmed, revised, or retired at or before that time.

Ethical Considerations in Research With Socially Identifiable Populations

• *Policy Statement*

AMERICAN ACADEMY OF PEDIATRICS

POLICY STATEMENT
Organizational Principles to Guide and Define the Child Health Care System and/or Improve the Health of All Children

Committee on Native American Child Health and Committee on Community Health Services

Ethical Considerations in Research With Socially Identifiable Populations

ABSTRACT. Community-based research raises ethical issues not normally encountered in research conducted in academic settings. In particular, conventional risk-benefits assessments frequently fail to recognize harms that can occur in socially identifiable populations as a result of research participation. Furthermore, many such communities require more stringent measures of beneficence that must be applied directly to the participating communities. In this statement, the American Academy of Pediatrics sets forth recommendations for minimizing harms that may result from community-based research by emphasizing community involvement in the research process.

ABBREVIATIONS. IRB, institutional review board; NARCH, Native American Research Centers for Health; IHS, Indian Health Service.

The term "community-based research" is used to describe the conduct of research in community settings (in contrast to research conducted primarily in hospitals, clinics, or institutions specifically dedicated to medical research). Within the specialty of pediatrics, the Muscatine Study examining the natural history of childhood obesity in a small Iowa town is a well-known example.[1] Generally, such projects are embraced by communities because of the perception in European cultures that scientific enterprise is likely to yield information that is potentially beneficial. However, there are communities in North America in which cultural perceptions and historical experience create a different, somewhat hostile view of Western science and research. Such communities commonly comprise persons of ethnic minorities who may be economically disadvantaged, culturally isolated, or politically underrepresented. They may include people with strong ethnic/tribal affinity living in relative geographic isolation (eg, American Indian/Alaska Native individuals living on reservations) or immigrants of common national origin living within a specific urban neighborhood. Although institutional review boards (IRBs) have developed well-recognized procedures to minimize risk to individuals who participate in research studies, collective risks to members of specific geographic, racial, religious, or ethnic communities may

be overlooked. The purpose of this statement is to outline the special research-related concerns of such communities and to suggest means by which investigators working with socially identifiable communities can minimize risks and maximize benefits involved with research. The considerations discussed apply to the broad spectrum of research pursuits that may take place in such communities.

SPECIAL RISKS TO SOCIALLY IDENTIFIABLE POPULATIONS

Risks to socially identifiable populations or communities generally can be subdivided into 2 areas: external risks and intracommunity risks. Although most researchers and IRB members have some familiarity with the former, the latter are seldom understood or regarded outside the community of interest.[2]

External Risks

Harms inflicted by outsiders are the best-known collective risk to people with a shared social or cultural identity. Racism, with all its negative components, is an obvious example of this sort of external risk. However, investigators seldom appreciate that the research enterprise may have unintended harms on the ethnic, religious, and social well-being of isolated or socially identifiable communities. These unintended harms may affect economic, social, legal, and political life within such communities.

Economic Risks

The lay press and professional journals have given considerable attention to the potential for employment and insurance discrimination on the basis of genetic information uncovered in the course of genetic research studies. Theoretically, individual research participants and their communities may be placed at risk by such activities. Although few cases of genetic discrimination have been documented, it continues to be a major concern.[3] The same can be said for other kinds of community-based research. For example, documentation of a high prevalence of human immunodeficiency virus infection or domestic violence within a community could have important adverse economic effects on that community, ranging from increased insurance rates for community members to decisions by businesses to move into or remain in that community.[4]

Social Risks

Studies that focus on community problems (eg, drug abuse, human immunodeficiency virus infection, teen pregnancy, youth violence) run the risk of stigmatizing such communities or inadvertently reinforcing common misconceptions about such communities within the dominant culture. Community members also may be harmed by the way they see themselves or one another in light of data that emphasize negative aspects of community life and neglect positive aspects of the community or culture. In each case, these harms may disproportionately affect children, whose cultural identity and self-esteem may be closely linked. Genetic studies inadvertently may limit community members in their opportunities for social interactions including marriage, adoption efforts, and child-custody claims.

Legal and Political Risks

In the United States, American Indian and Alaska Native persons share special social and political status on the basis of their descent from the people who inhabited the land before European contact. Issues of tremendous social, political, and economic complexity may be raised by research (including but not limited to genetic studies) that challenges claims of descent or status as original inhabitants of a specific region (eg, the "Kennewick Man" discovered in Washington state[5]). Thus, research findings or interpretations that might be innocuous to some communities may threaten the existence of others.

Intracommunity Risks

As noted previously, intracommunity risks may not be considered when IRBs review research involving human subjects, in part because intracommunity harms are highly localized and often not evident to those outside the community. Nonetheless, outside involvement in local communities—even seemingly beneficial interventions—can be highly disruptive to existing social relationships. Although the involvement of local community members on university IRBs, encouraged by federal regulation, may reduce the occurrence of such harms, it is unusual for communities geographically removed from university centers to have representation on university IRBs. Perhaps the most important consideration from the point of view of socially identifiable communities is the risk to cultural and moral authority that may be engendered by community members' participation in research.

Although informed consent by individuals participating in research is the standard by which many Europeans and Americans judge the ethical propriety of research activities, many societies require collective consensus and assent. Such considerations were, for example, at the heart of the establishment of the Iroquois Confederacy more than 500 years ago.[6] Collective assent is especially important when research activities or findings may affect the whole community. IRB standards and procedures that govern the protection of human subjects in scientific research are based on the rights of individuals. Research cannot be conducted without the informed consent of individuals (or in the case of children, the consent of their parents). However, in many instances of community research, there are other ethical considerations of collective consensus and assent that should be carefully considered and, where appropriate, documented. For example, the University of Washington's IRB requires documentation that appropriate letters of tribal support be presented for research projects involving American Indian/Alaska Native communities. Area offices of the Indian Health Service (IHS), which also sponsor IRBs for research conducted in their areas, maintain the same requirement.

None of these considerations should be construed to indicate that community consent may properly override the autonomy of an individual who does not wish to participate in research.

Involving community members and groups on the research team from planning, through analysis, and to dissemination of the results will help the research team recognize potential risks to the community and identify how best to avoid or minimize them.[7]

SPECIAL POTENTIAL BENEFITS TO SOCIALLY IDENTIFIABLE POPULATIONS

In addition to having to consider unique aspects of informed consent in socially recognizable communities, many indigenous populations desire a rethinking of the concept of beneficence, that is, of doing no harm while maximizing potential benefits.[8] In conventional views of research, an acceptable understanding of beneficence includes the notion that, although the research may not directly benefit study participants, it has significant potential to benefit society as a whole or to benefit some portion of the society (eg, people with a specific disease). Many indigenous populations have expressed dissatisfaction with this interpretation of beneficence and have required, instead, that research proposals contain concrete, well-defined plans for how the research findings will be used to directly benefit the community.[9] In many instances, such requirements include involvement by researchers in the community even after the data-gathering phase of the research is complete. Thus, for example, a study examining the impact of violence in a neighborhood's public schools might be considered unacceptable if the investigators proposing the study could not articulate clearly how study results might be used to ameliorate the problem.

The early and continuing involvement of community members and groups on the research team will help the team recognize potential benefits to the community and identify how best to maximize them.[7] The medical and public health literature contains numerous examples of successful research partnerships established between academic organizations and socially identifiable communities. The Kahnawake Schools Diabetes Prevention Project in a Mohawk community in Canada is an excellent example of the mutual benefits researchers and communities derive from ethically sound community-based research.[7] Successful research projects have been undertaken with community participation from the onset of the project, including writing the research proposal and grant application.[10] The establishment of community members as principal investigators in research projects was given further strength and credibility by the recently combined IHS/National Institutes of Health program for establishing Native American Research Centers for Health (NARCH). The NARCH initiative, which partners American Indian and Alaska Native tribes with academic centers and other research institutions, identifies tribes as the investigators and research institutions as partners, a direct reversal of what has been common practice until now. The National Institutes of Health-funded Excellence in Partnerships for Community Outreach, Research on Health Disparities and Training (Project EXPORT) encourages the same approach with other minority communities. The NARCH and Project EXPORT initiatives have the potential to promote the benefits of national, multisite research partnerships between academia and communities and to further the impact of community-based, socially responsible research.

In summary, the ethical conduct of research in socially identifiable communities requires application of standards not commonly used in biomedical or social sciences research. These special considerations are based on the cultural views of many such communities, their historical experience with European-dominated cultures, and in many cases, the unique political statuses of these communities. Important elements of the responsible conduct of research in and with such communities include engaging indigenous or other socially identifiable communities as partners in the research enterprise, developing common goals for researchers and community members, recognizing potential risks and identifying how best to avoid or minimize them, recognizing potential benefits and identifying how to maximize and achieve them, and using knowledge gained from the research to assist communities in need. Investigators who are meticulous in observing these standards almost invariably find that their research goals are met while they are enriched by a deeper knowledge of the unique histories and cultures of their community partners.

CONSIDERATIONS

In addition to the aforementioned points, the following concepts should be considered by researchers seeking to engage socially identifiable communities in research activities.

1. Members of the research team and, where appropriate, research sponsors should strive to assist community organizations in the designing and implementing of interventions based on their research findings. If, for example, the project has examined the prevalence of hypertension among obese adolescents in an inner-city community, researchers should be encouraged to follow their study with concrete assistance to the community in addressing this problem.
2. Efforts should be made to include persons of ethnic minorities as researchers on these teams. Given the small proportion of researchers of ethnic minorities, it is critical that mentorship opportunities be created for these individuals.
3. Researchers should offer their expertise to individuals in the community who may want to develop their own research to address questions raised by the original study.
4. Individual researchers are supported by academic institutions that also have responsibilities to communities. Institutions are strongly urged to create and maintain educational, training, and funding opportunities that facilitate the mentoring relationships necessary to enable communities to cultivate researchers, particularly those of ethnic minorities.

RECOMMENDATIONS

Several steps can be taken during the planning phase of a community-based research project to minimize the aforementioned risks.[11,12] It should be noted that these recommendations may not be applicable to every community. Communities sharing identical views as the dominant culture (eg, a project conducted in a neighborhood in suburban Boston) may not require the same cautious and painstaking approach. Thus, "community" here will refer to socially identifiable groups (not necessarily living in the same geographic region) for which there is a reasonable possibility that group ethos concerning research and/or community responsibility may differ from the dominant culture.

1. Members of the community should be consulted in the planning of the research and the definition of research objectives. Potential benefits to the community should be articulated clearly and unambiguously.[13]
2. Research participants should be considered partners, not research subjects. Responsible members of the community (eg, tribal health care leaders, planners) should have ongoing oversight of the project and be given responsibility for ensuring adherence to the original goals of the project and procedures designed to protect the community. (Research that expects to use any resources of the IHS [eg, IHS personnel, review charts, blood work] must first comply with the IHS requirement that the tribal government explicitly approve the research.)
3. Community members should be the first to be informed of study results. They should be active participants in the analysis and interpretation of data. To provide community members the opportunity to articulate their interpretation of study findings, community members also should be consulted about proper methods for publishing and disseminating the data gathered in their community.
4. If there is potential that the results could be damaging to a specific community, research investiga-

tors should keep the community anonymous when publishing and presenting the results.

5. Human research protection programs and IRBs should utilize appropriate options provided within the federal regulations (45 CFR 46) to guarantee that proper representation of community interests is part of the ethical review process. This often will require the recruitment of experts from outside of the IRB to help in the review of community-based studies. Appropriate IRB review of community-based research should also be promoted and enforced within human research protection accreditation standards.

COMMITTEE ON NATIVE AMERICAN CHILD HEALTH, 2002–2003
David C. Grossman, MD, MPH, Chairperson
Indu Agarwal, MD
Vincent M. Biggs, MD
George Brenneman, MD
Sheila Gahagan, MD
*James N. Jarvis, MD
Harold S. Margolis, MD

LIAISONS
Joseph T. Bell, MD
    Association of American Indian Physicians
J. Chris Carey, MD
    American College of Obstetricians and
    Gynecologists
James B. Carson, MD
    Canadian Paediatric Society
Kelly R. Moore, MD
    Indian Health Service
Michael Storck, MD
    American Academy of Child and Adolescent
    Psychiatry

COMMITTEE ON COMMUNITY HEALTH SERVICES, 2002–2003
Helen M. DuPlessis, MD, MPH, Chairperson
Wyndolyn C. Bell, MD
Suzanne C. Boulter, MD
Denice Cora-Bramble, MD
Charles Feild, MD, MPH
Gilbert A. Handal, MD
Murray L. Katcher, MD, PhD
Francis E. Rushton, Jr, MD
David L. Wood, MD, MPH

LIAISONS
Jose H. Belardo, MSW, MS
    Maternal and Child Health Bureau
Lance E. Rodewald, MD
    Ambulatory Pediatric Association

CONSULTANTS
Morris Foster, PhD
William L. Freeman, MD, MPH, CIP
Richard Sharp, PhD

*Lead author

REFERENCES

1. Clarke WR, Woolson RF, Lauer RM. Changes in ponderosity and blood pressure in childhood: the Muscatine study. *Am J Epidemiol.* 1986;124:195–206
2. Foster MW, Sharp RR. Genetic research and culturally specific risks: one size does not fit all. *Trends Genet.* 2000;16:93–95
3. Alper JS, Geller LN, Barash CI, Billings PR, Laden V, Natowicz MR. Genetic discrimination and screening for hemochromatosis. *J Public Health Policy.* 1994;15:345–358
4. University of Colorado Health Sciences Center. *Am Indian Alsk Native Ment Health Res.* 1989;2:1–88
5. Morell V. Kennewick Man's trials continue. *Science.* 1998;280:190–192
6. Richter DK. *The Ordeal of the Longhouse: The Peoples of the Iroquois League in the Era of European Colonization.* Chapel Hill, NC: University of North Carolina Press; 1992
7. Macaulay AC, Paradis G, Potvin L, et al. The Kahnawake Schools Diabetes Prevention Project: intervention, evaluation, and baseline results of a diabetes primary prevention program with a native community in Canada. *Prev Med.* 1997;26:779–790
8. Dunn CM, Chadwick G. *Protecting Study Volunteers in Research. A Manual for Investigative Sites.* Boston, MA: CenterWatch Inc; 1999
9. Kone A, Sullivan M, Senturia KD, Chrisman NJ, Ciske SJ, Krieger JW. Improving collaboration between researchers and communities. *Public Health Rep.* 2000;115:243–248
10. Matsunaga DS, Enos R, Gotay CC, et al. Participatory research in a native Hawaiian community: the Wai'anae Cancer Research Project. *Cancer.* 1996;78(7 suppl):1582–1586
11. Macaulay AC, Commanda LE, Freeman WL, et al. Participatory research maximises community and lay involvement. North American Primary Care Research Group. *BMJ.* 1999;319:774–778
12. Foster MW, Bernsten D, Carter TH. A model agreement for genetic research in socially identifiable populations. *Am J Hum Genet.* 1998;63:696–702
13. Strauss RP, Sengupta S, Quinn SC, et al. The role of community advisory boards: involving communities in the informed consent process. *Am J Public Health.* 2001;91:1938–1943

All policy statements from the American Academy of Pediatrics automatically expire 5 years after publication unless reaffirmed, revised, or retired at or before that time.

Evaluation and Treatment of the Human Immunodeficiency Virus-1–Exposed Infant

- *Clinical Report*

AMERICAN ACADEMY OF PEDIATRICS

Susan M. King, MD, MSc; and the Committee on Pediatric AIDS

CANADIAN PAEDIATRIC SOCIETY

Infectious Diseases and Immunization Committee

CLINICAL REPORT
Guidance for the Clinician in Rendering Pediatric Care

Evaluation and Treatment of the Human Immunodeficiency Virus-1–Exposed Infant

ABSTRACT. In developed countries, care and treatment are available for pregnant women and infants that can decrease the rate of perinatal human immunodeficiency virus type 1 (HIV-1) infection to 2% or less. The pediatrician has a key role in prevention of mother-to-child transmission of HIV-1 by identifying HIV-exposed infants whose mothers' HIV infection was not diagnosed before delivery, prescribing antiretroviral prophylaxis for these infants to decrease the risk of acquiring HIV-1 infection, and promoting avoidance of HIV-1 transmission through human milk. In addition, the pediatrician can provide care for HIV-exposed infants by monitoring them for early determination of HIV-1 infection status and for possible short- and long-term toxicities of antiretroviral exposure, providing chemoprophylaxis for *Pneumocystis* pneumonia, and supporting families living with HIV-1 infection by providing counseling to parents or caregivers. *Pediatrics* 2004;114:497–505; *HIV-1, mother-to-child transmission, HIV-exposed infants, antiretroviral, diagnosis.*

ABBREVIATIONS. HIV, human immunodeficiency virus; AAP, American Academy of Pediatrics; EIA, enzyme immunoassay; ZDV, zidovudine; NVP, nevirapine; 3TC, lamivudine; TB, tuberculosis; PCR, polymerase chain reaction; PCP, *Pneumocystis* pneumonia.

INTRODUCTION

The epidemiology of perinatal human immunodeficiency virus type 1 (HIV-1) infection in North America has changed drastically with implementation of strategies to prevent perinatal HIV-1 transmission. Prevention of 98% of perinatal HIV-1 infections is a realizable goal. HIV-1 testing and interventions to decrease the rate of HIV-1 transmission during pregnancy are detailed in an American Academy of Pediatrics (AAP) technical report.[1] Prevention of perinatal HIV infection requires coordinated efforts from health care professionals caring for both the mother and the child. Those caring for infants born to HIV-1–infected mothers should en-

sure that strategies for prevention are continued after delivery, that infants are followed and tested for early determination of their HIV infection status, and that appropriate steps are taken for treatment or prevention of other congenital and perinatal infections associated with HIV-1 infection. The pediatrician has a key role in counseling parents, identifying families' needs, and linking them with additional support services.

Identification of Maternal HIV-1 Infection

Failure to identify HIV-1 infection of the mother before delivery is clearly suboptimal for prevention of perinatal transmission and for care of the mother. Therefore, programs to identify and initiate care for HIV-1 infection before or during pregnancy should be a priority.[2,3] However, identification of HIV-1 exposure even during labor or at birth rather than later allows for improved care of the HIV-exposed infant.

HIV Testing of the Infant if the Mother's HIV-1-Infection Status Is Unknown

If the infant is born to a mother whose HIV-1 infection status is unknown, the mother or the infant should have HIV-1 testing with maternal consent.[1,4–7] Documented consent for maternal and/or newborn HIV testing may be obtained in a variety of ways, including by right of refusal (documented patient education with testing to take place unless rejected in writing by the patient). The AAP supports use of consent procedures that facilitate rapid incorporation of HIV education and testing into routine medical care settings.[1] Some states mandate HIV-1 testing of all infants whose mothers' HIV-1 infection status is unknown. To intervene with postnatal prophylaxis, the neonatal HIV-1 test result should be available as soon as possible after birth and certainly within 24 hours. This is feasible by using "expedited" HIV-1 enzyme immunoassay (EIA) or by using rapid testing kits. An expedited EIA uses the first step of the standard laboratory HIV-1 antibody testing, with both positive and negative test results being available within 24 hours. A rapid test is one using a kit designed to test a single specimen for HIV-1 antibodies, with a result available within minutes to 2 hours.

Two such tests, OraQuick Rapid HIV-1 Antibody Test (OraSure Technologies Inc, Bethlehem, PA) and Single Use Diagnostic System (SUDS) HIV-1 Test (Murex Corporation, Norcross, GA), are licensed in the United States.[8,9] Clinical testing of a comparable kit is underway in Canada.

The rapid test result should be confirmed by standard HIV-1 testing. If the expedited EIA or the rapid test result is positive, then a confirmatory supplemental test is required to diagnose HIV-1 seropositivity definitively. Starting antiretroviral infant prophylaxis as soon as possible after birth (before 24 hours of age) is critical to prevent perinatal transmission. Therefore, if antiretroviral prophylaxis is given to an infant born to a mother with a positive EIA or rapid test result, it should be initiated pending results of her confirmatory test. The decision whether to start antiretroviral prophylaxis would take into consideration the positive predictive value of the screening test and the potential benefits and risks of the prophylactic agents.[10]

INTERVENTIONS FOR PREVENTION OF PERINATAL HIV-1 TRANSMISSION

Antiretroviral Prophylaxis When Initiated During Pregnancy

In North America, most HIV-1–infected pregnant women receive care for HIV infection during the prenatal period, in which case most receive combination antiretroviral therapy with 3 or more drugs, have a low viral load, have access to obstetric interventions such as scheduled cesarean section at 38 weeks' gestation, and plan not to breastfeed. Perinatal HIV-1 transmission rates as low as 1% have been observed in such circumstances.[11,12] When prenatal and intrapartum maternal antiretroviral therapy have been received, administration of zidovudine (ZDV) for 6 weeks to the infant remains the preferred prophylactic regimen for most infants.[1,13] Two stud-

ies conducted in developing countries have suggested that a single maternal intrapartum dose and a single neonatal dose of nevirapine (NVP) in addition to short-course maternal ZDV (with oral ZDV during labor and either no infant prophylaxis or 1 week of infant ZDV prophylaxis) may provide increased efficacy in decreasing perinatal transmission compared with short-course maternal ZDV alone.[14,15] In contrast to these studies, a clinical trial in the United States, Europe, Brazil, and the Bahamas (PACTG 316) evaluated whether the addition of a single dose of NVP to the regimens of both the mother and infant compared with placebo added to standard antiretroviral therapy for both would provide additional benefits in lowering transmission; at a minimum, women received prenatal and intrapartum ZDV, and 75% of women received combination therapy. All infants received standard 6-week ZDV prophylaxis. In this study, transmission rates were very low in both groups (1.5%), and the addition of NVP did not demonstrate any additional protection against perinatal transmission but was associated with the development of NVP-resistance mutations 6 weeks after birth in 15% of the women who received NVP.[16,17] Thus, currently, addition of NVP as a single maternal intrapartum dose with a single neonatal dose is not recommended for women who have received highly active antiretroviral therapy during pregnancy.[11]

Antiretroviral Prophylaxis When Initiated During Labor

If the woman's HIV-1 infection status is determined only at the time of labor and delivery, several effective regimens for prevention of perinatal transmission are available (Table 1). These regimens include:

TABLE 1. Maternal Intrapartum and Infant Prophylactic Antiretroviral Drug Regimens When an HIV-1—Infected Mother Has Not Received Prenatal Antiretroviral Therapy

Drug	Maternal Dosing, Intrapartum	Infant Dosing	Infant Schedule
NVP	Single 200-mg dose PO at onset of labor	2 mg/kg PO single dose	Single dose at 48–72 h
ZDV with 3TC	ZDV, 600 mg PO at onset of labor followed by 300 mg PO every 3 h until delivery; and 3TC, 150 mg PO at onset of labor followed by 150 mg PO every 12 h until delivery	ZDV, 4 mg/kg PO every 12 h; and 3TC, 2 mg/kg PO every 12 h	For 1 wk
ZDV	2 mg/kg, IV bolus followed by continuous infusion of 1 mg/kg per h until delivery	2 mg/kg PO 4 times per day; If unable to tolerate oral therapy, 1.5 mg/kg IV every 6 h; If infant is preterm, 1.5 mg/kg every 12 hours for 2 weeks and then increase to 2 mg/kg every 8 h	Beginning 8–12 h after birth and continuing through 6 wk of age
ZDV with NVP	ZDV, 2 mg/kg IV bolus followed by continuous infusion of 1 mg/kg per h until delivery; and NVP, single 200-mg dose, PO, at onset of labor	ZDV, 2 mg/kg PO 4 times per day; and NVP, 2 mg/kg PO single dose	Start ZDV beginning 8–12 h after birth and continuing through 6 wk of age; and single dose of NVP at 48–72 h of age

IV indicates intravenous; PO, oral.

1. One oral dose of NVP at the onset of labor followed by 1 oral dose of NVP for the infant 48 to 72 hours after birth
2. Intrapartum oral ZDV and lamivudine (3TC) followed by 1 week of oral ZDV and 3TC for the infant
3. Intrapartum intravenous ZDV followed by 6 weeks of ZDV for the infant
4. The ZDV with NVP regimen, 1 oral dose of NVP at the onset of labor, followed by 1 oral dose of NVP for the infant, combined with intrapartum intravenous ZDV, followed by 6 weeks of ZDV for the infant

In randomized, clinical trials among breastfeeding populations, the NVP regimen and the ZDV-with-3TC regimen have been shown to decrease the rate of perinatal transmission by 38% to 47%.[1,13,18–21] Observational data from populations of HIV-1–infected women in which breastfeeding is uncommon suggest that the third regimen, maternal intrapartum and infant ZDV alone, is associated with lower transmission rates when compared with no intervention (10% vs 27%, respectively, in New York state and 11% vs 31%, respectively, in North Carolina).[22,23] The fourth regimen of ZDV with NVP is theoretically appealing, but limited data are available to address whether the combination regimen offers added benefit to either drug alone.[13] Conflicting data are available from a study conducted in Malawi of women first identified as HIV-1 infected during labor, in which the effect of a single maternal intrapartum and single neonatal dose of NVP was compared with the same NVP regimens plus 1 week of ZDV for the infant.[24] When the mother received intrapartum NVP, there was no difference between the NVP and NVP-plus-ZDV groups; however, when the woman did not receive intrapartum NVP, the combination regimen seemed to have greater efficacy.[24] Thus, at the present time, any of the 4 potential intrapartum/ postnatal regimens are reasonable to consider in the circumstance in which the woman had not received antiretroviral therapy during pregnancy.

Postnatal Antiretroviral Prophylaxis

When the mother's or infant's HIV-1 infection status is known only after the infant's birth and, thus, maternal prenatal and intrapartum antiretroviral therapy is not received, observational data suggest that 6 weeks of antiretroviral prophylaxis with ZDV given to the infant may provide some protection against transmission if initiated within 24 hours of birth.[13,22] This 6-week ZDV regimen is considered standard for prophylaxis in this circumstance in developed countries.[13] Results from the Malawi study comparing single-dose infant NVP to single-dose infant NVP plus 1 week of infant ZDV to infants whose mothers did not receive antiretroviral therapy during pregnancy suggest that the combination regimen is more effective than single-dose infant NVP alone, but only if the mother did not receive intrapartum NVP.[24] However, whether this combination would be more effective than the standard 6-week course of ZDV prophylaxis used in developed countries is unknown. Although data to demonstrate superior efficacy of combination regimens are lacking, when only infant prophylaxis can be provided, some clinicians combine the 6-week infant ZDV prophylaxis regimen with 1 or more additional antiretroviral drugs, viewing the situation as analogous to postexposure prophylaxis in other circumstances.

Data from studies of animals indicate that the longer the delay in institution of prophylaxis, the less likely that infection will be prevented. In most studies of animals, antiretroviral prophylaxis initiated 24 to 36 hours after exposure usually is not effective for preventing infection.[25–27] HIV-1 infection is established in most perinatally infected infants by 1 to 2 weeks of age. Initiation of postexposure prophylaxis after 2 days of age is not likely to be efficacious in preventing transmission, and by 14 days of age infection would be established in most infants.

Avoidance of HIV-1 Infection From Human Milk

Postnatal HIV-1 transmission can occur from ingestion of human milk from HIV-1–infected women. The literature on breastfeeding and HIV-1 transmission is detailed in the AAP technical report "Human Milk, Breastfeeding, and Transmission of Human Immunodeficiency Virus-1 Infection in the United States."[28] In the United States and Canada, where infant formulas are safe and readily available, an HIV-1–infected mother should be advised not to breastfeed even if she is receiving antiretroviral therapy.[1,13] Complete avoidance of breastfeeding (and milk donation) by HIV-1–infected women remains the only mechanism by which prevention of human milk transmission of HIV-1 can be ensured.

CARE OF THE HIV-1–EXPOSED INFANT

Assessment at Birth

At the time of the initial assessment of the infant (see Table 2), maternal health information should be reviewed to determine if the infant may have been exposed to maternal coinfections such as tuberculosis (TB), syphilis, toxoplasmosis, hepatitis B or C, cytomegalovirus, or herpes simplex virus.[29] Although there is little information as to the relative transmission or infection rates of these agents in infants of mothers with and without HIV-1 infection, there is theoretic concern that latent infections may reactivate in immunocompromised pregnant women and be transmitted to their infants. Diagnostic testing and treatment of the infant are based on maternal findings.

Determination of the Infant's HIV-1 Infection Status

Determining as soon as possible whether the HIV-1–exposed infant is infected is important to allow early initiation of antiretroviral therapy and adjunctive therapies as needed. The types of virologic assays that detect the virus include the following.

- HIV-1 DNA polymerase chain reaction (PCR): these PCR assays detect HIV-1 DNA within the peripheral blood mononuclear cells. For HIV-1 subtype B, the most common subtype in North America, the sensitivity and specificity of HIV-1

TABLE 2.   Care of the HIV-1–Exposed Infant (Birth to 6 Months of Age)

	Infant Age						
	Birth	4 wk	6 wk	2 mo	3 mo	4 mo	6 mo
History and physical examination	X	X		X			X
Assess risk of other infections*	X						
Antiretroviral prophylactic regiment	←———————————→						
CBC and differential leukocyte counts	X	X		X			
HIV-1 DNA PCR or other virologic assays for HIV-1‡	X	←———→		←————————→			
Initiate prophylaxis for PCP§				←————→			

If during this period the infant is diagnosed as HIV-1 infected, then laboratory monitoring and immunizations should follow the guidelines for treatment of pediatric HIV-1 infection.[27] CBC indicates complete blood cell; arrows indicate the time intervals over which the procedure may be performed.
* Review maternal health information to assess for possible exposure to coinfections (see text).
† ZDV is usually the preferred prophylactic agent, although alternatives are: 1) ZDV with 3TC; 2) NVP; or 3) ZDV with NVP when the mother did not receive prenatal antiretroviral therapy (see Table 1). The arrow indicates treatment spanning from birth to 6 weeks of age.
‡ See text for discussion of HIV-1 virologic assays. If a test result is positive, repeat HIV-1 DNA PCR assay immediately to confirm infection. Some HIV-1 specialists suggest an additional HIV-1 DNA PCR test at 2 weeks of age. If clinical status or other laboratory parameters suggest HIV-1 infection, repeat testing as soon as possible. If by 4 months of age the test results are all negative for infection, testing for HIV-1 seroreversion at 12 to 18 months of age is indicated to definitively exclude HIV-1 infection.
§ The preferred prophylactic agent is trimethoprim-sulfamethoxazole; alternatives are dapsone, pentamidine, and atovaquone (Table 3). The arrow indicates the time interval over which the procedure may be performed.

DNA PCR assays approach 96% and 99%, respectively, by 28 days of age.[30] However, the currently available HIV-1 DNA PCR assays have less sensitivity for detection of non-B subtype, and false-negative DNA PCR assay results have been reported for infants infected with non-B subtype virus infection.[31–33]

- HIV-1 RNA assays: these assays detect viral RNA in the plasma by using a variety of methodologies including PCR, in vitro signal amplification nucleic probes (branched DNA, also known as bDNA), and nucleic acid sequence-based amplification (NASBA). RNA assays may be at least as sensitive or more sensitive than HIV-1 DNA PCR assays and are as specific.[34–37] Some HIV-1 RNA assays may be more sensitive than HIV-1 DNA PCR assays for detection of non-B subtype.[37] Although the sensitivity of HIV-1 RNA assays has been shown not to be affected by the use of ZDV alone as prophylaxis,[37,38] it is not known if it would be affected by the use of additional antiretroviral agents.
- HIV-1 peripheral blood cell culture: HIV-1 culture has largely been replaced by HIV-1 DNA PCR assays. HIV-1 culture is expensive, is available in only a few laboratories, and may require up to 28 days for positive results.
- HIV-1 immune complex-dissociated p24 antigen: HIV-1 p24 antigen is not recommended for diagnosis in infants because of its low sensitivity.

In general, HIV-1 DNA PCR assay is the preferred diagnostic test in North America.[1,3] However, women who acquired their HIV-1 infection outside North America or Western Europe may be infected with an HIV-1 non-B subtype.[39] For infants born to women known or suspected to be infected with

non-B subtypes, consultation with an HIV-1 specialist is recommended for advice on diagnostic investigations. The birth specimen must be a neonatal, not cord blood, sample. Cord-blood sampling is associated with an unacceptably high rate of false-positive test results. For infants born in North America who have not been breastfed, if the HIV-1 DNA PCR assay results (obtained at birth, at 4–7 weeks of age, and at 8–16 weeks of age) are negative, then HIV-1 infection has been reasonably excluded.[40]

If the mother is HIV-2 infected, then the laboratory HIV antibody tests, but not all rapid tests, will detect both HIV-1 and HIV-2. In these circumstances, a specific request must be made for HIV-2 PCR testing for diagnosis of HIV-2 infection in the infant.

Management if an HIV-1 Virologic Assay Result Is Positive

A positive HIV-1 virologic assay result should be repeated immediately for confirmation. If infection is confirmed, an HIV-1 specialist should be consulted for advice regarding antiretroviral therapy. It is currently recommended that treatment be initiated in all HIV-infected infants younger than 12 months who have HIV-associated clinical or immunologic abnormalities regardless of HIV-1 RNA level, and that therapy be considered for HIV-infected infants younger than 12 months who are asymptomatic and have normal immune parameters.[41] This recommendation is based on the substantial risk of rapid disease progression in infants and the inability to predict those at risk of rapid disease progression.[42–44]

Role of HIV-1 Antibody Testing in HIV-1–Exposed Infants

Serologic testing after 12 months of age is used to confirm that maternal HIV-1 antibodies transferred to the infant in utero have disappeared. If the child is still antibody positive at 12 months of age, then testing should be repeated at 18 months of age.[3,40] Loss of HIV-1 antibody in a child with previously negative HIV-1 DNA PCR test results definitively confirms that the child is HIV-1 uninfected. Positive HIV-1 antibodies at ≥18 months of age indicates HIV-1 infection. Repeat HIV-1 antibody testing at 24 months of age is no longer recommended.

Prevention of *Pneumocystis* Pneumonia

Pneumocystis pneumonia (PCP) is the most common serious opportunistic infection in HIV-1–infected children. This condition is caused by *Pneumocystis jiroveci* (formerly *Pneumocystis carinii*). It is recommended that PCP prophylaxis be started at or near the completion of ZDV prophylaxis (4–6 weeks of age) but discontinued when HIV-1 infection is reasonably excluded. PCP prophylaxis would be discontinued, therefore, when results of 2 virologic assays performed on 2 separate samples, 1 after 1 month of age and the other after 2 to 4 months of age, are known to be negative (see Table 2). Drugs and dosing regimens for PCP prophylaxis in the infant are listed in Table 3. Infants who are HIV-1 infected should remain on PCP prophylaxis until 12 months of age, at which time they should receive PCP prophylaxis according to guidelines from the US Public Health Service/Infectious Diseases Society of America for prevention of opportunistic infections.[45]

Prevention of TB

The populations at risk of infection with HIV-1 and TB overlap. Therefore, for the infant born to an HIV-1–infected mother, information should be obtained regarding the TB infection status of the mother and other household members. If the mother has hematogenous dissemination of TB, the infant should be evaluated for congenital TB as outlined in US or Canadian TB guidelines.[46–48] If the mother or a household member has active TB that is of a contagious form, the infant should be separated from that person, if possible, until the person is considered noncontagious. If the infant is exposed to TB, the infant should be managed as outlined in US or Canadian TB guidelines.[46–48] Although the BCG vaccine is widely used in infants around the world for prevention of TB, it is rarely used in most of North America and is contraindicated in infants who are HIV-1 infected or are of unknown HIV-1 status.[49]

Immunizations

All routine infant immunizations should be given to HIV-1–exposed infants.[50,51] However, if HIV-1 infection is confirmed, then guidelines for the HIV-1–infected child should be followed.[50–54]

Monitoring for Toxicity From Exposure to Antiretroviral Drugs in Utero and During Infancy

Infants born to HIV-1–infected mothers who have received prenatal care and are receiving therapy according to the US Public Health Service guidelines for treatment of HIV-1 infection will be exposed to antiretroviral agents in utero and as infants.[1,13,55,56] Some studies suggest that combination antiretroviral therapy during pregnancy increases the risk of preterm birth and other adverse outcomes of pregnancy.[57] However, a review of outcomes in 7 studies in which 3266 HIV-1–infected pregnant women were enrolled suggests that combination therapy is not associated with increased rates of preterm birth, low birth weight, low Apgar scores, or stillbirth.[58]

The data available on the short- and long-term toxicity for the infant exposed to combinations of antiretroviral drugs in utero are limited.[10,59] The most common short-term adverse consequence with ZDV prophylaxis is anemia.[10,59] Therefore, infants receiving ZDV should have a complete blood cell count at birth, 1 month of age, and 2 months of age (Tables 1 and 2). Transient lactatemia also has been observed, but the significance of this is not known.[60,61] Mitochondrial dysfunction was described in 8 of 1754 (0.46%) uninfected infants in a French cohort with in utero exposure to ZDV with 3TC or to ZDV alone.[62] Two of these infants developed severe neurologic disease and died (both exposed to ZDV with 3TC); 3 had mild-to-moderate symptoms (including a transient cardiomyopathy); and 3 had no symptoms but transient laboratory abnormalities including high lactate concentration.[62] Another evaluation of mitochondrial toxicity was conducted in 4392 uninfected or HIV-indeterminate children (2644 with perinatal antiretroviral exposure) followed within the French Pediatric Cohort or identified within a France National Register developed for reporting possible mitochondrial dysfunction in

TABLE 3.   Regimens for PCP Prophylaxis in Infants

Drug	Dose	Route	Schedule
Trimethoprim-sulfamethoxazole	Trimethoprim 150 mg/m² per day, with sulfamethoxazole 750 mg/m² per day	PO	Twice daily for 3 days per wk (consecutive days, eg, Monday, Tuesday and Wednesday) or alternate days (every Monday, Wednesday, and Friday) Alternatives: once daily for 3 days per wk or twice daily for 7 days per wk
Dapsone	2 mg/kg	PO	Once daily
	4 mg/kg	PO	Once weekly
Pentamidine	4 mg/kg	IV	Every 2–4 weeks
Atovaquone			
Infants 1–3 mo of age	30 mg/kg	PO	Once daily
Infants 4–24 mo of age	45 mg/kg	PO	Once daily

IV indicates intravenous; PO, oral.

HIV-exposed children. Evidence of mitochondrial dysfunction was identified in 12 children (including the previous 8 reported cases), all of whom had perinatal antiretroviral exposure, an 18-month incidence of 0.26%.[63] Similar findings have not been reported from other cohorts.[10,64] The French Perinatal Cohort Study Group has also reported a potential increase in the rate of early febrile seizures in uninfected infants with antiretroviral exposure (cumulative risk of first febrile seizure by 18 months of age of 1.1% in antiretroviral-exposed infants, compared with 0.4% in unexposed infants).[65] The strength of the association of these clinical and laboratory findings with in utero antiretroviral exposure is controversial.[59,64] However, if causal, significant disease or death seem to be extremely rare, and the potential morbidity or mortality needs to be compared with the proven benefit of ZDV in decreasing the risk of mother-to-child transmission of a fatal infection by nearly 70%. These data emphasize the importance of long-term follow-up for any child with exposure to antiretroviral drugs regardless of infection status.[13]

Although the use of ZDV monotherapy does not seem to be teratogenic, in utero exposure to multiple antiretroviral drugs is increasingly frequent, and little is known of the teratogenic risk of such exposures.[13,56,66,67] For example, efavirenz, a nonnucleoside reverse-transcriptase inhibitor, is teratogenic in monkeys, causing significant central nervous system malformations in infant cynomolgus monkeys.[56] There has been a case report of myelomeningocele in a human infant born to a woman who was receiving efavirenz at conception and during the first trimester.[67,68] Exposure of fetal monkeys to tenofovir was not associated with gross structural abnormalities, but lower circulating concentrations of growth factors, a 13% decrease in birth weight, and a transient decrease in bone porosity were observed.[56] Hydroxyurea is another antiretroviral agent for which teratogenicity has been observed in several animal species, but information in human pregnancies is limited.[69–71] Other medications given to the mother for complications associated with HIV-1 infection also can be teratogenic. For example, fluconazole has been associated with congenital craniofacial, skeletal, and cardiac anomalies in infants, but the strength of this association remains controversial.[72–74]

Until there are more data on the safety of in utero antiretroviral exposure, infants should be monitored by examination at birth for congenital anomalies[13,56] and assessed at 6 months of age and at annual visits for long-term adverse effects of drug exposure. The assessment at follow-up includes evaluation for symptoms and signs suggestive of mitochondrial toxicity.[75,76] Symptoms and signs of mitochondrial toxicity are varied and generally nonspecific, but serious signs and symptoms would include neurologic manifestations including encephalopathy, afebrile seizures or developmental delay, cardiac symptoms attributable to cardiomyopathy, and gastrointestinal symptoms attributable to hepatitis. The physical examination should include a developmental assessment. If abnormalities suggestive of mitochondrial toxicity are observed, then consultation should be obtained with a specialist knowledgeable in this field. There will be regional variation in the specialists knowledgeable in this topic; they may be neurologists, specialists in metabolic disorders, or HIV-1–infection specialists.

Testing Family Members

The infant's father and all siblings should be offered testing for HIV-1 infection. Testing should be strongly recommended. The age of the sibling should not be a deterrent to testing, because it is possible that perinatally infected children may remain asymptomatic for many years, even into adolescence.

Counseling and Support

When counseling the mother of an HIV-1–exposed infant, the pediatrician should take into account that the diagnosis may be recent for the mother, whose infection may have been identified during or after pregnancy. The diagnosis has profound implications for the mother and the family. If the mother is not already receiving care, she should be referred for HIV-1 care for herself. Some families may require additional support because of HIV-1 illness or death in other family members. Other social factors that may lead to an increased need for social services are poverty, substance abuse, depression, lack of health care, unemployment, difficulty finding housing, domestic violence, and fear of loss of existing supports and services, such as loss of support from partner or loss of employment, insurance, or health care coverage. Pregnant adolescents are a particularly vulnerable group, especially early adolescents (10–14 years of age). For women and their families from other countries, there are frequently additional factors related to their culture and concerns about their immigration status.

When counseling new parents or caregivers of an HIV-1–exposed infant, the pediatrician should provide an outline of plans for medical care (Table 2). Important topics to cover are medications to prevent perinatal acquisition of HIV-1 infection and opportunistic infections such as PCP, as well as the schedule of follow-up visits for assessment and laboratory assays (both for the diagnosis of HIV-1 and to check for any adverse effects associated with exposure to antiretroviral drugs). Mothers should be advised not to breastfeed.[28] Parents and caregivers should be advised of the importance of prompt assessment if the infant becomes ill. For the infant in foster care, caregivers should have sufficient information about the infant's health, including HIV-1 infection status, to ensure appropriate health care. The necessity of maintaining confidentiality should be emphasized.[77] HIV-1 infection is not a reason for exclusion from child care.[78] Pediatricians should discuss the need for planning for future care if the mother were to become ill with her HIV-1 infection.[79]

SUMMARY

1. Whenever possible, maternal HIV-1 infection should be identified before or during pregnancy, because this allows for earlier initiation of care

for the mother and for more effective interventions to prevent perinatal transmission.

2. If the maternal HIV-1 infection status is unknown at the time of the infant's birth, then HIV-1 testing of the mother or the infant is recommended with maternal consent and with results available within 24 hours of birth. The expedited EIA and rapid HIV-1 test are screening tests that may be used in this setting.

3. If the test result for HIV-1 is positive, prophylactic antiretroviral therapy should be started promptly in the infant and confirmatory HIV-1 testing should be performed.

4. HIV-1–infected mothers should not breastfeed their infants and should be educated about safe alternatives.[28]

5. Maternal health information should be reviewed to determine if the HIV-1–exposed infant may have been exposed to maternal coinfections including TB, syphilis, toxoplasmosis, hepatitis B or C, cytomegalovirus, and herpes simplex virus. Diagnostic testing and treatment of the infant are based on maternal findings.

6. Pediatricians should provide counseling to parents and caregivers of HIV-1–exposed infants about HIV-1 infection, including anticipatory guidance on the course of illness, infection-control measures, care of the infant, diagnostic tests, and potential drug toxicity.

7. All HIV-1–exposed infants should undergo virologic testing for HIV-1 at birth, at 4 to 7 weeks of age, and again at 8 to 16 weeks of age to reasonably exclude HIV-1 infection as early as possible. If any test result is positive, the test should be repeated immediately for confirmation. If all test results are negative, the infant should have serologic testing repeated at 12 months of age or older to document disappearance of the HIV-1 antibody, which definitively excludes HIV-1 infection.

8. All infants exposed to antiretroviral agents in utero or as infants should be monitored for short- and long-term drug toxicity.

9. Prophylaxis for PCP should be started at 4 to 6 weeks of age in HIV-1–exposed infants in whom infection has not been excluded. PCP prophylaxis may be discontinued when HIV-1 infection has been reasonably excluded.

10. Immunizations and TB screening should be provided for HIV-1–exposed infants in accordance with national guidelines. In the United States, immunization guidelines are established by the AAP, the Advisory Committee on Immunization Practices of the Centers for Disease Control and Prevention, and the American Academy of Family Physicians; in Canada, guidelines are established by the National Advisory Committee for Immunizations.

11. HIV-1 testing should be offered and recommended to family members.

12. The practitioner providing care for the HIV-1–exposed or HIV-1–infected infant should consult with a pediatric HIV-1 specialist and, if the HIV-1–infected mother is an adolescent, also consult with a practitioner familiar with the care of adolescents.

REFERENCES

1. Mofenson LM, and American Academy of Pediatrics, Committee on Pediatric AIDS. Technical report: perinatal human immunodeficiency virus testing and prevention of transmission. *Pediatrics.* 2000:106(6). Available at: www.pediatrics.org/cgi/content/full/106/6/e88

2. Centers for Disease Control and Prevention. Revised guidelines for HIV counseling, testing, and referral. *MMWR Recomm Rep.* 2001;50(RR-19): 1–57

3. Centers for Disease Control and Prevention. Revised recommendations for HIV screening of pregnant women. *MMWR Recomm Rep.* 2001; 50(RR-19):63–85

4. Minkoff H, O'Sullivan MJ. The case for rapid HIV testing during labor. *JAMA.* 1998;279:1743–1744

5. Grobman WA, Garcia PM. The cost-effectiveness of voluntary intrapartum rapid human immunodeficiency virus testing for women without adequate prenatal care. *Am J Obstet Gynecol*. 1999;181:1062–1071

6. Kane B. Rapid testing for HIV: why so fast? *Ann Intern Med*. 1999;131:481–483

7. Stringer JS, Rouse DJ. Rapid testing and zidovudine treatment to prevent vertical transmission of human immunodeficiency virus in unregulated parturients: a cost-effectiveness analysis. *Obstet Gynecol*. 1999;94:34–40

8. Centers for Disease Control and Prevention. Approval of a new rapid test for HIV antibody. *MMWR Morb Mortal Wkly Rep*. 2002;51:1051–1052

9. Kassler WJ, Haley C, Jones WK, Gerber AR, Kennedy EJ, George JR. Performance of a rapid, on-site human immunodeficiency virus antibody assay in a public health setting. *J Clin Microbiol*. 1995;33:2899–2902

10. Mofenson LM, Munderi P. Safety of antiretroviral prophylaxis of perinatal transmission for HIV-infected pregnant women and their infants. *J Acquir Immune Defic Syndr*. 2002;30:200–215

11. Cooper ER, Charurat M, Mofenson L, et al. Combination antiretroviral strategies for the treatment of pregnant HIV-1-infected women and prevention of perinatal HIV-1 transmission. *J Acquir Immune Defic Syndr*. 2002;29:484–494

12. Ioannidis JP, Abrams EJ, Ammann A, et al. Perinatal transmission of human immunodeficiency virus type 1 by pregnant women with RNA virus loads <1000 copies/ml. *J Infect Dis*. 2001;183:539–545

13. US Public Health Service. Public Health Service Task Force recommendations for the use of antiretroviral drugs in pregnant HIV-1-infected women for maternal health and interventions to reduce perinatal HIV-1 transmission in the United States. *MMWR Recomm Rep*. 2002;51(RR-18):1–40. Revised August 30, 2002. Available at: www.aidsinfo.nih.gov/guidelines. Accessed June 3, 2003

14. Dabis F, Leroy V, Bequet L, et al. Effectiveness of a short course of zidovudine + nevirapine to prevent mother-to-child transmission (PMTCT) of HIV-1: the Ditrame Plus ANRS 1201 Project in Abidjan, Côte d'Ivore [abstract ThOrD1428]. Presented at: XIV International AIDS Conference; July 7–12, 2002; Barcelona, Spain

15. Lallemant M, Jourdain G, Le Coeur S, et al. Nevirapine (NVP) during labor and in the neonate significantly improves zidovudine (ZDV) prophylaxis for the prevention of perinatal HIV transmission: results of PHPT-2 first interim analysis [abstract LbOr22]. Presented at: XIV International AIDS Conference; July 7–12, 2002; Barcelona, Spain

16. Dorenbaum A, Cunningham CK, Gelber RD, et al. Two-dose intrapartum/infant nevirapine and standard antiretroviral therapy to reduce perinatal HIV transmission: a randomized trial. *JAMA*. 2002;288:189–198

17. Cunningham CK, Chaix ML, Rekacewicz C, et al. Development of resistance mutations in women receiving standard antiretroviral therapy who received intrapartum nevirapine to prevent perinatal human immunodeficiency virus type 1 transmission: a substudy of pediatric AIDS clinical trials group protocol 316. *J Infect Dis*. 2002;186:181–188

18. Guay LA, Musoke P, Fleming T, et al. Intrapartum and neonatal single-dose nevirapine compared with zidovudine for prevention of mother-to-child transmission of HIV-1 in Kampala, Uganda: HIV-NET 012 randomised trial. *Lancet*. 1999;354:795–802

19. Owor M, Deseyve M, Duefield C, et al. The one year safety and efficacy data of the HIVNET 012 trial [abstract LbOr1]. Presented at: XIII International AIDS Conference; July 9–14, 2000; Durban, Natal, South Africa

20. Moodley D, Moodley J, Coovadia H, et al. A multicenter randomized controlled trial of nevirapine versus a combination of zidovudine and lamivudine to reduce intrapartum and early postpartum mother-to-child transmission of human immunodeficiency virus type 1. *J Infect Dis*. 2003;187:725–735

21. The Petra Study Team. Efficacy of three short-course regimens of zidovudine and lamivudine in preventing early and late transmission of HIV-1 from mother to child in Tanzania, South Africa, and Uganda (Petra study): a randomised, double-blind, placebo-controlled trial. *Lancet*. 2002;359:1178–1186

22. Wade NA, Birkhead GS, Warren BL, et al. Abbreviated regimens of zidovudine prophylaxis and perinatal transmission of the human immunodeficiency virus. *N Engl J Med*. 1998;339:1409–1414

23. Fiscus SA, Adimora AA, Schoenbach VJ, et al. Trends in human immunodeficiency virus (HIV) counseling, testing, and antiretroviral treatment of HIV-infected women and perinatal transmission in North Carolina. *J Infect Dis*. 1999;180:99–105

24. Taha TE, Kumwenda N, Gibbons A, et al. Neonatal post-exposure prophylaxis with nevirapine and zidovudine reduces mother-to-child transmission of HIV [abstract ThOrD1427]. Presented at: XIV International AIDS Conference; July 7–12, 2002; Barcelona, Spain

25. Van Rompay KK, Otsyula MG, Marthas ML, Miller CJ, McChesney MB, Pedersen NC. Immediate zidovudine treatment protects simian immunodeficiency virus-infected newborn macaques against rapid onset of AIDS. *Antimicrob Agents Chemother*. 1995;39:125–131

26. Tsai CC, Follis KE, Sabo A, et al. Prevention of SIV infection in macaques by (R)-9-(2-phosphonylmethoxypropyl)adenine. *Science*. 1995;270:1197–1199

27. Bottiger D, Johansson NG, Samuelsson B, et al. Prevention of simian immunodeficiency virus, SIVsm, or HIV-2 infection in cynomolgus monkeys by pre- and postexposure administration of BEA-005. *AIDS*. 1997;11:157–162

28. Read JS, and American Academy of Pediatrics, Committee on Pediatric AIDS. Technical report: human milk, breastfeeding, and the transmission of HIV-1 infection in the United States. *Pediatrics*. 2003;112:1196–1205

29. American Academy of Pediatrics, Committee on Infectious Diseases. Hepatitis C virus infection. *Pediatrics*. 1998;101:481–485

30. Dunn DT, Brandt CD, Krivine A, et al. The sensitivity of HIV-1 DNA polymerase chain reaction in the neonatal period and the relative contributions of intra-uterine and intra-partum transmission. *AIDS*. 1995;9:F7–F11

31. Kline NE, Schwarzwald H, Kline MW. False negative DNA polymerase chain reaction in an infant with subtype C human immunodeficiency virus 1 infection. *Pediatr Infect Dis J*. 2002;21:885–886

32. Haas J, Geiss M, Bohler T. False-negative polymerase chain reaction-based diagnosis of human immunodeficiency virus (HIV) type 1 in children infected with HIV strains of African origin. *J Infect Dis*. 1996;174:244–245

33. Zaman MM, Recco RA, Haag R. Infection with non-B subtype HIV type 1 complicates management of established infection in adult patients and diagnosis of infection in infant infants. *Clin Infect Dis*. 2002;34:417–418

34. Cunningham CK, Charbonneau TT, Song K, et al. Comparison of human immunodeficiency virus 1 DNA polymerase chain reaction and qualitative and quantitative RNA polymerase chain reaction in human immunodeficiency virus 1-exposed infants. *Pediatr Infect Dis J*. 1999;18:30–35

35. Simonds RJ, Brown TM, Thea DM, et al. Sensitivity and specificity of a qualitative RNA detection assay to diagnose HIV infection in young infants. *Perinatal AIDS Collaborative Transmission Study. AIDS*. 1998;12:1545–1549

36. Rouet F, Montcho C, Rouzioux C, et al. Early diagnosis of paediatric HIV-1 infection among African breast-fed children using a quantitative plasma HIV RNA assay. *AIDS*. 2001;15:1849–1856

37. Young NL, Shaffer N, Chaowanachan T, et al. Early diagnosis of HIV-1-infected infants in Thailand using RNA and DNA PCR assays sensitive to non-B subtypes. *J Acquir Immune Defic Syndr*. 2000;24:401–407

38. Mofenson L, Harris R, Steihm ER, et al. Performance characteristics of HIV-1 culture, DNA PCR and quantitative RNA for early diagnosis of perinatal HIV-1 infection [abstract 713]. Presented at: 7th Conference on Retroviruses and Opportunistic Infection; January 30–February 2, 2000; San Francisco, CA

39. Lapointe N, Samson J, Boucher M. Facing a new epidemic: molecular epidemiology of HIV among mother and child cohort in Montreal [abstract 252P]. Presented at: 11th Annual Canadian Conference on HIV/AIDS Research; April 25–28, 2002; Winnipeg, Manitoba. Available at: www.pulsus.com/cahr2002/abs/abs252P.htm. Accessed June 3, 2003

40. Centers for Disease Control and Prevention. Guidelines for national human immunodeficiency virus case surveillance, including monitoring for human immunodeficiency virus infection and acquired immunodeficiency syndrome. *MMWR Recomm Rep*. 1999;48(RR-13):1–27, 29–31

41. National Institutes of Health, Health Resources and Services Administration, Working Group on Antiretroviral Therapy and Medical Management of HIV-Infected Children. *Guidelines for the Use of Antiretroviral Agents in Pediatric HIV Infection*. Rockville, MD: AIDSinfo, National Institutes of Health; 2001. Available at: www.aidsinfo.nih.gov/guidelines. Accessed January 17, 2004

42. Scott GB, Hutto C, Makuch RW, et al. Survival in children with perinatally acquired human immunodeficiency virus type 1 infection. *N Engl J Med*. 1989;321:1791–1796

43. Barnhart HX, Caldwell MB, Thomas P, et al. Natural history of human immunodeficiency virus disease in perinatally infected children: an analysis from the Pediatric Spectrum of Disease Project. *Pediatrics*. 1996;97:710–716

44. Blanche S, Newell ML, Mayaux MJ, et al. Morbidity and mortality in European children vertically infected by HIV-1. The French Pediatric HIV Infection Study Group and European Collaborative Study. *J Acquir Immune Defic Syndr Hum Retrovirol*. 1997;14:442–450

45. US Public Health Service, Infectious Diseases Society of America, Prevention of Opportunistic Infections Working Group. *2001 USPHS/IDSA Guidelines for the Prevention of Opportunistic Infections in Persons Infected With Human Immunodeficiency Virus.* Rockville, MD: AIDSinfo, National Institutes of Health; 2001. Available at: www.aidsinfo.nih.gov/guidelines. Accessed June 3, 2003

46. American Academy of Pediatrics. Tuberculosis. In: Pickering LK, ed. *Red Book: 2003 Report of the Committee on Infectious Diseases.* 26th ed. Elk Grove Village, IL: American Academy of Pediatrics; 2003:642–660

47. Canadian Lung Association/Canadian Thoracic Society and Tuberculosis Prevention and Control, Centre for Infectious Disease Prevention and Control, Health Canada. *Canadian Tuberculosis Standards.* 5th ed. Ottawa, Ontario, Canada: Canadian Lung Association; 2002

48. American Thoracic Society/Centers for Disease Control and Prevention. Supplement: targeted tuberculin testing and treatment of latent tuberculosis infection. *Am J Respir Crit Care Med.* 2000;161:S221–S247 (endorsed by the American Academy of Pediatrics at: www.aap.org/policy/tuberculosis.html. Accessed June 3, 2003)

49. World Health Organization. BCG vaccine. Available at: www.who.int/vacines/en/tuberculosis.shtml. Accessed June 3, 2003

50. American Academy of Pediatrics, Advisory Committee on Immunization Practices, American Academy of Family Physicians. Recommended childhood immunization schedule—United States, 2002. *Pediatrics.* 2002;109:162–164

51. National Advisory Committee on Immunizations. Recommended immunization for infants, children and adults. In: *Canadian Immunization Guide.* 6th ed. Ottawa, Ontario, Canada: Health Canada; 2002:55–70. Available at: www.hc-sc.gc.ca/pphb-dgspsp/publicat/cig-gci. Accessed June 3, 2003

52. American Academy of Pediatrics, Committee on Infectious Diseases and Committee on Pediatric AIDS. Measles immunization in HIV-infected children. *Pediatrics.* 1999;103:1057–1060

53. American Academy of Pediatrics, Committee on Infectious Diseases. Varicella vaccine update. *Pediatrics.* 2000;105:136–141

54. American Academy of Pediatrics. Human immunodeficiency virus infection. In: Pickering LK, ed. *Red Book: 2003 Report of the Committee on Infectious Diseases.* Elk Grove Village, IL: American Academy of Pediatrics; 2003:360–382

55. US Department of Health and Human Services and Henry J. Kaiser Family Foundation. *Guidelines for the Use of Antiretroviral Agents in HIV-Infected Adults and Adolescents.* Rockville, MD: AIDSinfo, National Institutes of Health; 2002. Available at: www.aidsinfo.nih.gov/guidelines. Accessed June 3, 2003

56. Centers for Disease Control and Prevention. *Guidelines for the Use of Antiretroviral Agents in HIV-Infected Adults and Adolescents. Supplement: Safety and Toxicity of Individual Antiretroviral Agents in Pregnancy.* Rockville, MD: 2002. Available at: www.aidsinfo.nih.gov/guidelines. Accessed June 3, 2003

57. Lorenzi P, Spicher VM, Laubereau B, et al. Antiretroviral therapies in pregnancy: maternal, fetal and neonatal effects. Swiss HIV Cohort Study, the Swiss Collaborative HIV and Pregnancy Study, and the Swiss Neonatal HIV Study. *AIDS.* 1998;12:F241–F247

58. Tuomala RE, Shapiro DE, Mofenson LM, et al. Antiretroviral therapy during pregnancy and the risk of an adverse outcome. *N Engl J Med.* 2002;346:1863–1870

59. European Collaborative Study. Exposure to antiretroviral therapy in utero or early life: the health of uninfected children born to HIV-infected women. *J Acquir Immune Defic Syndr.* 2003;32:380–387

60. Alimenti A, Burdge DR, Ogilvie GS, Money DM, Forbes JC. Lactic acidemia in human immunodeficiency virus-uninfected infants exposed to perinatal antiretroviral therapy. *Pediatr Infect Dis J.* 2003;22:782–789

61. Giaquinto C, De Romeo A, Giacomet V, et al. Lactic acid levels in children perinatally treated with antiretroviral agents to prevent HIV transmission. *AIDS.* 2001;15:1074–1075

62. Blanche S, Tardieu M, Rustin P, et al. Persistent mitochondrial dysfunction and perinatal exposure to antiretroviral nucleoside analogues. *Lancet.* 1999;354:1084–1089

63. Barret B, Tardieu M, Rustin P, et al. Persistent mitochondrial dysfunction in HIV-1–exposed but uninfected infants: clinical screening in a large prospective cohort. *AIDS.* 2003;17:1769–1785

64. The Perinatal Safety Review Working Group. Nucleoside exposure in the children of disease in children who died before 5 years of age in five United States cohorts. *J Acquir Immune Defic Syndr.* 2000;25:261–268

65. Landreau-Mascaro A, Barret B, Mayaux MJ, Tardieu M, Blanche S. Risk of early febrile seizures with perinatal exposure to nucleoside analogues. French Perinatal Cohort Study Group. *Lancet.* 2002;359:583–584

66. Garcia PM, Beckerman K, Watts H, et al. Assessing the teratogenic potential of antiretroviral drugs: data from the Antiretroviral Pregnancy Registry [abstract I-1325]. Presented at: 41st Conference on Antimicrobial Agents and Chemotherapy; December 16–19, 2001; Chicago, IL

67. Antiretroviral Pregnancy Registry Steering Committee. *Antiretroviral Pregnancy Registry International Interim Report for 1 January 1989 through 31 July 2002.* Wilmington, NC: Registry Project Office; 2002

68. De Santis M, Carducci B, De Santis L, Cavaliere AF, Straface G. Periconceptional exposure to efavirenz and neural tube defects. *Arch Intern Med.* 2002;162:355

69. Fundaro C, Genovese O, Rendeli C, Tamburrini E, Salvaggio E. Myelomeningocele in a child with intrauterine exposure to efavirenz. *AIDS.* 2002;16:299–300

70. Wilson JG, Scott WJ, Ritter EJ, Fradkin R. Comparative distribution and embryotoxicity of hydroxyurea in pregnant rats and rhesus monkeys. *Teratology.* 1975;11:169–178

71. Khera KS. A teratogenicity study on hydroxyurea and diphenylhydantoin in cats. *Teratology.* 1979;20:447–452

72. Pursley TJ, Blomquist IK, Abraham J, Andersen HF, Bartley JA. Fluconazole-induced congenital anomalies in three infants. *Clin Infect Dis.* 1996;22:336–340

73. Jick SS. Pregnancy outcomes after maternal exposure to fluconazole. *Pharmacotherapy.* 1999;19:221–222

74. Mastroiacovo P, Mazzone T, Botto LD, et al. Prospective assessment of pregnancy outcomes after first-trimester exposure to fluconazole. *Am J Obstet Gynecol.* 1996;175:1645–1650

75. Johns DR. Seminars in medicine of the Beth Israel Hospital, Boston. Mitochondrial DNA and disease. *N Engl J Med.* 1995;333:638–644

76. Wallace DC. Mitochondrial diseases in man and mouse. *Science.* 1999;283:1482–1488

77. American Academy of Pediatrics, Committee on Pediatric AIDS. Identification and care of HIV-exposed and HIV-infected infants, children, and adolescents in foster care. *Pediatrics.* 2000;106:149–153

78. American Academy of Pediatrics, Committee on Pediatric AIDS and Committee on Infectious Diseases. Issues related to human immunodeficiency virus transmission in schools, child care, medical settings, the home, and community. *Pediatrics.* 1999;104:318–324

79. American Academy of Pediatrics, Committee on Pediatric AIDS. Planning for children whose parents are dying of HIV/AIDS. *Pediatrics.* 1999;103:509–511

All clinical reports from the American Academy of Pediatrics automatically expire 5 years after publication unless reaffirmed, revised, or retired at or before that time.

Fathers and Pediatricians: Enhancing Men's Roles in the Care and Development of Their Children

- *Clinical Report*

AMERICAN ACADEMY OF PEDIATRICS

CLINICAL REPORT
Guidance for the Clinician in Rendering Pediatric Care

William L. Coleman, MD, Craig Garfield, MD, and the Committee on Psychosocial Aspects of
Child and Family Health

Fathers and Pediatricians: Enhancing Men's Roles in the Care and Development of Their Children

ABSTRACT. Research substantiates that fathers' interactions with their children can exert a positive influence on their children's development. This report suggests ways pediatricians can enhance fathers' caregiving involvement by offering specific, culturally sensitive advice and how pediatricians might change their office practices to support and increase fathers' active involvement in their children's care and development. *Pediatrics* 2004;113:1406–1411; *father's roles, families, child care, pediatrician's roles.*

O ver the last 30 years, fathers' roles in caring for their children have been expanded by rapid and profound socioeconomic changes and by society's evolving perceptions and expectations of fathers' roles. "Father" in the United States means more than "wage earner" or "provider" and now can include stay-at-home dad, caregiver of child, and sharer of child care responsibilities. It even may include a grandfather caring for his grandchild. There is increasing recognition of the benefit to the child of the father's role in providing love and support to the mother or, when the spouse is not the biological mother, the partner. Recent increases in immigration and growing cultural diversity are 2 more sources of change in the roles, expectations, and involvement of fathers. A father may be a biological, foster, or adoptive father; he may be a stepfather, grandfather, adolescent father, father figure, or coparent father in a gay relationship; and he may be custodial or noncustodial, resident or nonresident, near or far. For purposes of this report, father is defined broadly as the male identified as most involved in caregiving and committed to the well-being of the child regardless of living situation or biological relation.

In response to changing expectations, diversity, and changing demographics (ie, more fathers assuming increased child care responsibilities), pediatricians need to broaden their understanding of fathers' roles and fathers' own expectations and appropriately modify their clinical style and office practices to accommodate and support fathers' expanding roles.

A substantial proportion of children in America (ie, 30% of white children, 42% of Hispanic children, and 69% of black children) are born to unwed mothers.[1] In these cases, pediatricians especially need to remind mothers of fathers' unique influence on a child's development, regardless of whether the parents are married, and encourage mothers to include fathers in the next visit(s) and in the care of the child. In addition to the common caregiving tasks, each father makes different and unique contributions to the child-father relationship and to family functioning. Validating, nurturing, and capitalizing on the father's contributions to the child's well-being and to the parents' relationship are major goals for those involved in caring for children.

Despite new expectations, related responsibilities, and evidence-based knowledge (scientific studies) regarding fatherhood, many men still enter fatherhood with little idea of their new role and how it will affect their own lives. They may be unprepared for the challenges of fatherhood yet excited to take up the task. Some may lack role models or previous experience with caregiving responsibilities; others may fail to realize the importance of their involvement to their children and families. Consequently, fathers may or may not be motivated to learn. With appropriate encouragement and specific supports, however, many fathers may become avid, successful learners and providers. Pediatricians are perceived as ideal teachers, role models, moral authorities, and supporters of families in this stage of the family life cycle at which men become fathers.

Pediatricians are necessarily concerned with both the child's and family's well-being, knowing full well that families are the single greatest and most enduring influence on children. They are uniquely positioned to enhance the father's involvement, inform the family about the father's special influence on his children's development, and encourage the father to support the other parent. In so doing, pediatricians enhance and support the multiple roles of fathers in their child's development, the father-child relationship, and healthy family functioning and well-being.

GOALS

The goals of this clinical report are to:
1. Describe the socioeconomic forces that have changed society's expectations of fathers' roles;

2. Explain how fathers' interactions with their children uniquely influence their children's development; and

3. Offer pediatricians specific advice on:
   • How to help fathers increase their caregiving and involvement;
   • How to help fathers and mothers support each other's roles as parents; and
   • How to change their clinical styles and office practices to promote, support, and increase fathers' active involvement in their children's care and development.

THE INCREASING PRESENCE OF FATHERS IN THE LIVES OF CHILDREN: SOCIOECONOMIC FORCES

Pediatricians see more fathers today than they have in the past as more fathers in 2-parent families or in shared-custody arrangements are spending more time with their children and beginning to attend more office visits. This national trend has the potential to strengthen the father-child relationship, stimulate the child's development, ease the mother's or partner's workload, and strengthen the overall family functioning. Several factors contribute to this trend.

• The number of father-only households (no wife or partner in the home) increased almost 25% from 1995 to 1998, to 2.1 million households.[2] The 2000 US Census revealed father-only households increased to 4.3 million, or 4.2% of US households. In Illinois alone, the number of children living in father-only households increased by 109%, from 47 000 in 1985 to 98 000 in 1995.[3] Although the total number is small, the rate of change is significant. Additionally, father-only households seem to be headed by fathers who are highly involved in their children's lives at home and school.[4]

• Economic shifts over the past 30 years increasingly place women in the workplace, often in higher paying jobs than their male partners. Subsequently, many men spend more time at home taking care of their children. For example, most mothers prefer the father to be the child care provider if the mother cannot provide the care.[5] Additionally, married men are likely to be the primary caregivers of their children during the mother's working hours if the family is poor, if the father is unemployed or working part-time, or if the children are younger.[6]

• The average amount of time fathers in 2-parent families spend with their children, directly engaged or accessible, has increased in the last decade to 2.5 hours per weekday and 6.3 hours per weekend.[7]

• In divorced families, a plan for shared-custody arrangements developed by both parents during divorce proceedings increases opportunities for the father to be more involved in his children's care.

• Changing technology in the marketplace, telecommuting from home, and making use of flexible work hours provides more opportunities for fathers to spend more time with their children and families.

• The media and popular culture reflect and positively reinforce fathers' increased involvement in the care and development of their children. Father birthing classes have sprung up in hospitals across the country. General parent magazines, special magazines, Web sites, and newspapers (both paper and Web based) increasingly are targeted at fathers and champion men who have taken to the "daddy track." Many daily and Sunday newspapers feature comic strips based on fathers' involvement and good-hearted foibles at home. Several celebrities, Paul Reiser, Bill Cosby, and Al Roker included, have written books describing their experiences.[8–10] This media emphasis, coupled with cultural image changes and products such as infant-joggers and snugglies that encourage men's participation, reflect the growing trend of fathers caring for and interacting with their children. Meanwhile, scholarly works continue focusing attention on the role and importance of fathers in their children's social and emotional well-being.[11–19]

FATHERS' INFLUENCE ON THEIR CHILDREN'S DEVELOPMENT: SCIENTIFIC EVIDENCE

Fathers' interactions exert a powerful influence on every domain of their children's functioning beginning at infancy. Recent research substantiates how fathers impact their children's social, emotional, and cognitive development. For example, in the first few days of life, many newborn infants turn their heads preferentially to their father's voices versus the voice of a stranger.[20] Premature infants who experience increased visits from their fathers have improved weight gain during hospitalization and score higher during the first 18 months of life on adaptive-behavior and social-development tests, even after controlling for levels of prematurity and hospital stay.[21] In a study of premature black infants, the father's involvement enhanced the child's cognitive and behavioral outcomes.[22]

Mothers and fathers influence their children in similar ways with regard to development of morality, competence in social interactions, academic achievement, and mental health. However, father involvement is of a different nature than mother involvement. In terms of relative frequency, fathers devote more time to playing with their children than do mothers. When children are young (0-4 years old), fathers tend to engage in more tactile physical and stimulating activities. As children enter middle childhood (the school-aged years), fathers engage in more recreational activities such as walks and outings as well as private talks. Fathers also have a strong influence on their children's gender role development and are important role models for both girls and boys.[23,24]

The long-term effects of fathers' direct involvement in the care of their children manifest through childhood and adolescence. For children with a father figure, those who described greater father support had a stronger sense of social competence and fewer depressive symptoms.[25] Although time spent with children is usually less for fathers compared with mothers, studies show that shared activities between fathers and their children are independently associated with improved academic performance.[7,26] Adolescents who perceive their fathers as encouraging and involved in their lives have higher college entrance examination scores, reach higher economic and educational attainment, show less delinquent behavior, and possess greater psychologic well-being.[27,28]

THE FATHER'S ROLE IN FAMILY FUNCTIONING

Fathers positively influence the behavior and relationships of the mother or other parent, siblings, and other family members. For example, fathers play an important role in the initiation, support, continuation, and ultimate ongoing success of breastfeeding.[29–35] Father involvement also stabilizes and promotes healthy family functioning. Fathers, as much as mothers, can and often do provide affection, nurturing, and comfort to their children. As teachers, disciplinarians, and role models, fathers assume some of the responsibility for teaching their children what they need to know for life-survival skills and for school learning. These lessons may come in the form of teaching about letters, numbers, and shapes; helping the school-aged child with homework; coaching the child in an athletic skill or hobby; teaching manners and social skills; and encouraging a healthy lifestyle. Rituals that involve special time with fathers, such as homework, play, sports activities, bathing routines, bedtime rituals, household chores, shopping, or reading together, also help strengthen the father-child bond. Such involvement may even prove to be protective. In families in which even mild levels of maternal depression exist, for example, a nurturing father-child relationship counteracts behavioral and interactional problems often associated with maternal depression.[36–38]

THE FATHER'S ROLE IN SUPPORTING THE OTHER PARENT IN THEIR RELATIONSHIP

The emotional support a father provides to the other parent helps in practical ways with the care of children. Parents who feel loved, appreciated, and supported as spouses or partners tend to parent with more demonstrations of love, approval, and support and communicate better with their children. Maintaining and nourishing the spousal or partner relationship helps improve the marriage and parenthood (eg, remembering special occasions, bestowing compliments, demonstrating affection, and taking time together as partners).[39–43] When parents are separated or unmarried, a positive, supportive relationship with the mother or other parent is an important predictor of children's successful adjustment to their family structure.

In general, mothers' support and encouragement of fathers is a key predictor of fathers' involvement with their children.[44,45] Mothers may actively oppose or quietly resist involvement or sharing household responsibilities for reasons of efficiency (things are done faster if she does it), quality (she does a better job), sympathy (not wanting to bother the father), admiration (he has done enough), anger (a by-product or after-effect of marital estrangement), or cultural beliefs in gender roles.[45] Thus, in some cases, fathers may desire more involvement, but mothers themselves may discourage greater paternal involvement. Mothers who feel supported themselves as mothers are more likely to support and encourage the father's involvement in the care of the child.

In families experiencing divorce, the relationships between father, mother, and children can become especially strained.[46] Divorce affects children's relationships with their parents and their sense of trust, acceptance, and support, creating feelings of loss and sadness.[47] The quality of the parents' pre- and post-divorce relationship plays a significant role in the child's emotional and social response and the father's involvement with his children. The quality of a father's parenting has been found to be inversely related to sibling conflict, adolescent depression, delinquent behavior, and affiliation with deviant peers.[48] Yet, there is a negative relationship between divorce and the quality of father's parenting; in other words, divorce can lead to less quality parenting by fathers, compounding the aforementioned problems.

There are situations, however, in which divorce can improve paternal involvement. In these situations, positive changes in the father-child bond are a result of increased opportunities to relate to the child in a conflict-free atmosphere.[49] Fathers may find themselves in the role of primary caregiver and, for the first time, engaging the health care system. Keeping both parents apprised of the child's health and involved in the child's life as well as keeping track of the emerging important adult figures in the child's life becomes part of the pediatrician's responsibilities.

THE PEDIATRICIAN'S ROLE

Many fathers want to be more involved in caring for their children. Pediatricians can help fathers learn to play a variety of roles in the family. Expanding on more than the stereotypical roles of the father as financial supporter and offering glimpses into the possibility and benefit of more roles for fathers suggests to the family that these roles are not in competition with those of mothers. In fact, these fathers' roles enhance and support mothers' roles. Furthermore, a father's additional roles serve to support the overall needs of the family and make parenthood more gratifying for both parents. Professionals caring for children need to be aware of these roles and of the greater social and cultural backdrops against which these roles may be played. A father from one family may be expected culturally to meet with the pediatrician and direct most conversations, and another father from a different culture may be expected to meet his child's pediatrician rarely or never. Given these family, social, and cultural variants, it is still largely true that pediatricians seldom get to know fathers as well as they do mothers.

Pediatricians usually see mothers and children in the office and may not be accustomed to or even comfortable with seeing fathers. Pediatricians can easily adapt their practices to accommodate fathers. The following advice will guide pediatricians in encouraging a father's involvement and participation in office visits by letting him know he is welcome in the office and the health care system more generally. Pediatricians are encouraged to make special efforts to engage fathers who are separated from the family.

Pediatricians who understand parental expectations and the family's cultural traditions and values and who respectfully explore and encourage the father-child relationship in pediatric visits are more likely to form a good rapport with fathers and make them feel welcome, which in turn conveys to fathers that they are important to their child's development and encourages them to be more active in the care and activities of their children. Encouragement from the child's advocate, the pediatrician, is a powerful message to fathers about their expanded and critical roles in their children's lives.

In this report we have explained some of the socioeconomic factors that place fathers in a changing, often more prominent position in the care and development of their children and in their support of the spousal or partner relationship. Compelling recent evidence reveals that fathers' involvement with their children will continue to increase as more women enter the workforce and men seek greater involvement at home. Pediatricians are uniquely qualified and placed to help fathers by encouragement, by practical advice, and by educating men, women, and their families about the benefits of positive father involvement for 1) the care and development of their children, 2) the other parent's well-being, and 3) healthy family functioning.

ADVICE FOR PEDIATRICIANS

Make Your Practice More Father-Friendly

1. Offer flexible and extended office hours (eg, late afternoons, evenings, weekends, and early mornings) to accommodate parents and encourage their attendance.

2. Actively encourage fathers to come in for at least one of the initial well-infant or acute-illness visits in the infant's first 2 months of life and more if possible.

3. Welcome fathers and express appreciation for their attendance. Speak directly to the father as well as the mother or partner and solicit his opinions. Encourage office staff and nurses to include fathers in the office-visit appointment.

4. Introduce yourself to the father and the mother or other parent. Politely explore the father's relationship to the other parent (eg, married, living together), his cultural traditions, and his own personal beliefs about his role in caring for the child. Assess differences in parenting beliefs and help them negotiate if necessary.

5. Learn something about the father's role and beliefs (eg, how he was parented, expectations and hopes for his children, his previous marriages, other children and how he parented them). Keep the discussions focused on the parenting context and the father's roles and beliefs; minimize small talk.

6. Actively engage the father in the office. For example, tell the father: "As your child's pediatrician, I want to know you and work with you and your child's [mother or other parent] to offer the best care for your child."

7. If the father is not involved in the dialogue, address him directly, asking him if he has specific questions or concerns. Solicit his opinions about child rearing, sharing responsibilities, and his perceived roles. Ask each parent about his or her transition to parenthood. For example, ask: "How is parenting going for each of you?"

8. Ask the parents how they support each other as parents, spouses or partners, and individuals.

9. Recognize that mothers and fathers may not always agree on how best to raise a child. For example, parents may disagree on the approach to discipline or issues of firearm safety. Pediatricians can serve as a mediator in such discussions, meeting with both parents or caregivers together to discuss these and other behavior-management issues and should avoid (whenever possible) siding with one parent or the other on important parenting issues.

10. Participate in educational opportunities (eg, courses, continuing medical education activities, medical literature) devoted to fathers' role issues, parental depression, and family functioning to enhance training and education in this area.

Understand the Family

1. Explore the family composition, cultural beliefs, overall mental and physical health, and delegation and discussions of child care tasks within the family. If parents are not both in the household, discuss living and custody arrangements as well.

2. In addition to discussing the feelings of joy and fulfillment having a child can bring, also be prepared to discuss issues of the allocation of child and sibling care and the common experiences that siblings and parents encounter with conflict, jealousy, and normal disappointments in connection with the arrival of a new infant.

3. Be sensitive to and informed about diverse cultural and ethnic values and customs, especially "traditional" father roles. Pediatricians can determine the extent of the father's responsibilities and presence at home by respectfully exploring these issues with parents.

4. Use a "parenting history" to help parents understand their behaviors by understanding how they themselves were parented. Parents often adopt a parenting style to compensate for their own childhood deficiencies or to emulate childhood experiences depending on their own parenting experiences.

5. Discuss how the couple is adapting to parenthood (with each child). Asking questions such as "How is your relationship (or the family) adjusting to the new infant?" or "How is it living with a teenager?" opens the door to reflection and discussion and can remind parents of the importance of their own partner relationship and the need to nurture and maintain it. Encourage parents to continue to dedicate time for adult activities without children.

Empower, Engage, and Inform Fathers of the Importance of Their Involvement

1. Remind the family that fathers are not only workers or breadwinners and mothers or partners are not only nurturers or primary providers of child care. They share these roles, complementing one another, often to the benefit of the child.
2. As early as in the delivery room or nursery and if culturally appropriate, fathers can be given responsibilities for caring for and making decisions regarding the child.
3. Encourage fathers to assume some roles in the care of the child, and encourage the mother to let the father be involved and learn from his own mistakes. Early time alone with the child helps a father gain confidence and develop his own style of interaction and provides a mother or other parent with much-needed time alone.
4. Determine how comfortable the father is with his parenting skills and whether he has concerns.
5. Explore with the father ways to decrease maternal stress. This might include his helping with meals or household chores, the involvement of other family members with household tasks, or the hiring of household help.
6. Identify institutions and policies that facilitate fathers' involvement and work-family balance. Encourage child care centers, support groups, and schools to involve and include fathers. Promote the use of policies such as the Family Medical Leave Act (codified at 29 CFR §825 [1993]) and flexible work schedules as ways to balance employment and family responsibilities.

Reinforce the Father's Support of the Mother or Partner

1. Inform the family about the normal elation, fatigue, and challenges of being a father. Discuss openly the usual interruptions in sleep for the whole family, the decreases in energy, the alterations in time together as a couple and individual free time, and the changes in intimacy and the sexual relationship. This may be the first time some fathers will have discussed these issues openly.
2. Look for signs of maternal depression (postpartum depression in the newborn period) and be able to offer resources to help.
3. Explore marital stress and inquire about the marriage or partner relationship. For example, you may ask: "How has the birth of this infant affected your relationship?"; "To whom do you turn for advice and support?"; and/or "Would you like a referral to talk to someone else who can help (individual or couples therapy and/or medication)?"
4. Educate fathers about the practicalities of breastfeeding and how to support mothers' nursing.
5. Encourage fathers to provide or protect time for mothers to have time to be alone, exercise, meet friends, or simply relax.

COMMITTEE ON PSYCHOSOCIAL ASPECTS OF CHILD AND FAMILY HEALTH, 2001–2002
Joseph F. Hagan, Jr, MD, Chairperson

William L. Coleman, MD
Jane Meschan Foy, MD
Edward Goldson, MD
Barbara J. Howard, MD
Ana Navarro, MD
Thomas J. Sullivan, MD
J. Lane Tanner, MD

INVITED CONTRIBUTOR
Craig F. Garfield, MD

LIAISONS
F. Daniel Armstrong, PhD
  Society of Pediatric Psychology
Peggy Gilbertson, RN, MPH, CPNP
  National Association of Pediatric Nurse Practitioners
Sally E. A. Longstaffe, MD
  Canadian Paediatric Society
Frances J. Wren, MD
  American Academy of Child and Adolescent Psychiatry

CONSULTANTS
George J. Cohen, MD
  National Consortium for Child and Adolescent Mental Health Services

STAFF
Karen Smith

REFERENCES

1. Ventura SJ, Bachrach CA. Nonmartial childbearing in the United States, 1940-99. Natl Vital Stat Rep. 2000,48:1–40. Available at: www.cdc.gov/nchs/data/nvsr/nvsr48/nvs48_16.pdf. Accessed January 30, 2003
2. Cabrera NJ, Tamis-LeMonda CS, Bradley RH, Hofferth S, Lamb ME. Fatherhood in the twenty-first century. Child Dev. 2000,71:127–136
3. Chapin Hall Center for Children. State of the Child in Illinois. Chicago, IL: Chapin Hall Center for Children; 2000
4. Winquist Nord C, West J. Fathers' and Mothers' Involvement in Their Children's Schools by Family Type and Resident Status. Washington, DC: US Department of Education, Office of Educational Research and Improvement; 2001
5. Riley LA, Glass JL. You can't always get what you want—infant care preferences and use among employed mothers. J Marriage Fam. 2002,64:2–15
6. Casper LM, O'Connell M. Work, income, the economy, and married fathers as childcare providers. Demography. 1998,35:243–250
7. Yeung WJ, Sanderberg JF, Davis-Kean PE, Hofferth SL. Children's time with fathers in intact families. J Marriage Fam. 2001,63:136–154
8. Reiser P. Babyhood. New York, NY: Rob Weisbach Books; 1997
9. Cosby B. Fatherhood. Garden City, NY: Doubleday; 1986
10. Roker A. Don't Make Me Stop this Car: Adventures in Fatherhood. New York, NY: Scribner; 2000
11. Blankenhorn D. Fatherless America: Confronting Our Most Urgent Social Problem. New York, NY: Basic Books; 1995
12. Jacobs EH. Fathering the ADHD Child: A Book for Fathers, Mothers, and Professionals. Northvale, NJ: J. Aronson; 1998
13. Griswold RL. Fatherhood in America: A History. New York, NY: Basic Books; 1993
14. Osherson S. Finding Our Fathers: How a Man's Life Is Shaped by His Relationship With His Father. Chicago, IL: Contemporary Books; 2001
15. Popenoe D. Life Without Father: Compelling New Evidence That Fatherhood and Marriage Are Indispensable for the Good of Children and Society. New York, NY: Martin Kessler Books; 1996
16. Parke RD. Fatherhood. Cambridge, MA: Harvard University Press; 1996
17. Osterman R, Spurrell C, Chubert CT. Father and Child: Practical Advice for Today's Dad. Allentown, PA: Longmeadow Press; 1991
18. Newberger EH. The Men They Will Become: The Nature and Nurture of Male Character. Cambridge, MA: Perseus Publishing; 2000
19. Kindlon DJ, Thompson M. Raising Cain: Protecting the Emotional Life of Boys. New York, NY: Ballantine Books; 1999
20. Brazelton TB. Touchpoints: Your Child's Emotional and Behavioral Development. Reading, MA: Addison-Wesley; 1992

21. Levy-Shiff R, Hoffman MA, Mogilner S, Levinger S, Mogilner MB. Fathers' hospital visits to their preterm infants as a predictor of father-infant relationship and infant development. *Pediatrics*. 1990,86:289–293

22. Yogman MW, Kindlon D, Earls F. Father involvement and cognitive/behavioral outcomes of preterm infants. *J Am Acad Child Adolesc Psychiatry*. 1995,34:58–66

23. Williams E, Radin N. Effects of father participation in child rearing: twenty-year follow up. *Am J Orthopsychiatry*. 1999,69:328–336

24. Lamb M, ed. *The Role of the Father in Child Development*. New York, NY: Wiley; 1997

25. Dubowitz H, Black MM, Cox CE, et al. Father involvement and children's functioning at age 6 years: a multisite study. *Child Maltreat*. 2001,6:300–309

26. Cooksey EC, Fondell MM. Spending time with his kids: effects of family structure on fathers and children's lives. *J Marriage Fam*. 1996,58:693–707

27. Furr LA. Fathers' characteristics and their children's scores on college entrance exams: a comparison of intact and divorced families. *Adolescence*. 1998,33:533–542

28. Harris KM, Furstenberg FF Jr, Marmer JK. Paternal involvement with adolescents in intact families: the influence of fathers over the life course. *Demography*. 1998,35:201–216

29. Littman H, Medendorp SV, Goldfarb J. The decision to breastfeed. The importance of father's approval. *Clin Pediatr (Phila)*. 1994,33:214–219

30. Jordan PL, Wall VR. Breastfeeding and fathers: illuminating the darker side. *Birth*. 1990,17:210–213

31. Bar-Yam NB, Darby L. Fathers and breastfeeding: a review of the literature. *J Hum Lact*. 1997,13:45–50

32. Sharma M, Petosa R. Impact of expectant fathers in breast-feeding decisions. *J Am Diet Assoc*. 1997,97:1311–1313

33. Freed GL, Fraley JK. Effect of expectant mothers' feeding plan on prediction of fathers' attitudes regarding breast-feeding. *Am J Perinatol*. 1993,10:300–303

34. Freed GL, Fraley JK, Schanler RJ. Attitudes of expectant fathers regarding breast-feeding. *Pediatrics*. 1992,90:224–227

35. Freed GL, Fraley JK, Schanler RJ. Accuracy of expectant mothers' predictions of fathers' attitudes regarding breast-feeding. *J Fam Pract*. 1993,37:148–152

36. Tannenbaum L, Forehand R. Maternal depressive mood: the role of the father in preventing adolescent problem behaviors. *Behav Res Ther*. 1994,32:321–325

37. Murray L. The impact of postnatal depression on infant development. *J Child Psychol Psychiatry*. 1992,33:543–561

38. Hart S, Field T, del Valle C, Pelaez-Nogueras M. Depressed mothers' interactions with their one year old infants. *Infant Behav Dev*. 1998,21:519–525

39. Gottman JM, deClaire J. *The Heart of Parenting: How to Raise an Emotionally Intelligent Child*. New York, NY: Simon & Schuster; 1997

40. Gottman JM, Silver N. *The Seven Principles for Making Marriage Work*. New York, NY: Crown Publishers; 1999

41. Gottman JM, de Claire J. *The Relationship Cure: A Five-Step Guide for Building Better Connections With Family, Friends, and Lovers*. New York, NY: Crown Publishers; 2001

42. Gottman JM, Silver N. *Why Marriages Succeed or Fail: What You Can Learn From the Breakthrough Research to Make Your Marriage Last*. New York, NY: Simon & Schuster; 1994

43. Wallerstein JS, Blakeslee S. *The Good Marriage: How and Why Love Lasts*. Boston, MA: Houghton Mifflin; 1995

44. De Luccie MF. Mothers: influential agents in father-child relations. *Genet Soc Gen Psychol Monogr*. 1996,122:285–307

45. Coleman WL. *Family-Focused Behavioral Pediatrics*. Philadelphia, PA: Lippincott Williams and Wilkins; 2001

46. American Academy of Pediatrics, Committee on Psychosocial Aspects of Child and Family Health. The pediatrician's role in helping children and families deal with separation and divorce. *Pediatrics*. 1994,94:119–121

47. Arditti JA, Prouty AM. Change, disengagement, and renewal: relationship dynamics between young adults and their fathers after divorce. *J Marital Fam Ther*. 1999,25:61–81

48. Sims RL. *Understanding Differences Between Divorced and Intact Families: Stress, Interaction, and Child Outcome*. Thousand Oaks, CA: Sage Publications; 1996

49. Friedman HJ. The father's parenting experience in divorce. *Am J Psychiatry*. 1980,137:1177–1182

All clinical reports from the American Academy of Pediatrics automatically expire 5 years after publication unless reaffirmed, revised, or retired at or before that time.

SUGGESTED WEB SITE RESOURCES ON FATHERING

US Dept of Health and Human Services Fatherhood Initiative. Available at: http://fatherhood.hhs.gov/index.shtml

Fathering Magazine. Available at: www.fathermag.com

National Fatherhood Initiative. Available at: www.fatherhood.org

Center for Successful Fathering. Available at: www.fathering.org

National Center for Fathering. Available at: www.fathers.com

Slowlane.com: The Online Resource for Stay at Home Dads. Available at: www.slowlane.com

Bootcamp for New Dads. Available at: www.newdads.com

Dads Can. Available at: www.dadscan.org

National Center on Fathers and Families. Available at: www.ncoff.gse.upenn.edu

Illinois Fatherhood Initiative. Available at: www.4fathers.org

Guidelines and Levels of Care for Pediatric Intensive Care Units

- *Clinical Report*

AMERICAN ACADEMY OF PEDIATRICS

SOCIETY OF CRITICAL CARE MEDICINE

CLINICAL REPORT
Guidance for the Clinician in Rendering Pediatric Care

David I. Rosenberg, MD; M. Michele Moss, MD; and the Section on Critical Care and Committee on Hospital Care

Guidelines and Levels of Care for Pediatric Intensive Care Units

ABSTRACT. The practice of pediatric critical care medicine has matured dramatically during the past decade. These guidelines are presented to update the existing guidelines published in 1993. Pediatric critical care services are provided in level I and level II units. Within these guidelines, the scope of pediatric critical care services is discussed, including organizational and administrative structure, hospital facilities and services, personnel, drugs and equipment, quality monitoring, and training and continuing education. *Pediatrics* 2004;114: 1114–1125; *pediatric intensive care unit, PICU, critical care services.*

ABBREVIATIONS. PICU, pediatric intensive care unit, EMS, emergency medical services, PALS, pediatric advanced life support.

INTRODUCTION

The practice of pediatric critical care has matured dramatically throughout the past 3 decades. Knowledge of the pathophysiology of life-threatening processes and the technologic capacity to monitor and treat pediatric patients suffering from them has advanced rapidly during this period. Along with the scientific and technical advances has come the evolution of the pediatric intensive care unit (PICU), in which special needs of critically ill or injured children and their families can be met by pediatric specialists. All critically ill infants and children cared for in hospitals, regardless of the physical setting, are entitled to receive the same quality of care.

In 1985, the American Board of Pediatrics recognized the subspecialty of pediatric critical care medicine and set criteria for subspecialty certification. The American Boards of Medicine, Surgery, and Anesthesiology gave similar recognition to the subspecialty. In 1990, the Residency Review Committee of the Accreditation Council for Graduate Medical Education completed its first accreditation of pediatric critical care medicine training programs. In 1986, the

American Association of Critical Care Nurses developed a certification program for pediatric critical care, and in 1999, a certification program for clinical nurse specialists in pediatric critical care was initiated.

In view of recent developments, the Pediatric Section of the Society of Critical Care Medicine and the Section on Critical Care Medicine and Committee on Hospital Care of the American Academy of Pediatrics believe that the original guidelines for levels of PICU care from 1993[1] should be updated. This report represents the consensus of the 3 aforementioned groups and presents those elements of hospital care that are necessary to provide high-quality pediatric critical care. The concept of level I and level II PICUs as established in the guidelines set forth in 1993 will be continued in this report. Individual states may have PICU guidelines, and it is not the intent of this report to supersede already established state rules, regulations, or guidelines; however, these guidelines represent the consensus report of critical care experts.

Pediatric critical care is ideally provided by a PICU that meets level I specifications. The level I PICU must provide multidisciplinary definitive care for a wide range of complex, progressive, and rapidly changing medical, surgical, and traumatic disorders occurring in pediatric patients of all ages, excluding premature newborns. Most, but not all, level I PICUs should be located in major medical centers or within children's hospitals. It is also recognized that in the appropriate clinical setting and as a result of many forces including but not limited to the presence of managed care, the insufficient supply of trained pediatric intensivists, and geographic and transport limitations, level II PICUs may be an appropriate alternative to the transfer of all critically ill children to a level I PICU.

The level I PICU should provide care to the most severely ill patient population. Specifications for level I PICUs are discussed in detail in the text and are summarized in Table 1. Level I PICUs will vary in size, personnel, physical characteristics, and equipment, and they may differ in the types of specialized care that are provided (eg, transplantation or cardiac surgery). Physicians and specialized services

The guidance in this report does not indicate an exclusive course of treatment or serve as a standard of medical care. Variations, taking into account individual circumstances, may be appropriate.

doi:10.1542/peds.2004-1599

PEDIATRICS (ISSN 0031 4005). Copyright © 2004 by the American Academy of Pediatrics.

TABLE 1.　　Minimum Guidelines and Levels of Care for PICUs

	Level I	Level II
I. Organization and administrative structure		
A. Category I facility	E	E
B. Organization		
1. PICU committee	E	E
2. Distinct administrative unit	E	E
3. Delineation of physician and nonphysician privilege	E	E
C. Policies		
1. Admission and discharge	E	E
2. Patient monitoring	E	E
3. Safety	E	E
4. Nosocomial infection	E	E
5. Patient isolation	E	E
6. Family-centered care	E	E
7. Traffic control	E	E
8. Equipment maintenance	E	E
9. Essential equipment breakdown	E	E
10. System of record keeping	E	E
11. Periodic review		
a. Morbidity and mortality	E	E
b. Quality of care	E	E
c. Safety	E	E
d. Critical care consultation	E	E
e. Long-term outcomes	D	D
f. Supportive care	D	D
D. Physical facility—external		
1. Distinct, separate unit	E	D
2. Distinct unit (not necessarily physically separate) with auditory and visual separation	E	E
3. Controlled access (no through-traffic)	E	E
4. Located near:		
a. Elevators	E	D
b. Operating room	D	D
c. Emergency room	D	D
d. Recovery room	D	D
e. Physician on-call room	E	D
f. Nurse manager's office	D	D
g. Medical director's office	D	D
h. Waiting room	E	D
5. Separate rooms available		
a. Family counseling room	E	D
b. Conference room	D	D
c. Staff lounge	D	D
d. Staff locker room	D	D
e. Storage lockers for patients' personal effects (may be internal)	E	E
f. Family sleep area and shower	E	D
E. Physical facility—internal		
1. Patient isolation capacity	E	E
2. Patient privacy provision	E	E
3. Satellite pharmacy	D	O
4. Medication station with drug refrigerator and locked narcotics cabinet	E	E
5. Emergency equipment storage	E	E
6. Clean utility (linen) room	E	E
7. Soiled utility (linen) room	E	E
8. Nourishment station	E	E
9. Counter and cabinet space	E	E
10. Staff toilet	E	E
11. Patient toilet	E	E
12. Hand-washing facility	E	E
13. Clocks	E	E
14. Televisions, radios, toys	E	E
15. Easy, rapid access to head of bed	E	E
16. 12 or more electrical outlets per bed	E	E
17. 2 or more oxygen outlets per bed	E	E
18. 2 or more compressed air outlets per bed	E	E
19. 2 vacuum outlets per bed	E	E
20. Computerized laboratory reporting or efficient equivalent	E	D
21. Building code or federal code conforming for:		
a. Heating, ventilation, and air conditioning	E	E
b. Fire safety	E	E
c. Electrical grounding	E	E
d. Plumbing	E	E
e. Illumination	E	E

TABLE 1. Continued

	Level I	Level II
II. Personnel		
A. Medical director		
1. Appointed by appropriate hospital authority and acknowledged in writing	E	E
2. Qualifications		
a. Board certified or actively pursuing certification in 1 of the following:		
i. Pediatric critical care medicine	E	E
• Initial board certification in pediatrics	E	E
• Codirector if director is not a pediatrician	E	D
ii. Anesthesiology with practice limited to infants and children and special qualifications in critical care medicine	E	E
iii. Pediatric surgery with added qualification in surgical critical care medicine	E	E
3. Responsibilities documented in writing	E	E
a. Acts as primary attending physician	D	D
b. Has authority to provide consultation when physician is not available	E	E
c. Assumes patient care if primary attending physician is not available	E	E
d. Participates in development, review, and implementation of PICU policies*	E	E
e. Maintenance of database and/or vital statistics*	E	E
f. Supervises quality-control and quality-assessment activities (including morbidity and mortality reviews)*	E	E
g. Supervises resuscitation techniques (including educational component)*	E	E
h. Ensures policy implementation*	E	E
i. Coordinates staff education*	E	E
j. Participates in budget preparation*	E	E
k. Coordinates research*	E	D
4. Substitute physician available to act as attending physician in medical director's absence	E	E
B. Physician staff		
1. A physician in-house 24 h per day	E	E
a. A physician at the postgraduate year 2 level or above assigned to the PICU	E	D
b. A physician at the postgraduate year 2 level or above available to the PICU (advanced practice nurse or physician assistant may be used)	E	E
c. A physician at the postgraduate year 3 level or above (in pediatrics or anesthesiology) in-house 24 h per day	E	O
2. Available in 30 min or less (24 h per day)		
a. Pediatric intensivist or equivalent	E	D
3. Available in 1 h or less		
a. Anesthesiologist	E	E
i. Pediatric anesthesiologist	E	D
b. General surgeon	E	E
c. Surgical subspecialists		
i. Pediatric surgeon	E	D
ii. Cardiovascular surgeon	E	O
• Pediatric cardiovascular surgeon	D	O
iii. Neurosurgeon	E	E
• Pediatric neurosurgeon	E	O
iv. Otolaryngologist	E	D
• Pediatric otolaryngologist	D	O
v. Orthopedic surgeon	E	D
• Pediatric orthopedic surgeon	D	O
vi. Craniofacial, oral surgeon	D	O
4. Pediatric subspecialists		
a. Intensivist	E	E
b. Cardiologist	E	D
c. Nephrologist	E	D
d. Hematologist/oncologist	D	D
e. Pulmonologist	D	D
f. Endocrinologist	D	D
g. Gastroenterologist	D	D
h. Allergist	D	D
i. Neonatologist	E	E
j. Neurologist	E	D
k. Geneticist	D	D
5. Radiologist	E	E
a. Pediatric radiologist	E	O
6. Psychiatrist or psychologist	E	D
C. Nursing staff		
1. Manager/director	E	E
a. Training and clinical experience in pediatric critical care	E	E
b. Master's degree in pediatric nursing or nursing administration	D	D
2. Nurse-to-patient ratio based on patient need	E	E
3. Nursing policies and procedures in place	E	E
4. Orientation to PICU	E	E
5. Completion of clinical and didactic critical care course	E	E
6. Address psychosocial needs of patient and family	E	E

TABLE 1. Continued

	Level I	Level II
7. Participate in continuing education	E	E
8. Completion of critical care registered nurse (pediatric) certification	D	D
9. Completion of PALS or an equivalent course	D	D
10. Nurse educator on staff (clinical nurse specialist)	E	D
a. Responsible for pediatric critical care in-service education	E	D
11. Nurse coordinator for regional continuing education	O	O
D. Respiratory therapy staff		
1. Supervisor responsible for training registered respiratory therapy staff	E	E
2. Maintenance of equipment and quality control and review	E	E
3. Respiratory therapist in-house 24 h per day assigned primarily to PICU	E	D
4. Respiratory therapist in-house 24 h per day	E	E
5. Respiratory therapists familiar with management of pediatric patients with respiratory failure	E	E
6. Respiratory therapists competent with pediatric mechanical ventilators	E	E
7. Completion of PALS or an equivalent course	D	D
E. Other team members		
1. Biomedical technician (in-hospital or available within 1 h, 24 h per day)	E	E
2. Unit clerk on staff 24 h per day with a written job description	E	D
3. Child life specialist	E	D
4. Clergy	E	E
5. Social worker	E	E
6. Nutritionist or clinical dietitian	E	E
7. Physical therapist	E	E
8. Occupational therapist	E	E
9. Pharmacist (24 h per day)	E	E
10. Pediatric clinical pharmacist	D	D
11. Radiology technician	E	E
12. Bereavement coordinator	D	D
III. Hospital facilities and services		
A. Emergency department		
1. Covered entrance	E	E
2. Separate entrance	E	D
3. Adjacent helipad	D	D
4. Staffed by physician 24 h per day	E	E
a. Trained in pediatric emergency medicine	D	D
5. Resuscitation area		
a. 2 or more areas with capacity and equipment to resuscitate medical, surgical, and trauma pediatric patients	E	D
b. 1 or more areas as described above	E	E
B. Intermediate care unit or step-down unit separate from PICU and pediatric acute care unit	D	D
C. Pediatric rehabilitation unit	D	D
D. Blood bank		
1. Comprehensive (all blood components)	E	E
2. Type and cross match within 1 h	E	E
E. Radiology services and nuclear medicine		
1. Portable radiograph	E	E
2. Fluoroscopy	E	D
3. Computed tomography scan	E	E
4. Magnetic resonance imaging	E	D
5. Ultrasound	E	E
6. Angiography	E	O
7. Nuclear scanning	E	O
8. Radiation therapy	D	O
F. Laboratory with microspecimen capability		
1. Available within 15 min		
a. Blood gases	E	E
2. Available within 1 h		
a. Complete blood cell, platelet, and differential counts	E	E
b. Urinalysis	E	E
c. Chemistry profile (electrolytes, serum urea nitrogen, glucose, calcium, and creatinine)	E	E
d. Clotting studies	E	E
e. Cerebrospinal fluid analysis	E	E
3. Available within 3 h		
a. Ammonia concentration	E	E
b. Drug screening	E	E
c. Osmolality	E	E
d. Magnesium and phosphorus concentrations	E	E
e. Toxicology screen	E	D
4. Preparation available 24 h per day		
a. Bacteriology (culture and Gram-stain)	E	E
5. Point-of-care diagnostic testing	D	D

TABLE 1. Continued

	Level I	Level II
G. Department of surgery		
1. Operating room available within 30 min, 24 h per day	E	E
2. Second operating room available within 45 min, 24 h per day	E	D
3. Capabilities		
a. Cardiopulmonary bypass	E	D
b. Bronchoscopy (pediatric)	E	D
c. Endoscopy (pediatric)	E	D
d. Radiograph in operating room	E	E
H. Cardiology department with pediatric capability		
1. Electrocardiography	E	E
2. Echocardiography		
a. Two-dimensional echocardiography with Doppler	E	E
3. Catheterization laboratory (pediatric)	D	O
I. Neurodiagnostic laboratory		
1. EEG	E	E
2. Evoked potentials	D	D
3. Transcranial Doppler flow	D	O
J. Hemodialysis	E	O
K. Peritoneal dialysis or continuous renal replacement therapy	E	O
L. Pharmacy with pediatric capability	E	E
1. Available 24 h per day for all requests	E	E
2. Located near PICU and pediatric acute care unit	D	O
3. Urgent drug-dosage form at bedside	E	E
4. Satellite pharmacy located in PICU	D	O
5. Pediatric pharmacist available for medical rounds	D	O
M. Rehabilitation department with pediatric capability		
1. Physical therapy	E	E
2. Speech therapy	E	E
3. Occupational therapy	E	E
IV. Drugs and equipment		
A. Emergency drugs	E	E
B. Portable equipment		
1. Emergency cart	E	E
2. Procedure lamp	E	E
3. Doppler ultrasonography device	E	E
4. Infusion pumps (with microinfusion capability)	E	E
5. Defibrillator and cardioverter	E	E
6. Electrocardiography machine	E	E
7. Suction machine (in addition to bedside)	E	E
8. Thermometers	E	E
9. Expanded scale electronic thermometer	E	E
10. Automated blood pressure apparatus	E	E
11. Otoscope and ophthalmoscope	E	E
12. Automatic bed scale	E	D
13. Patient scales	E	E
14. Cribs (with head access)	E	E
15. Beds (with head access)	E	E
16. Infant warmers, incubators	E	E
17. Heating and cooling blankets	E	E
18. Bilirubin lights	E	E
19. Transport monitor	E	D
20. EEG machine	E	E
21. Isolation cart	E	E
22. Blood warmer	E	E
23. Pacer (transthoracic or transvenous)	E	E
C. Small equipment		
1. Tracheal intubation equipment	E	E
2. Endotracheal tubes (all pediatric sizes)	E	E
3. Oropharyngeal and nasopharyngeal airways	E	E
4. Vascular access equipment	E	E
5. Cut-down trays	E	E
6. Tracheostomy tray	E	E
7. Flexible bronchoscope	E	D
8. Cricothyroidotomy tray	E	E
D. Respiratory support equipment		
1. Bag-valve-mask resuscitation devices	E	E
2. Oxygen tanks	E	E
3. Respiratory gas humidifiers	E	E
4. Air compressor	E	E
5. Air-oxygen blenders	E	E
6. Ventilators of all sizes for pediatric patients	E	E
7. Inhalation therapy equipment	E	E
8. Chest physiotherapy and suctioning	E	E
9. Spirometers	E	E
10. Continuous oxygen analyzers with alarms	E	E

TABLE 1.   Continued

	Level I	Level II
E. Monitoring equipment		
1. Capability of continuous monitoring of:		
a. Electrocardiography, heart rate	E	E
b. Respiration	E	E
c. Temperature	E	E
d. Systemic arterial pressure	E	E
e. Central venous pressure	E	E
f. Pulmonary arterial pressure	E	D
g. Intracranial pressure	E	D
h. Esophageal pressure	D	O
i. Capability to measure 4 pressures simultaneously	E	D
j. Capability to measure 5 pressures simultaneously	D	D
k. Arrhythmia detection and alarm	E	E
l. Pulse oximetry	E	E
m. End-tidal CO_2	E	E
2. Monitor characteristics		
a. Visible and audible high and low alarms for heart rate, respiratory rate, and all pressures	E	E
b. Hard-copy capability	E	E
c. Routine testing and maintenance	E	E
d. Patient isolation	E	E
e. Central station	E	E
V. Prehospital care		
A. Integration and communication with EMS system	E	E
B. Transfer arrangements with referral hospital	E	E
C. Transfer arrangement with level I PICU	NA	E
D. Educational programs in stabilization and transportation for EMS personnel	E	D
E. Transport system (including transport team)	E	O
F. Emergency communication into PICU and pediatric acute care unit (eg, phone, radio) 24 h per day	E	E
G. Communication link to poison control center	E	E
VI. Quality improvement		
1. Collaborative quality assessment	E	E
2. Morbidity and mortality review	E	E
3. Utilization review	E	E
4. Medical records review	E	E
5. Discharge criteria (planning)	E	E
6. Safety review	E	E
7. Long-term follow-up of patients and family	D	D
VII. Training and continuing education		
A. Physician training		
1. Unit in facility with accredited pediatric residency program	D	O
2. Unit provides clinical rotation for pediatric residents in pediatric critical care	D	O
3. Fellowship program in pediatric critical care	D	O
4. Cardiopulmonary resuscitation certification	E	E
5. PALS or advanced pediatric life support	E	E
6. Ongoing continuing medical education for physicians specific to pediatric critical care	E	E
7. Staff physicians to attend and participate in pediatric critical care	E	E
B. Unit personnel		
1. Cardiopulmonary resuscitation certification for nurses and respiratory therapists	E	E
2. Resuscitation practice sessions	E	E
3. Ongoing continuing education (on-site and/or off-site workshops and programs for nurses respiratory therapists, clinical pharmacists)	E	E
4. Certified by the American Association of Critical Care Nurses	D	D
5. PALS or advanced pediatric life support certification	E	E
6. Critical care registered nurse certification	D	D
C. Regional education		
1. Participation in regional pediatric critical care education	E	O
2. Service as educational resource center for public education in pediatric critical care	D	D
3. Prehospital care and interhospital transport	D	O

E indicates essential; D, desired; O, optional; NA, not applicable.
* In conjunction with nurse manager.

may differ between levels, such that level I PICUs will have a full complement of medical and surgical subspecialists including pediatric intensivists. Each level I and level II PICU should be able to address the physical, psychosocial, emotional, and spiritual needs of patients with life-threatening conditions and their families.

Some pediatric patients with moderate severity of illness can be managed in level II PICUs. Level II PICUs may be necessary to provide stabilization of critically ill children before transfer to another center or to avoid long-distance transfers for disorders of less complexity or lower acuity. It is imperative that the same standards of quality care be applied to patients managed in level II PICUs and level I PICUs. Requirements for level II PICUs differ from those for level I PICUs primarily with respect to the type and immediacy of physician presence and hospital resources. A level II PICU does not require a full spectrum of subspecialists, as outlined in Table 1. Level II units should be located according to documented demand or need and in concert with accepted principles of regionalization of medical care.[2] Each level II unit must have a well-established communications system with a level I unit to allow for timely referral of patients who need care that is not available in the level II PICU. Although other special care units may be appropriate for hospitals with small pediatric inpatient services, they should not be considered PICUs.

Cooperation among hospitals and professionals within a given region is essential to ensure that the appropriate numbers of level I and level II units are designated. Duplication of services may lead to underutilization of resources and inadequate development of skills by clinical personnel and may be costly. Detailed discussion of the importance of regionalization of critical care services has been provided by the American College of Critical Care Medicine and the American Academy of Pediatrics.[3]

This report provides the minimum acceptable guidelines for the following aspects of pediatric critical care: organization and administrative structure; personnel; hospital facilities and services; drugs and equipment; prehospital care; quality improvement; and training and continuing education (Table 1). These guidelines are intended to assist: (1) hospitals, in properly determining resource allocation and equipment needs; (2) physicians, as a reference for referral and care of critically ill infants and children; (3) emergency medical services (EMS) personnel, for proper prehospital triage; and (4) level I and II PICUs, as a means of ensuring proper patient care.

In preparing this report, significant efforts were made to build on previous work describing regional and national guidelines and standards that apply to these guidelines and, when possible, to incorporate those previous recommendations. The existing guidelines for PICUs established by the American Academy of Pediatrics and the Society of Critical Care Medicine were used as the major reference source.[1] In addition, this report incorporates the experience, expertise, and opinions of pediatric care givers including pediatric critical care physicians and nurses representing diverse regions of the country and types of practice.

ORGANIZATION AND ADMINISTRATIVE STRUCTURE

The level I and level II PICU will be a distinct, separate unit within the hospital that is equal in status to all other special care units. There should be a distinct administrative structure and staff for the PICU regardless of its location. A PICU committee will be established as a standing (interdisciplinary) committee within the hospital, with membership including physicians, nurses, respiratory therapists, clinical pharmacists, social workers, child life specialists, and others directly involved in PICU activities. The committee should provide input regarding the delineation of privileges for all personnel (physician and nonphysician) working in the PICU, consistent with hospital policies.

The medical director and nurse manager/nursing director should establish policies in collaboration with the PICU committee. Such policies shall govern matters including but not limited to safety procedures, nosocomial infection, patient isolation, visitation, traffic control, admission and discharge criteria, patient monitoring, equipment maintenance, patient record keeping, family care management (including family meetings, support groups, and sibling support), and bereavement care. A manual of these policies will be available for reference in the PICU.

Physical Design and Facilities

The physical facilities for PICUs will vary as a result of differences in hospital architecture, size, space, and design. Access to the PICU should be monitored to maintain patient and staff safety and confidentiality. The PICU should be located in proximity to elevators for patient transport, to the physicians' on-call room, and to family waiting and sleep areas. Proximity to the emergency department, operating room, and recovery room is desirable. Access to the medical and nursing directors will be improved by having their offices located near the PICU. When designing a PICU, the psychological, spiritual, cultural, and social needs of the patient and family should be taken into consideration, and policies should reflect a patient- and family-centered approach.

Floor Plan

Several distinct room types are required within the PICU, including rooms for patient isolation and separate rooms for clean and soiled linens and equipment. A laboratory area for rapid determination of blood gases and other essential studies is desirable, assuming compliance with national, state, and local regulations.

Space will be allocated for a medication station (including a refrigerator and a narcotics locker), a nourishment station, counters, and cabinets. It is desirable to have a satellite pharmacy within the PICU that is capable of providing routine and emergency medications at the point of ordering. A computerized link to the laboratory or another rapid and reliable system should be available for reporting laboratory results.

A separate room for family counseling is necessary for private discussions between the staff and the family. An area for storing patients' personal effects is also desirable. A conference area for staff personnel is highly desirable and should be located near the unit. A staff toilet is essential. Separate facilities for patient's families, including space for sleeping and bathing, are essential for level I and level II PICUs.

Bedside Facilities

PICUs with individual patient rooms should allow at least 250 ft^2 per room (assuming there is 1 patient per room), and ward-type PICUs should allow at least 225 ft² per patient. The head of each bed or crib shall be rapidly accessible for emergency airway management. Electrical power, oxygen, medical compressed air, and vacuum outlets sufficient in number to supply all necessary equipment should meet local code and other accrediting requirements. In most cases, 12 or more electrical outlets and a minimum of 2 compressed air outlets, 2 oxygen outlets, and 2 vacuum outlets will be necessary per bed space. Reserve emergency power and gas supply (oxygen, compressed air) are essential. All outlets, heating, ventilation, air conditioning, fire-safety procedures and equipment, electrical grounding, plumbing, and illumination must adhere to appropriate local, state, and national codes. Walls or curtains must be provided to ensure patient privacy.

PERSONNEL

Medical Director

A medical director will be appointed. A record of the appointment and acceptance should be made in writing. Medical directors of level I and II PICUs must be:

1. Initially board certified in pediatrics and board certified or in the process of certification in pediatric critical care medicine; or
2. Board certified in anesthesiology with practice limited to infants and children and with special qualifications (as defined by the American Board of Anesthesiology) in critical care medicine; or
3. Board certified in pediatric surgery with added qualifications in surgical critical care medicine (as defined by the American Board of Surgery).

If the medical director is not a pediatrician, a pediatric intensivist will be appointed as codirector. This is essential for level I PICUs and desirable for level II PICUs. Medical directors must achieve certification within 5 years of their initial acceptance into the certification process and must maintain active certification in critical care medicine.

The medical director, in conjunction with the nurse manager, should participate in developing and reviewing multidisciplinary PICU policies, promote policy implementation, participate in budget preparation, help coordinate staff education, maintain a database that describes unit experience and performance, ensure communication between the intensivists and referring primary care and/or subspecialty physicians, supervise resuscitation techniques, and, in coordination with the nurse manager, lead quality-improvement activities and coordinate medical research. Others may supervise these activities, but the medical director shall participate in each.

The medical director will name a qualified physician to fulfill his or her duties during absences. The medical director or designated substitute will often serve as the attending physician on patients in the unit. In addition, the medical director or designated substitute should have the institutional authority to provide primary or consultative care for all PICU patients. This authority should be codified in institutional policy and will also include providing daily consultation and intervention in the event that the primary attending physician is not available. Direct physician-to-physician contact should be made for all patients admitted to the PICU, including patients transferred from other institutions, as well as patients admitted from the emergency department or operating room.

Physician Staff

Studies suggest that having a full-time pediatric intensivist in the PICU improves patient care and efficiency.[4–8] At certain times of the day, the attending physician in the PICU may delegate the care of patients to a physician of at least the postgraduate year 2 level (in a level I PICU, this physician must be assigned to the PICU, and in a level II PICU, this physician must be available to the PICU) or to an advanced practice nurse or physician's assistant with specialized training in pediatric critical care. These nonphysician providers must receive credentials and privileges to provide care in the PICU only under the direction of the attending physician, and the credentialing process must be made in writing and approved by the medical director. An in-house physician at the postgraduate year 3 level or above in pediatrics or anesthesiology is essential for all level I PICUs. In addition, all hospitals with PICUs must have a physician in-house 24 hours per day who is available to provide bedside care to patients in the PICU. This physician must be skilled in and have credentials to provide emergency care to critically ill children.

Depending on the unit size and patient population, more physicians at higher training levels may be required. Other physicians, including the attending physician or his or her designee, should be available within 30 minutes to assist with patient management. For level I units, available physicians must include a pediatric intensivist, a pediatric anesthesiologist, a pediatric cardiologist, a pediatric neurologist, a pediatric radiologist, a psychiatrist or psychologist, a pediatric surgeon, a pediatric neurosurgeon, an otolaryngologist (pediatric subspecialist desired), an orthopedic surgeon (pediatric subspecialist desired), and a cardiothoracic surgeon (pediatric subspecialist desired). For level II PICUs, pediatric subspecialists (with the exception of the pediatric intensivist) are not essential but are desirable, a general surgeon and neurosurgeon are essential, and an otolaryngologist and orthopedic surgeon are desirable (pediatric subspecialists optional). For level II PICUs, a cardiovascular surgeon is also optional.

For level I PICUs, it is desirable to have available on short notice a craniofacial (plastic) surgeon, an oral surgeon, a pediatric pulmonologist, a pediatric hematologist/oncologist, a pediatric endocrinologist, a pediatric gastroenterologist, and a pediatric allergist or immunologist. These physicians should be available for patients in level II PICUs within a 24-hour period.

Nursing Staff

A nurse manager with substantial pediatric expertise should be designated for level I and II PICUs. A master's degree in pediatric nursing or nursing administration is desirable. In collaboration with the nursing leadership team, the nurse manager is responsible for assuring a safe practice environment consisting of appropriate nurse staffing, skill-level mix, and supplies and equipment. The nurse manager shall participate in the development and review of written policies and procedures for the PICU; coordinate multidisciplinary staff education, quality assurance, and nursing research; and prepare budgets together with the medical director. These responsibilities can be shared or delegated to advanced practice nurses, but the nurse manager has responsibility for the overall program. The nurse manager shall name qualified substitutes to fulfill his or her duties during absences.

An advanced practice nurse (clinical nurse specialist or nurse practitioner) should be available to provide clinical leadership in the nursing care management of patients. This is recommended for level I PICUs and optional for level II PICUs. The clinical nurse specialist should possess a master's degree in nursing, pediatric critical care nurse specialist certification, and clinical expertise in pediatric critical care. The nurse practitioner should hold a master's degree in nursing and national pediatric nurse practitioner certification and have completed a preceptorship in the management of critically ill pediatric patients. Expanded role components of the advanced practice nurse should match the clinical needs of patients within the particular PICU and health care system.

The department of nursing or patient care services should establish a program for nursing orientation, yearly competency review of high-risk low-frequency therapies, core competencies based on patient population, and an ongoing educational program specific for pediatric critical care nursing. Program content should match the diverse needs of each unit's patient population. It is desirable that most nursing staff working in level I and II PICUs obtain pediatric critical care certification.

Patient care in level I and II PICUs should be conducted or supervised by a pediatric critical care nurse. All nurses working in level I and II PICUs should complete a clinical and didactic pediatric critical care orientation before assuming full responsibility for patient care. Pediatric advanced life support (PALS) or an equivalent course should be required. Nurse-to-patient ratios should be based on patient acuity, usually ranging from 2:1 to 1:3.

Respiratory Therapy Staff

The respiratory therapy department should have a supervisor responsible for performance and training of staff, maintaining equipment, and monitoring multidisciplinary quality improvement and review. Under the supervisor's direction, respiratory therapy staff primarily designated and assigned to the level I PICU shall be in-house 24 hours per day. Hospitals with level II PICUs must have respiratory therapy staff in-house at all times; however, this staff need not be dedicated to the PICU (unless patient acuity so dictates). All respiratory therapists who care for children in level I and II PICUs should have clinical experience managing pediatric respiratory failure and pediatric mechanical ventilators and should have training in PALS or an equivalent course.

Ancillary Support Personnel

An appropriately trained and qualified clinical pharmacist should be assigned to the level I PICU; this is desirable for the level II PICU. Staff pharmacists must be in-house 24 hours per day in hospitals with level I PICUs, and this is desirable in hospitals with level II PICUs.

Biomedical technicians must be available within 1 hour, 24 hours per day for level I and II PICUs. For level I PICUs, unit secretaries (clerks) should have primary assignment in the PICU 24 hours per day. A radiology technician (preferably with advanced pediatric training) must be in-house 24 hours per day in hospitals with level I PICUs, and this is strongly recommended for those with level II units. In addition, social workers; physical, occupational, and speech therapists; nutritionists; child life specialists; clinical psychologists; and clergy must be available (this is essential for level I and desirable for level II PICUs).

HOSPITAL FACILITIES AND SERVICES

The level I or II PICU should be located in a category I facility as defined by the American Hospital Association. The emergency department should have a separate, covered entrance. An adjacent helipad is desirable. For hospitals with level I PICUs, 2 or more areas within the emergency department will have the capacity and equipment to resuscitate any pediatric patient with medical, surgical, or traumatic illness. Hospitals with level II units need to have only 1 such area. The emergency department will be staffed by physicians 24 hours per day in all hospitals with PICUs. Hospitals with level I PICUs should have separate pediatric emergency departments and should have physicians trained in pediatric emergency medicine in-house 24 hours per day.

The department of surgery in hospitals with a level I or level II PICU will have at least 1 operating room available within 30 minutes, 24 hours per day, and a second room available within 45 minutes. Capabilities in the operating room in hospitals with level I PICUs must include cardiopulmonary bypass, pediatric bronchoscopy, endoscopy, and radiography.

The blood bank must have all blood components available 24 hours per day in hospitals with a level I or II PICU. Unless unusual cross-matching issues are encountered, blood typing and cross matching shall allow transfusion within 1 hour.

Pediatric radiology services in hospitals with a level I or II PICU must include portable radiography, fluoroscopy, computerized tomography scanning, and ultrasonography. Nuclear scanning angiography and magnetic resonance imaging should be available at all times in hospitals with level I PICUs and must be available within 4 hours in hospitals with level II

PICUs. Facilities must be able to provide for the age-adjusted needs of pediatric patients (thermal homeostasis, sedation, etc). The availability of radiation therapy is desirable for level I PICUs and optional for level II PICUs.

Clinical laboratories in hospitals with a level I or II PICU will have microspecimen capability and 1-hour turnaround time for complete blood cell, differential, and platelet counts; urinalysis; measurement of electrolytes, blood urea nitrogen, creatinine, glucose, and calcium concentrations and prothrombin and partial thromboplastin time; and cerebrospinal fluid analysis. Blood gas values must be available within 15 minutes. Results of drug screening and levels of serum ammonia, serum and urine osmolarity, phosphorus, and magnesium should all be available within 3 hours for level I PICUs. Results of Gram stains and bacteriologic cultures should be available 24 hours per day. Point-of-care diagnostic testing capabilities are desirable for level I and II PICUs.[9]

The hospital pharmacy must be capable of dispensing all necessary medications for pediatric patients of all types and ages 24 hours per day. A satellite pharmacy close to the unit is desirable. A qualified pediatric clinical pharmacist is highly desirable for hospitals with level I PICUs and optional for hospitals with level II PICUs. A pharmacist should be available for participation in medical rounds, monitoring of drug therapy, the provision of drug information to PICU practitioners, and the evaluation of pertinent drug-related issues.[10] At each bedside, there should be a reference that lists urgent and resuscitation drugs with dosages appropriate for the individual patient.

Diagnostic cardiac and neurologic studies will be available for infants and children in hospitals with level I PICUs and are optional for hospitals with level II PICUs. Technicians with special training in pediatrics should be available to perform these studies. Electrocardiograms, 2-dimensional echocardiograms with color Doppler, and electroencephalograms should be available 24 hours per day for level I and II PICUs. A catheterization laboratory or angiography suite equipped to perform studies in pediatric patients should be present in hospitals with level I PICUs and is optional in hospitals with level II PICUs. Doppler ultrasonography devices and evoked potential monitoring equipment are desirable in hospitals with a level I or II PICU.

Hemodialysis equipment and technicians with pediatric experience should be available 24 hours per day in hospitals with level I PICUs and are optional for hospitals with level II PICUs.

Hospital facilities should include a comfortable waiting room, private consultation areas, dining facilities, a conference area, and sleeping accommodations and telephone, shower, and laundering facilities for patients' families. Facilities and personnel should also be available to meet the psychological and spiritual needs of patients and their families. Medical staff, patients, and patient families must have 24-hour-a-day access to competent, non-family member, language-interpreter services for non–English-speaking patients and families.

DRUGS AND EQUIPMENT

Drugs for resuscitation and advanced life support must be present and immediately available for any patient in the PICU. These drugs should be available in accordance with advanced cardiac life support and PALS guidelines and should include all those necessary to support the patient population that the PICU serves. The life-saving, therapeutic, and monitoring equipment detailed in this section must be present or immediately available in each level I and level II PICU.

Portable Equipment

Portable equipment will include an emergency ("code" or "crash") cart; a procedure lamp; pediatric-sized blood pressure cuffs for systemic arterial pressure determination; a Doppler ultrasonography device; an electrocardiograph; a defibrillator or cardioverter with pediatric paddles and preferably with pacing capabilities; thermometers with a range sufficient to identify extremes of hypothermia and hyperthermia; an automated blood pressure apparatus; transthoracic pacer with pediatric pads; devices for accurately measuring body weight; cribs and beds with head access; infant warmers; heating and cooling devices; lights for photograph therapy; temporary pacemakers; a blood-warming apparatus; and a transport monitor. A suitable number of infusion pumps with microcapability (0.1 mL/hour) must be available. Oxygen tanks are needed for transport and backup of the central oxygen supply. Similarly, portable suction machines are needed for transport and backup.

Additional equipment that must be available includes volumetric infusion pumps, air-oxygen blenders, an air compressor, gas humidifiers, bag-valve-mask resuscitators, an otoscope and ophthalmoscope, and isolation carts. A portable electroencephalography machine must be available in the hospital for bedside recordings in level I and II PICUs. Televisions, radios, and chairs should be available for patients and families who would benefit from their use.

Small Equipment

Certain small equipment appropriately sized for pediatric patients must be immediately available at all times. Such equipment includes suction catheters; tracheal intubation equipment (laryngoscope handles, sizes and types of blades adequate to intubate patients of all ages, and Magill forceps); endotracheal tubes of all sizes (cuffed and uncuffed); oropharyngeal and nasopharyngeal airways; laryngeal mask airways; central catheters for vascular access; catheters for arterial access; pulmonary artery catheters; thoracostomy tubes; transvenous pacing catheters; and surgical trays for vascular cut-downs, open-chest procedures, cricothyroidotomy, and tracheostomy. Hospitals with level I and II PICUs should have pediatric-sized equipment for flexible bronchoscopy available. This is essential for level I PICUs and desirable for level II PICUs.

Respiratory Equipment

Mechanical ventilators suitable for pediatric patients of all sizes must be available for each level I and level II PICU bed. Equipment for chest physiotherapy and suctioning, spirometers, and oxygen analyzers must always be available for every patient. Oxygen monitors (pulse oximeters and transcutaneous oxygen monitors) and CO_2 monitors (transcutaneous and end-tidal) are required; portable (transport) ventilators are desired.

Bedside Monitors

Bedside monitors in all PICUs must have the capability for continuously monitoring heart rate and rhythm, respiratory rate, temperature, 1 hemodynamic pressure, oxygen saturation, end-tidal CO_2, and arrhythmia detection. Bedside monitoring in level I PICUs must be capable of simultaneously monitoring systemic arterial, central venous, pulmonary arterial, and intracranial pressures. The capability for a fifth simultaneous pressure measurement is desirable but not essential. Monitors must have high and low alarms for heart rate, respiratory rate, and all pressures. The alarms must be audible and visible. A permanent hard copy of the rhythm strip must be available in level I and II PICUs. Hard copy and trending capability for all monitored variables is desirable. All monitors must be maintained and tested routinely.

PREHOSPITAL CARE

Often, patients requiring admission to a PICU are transported from the scene of an injury or from another hospital. Accordingly, PICUs shall be integrated with the regional EMS system. The method of communication may vary, but a standard written approach to emergencies involving the EMS system and the PICU should be prepared. All level I and II PICUs must have multiple telephone lines so that outside calls can be received even at very busy times. Rapid access to a poison control center is essential. A fax machine is essential for level I and II PICUs.

Each level I and level II PICU must endeavor to meet the needs of other hospitals less well-equipped to handle certain types of care. Formal transfer arrangements are encouraged. Each PICU will have or be affiliated with a transport system and team with advanced pediatric training to assist other hospitals in arranging safe patient transport.[11,12] Ideally, such transport teams should be able to deliver PICU care during transport. Supervisory physicians must be available for consultation during the interfacility transport process. These transport teams must have appropriately sized pediatric equipment to anticipate and manage the diverse health care needs of pediatric patients in this environment.[11,12] Telemedicine capabilities should be considered and will be desirable as technology becomes more widely available.

Policies should describe mechanisms that achieve smooth and timely exchange of patients between the emergency department, operating rooms, imaging facilities, special procedure areas, regular inpatient care areas, and the PICU.

QUALITY IMPROVEMENT

The PICU must use a multidisciplinary collaborative quality assessment process. Objective methods should be used to compare observed and predicted morbidity and mortality rates for the severity of illness in the population examined. Benchmarking methods should be used to compare outcomes between similar PICUs.

TRAINING AND CONTINUING EDUCATION

Each PICU should train health care professionals in basic aspects of, and serve as a focus for, continuing education programs in pediatric critical care. In addition, all health care providers working in the PICU should routinely attend or participate in regional and national meetings with course content pertinent to pediatric critical care.

Many level I PICUs and some level II PICUs will possess sufficient patient volume, teaching expertise, and research capability to support a fellowship program in pediatric critical care medicine. Programs providing subspecialty training in pediatric critical care medicine must possess approval by the Residency Review Committee of the Accreditation Council on Graduate Medical Education.

Nurses, respiratory therapists, and physicians must have basic life support certification and participate in resuscitation practice sessions and should be encouraged and supported to attend appropriate onsite or off-site educational programs. Successful completion and current reaffirmation of PALS or a similar course should be required.

It is desirable for level I PICU personnel to participate in regional pediatric critical care education for EMS providers, for emergency department and transport personnel, and for the general public. Some level I and II PICUs will be suited to serve as an educational resource for public education in areas pertinent to pediatric critical care.

Research is essential for improving the understanding of the pathophysiology affecting vital organ systems as well as appropriate symptom management and psychosocial supportive interventions for the patient, family, and bereaved survivors. Such knowledge is a vital component in improving patient care techniques and therapies, thereby decreasing morbidity and mortality. All level I PICUs and some level II PICUs can serve as laboratories for clinical research.

Section on Critical Care, 2001–2002
M. Michele Moss, MD, Chairperson
Alice D. Ackerman, MD
Thomas Bojko, MD, MS
Brahm Goldstein, MD
Stephanie A. Storgion, MD
Otwell D. Timmons, MD
Timothy S. Yeh, MD, Immediate Past Chairperson

Liaisons
Richard J. Brilli, MD
　Society of Critical Care Medicine
Lynda J. Means, MD
　Section on Anesthesiology and Pain Medicine

Anthony L. Pearson-Shaver, MD
  Section on Transport Medicine
Stephanie A. Storgion, MD
  Committee on Coding and Reimbursement
Loren G. Yamamoto, MD, MPH, MBA
  National Conference and Exhibition Planning
  Group
Timothy S. Yeh, MD
  Committee on Pediatric Emergency Medicine

STAFF
Susan Tellez

COMMITTEE ON HOSPITAL CARE, 2001–2002
John M. Neff, MD, Chairperson
Jerrold M. Eichner, MD
David R. Hardy, MD
Jack M. Percelay, MD, MPH
Ted D. Sigrest, MD
Erin R. Stucky, MD

LIAISONS
Susan Dull, RN, MSN, MBA
  National Association of Children's Hospitals
  and Related Institutions
Mary T. Perkins, RN, DNSc
  American Hospital Association
Jerriann M. Wilson, CCLS, MEd
  Child Life Council

CONSULTANTS
Timothy E. Corden, MD
Michael Klein, MD, Section on Surgery
Mary O'Connor, MD, MPH
Theodore Striker, MD, Section on Anesthesiology
  and Pain Medicine

STAFF
Stephanie Mucha

SOCIETY OF CRITICAL CARE MEDICINE
  TASK FORCE ON LEVELS OF CARE FOR PICUs
David I. Rosenberg, MD, Chairperson
Richard Brilli, MD
Martha A.Q. Curley, RN
Lucian DeNicola, MD
Alan Fields, MD
Barry Frank, MD
Lorry Frankel, MD
Christa Joseph, RN

Gregory L. Kearns, PharmD, PhD
M. Michele Moss, MD
Daniel Notterman, MD
Thomas Rice, MD
Robert Seigler, MD
Curt Steinhart, MD, MBA
Ralph Vardis, MD
Timothy S. Yeh, MD

REFERENCES

1. American Academy of Pediatrics, Committee on Hospital Care and Pediatric Section of the Society of Critical Care Medicine. Guidelines and levels of care for pediatric intensive care units. *Pediatrics.* 1993;92:166–175
2. Society of Critical Care Medicine. Consensus report for regionalization of services for critically ill or injured children. *Crit Care Med.* 2000;28:236–239
3. American College of Critical Care Medicine, Society of Critical Care Medicine. Critical care services and personnel: recommendations based on a system of categorization into two levels of care. *Crit Care Med.* 1999;27:422–426
4. Pollack MM, Cuerdon TT, Patel KM, Ruttiman UE, Getson PR, Levetown M. Impact of quality-of-care factors on pediatric intensive care unit mortality. *JAMA.* 1994;272:941–946
5. Pollack MM, Patel KM, Ruttiman E. Pediatric critical care training programs have a positive effect on pediatric intensive care mortality. *Crit Care Med.* 1997;25:1637–1642
6. Pollack MM, Cuerdon TC, Getson PR. Pediatric intensive care units: results of a national survey. *Crit Care Med.* 1993;21:607–614
7. Pollack MM, Alexander SR, Clarke N, Ruttiman UE, Tesselaar HM, Bachulis AC. Improved outcomes from tertiary center pediatric intensive care: a statewide comparison of tertiary and nontertiary care facilities. *Crit Care Med.* 1991;19:150–159
8. Reynolds HN, Haupt MT, Thill-Baharozian MC, Carlson RW. Impact of critical care physician staffing on patients with septic shock in a university hospital medical intensive care unit. *JAMA.* 1988;260:3446–3450
9. Halpern NA. Point of care diagnostics and networks. *Crit Care Clin.* 2000;16:623–640
10. Mann HJ. Pharmacy technology of the ICU: today and tomorrow. *Crit Care Clin.* 2000;16:641–658
11. American Academy of Pediatrics, Task Force on Interhospital Transport. *Guidelines for Air and Ground Transport of Neonatal and Pediatric Patients.* MacDonald MG, Ginzburg HM, eds. Elk Grove Village, IL: American Academy of Pediatrics; 1999
12. American Academy of Pediatrics, Committee on Pediatric Emergency Medicine. *Emergency Medical Services for Children: The Role of the Primary Care Provider.* Singer J, Ludwig S, eds. Elk Grove Village, IL: American Academy of Pediatrics; 1992

All clinical reports from the American Academy of Pediatrics automatically expire 5 years after publication unless reaffirmed, revised, or retired at or before that time.

Guidelines for Pediatric Cancer Centers

- *Policy Statement*

AMERICAN ACADEMY OF PEDIATRICS

POLICY STATEMENT
Organizational Principles to Guide and Define the Child Health Care System and/or Improve the Health of All Children

Section on Hematology/Oncology

Guidelines for Pediatric Cancer Centers

ABSTRACT. Since the American Academy of Pediatrics published guidelines for pediatric cancer centers in 1986 and 1997, significant changes in the delivery of health care have prompted a review of the role of tertiary medical centers in the care of pediatric patients. The potential effect of these changes on the treatment and survival rates of children with cancer led to this revision. The intent of this statement is to delineate personnel and facilities that are essential to provide state-of-the-art care for children and adolescents with cancer. This statement emphasizes the importance of board-certified pediatric hematologists/oncologists, pediatric subspecialty consultants, and appropriately qualified pediatric medical subspecialists and pediatric surgical specialists overseeing the care of all pediatric and adolescent cancer patients and the need for facilities available only at a tertiary center as essential for the initial management and much of the follow-up for pediatric and adolescent cancer patients. *Pediatrics* 2004;113:1833–1835; *cancer, pediatrics, hematology, oncology, cancer center.*

INTRODUCTION

A pediatric cancer center must have the staff and facilities to ensure that the pediatric patient with cancer will receive the best care that is available for his or her diagnosis. The medical staff at such a center is composed of the primary care pediatrician, pediatric medical subspecialists, and pediatric surgical specialists—hematologists/oncologists, surgeons, urologists, neurologists, neurosurgeons, orthopedic surgeons, radiation oncologists, pathologists, child life specialists, and diagnostic radiologists. These physicians and nurse practitioners, pediatric nurses, social workers, pharmacists, nutritionists, and other allied health professionals serve as a multidisciplinary team committed to the care of the child or adolescent with cancer.

In the United States, the oncologic care of the child or adolescent with cancer should be coordinated by a pediatric hematologist/oncologist who is board certified in the subspecialty of pediatric hematology and oncology by the American Board of Pediatrics. Other subspecialists should be similarly board certified when applicable.

Oncologic care should be provided in a pediatric center that has the following personnel, facilities, and capabilities.

Personnel

- Communication with the primary pediatrician, which is essential in the provision of family-centered supportive care
- Board-certified pediatric hematologists/oncologists
- Pediatric oncology nurses who are certified in chemotherapy, knowledgeable about pediatric protocols, and experienced in the management of complications of therapy
- Board-certified radiologists with specific expertise in the diagnostic imaging of infants, children, and adolescents
- Board-certified surgeons with expertise in pediatric general surgery
- Surgical specialists with pediatric expertise (ie, training and certification, if available) in neurosurgery, urology, orthopedics, ophthalmology, otolaryngology, dentistry, and gynecology
- A board-certified radiation oncologist trained and experienced in the treatment of infants, children, and adolescents
- A board-certified pathologist with special training in the pathology of hematologic malignancies and solid tumors of children and adolescents
- Board-certified pediatric subspecialists available to participate actively in all areas of the care of the child with cancer, including anesthesiology, intensive care, infectious diseases, cardiology, neurology, endocrinology and metabolism, genetics, gastroenterology, child and adolescent psychiatry, nephrology, and pulmonology
- Pediatric physical and mental rehabilitation services including pediatric physiatry
- Pediatric (oncology) social worker(s), pediatric psychologists, child life specialists, and access to family support group services
- Pediatric nutrition experts with the capability of preparing, administering, and monitoring total parenteral nutrition

Facilities

- An immediately accessible and fully staffed, on-site pediatric intensive care unit
- Up-to-date diagnostic imaging facilities to perform radiography, computed tomography, magnetic resonance imaging, ultrasonography, radionuclide imaging, and angiography; positron-emission tomography scanning and other emerging technologies are desirable

PEDIATRICS (ISSN 0031 4005). Copyright © 2004 by the American Academy of Pediatrics.

- Up-to-date radiation-therapy equipment with facilities for treating pediatric patients
- A hematopathology laboratory capable of performing cell-phenotype analysis using flow cytometry, immunohistochemistry, molecular diagnosis, and cytogenetics and access to blast colony assays and polymerase chain reaction-based methodology
- Access to hemodialysis and/or hemofiltration and apheresis for collection and storage of hematopoietic progenitor cells

Capabilities

- A clinical chemistry laboratory with the capability to monitor antibiotic and antineoplastic drug levels
- A blood bank capable of providing a full range of products including irradiated, cytomegalovirus-negative, and leucodepleted blood components
- A pharmacy capable of accurate, well-monitored preparation and dispensing of antineoplastic agents and investigational agents
- Capability of providing sufficient isolation of patients from airborne pathogens, which could include high-efficiency particulate air (HEPA) filtration or laminar flow and positive/negative pressure rooms
- Access to stem cell transplant services
- Educational and training programs for health care professionals including the primary care physician
- Coordination of services including home health, pain management, palliative, and end-of-life care
- A regularly scheduled multidisciplinary pediatric tumor board
- An established program designed to provide long-term, multidisciplinary follow-up of successfully treated patients at the original treatment center or by a team of health care professionals who are familiar with the potential adverse effects of treatment for childhood cancer
- Membership or affiliation with the Children's Oncology Group to provide access to state-of-the-art clinical trials; availability of support for coordination to track patients' progress and maintain clinical trials data
- Capability of providing parent, caregiver, and patient education
- Full-time access to translation services to ensure accurate translation and effective communication among all health care professionals and the patient and family
- An ongoing program of assessment of care for continuing quality improvement and safety
- A formal program for cancer education for the family and instruction on self-management

ROLE OF CENTERS IN DIAGNOSIS AND TREATMENT

Approximately 12 000 new cases of cancer are diagnosed in children younger than 20 years annually in the United States.[1,2] Cancer remains the second most frequent cause of death, after injury, in children older than 3 months.[3]

Great progress has been made in the development of successful treatment programs for children and adolescents with cancer. These improvements have been possible because of the availability of pediatric cancer treatment centers with collective expertise in the clinical management of children with cancer and the existence of a network of experienced investigators and allied health professionals who recognize the central importance of randomized clinical trials as the best available method for identifying more successful treatment strategies and who have the resources to evaluate new treatment modalities as they become available.

The importance of comprehensive, multidisciplinary treatment in improving patient outcome in a cost-effective manner has been well documented for children with acute lymphoblastic leukemia,[4] non–Hodgkin lymphoma,[5,6] brain tumors,[7,8] rhabdomyosarcoma,[5,8] Wilms' tumor,[9,10] and Ewing sarcoma.[5] Almost 80% of these children can be treated successfully if modern diagnostic and therapeutic approaches are initiated expeditiously.[2] Early detection, accurate diagnosis, and appropriate treatment depend on a multidisciplinary treatment approach to children and adolescents with cancer, an approach that is uniquely available at a pediatric cancer center. The roles of specialized nursing, pharmacy, rehabilitation, and paramedical personnel and access to increasingly complex equipment and facilities are critical to improving long-term survival and quality of life.

The center-based pediatric hematologist/oncologist is the coordinator for the diagnosis and treatment of most children and adolescents with cancer. Pediatric hematology/oncology is an established specialty with specific training requirements that lead to subspecialty board eligibility. Because most pediatric tumors show a striking response to specific regimens of intensive chemotherapy, pediatric hematologists/oncologists are necessarily resolute in carrying out therapies that can have devastating morbidity and appreciable mortality. For these therapies to be administered safely, a pediatric hematologist/oncologist who is trained and experienced in the management of children and adolescents with cancer and who has extensive knowledge of the relevant drug indications and toxicities must coordinate this care.

The pediatric hematologist/oncologist must be assisted by skilled nurses, social workers, pharmacists, nutritionists, and psychologists who specialize in pediatric oncology. Professional organizations such as the Association of Pediatric Oncology Nurses and Association of Pediatric Oncology Social Workers facilitate the professional growth and education of these individuals. Diagnostic radiologists and radiation oncologists with specific training and interest in pediatric oncology should be available at the pediatric cancer center. Principles of surgery that are unique to childhood tumors have evolved, and in fields such as general (pediatric) surgery, urology, neurology, and orthopedics, the presence of surgeons whose sole (or major) effort is directed toward pediatric oncology has become indispensable in achieving maximum survival.

A pathologist experienced in pediatric oncology is an essential member of the multidisciplinary team at the pediatric cancer center. State-of-the-art diagnosis of many pediatric hematologic malignancies and tumors requires immunochemistry and/or molecular techniques. Because solid tumors in children and adolescents are rare in the experience of most pathologists, an incorrect histologic diagnosis may be given when initial surgical management occurs at a nonspecialized hospital. Ideally, the diagnostic biopsy should be performed at the cancer center, at which the facilities are available to order and obtain all the special studies that would be appropriate and would obviate the need for subjecting the patient to repeat procedures.

PRACTICE OF PEDIATRIC ONCOLOGY OUTSIDE RECOGNIZED CENTERS

The clinical results in children with cancer have been shown to be superior when specialized diagnostic, supportive, and specific care is given at a pediatric cancer center.[4–10] After diagnosis has been established and the treatment plan has been determined by the pediatric cancer center, certain aspects of care may be continued in the office of a primary care pediatrician for selected children. When such a plan for shared treatment is undertaken, it must be with the understanding that the child will be referred back to the pediatric cancer center if complications develop or there is recurrence of the tumor. For many children, the facilities and expertise available at the pediatric cancer center are required for all aspects of therapy. However, it must be emphasized that the primary care pediatrician should retain an important supportive role for the patient with cancer and his or her family, which requires excellent regular communication between the oncologist and the pediatrician.

SUMMARY

On the basis of the effectiveness of pediatric cancer centers in treating children and adolescents with cancer, the American Academy of Pediatrics recommends the following:

- Children and adolescents with newly suspected and/or recurrent malignancy should be referred to a pediatric cancer center for prompt and accurate diagnosis and management.
- Children and adolescents with newly diagnosed and/or recurrent malignancies should have their treatment coordinated by a board-certified pediatric hematologist/oncologist; treatment should be prescribed and initiated at a pediatric cancer center but may be continued at a center not specialized in the care of the pediatric oncology patient under the continuing oversight of the center's multidisciplinary team.
- Multidisciplinary team members should have pediatric expertise within their specialty area.

Section on Hematology/Oncology, 2003–2004
Roger L. Berkow, MD, Chairperson
*James J. Corrigan, MD
*Stephen A. Feig, MD
F. Leonard Johnson, MD
Peter A. Lane, MD
John J. Hutter, Jr, MD

Liaisons
Edwin N. Forman, MD
   Childhood Cancer Alliance
Naomi L. Luban, MD
   American Association of Blood Banks

Staff
Laura Laskosz, MPH

*Lead authors

REFERENCES

1. Kosary CL, Ries LAG, Miller BA, Hankey BF, Harras A, Edwards BK, eds. *SEER Cancer Statistics Review, 1973–1992: Tables and Graphs.* Bethesda, MD: US Department of Health and Human Services, Public Health Service, National Institutes of Health; 1995. DHHS Publication No. NIH 96-2789
2. Bleyer WA. What can be learned about childhood cancer from "Cancer Statistics Review 1973–1988." *Cancer.* 1993;71(10 suppl):3229–3236
3. Wegman ME. Annual summary of vital statistics—1993. *Pediatrics.* 1994;94:792–803
4. Meadows AT, Kramer S, Hopson R, Lustbader E, Jarrett P, Evans AE. Survival in childhood acute lymphocytic leukemia: effect of protocol and place of treatment. *Cancer Invest.* 1983;1:49–55
5. Stiller CA. Centralisation of treatment and survival rates for cancer. *Arch Dis Child.* 1988;63:23–30
6. Wagner HP, Dingeldein-Bettler I, Berchthold W, et al. Childhood NHL in Switzerland: incidence and survival of 120 study and 42 non-study patients. *Med Pediatr Oncol.* 1995;24:281–286
7. Duffner PK, Cohen ME, Flannery JT. Referral patterns of childhood brain tumors in the state of Connecticut. *Cancer.* 1982;50:1636–1640
8. Kramer S, Meadows AT, Pastore G, Jarrett P, Bruce D. Influence of place of treatment on diagnosis, treatment, and survival in three pediatric solid tumors. *J Clin Oncol.* 1984;2:917–923
9. Lennox EL, Stiller CA, Jones PH, Wilson LM. Nephroblastoma: treatment during 1970–3 and the effect on survival of inclusion in the first MRC trial. *Br Med J.* 1979;2(6190):567–569
10. Green DM, Breslow NE, Evans I, et al. The relationship between dose schedule and charges for treatment on National Wilms' Tumor Study-4. A report from the National Wilms' Tumor Study Group. *J Natl Cancer Inst Monogr.* 1995;19:21–25

SELECTED READINGS

Bleyer WA. Cancer in older adolescents and young adults: epidemiology, diagnosis, treatment, survival, and importance of clinical trials. *Med Pediatr Oncol.* 2002;38:1–10
Carter TL, Watt PM, Kumar R, et al. Hemizygous p16 (INK4A) deletion in pediatric acute lymphoblastic leukemia predicts independent risk of relapse. *Blood.* 2001;97:572–274
Coffin CM, Dehner LP. Pathologic evaluation of pediatric soft tissue tumors. *Am J Clin Pathol.* 1998;109:S38–S52
Dayton V, Nguyen PL, Jaszcz V. Interpreting flow cytometry for hematologic neoplasms. *Am J Clin Pathol.* 2000;114:151–153
Gurney JG, Severson RK, Davis S, Robison LL. Incidence of cancer in children in the United States: sex-, race-, and 1-year age-specific rates by histologic type. *Cancer.* 1995;75:2186–2195
Lo Coco FL, De Santis S, Esposito A, Divona M, Diverio D. Molecular monitoring of hematologic malignancies: current and future issues. *Semin Hematol.* 2002;39:14–17
Rowley JD. Cytogenetic analysis in leukemia and lymphoma: an introduction. *Semin Hematol.* 2000;37:315–319
Rowley JD. Molecular genetics in leukemia. *Leukemia.* 2000;14:513–517
Shochat SJ, Fremgen AM, Murphy SB, et al. Childhood cancer: patterns of protocol participation in a national survey. *CA Cancer J Clin.* 2001;51:119–130

All policy statements from the American Academy of Pediatrics automatically expire 5 years after publication unless reaffirmed, revised, or retired at or before that time.

Hospital Stay for Healthy Term Newborns

• *Policy Statement*

AMERICAN ACADEMY OF PEDIATRICS

POLICY STATEMENT
Organizational Principles to Guide and Define the Child Health Care System and/or Improve the Health of All Children

Committee on Fetus and Newborn

Hospital Stay for Healthy Term Newborns

ABSTRACT. Decisions regarding the length of hospital stays for newborns and their mothers became driven by financial reimbursement from third-party payers in the 1990s. The Newborns' and Mothers' Health Protection Act of 1996 and a report from the Secretary's Advisory Committee on Infant Mortality acknowledge the importance of physician assessment in determining the timing of each newborn's discharge. The pediatrician's primary role is to ensure the health and well-being of the newborn in the context of the family. It is within this context that this revised statement addresses the short hospital stay (<48 hours after birth) for healthy term newborns. *Pediatrics* 2004;113:1434–1436; *newborn, hospital, discharge.*

BACKGROUND

Early newborn discharge began as a consumer-initiated movement and as an alternative to home delivery in the 1980s. In the 1990s, it became driven by third-party payers refusing payment for hospital stays extending beyond 24 hours after an uncomplicated vaginal delivery.[1] Congress responded by signing into law the Newborns' and Mothers' Health Protection Act of 1996,[2] which prohibited payers from restricting benefits for hospital stays to <48 hours for a vaginal delivery or <96 hours after birth by cesarean section. The act, however, did not prohibit earlier discharge of a mother and her newborn if she and her attending health care professional are in agreement that it is appropriate. Reports of recent experience with early discharge have documented both problems and successful programs.[3–8] The Secretary's Advisory Committee on Infant Mortality recently published its recommendations from a preliminary report to Congress. The report emphasized that "the goal of postnatal and postpartum care should be good health and well-being, not only the prevention of rare and catastrophic events."[9]

The pediatrician's primary role is to ensure the health and well-being of the infant in the context of the family. It is within this context that this revised statement addresses the short hospital stay (<48 hours after birth) for healthy term newborns.

The hospital stay of the mother-infant dyad should be long enough to allow identification of early problems and to ensure that the family is able and prepared to care for the infant at home. Many cardio-

pulmonary problems related to the transition from an intrauterine to an extrauterine environment usually become apparent during the first 12 hours after birth.[10] However, detection of jaundice,[11] ductal-dependent cardiac lesions,[12,13] gastrointestinal obstruction,[14] and other problems[15] may require a longer period of observation by skilled and experienced health care professionals. Furthermore, the length of stay should be based on the unique characteristics of each mother-infant dyad, including the health of the mother, the health and stability of the infant, the ability and confidence of the mother to care for her infant, the adequacy of support systems at home, and access to appropriate follow-up care.[16,17] All efforts should be made to keep mothers and infants together to promote simultaneous discharge.

RECOMMENDATIONS

It is recommended that the following minimum criteria be met before any newborn discharge. It is unlikely that fulfillment of these criteria and conditions can be accomplished in <48 hours. If discharge is considered before 48 hours, it should be limited to infants who are of singleton birth between 38 and 42 weeks' gestation, who are of birth weight appropriate for gestational age, and who meet other discharge criteria as follows:

1. The antepartum, intrapartum, and postpartum courses for mother and infant are uncomplicated.
2. Delivery is vaginal.
3. The infant's vital signs are documented as being within normal ranges and stable for the last 12 hours preceding discharge, including a respiratory rate below 60 per minute, a heart rate of 100 to 160 beats per minute,[18] and axillary temperature of 36.5°C to 37.4°C (97.7°F to 99.3°F),[19,20] measured properly in an open crib with appropriate clothing.
4. The infant has urinated and passed at least 1 stool spontaneously.
5. The infant has completed at least 2 successful feedings, with documentation that the infant is able to coordinate sucking, swallowing, and breathing while feeding.
6. Physical examination reveals no abnormalities that require continued hospitalization.
7. There is no evidence of excessive bleeding at the circumcision site for at least 2 hours.
8. The clinical significance of jaundice, if present before discharge, has been determined, and ap-

propriate management and/or follow-up plans have been put in place.[21,22]

9. The mother's knowledge, ability, and confidence to provide adequate care for her infant are documented by the fact that she has received training and demonstrated competency regarding:
   - Breastfeeding or bottle feeding (the breastfeeding mother and infant should be assessed by trained staff regarding breastfeeding position, latch-on, and adequacy of swallowing)
   - Appropriate urination and defecation frequency for the infant
   - Cord, skin, and genital care for infant
   - Ability to recognize signs of illness and common infant problems, particularly jaundice
   - Proper infant safety (eg, proper use of a car safety seat and supine positioning for sleeping)

10. Family members or other support persons, including health care professionals such as the family pediatrician or his or her designees, who are familiar with newborn care and knowledgeable about lactation and the recognition of jaundice and dehydration are available to the mother and her infant after discharge.

11. Maternal and infant blood test results are available and have been reviewed, including:
    - Maternal syphilis and hepatitis B surface antigen status
    - Cord or infant blood-type and direct Coombs test results, as clinically indicated[22]
    - Screening tests performed in accordance with state regulations, including screening for human immunodeficiency virus infection[23]

12. Initial hepatitis B vaccine is administered as indicated by the infant's risk status and according to the current immunization schedule.[24]

13. Hearing screening has been completed per hospital protocol and state regulations.[25]

14. Family, environmental, and social risk factors have been assessed. These risk factors may include but are not limited to:
    - Untreated parental substance abuse or positive urine toxicology results in the mother or newborn
    - History of child abuse or neglect
    - Mental illness in a parent who is in the home
    - Lack of social support, particularly for single, first-time mothers
    - No fixed home
    - History of untreated domestic violence, particularly during this pregnancy
    - Adolescent mother, particularly if other conditions above apply

    When these or other risk factors are identified, discharge should be delayed until they are resolved or a plan to safeguard the infant is in place.

15. Barriers to adequate follow-up care for the newborn such as lack of transportation to medical care services, lack of easy access to telephone communication, and non–English-speaking parents have been assessed and, wherever possible, assistance has been given the family to make suitable arrangements to address them.

16. A physician-directed source of continuing medical care for the mother and the infant is identified. For newborns discharged <48 hours after delivery, a definitive appointment has been made for the infant to be examined within 48 hours of discharge. It is essential that all infants having a short hospital stay be examined by experienced health care professionals. If this cannot be ensured, discharge should be deferred until a mechanism for follow-up evaluation is identified. The follow-up visit can take place in a home or clinic setting as long as the health care professionals examining the infant are competent in newborn assessment and the results of the follow-up visit are reported to the infant's physician or his or her designees on the day of the visit.[26,27]

The purpose of the follow-up visit is to:

- Weigh the infant; assess the infant's general health, hydration, and degree of jaundice; identify any new problems; review feeding pattern and technique, including observation of breastfeeding for adequacy of position, latch-on, and swallowing; and obtain historical evidence of adequate urination and defecation patterns for the infant
- Assess quality of mother-infant interaction and details of infant behavior
- Reinforce maternal or family education in infant care, particularly regarding infant feeding
- Review the outstanding results of laboratory tests performed before discharge
- Perform screening tests in accordance with state regulations and other tests that are clinically indicated, such as serum bilirubin
- Verify the plan for health care maintenance, including a method for obtaining emergency services, preventive care and immunizations, periodic evaluations and physical examinations, and necessary screenings

The follow-up visit should be considered an independent service to be reimbursed as a separate package and not as part of a global fee for maternity-newborn labor and delivery services.

CONCLUSIONS

The fact that a short hospital stay (<48 hours after birth) for term healthy infants can be accomplished does not mean that it is appropriate for every mother and infant. Each mother-infant dyad should be evaluated individually to determine the optimal time of discharge. The timing of discharge should be the decision of the physician caring for the infant and should not be based on arbitrary policy established by third-party payers. Local institution of these guidelines is best accomplished through the collaborative efforts of all parties concerned. Institutions should develop guidelines through their professional staff in collaboration with appropriate community agencies, including third-party payers, to establish hospital-stay programs for healthy term infants that implement these recommendations. State and local public health agencies also should be involved in the oversight of existing hospital-stay programs for quality assurance and monitoring. Additional research results from the Pediatric Research in Office Settings network study of the various issues of care of newborns and their mothers in the early postnatal weeks, including postdischarge follow-up, are anticipated to provide additional understanding of safe and appropriate practices.[28]

COMMITTEE ON FETUS AND NEWBORN, 2002–2003
Lillian R. Blackmon, MD, Chairperson
Daniel G. Batton, MD
Edward F. Bell, MD
William A. Engle, MD
William P. Kanto, Jr, MD
Gilbert I. Martin, MD
Warren Rosenfeld, MD
Ann Stark, MD

Carol Miller, MD*
    Past Committee Member

LIAISONS
Keith J. Barrington, MD
    Canadian Paediatric Society
Jenny Ecord, MS, RNC, NNP, PNP
    American Nurses Association
Association of Women's Health, Obstetric, and
    Neonatal Nurses
National Association of Neonatal Nurses
Solomon Iyasu, MBBS, MPH
    Centers for Disease Control and Prevention
Laura E. Riley, MD
    American College of Obstetricians and
    Gynecologists
Linda L. Wright, MD
    National Institutes of Health

STAFF
Jim Couto, MA

Lead author

REFERENCES

1. Hospital stays continue 10-year decline. *Am J Public Health.* 1992;82:54–
2. Bradley W. Newborns' and Mothers' Health Protection Act of 1996. Pub L No. 104-204
3. Welt SI, Cole JS, Myers MS, Sholes DM Jr, Jelovsek FR. Feasibility of postpartum rapid hospital discharge: a study from a community hospital population. *Am J Perinatol.* 1993;10:384–387
4. Soskolne EI, Schumacher R, Fyock C, Young ML, Schork A. The effect of early discharge and other factors on readmission rates of newborns. *Arch Pediatr Adolesc Med.* 1996;150:373–379
5. Danielsen B, Castles AG, Damberg CL, Gould JB. Newborn discharge timing and readmissions: California, 1992–1995. *Pediatrics.* 2000;106:31–39
6. Malkin JD, Garber S, Broder MS, Keeler E. Infant mortality and early postpartum discharge. *Obstet Gynecol.* 2000;96:183–188
7. Liu LL, Clemens CJ, Shay DK, Davis RL, Novack AH. The safety of newborn early discharge: the Washington State experience. *JAMA.* 1997;278:293–298

8. Braveman P, Egerter S, Pearl M, Marchi K, Miller C. Problems associated with early discharge of newborn infants. Early discharge of newborns and mothers: a critical review of the literature. *Pediatrics.* 1995;96:716–726
9. Eaton AP. Early postpartum discharge: recommendations from a preliminary report to Congress. *Pediatrics.* 2001;107:400–403
10. Desmond MM, Rudolph AJ, Phitaksphraiwan P. The transitional care nursery: a mechanism for preventive medicine in the newborn. *Pediatr Clin North Am.* 1966;13:651–668
11. American Academy of Pediatrics, Provisional Committee on Quality Improvement and Subcommittee on Hyperbilirubinemia. Practice parameter: management of hyperbilirubinemia in the healthy term newborn. *Pediatrics.* 1994;94:558–565
12. Gentile R, Stevenson G, Dooley T, Franklin D, Kawabori I, Pearlman A. Pulsed Doppler echocardiographic determination of time of ductal closure in normal newborn infants. *J Pediatr.* 1981;98:443–448
13. Lambert EC, Canent RV, Hohn AR. Congenital cardiac anomalies in the newborn. A review of conditions causing death or severe distress in the first month of life. *Pediatrics.* 1966;37:343–351
14. Lister J, Irving IM, eds. *Neonatal Surgery.* 3rd ed. London, England: Butterworths; 1990
15. Jackson GL, Kennedy KA, Sendelbach DM, et al. Problem identification in apparently well neonates: implications for early discharge. *Clin Pediatr (Phila).* 2000;39:581–590
16. Britton JR, Baker A, Spino C, Bernstein HH. Postpartum discharge preferences of pediatricians: results from a national survey. *Pediatrics.* 2002;110:53–60
17. Bernstein HH, Spino C, Baker A, Slora EJ, Touloukian CL, McCormick MC. Postpartum discharge: do varying perceptions of readiness impact health outcomes? *Ambul Pediatr.* 2002;2:388–395
18. Southall DP, Richards J, Mitchell P, Brown DJ, Johnston PG, Shinebourne EA. Study of cardiac rhythm in healthy newborn infants. *Br Heart J.* 1980;43:14–20
19. Eoff MJ, Meier RS, Miller C. Temperature measurement in infants. *Nurs Res.* 1974;23:457–460
20. Mayfield SR, Bhatia J, Nakamura KT, Rios GR, Bell EF. Temperature measurement in term and preterm neonates. *J Pediatr.* 1984;104:271–275
21. Bhutani VK, Johnson L, Sivieri EM. Predictive ability of a predischarge hour-specific serum bilirubin for subsequent significant hyperbilirubinemia in healthy term and near-term newborns. *Pediatrics.* 1999;103:6–14
22. American Academy of Pediatrics, Subcommittee on Neonatal Hyperbilirubinemia. Neonatal jaundice and kernicterus. *Pediatrics.* 2001;108:763–765
23. American Academy of Pediatrics, American College of Obstetricians and Gynecologists. Human immunodeficiency virus screening. *Pediatrics.* 1999;104:128
24. American Academy of Pediatrics, Committee on Infectious Diseases, Advisory Committee on Immunization Practices of the Centers for Disease Control and Prevention, American Academy of Family Physicians. Recommended childhood and adolescent immunization schedule—United States, January–June 2004. *Pediatrics.* 2004;113:142–147
25. American Academy of Pediatrics, Task Force on Newborn and Infant Hearing. Newborn and infant hearing loss: detection and intervention. *Pediatrics.* 1999;103:527–530
26. Nelson VR. The effect of newborn early discharge follow-up program on pediatric urgent care utilization. *J Pediatr Health Care.* 1999;13:58–61
27. Escobar GJ, Braveman PA, Ackerson L, et al. A randomized comparison of home visits and hospital-based group follow-up visits after early postpartum discharge. *Pediatrics.* 2001;108:719–727
28. American Academy of Pediatrics. PROS LAND Study. Available at: www.aap.org/pros/landmain.htm. Accessed February 24, 2004

Injury Risk of Nonpowder Guns

- *Technical Report*

AMERICAN ACADEMY OF PEDIATRICS

TECHNICAL REPORT

Danielle Laraque, MD, and the Committee on Injury, Violence, and Poison Prevention

Injury Risk of Nonpowder Guns

ABSTRACT. Nonpowder guns (ball-bearing [BB] guns, pellet guns, air rifles, paintball guns) continue to cause serious injuries to children and adolescents. The muzzle velocity of these guns can range from approximately 150 ft/second to 1200 ft/second (the muzzle velocities of traditional firearm pistols are 750 ft/second to 1450 ft/second). Both low- and high-velocity nonpowder guns are associated with serious injuries, and fatalities can result from high-velocity guns. A persisting problem is the lack of medical recognition of the severity of injuries that can result from these guns, including penetration of the eye, skin, internal organs, and bone. Nationally, in 2000, there were an estimated 21840 (coefficient of variation: 0.0821) injuries related to nonpowder guns, with approximately 4% resulting in hospitalization. Between 1990 and 2000, the US Consumer Product Safety Commission reported 39 nonpowder gun–related deaths, of which 32 were children younger than 15 years. The introduction of high-powered air rifles in the 1970s has been associated with approximately 4 deaths per year. The advent of war games and the use of paintball guns have resulted in a number of reports of injuries, especially to the eye. Injuries associated with nonpowder guns should receive prompt medical management similar to the management of firearm-related injuries, and nonpowder guns should never be characterized as toys. *Pediatrics* 2004;114:1357–1361; *nonpowder guns, BB guns, pellet guns, air rifles, paintball guns.*

ABBREVIATIONS. BB, ball bearing; CPSC, US Consumer Product Safety Commission; NEISS, National Electronic Injury Surveillance System; EPD, eye-protective device; ASTM, American Society for Testing and Materials.

BACKGROUND

A traditional firearm gun is one that launches a projectile (ie, a bullet) by using the energy generated by burning of gunpowder. Nonpowder guns utilize the power of compressed air to launch a projectile. Nonpowder guns can be classified by the type of projectile they fire, the propulsion mechanism, or the type of barrel.[1–4] The type of projectile can be lead, brass, steel, copper, or, most recently, a paintball. Paintballs are small gelatin projectiles that are 17 mm in diameter, filled with nontoxic, water-soluble paint, and intended to explode on contact with an object.[5,6] This type of projectile is

used in war games designed to mark the player with paint when he or she is hit. Air guns have been used since the 16th century[7,8] in warfare and to kill game as large as deer.

The caliber of a projectile refers to its diameter and is measured in hundredths of an inch or millimeters. The caliber affects how much energy the projectile acquires before leaving the muzzle, or the end of the barrel. Tight-fitting missiles, those with little discrepancy between the diameter of the projectile and that of the muzzle, lead to higher velocities. In older nonpowder guns, the projectile was smaller than the barrel size, leading to dissipating of compressed air and an inefficient, low-velocity gun. Technical modifications of these guns have resulted in higher-velocity weapons.[9] Standard pellet guns fire a pellet or spherical ball bearing (BB) with a diameter of less than 0.18 in (4.57 mm). Pellets have several designs, such as wad cutter, sharp pointed, round nosed, and hollow point. Each is suited for a different purpose. Hollow points are used for hunting, and the pellet's diameter increases on impact to cause maximum damage. Ballistic studies have shown that a larger caliber pellet will penetrate the body (eg, skin, bone) at lower velocities because of its increased mass. Skin penetration can be achieved, for example, at a velocity of approximately 331 ft/second with a 0.177-caliber pellet but at 245 ft/second with a 0.22-caliber pellet. Ocular penetration can occur at velocities as low as 130 ft/second.[7,10] Polishing steel pellets with a plastic skirt increases velocity, accuracy, and range and is designed to increase penetration. Typically, high-velocity guns are classified as those with muzzle velocities higher than 350 ft/second (D. Tinsworth, MS, US Consumer Product Safety Commission [CPSC], written communication, November 26, 2001).[7,9,11–13]

Projectiles can be fired by 3 propulsion mechanisms. The spring-piston type is a powerful spring that is cocked manually and released, driving the piston that shoots a stream of air. Use of the spring-piston can result in muzzle velocities between 250 and 350 ft/second. The carbon dioxide–powered gun uses a gas cartridge to generate a propulsive force that can produce muzzle velocities of 350 to 450 ft/second. Muzzle velocities ranging, on average, from 300 to 950 ft/second can be generated depending on the number of times the weapon is pumped, although velocities in excess of 1200 ft/second have been reported in the literature. This range of velocity

The guidance in this report does not indicate an exclusive course of treatment or serve as a standard of medical care. Variations, taking into account individual circumstances, may be appropriate.

doi:10.1542/peds.2004-1799

PEDIATRICS (ISSN 0031 4005). Copyright © 2004 by the American Academy of Pediatrics.

overlaps velocities reached by traditional firearm pistols that have muzzle velocities from 750 ft/second to 1450 ft/second.[1,3,9]

The longer the gun barrel is, the higher the velocity. Gun barrels can be smooth or rifled. Rifled weapons produce a spin in the projectile, giving it more stability in flight. Dieseling of the barrel is achieved when oil placed in the barrel is combusted by the heat generated from friction, leading to an explosion. This is used to increase the speed of the projectile. Piggybacking entails simultaneously loading 2 pellets into the firing chamber, increasing the momentum and energy of the missile.[9] A "zip gun" is a modified gun using homemade powder ammunition.[8] These modifications of nonpowder guns can result in increased ability of these guns to cause serious injury, not unlike traditional powder guns.

EXPOSURE AND INJURY PROFILE

The CPSC estimates that there are approximately 3.2 million nonpowder guns sold yearly.[12–14] Nonpowder guns are sold in many department stores, including toy stores.[9] Eighty percent have muzzle velocities over 350 ft/second, and 50% have muzzle velocities between 500 and 930 ft/second. In 2000, the National Electronic Injury Surveillance System (NEISS), operated by the CPSC, collected information from a nationally representative sample of 100 US hospital emergency departments that included information on nonpowder gun injuries.

According to data from the Centers for Disease Control and Prevention (http://webapp.cdc.gov/sasweb/ncipc/nfirates.html and www.cdc.gov/ncipc/wisqars/nonfatal/datasources.htm) and the CPSC,[12] in 2000 the overall nonfatal age-adjusted rate of injury from BB or pellet guns was 7.71 per 100000 population. In 2000, there were an estimated 21840 (coefficient of variation: 0.0821) nonpowder gun–related injuries treated in emergency departments (D. Tinsworth, MS, CPSC, written communication, November 26, 2001). Of these, 2% occurred in children 0 to 4 years of age; 49% occurred in children 5 to 14 years of age; 33% occurred in those 15 to 24 years of age; and the balance occurred in adults 25 years and older. Approximately 12% of injuries were to the eye; 24% were to the head and neck, excluding the eye; 63% were to extremities; and 1% were to other body areas. With the exception of the age group of 0 to 4 years, most victims were males. Sixty-six percent of injuries were diagnosed as either foreign-body lodgments or puncture wounds. There were no clear seasonal variations in the injury incidence. Nguyen et al[15] provided a review of trends in BB or pellet gun injuries in children and adolescents in the United States from 1985 to 1999 derived from a special study using the NEISS, which focused specifically on injuries associated with penetrating gunshot wounds. On the basis of data from this study, in 1999 an estimated 14313 (95% confidence interval: 12025-16601) children and adolescents had BB or pellet gun–related injuries.

Many articles have been written detailing the clinical manifestations of children injured by nonpowder guns.[3–10,16–31] Some striking observations have been made. Lawrence[3] reported on a series of 10 fatalities, 1 of which was a shot through the medial canthus of the eye in a 6-year-old. The weapon was a carbon dioxide–powered BB pistol. Bond et al[10] described 16 children, 57% of whom required intraoperative treatment, and 19% of whom required other invasive procedures such as arteriogram or ventriculostomy. Thoracic injuries were associated with high morbidity and mortality when penetration of the chest wall occurred. Abdominal wounds were frequently associated with visceral injury and multiple perforations, usually of the small bowel. Peritoneal penetration was associated with a more than 80% chance of visceral injury. Transtracheal and brain injuries were also reported. These authors warn that the wound itself may seem trivial, but if not appreciated for their potential for tissue disruption, nonpowder gun injuries to the head, chest, and abdomen may have catastrophic results. They also note that the pellets from air guns have a propensity to embolize if the missile enters a blood vessel or the heart. The light weight of air gun pellets allows the missile to be swept by the blood flow more readily than heavier, higher-energy projectiles. Friedman et al[7] report that the potential seriousness of pneumatic weapon injury is frequently underestimated. These authors concluded that injuries from air guns should be treated in a manner similar to those from low-velocity powder firearms. Bratton et al[4] reviewed the clinical course of 101 children injured by nonpowder guns between 1988 and 1996 from Cincinnati, Ohio; Kansas City, Missouri; and Seattle, Washington. The case fatality rate for intracranial injuries was 30%, and 56% of patients required at least 1 surgical procedure. Amirjamshidi et al[16] noted that air-gun pellet injuries are rare but catastrophic, with entrance usually through the orbit or the neck and the entry wound being so small that it may be disregarded on physical examination in the emergency department. They concluded that early recognition and correct management of possible complications is important to improve outcomes. Bhattacharyya et al[17] reported on 42 children admitted to a level I pediatric trauma center for air-gun injuries over a 7-year period (1988-1995). They had a mean hospital stay of 7 days (range: 1-136 days) and a mean injury severity score of 8.3. Half of the children underwent operative procedures, and 38% had serious long-term disability. They concluded that these guns are not toys but are weapons, and injuries related to their use should be evaluated and managed in a similar fashion to powder-weapon injuries. These findings were similar to those of Walsh et al.[18] In 1 study, the predominant risk factors for ocular injury from an air gun were lack of adult supervision, use of the gun for a purpose other than target practice, and being at a friend's home or yard.[20] Hearing loss has been reported from nonpowder gun use,[23] and suicides from the use of air guns have been documented.[8,28] Concurrent use of alcohol has been noted also and probably contributes to misuse.

Paintballs used in war games are a relatively new phenomenon.[5,6,21,25] Semiautomatic and fully automatic paintball pistols are available for purchase. The sport typically involves a team, designated fields, and referees used to ensure fair and "safe" play. Players should be 18 years and older, but younger adolescents are allowed to play with the consent of their parent(s). Private games also occur. The players often wear camouflage, and start-up costs for the weapon, goggles, and paintballs total $100 to $150. The paintballs consist of spherical shells filled with sorbitol, glycol, and food dye. The propulsion mechanism is usually a carbon dioxide canister, and muzzle velocities between 60 and 250 ft/second can be achieved. Given the size of the projectile, the resulting injuries are nonpenetrating. Locally manufactured paintballs are harder than the more expensive imported varieties and may be responsible for the severity of injuries reported in the United States. Importantly, the increasing popularity of war games has been associated with a number of reports in the literature of ocular injuries. These injuries have included but are not limited to hyphemas, commotio retinae, glaucoma, cataracts, choroidal rupture, corneal abrasion, conjunctival laceration, dislocation of the crystalline lens, macular hole, and retinal detachments.[5,6,25,32,33] The visual outcome for many of these injuries is poor. Injuries have occurred even with eye-protective devices (EPDs), but no case of a player injured while properly wearing an EPD meeting the current American Society for Testing and Materials (ASTM) standards has been reported.[6] Some players have sustained injuries to the eye when they have removed their goggles because of fogging. Current antifog inserts with a polycarbonate lens with a urethane-based hydroscopic coating can help prevent fogging. The current ASTM specifications do not involve testing EPDs for their ability to resist fogging but do require manufacturers to attach a warning to EPDs without antifog treatment noting that fogging may occur and recommending the use of an antifog solution. There have been no reported deaths directly related to paintballs, but the CPSC issued a warning on March 24, 2004, because of its investigation of 2 deaths caused by carbon dioxide canisters flying off paintball guns (www.cpsc.gov/CPSCPUB/PREREL/prhtml04/04105.html).

Before 1972, only 2 nonpowder gun–related fatalities were reported in the literature. However, between 1972 and 1982, the decade after the introduction of high-powered air rifles, 10 more fatalities were recorded by the CPSC.[10] The number of deaths per year has increased since then. From 1990 to 2000, the CPSC reported 39 nonpowder gun–related deaths, of which 32 were children younger than 15 years, with an average of 4 deaths per year.[11] The highest number of deaths occurred in 1989, 1990, and 1991.[15] The trends in nonpowder gun fatalities and nonfatal injuries parallel the epidemic of firearm-related injuries and deaths of the past 2 decades.[34]

SAFETY STANDARDS

An ASTM voluntary safety standard was originally published in 1978. The current edition was published in December 1992 (ASTM F589, Standard Consumer Safety Specification for Non-Powder Guns).[35] This standard contains performance requirements to ensure the proper functioning of these products as well as provisions to address instructions, labeling, and marketing. The guns are general-purpose guns not classified as precision, adult, or training guns. For higher-power guns, the minimum labeled age is 16 years, and the potential for serious injury or death is indicated. For lower-power guns, the minimum labeled age is 10 years, and the risk of serious injury, particularly to the eye, is indicated, but not the risk of death. In the pediatric literature as early as 1984, Christoffel et al[36,37] pointed to the dangers of nonpowder guns, noting that they were loosely regulated and could be legally purchased by young adolescents in most jurisdictions. They also emphasized the inadequacy of voluntary standards and proposed stricter regulations.

From June 1 through July 31, 1994, the CPSC conducted a limited study using follow-up telephone investigation of the circumstances of 55 cases of nonpowder gun–related injuries reported to the NEISS. Percentages provided in the analysis were based on national estimates projected from the 55 cases for the 2 months of the survey. Additionally, information on deaths was obtained from the CPSC Death Certificate, In-Depth Investigation, and Injury or Potential Injury Incident files for the period of January 1, 1985, through September 1, 1994. Information on 37 deaths was included (D. Tinsworth, MS, CPSC, written communication, November 26, 2001). Respondents were victims or parents or guardians of victims. The injury epidemiology mirrored that described for the 2000 data, with most injuries occurring in males younger than 16 years. Individuals who fired the guns ranged in age from 8 to 32 years, with most reported to be younger than 16 years. When the gun operator was younger than 16 years, there was no one 18 years or older present at the time of the incident in more than two thirds of the cases. The gun was most often reported to be a rifle and received as a gift, and two thirds were high-powered guns. As reported by the respondents, 51% of the hazard patterns were unintentional shootings, with victims coming into the line of fire during practice, discharges during loading of the gun, or incidents in which the gun "accidentally fired." Fourteen percent were of unknown intent, 7% were intentional shootings, and 28% involved a gun thought to be unloaded, guns that discharged unexpectedly, ammunition that ricocheted, or fingers that became pinched in gun components. Ninety percent of those who died were younger than 16 years. Most fatalities resulted from wounds to the head or chest.

The CPSC report concluded that the effectiveness of age-specific warnings on packaging and instructions needed additional study and that adult supervision was often lacking. It was unclear from the data whether product modification to reduce hazards would be effective.

LEGISLATIVE EFFORTS

Almost 30 states have regulations, ordinances, or laws covering nonpowder guns.[9,38] Two of the strongest are in New York City and New York State. In New York City, air rifles and BB guns are prohibited, and licenses are not available. In New York State, no purchase or unsupervised use by someone younger than 16 years is permitted, and adult supervision is required at a shooting range or when hunting for someone of this age. Florida also has a strong law similar to the New York State law. In Florida, it is a second-degree misdemeanor for a minor younger than 16 years to use a BB gun, air gun, or gas-operated gun unless an adult is supervising the possession and the minor's parent has consented to such possession.

However, much variability exists, with some states regarding nonpowder guns as firearms and others not.[15] Some state laws do not address nonpowder guns at all. Many authors have called for restrictions in sales and use of nonpowder guns, especially in light of the technologic advances that have resulted in much more powerful and dangerous weapons that are capable of killing and maiming.[9,19,31,39]

SUMMARY/CONCLUSIONS

This technical report is focused mainly on the potential for injury and death associated with the use of nonpowder guns. Although some comments have been made on risk factors for injury, this report is not meant to be an exhaustive review of the behavioral risk factors for injury, nor does the report summarize the literature regarding the psychological implications or effects of the use of these weapons. The data presented do allow the following conclusions:

- Nonpowder guns pose a serious risk of injury, permanent disability, and even death.
- Since the 1980s, the use of high-powered air rifles has been associated with approximately 4 deaths per year.
- The range of muzzle velocities for nonpowder guns overlaps velocities reached by traditional firearms.
- Data suggest that lack of supervision and unstructured use may be risk factors contributing to the incidence of injury from nonpowder guns.
- EPDs can be useful in decreasing, but not fully eliminating, the incidence of ocular injuries associated with paintball use.
- Injuries associated with nonpowder guns should receive prompt medical management similar to the management of firearm-related injuries.
- Nonpowder guns (BB guns, pellet guns, air rifles, paintball guns) are weapons and should never be characterized as toys.

COMMITTEE ON INJURY, VIOLENCE, AND POISON
    PREVENTION, 2002–2003
Marilyn J. Bull, MD, Chairperson
Phyllis Agran, MD, MPH
M. Denise Dowd, MD, MPH
Victor Garcia, MD
H. Garry Gardner, MD
Gary A. Smith, MD, DrPH
Milton Tenenbein, MD
Jeffrey C. Weiss, MD
Joseph L. Wright, MD, MPH

LIAISONS
Ruth A. Brenner, MD
    National Institute of Child Health and
    Human Development
Stephanie Bryn, MPH
    Health Resources and Services
    Administration/Maternal and Child Health
    Bureau
Richard A. Schieber, MD, MPH
    Centers for Disease Control and Prevention
Alexander (Sandy) Sinclair
    National Highway Traffic Safety
    Administration
Deborah Tinsworth
    US Consumer Product Safety Commission
Lynne J. Warda, MD
    Canadian Paediatric Society

STAFF
Rebecca Levin-Goodman, MPH

REFERENCES

1. Karlson TA, Hargarten SW. *Reducing Firearm Injury and Death: A Public Health Sourcebook on Guns.* New Brunswick, NJ: Rutgers University Press; 1997
2. Milne JS, Hargarten SW, Withers RL. *A Glossary of Handgun and Handgun Safety Terminology.* Milwaukee, WI: Firearm Injury Center, Department of Emergency Medicine, Medical College of Wisconsin; 1997
3. Lawrence HS. Fatal nonpowder firearm wounds: case report and review of the literature. *Pediatrics.* 1990;85:177–181
4. Bratton SL, Dowd MD, Brogan TV, Hegenbarth MA. Serious and fatal air gun injuries: more than meets the eye. *Pediatrics.* 1997;100:609–612
5. Fineman MS, Fischer DH, Jeffers JB, Buerger DG, Repke C. Changing trends in paintball sport-related ocular injuries. *Arch Ophthalmol.* 2000;118:60–64
6. Wrenn KD, White SJ. Injury potential in "paintball" combat simulation games: a report of two cases. *Am J Emerg Med.* 1991;9:402–404
7. Friedman D, Hammond J, Cardone J, Sutyak J. The air gun: toy or weapon? *South Med J.* 1996;89:475–478
8. Milroy CM, Clark JC, Carter N, Rutty G, Rooney N. Air weapon fatalities. *J Clin Pathol.* 1998;51:525–529
9. Naude GP, Bongard FS. From deadly weapon to toy and back again: the danger of air rifles. *J Trauma.* 1996;41:1039–1043
10. Bond SJ, Schnier GC, Miller FB. Air-powered guns: too much firepower to be a toy. *J Trauma.* 1996;41:674–678
11. Tinsworth DK, Cassidy SP. *Injuries and Deaths Involving Non-Powder Guns.* Washington, DC: US Consumer Product Safety Commission, Division of Hazard Analysis Directorate for Epidemiology; 1994
12. Consumer Product Safety Commission. BB guns can kill. Available at: www.cpsc.gov/cpscpub/pubs/5089.html. Accessed November 12, 2003
13. The HELP Network. *HELP Fact Sheet: Non-Powder Gun Injuries.* Chicago, IL: The HELP Network. Available at: www.helpnetwork.org/frames/resources_factsheets_nonpowder.html. Accessed November 12, 2003
14. Centers for Disease Control and Prevention. BB and pellet gun-related injuries—United States, June 1992-May 1994. *MMWR Morb Mortal Wkly Rep.* 1995;44:909–913
15. Nguyen MH, Annest JL, Mercy JA, Ryan GW, Fingerhut LA. Trends in BB/pellet gun injuries in children and teenagers in the United States, 1985–99. *Inj Prev.* 2002;8:185–191
16. Amirjamshidi A, Abbassioun K, Roosbeh H. Air-gun pellet injuries to the head and neck. *Surg Neurol.* 1997;47:331–338
17. Bhattacharyya N, Bethel CA, Caniano DA, Pillai SB, Deppe S, Cooney DR. The childhood air gun: serious injuries and surgical interventions. *Pediatr Emerg Care.* 1998;14:188–190
18. Walsh IR, Eberhart A, Knapp JF, Sharma V. Pediatric gunshot wounds—powder and nonpowder weapons. *Pediatr Emerg Care.* 1988;4:279–283
19. DeCou JM, Abrams RS, Miller RS, Touloukian RJ, Gauderer MW. Life-threatening air rifle injuries to the heart in three boys. *J Pediatr Surg.* 2000;35:785–787

20. Enger C, Schein OD, Tielsch JM. Risk factors for ocular injuries caused by air guns. *Arch Ophthalmol.* 1996;114:469–474

21. Farr AK, Fekrat S. Eye injuries associated with paintball guns. *Int Ophthalmol.* 1998–99;22:169–173

22. Ford EG, Senac MO Jr, McGrath N. It may be more significant than you think: BB air rifle injury to a child's head. *Pediatr Emerg Care.* 1990;6: 278–279

23. Gupta D, Vishwakarma SK. Toy weapons and firecrackers: a source of hearing loss. *Laryngoscope.* 1989;99:330–334

24. Kitchens JW, Danis RP. Increasing paintball related eye trauma reported to a state eye injury registry. *Inj Prev.* 1999;5:301–302

25. Kruger LP, Acton JK. Paintball ocular injuries. *S Afr Med J.* 1999;89: 265–268

26. Lamb RK, Pawade A, Prior AL. Intravascular missile: apparent retrograde course from the left ventricle. *Thorax.* 1988;43:499–500

27. Mamalis N, Monson MC, Farnsworth ST, White GL Jr. Blunt ocular trauma secondary to "war games." *Ann Ophthalmol.* 1990;22:416–418

28. Pottker TI, Dowd MD, Howard J, DiGiulio G. Suicide with an air rifle. *Ann Emerg Med.* 1997;29:818–820

29. Radhakrishnan J, Fernandez L, Geissler G. Air rifles—lethal weapons. *J Pediatr Surg.* 1996;31:1407–1408

30. Senturia YD, Binns HJ, Christoffel KK, Tanz RR. In-office survey of children's hazard exposure in the Chicago area: age-specific exposure information and methodological lessons. Pediatric Practice Research Group. *J Dev Behav Pediatr.* 1993;14:169–175

31. Shanon A, Feldman W. Serious childhood injuries caused by air guns. *CMAJ.* 1991;144:723–725

32. Karel I, Pitrova S, Lestak J, Zahlava J. Eye injury from a paintball projectile[in Czechoslovakian]. *Cesk Slov Oftalmol.* 2002;58:171–175

33. Thach AB, Ward TP, Hollifield RD, et al. Ocular injuries from paintball pellets. *Ophthalmology.* 1999;106:533–537

34. American Academy of Pediatrics, Committee on Injury and Poison Prevention. Firearm-related injuries affecting the pediatric population. *Pediatrics.* 2000;105:888–895

35. American Society for Testing and Materials, Committee on Standards. *Standard Consumer Safety Specification for Non-Powder Guns.* Conshohocken, PA: American Society for Testing and Materials; 1992

36. Christoffel KK, Tanz R, Sagerman S, Hahn Y. Childhood injuries by nonpowder firearms. *Am J Dis Child.* 1984;138:557–561

37. Christoffel T, Christoffel K. Nonpowder firearm injuries: whose job is it to protect children? *Am J Public Health.* 1987;77:735–738

38. Department of Treasury Bureau of Alcohol, Tobacco and Firearms. *State Laws and Published Ordinances—Firearms.* 22nd ed. Available at: www.atf.gov/firearms/statelaws/22edition.htm. Accessed November 12, 2003

39. Sharif KW, McGhee CN, Tomlinson RC. Ocular trauma caused by air-gun pellets: a ten year survey. *Eye.* 1990;4:855–860

All technical reports from the American Academy of Pediatrics automatically expire 5 years after publication unless reaffirmed, revised, or retired at or before that time.

Legalization of Marijuana: Potential Impact on Youth

- *Policy Statement*
- *Technical Report*

AMERICAN ACADEMY OF PEDIATRICS

POLICY STATEMENT
Organizational Principles to Guide and Define the Child Health Care System and/or Improve the Health of All Children

Committee on Substance Abuse and Committee on Adolescence

Legalization of Marijuana: Potential Impact on Youth

ABSTRACT. As experts in the health care of children and adolescents, pediatricians may be called on to advise legislators concerning the potential impact of changes in the legal status of marijuana on adolescents. Parents, too, may look to pediatricians for advice as they consider whether to support state-level initiatives that propose to legalize the use of marijuana for medical purposes or to decriminalize possession of small amounts of marijuana. This policy statement provides the position of the American Academy of Pediatrics on the issue of marijuana legalization, and the accompanying technical report (available online) reviews what is currently known about the relationship between adolescents' use of marijuana and its legal status to better understand how change might influence the degree of marijuana use by adolescents in the future. *Pediatrics* 2004;113:1825–1826; *marijuana, legalization, substance abuse, decriminalization.*

INTRODUCTION

Substance abuse by adolescents is an ongoing concern of pediatricians. Marijuana is the illicit substance most commonly abused by adolescents.[1] Any change in the legal status of marijuana, even if limited to adults, could affect the prevalence of use among adolescents.[2] For example, tobacco and alcohol products, both legal for adults 18 and 21 years of age, respectively, are the psychoactive substances most widely abused by adolescents.

Marijuana currently is classified by the US Drug Enforcement Agency as a schedule I drug, which means that it has a high potential for abuse, has no currently accepted medical use in the United States, and lacks accepted safety for use under supervision by a physician. Rigorous scientific research to determine whether marijuana, especially cannabinoids, has any potential therapeutic effect is just beginning. In contrast, the significant neuropharmacologic, cognitive, behavioral, and somatic consequences of acute and long-term marijuana use are well known and include negative effects on short-term memory, concentration, attention span, motivation, and problem solving, which clearly interfere with learning; adverse effects on coordination, judgment, reaction time, and tracking ability, which contribute substantially to unintentional deaths and injuries among adolescents (especially those associated with motor vehicles); and negative health effects with repeated use similar to effects seen with smoking tobacco.[3]

More information, including historical perspectives on the legal status of marijuana as well as concerns surrounding medicinal use of marijuana, is available in the accompanying technical report (available online).[2]

RECOMMENDATIONS

1. The American Academy of Pediatrics opposes the legalization of marijuana.
2. The American Academy of Pediatrics supports rigorous scientific research regarding the use of cannabinoids for the relief of symptoms not currently ameliorated by existing legal drug formulations.

COMMITTEE ON SUBSTANCE ABUSE, 2001–2002
Edward A. Jacobs, MD, Chairperson
*Alain Joffe, MD, MPH
John R. Knight, MD
John Kulig, MD, MPH
Peter D. Rogers, MD, MPH
Janet F. Williams, MD

LIAISON
Deborah Simkin, MD
   American Academy of Child and Adolescent Psychiatry

STAFF
Karen S. Smith

COMMITTEE ON ADOLESCENCE, 2001–2002
David W. Kaplan, MD, MPH, Chairperson
Angela Diaz, MD
Ronald A. Feinstein, MD
Martin M. Fisher, MD
Jonathan D. Klein, MD, MPH
Ellen S. Rome, MD, MPH
*W. Samuel Yancy, MD

LIAISONS
Ann J. Davis, MD
   American College of Obstetricians and Gynecologists
Glen Pearson, MD
   American Academy of Child and Adolescent Psychiatry
Jean-Yves Frappier, MD
   Canadian Paediatric Society

STAFF
Karen S. Smith

Lead authors

REFERENCES

1. Schydlower M. Preface. In: Schydlower M, ed. *Substance Abuse: A Guide for Health Professionals*. 2nd ed. Elk Grove Village, IL: American Academy of Pediatrics; 2002:viii–x
2. American Academy of Pediatrics, Committee on Substance Abuse and Committee on Adolescence. Technical report: legalization of marijuana: potential impact on youth. *Pediatrics*. 2004;113(6). Available at: www.pediatrics.org/cgi/content/full/113/6/e632
3. American Academy of Pediatrics, Committee on Substance Abuse. Marijuana: a continuing concern for pediatricians. *Pediatrics*. 1999;104: 982–985

All policy statements from the American Academy of Pediatrics automatically expire 5 years after publication unless reaffirmed, revised, or retired at or before that time.

AMERICAN ACADEMY OF PEDIATRICS

TECHNICAL REPORT

Alain Joffe, MD, MPH, and W. Samuel Yancy, MD, the Committee on Substance Abuse
and Committee on Adolescence

Legalization of Marijuana: Potential Impact on Youth

ABSTRACT. This technical report provides historical perspectives and comparisons of various approaches to the legal status of marijuana to aid in forming public policy. Information on the impact that decriminalization and legalization of marijuana could have on adolescents, in addition to concerns surrounding medicinal use of marijuana, are also addressed in this report. Recommendations are included in the accompanying policy statement. *Pediatrics* 2004;113:e632–e638. URL: http://www.pediatrics.org/cgi/content/full/113/6/e632; *marijuana, legalization, substance abuse, decriminalization.*

ABBREVIATIONS. AAP, American Academy of Pediatrics; IOM, Institute of Medicine.

BACKGROUND

Over the last 40 years, the legal status of marijuana has been debated vigorously. Proponents of policies that would permit individual possession of small amounts of marijuana argue that it is a safe drug and that criminal sanctions against personal use and possession represent at worst excessively harsh and at best unnecessary penalties. Echoing these sentiments, editors of *The Lancet* have concluded that "cannabis per se is not a hazard to society but driving it further underground may well be."[1] Advocates for legalization also point out that the morbidity, mortality, and economic costs to society associated with alcohol and tobacco use in the United States dwarf those associated with marijuana use.

Those opposing liberalization of current laws counter that marijuana is not a benign drug, especially in light of new psychopharmacologic information demonstrating that marijuana shares many features with other illicit drugs. They also contend that legalization or decriminalization of personal use of marijuana likely would trigger a substantial increase in use, with foreseeable increases in the social, economic, and health costs.

Most recently, the debate has focused on the medical use of marijuana (that is, the use of smoked marijuana to treat a variety of medical conditions). Eight states (Alaska, Arizona, California, Colorado, Maine, Nevada, Oregon, and Washington) have

passed ballot initiatives that provide for medical use of marijuana under certain circumstances; one other state (Hawaii) has enacted state legislation permitting medical marijuana use.[2] The federal government has opposed vigorously any efforts to permit physicians to prescribe marijuana for medical purposes, an approach characterized by the former editor of the *New England Journal of Medicine* as "misguided, heavy-handed, and inhumane."[3]

Controversy regarding marijuana is not limited to the United States. Australia has decriminalized the use of marijuana in some territories, and Canada[4] as well as Switzerland and other European countries[5] are reconsidering their approach to marijuana. However, the most widely publicized approach to regulation of marijuana is that of The Netherlands. Under a complex system of "law-on-the-books" and "law-in-action," Dutch law permits personal use of marijuana but outlaws possession.[6]

Pediatricians, too, are not of one mind in their views regarding the legal status of marijuana. In a periodic survey of fellows of the American Academy of Pediatrics (AAP) conducted in 1995,[7] only a minority (18%) favored legalization, and 26% believed that possession or sale should be a felony; 31% felt that marijuana should be available by prescription for medical purposes to a certain class of patients, and 24% believed that marijuana should remain illegal but penalties for personal possession should be reduced or eliminated.

Since the periodic survey was conducted, much more has been learned about the psychopharmacologic properties of marijuana. Scientists have demonstrated that the emotional stress caused by withdrawal from marijuana is linked to corticotropin-releasing factor, the same brain chemical that has been linked to anxiety and stress during opiate, alcohol, and cocaine withdrawal.[8] Others report that tetrahydrocannabinol, the active ingredient in marijuana, stimulates release of dopamine in the mesolimbic area of the brain, the same neurochemical process that reinforces dependence on other addictive drugs.[9] Current scientific information about marijuana has been summarized in the AAP policy statement "Marijuana: A Continuing Concern for Pediatricians."[10] Some of the significant neuropharmacologic, cognitive, behavioral, and somatic consequences of acute and long-term marijuana use are well known and include negative effects on short-term memory, concentration, attention span, motivation, and problem solving, which clearly interfere with learning; adverse effects on coordination, judgment, reaction time, and tracking ability, which contribute substantially to unintentional deaths and injuries among adolescents (especially those associated with motor vehicles); and negative health effects with repeated use similar to effects seen with smoking tobacco. Three recent studies[11-13] demonstrate an association between marijuana use and the subsequent development of mental health problems; however, a small study of 56 monozygotic cotwins discordant for marijuana use did not find any such associations.[14]

DEFINITION OF TERMS

There are 3 general policy perspectives concerning the status of marijuana in the United States: prohibition, decriminalization, and legalization. Prohibition describes current federal policy toward marijuana use, which seeks to minimize or prevent use of marijuana with strong legal sanctions and aggressive interdiction of supply routes. Decriminalization and depenalization (used interchangeably in this report) refer to the elimination, reduction, and/or nonenforcement of penalties for the sale, purchase, or possession of marijuana although such activities remain illegal. Under decriminalization, penalties for use or distribution are at least possible theoretically, and advertising would be banned. Legalization, one step beyond decriminalization, would fundamentally change the status of marijuana in society. It is an acknowledgment that the government has no fundamental interest in an individual's use of a drug, although it may still seek to regulate its sale, distribution, use, and advertisement to safeguard the public's health. Such is the case with alcohol and tobacco. Of the 3 approaches, only the prohibitionist approach has reducing or limiting drug use as its explicit goal.

HISTORICAL PERSPECTIVES ON DRUG POLICIES IN THE UNITED STATES

Important perspectives on how changing the status of marijuana could affect use by adolescents can be gleaned from an examination of this country's experience with drugs over the last 200 years. During the 19th century, opiate drugs were legal and widely available. Opium use was common, especially among middle-class white women.[15] Use of morphine also was extensive, and heroin was marketed as a "sedative for coughs." Cocaine, which routinely was added to patent medicines and beverages, also was legal; it was prized for its local anesthetic effect and its ability to counteract the effects of morphine. The national opiate addiction rate increased from 0.72 per 1000 in 1840 to 4.59 per 1000 in the 1890s, thereafter beginning a sustained decline.[16(p28)]

Another wave of drug use began in the mid-1960s as enforcement of marijuana laws by police became lax and adolescent and layperson perceptions of the risk of regular use declined. Officials from the US Drug Enforcement Agency expressed the view that the fight against marijuana detracted from the more important work of combating heroin use.[16(p174)] Drug incarcerations per 1000 arrests began to drop in 1960 and remained low through 1979. The Carter administration (1977–1981) proposed removing criminal sanctions for possessing small amounts of marijuana.[16(p175)] In 1975, 6% of high school seniors reported using marijuana daily during the previous 30 days. By 1978, the same year during which perceived risk of regular use of marijuana reached its lowest point ever, 10.7% of high school seniors reported using the drug daily.[17]

Drug use in America tends to follow cycles, often with one generation having to relearn the experiences of previous ones. Ninety years after the first cocaine epidemic, cocaine use began to increase in the 1970s and escalated substantially from 1980 to 1995. Because it had been so long since the previous epidemic, cocaine was perceived to be a safe drug. In a chapter on cocaine in the 1980 edition of a prominent textbook of psychiatry, the authors wrote: "If it is used no more than two or three times a week, cocaine creates no serious problems."[18] In 1977, 10% of 18- to 25-year-olds had used cocaine; that proportion doubled to 20% in 1979. By 1985, one third of 18- to 25-year-olds had used cocaine, as had 17.3% of 12th graders.[15] Only with subsequent widespread publicity about the health risks and addictive properties of cocaine and the epidemic of crack cocaine did cocaine use among young people begin to wane.

US AND INTERNATIONAL EXPERIENCES WITH MARIJUANA LEGALIZATION AND DEPENALIZATION

Because to our knowledge no country has completely legalized the sale, possession, and advertising of marijuana, there are no studies that examine the effect of legalization on marijuana use by young people. Hence, we examine data on adolescents' use of marijuana in states and countries that have, to a greater or lesser extent, decriminalized use and possession of this drug.

Analyzing data from the annual Monitoring the Future survey, Johnston et al[19] concluded that decriminalization of marijuana in a number of states from 1975 to 1980 apparently had no effect on high school students' beliefs and attitudes about marijuana or on their use of the drug during those years. In contrast, Chaloupka et al,[20] analyzing data from the 1992–1994 Monitoring the Future surveys, found that "youths living in decriminalized states are significantly more likely to report currently using marijuana and may consume more frequently."

There are several possible explanations for these disparate findings. Although the study by Johnston et al did not find any effect of decriminalization, baseline marijuana use was higher in states that changed their laws compared with states that did not, although the subsequent rate of increase in all states was the same. It is possible that the higher baseline rates of use in the states that decriminalized marijuana use may have reflected a more lax or tolerant approach to marijuana use before decriminalization. Hence, decriminalization would not have resulted in any significant lessening of enforcement, and the observed rate of increase would parallel but not exceed changes in the states that did not alter their laws. Also, because the Monitoring the Future survey is administered in schools, any effect of decriminalization on marijuana use by out-of-school youth (who typically have higher levels of drug use[21]) would not have been reflected.

An additional explanation is provided by a recent analysis of marijuana decriminalization laws in the United States by Pacula et al.[22] They found that some states that are viewed as having decriminalized marijuana use have in fact retained a first-time marijuana offense as a criminal offense. In addition, many states that are characterized as not having decriminalized laws pertaining to marijuana use specify first-time marijuana possession offenses as noncriminal. These same authors found that youth living in states that lowered offenses for marijuana possession to below the felony level were more likely to report use of marijuana in the past month.[22]

Several territories in Australia have decriminalized use of marijuana. Studies comparing use in these territories with use in those that did not reduce penalties found no appreciable differences in use.[23,24]

The most widely scrutinized large-scale change in the legal status of marijuana occurred in The Netherlands. Dutch policy regarding decriminalization is very complex. Use of illegal drugs per se is not punishable by law, but possession for use is; drug dealing also is considered a felony.[25] Theoretically, one can be imprisoned for up to 1 month for possession of 5 g or less of cannabis, and promotion of marijuana through advertisements is forbidden also.

From 1984 to 1996, the period during which Dutch prosecution of marijuana-related offenses became virtually nonexistent, marijuana use increased consistently and substantially until 1992 while decreasing or remaining stable in other countries.[26,27] Among 18- to 20-year-olds, the proportion who reported ever having used marijuana increased from 15% to 44%, and the proportion who reported using it within the previous 30 days increased from 8.5% to 18.5%. Use among adolescents in the United States decreased steadily from 1979 to 1992. In Norway, which also forbids the sale of marijuana, use remained constant until 1992 and then increased. Use remained steady or decreased in Catalunya (Spain), Stockholm, Hamburg, and Denmark during this period. These figures strongly suggest that marijuana use was influenced by changes in Dutch policy during this period. However, the United States and Norway (Oslo) also experienced increases in use of marijuana from 1992 to 1996, and thus it is difficult to attribute any change in use among Dutch youth after 1992 to the country's drug policies.

The 1999 European School Survey Project on Alcohol and Drugs, specifically developed to provide data on European drug use comparable with that obtained by the Monitoring the Future surveys, revealed that the proportion of adolescents in The Netherlands who reported ever having used marijuana (28%) was substantially lower than that of 10th graders in the United States (41%). However, the European survey also indicated that Dutch use was higher than any other European country except Ireland, the United Kingdom, France, and the Czech Republic.[28]

MEDICAL MARIJUANA

Considerable anecdotal evidence suggests that marijuana may be effective in treating a number of medical conditions. This perspective has been an important force behind efforts to change the legal status of marijuana. Marijuana has been touted as ameliorating chemotherapy-induced nausea, wasting and anorexia associated with AIDS, intraocular pressure in glaucoma, and muscle spasticity arising from such conditions as multiple sclerosis. Two comprehensive reviews evaluating the scientific basis for these claims, one conducted by the Institute of Medicine (IOM) and the other by the American Medical Association, have been published recently.[29,30] Both reports acknowledge the lack of rigorous data to support the use of smoked marijuana as medicine while calling for additional research into the medical use of cannabinoids, especially those that could be delivered rapidly in a smoke-free manner. The IOM report noted that marijuana smoke delivers "harmful substances" as well as tetrahydrocannabinol to the body and that marijuana "plants cannot be expected to provide a precisely defined drug effect." "For these reasons," the IOM report concluded, "there is very little future in smoked marijuana as a medically approved medication. If there is any future in cannabinoid development, it lies with agents of more certain, not less certain, composition."

POTENTIAL EFFECT OF DECRIMINALIZATION OR LEGALIZATION ON US ADOLESCENTS

Although efforts to legalize marijuana are focused solely on adults (no one is proposing that use or possession of marijuana by adolescents should be legalized), any change in its legal status could nonetheless have an effect on adolescents. Alcohol (illegal for those under 21 years of age) and tobacco products (illegal under 18 years of age) are nonetheless the psychoactive substances most widely abused by adolescents. During 2003, 47.5% of 12th graders reported using alcohol in the past 30 days and 24.4% reported smoking cigarettes in the past 30 days.[31]

Legalization of marijuana could result in advertising campaigns for its use, some of which might be directed toward adolescents. Control measures to prevent advertising to young people, as recent experience demonstrates, may be difficult to implement. As revealed during the course of the Comprehensive Tobacco Settlement negotiations, tobacco companies systematically have marketed their products to young people even while disavowing any efforts to do so. Even after the Comprehensive Tobacco Settlement was implemented (which prohibited any youth-oriented advertising), tobacco companies continued marketing to young people. A recent study noted that cigarette advertising in youth-oriented magazines increased by $54 million after the Tobacco Master Settlement Agreement.[32] Another study showed that advertising of youth brands of cigarettes (defined as those smoked by >5% of 8th, 10th, and 12th graders in 1998) in youth-oriented magazines increased from 1995 to 2000, as did expenditures for adult brands in youth-oriented magazines.[33] The Supreme Court recently struck down several Massachusetts regulations aimed at protecting schoolchildren from tobacco advertising (including bans on tobacco ads within 1000 feet of a school or playground). "The state's interest in preventing underage tobacco use is substantial and even compelling, but it is no less true that the sale and use of tobacco by adults is a legal activity," wrote Justice Sandra Day O'Connor for the majority. She continued, ". . . tobacco retailers and manufacturers have an interest in conveying truthful information about their products to adults, and adults have a corresponding interest in receiving truthful information about tobacco products."[34] Presumably, these same interests in regard to advertising for marijuana products also would be protected.

DiFranza[35] has demonstrated that both the states and the federal government are poorly enforcing the Synar Amendment, which requires states to control the sale of tobacco products to those younger than 18 years. Legalization of marijuana for adults but not adolescents would necessitate additional law en-

forcement burdens on a system that currently is not meeting its regulatory obligations.

Similarly, the alcoholic-beverage industry continues to portray drinking in terms that clearly appeal to young people. Drinking is associated with being sexy, popular, and fun and as an ideal means to "break the ice" in social settings.[36] These portrayals are extremely enticing to adolescents, who are in the process of developing their own identities as well as refining their social skills. One can speculate that distributors of marijuana quickly would recognize the profitability of portraying marijuana in a similar manner (thereby maximizing sales), all the while protesting that their marketing attempts seek only to induce adults to change brands.

How adolescents would perceive a change in the legal status of marijuana, even if only for adults, also is difficult to determine. However, recent studies have shown that prevalence of adolescent marijuana use is inversely proportional to the perceived risk associated with use (Fig 1).[37] The proportion of 12th graders who reported using marijuana in the past 30 days peaked in 1978 and again in 1997, exactly the years in which the perceived risk of regular use was at its lowest.

Some research suggests that legal sanctions may

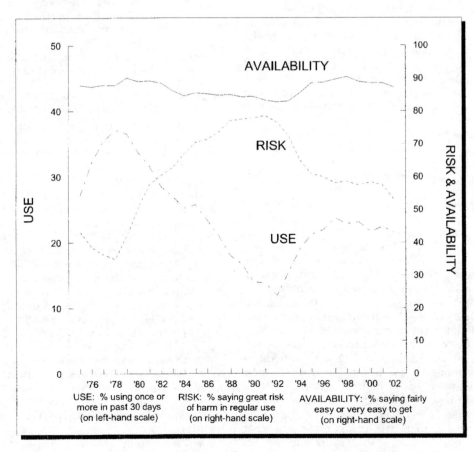

Source: Johnston LD, O'Malley PM, Bachman JG. Monitoring the Future: National Survey Results on Drug Use, 1975-2002. Vol I: Secondary School Students. Bethesda, MD: National Institute on Drug Abuse; 2003

Fig 1. Marijuana: trends in perceived availability, perceived risk of regular use, and prevalence of use in past 30 days for 12th graders

influence the initial decision to use drugs and that this influence diminishes as drug use by individuals progresses.[38] If so, it is the youngest adolescents (those who have not yet tried marijuana or are in the experimentation phase) who would be affected most by changes in marijuana laws. Age at first use is, in turn, a risk factor for problem use in the future.[39]

Moral development in children and adolescents assumes a developmental trajectory. Early adolescents have a concrete approach to morality: laws are obeyed to avoid punishment. As such, young adolescents would be most susceptible to the deterrent effects of drug laws. This deterrent effect could disappear or lessen with legalization of marijuana. Once adolescents gain the ability to think abstractly, challenges to the apparent hypocrisy of "do as I say, not as I do" can be anticipated.

Parental drug use is an important influence on adolescents' drug use.[40] Recent data indicate that easy household access to illicit substances is associated with greater risk of marijuana use among both younger and older adolescents.[41] Some adults may choose not to use marijuana (however they may feel about the law), because the potential risk of criminal sanctions outweighs any perceived benefit from using the drug. With the demise of legal sanctions against use, some parents may choose to begin using marijuana, acting as an important new source of exposure for their adolescents. Parental use of marijuana in the last year is associated with their adolescent's use during the same period.[42]

Availability of marijuana, which might increase if the drug were legalized, clearly has been shown to affect adolescents' use. Adolescents who have been offered marijuana are 7 times more likely to use it than are those who have not been offered marijuana. Similarly, those who report that marijuana is easy to get are approximately 2.5 times more likely to use it than those who consider it hard to get.[43]

Marijuana is cheap and easy to produce; if it were legalized, its price likely would decrease below current levels. Work by Pacula et al[44] in the United States and Williams[45] in Australia demonstrates clearly that a decrease in the price of marijuana is associated with a significant increase in the prevalence of use among adolescents.

Some advocates for the legalization of marijuana argue that it is safer than alcohol. They suggest that increased use of marijuana by young people might have a positive effect if some adolescents switched from alcohol to marijuana (a substitution effect). This theory cannot be supported by recent studies on adolescent marijuana and alcohol use that incorporated the price of marijuana into the analysis. These studies conclude that an increase in use of marijuana by adolescents would result in an increased use of alcohol (ie, that the 2 drugs are economic complements).[46]

From a public health perspective, even a small increase in use, whether attributable to increased availability or decreased perception of risk, would have significant ramifications. For example, if only an additional 1% of 15- to 19-year-olds in the United States began using marijuana, there would be approximately 190 000 new users.[47]

COMPARISONS BETWEEN MARIJUANA, ALCOHOL, AND TOBACCO

Proponents of legalization of marijuana argue that in terms of costs to society, both financial and health-related, alcohol and tobacco cause far more harm than does marijuana. They argue that classifying a relatively benign drug (marijuana) as schedule I and vigorously prosecuting its sale and possession while permitting the legal use of substances that cause far more damage are inconsistent and illogical practices or policies. That alcohol and tobacco cause far more harm in our society than marijuana is undeniable, but it does not follow logically that yet a third addictive psychoactive drug (marijuana) should be legalized. Many of the harms associated with alcohol and tobacco use stem from the widespread acceptability, availability, and use of these substances. Still other harms result from lax enforcement of current laws regulating their use or sale, especially to underage youth. Rather than legalizing marijuana, an equally compelling approach would be vigorously enforcing current regulations regarding sale and use of alcohol and tobacco products to minimize health-related problems attributable to their consumption. Recent examples include lowering the blood alcohol concentration that defines whether an individual is driving while intoxicated to 0.08 mg/dL (0.02 mg/dL for youth), limiting or banning smoking in public places, and banning cigarette advertisements targeted toward young people.

SUMMARY

Several recent studies concerning American adolescents, the Dutch experience with decriminalization (from 1984 to 1992), and the relationship between cheaper marijuana and use by adolescents suggest that decriminalization increases marijuana use by adolescents. Because no country has legalized use of marijuana outright, there are no studies available to evaluate the potential effect of legalization in the United States. Legalization of marijuana could decrease adolescents' perceptions of the risk of use and increase their exposure to this drug. Furthermore, data concerning adolescents' use of the 2 drugs that are legal for adults (alcohol and tobacco) suggest strongly that legalization of marijuana would have a negative effect on youth. Alcohol and tobacco are the drugs most widely abused by adolescents, although their sale to adolescents (younger than 18 years for tobacco and younger than 21 years for alcohol) is illegal. Research demonstrates that manufacturers of alcohol and tobacco market their products to young people, and the recent Supreme Court decision and experience with the Synar Amendment suggest that, if marijuana were legalized, restrictions on the sale and advertising of the substance to young people would prove daunting. Finally, two in-depth reviews of medical marijuana conclude that future research should focus on the medical use of cannabinoids, not smoked marijuana.

Recommendations from the AAP are included in the accompanying policy statement.[48]

COMMITTEE ON SUBSTANCE ABUSE, 2001–2002
Edward A. Jacobs, MD, Chairperson
Alain Joffe, MD, MPH
John R. Knight, MD
John Kulig, MD, MPH
Peter D. Rogers, MD, MPH
Janet F. Williams, MD

LIAISON
Deborah Simkin, MD
  American Academy of Child and Adolescent
  Psychiatry

STAFF
Karen S. Smith

COMMITTEE ON ADOLESCENCE, 2001–2002
David W. Kaplan, MD, MPH, Chairperson
Angela Diaz, MD
Ronald A. Feinstein, MD
Martin M. Fisher, MD
Jonathan D. Klein, MD, MPH
Ellen S. Rome, MD, MPH
W. Samuel Yancy, MD

LIAISONS
Ann J. Davis, MD
  American College of Obstetricians and
  Gynecologists
Glen Pearson, MD
  American Academy of Child and Adolescent
  Psychiatry
Jean-Yves Frappier, MD
  Canadian Paediatric Society

STAFF
Karen S. Smith

REFERENCES

1. Deglamorising cannabis [editorial]. *Lancet.* 1995;346:1241
2. National Drug Intelligence Center. *Marijuana. National Drug Threat Assessment 2003.* Johnstown, PA: National Drug Intelligence Center; 2003. Available at: www.usdoj.gov/ndic/pubs3/3300/marijuan.htm. Accessed February 4, 2004
3. Kassirer JP. Federal foolishness and marijuana. *N Engl J Med.* 1997;336:366–367
4. Canada Senate. *Cannabis: Our Position for a Canadian Public Policy. Report of the Senate Special Committee on Illegal Drugs.* Available at: www.medicalmarihuana.ca/pdfiles/senatesummary.pdf. Accessed February 4, 2004
5. Katz G. Europe loosens its pot laws. *Roll Stone.* 2002,(899–900):55–57
6. Silvis J. Enforcing drug laws in The Netherlands. In: Leuw E, Marshall IH, eds. *Between Prohibition and Legalization. The Dutch Experiment in Drug Policy.* Amsterdam, The Netherlands: Kugler Publications; 1994: 41–58
7. American Academy of Pediatrics, Division of Child Health Research. *AAP Periodic Survey of Fellows No. 31: Issues Surrounding Drug Legalization.* Elk Grove Village, IL: American Academy of Pediatrics; 1995
8. Rodriguez de Fonseca F, Carrera MR, Navarro M, Koob GF, Weiss F. Activation of corticotropin-releasing factor in the limbic system during cannabinoid withdrawal. *Science.* 1997;276:2050–2054
9. Tanda G, Pontieri FE, Di Chiara G. Cannabinoid and heroin activation of mesolimbic dopamine transmission by a common μ_1 opioid receptor mechanism. *Science.* 1997;276:2048–2050
10. American Academy of Pediatrics, Committee on Substance Abuse. Marijuana: a continuing concern for pediatricians. *Pediatrics.* 1999;104:982–985
11. Patton GC, Coffey C, Carlin JB, Degenhardt L, Lynskey M, Hall W. Cannabis use and mental health in young people: cohort study. *BMJ.* 2002;325:1195–1198
12. Zammit S, Allebeck P, Andreasson S, Lundberg I, Lewis G. Self reported cannabis use as a risk factor for schizophrenia in Swedish conscripts of 1969: historical cohort study. *BMJ.* 2002;325:1199–1203
13. Arseneault L, Cannon M, Poulton R, Murray R, Caspi A, Moffitt TE. Cannabis use in adolescence and risk for adult psychosis: longitudinal prospective study. *BMJ.* 2002;325:1212–1213
14. Eisen SA, Chantarujikapong S, Xian X, et al. Does marijuana use have residual effects on self-reported health measures, socio-demographics and quality of life? A monozygotic co-twin control study in men. *Addiction.* 2002;97:1137–1144
15. Jonnes J. *Hep-Cats, Narcs, and Pipe Dreams: A History of America's Romance With Illegal Drugs.* New York, NY: Scribner; 1996
16. Courtwright DT. *Dark Paradise: A History of Opiate Addiction in America.* Cambridge, MA: Harvard University Press; 2001
17. Johnston LD, O'Malley PM, Bachman JG. *Monitoring the Future: National Survey Results on Drug Abuse, 1975–2001. Volume I: Secondary School Students.* Bethesda, MD: National Institute on Drug Abuse, Department of Health and Human Services; 2002. NIH Publication No. 02-5106. Available at: www.monitoringthefuture.org/pubs/monographs/vol1_2001.pdf. Accessed May 13, 2003
18. Grinspoon L, Bakalar JB. Drug dependence: nonnarcotic agents. In: Kaplan HL, Freedman AM, Sadock BJ, eds. *Comprehensive Textbook of Psychiatry.* 3rd ed. Baltimore, MD: Williams & Wilkins; 1980:1621
19. Johnston LD, O'Malley PM, Bachman JG. *Marijuana Decriminalization: The Impact on Youth 1975–1980.* Monitoring the Future Occasional Paper No. 13. Ann Arbor, MI: Institute for Social Research, University of Michigan; 1981
20. Chaloupka FJ, Pacula RL, Farrelly MC, Johnston LD, O'Malley PM. *Do Higher Cigarette Prices Encourage Youth to Use Marijuana?* NBER Working Paper No. w6939. Cambridge, MA: National Bureau of Economic Research; 1999. Available at: www.nber.org/papers/w6939. Accessed May 7, 2003
21. Swaim RC, Beauvais F, Chavez EL, Oetting ER. The effect of school dropout rates on estimates of adolescent substance abuse among three racial/ethnic groups. *Am J Public Health.* 1997;87:51–55
22. Pacula RL, Chriqui JF, King J. *Marijuana Decriminalization: What Does it Mean in the United States?* Available at: www.impacteen.org/generalarea_PDFs/mjdecriminal_paculaJuly2002.pdf. Accessed January 27, 2004
23. Donnelly N, Hall W, Christie P. The effects of partial decriminalisation on cannabis use in South Australia, 1985 to 1993. *Aust J Public Health.* 1995;19:281–287
24. McGeorge J, Aitken CK. Effects of cannabis decriminalization in the Australian Capital Territory on university students' pattern of use. *J Drug Issues.* 1997;27:785–793
25. Korf DJ. *Dutch Treat: Formal Control and Illicit Drug Use in The Netherlands.* Amsterdam, The Netherlands: Thesis Publishers; 1995
26. MacCoun R, Reuter P. Interpreting Dutch cannabis policy: reasoning by analogy in the legalization debate. *Science.* 1997;278:47–52
27. MacCoun R, Reuter P. Evaluating alternative cannabis regimes. *Br J Psychiatry.* 2001;178:123–128
28. State University of New York at Albany. Press Release February 20, 2001. Available at: http://monitoringthefuture.org/pubs/espad_pr.pdf. Accessed December 17, 2003
29. Institute of Medicine. Introduction. In: Joy JE, Watson SJ, Benson JA, eds. *Marijuana and Medicine: Assessing the Science Base.* Washington, DC: National Academies Press; 1999:13–31
30. American Medical Association. *Medical Marijuana.* Report of the Council on Scientific Affairs (A-01). Chicago, IL: American Medical Association; 2001. Available at: www.ama-assn.org/ama/pub/article/2036-4971.html. Accessed May 7, 2003
31. Johnston LD, O'Malley PM, Bachman JG. Table 2: Trends in annual and 30-day prevalence of use of various drugs for eighth, tenth, and twelfth graders. Available at: www.monitoringthefuture.org/data/03data/pr03t2.pdf. Accessed January 27, 2004
32. Center for Substance Abuse Research. Cigarette advertisements in youth magazines increased by $54 million after Tobacco Master Settlement Agreement. In: *CESAR Fax.* Vol. 9. College Park, MD: Center for Substance Abuse Research, University of Maryland; 2000. Available at: www.cesar.umd.edu/cesar/cesarfax/vol9/9-26.pdf. Accessed May 7, 2003
33. King C III, Siegel M. The Master Settlement Agreement with the tobacco industry and cigarette advertising in magazines. *N Engl J Med.* 2001;345:504–511
34. *Lorillard Tobacco Company v Reilly.* 218 F3d 30 (US Supreme Court 2001)
35. DiFranza JR. State and federal compliance with the Synar Amendment: federal fiscal year 1998. *Arch Pediatr Adolesc Med.* 2001;155:572–578

36. Austin SB, Rich M. Consumerism: its impact on the health of adolescents. *Adolesc Med.* 2001,12:389–409

37. Johnston LD, O'Malley PM, Bachman JG. *Monitoring the Future National Survey Results on Drug Use, 1975–2002. Volume I: Secondary School Students.* Bethesda, MD: National Institute on Drug Abuse; 2003. NIH Publication No. 03-5375

38. MacCoun RJ. Drugs and the law: a psychological analysis of drug prohibition. *Psychol Bull.* 1993,113:497–512

39. Hawkins JD. Risk and protective factors and their implications for preventive interventions for the health care professional. In: Schydlower M, ed. *Substance Abuse: A Guide for Health Professionals.* 2nd ed. Elk Grove Village, IL: American Academy of Pediatrics; 2002:1–19

40. Hawkins JD, Catalano RF, Miller JY. Risk and protective factors for alcohol and other drug problems in adolescence and early adulthood: implications for substance abuse prevention. *Psychol Bull.* 1992,112:64–105

41. Resnick MD, Bearman PS, Blum RW, et al. Protecting adolescents from harm. Findings from the National Longitudinal Study on Adolescent Health. *JAMA.* 1997,278:823–832

42. Kandel DB, Griesler PC, Lee G, Davies M, Schaffren C. *Parental Influences on Adolescent Marijuana Use and the Baby Boom Generation: Findings From the 1979–1996 Household Surveys on Drug Abuse.* Rockville, MD: Office of Applied Studies, Substance Abuse and Mental Health Services Administration, Department of Health and Human Services; 2001. Available at: www.SAMHSA.gov/OAS/NHSDA/BabyBoom/cover.htm. Accessed May 7, 2003

43. Lane J, Gerstein D, Huang L, Wright D. *Risk and Protective Factors for Adolescent Drug Use: Findings From the 1997 National Household Survey on Drug Abuse.* Rockville, MD: Office of Applied Studies, Substance Abuse and Mental Health Services Administration, Department of Health and Human Services; 2001. Available at: www.samhsa.gov/oas/NHSDA/NAC97/Table_of_Contents.htm. Accessed May 7, 2003

44. Pacula RL, Grossman M, Chaloupka FJ, O'Malley PM, Johnston LD, Farrelly MC. Marijuana and youth. In: Gruber J, ed. *Risky Behavior Among Youths. An Economic Analysis.* Chicago, IL: University of Chicago Press; 2001:271–326

45. Williams J. The effects of price and policy on marijuana use: what can be learned from the Australian experience? *Health Economics* [serial online]. Available at: www3.interscience.wiley.com/cgi-bin/abstract/103520930/START. Accessed May 13, 2003

46. Hall W, Pacula RL. *Cannabis Use and Dependence: Public Health and Public Policy.* Victoria, Australia: Cambridge University Press; 2003

47. Census 2000 supplementary survey profile for United States. Available at: www.census.gov/acs/www/Products/Profiles/Single/2002/ACS/Tabular/010/01000US1.htm. Accessed May 13, 2003

48. American Academy of Pediatrics, Committee on Substance Abuse and Committee on Adolescence. Policy statement: legalization of marijuana: potential impact on youth. *Pediatrics.* 2004,113:1825–1826

All technical reports from the American Academy of Pediatrics automatically expire 5 years after publication unless reaffirmed, revised, or retired at or before that time.

Levels of Neonatal Care

• *Policy Statement*

AMERICAN ACADEMY OF PEDIATRICS

POLICY STATEMENT

Organizational Principles to Guide and Define the Child Health Care System and/or Improve the Health of All Children

Committee on Fetus and Newborn

Levels of Neonatal Care

ABSTRACT. The concept of designations for hospital facilities that care for newborn infants according to the level of complexity of care provided was first proposed in 1976. Subsequent diversity in the definitions and application of levels of care has complicated facility-based evaluation of clinical outcomes, resource allocation and utilization, and service delivery. We review data supporting the need for uniform nationally applicable definitions and the clinical basis for a proposed classification based on complexity of care. Facilities that provide hospital care for newborn infants should be classified on the basis of functional capabilities, and these facilities should be organized within a regionalized system of perinatal care. *Pediatrics* 2004;114:1341–1347; *neonatal intensive care, high-risk infant, regionalization, health policy, very low birth weight infant, nurseries, hospital newborn care services.*

ABBREVIATIONS. NICU, neonatal intensive care unit; TIOP, *Toward Improving the Outcome of Pregnancy*; TIOP II, *Toward Improving the Outcome of Pregnancy: The 90s and Beyond*; VLBW, very low birth weight; OR, odds ratio; ECMO, extracorporeal membrane oxygenation.

OBJECTIVES

The objectives of this statement are to review the current status of the designation of neonatal intensive care units (NICUs) in the United States and the association of the designated level of care of the site with neonatal outcomes and to make recommendations for uniform nationally applicable definitions of levels of neonatal intensive care that are based on the capability of facilities to provide increasing complexity of quality care.

BACKGROUND

The availability of neonatal intensive care has improved outcomes for high-risk infants including those born preterm or with serious medical or surgical conditions. The concept of regionalized perinatal care was articulated in the 1976 March of Dimes report *Toward Improving the Outcome of Pregnancy* (TIOP).[1] The report included criteria that stratified maternal and neonatal care into 3 levels of complexity and recommended referral of high-risk patients to centers with the personnel and resources needed for their degree of risk and severity of illness. At the time, resources for the most complex care were relatively scarce and concentrated in academic medical centers.[2]

During the past 2 decades, the number of neonatologists in the United States has increased and NICUs have proliferated.[2] However, no consistent relationship seems to exist between neonatal mortality and the number of NICU beds within a service area.[2] The effect of the availability of highly specialized personnel and resources on other neonatal outcomes is not known. In addition, no standard definitions exist for the graded levels of complexity of care that NICUs provide, making it difficult to compare outcomes of care.

Development of uniform definitions of levels of care offers at least 4 advantages that may improve the assessment of outcomes for high-risk newborn infants and provide the basis for policy decisions that affect allocation of resources. First, standard definitions will permit comparisons for health outcomes, resource utilization, and costs among institutions. Second, standardized nomenclature will be informative to the public, especially high-risk maternity patients who may seek an active role in selecting a delivery service. Third, uniformity in definitions of levels of care published by a professional organization will minimize the perceived need for businesses that purchase health insurance for their employees to develop their own standards.[3,4] Finally, uniform definitions will facilitate the development and implementation of consistent standards of service provided for each level of care.

Regionalized Neonatal Care

In 1993, *Toward Improving the Outcome of Pregnancy: The 90s and Beyond*[5] (TIOP II) reaffirmed the importance of an integrated system of regionalized care. The designations were changed from levels I, II, and III to basic, specialty, and subspecialty, respectively, and the criteria were expanded. These definitions are included in the fifth edition of *Guidelines for Perinatal Care.*[6]

Within the regionalized system, personnel and technology at each level should be appropriate for patient needs to facilitate optimal outcomes. Level I, or basic neonatal care, is the minimum requirement for any facility that provides inpatient maternity care. The institution must have the personnel and equipment to perform neonatal resuscitation, evaluate healthy newborn infants and provide postnatal care, and stabilize ill newborn infants until transfer

doi:10.1542/peds.2004-1697
PEDIATRICS (ISSN 0031 4005). Copyright © 2004 by the American Academy of Pediatrics.

to a facility that provides intensive care. Level II, or specialty care nurseries, in addition to providing basic care, can provide care to infants who are moderately ill with problems that are expected to resolve rapidly[6] or who are recovering from serious illness treated in a level III (subspecialty) NICU. Level III, or subspecialty NICUs, can care for newborn infants with extreme prematurity or who are critically ill or require surgical intervention.

Variation in Definition and Enforcement

Although the TIOP designations provide a general framework for classification of NICUs, both interpretation and application vary widely within the United States, and no national definition exists.[7,8] In late 2003, 15 states and the District of Columbia had no formal definitions. An independent survey performed by the Section on Perinatal Pediatrics of the American Academy of Pediatrics that included corroboration by neonatologists within each state found that only 32 states had published definitions of levels of care. Great diversity exists among states (D. Bhatt, MD, Report to the Section on Perinatal Pediatrics Executive Committee, October 2002). In 11 states, 3 levels of care are defined based on TIOP I, TIOP II, or *Guidelines for Perinatal Care*, 3rd or 4th editions. In the remaining states, additional levels were added above or below the original highest level (level III or subspecialty). Nine states name a level above level III delegating regional responsibilities in addition to the level III designation for NICU services.

In states that have defined levels of care, the process for designating NICU levels and enforcing NICU-related regulations varies. NICU levels at specific hospitals may be designated by the state through the official process of licensing or granting a certificate of need or state-administered health care funding. In 9 states, formal definitions have been established through programs either supported by or affiliated with maternal child health programs of the state health department. More than 1 of these mechanisms is used in 12 states.

Policies regarding monitoring of compliance also vary (D. Bhatt, MD, Report to the Section on Perinatal Pediatrics Executive Committee, October 2002). Furthermore, only 14 states have minimum standards for utilization. These standards are based variously on NICU occupancy rates, annual births or NICU admissions, or capacity. Definitions include specific language regarding birth weight and/or gestational age as criteria for a given level of care in only 15 states.

A source of confusion has been that designations for levels of care are variably applied to units caring for newborn infants and to the hospitals themselves. Facilities are usually designated by the highest level of care they provide, although they may provide less complex care as well. One exception may be freestanding children's hospitals, which may provide specialty and subspecialty care but transfer newborn infants to other facilities (often the hospital of birth) for lower levels of care as their medical conditions improve. Some hospitals have single units that integrate specialty and subspecialty care, and others

have separate units for each level. Regional centers are hospitals that include the highest level of NICU care and serve regional needs through education, data collection, and transport services. Some perinatal centers with large delivery services have NICUs but depend on agreements with neighboring institutions for pediatric subspecialty services including advanced imaging and operating rooms. In some regions, perinatal centers may be great distances from pediatric subspecialty care. Furthermore, hospitals with specific designations may vary in the types of neonatal services that are provided. In a survey of California hospitals, for example, facilities that were designated by the state as regional, community, and intermediate newborn units varied considerably within these categories in the services available (L.J. Van Marter, MD, MPH, Report to the Section on Perinatal Pediatrics Executive Committee, October 2001).

Level of Care, Patient Volume, and Outcome

Most studies that link neonatal outcomes with levels of perinatal care indicate that morbidity and mortality for very low birth weight (VLBW) infants are improved when delivery occurs in a subspecialty facility rather than a basic or specialty facility even after adjustments for severity of illness.[9] Contributing factors include the increased experience available at tertiary centers and the potential negative effect of the transport process. One report examined outcomes of 3769 singleton infants born at less than 32 weeks' gestation admitted to 17 Canadian NICUs during 1996–1997.[10] Outborn infants (those born outside the centers and requiring transfer) had significantly greater risk of mortality (odds ratio [OR]: 1.7), severe intraventricular hemorrhage (OR: 2.2), respiratory distress syndrome (OR: 4.8), patent ductus arteriosus (OR: 1.6), and nosocomial infection (OR: 2.5), compared with infants born at tertiary care centers. In a separate report from the same database, the advantage of preterm birth at tertiary centers was inversely related to gestational age.[11] The risk-adjusted incidence was significantly greater for outborn than inborn infants for mortality (OR: 2.2) and grade 3 or 4 intraventricular hemorrhage (OR: 2.1) at 26 weeks' gestation or less and for chronic lung disease (OR: 1.7) at 27 to 29 weeks' gestation. Another study analyzed neonatal mortality rates of 2375 infants with VLBW in South Carolina in 1993–1995 by level of perinatal services at the hospital of birth.[12] Neonatal mortality rate, adjusted for birth weight and race, was significantly higher for infants born at level I and II hospitals and for level II hospitals with 24-hour neonatology coverage (267, 232, and 213 deaths per 1000 live births, respectively), compared with level III centers (146 deaths per 1000 live births). When a similar analysis of VLBW infants in South Carolina in 1991–1995 was restricted to Medicaid recipients (64% of VLBW births), the risk of death was also greater in level I and II hospitals (relative risk: 1.9; 95% confidence interval: 1.6–2.2), compared with level III hospitals, although not in level II hospitals with neonatology coverage.[13]

Even transfer between tertiary centers may increase the risk of mortality. In a study in Australia, 25% of infants less than 30 weeks' gestational age born at a tertiary care center during an 18-month period required transfer to another tertiary care center because the initial NICU was fully occupied.[14] After exclusion of lethal malformations and adjustment for confounding variables, mortality in the transferred infants was significantly greater than in those who remained at the birth hospital. Thus, to the extent possible, delivery of a high-risk infant should be planned to occur in a facility capable of providing the anticipated appropriate level of NICU care. If delivery in a facility without the necessary capabilities cannot be avoided, the infant should be stabilized and transferred to a NICU with the appropriate capabilities to ensure optimal outcome.

In addition to level of care, patient volume in the NICU seems to influence outcome. However, it must be acknowledged that the relationship between volume and outcome tends to be true on the average, and considerable variability exists among individual hospitals and physicians.[15,16] In a study of hospitals in California in 1990, risk-adjusted neonatal mortality based on linked birth and death certificate data were significantly lower for births that occurred in hospitals with level III NICUs that had an average daily census of at least 15 patients, compared with lower-volume centers.[17] In another study using linked birth and death certificate data in California for 1992 and 1993, the effect on mortality of the level of care provided at the hospital of birth was examined for low birth weight infants.[18] Compared with birth in a hospital with a regional NICU, risk-adjusted mortality for infants with birth weight less than 2000 g was significantly higher at a hospital with no NICU, an intermediate NICU, or a community NICU with an average census less than 15 patients (OR: 2.38, 1.92, and 1.42, respectively). The ORs were larger when the analysis was restricted to infants with birth weight less than 1500 g or less than 1250 g. However, risk-adjusted mortality in a community hospital NICU with an average census of more than 15 was not significantly different from a hospital with a regional NICU.

No specific data are available on the influence on outcomes of the volume of complex procedures performed in newborn infants at hospitals or by physicians. However, these data are available for adults and older children.[16] Numerous studies have documented the inverse relationship between the volume of patients treated and mortality for surgical procedures[19,20] or medical conditions such as acute myocardial infarction in adults.[21] A similar relationship of patient volume to mortality has been demonstrated in children. Among 16 pediatric intensive care units with an annual volume ranging from 147 to 1378 patients, an increase in volume of 100 patients was associated with a significantly reduced risk-adjusted mortality and length of stay.[22] Other pediatric intensive care unit characteristics including number of beds, affiliation with a university or children's hospital, or fellowship training program did not affect mortality or duration of hospitalization. Similarly, a higher volume of pediatric cardiac sur-

gical procedures performed by a hospital and/or surgeon was associated with lower in-hospital mortality.[23,24] In 1 study, adjusted mortality rates of higher-volume hospitals (those that performed more than 100 procedures annually) were decreased (5.95% vs 8.26%), compared with lower volume hospitals.[23] Mortality rates were lower also for surgeons with annual volumes of 75 or more compared with lower volumes (5.9% vs 8.77%).

Some reports have not shown a consistent association of NICU volume and neonatal mortality, although the conclusions were likely influenced by the characteristics of the NICUs included in the study and aspects of the analysis. One study examined 28-day mortality of 7672 infants with birth weights of 501 to 1500 g in 62 NICUs participating in the Vermont Oxford Network in 1991–1992.[25] The median annual patient volume was 76 (interquartile range: 47–113). The standardized mortality ratio (ratio of observed to predicted deaths) varied among NICUs. However, differences in the mortality rate or standardized mortality ratio were not explained by differences in patient volume. This may be explained, in part, because most of the NICUs had annual admissions of 47 or more VLBW infants. In another study of 54 NICUs in the United Kingdom in 1998–1999, risk-adjusted mortality was not associated with patient volume, although mortality rate increased inversely with nurse-to-patient ratio, which reflected increasing nursing workload.[26] However, 8 of the 12 NICUs included in this study admitted 57 or fewer VLBW infants per year. In both the Vermont Oxford and United Kingdom studies, deaths were attributed to the NICU rather than the hospital of birth. Additional studies are needed to examine other characteristics of NICUs and specific care practices that affect the quality of care and rates of mortality and morbidity.[15,27,28] Comparisons among centers will be facilitated by more precise definitions of levels of care provided by NICUs.

Risk of Complications

Appropriate matching of levels of complexity of neonatal care to patient needs requires recognition of risk factors. Mortality and morbidity are highest in infants of the lowest birth weights and gestational ages. For example, in centers of the National Institute of Child Health and Human Development Neonatal Research Network in 1995–1996, survival to discharge was 97% at birth weight of 1251 to 1500 g, 94% at birth weight of 1001 to 1250 g, 86% at birth weight of 751 to 1000 g, and 54% at birth weight of 501 to 750 g.[29] Similarly, the incidence in survivors of major morbidity, defined as chronic lung disease, severe intracranial hemorrhage, and/or proven necrotizing enterocolitis, was 10%, 23%, 42%, and 63% at birth weights of 1251 to 1500, 1001 to 1250, 751 to 1000, and 501 to 750 g, respectively.

However, any degree of prematurity confers some risk. Compared with those born at term, infants born at 34 to 37 weeks' gestation are at increased risk of complications because of their physiologic immaturity. Biological variability exists in the time of attainment of independent thermoregulation[30]; resolution of apnea, bradycardia, and/or hypoxemic episodes[31–33]; and oral feedings.[34] Near-term infants (35–37 weeks' gestation) are at increased risk of hyperbilirubinemia and kernicterus.[35] Thus, proposed definitions for levels of care should take into account the increased risk along the continuum of decreasing gestational ages.

Expanded Definitions of Levels of Care

Expansion of the definitions of levels of care should be based on the capability to provide increasing complexity of care. The need for mechanical ventilation is a reasonable indication of a minimum level of subspecialty intensive care. In the revised US Standard Certificate of Birth, the National Center for Health Statistics defined a NICU as a "hospital facility or unit staffed and equipped to provide continuous mechanical ventilatory support for a newborn infant."[36]

In 2001, the Section on Perinatal Pediatrics performed a survey of hospital-based newborn services in the United States. A NICU was identified as a unit providing care for newborn infants in which a neonatologist provided primary care, as indicated by the results of a previous survey that identified all US neonatologists and their site of practice.[37] The survey instrument was a modified version of the classification of NICU levels used by the Vermont Oxford Network.[38] The classification consisted of basic care (level I), specialty care (level II), and subspecialty intensive care (level III) (Table 1). Subspecialty care was divided further into 4 categories (IIIA–IIID) based on whether the use of mechanical ventilation

TABLE 1. Definitions of Hospital-Based Newborn Services Used for Survey Performed by Section on Perinatal Pediatrics

Basic neonatal care (level I)
  Well-newborn nursery
  Evaluation and postnatal care of healthy newborns
  Neonatal resuscitation
  Stabilization of ill newborns until transfer to a facility at
    which specialty neonatal care is provided
Specialty neonatal care (level II)
  Special care nursery
  Care of preterm infants with birth weight ≥1500 g
  Resuscitation and stabilization of preterm and/or ill infants
    before transfer to a facility at which newborn intensive care
    is provided
Subspecialty neonatal intensive care (level III)
  Level IIIA
    Hospital or state-mandated restriction on type and/or
      duration of mechanical ventilation
  Level IIIB
    No restrictions on type or duration of mechanical
      ventilation
    No major surgery
  Level IIIC
    Major surgery performed on site (eg, omphalocele repair,
      tracheoesophageal fistula or esophageal atresia repair,
      bowel resection, myelomeningocele repair,
      ventriculoperitoneal shunt)
    No surgical repair of serious congenital heart anomalies
      that require cardiopulmonary bypass and /or ECMO for
      medical conditions
  Level IIID
    Major surgery, surgical repair of serious congenital heart
      anomalies that require cardiopulmonary bypass, and/or
      ECMO for medical conditions

was restricted and the availability of major surgery, cardiovascular surgery, or extracorporeal membrane oxygenation (ECMO). A total of 880 NICUs were identified, of which 120 were level II and 760 were level III by survey definition.

Proposed Definitions

The results of the survey have been used to refine the definitions of levels of care on the basis of a more comprehensive assessment of patient needs and distinction among low, moderate, and high levels of complexity and risk. These definitions reflect the capability to provide increasingly complex care, reflected in appropriate personnel, equipment, and organization. In the future, standards can be developed that delineate the specific components required for each capability (Table 2).

According to these definitions, level I units (well-newborn nurseries) provide a basic level of newborn care to infants at low risk. They have the capabilities to perform neonatal resuscitation at every delivery and to evaluate and provide routine postnatal care of healthy newborn infants. In addition, they can stabilize and care for near-term infants (35–37 weeks' gestation) who remain physiologically stable and can stabilize newborn infants who are less than 35 weeks' gestation or ill until they can be transferred to a facility at which specialty neonatal care is provided.

Level II (specialty) special care nurseries can provide care to infants who are moderately ill with problems that are expected to resolve rapidly.[6] These patients are at moderate risk of serious complications related to immaturity, illness, and/or their management. In general, care in this setting should be limited to newborn infants who are more than 32 weeks' gestational age and weigh more than 1500 g at birth or who are recovering from serious illness treated in a level III (subspecialty) NICU. Level II units are differentiated into 2 categories, IIA and IIB, on the basis of their ability to provide assisted ventilation.

Level IIA nurseries do not have the capabilities to provide assisted ventilation except on an interim basis until the infant can be transferred to a higher-level facility. Level IIB nurseries can provide mechanical ventilation for brief durations (less than 24 hours) or continuous positive airway pressure. They must have equipment (eg, portable chest radiograph, blood gas laboratory) and personnel (eg, physician, specialized nurses, respiratory therapists, radiology technicians, and laboratory technicians) continuously available to provide ongoing care as well as to address emergencies.[6]

Level III (subspecialty) NICUs are defined by having continuously available personnel (neonatologists, neonatal nurses, respiratory therapists) and equipment to provide life support for as long as needed. Level III NICUs are differentiated by their ability to provide care to newborn infants with differing degrees of complexity and risk. Newborn infants with birth weight of more than 1000 g and gestational age of more than 28 weeks can be cared for in level IIIA NICUs. These facilities have the

TABLE 2. Proposed Uniform Definitions for Capabilities Associated With the Highest Level of Neonatal Care Within an Institution (See Text for Details)

Level I neonatal care (basic)
  Well-newborn nursery: has the capabilities to
    Provide neonatal resuscitation at every delivery
    Evaluate and provide postnatal care to healthy newborn infants
    Stabilize and provide care for infants born at 35 to 37 weeks' gestation who remain physiologically stable
    Stabilize newborn infants who are ill and those born at <35 weeks' gestation until transfer to a facility that can provide the appropriate level of neonatal care
Level II neonatal care (specialty)
  Special care nursery: level II units are subdivided into 2 categories on the basis of their ability to provide assisted ventilation including continuous positive airway pressure
    Level IIA: has the capabilities to
      Resuscitate and stabilize preterm and/or ill infants before transfer to a facility at which newborn intensive care is provided
      Provide care for infants born at >32 weeks' gestation and weighing ≥1500 g (1) who have physiologic immaturity such as apnea of prematurity, inability to maintain body temperature, or inability to take oral feedings or (2) who are moderately ill with problems that are anticipated to resolve rapidly and are not anticipated to need subspecialty services on an urgent basis
      Provide care for infants who are convalescing after intensive care
    Level IIB has the capabilities of a level IIA nursery and the additional capability to provide mechanical ventilation for brief durations (<24 hours) or continuous positive airway pressure
Level III (subspecialty) NICU: level III NICUs are subdivided into 3 categories
  Level IIIA: has the capabilities to
    Provide comprehensive care for infants born at >28 weeks' gestation and weighing >1000 g
    Provide sustained life support limited to conventional mechanical ventilation
    Perform minor surgical procedures such as placement of central venous catheter or inguinal hernia repair
  Level IIIB NICU: has the capabilities to provide
    Comprehensive care for extremely low birth weight infants (≤1000 g and ≤28 weeks' gestation)
    Advanced respiratory support such as high-frequency ventilation and inhaled nitric oxide for as long as required
    Prompt and on-site access to a full range of pediatric medical subspecialists
    Advanced imaging, with interpretation on an urgent basis, including computed tomography, magnetic resonance imaging, and echocardiography
    Pediatric surgical specialists and pediatric anesthesiologists on site or at a closely related institution to perform major surgery such as ligation of patent ductus arteriosus and repair of abdominal wall defects, necrotizing enterocolitis with bowel perforation, tracheoesophageal fistula and/or esophageal atresia, and myelomeningocele
  Level IIIC NICU: has the capabilities of a level IIIB NICU and also is located within an institution that has the capability to provide ECMO and surgical repair of complex congenital cardiac malformations that require cardiopulmonary bypass

capability to provide conventional mechanical ventilation for as long as needed but do not use more advanced respiratory support such as high-frequency ventilation. Other capabilities that may be available are minor surgical procedures such as placement of a central venous catheter or inguinal hernia repair.

Newborn infants with extreme prematurity (28 weeks' gestation or less) or extremely low birth weight (1000 g or less) or who have severe and/or complex illness are in the highest risk group and have the most specialized needs. These infants require a more advanced level III unit (designated level IIIB) with a broad range of pediatric medical subspecialists and pediatric surgical specialists, highly skilled nursing and respiratory care staff, advanced respiratory support and physiologic monitoring equipment, laboratory and imaging facilities, nutrition and pharmacy support with pediatric expertise, social services, and pastoral care. Advanced respiratory care should include high-frequency ventilation and inhaled nitric oxide. For example, extremely low birth weight infants typically require sustained ventilator support, parenteral nutrition, and neuroimaging and may need surgical ligation of a patent ductus arteriosus, surgical treatment of necrotizing enterocolitis, or neurosurgical management of hydrocephalus. A level IIIB unit should have the capability to perform major surgery (including anesthesiologists with pediatric expertise) on site or at a closely related institution for patients with congenital malformations (such as abdominal wall defect, tracheoesophageal fistula and/or esophageal atresia, or meningomyelocele) or acquired conditions (such as bowel perforation, retinopathy of prematurity, or hydrocephalus secondary to intraventricular hemorrhage). A closely related institution would ideally be in geographic proximity and share coordinated care such as physician staff. Outcomes of less complex surgical procedures in children, such as appendectomy or pyloromyotomy, are better when performed by pediatric surgical subspecialists compared with general surgeons.[39–41] Thus, it is recommended that pediatric surgical specialists perform more complex procedures in newborn infants.

The most advanced level III units, designated level IIIC, which may be located at children's hospitals, have additional capabilities within the institution, including ECMO and surgical repair of serious congenital cardiac malformations that require cardiopulmonary bypass.[42–44] It is logical to assume that substantial experience is needed for the best outcomes in patients who require the most advanced support.[23,24,45] However, data are not currently available to define this requirement. Concentrating the care of infants with conditions that occur infrequently and require the highest level of intensive care at designated level III centers allows these centers to develop the expertise needed to achieve optimal outcomes and avoids costly duplication of services in multiple institutions within close proximity.

Level IIIB and IIIC units care for the most complex and critically ill patients and should have immediate and on-site access to pediatric medical subspecialty consultants. These facilities should have the capability to perform advanced imaging with interpretation on an urgent basis, including computed tomography, magnetic resonance imaging, and echocardiography. Data are unavailable on the relationship between availability of these consultants or of imaging capability and neonatal outcomes.

Large regional differences exist in the numbers of neonatologists and NICU beds, and the availability of these resources is not consistently related to the number of high-risk newborn infants.[2] Regional differences also exist in the numbers of other pediatric subspecialists and in the distances patients must travel to receive care for serious illness.[46] Limitation of all complex neonatal care to high-volume centers distant from the homes of some patients must be weighed against developing other approaches to improve outcomes in institutions with lower volumes. In a theoretic analysis of regionalization of pediatric cardiac surgery in California, for example, referral of all cases to high-volume centers would reduce surgical mortality from 5.34% to 4.08% but would increase average travel distance from 45.4 to 58.1 miles.[47]

RECOMMENDATIONS

1. Regionalized systems of perinatal care are recommended to ensure that each newborn infant is delivered and cared for in a facility appropriate for his or her health care needs and to facilitate the achievement of optimal outcomes.
2. The functional capabilities of facilities that provide inpatient care for newborn infants should be classified uniformly, as follows:
   - Level I (basic): a hospital nursery organized with the personnel and equipment to perform neonatal resuscitation, evaluate and provide postnatal care of healthy newborn infants, stabilize and provide care for infants born at 35 to 37 weeks' gestation who remain physiologically stable, and stabilize newborn infants born at less than 35 weeks' gestational age or ill until transfer to a facility that can provide the appropriate level of neonatal care.
   - Level II (specialty): a hospital special care nursery organized with the personnel and equipment to provide care to infants born at more than 32 weeks' gestation and weighing more than 1500 g who have physiologic immaturity such as apnea of prematurity, inability to maintain body temperature, or inability to take oral feedings; who are moderately ill with problems that are expected to resolve rapidly and are not anticipated to need subspecialty services on an urgent basis; or who are convalescing from intensive care. Level II care is subdivided into 2 categories that are differentiated by those that do not (level IIA) or do (level IIB) have the capability to provide mechanical ventilation for brief durations (less than 24 hours) or continuous positive airway pressure.
   - Level III (subspecialty): a hospital NICU organized with personnel and equipment to provide continuous life support and comprehensive care for extremely high-risk newborn infants and those with complex and critical illness. Level III is subdivided into 3 levels differentiated by the capability to provide advanced medical and surgical care.
   Level IIIA units can provide care for infants with birth weight of more than 1000 g and gestational age of more than 28 weeks. Continuous life support can be provided but is limited to conventional mechanical ventilation.
   Level IIIB units can provide comprehensive care for extremely low birth weight infants (1000 g birth weight or less and 28 or less weeks' gestation); advanced respiratory care such as high-frequency ventilation and inhaled nitric oxide; prompt and on-site access to a full range of pediatric medical subspecialists; and advanced imaging with interpretation on an urgent basis, including computed tomography, magnetic resonance imaging, and echocardiography and have pediatric surgical specialists and pediatric anesthesiologists on site or at a closely related institution to perform major surgery.
   Level IIIC units have the capabilities of a level IIIB NICU and are located within institutions that can provide ECMO and surgical repair of serious congenital cardiac malformations that require cardiopulmonary bypass.
3. Uniform national standards such as requirements for equipment, personnel, facilities, ancillary services, and training, and the organization of services (including transport) should be developed for the capabilities of each level of care.
4. Population-based data on patient outcomes, including mortality, specific morbidities, and long-term outcomes, should be obtained to provide level-specific standards for volume of patients requiring various categories of specialized care, including surgery.

COMMITTEE ON FETUS AND NEWBORN, 2003–2004
Lillian Blackmon, MD, Chairperson
Daniel G. Batton, MD
Edward F. Bell, MD
Susan E. Denson, MD
William A. Engle, MD
William P. Kanto, Jr, MD
Gilbert I. Martin, MD
*Ann R. Stark, MD

LIAISONS
Keith J. Barrington, MD
   Canadian Paediatric Society
Tonse Raju, MD, DCH
   National Institutes of Health
Laura E. Riley, MD
   American College of Obstetricians and
   Gynecologists
Kay M. Tomashek, MD
   Centers for Disease Control and Prevention
Carol Wallman, MSN, RNC, NNP
   National Association of Neonatal Nurses

CONSULTANTS
Jeffrey D. Horbar, MD
Ciaran Phibbs, MD
Paul M. Seib, MD

STAFF
Jim Couto, MA

*Lead author

REFERENCES

1. Committee on Perinatal Health. *Toward Improving the Outcome of Pregnancy: Recommendations for the Regional Development of Maternal and Perinatal Health Services*. White Plains, NY: March of Dimes National Foundation; 1976
2. Goodman DG, Fisher ES, Little GA, Stukel TA, Chang CH, Schoendorf KS. The relation between the availability of neonatal intensive care and neonatal mortality. *N Engl J Med*. 2002;346:1538–1544
3. Castles AG, Milstein A, Damberg CL. Using employer purchasing power to improve the quality of perinatal care. *Pediatrics*. 1999;103:248–254
4. Cors WK. Physician executives must leap with the frog. Accountability for safety and quality ultimately lie with the doctors in charge. *Physician Exec*. 2001;27(6):14–16
5. Committee on Perinatal Health. *Toward Improving the Outcome of Pregnancy: The 90s and Beyond*. White Plains, NY: March of Dimes Birth Defects Foundation; 1993
6. Oh W, Gilstrap L, eds. *Guidelines for Perinatal Care*. 5th ed. Elk Grove Village, IL: American Academy of Pediatrics, American College of Obstetricians and Gynecologists; 2002
7. Shaffer ER. *State Policies and Regional Neonatal Care: Progress and Challenges 25 Years After TIOP*. White Plains, NY: March of Dimes; 2001
8. Van Marter LJ. Perinatal section surveys and databases. *Perinat Sect News*. 2000;26:8–9
9. Blackmon L. The role of the hospital of birth on survival of extremely low birth weight, extremely preterm infants. *NeoReviews*. 2003;4:e147–e157
10. Chien LY, Whyte R, Aziz K, Thiessen P, Matthew D, Lee SK. Improved outcome of preterm infants when delivered in tertiary care centers. *Obstet Gynecol*. 2001;98:247–252
11. Lee SK, McMillan DD, Ohlsson A, et al. The benefit of preterm birth at tertiary care centers is related to gestational age. *Am J Obstet Gynecol*. 2003;188:617–622
12. Menard MK, Liu Q, Holgren EA, Sappenfield WM. Neonatal mortality for very low birth weight deliveries in South Carolina by level of hospital perinatal service. *Am J Obstet Gynecol*. 1998;179:374–381
13. Sanderson M, Sappenfield WM, Jespersen KM, Liu Q, Baker SL. Association between level of delivery hospital and neonatal outcomes among South Carolina Medicaid recipients. *Am J Obstet Gynecol*. 2000;183:1504–1511
14. Bowman E, Doyle LW, Murton LJ, Roy RN, Kitchen WH. Increased mortality of preterm infants transferred between tertiary perinatal centers. *BMJ*. 1988;297:1098–1100
15. Hannan EL. The relation between volume and outcome in health care. *N Engl J Med*. 1999;340:1677–1679
16. Halm EA, Lee C, Chassin MR. Is volume related to outcome in health care? A systematic and methodologic critique of the literature. *Ann Intern Med*. 2002;137:511–520
17. Phibbs CS, Bronstein JM, Buxton E, Phibbs RH. The effects of patient volume and level of care at the hospital of birth on neonatal mortality. *JAMA*. 1996;276:1054–1059
18. Cifuentes J, Bronstein J, Phibbs CS, Phibbs RH, Schmitt SK, Carlo WA. Mortality in low birth weight infants according to level of neonatal care at hospital of birth. *Pediatrics*. 2002;109:745–751
19. Birkmeyer JD, Siewers AE, Finlayson EV, et al. Hospital volume and surgical mortality in the United States. *N Engl J Med*. 2002;346:1128–1137
20. Begg CB, Riedel ER, Bach PB, et al. Variations in morbidity after radical prostatectomy. *N Engl J Med*. 2002;346:1138–1144
21. Thiemann DR, Coresh J, Oetgen WJ, Powe NR. The association between hospital volume and survival after acute myocardial infarction in elderly patients. *N Engl J Med*. 1999;340:1640–1648
22. Tilford JM, Simpson PM, Green JW, Lensing S, Fiser DH. Volume-outcome relationships in pediatric intensive care units. *Pediatrics*. 2000;106:289–294
23. Hannan EL, Racz M, Kavey RE, Quaegebeur JM, Williams R. Pediatric cardiac surgery: the effect of hospital and surgeon volume on in-hospital mortality. *Pediatrics*. 1998;101:963–969
24. Spiegelhalter DJ. Mortality and volume of cases in paediatric cardiac surgery: retrospective study based on routinely collected data. *BMJ*. 2002;324:261–263
25. Horbar JD, Badger GJ, Lewit EM, Rogowski J, Shiono PH. Hospital and patient characteristics associated with variation in 28-day mortality rates for very low birth weight infants. *Pediatrics*. 1997;99:149–156
26. Tucker J, UK Neonatal Staffing Study Group. Patient volume, staffing, and workload in relation to risk-adjusted outcomes in a random stratified sample of UK neonatal intensive care units: a prospective evaluation. *Lancet*. 2002;359:99–107
27. Pollack MM, Patel KM. Need for shift in focus in research into quality of intensive care. *Lancet*. 2002;359:95–96
28. Pollack MM, Koch M. The NIH-DC Neonatal Network. Good management improves outcomes: the association of organizational characteristics and neonatal outcomes [abstract]. *Pediatr Res*. 2001;49:316A
29. Lemons JA, Bauer CR, Oh W, et al. Very low birth weight outcomes of the National Institute of Child Health and Human Development Neonatal Research Network, January 1995 through December 1996. *Pediatrics*. 2001;107(1). Available at: www.pediatrics.org/cgi/content/full/107/1/e1
30. Sinclair JC, ed. *Temperature Regulation and Energy Metabolism in the Newborn*. New York, NY: Grune and Stratton; 1978
31. Hodgman JE, Gonzalez F, Hoppenbrouwers T, Cabal LA. Apnea, transient episodes of bradycardia, and periodic breathing in preterm infants. *Am J Dis Child*. 1990;144:54–57
32. Poets CF, Stebbens VA, Richard D, Southall DP. Prolonged episodes of hypoxemia in preterm infants undetectable by cardiorespiratory monitors. *Pediatrics*. 1995;95:860–863
33. Merchant JR, Worwa C, Porter S, Coleman JM, deRegnier RA. Respiratory instability of term and near-term healthy newborn infants in car safety seats. *Pediatrics*. 2001;108:647–652
34. Eichenwald EC, Blackwell M, Lloyd JS, Tran T, Wilker RE, Richardson DK. Inter-neonatal intensive care unit variation in discharge timing: influence of apnea and feeding management. *Pediatrics*. 2001;108:928–933
35. American Academy of Pediatrics Subcommittee on Neonatal Hyperbilirubinemia. Neonatal jaundice and kernicterus [commentary]. *Pediatrics*. 2001;108:763–765
36. National Center of Health Statistics, Division of Vital Statistics. Guide to completing the facility worksheets for the certificate of live birth and report of fetal death (2003 revision). Available at: www.cdc.gov/nchs/data/dvs/GuidetoCompleteFacilityWks.pdf. Accessed September 28, 2004
37. Bhatt D. Towards a unified definition of NICU levels of care. *Perinat Sect News*. 2001;7:12
38. Horbar JD, Carpenter J, eds. *Vermont Oxford Network 2001 Database Summary*. Burlington, VT: Vermont Oxford Network; 2002
39. Kokoska ER, Minkes RK, Silen ML, et al. Effect of pediatric surgical practice on the treatment of children with appendicitis. *Pediatrics*. 2001;107:1298–1301
40. Pranikoff T, Campbell BT, Travis J, Hirschl RB. Differences in outcome with subspecialty care: pyloromyotomy in North Carolina. *J Pediatr Surg*. 2002;37:352–356
41. Brain AJ, Roberts DS. Who should treat pyloric stenosis: the general or specialist pediatric surgeon? *J Pediatr Surg*. 1996;31:1535–1537
42. American Academy of Pediatrics, Committee on Fetus and Newborn. Use of inhaled nitric oxide. *Pediatrics*. 2000;106:344–345
43. Aharon AS, Drinkwater DC Jr, Churchwell KB, et al. Extracorporeal membrane oxygenation in children after repair of congenital cardiac lesions. *Ann Thorac Surg*. 2001;72:2095–2101
44. Shen I, Giacomuzzi C, Ungerleider RM. Current strategies for optimizing the use of cardiopulmonary bypass in neonates and infants. *Ann Thorac Surg*. 2003;75:S729–S734
45. Jenkins KJ, Newburger JW, Lock JE, Davis RB, Coffman GA, Iezzoni LI. In-hospital mortality for surgical repair of congenital heart defects: preliminary observations of variation by hospital caseload. *Pediatrics*. 1995;95:323–330
46. Stoddard JJ, Cull WL, Jewett EA, Brotherton SE, Mulvey HJ, Alden ER; for the American Academy of Pediatrics Committee on Pediatric Workforce Subcommittee on Subspecialty Workforce. Providing pediatric subspecialty care: a workforce analysis. *Pediatrics*. 2000;106:1325–1333
47. Chang RR, Klitzner TS. Can regionalization decrease the number of deaths for children who undergo cardiac surgery? A theoretical analysis. *Pediatrics*. 2002;109:173–181

All policy statements from the American Academy of Pediatrics automatically expire 5 years after publication unless reaffirmed, revised, or retired at or before that time.

Managed Care and Children With Special Health Care Needs

- *Clinical Report*

AMERICAN ACADEMY OF PEDIATRICS

CLINICAL REPORT
Guidance for the Clinician in Rendering Pediatric Care

Theodore A. Kastner, MD; and the Committee on Children With Disabilities

Managed Care and Children With Special Health Care Needs

ABSTRACT. The implementation of managed care for children with special health care needs is often associated with apprehension regarding new barriers to health care services. At times, these barriers may overshadow opportunities for improvement. This statement discusses such opportunities, identifies challenges, and proposes active roles for pediatricians and families to improve managed care for children with special health care needs. *Pediatrics* 2004;114:1693–1698; *managed care, children with special health care needs, chronic illness, disease management, Medicaid.*

ABBREVIATIONS. MCO, managed care organization; SCHIP, State Children's Health Insurance Program; AAP, American Academy of Pediatrics; CHCS, Center for Health Care Strategies.

INTRODUCTION

Managed care has been expanding to include coverage for children* with special health care needs, most of whom have previously received health services through a combination of fee-for-service plans and public programs including Medicaid and state and federal maternal and child health programs. Many managed care plans focus on the provision of efficient services to generally healthy populations and are not routinely designed to respond to the special needs of children who have disabilities and chronic illnesses. Managed care could benefit these children and their families by improving access and coordination of services. However, there is potential for the difficulties that families face in obtaining the full range of child and family services necessary to ensure the child's good health and proper development to increase.[1,2] Aspects of managed care are reviewed as they relate to children with special health care needs, and steps for improving managed care services for these children are suggested, including recommendations to assist pediatricians in improving their ability to be reimbursed for providing services to children with special health care needs who are enrolled in managed care organizations (MCOs).

The guidance in this report does not indicate an exclusive course of treatment or serve as a standard of medical care. Variations, taking into account individual circumstances, may be appropriate.

doi:10.1542/peds.2004-2148

*In accordance with the policies of the American Academy of Pediatrics, references to "child" and "children" in this document include infants, children, adolescents, and young adults up to age 21.

PEDIATRICS (ISSN 0031 4005). Copyright © 2004 by the American Academy of Pediatrics.

WHAT IS MANAGED CARE?

Freund and Lewit[3] define managed care as a delivery system that integrates financing and delivery of specified health care services by means of 4 key elements:

1. Arrangement with selected clinicians to furnish health care services to members of the plan for preset fees.
2. Explicit standards for the selection of clinicians.
3. Formal programs of quality assurance and utilization review.
4. Substantial incentives for members to use clinicians associated with the plan.

Managed care aims to provide quality health services through utilization-control and cost-containment mechanisms. Achieving these goals for children with special health care needs requires special attention to several key issues. These concerns operate throughout the system of care, including the pediatrician, the family and child, the MCO, and the payor (parent's employer, Medicaid, Medicare, etc). A more thorough discussion of managed care can be found in *The Pediatrician's Guide to Managed Care.*[4]

WHO ARE CHILDREN WITH SPECIAL HEALTH CARE NEEDS?

Children with special health care needs represent a diverse population.[5,6] Recently, the federal Maternal and Child Health Bureau's Division of Services for Children With Special Health Care Needs convened a workgroup to develop a definition:

> Children with special health care needs are those who have or are at increased risk for a chronic physical, developmental, behavioral, or emotional condition and who also require health and related services of a type or amount beyond that required by children generally.[7(p138)]

Studies indicate that 6%[3] to 35%[8] (depending on what is included among the disabling conditions) of children have special health care needs and require special health care services. Children with special health care needs utilize significantly more health care services than other children.[9] These children have more complicated disabilities (eg, multiple, lifelong, and/or technology dependent) that compound their needs. Subspecialty and inpatient care, often at tertiary facilities, as well as ongoing complex outpatient management, community-based services, home nursing services, and medical supplies make it difficult to devise realistic strategies for cost containment.

This subset of the pediatric population, children with special health care needs and their families, faces an important challenge with the growth of managed care in being able to access all services described.

Children with special health care needs differ from adults with disabilities in a managed care environment in a variety of ways. Three major differences include: (1) the changing dynamics of child development affect the needs of these children at different developmental stages and alter their expected outcomes; illness and disability can delay, sometimes irreversibly, a child's normal development; (2) the epidemiology and prevalence of childhood disabilities, with many rare or low-incidence conditions and few common ones, differ markedly from those of adults, in which there are few rare conditions and several common ones; and (3) because of children's need for adult protection and guidance, their health and development depend greatly on their families' health and socioeconomic status.[1] Strategies that optimize child health outcomes, minimize the potential for developmental delay, and address these differences must be an integral part of any system that presumes to manage care for this special population.

PEDIATRICIANS, MANAGED CARE, AND THE MEDICAL HOME

The medical home is characterized as "accessible, continuous, comprehensive, family centered, coordinated, compassionate, and culturally effective. It should be delivered or directed by well-trained physicians who provide primary care and help to manage and facilitate essentially all aspects of pediatric care. The physician should be known to the child and family and should be able to develop a partnership of mutual responsibility and trust with them."[10(p184)]

Incentives of managed care that focus on primary care, care coordination, and community-based services based on the principles of the medical home are generally more effective than costly uncoordinated care, such as relying on episodic care in emergency departments. As a result, the pediatrician serving children with special health care needs in managed care must focus on preserving the medical home and enhancing the capacity of the family to care for the child in the community.

Given this need, it is particularly important to gather objective data to evaluate important process and outcome measures in managed care.[11,12] Managed care, because it aggregates cost, utilization, and outcomes data, provides a unique opportunity to assess the quality of care received by children with special health care needs. Newacheck et al[13] outlined the necessary attributes for such a system. Effective monitoring of managed care for children with special health care needs requires the capability to identify various categories of children with chronic conditions in the target population. Uniform definitions and coding mechanisms may also need to be established to retrieve data for these children. The system should be comprehensive enough to monitor a variety of factors pertinent to families with children with special health care needs, such as child health, family influences, access, utilization, expenditures, cost-ef-

fectiveness, quality, satisfaction, and short- and long-term effects. "Managed Care and Children With Special Health Care Needs: Creating a Medical Home" is an excellent review of this topic and can be found at www.aap.org/advocacy/mmcmdhom.htm.

FOCUS ON THE FAMILY OF CHILDREN WITH SPECIAL HEALTH CARE NEEDS

As families change from fee-for-service to managed care, long-term relationships may change abruptly. At times, the change is from physicians with whom the family feels familiarity and comfort based on common experience and understanding to physicians in another plan who may lack the experience or desire to care for children with special needs. Other factors such as unfamiliarity with the child and family, lack of resources available to families and children with special health care needs, or the inability to coordinate care may result in a decrease in the quality of care.[14]

Managed care may also pose other risks for children with special health care needs. First, "risk avoidance" may motivate health plans to "cherry pick," thereby leading to the exclusion of high-risk populations from many managed care initiatives. In addition, capitation contracts, particularly those that include financial risk, may create disincentives for primary care pediatricians to take on high-cost patients, especially without agreement as to what constitutes "fair" payment rates or adequate risk adjustment. Paradoxically, managed care can also lead to fragmentation of care. For example, the use of carve-outs for behavioral and other services often prevent pediatricians from being reimbursed for services, which can lead to difficulties in coordinating care between pediatricians and behavioral health care professionals. Finally, few data currently provide information on the relationship between managed care and other vitally important supports for the child and family. For example, states implementing Medicaid managed care for children with special health care needs need to ensure that "medically necessary services" include habilitative services, the goals of which are to improve function, including physical therapy, speech therapy, occupational therapy, durable medical equipment, specialized nursing services, telemedicine, and other similar services.[15] These services need to be closely coordinated with additional guidance provided through the Individuals With Disabilities Education Act (Pub L No. 101-476 [1990]), the Home and Community Based Services Waiver (Pub L No. 97-35 §2176 §1915), the "Katie Beckett" Waiver, and Early and Periodic Screening, Diagnostic, and Treatment program services.

MAKING MANAGED CARE WORK

Pediatricians are in a unique position to have a significant role in ensuring the appropriate design and implementation of managed care for children with special health care needs, particularly when public programs such as Medicaid and the State Children's Health Insurance Program (SCHIP) are involved. The American Academy of Pediatrics

(AAP) offers a wealth of information to pediatricians interested in contracting with Medicaid MCOs. Particularly useful are "Medicaid Policy Statement," "Medicaid Managed Care Contracts: Key Issues for Pediatricians," (see "Resources") and "Guiding Principles for Managed Care Arrangements for the Health Care of Newborns, Infants, Children, Adolescents, and Young Adults."[12]

The following section is not a comprehensive review but represents a brief discussion of selected topics related to children with special health care needs.

At the state level, individual pediatricians can work closely with state agencies that contract with and/or regulate health plans. In many instances, pediatricians will find that their interests are aligned with those of other health care professionals, advocates, and consumers who see opportunities in the changing marketplace. For example, as states implement Medicaid managed care, pediatricians can play an important role at the state and plan levels in strengthening the capacity of MCOs to address special needs of children, including recruitment and retention of general and subspecialty pediatricians. They also can assist in establishing appropriate utilization review mechanisms and quality improvement activities. Finally, they can be important partners in ensuring cost-effective systems of care for children with special health care needs. The AAP has numerous policy statements and, along with state chapters, other resources available to states and plans. For example, the AAP is working with health plans to ensure that a definition of medical necessity be sensitive to the needs of children, particularly children with special health care needs.[15]

At the MCO level, pediatricians can support health plans by advocating for adequate capitation by payors. This may be an important step in building good will between pediatricians and health plans. Capitation systems that include managing the care of children with special health care needs should recognize the need for increased pediatrician time required for service coordination, an increased number of office visits, lengthy counseling, and the potential for increased communication associated with referral for community, subspecialty, and hospital services. If capitation is to be realistic in relation to the care of children with special health care needs, methods to determine fair and appropriate capitation rates need to be developed, including application of an empirically sound and methodologically valid risk-adjustment payment system based on health status. State AAP chapters and their member pediatricians can assist MCOs in negotiating with government or commercial payors.

The Center for Health Care Strategies (CHCS) offers a number of resources for pediatricians. The CHCS works with state officials, health plan leaders, and consumer organizations across the country to improve health services for low-income families and for people with severe illnesses and disabilities whose needs cross over from the routine to the highly specialized. These resources include training and technical assistance to help states, health plans, and consumer organizations effectively use managed care to improve the quality of services for beneficiaries, reduce racial and ethnic health disparities, and increase community options for people with disabilities. CHCS recently concluded a program titled "Improving Managed Care for Children With Special Needs" to develop and pilot strategies to improve the quality of care for children with special needs enrolled in Medicaid and SCHIP. The workgroup, consisting of chief medical officers and decision makers from leading Medicaid health plans across the country, identified and piloted best practices for children with special needs. Plans focused on creating a "Medical Home," cultural competency, risk adjustment, and consumer relations. A toolkit summarizing best practices learned by workgroup plans is available online at www.chcs.org.

PEDIATRICIANS CAN ADVOCATE FOR THEMSELVES IN THIS PROCESS

As noted above, pediatricians contracting with health plans are paid through a variety of means such as fee-for-service reimbursement, capitation, and/or administrative fees. It is certain that providing care to children with special health care needs is more expensive than providing care to average healthy children. As a result, it is most important that pediatricians contracting with health care plans have specific knowledge about how much it costs their practices to provide care to specific types of patients. Pediatricians who contract with MCOs at rates that are below cost will ultimately shortchange themselves, their patients, and their patients' families and be frustrated by what they perceive as a poor relationship with their MCO partners. As a result, all negotiations for reimbursement must be guided by and based on knowledge of the practice's internal cost structure. Fee-for-service options are most appropriate for pediatricians in smaller practices that have small numbers of children with special health care needs. In this scenario, the practice is protected against cost overruns associated with unexpected patterns of utilization (adverse events). In contrast, pediatricians in larger practices may consider capitation as a means of reimbursement. When appropriate, capitation can improve cash flow, thereby enabling pediatricians to make investments in necessary support services. More importantly, capitation may allow pediatricians to negotiate to provide an expanded array of services that may include mental health and care management services. For example, reimbursement through capitation may be used to pay for care coordination services that may not be paid for in a fee-for-service system. In addition, capitation that includes primary care and behavioral services may protect pediatricians and their patients from the negative effects of aforementioned behavioral carve-outs, which may be particularly useful for pediatricians whose practices are focused on neurodevelopmental disabilities or developmental and behavioral pediatrics.

Finally, pediatricians should seek opportunities to

work with utilization management and quality improvement committees of MCOs. Pediatricians may be assisted in this effort by their AAP chapters. Many chapters operate practice-management committees that work closely with pediatricians to monitor contracting issues between pediatricians and MCOs. These forums provide opportunities for pediatricians to educate MCO personnel about standards of care for children with and without special health care needs and to address issues including Early and Periodic Screening, Diagnostic, and Treatment program services, clinical practice, and transition planning.

CARE COORDINATION

Care coordination has emerged as a vitally important part of successful managed care for children with special health care needs.[16] In this regard, care coordination is not focused solely on utilization management but rather represents a collaborative process that assesses, plans, implements, coordinates, and monitors and evaluates available services that may be required to meet an individual's health needs. Care coordination can occur at several levels including state systems such as Title V. Care coordination can occur within the MCO through models such as those used in Oregon or New Jersey. For example, New Jersey requires that all contracting MCOs provide care management services to persons with "special needs." These individuals receive a comprehensive needs assessment, an individual care plan, and monthly case management support. In addition, case management can occur through carve-out organizations, including disease management companies or behavioral health care organizations, or at the level of the individual physician. The best known carve-out models relate to the provision of mental health services. Most pediatricians find these arrangements uncomfortable because they encourage fragmentation in contracting and service delivery.

MCOs recently began to explore the role of care management programs targeted at special-needs populations. These programs are generally modeled after disease management programs demonstrated to have been successful in addressing issues related to chronic illness (eg, asthma, diabetes, depression, congestive heart failure) in managed care. Programs include Community Medical Alliance (Neighborhood Health Plan), which focuses on human immunodeficiency virus infection and physical disabilities; Independent Care (Humana), serving all persons with special health care needs; and Developmental Disabilities Health Alliance Inc (University Health Plan),[17] addressing children and adults with developmental disabilities. Care management takes time and requires financial support. Pediatricians should advocate for adequate funding of care management. For pediatricians who want to provide these services, reimbursement for care management is occasionally available in the form of enhanced fee-for-service reimbursement, capitation, and/or administrative fees.

CHARACTERISTICS OF SUCCESSFUL PEDIATRIC PRACTICES FOR CHILDREN WITH SPECIAL HEALTH CARE NEEDS

Satisfaction for pediatricians working with MCOs to provide care to children with special health care needs can be enhanced. Negotiating for adequate compensation is strengthened if pediatricians can demonstrate that primary care and preventive health interventions decrease hospitalizations, emergency department utilization, and pharmaceutical costs. For the individual clinician, collection of utilization data on all patients with special health care needs in the practice is useful. For example, Developmental Disabilities Health Alliance Inc has demonstrated that appropriate outpatient care and care management services can decrease inpatient utilization and costs by ~25% for persons with developmental disabilities,[18–20] and Children's Hospital at Strong in Rochester, New York, demonstrated an eightfold decrease in length of stay for selected children.[21,22] In general, it is more efficient for a practice to serve a larger volume of patients through a smaller number of payors. Once a practice has chosen to work with a specific payor, it should also discuss methods of ensuring that an adequate volume of patients be referred for care.

It should be cautioned that partially or fully capitated reimbursement strategies could also create disincentives for appropriate subspecialty referral. In fully capitated plans, the primary care physician assumes financial risk for all care. Consequently, the reimbursement to the primary care physician decreases with increasing need for subspecialty care and hospital services. Children with disabilities and other chronic conditions that may lead to disability require the services of pediatric medical subspecialists and pediatric surgical specialists in addition to primary care pediatricians. Access to and availability of pediatric medical subspecialty and pediatric surgical services must not be significantly impeded by managed care arrangements. Although it is ideal for the primary care physician to manage and coordinate care for a child's health needs, the complex or rare nature of a particular child's condition may make it difficult for the primary care physician to meet all the needs of the child and family adequately without the expertise of pediatric medical and surgical consultants. As presented in the AAP policy statement "Guiding Principles for Managed Care Arrangements for the Health Care of Newborns, Infants, Children, Adolescents, and Young Adults,"[12] access to pediatric medical subspecialty and pediatric surgical specialty care should exist without the burden of additional financial barriers and with appropriate referral processes and criteria in place. Adult-oriented physician medical subspecialists and surgeons should not be expected to have the expertise necessary to care for children with special health care needs. Likewise, pediatric therapy providers (physical therapy, occupational therapy, speech-language pathology, etc) should have significant pediatric specialty training and experience. Furthermore, child-specific technologic services should be accessible and affordable. Finally, pediatricians may also benefit from education guidelines related to specific conditions, such as those published by the Center for Health Improvement (available at www.ddhealthinfo.org).

All persons involved in managed care, including pediatricians and families, must fully understand how managed care works and how to advocate effectively for services. When plans for managed care are designed and implemented, planners and policy makers need to monitor them closely for unintended or unanticipated negative effects on children with special health care needs, their families, and their pediatricians. Flexibility and openness to promptly modifying these plans is called for when significant ineffectiveness, unnecessary costs, or a reduction in the quality of patient care is evident. Effective systems management and the use of predictable points of intervention can facilitate management in an already complex delivery system. If managed care is to demonstrate the capacity and flexibility to serve children with special health care needs adequately, pediatricians and families must hold MCOs to standards of conduct and service that parallel their own obligations to children.[14]

In conclusion, it is possible to make managed care work for children with special health care needs, their families, and their pediatricians. Successful models of managed care can be adapted to meet local market conditions. Partnerships among children with special health care needs, their families, and their pediatricians can be successful in creating a medical home for children with special health care needs in managed care.

IMPORTANT POINTS FOR THE PEDIATRICIAN

Opportunities exist for improving care for children with special health care needs in managed care systems. They can be facilitated by exercising the following strategies:

1. Creating partnerships among pediatricians, families of children with special health care needs, advocates, and payors, particularly state Medicaid and SCHIP programs, to address the needs of children with special health care needs in managed care.
2. Creating an understanding of major differences in disabilities between adults and children and the resulting need for managed care models to be sufficiently flexible to serve children with special health care needs and their families.
3. Ensuring access to care for all children through understanding and use of the medical home concept.
4. Adapting successful models of managed care to meet local market conditions through negotiation with payors and regulatory and licensing agencies.
5. Establishing fair reimbursement rates to compensate the physician for the increased time and complexity associated with providing health care services to children with special health care needs

and their families. At the MCO level, this translates into risk adjustment for capitated systems.
6. Obtaining additional funding for care coordination functions required by children with special health care needs and their families. These funds could be used to support social workers, nurses, or nurse practitioners in pediatric care settings.
7. Ensuring access to and appropriate use of pediatric medical subspecialists and pediatric surgical specialists with defined roles and open lines of communication between secondary and tertiary care and the medical home.
8. Creating viable systems of quality improvement capable of evaluating process and outcome data from which appropriate adjustments in the system are made to refine care to benefit children with special health care needs and their families.
9. Advocating at the federal level to protect children with special health care needs by ensuring access to adequate benefits, appropriate specialty services, and habilitative care.

COMMITTEE ON CHILDREN WITH DISABILITIES,
2003–2004
Adrian D. Sandler, MD, Chairperson
J. Daniel Cartwright, MD
John C. Duby, MD
Chris Plauché Johnson, MD, MEd
Lawrence Kaplan, MD
Eric B. Levey, MD
Nancy A. Murphy, MD
Ann Henderson Tilton, MD
W. Carl Cooley, MD
    Past Committee Member
David Hirsch, MD
    Past Committee Member
Theodore A. Kastner, MD
    Past Committee Member
Marian E. Kummer, MD
    Past Committee Member

LIAISONS
Bev Crider
    Family Voices
Merle McPherson, MD, MPH
    Maternal and Child Health Bureau
Donald Lollar, EdD
    Centers for Disease Control and Prevention
Paul Burgan, MD, PhD
    Past Liaison, Social Security Administration
Linda Michaud, MD
    Past Liaison, American Academy of Physical
    Medicine and Rehabilitation
Marshalyn Yeargin-Allsopp, MD
    Past Liaison, Centers for Disease Control and
    Prevention

STAFF
Stephanie Mucha, MPH

REFERENCES

1. Jameson EJ, Wehr E. Drafting national health care reform legislation to protect the health interests of children. *Stanford Law Pol Rev.* 1993;51: 152–176
2. Cooper WO, Kuhlthau K. Evaluating Medicaid managed care programs for children. *Ambul Pediatr.* 2001;1:112–116
3. Freund DA, Lewit EM. Managed care for children and pregnant women: promises and pitfalls. *Future Child.* 1993;3:92–122

4. American Academy of Pediatrics. *The Pediatrician's Guide to Managed Care.* 2nd ed. Elk Grove Village, IL: American Academy of Pediatrics; 2001

5. Newacheck PW, Strickland B, Shonkoff JP, et al. An epidemiologic profile of children with special health care needs. *Pediatrics.* 1998;102: 117–123

6. Perrin EC, Newacheck P, Bless IB, et al. Issues involved in the definition and classification of chronic health conditions. *Pediatrics.* 1993;91: 787–793

7. McPherson MP, Arango P, Fox H, et al. A new definition of children with special health care needs. *Pediatrics.* 1998;102:137–140

8. Newacheck PW, Hughes DC, Stoddard JJ, Halfon N. Children with chronic illness and Medicaid managed care. *Pediatrics.* 1994;93:497–500

9. Weller WE, Minkovitz CS, Anderson GF. Utilization of medical and health-related services among school-age children and adolescents with special health care needs (1994 National Health Interview Survey on Disability [NHIS-D] Baseline Data). *Pediatrics.* 2003;112:593–603

10. American Academy of Pediatrics, Medical Home Initiatives for Children With Special Needs Project Advisory Committee. The medical home. *Pediatrics.* 2002;110:184–186

11. Walsh KK, Kastner TA. Quality of health care for people with developmental disabilities: the challenge of managed care. *Ment Retard.* 1999; 37:1–15

12. American Academy of Pediatrics, Committee on Child Health Financing. Guiding principles for managed care arrangements for the health care of newborns, infants, children, adolescents, and young adults. *Pediatrics.* 2000;105:132–135

13. Newacheck PW, Stein RE, Walker DK, Gortmaker SL, Kuhlthau K, Perrin JM. Monitoring and evaluating managed care for children with chronic illnesses and disabilities. *Pediatrics.* 1996;98:952–958

14. Family Voices. *Managed Care: How Will Children With Special Health Care Needs Fare in Managed Care? Questions to Ask and Answer.* Algodones, NM: Family Voices; 1995. Available at: www.familyvoices.org/Information/mcqanda.htm. Accessed August 27, 2004

15. Berman S. A pediatric perspective on medical necessity. *Arch Pediatr Adolesc Med.* 1997;151:858–859

16. American Academy of Pediatrics, Committee on Children With Disabilities. Care coordination: integrating health and related systems of care for children with special health care needs. *Pediatrics.* 1999;104:978–981

17. US Public Health Service. *Closing the Gap: A National Blueprint to Improve the Health of Persons With Mental Retardation. Report of the Surgeon General's Conference on Health Disparities and Mental Retardation.* Washington, DC: US Public Health Service; 2002

18. Criscione T, Walsh KK, Kastner TA. An evaluation of care coordination in controlling inpatient hospital utilization of people with developmental disabilities. *Ment Retard.* 1995;33:364–373

19. Criscione T, Kastner TA, O'Brien D, Nathanson. Replication of a managed health care initiative for people with mental retardation living in the community. *Ment Retard.* 1994;32:43–52

20. Criscione T, Kastner TA, Walsh KK, Nathanson R. Managed health care services for people with mental retardation: impact on inpatient utilization. *Ment Retard.* 1993;31:297–306

21. Liptak GS, Burns CM, Davidson PW, McAnarney ER. Effects of providing comprehensive ambulatory services to children with chronic conditions. *Arch Pediatr Adolesc Med.* 1998;152:1003–1008

22. Kastner T, Walsh K. Cost of care coordination for children with special health care needs. *Arch Pediatr Adolesc Med.* 1999;153:1003–1004

RESOURCES

American Academy of Pediatrics. Managed care and children with special health care needs: creating a medical home. Available at: www.aap.org/advocacy/mmcmdhom.htm. Accessed August 27, 2004

American Academy of Pediatrics. Medicaid managed care contracts: key issues for pediatricians. Available at: www.aap.org/advocacy/mmcstrat.htm. Accessed August 27, 2004

American Academy of Pediatrics, Committee on Child Health Financing. Medicaid policy statement. *Pediatrics.* 1999;104:344–347

Hirsch D. Managing managed care: special care for special needs. *Pediatr News.* December 2000;42

Institute for Child Health Policy. *Evaluating Managed Care Plans for Children With Special Care Needs: A Purchaser's Tool.* Gainesville, FL: Institute for Child Health Policy; March 1998

Lewit EM, Monheit AC. Expenditures on health care for children and pregnant women. *Future Child.* 1992;2:95–114

Managed care for children with special needs: are medical homes provided? A self-evaluation tool for managed care companies [insert]. *AAP News.* March 1998

White P. Access to health care: insurance considerations for young adults with special health care needs/disabilities. *Pediatrics.* 2002;110:1328–1335

Nontherapeutic Use of Antimicrobial Agents in Animal Agriculture: Implications for Pediatrics

- *Technical Report*

AMERICAN ACADEMY OF PEDIATRICS

TECHNICAL REPORT

Katherine M. Shea MD, MPH, and the Committee on Environmental Health and
Committee on Infectious Diseases

Nontherapeutic Use of Antimicrobial Agents in Animal Agriculture: Implications for Pediatrics

ABSTRACT. Antimicrobial resistance is widespread. Overuse or misuse of antimicrobial agents in veterinary and human medicine is responsible for increasing the crisis of resistance to antimicrobial agents. The American Academy of Pediatrics, in conjunction with the US Public Health Service, has begun to address this problem by disseminating policies on the judicious use of antimicrobial agents in humans. Between 40% and 80% of the antimicrobial agents used in the United States each year are used in food animals; many are identical or very similar to drugs used in humans. Most of this use involves the addition of low doses of antimicrobial agents to the feed of healthy animals over prolonged periods to promote growth and increase feed efficiency or at a range of doses to prevent disease. These nontherapeutic uses contribute to resistance and create health dangers for humans. This report will describe how antimicrobial agents are used in animal agriculture and review the mechanisms by which such uses contribute to resistance in human pathogens. Although therapeutic use of antimicrobial agents in agriculture clearly contributes to the development of resistance, this report will concentrate on nontherapeutic uses in healthy animals. *Pediatrics* 2004; 114:862–868; *antibiotic, antimicrobial, resistance, child, infant, agriculture, foodborne, epidemiology.*

ABBREVIATIONS. NARMS, National Antimicrobial Resistance Monitoring System; VRE, vancomycin-resistant enterococci; Q-D, quinupristin-dalfopristin.

ANTIMICROBIAL USE IN ANIMAL FEEDS

Rationale for Use

In livestock and poultry production, antimicrobial agents are used therapeutically, prophylactically, and to promote growth and improve feed efficiency.[1] Therapeutic use in clinically ill animals involves using curative doses of antimicrobial agents for a relatively short period of time. However, antimicrobial agents used for acute illness may be delivered not just to sick individuals but to the entire group of animals to which the sick individuals belong. Many therapeutic antimicrobial agents are administered in water to animals raised in large numbers under industrial conditions, which may result in individual animals or birds receiving inadequate doses. The nature of swine and poultry production makes it difficult to treat individual animals; if a few birds show signs of clinical illness, the entire house (10 000–30 000 birds) is treated. Of the wide variety of agents approved for therapeutic use in animals, many are identical or similar to drugs used in human medicine[2] (Table 1). Only some require a veterinarian's prescription. Although the therapeutic uses of antimicrobial agents in agriculture have significant impact on the development of resistant organisms, they are not the focus of this report.

Antimicrobial agents are also used in animal production to promote growth, primarily by enhancing feed efficiency; the mechanism of action is not known. When used for this purpose, low doses of antimicrobial agents are added to the feed of healthy animals for much of their life span. In addition, prophylactic antimicrobial agents are used to control the dissemination of clinically diagnosed infectious diseases identified within a group of animals or to prevent an infectious disease that has not yet been clinically diagnosed.[1] Prophylactic antimicrobial agents may be used at either low doses or therapeutic doses. These uses generate selection pressure on microbial populations that is similar to growth-promotion use and will be discussed under the common term "nontherapeutic use" to denote their use in healthy animals. Prophylactic antimicrobial agents are used to prevent diseases common to animals grown under industrial conditions.[1] Feed efficiency refers to the ability to grow animals faster with less food. This results in shorter time to slaughter at less expense to the producer, improving profits and decreasing consumer costs.[3] Addition of subtherapeutic doses of antimicrobial agents to feed also results in bigger animals, an effect known as growth promotion.

Scope of Use

Manufacturers and users of antimicrobial agents are not required to report data on production or use for human or food-animal applications. Annual production estimates range from 35 million[4] to 50 million[5] pounds per year. The major nonhuman use of antimicrobial agents is in food-animal production. The Institute of Medicine estimates that 40% of an-

The guidance in this report does not indicate an exclusive course of treatment or serve as a standard of medical care. Variations, taking into account individual circumstances, may be appropriate.
DOI: 10.1542/peds.2004-1233

TABLE 1. Major Antimicrobial Agent Classes Approved for Nontherapeutic Use in Animals

Antimicrobial Class	Species	Prophylaxis	Growth Promotion
Aminoglycoside	Beef cattle, goats, poultry, sheep, swine	Yes	No
β-Lactam (penicillin)	Beef cattle, dairy cows, fowl, poultry, sheep, swine	Yes	Yes
β-Lactam (cephalosporin)	Beef cattle, dairy cows, poultry, sheep, swine	Yes	No
Ionophore	Beef cattle, fowl, goats, poultry, rabbits, sheep	Yes	Yes
Lincosamide	Poultry, swine	Yes	Yes
Macrolide	Beef cattle, poultry, swine	Yes	Yes
Polypeptide	Fowl, poultry, swine	Yes	Yes
Streptogramin	Beef cattle, poultry, swine	Yes	Yes
Sulfonamide	Beef cattle, poultry, swine	Yes	Yes
Tetracycline	Beef cattle, dairy cows, fowl, honey bees, poultry, sheep, swine	Yes	Yes
Other			
Bambermycins	Beef cattle, poultry, swine	Yes	Yes
Carbadox	Swine	Yes	Yes
Novobiocin	Fowl, poultry	Yes	No
Spectinomycin	Poultry, swine	Yes	No

Source: US General Accounting Office. *The Agricultural Use of Antibiotics and Its Implications for Human Health.* Washington, DC: General Accounting Office; 1999. Publication no. GAO-RCED 99–74

nual antimicrobial use in the United States is veterinary, and approximately three fourths of this use is categorized as nontherapeutic "supplements" in food animals.[5] Other estimates of nontherapeutic use in livestock are as high as 78%[4] of the total annual use of antimicrobial agents in the United States.

EVIDENCE OF SELECTION FOR ANTIMICROBIAL RESISTANCE ATTRIBUTABLE TO AGRICULTURAL USES OF ANTIMICROBIAL AGENTS

One of the most efficient ways to select for resistance genes in bacteria is to expose bacteria chronically to low doses of broad-spectrum antimicrobial agents. Levy et al[6] examined the effect of low-dose tetracycline in feed on the intestinal flora of chickens. Chickens were divided into experimental and control groups; the experimental group received feed containing oxytetracycline at concentrations similar to those used for therapy or prophylaxis; the control group received feed without oxytetracycline. The baseline resistance to tetracycline was generally less than 10%, with many samples exhibiting less than 0.1% resistance. Within 36 hours, resistance began to increase, and after 2 weeks, 90% of the chickens in the experimental group were excreting bacteria that were 100% resistant to tetracycline. Chickens in the control group did not exhibit an increase in resistant organisms during this same time period. Although the chickens were exposed only to tetracycline, multidrug resistance developed (to tetracycline, sulfonamides, streptomycin, ampicillin, and carbenicillin) through plasmid transfer. By 12 weeks, almost two thirds of the chickens in the experimental group excreted organisms resistant to tetracycline and at least 1 additional antimicrobial agent, and more than one quarter were resistant to 4 antimicrobial agents (tetracycline, ampicillin, streptomycin, and carbenicillin). Over time, chickens in the control group, despite isolation in different pens, also developed resistance, although at lower levels. One third of chickens in the control group were excreting more than 50% resistant organisms after 4 months. Transfer of resistance to humans also occurred, although

more slowly and at lower levels than in the control-group chickens. Within 6 months, more than 30% of fecal samples from farm dwellers contained more than 80% tetracycline-resistant bacteria versus 6.8% from control neighbors ($P < .001$). A 4-drug resistance pattern was found in farm families corresponding to that of the experimental-group chickens but was not found in neighborhood controls. Six months after the removal of all tetracycline feed from the farm, no tetracycline-resistant organisms were isolated from stool samples in 8 of 10 farm dwellers tested. This experiment demonstrated that resistance can develop quickly in the presence of antimicrobial pressure, that single-drug resistance becomes multidrug resistance, that resistance spreads beyond individuals exposed to the antimicrobial agent to other members of their species within the environment and to humans living and working on the farm, and that stopping feed supplementation with oxytetracycline leads to decreased incidence of resistance.

MECHANISMS OF SPREAD OF RESISTANT BACTERIA TO HUMANS

When animals become colonized with resistant organisms, these organisms can eventually reach humans through the food chain, direct contact, or contamination of water or crops from animal excreta.[7] Increasingly, food animals are raised in large numbers under close confinement, transported in large groups to slaughter, and processed very rapidly.[8] These stressful conditions cause increased bacterial shedding and inevitable contamination of hide, carcass,[9] and meat[10] with fecal bacteria. Dissemination of resistant pathogens via the food chain is facilitated further by centralized food processing and packaging, particularly of ground meat products, and broad distribution through food wholesalers and retail chains.[11] Farmers, farm workers, and farm families[6] as well as casual visitors[12] are at risk of infection with resistant organisms.

Environmental reservoirs may also contribute to the movement of resistance genes. Active antimicrobial agents have been detected in water near animal waste lagoons,[13] surface waters, and river sediments,[14] giving rise to concerns that environmental contamination with antimicrobial agents from agricultural and human use could present microbial populations with selective pressure, stimulate horizontal gene transfer, and amplify the number and variety of organisms that are resistant to antimicrobial agents. Supporting this concern, investigators recently found resistance genes identical to those found in swine waste lagoons in groundwater and soil microbes hundreds of meters downstream.[15]

Finally, there may also be direct human exposure to antimicrobial agents. Because many antimicrobial agents used in food-animal production can be obtained without a veterinarian's prescription, they are available for direct purchase and are often manually added to feed or water at farm level. This may be another pathway leading to development of resistance in occupationally exposed individuals, their families, and neighbors.[6]

EFFECT ON TREATMENT OF INFECTIONS IN CHILDREN

This section of the report reviews evidence that links agricultural use of antimicrobial agents to disease in infants and children for 2 major foodborne pathogens, *Campylobacter* species and *Salmonella* species, and for the opportunistic pathogen *Enterococcus* species.

Campylobacter Species

Campylobacter organisms cause approximately 2.5 million cases of foodborne illness annually in the United States and are the leading cause of bacterial foodborne illness.[16] The incidence of *Campylobacter* infections in infants younger than 1 year is twice that in the general population (54.1 vs 21.7 per 100 000 population).[17] Almost 20% of all reported cases of *Campylobacter* infections occur in children younger than 10 years.[18]

Erythromycin or another macrolide is the drug of choice for *Campylobacter* infections in infants and children; fluoroquinolones and tetracyclines are used frequently in adults. Antimicrobial resistance in *Campylobacter* species is an increasing problem.[19] Currently, macrolide resistance in human isolates of *Campylobacter jejuni*, the species causing 90% of human infections, is stable and usually less than 5%.[19] *Campylobacter coli*, which causes approximately 10% of human infections, has a much higher resistance rate, reaching 70%.[20] The major reservoirs are poultry for *C jejuni* and turkeys and swine for *C coli*.[21] Differences in resistance rates may reflect differences in the use of antimicrobial agents.[20] Erythromycin and tetracyclines are approved for use in food-producing animals for therapeutic and growth-promotion purposes.

Fluoroquinolone resistance in *Campylobacter* species demonstrates the links among agricultural use of antimicrobial agents, selection of resistance, and dissemination of resistant infections through the food chain. Fluoroquinolones were approved for use by prescription in diseased poultry flocks in the United States in 1995.[22] In Minnesota between 1996 and 1998, infections in humans caused by fluoroquinolone-resistant organisms increased, parallel with the prevalence of retail domestic chicken products contaminated with fluoroquinolone-resistant organisms. Data from the National Antimicrobial Resistance Monitoring System (NARMS) demonstrate that fluoroquinolone resistance among *Campylobacter* isolates from humans began to increase nationwide in the late 1990s, from 13% in 1997 to 20.5% in 1999.[23] A 1999 survey of grocery store chicken found that 44% of samples were contaminated with *Campylobacter* species; 24% of the isolates were resistant to ciprofloxacin, and 32% were resistant to nalidixic acid.[24] Increasing resistance is even more worrisome, because data suggest that strains of resistant *Campylobacter* species may be more virulent than sensitive strains. In a case-control telephone study, investigators found that untreated patients with fluoroquinolone-resistant *Campylobacter* infection had an average of 12 days of diarrhea versus 6 days in patients with sensitive strains ($P = .02$).[25] For patients who were treated with fluoroquinolones, the duration of diarrhea was significantly longer in those infected with resistant versus sensitive strains (8 vs 6 days [$P = .02$]).

Salmonella Species

Nontyphoidal *Salmonella* organisms cause 1.4 million illnesses annually, 95% of which are thought to be foodborne.[16] It is estimated that 600 deaths occur annually from *Salmonella* infections, primarily among the elderly and very young.[16] More than one third of all cases occur in children younger than 10 years,[18] and the incidence in children younger than 1 year is 10 times higher than in the general population (128.9 vs 12.4 per 100 000).[17] Ten percent of blood and central nervous system infections caused by *Salmonella* species as reported to the Centers for Disease Control and Prevention occur in children younger than 1 year.[26] Children of all ages with chronic conditions such as sickle cell anemia are at high risk of serious complications from infections with *Salmonella* species.[27]

The dissemination of resistant *Salmonella* infections through the food chain is well documented. A 6-state outbreak of plasmid-mediated, multidrug-resistant *Salmonella newport* infection attributed to consumption of contaminated beef was traced back to a feedlot that used nontherapeutic doses of chlortetracycline as a growth promoter in feed.[28] Investigators found the outbreak organism in isolates from both animals and humans on an adjacent dairy farm. An increased risk of illness caused by a resistant strain was observed in patients who were taking antimicrobial agents for other infections (odds ratio, 51.3; $P = .001$), suggesting that asymptomatic carriage was converted to symptomatic infection by the use of antimicrobial agents. Of 3 children younger than 10 years, 2 had received antimicrobial agents before onset of their illness.

Neonatal infections caused by *Salmonella* species also have been attributed to indirect exposure to foodborne sources. Bezanson et al[29] described a plasmid-mediated, 6-drug–resistant strain of *Salmonella* serotype Typhimurium acquired asymptomatically by a pregnant woman from raw milk and passed to her infant at birth. The infant became ill within 24 hours with septicemia and meningitis. Three to 4 days later, several other infants in the newborn nursery developed diarrhea with the same resistant organism. In another newborn nursery outbreak, *Salmonella heidelberg* resistant to chloramphenicol, sulfamethoxazole, and tetracycline caused bloody diarrhea in 3 infants.[30] The index case was a term infant born by cesarean delivery after 18 hours of ruptured membranes. The mother was a farmer's daughter who, until shortly before delivery, had been working with new calves from a herd containing several sick calves.

The treatment of *Salmonella* infections, especially in young children, has become increasingly difficult because of antimicrobial resistance. In the early 1980s, the prevalence of multidrug-resistant *Salmonella* species began to increase and by 1995 had reached 19% in the United States.[31] Some strains, particularly *Salmonella* serotype Typhimurium DT104, cause invasive disease that frequently requires treatment but may be resistant to 5 or more classes of antimicrobial agents.[32,33] Currently, extended-spectrum cephalosporins have become the preferred drugs for empiric treatment in pediatrics, and fluoroquinolones are preferred in adults. The efficacy of these drugs may now be threatened. In 1999, Molbak et al[34] described an outbreak in Denmark of *Salmonella* serotype Typhimurium DT104 resistant to ampicillin, chloramphenicol, streptomycin, sulfonamides, tetracycline, and quinolones, linked by molecular fingerprinting (the process of identifying unique clones by DNA typing) to 2 swine herds. Two patients died in this outbreak, and therapeutic failure was considered related to antimicrobial resistance. Of 4 children, 1 was an infant who was hospitalized and treated with cefotaxime. Fey et al[35] reported on a child from Nebraska who became infected with *Salmonella* serotype Typhimurium DT104 resistant to ampicillin, chloramphenicol, tetracycline, sulfisoxazole, kanamycin, streptomycin, several classes of cephalosporins, aztreonam, cefoxitin, gentamicin, and tobramycin. An analysis of recent NARMS data revealed that 77% of patients with culture-proven ceftriaxone-resistant *Salmonella* infection between 1997 and 1998 were younger than 18 years and that the prevalence of ceftriaxone-resistant human isolates increased fivefold from 0.1% in 1996 to 0.5% in 1999.[36] Human isolates of *Salmonella* species resistant to 8 or more agents increased almost sevenfold from 0.3% in 1996% to 2% in 1999. Decreased susceptibility to fluoroquinolones may also be emerging. According to NARMS data, the prevalence of resistance to ciprofloxacin among *Salmonella* isolates increased from 0.4% in 1996 to 1% in 1999.

Major reservoirs for *Salmonella* infection are food animals, including poultry, cattle, and swine. Nontherapeutic antimicrobial agents are routinely used, particularly in swine. One survey of 825 retail samples of raw chicken, turkey, pork, and beef revealed an overall rate of 3% contamination with *Salmonella* species.[37] White et al[38] recently reported that 20% of retail ground meat samples were contaminated with *Salmonella* species; 80% of these samples were resistant to at least 1 antimicrobial agent, 53% were resistant to at least 3 antimicrobial agents, and 16% were resistant to ceftriaxone.

Enterococci

Enterococci are normal flora in food animals, domesticated animals, wild animals, and humans. In the 1990s, vancomycin-resistant enterococci (VRE) became common bacterial pathogens responsible for an increasing number of nosocomial infection in the United States, including in children.[39] Hospitalized and seriously ill children are increasingly affected.[40,41] Patterns in the prevalence of VRE infection have developed differently in the United States and Europe, helping to elucidate the links between use of antimicrobial agents in animals and resistance in humans. Whereas the epidemic of VRE infection in the United States seems related to the large increase in vancomycin use in human medicine,[42] the increased incidence of VRE infection in Europe seems to be attributable to the use of antimicrobial agents in animals. Vancomycin has not been used widely in Europe in human medicine, but avoparcin, a related glycopeptide, has been used as a growth promoter for decades.[43] Avoparcin selects for cross resistance to vancomycin when used in farm animals.[44,45] In the United States, VRE is rarely cultured from healthy individuals in the community,[46] but it is often isolated from healthy community members in Europe.[47] In Europe, VRE can also be cultured from healthy poultry, pigs,[48] ponies, and dogs[49]; uncooked chicken meat[50] and minced pork; and raw sewage from urban and rural locations.[51] Molecular fingerprinting of these isolates shows much higher heterogeneity in European isolates compared with US isolates, suggesting that the prevalence of VRE in Europe is a response of multiple enterococcal populations to the presence of avoparcin in a variety of host species and locations.

Recent reports from the United States, however, suggest a strong and emerging link between VRE and agricultural use of antimicrobial agents. In response to the epidemic of VRE infection, quinupristin-dalfopristin (Q-D) was licensed for use in 1999 by the US Food and Drug Administration as treatment for highly resistant strains. Q-D is a streptogramin, a class of antimicrobials not used previously in humans because of unacceptable toxicity.[52] Virginiamycin is a related streptogramin that has been used in the United States as a growth promoter for poultry, swine, and cattle since 1974.[53] In a recent study, 58% of 407 retail chicken samples and 1% of human stool samples were found to harbor Q-D-resistant enterococci 1 year before its release for human use, and humans were also found to carry resistant organisms without previous exposure to Q-D.[54] This suggests that ingestion of resistant enterococci in retail meats resulted in colonization of the human gut by these foodborne pathogens; such colonization of the gut of humans has been documented for up to 14 days after ingestion.[55] It also demonstrates the potential risks of using antimicrobial agents thought not to be important to human medicine as growth promoters. As antimicrobial resistance increases, it is likely that more veterinary agents may be modified for human use. If resistance has already developed in animal populations, however, the period of their efficacy in human disease may be quite limited.

EUROPEAN EXPERIENCE

Sweden led Europe in banning antimicrobial growth promoters in 1986.[56] The ban in Sweden has resulted in decreased use of antimicrobial agents in food animals and, accompanied by improved animal husbandry practices, sustained productivity and profitability of the industry.[57] Denmark, which has a more industrialized animal production system similar to that in the United States, instituted a voluntary ban on antimicrobial growth promoters in 1998. Denmark has had a similar decrease in antimicrobial use and decreased prevalence of resistant organisms in food animals without loss of productivity or profitability.[58]

CONCLUSIONS

Resistance to antimicrobial agents is an increasing and serious problem. Judicious use of antimicrobial agents in humans will address only approximately 50% of use and will be insufficient to curb the accelerating upward trend in resistance. The largest nonhuman use of antimicrobial agents is in food-animal production, and most of this is in healthy animals to increase growth or prevent diseases. Evidence now exists that these uses of antimicrobial agents in food-producing animals have a direct negative impact on human health and multiple impacts on the selection and dissemination of resistance genes in animals and the environment. Children are at increased risk of acquiring many of these infections with resistant bacteria and are at great risk of severe complications if they become infected. Improved surveillance and continued documentation will elucidate the magnitude of the impact that these uses have on public health in general and children's health in particular.

COMMITTEE ON ENVIRONMENTAL HEALTH, 2003–2004
Michael W. Shannon, MD, MPH, Chairperson
Dana Best, MD, MPH
Helen J. Binns, MD, MPH
Christine L. Johnson, MD
Janice J. Kim, MD, MPH, PhD
Lynnette J. Mazur, MD, MPH
David W. Reynolds, MD
James R. Roberts, MD, MPH
William B. Weil, Jr, MD

PAST COMMITTEE MEMBERS
Katherine M. Shea, MD, MPH
Sophie J. Balk, MD
    Past Chairperson

LIAISONS
Robert H. Johnson, MD
    Agency for Toxic Substances and Disease Registry/
    Centers for Disease Control and Prevention
Elizabeth Blackburn, RN
    US Environmental Protection Agency

Martha Linet, MD
    National Cancer Institute
Walter Rogan, MD
    National Institute of Environmental Health
    Sciences

STAFF
Paul Spire

COMMITTEE ON INFECTIOUS DISEASES, 2003–2004
Margaret B. Rennels, MD, Chairperson
Carol J. Baker, MD
Robert S. Baltimore, MD
Joseph A. Bocchini, Jr, MD
Penelope H. Dennehy, MD
Robert W. Frenck, Jr, MD
Caroline B. Hall, MD
Sarah S. Long, MD
Julia A. McMillan, MD
H. Cody Meissner, MD
Keith R. Powell, MD
Lorry G. Rubin, MD
Thomas N. Saari, MD

PAST COMMITTEE MEMBERS
Jon S. Abramson, MD
    Past Chairperson
Gary D. Overturf, MD

LIAISONS
Joanne Embree, MD
    Canadian Paediatric Society
Marc A. Fischer, MD
    Centers for Disease Control and Prevention
Bruce G. Gellin, MD, MPH
    National Vaccine Program Office
Martin Mahoney, MD, PhD
    American Academy of Family Physicians
Mamodikoe Makhene, MD
    National Institutes of Health
Walter A. Orenstein, MD
    Centers for Disease Control and Prevention
Douglas R. Pratt, MD
    Food and Drug Administration
Jeffrey R. Starke, MD
    American Thoracic Society
Jack Swanson, MD
    Practice Action Group

CONSULTANT
Edgar O. Ledbetter, MD

EX OFFICIO
Larry K. Pickering, MD
    Red Book Editor

STAFF
Martha Cook, MS

REFERENCES

1. Institute of Medicine, Committee on Drug Use in Food Animals and National Research Council. *The Use of Drugs in Food Animals: Benefits and Risks.* Washington, DC: National Academy Press; 1999
2. US Department of Agriculture, Center for Veterinary Medicine. *2003 Online Green Book.* Rockville, MD: Center for Veterinary Medicine; 2003. Available at: www.fda.gov/cvm/greenbook/elecgbook.html. Accessed September 30, 2003
3. Mathews KJ. *Antimicrobial Drug Use and Veterinary Costs in U.S. Livestock Production.* Washington, DC: Economic Research Service, US Department of Agriculture; 2001. USDA Agricultural Information Bulletin 766.

Available at: www.ers.usda.gov/publications/aib766/aib766.pdf. Accessed September 30, 2003

4. Mellon M, Benbrook C, Lutz Benbrook K. *Hogging it! Estimates of Antimicrobial Abuse in Livestock.* Washington, DC: Union of Concerned Scientists; 2001

5. Institute of Medicine, Committee on Human Health Risk Assessment of Using Subtherapeutic Antibiotics in Animal Feeds. *Human Health Risks With the Subtherapeutic Use of Penicillin or Tetracyclines in Animal Feed.* Washington, DC: National Academy Press; 1989

6. Levy SB, FitzGerald GB, Macone AB. Changes in intestinal flora of farm personnel after introduction of a tetracycline-supplemented feed on a farm. *N Engl J Med.* 1976;295:583–588

7. Witte W. Medical consequences of antibiotic use in agriculture. *Science.* 1998;279:996–997

8. Center for Science in the Public Interest, Environmental Defense Fund, Food Animal Concerns Trust, Public Citizens Health Research Group, Union of Concerned Scientists. Petition to rescind approvals for the subtherapeutic uses in livestock of antibiotics used in (or related to those used in) human medicine. Available at: www.cspinet.org/ar/petition_3_99.html. Accessed September 30, 2003

9. Barkocy-Gallagher GA, Arthur TM, Siragusa GR, et al. Genotypic analysis of *Escherichia coli* O157:H7 and O157 nonmotile isolates recovered from beef cattle and carcasses at processing plants in the Midwestern states of the United States. *Appl Environ Microbiol.* 2001;67:3810–3818

10. Millemann Y, Gaubert S, Remy D, Colmin C. Evaluation of IS 200-PCR and comparison with other molecular markers to trace *Salmonella enterica* subsp. *enterica* serotype *Typhimurium* bovine isolates from farm to meat. *J Clin Microbiol.* 2000;38:2204–2209

11. Tauxe RV, Holmberg SD, Cohen ML. The epidemiology of gene transfer in the environment. In: Levy SB, Miller RV, eds. *Gene Transfer in the Environment.* New York, NY: McGraw-Hill Publishing Co; 1989:377–403

12. Centers for Disease Control and Prevention. Outbreaks of *Escherichia coli* O157:H7 infections among children associated with farm visits—Pennsylvania and Washington, 2000. *MMWR Morb Mortal Wkly Rep.* 2001;50:293–298

13. Meyer MT, Kolpin DW, Bumgarner JE, Varns JL, Daughtridge JV. Occurrence of antibiotics in surface and ground water near confined animal feeding operations and waste water treatment plants using radioimmunoassay and liquid chromatography/electrospray mass spectrometry [abstract 34].Presented at the 219th meeting of the American Chemical Society; March 26–30, 2000; San Francisco, CA

14. Halling-Sorensen B, Nors Nielsen S, Lanzky PF, Ingerslev F, Holten Lutzhoft HC, Jorgensen SE. Occurrence, fate and effects of pharmaceutical substances in the environment—a review. *Chemosphere.* 1998;36:357–393

15. Chee-Sanford JC, Aminov RI, Krapac IJ, Garrigues-Jeanjean N, Mackie RI. Occurrence and diversity of tetracycline resistance genes in lagoons and groundwater underlying two swine production facilities. *Appl Environ Microbiol.* 2001;67:1494–1502

16. Mead PS, Slutsker L, Dietz V, et al. Food-related illness and death in the United States. *Emerg Infect Dis.* 1999;5:607–625. Available at: www.cdc.gov/ncidod/EID/vol5no5/pdf/mead.pdf. Accessed September 30, 2003

17. US Department of Agriculture, Food Safety and Inspection Service. *Report to Congress. FoodNet: An Active Surveillance System for Bacterial Foodborne Diseases in the United States.* Washington, DC: Food Safety and Inspection Service; 1999. Available at: www.fsis.usda.gov/ophs/rpcong98/rpcong98.htm. Accessed September 30, 2003

18. US Department of Agriculture, Food Safety and Inspection Service. *Sentinel Site Study. The Establishment and Implementation of an Active Surveillance System for Bacterial Foodborne Diseases in the United States.* Washington, DC: Food Safety and Inspection Service; 1997. Available at: www.fsis.usda.gov/OPHS/fsisrep2.htm. Accessed September 30, 2003

19. Smith KE, Bender JB, Osterholm MT. Antimicrobial resistance in animals and relevance to human infections. In: Nachamkin I, Blaser MJ, eds. *Campylobacter.* 2nd ed. Washington, DC: ASM Press; 2000:483–495

20. Engberg J, Aarestrup FM, Taylor DE, Gerner-Smidt P, Nachamkin I. Quinolone and macrolide resistance in *Campylobacter jejuni* and *C coli*: resistance mechanisms and trends in human isolates. *Emerg Infect Dis.* 2001;7:24–34

21. Van Looveren M, Daube G, De Zutter L, et al. Antimicrobial susceptibilities of *Campylobacter* strains isolated from food animals in Belgium. *J Antimicrob Chemother.* 2001;48:235–240

22. Abbott Laboratories. *Sarafloxacin Water Soluble Powder (Sarafloxacin Hydrochloride) for the Control of Mortality Associated with E. coli in Growing Broiler Chickens and Turkeys.* North Chicago, IL: Abbott Laboratories; 1995. Available at: www.fda.gov/cvm/efoi/section2/141017081895.html. Accessed September 30, 2003

23. Rossiter S, Joyce K, Benson M, et al. High prevalence of fluoroquinolone-resistant *Campylobacter jejuni* in the FoodNet sites: a hazard in the food supply.Presented at the 2nd International Conference on Emerging Infectious Diseases; July 16–17, 2000; Atlanta, GA. Available at: www.cdc.gov/narms/pub/presentations/2000/rossiter_s_2.htm. Accessed September 30, 2003

24. Rossiter S, Joyce K, Benson J, et al. High prevalence of antimicrobial-resistant, including fluoroquinolone-resistant, *Campylobacter* on chicken in US grocery stores. Presented at the American Society for Microbiology 100th General Meeting; May 2000; Los Angeles, CA. Available at: www.cdc.gov/narms/pub/presentations/asm/2000/rossiter_s_3.htm. Accessed September 30, 2003

25. Marano N, Vugia D, Fiorentine T, et al. Fluoroquinolone-resistant *Campylobacter* causes longer duration of diarrhea than fluoroquinolone-susceptible *Campylobacter* strains in FoodNet sites. Presented at the 2nd International Conference on Emerging Infectious Diseases; July 2000; Atlanta, GA. Available at: www.cdc.gov/narms/pub/presentations/2000/marano_n_3.htm. Accessed September 30, 2003

26. Dunne EF, Fey PD, Kludt P, et al. Emergence of domestically acquired ceftriaxone-resistant *Salmonella* infections associated with AmpC beta-lactamase. *JAMA.* 2000;284:3151–3156

27. American Academy of Pediatrics. *Red Book: 2003 Report of the Committee on Infectious Diseases.* 26th ed. Pickering LK, ed. Elk Grove Village, IL: American Academy of Pediatrics; 2003

28. Holmberg SD, Osterholm MT, Senger KA, Cohen ML. Drug-resistant *Salmonella* from animals fed antimicrobials. *N Engl J Med.* 1984;311:617–622

29. Bezanson GS, Khakhria R, Bollegraaf E. Nosocomial outbreak caused by antibiotic-resistant strain of *Salmonella typhimurium* acquired from dairy cattle. *Can Med Assoc J.* 1983;128:426–427

30. Lyons RW, Samples CL, DeSilva HN, Ross KA, Julian EM, Checko PJ. An epidemic of resistant *Salmonella* in a nursery: animal-to-human spread. *JAMA.* 1980;243:546–547

31. Glynn MK, Bopp C, Dewitt W, Dabney P, Mokhtar M, Angulo FJ. Emergence of multidrug-resistant *Salmonella enterica* serotype Typhimurium DT104 infections in the United States. *N Engl J Med.* 1998;338:1333–1338

32. Cody SH, Abbott SL, Marfin AA, et al. Two outbreaks of multidrug-resistant *Salmonella* serotype Typhimurium DT104 infections linked to raw-milk cheese in northern California. *JAMA.* 1999;281:1805–1810

33. Villar RG, Macek MD, Simons S, et al. Investigation of multidrug-resistant *Salmonella* serotype Typhimurium DT104 infections linked to raw-milk cheese in Washington State. *JAMA.* 1999;281:1811–1816

34. Molbak K, Baggesen DL, Aarestrup FM, et al. An outbreak of multi-drug-resistant, quinolone-resistant *Salmonella enterica* serotype Typhimurium DT104. *N Engl J Med.* 1999;341:1420–1425

35. Fey PD, Safranek TJ, Rupp ME, et al. Ceftriaxone-resistant *Salmonella* infection acquired by a child from cattle. *N Engl J Med.* 2000;342:1242–1249

36. Stamey K, Baker R, Root T, et al. Emerging resistance to clinically important antimicrobial agents among human *Salmonella* isolates in the United States, 1996–1999. 40th Interscience Conference on Antimicrobial Agents and Chemotherapy; September 2000; Toronto, Ontario, Canada. Available at: www.cdc.gov/narms/pub/presentations/icaac/2000/Stamey_k.htm. Accessed September 30, 2003

37. Zhao C, Ge B, De Villena J, et al. Prevalence of *Campylobacter* spp., Escherichia coli, and Salmonella serovars in retail chicken, turkey, pork, and beef from the Greater Washington, D.C., area. *Appl Environ Microbiol.* 2001;67:5431–5436

38. White DG, Zhao S, Sudler R, et al. The isolation of antibiotic-resistant *Salmonella* from retail ground meats. *N Engl J Med.* 2001;345:1147–1154

39. Richards MJ, Edwards JR, Culver DH, Gaynes RP, National Nosocomial Infections Surveillance System. Nosocomial infections in pediatric intensive care units in the United States. *Pediatrics.* 1999;103(4). Available at: www.pediatrics.org/cgi/content/full/103/4/e39

40. Gray JW, George RH. Experience of vancomycin-resistant enterococci in a children's hospital. *J Hosp Infect.* 2000;45:11–18

41. McNeeley DF, Brown AE, Noel GJ, Chung M, DeLencastre H. An investigation of vancomycin-resistant *Enterococcus faecium* within the pediatric service of a large urban medical center. *Pediatr Infect Dis J.* 1998;17:184–188

42. Martone WJ. Spread of vancomycin-resistant enterococci: why did it happen in the United States? *Infect Control Hosp Epidemiol.* 1998;19:539–545

43. Wegener HC. Historical yearly usage of glycopeptides for animals and humans: the American-European paradox revisited [letter]. *Antimicrob Agents Chemother.* 1998;42:3049

44. Aarestrup FM. Occurrence of glycopeptide resistance among *Enterococcus faecium* isolates from conventional and ecological poultry farms. *Microb Drug Resist.* 1995;1:255–257

45. Aarestrup FM, Aherns P, Madsen M, Paleesen LV, Poulsen RL, Westin H. Glycopeptide susceptibility among Danish *Enterococcus faecium* and *Enterococcus faecalis* isolated from animal and human origin and PCR identification of genes within the VanA cluster. *Antimicrob Agents Chemother.* 1996;40:1938–1940

46. Silverman J, Thal LA, Perri MB, Bostic G, Zervox MJ. Epidemiologic evaluation of antimicrobial resistance in community-acquired enterococci. *J Clin Microbiol.* 1998;36:830–832

47. Van der Auwera P, Pensart N, Korten V, Murray BE, Leclercq R. Influence of oral glycopeptides on the fecal flora of human volunteers: selection of highly glycopeptide-resistant enterococci. *J Infect Dis.* 1996; 173:1129–1136

48. Jensen LB. Difference in the occurrence of two base pair variants of Tn1546 from vancomycin-resistant enterococci from humans, pigs, and poultry [letter]. *Antimicrob Agents Chemother.* 1998;42:2463–2464

49. Bates J, Jordens Z, Selkon JB. Evidence for an animal origin of vancomycin-resistant enterococci [letter]. *Lancet.* 1993;342:490–491

50. Bates J, Jordens JZ, Griffiths DT. Farm animals as a putative reservoir for vancomycin-resistant enterococcal infections in man. *J Antimicrob Chemother.* 1994;34:507–514

51. Klare I, Heier H, Claus H, et al. *Enterococcus faecium* strains with vanA-mediated high-level glycopeptide resistance isolated from animal food-stuffs and fecal samples of humans in the community. *Microb Drug Resist.* 1995;1:265–272

52. Quinupristin/dalfopristin. *Med Lett Drugs Ther.* 1999;41:109–110

53. Welton LA, Thal LA, Perri MB, et al. Antimicrobial resistance in enterococci isolated from turkey flocks fed virginiamycin. *Antimicrob Agents Chemother.* 1998;42:705–708

54. McDonald LC, Rossiter S, Mackinson C, et al. Quinupristin-dalfopristin-resistant *Enterococcus faecium* on chicken and in human stool specimens. *N Engl J Med.* 2001;345:1155–1160

55. Sorensen TL, Blom M, Monnet DL, Frimodt-Moller N, Poulsen RL, Espersen F. Transient intestinal carriage after ingestion of antibiotic-resistant *Enterococcus Faecium* from chicken and pork. *N Engl J Med.* 2001;345:1161–1166

56. Wierup M. The experience of reducing antibiotics used in animal production in the Nordic countries. *Int J Antimicrob Agents.* 2001;18:287–290

57. The Swedish Model of Animal Production. Ministry of Agriculture, Food and Fisheries, Stockholm, Sweden. September 1998. Available at: www.keepantibioticsworking.com/library/uploadedfiles/Swedish_Model_of_Animal_Production_The.pdf. Accessed September 30, 2003

58. Danish Integrated Antimicrobial Resistance Monitoring and Research Programme. *Danmap 2001: Use of Antimicrobial Agents and Occurrence of Antimicrobial Resistance in Bacteria From Food Animals, Foods, and Humans in Denmark.* Available at: www.vetinst.dk/file/Danmap%2001.pdf. Accessed September 30, 2003

All technical reports from the American Academy of Pediatrics automatically expire 5 years after publication unless reaffirmed, revised, or retired at or before that time.

Overcrowding Crisis in Our Nation's Emergency Departments: Is Our Safety Net Unraveling?

• *Policy Statement*

AMERICAN ACADEMY OF PEDIATRICS

POLICY STATEMENT
Organizational Principles to Guide and Define the Child Health Care System and/or Improve the Health of All Children

Committee on Pediatric Emergency Medicine

Overcrowding Crisis in Our Nation's Emergency Departments: Is Our Safety Net Unraveling?

ABSTRACT. Emergency departments (EDs) are a vital component in our health care safety net, available 24 hours a day, 7 days a week, for all who require care. There has been a steady increase in the volume and acuity of patient visits to EDs, now with well over 100 million Americans (30 million children) receiving emergency care annually. This rise in ED utilization has effectively saturated the capacity of EDs and emergency medical services in many communities. The resulting phenomenon, commonly referred to as ED overcrowding, now threatens access to emergency services for those who need them the most. As managers of the pediatric medical home and advocates for children and optimal pediatric health care, there is a very important role for pediatricians and the American Academy of Pediatrics in guiding health policy decision-makers toward effective solutions that promote the medical home and timely access to emergency care. *Pediatrics* 2004;114:878–888; *access to emergency care, ambulance diversion, emergency medical services for children, EMTALA, emergency department overcrowding.*

ABBREVIATIONS. ED, emergency department; EMS, emergency medical services; ACEP, American College of Emergency Physicians; AHA, American Hospital Association; GAO, US General Accounting Office; EMTALA, Emergency Medical Treatment and Active Labor Act; MSE, medical screening examination; SCHIP, State Children's Health Insurance Program; IOM, Institute of Medicine.

INTRODUCTION

Much has been written about the use of emergency services. A prophetic 1958 study examining a significant increase in emergency department (ED) utilization suggested that physicians and hospitals should plan for the future by increasing the number of emergency facilities.[1] Since that time, the number of ED visits in the United States has increased more than 600%, with an estimated 108 million ED visits in 2000.[2] Thirty million of those ED visits were for children 0 to 18 years of age.[2]

Over the past 2 decades, there has been increasing concern about this dramatic growth in ED visits. During the mid-1980s and early 1990s, many health care policy analysts viewed these increases as evidence of overutilization of EDs, specifically for nonemergent problems.[3,4] Armed with data suggesting that care provided in the ED was more expensive and perhaps less effective, policy-makers and managed care organizations worked to limit patients'

access to emergency care. This perception was perhaps best summarized in 1993 by President Clinton, who in a nationally televised speech to Congress and the nation referred to EDs as "the most expensive place of all" to get care.[5]

In the past decade, physicians and administrators responsible for the management of municipal emergency medical services (EMS) systems and hospital EDs have been voicing their concern regarding the capacity of their services. Their concern has been driven by an increasingly familiar phenomenon, overcrowding of EDs, which has worsened to the point of crisis in certain communities.[6–13] Surprisingly, this saturation of emergency services is not primarily a result of excessive, inappropriate use of the ED by those with nonemergent problems. It is a byproduct of increasing numbers of patients with serious illnesses or injuries requiring hospital and/or intensive care unit admission.[14,15] Evidence of the severity of the problem may be found in numerous articles in the lay press and in publications from the American College of Emergency Physicians (ACEP),[16–19] the Emergency Nurses Association,[20,21] and the American Hospital Association (AHA)[22–24] and in peer-reviewed journals such as *Academic Emergency Medicine*, which recently devoted an entire issue to this crisis and its related problems.[25] The US Senate has commissioned a study of ED overcrowding, as reported by the US General Accounting Office (GAO) in March 2003.[26] This problem has also garnered the attention of the Joint Commission on Accreditation of Healthcare Organizations, which developed a standard regarding overcrowding for publication in the *2004 Hospital Accreditation Manual*.[27]

So, how did this happen, what are the implications, and what can pediatric health care professionals do to help? ED overcrowding has evolved from a complex series of problems. An understanding of the key legislative, social, and health care economic factors that have led us to where we are today is warranted before considering potential solutions.

THE EMERGENCY MEDICAL TREATMENT AND ACTIVE LABOR ACT: THE UNDERFUNDED FEDERAL MANDATE FOR UNIVERSAL HEALTH CARE

The Emergency Medical Treatment and Active Labor Act (EMTALA) was enacted in 1985 as part of the

Consolidated Omnibus Budget Reconciliation Act. Its purpose was to protect the rights of indigent patients seeking emergency care.[28] The law was a response to the practice of patient "dumping," the refusal of a hospital (and/or hospital-based physicians) to provide emergency care for patients who could not pay for their care. This regulation requires all Medicare-participating hospitals to provide a medical screening examination (MSE) for all patients who present for care to the ED regardless of their ability to pay.[29-31]

Subsequent revisions, reinterpretation, and increased enforcement of this law over the past decade have expanded the reach of EMTALA, delineating the responsibility of hospitals, EDs, and their physicians to provide services to all patients who request them in a nondiscriminatory and consistent manner. The law specifies that the scope of the MSE should include all ancillary services routinely available to the ED, such as physician consultation and inpatient care, if required.[32] In the absence of a national universal health benefits program, hospital EDs are essentially the only place in our current health care system at which all patients are guaranteed medical care.[3,4,29,33]

Although clearly intended to promote the public good, EMTALA poses a profound economic challenge for hospitals and emergency care professionals, because this mandate for care does not carry with it a mandate for reimbursement for services rendered. Nationwide, EMTALA requirements are estimated to cost emergency care professionals more than $425 million annually.[17] Mitchell and Remmel[34] projected the financial impact of uncompensated emergency care in the state of Florida to reach an annual cost of $100 000 per emergency physician. This "free care" was estimated to be 5 times the amount provided by primary care physicians in that state. National data from 1998 suggest that the total direct expense for emergency physician services provided to uninsured patients approximated $1 billion.[17,35] Hospital facility costs for this same group of patients exceeded another $2 billion.[29,35] This incredible economic burden is exacerbated by insufficient Medicare reimbursement, which frequently fails to cover the direct costs of either the hospital facility or the emergency physician. In most states, services provided under Medicaid are reimbursed at 30% to 50% less than the same services provided under Medicare, creating an even greater funding gap for those providing care to our nation's 44.3 million Medicaid recipients.[36,37] It is little wonder that these financial stresses have resulted in the closure of nearly 500 hospitals and more than 1000 EDs over the past decade.[38]

More recently, the Centers for Medicare and Medicaid Services published a set of rule changes[39] that seem to be an effort at moving the law back toward its original intent as well as giving the courts clearer guidance for enforcement. The new rules clarify that a hospital must maintain an on-call physician list "that best meets the needs of the hospital's patients."[39] Physicians no longer have to be available all the time, but the hospital must have a written policy on how to deal with times when the on-call specialist is unavailable. Although this seems to be good news for rural and smaller hospitals and their medical staff members who have struggled to provide 24-hour coverage, this relaxation ultimately could contribute to a greater reliance on hospitals that suffer the most from overcrowding: large urban tertiary care centers, trauma centers, and academic medical centers.

Although EMTALA interpretation and enforcement has become increasingly punitive,[40,41] EMTALA is arguably more important today than when it was first enacted. With growing numbers of uninsured Americans, more physicians opting not to provide services to Medicaid and Medicare beneficiaries, and a failing public health and social welfare network, the ED has become one of the few reliable points of health care access in an unraveling safety net.[3,4,25,42-45]

THE EXPANDING ROLE OF THE ED IN A SHRINKING PUBLIC HEALTH SAFETY NET

Hospital EDs hold a very strategic position in the continuum of care in our society. Accessible and always open, the ED remains one of the few institutions available to aid all persons. Services are provided regardless of economic or social status and without an appointment. As previously noted, this societal responsibility has been both affirmed and mandated through federal legislation.

The importance of the ED's role has increased over the past decade as other public health and social care programs have eroded. Many people in need do not qualify for public support or are unable to take advantage of services to which they are entitled, including several million uninsured and underinsured children who could qualify for Medicaid or State Children's Health Insurance Program (SCHIP) benefits.[46,47] Disadvantaged Americans may pass through the entrance of an ED more than any other public institution. Some have suggested that this represents a remarkable opportunity for EDs to serve the needs of the disadvantaged by developing their full potential as social welfare institutions.[48-51]

In 2000, the Institute of Medicine (IOM) published a report titled *America's Health Care Safety Net: Intact but Endangered.*[52] The goal of the IOM was to "examine the impact of Medicaid managed care and other changes in health care coverage on the future viability of safety net providers operating primarily in ambulatory and primary care settings."[52] In its report, the IOM panel expressed grave concern for the current and future state of our nation's unraveling health care safety net and the vulnerable populations it serves. The report described several trends that seem to threaten the viability of safety net providers. These trends included inadequate monitoring of safety net viability and function, poor integration of services, financial instability of core safety net providers, and rapid shifts to Medicaid managed care.[44] Although this report did not specifically focus on the role played by EDs, it is clear that EDs meet the 2 defining characteristics of core safety net providers: 1) maintenance of an open-door policy, offering ser-

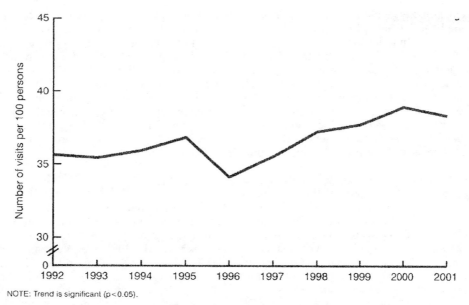

Fig. 1. Trend in ED visit rates: United States, 1992–2001. Source: McCaig LF, Burt CW. *National Hospital Ambulatory Medical Care Survey: 2001 Emergency Department Summary.* Hyattsville, MD: National Center for Health Statistics; 2003.

vices to patients regardless of their ability to pay; and 2) caring for a patient mix with a substantial share of Medicaid, uninsured, and other vulnerable populations.[52]

The number of uninsured Americans has grown steadily every year, even during the economic boom of the 1990s. In our nation of amazing wealth, there is also great poverty. There were approximately 43.6 million uninsured Americans in 2002, including 12.5 million children through 21 years of age. In fact, the proportion of the nonelderly American population (younger than 65 years) with health insurance coverage decreased in 2002 to a post-1987 low of 82.7%.[53] Although difficult to assess, there are between 4 and 13 million homeless persons in America.[54] More than 30% of children younger than 21 years (24.2 million) receive their health care benefits through the Medicaid program.[37] Although there are data showing that the Medicaid program has significantly improved the primary care access of impoverished children,[46,47,55,56] the program has fallen far short of creating equity between Medicaid beneficiaries and children living above the poverty line.[46,47,55–57]

An analysis of data from the 1988 National Health Interview Survey provides additional insight into the problem. Indigent children with Medicaid insurance were more likely to have a regular source of health care than those without Medicaid coverage. However, in comparison with children living above the poverty line, poor children with Medicaid were less likely to receive routine care in a physician's office, were more likely to lack continuity between their usual sources for sick and well care, and were more likely to identify hospital EDs as their preferred source for sick care.[46] In all, the survey determined that 6 million children lacked a usual source for primary care, and 12 million had not made a timely visit for preventive health care.[46] Although studies a decade later indicated significant improvement in

access to care for Medicaid beneficiaries, these children are still less likely to have a consistent source of health care and are 3 times more likely to have unmet health needs than are nonpoor children with private insurance.[57,58] Recent studies by the GAO indicate that less than half of Medicaid and SCHIP recipients have received early and periodic screening, diagnosis, and treatment services and that most states are doing little to monitor the use of primary or preventive health care services in this vulnerable population.[59,60]

Complaint urgency aside, inadequate or inaccessible sources of primary care are frequently cited as the most common reason for use of emergency services.[61–66] Studies examining the use of EDs by children for routine sick care have found several key demographic risk factors for "excessive" ED use, including black versus white race, single versus 2-parent family, parent with less than high school education versus education at the high school level or greater, poor versus nonpoor, and urban versus suburban location.[67] Children who receive their usual care in a neighborhood health clinic seem to be twice as likely as private-office practice patients to seek care in the ED. Furthermore, the absence of readily available primary care physicians is significantly associated (twofold increase) with ED use.[67]

What remains unclear is the role that health insurance plays in the use of emergency services. Data for 1998 from the National Center for Health Statistics indicate different utilization rates for commercially insured (19.9 visits per 100 individuals), Medicaid (64.2 visits per 100 individuals), and uninsured (34.2 visits per 100 individuals) patient groups.[29,68] Viewed as a proportion of total ambulatory care utilization, data from the 2001 National Ambulatory Medical Care Survey indicate that ED visits represented 25% of all outpatient use by the uninsured versus 17.5% by Medicaid recipients and nearly 8% by those with private insurance.[69] Although it would seem that Medicaid and uninsured patients are more likely to use the ED for acute episodic care, when one controls for confounding variables, this does not hold true.[70] Several studies have found that the lack of an established primary care relationship or the lack of accessible primary care services (not the lack of health insurance) are the primary risk factors for nonurgent ED visits.[61,67,71,72] In fact, it was the steady growth in the utilization of emergency services by privately insured patients that represented the largest segment of increased ED visits between 1996 and 2001 (Fig 1).[73]

A primary influence for the great attention and concern regarding ED utilization by these populations is the well-held perception of a relatively high cost for those services. Various studies have suggested cost differentials between ED care and the same care in a doctor's office to be between 50% and 100%.[3] Although charges are a poor reflection of true cost, the relative cost of ED care may be best understood through an analysis of marginal cost, or the cost of seeing 1 additional patient. In a study of 6 EDs in Michigan, Williams[35] found the marginal cost (the direct cost incurred from providing care for 1 additional patient) of an urgent ED visit to be $148, whereas for nonurgent visits, that cost was only $24, an amount likely less than the marginal cost associated with keeping a doctor's office open after regular office hours for nonurgent patient visits. In other words, EDs may be a cost-effective solution for certain components of after-hours ambulatory care.

DEFINING ED OVERCROWDING

Although the subjective assessment that a particular ED (or any public facility) is overcrowded may be inherently obvious to the average observer, objective and generalizable indicators of ED capacity and precise patient volume or acuity thresholds consistent with saturation of ED resources have proven to be difficult to define scientifically.[14] ED overcrowding is defined by the ACEP as a situation in which the identified need for emergency services outstrips available resources in the ED[16] (the Appendix contains a list of terms and metrics typically used in describing ED overcrowding and their definitions). In fact, part of the problem faced by those who manage emergency care systems is that there is not a universally held gold-standard definition for ED overcrowding.[43] Some have described overcrowding on the basis of excessive waiting times to see an ED physician or by treatment time delays in the ED. Others have based the definition on delays in the movement of admitted ED patients to inpatient beds. For some, the definition is based on the number of patients versus the number of available ED treatment stations (beds) or the forced use of nontreatment areas (eg, the ED hallway) to care for or hold ED patients. Others have attempted to define overcrowding on the basis of an assessment of patient acuity in the ED in relation to staffing resources. Finally, some link ED overcrowding to the need to divert incoming ambulance transports.[43]

Surveys of ED medical directors have identified a number of commonly held definitions for over-

crowding, including patients placed in hallways, all ED beds occupied for more than 6 hours per day, a full ED waiting room for 6 hours or more per day, physicians feeling rushed for 6 hours or more per day, and acutely ill patients who wait more than 60 minutes to see a physician.[7,74] To better understand increasing demand for emergency services, pursue multicenter or regional research on overcrowding, and plan for future ED resource needs, some have proposed the use of standard formulas to assess ED capacity (Table 1).[75]

STUDIES ON ED UTILIZATION AND OVERCROWDING

ED overcrowding is an obvious, almost predictable symptom of steadily growing demand that has exceeded available resources. ED visits have increased nearly 20% over the past decade. In 1988, 5200 US hospitals had 86 million ED visits. A decade later, emergency care was provided for 103 million encounters, but by this time only 4700 hospital EDs provided emergency care.[17] Many EDs are experiencing significant increases in their patient volumes because of regional population growth, an increasing number of visits from uninsured and underinsured patients, and decreased access to primary care services. In general, the pace and extent of facility and personnel resource expansion in the remaining EDs has not kept up with patient volume and acuity increases.

As the prevalence and severity of the phenomenon has grown, so have the number of descriptive reports and studies attempting to assess overcrowding. A decade ago, only a small percentage (less than 10%) of ED directors, mostly those from urban public hospitals, reported concerns about overcrowding.[19] More recent studies find nearly all ED medical directors reporting at least periodic ED saturation, with a steadily increasing number of directors reporting it as a frequent problem.[7,8,10,12,16,22,26,74,76,77]

Derlet et al[7] conducted a national random survey of 575 ED directors in 1998–1999 regarding the definition and extent of ED overcrowding and factors associated with it. Ninety-one percent of the responding medical directors reported ED overcrowding, with 53% reporting overcrowding occurring several times a week and 39% stating that it was a daily

---

TABLE 1.   Calculations to Assess ED Overcrowding[66]

Bed ratio (BR): the relationship between the number of ED patients and the number of treatment stations (beds) in the ED at any given time.
  BR = (number of patients in ED + predicted arrivals − predicted departures)/ED beds
Acuity ratio (AR): a measure of total patient acuity in the ED at a given point in time
  AR = sum of patient triage category/number of patients or sum of all triage scores/number of patients
Provider ratio (PR): the relationship between patient arrivals and ED physician staff, specifically the number of patients per hour (PPH) that each provider can manage
  PR = arrivals per hour/the sum of PPH for each physician
Demand value (DV): an overall measure of ED demand, including bed capacity, total patient acuity, and provider resources
  DV = (BR + PR) × AR

problem. Overcrowding problems were similar (more than 90%) in academic and private hospitals, although hospitals serving populations of greater than 250 000 had higher rates of overcrowding than did hospitals serving smaller populations (96% vs 87%). One third of the directors reported that patients had experienced poor outcomes as a result of overcrowding. Most frequently cited causes for overcrowding were high ED patient acuity, hospital bed shortage, high ED patient volume, ancillary service delays, and insufficient ED space.[7]

The AHA surveyed member hospitals regarding ED capacity and overcrowding in November 2001.[22] A total of 1500 hospitals responded. ED visit volume had grown by 5% over the previous year. Overall, 62% of respondents reported that they were either at or above the operating capacity of their ED, with 80% of teaching hospitals and urban hospitals and 90% of level I trauma centers experiencing this problem. One third of all hospitals experienced "ED diversion," with more than half of the urban hospitals reporting some time on diversion. One third of urban hospitals reported being on ambulance diversion at least 10% of the time, with 1 of 8 reporting time on diversion at 20% or greater. Lack of available, staffed critical care beds was the number one reason cited by hospitals for ED diversion.[22]

Lambe et al[76] conducted an analysis of the changes in California's hospital ED capacity between 1990 and 1999. Over the decade, the number of EDs in California decreased by 12%. The total number of ED treatment stations (ED beds) increased by 16%, but there was a 27% increase in visits per ED, with disproportionately greater volume increases in public versus private hospitals. In regard to patient acuity, critical care visits per ED increased by 59%, and nonurgent visits decreased by 8%.[76] The combination of volume and acuity increases was hypothesized to be the source of ED overcrowding. A 1999 survey of California ED medical directors found that 96% reported overcrowding as a problem, and 28% reported daily overcrowding.[74] The most frequently cited causes for overcrowding were increasing patient acuity and volume, hospital bed shortage, laboratory delays, and nursing shortage.

A 2001 survey of ED medical directors in the state of Washington revealed that 100% of large hospitals and 91% of small hospitals reporting overcrowding problems.[16] Frequent overcrowding (more than 3 times per week) was reported by 59% of large hospitals. On average, hospitals were on ambulance diversion 18 times per month, with an average time on diversion of 7.5 hours. The 3 most common reasons cited for overcrowding were volume overload, full hospital capacity, and nonphysician staff shortages.[16]

ED medical directors in Massachusetts were surveyed in 2000 regarding the causes of ambulance diversion.[77] Diversion was attributed most often to a lack of inpatient bed capacity and increased numbers of high-acuity patients in the ED. Nearly 90% reported facing a nursing shortage, which contributed to the problem. Seventy-two percent of the medical directors believed that patient care was compromised in some manner by overcrowding, and 21%

reported adverse patient outcomes directly attributable to overcrowding.[77]

In response to numerous anecdotal reports in the news media, the Committee on Government Reform of the US House of Representatives commissioned a study on ambulance diversion in 2000. In their report, *National Preparedness: Ambulance Diversions Impede Access to Emergency Rooms*,[13] the committee found ambulance diversion impeding timely access to metropolitan emergency services in 22 states, affecting nearly 75 million Americans residing in those areas.[13]

The GAO, commissioned by the US Senate Committee on Finance to study ED overcrowding, conducted a national survey of more than 2000 hospital EDs in 2001.[26] Two of every 3 EDs reported diversion at some point during that year. ED overcrowding and diversion was reported to be more common by hospitals located in areas with larger populations or those with high rates of population growth and by hospitals in areas with higher-than-average proportions of people without health insurance. Overcrowding was also more prevalent at trauma centers and teaching hospitals. Although no single factor stood out as the primary reason for ED overcrowding, the factor most commonly associated with crowding was the inability to transfer existing ED patients to hospital inpatient beds. Ninety percent of the surveyed hospitals reported "boarding" of admitted patients in their ED, with nearly 50% indicating an average boarding time of 2 hours or longer. Inpatient beds in greatest demand were intensive care unit and other monitored beds.[26]

KEY FACTORS CONTRIBUTING TO ED OVERCROWDING

Although increasing demand and fewer EDs are part of the problem, as indicated in the GAO report, many experts feel that the primary source of ED overcrowding is the increasing difficulty that most EDs face in moving acutely ill "admitted" patients from ED beds to inpatient beds. Intense economic pressures over the past 2 decades have forced most hospitals to decrease inpatient care capacity, leaving many with an inadequate number of inpatient beds or insufficient qualified nursing staff to handle fluctuating levels of demand. According to the AHA, there were 1.36 million inpatient beds in 6933 hospitals in 1981, 927 000 staffed beds in 5370 hospitals in 1991, and 829 000 beds in 4956 hospitals in 1999.[78]

With nearly all hospitals running at a higher census, it has become more difficult to admit patients. This seems especially true for patients (including children) who require admission on an unscheduled or emergency basis and compete for a limited number of beds with scheduled inpatient procedures and semielective admissions.[26] Tertiary and critical care beds are particularly in short supply. With no other place to move seriously ill or injured patients in need of admission, EDs must hold these patients for increasingly greater periods of time until an inpatient bed is available. These admitted patients, commonly referred to as "ED boarders," require ongoing care, consuming already taxed ED resources. Boarders essentially shrink the capacity of the ED and compromise its ability to provide timely care for incoming ambulance cases as well as acute patients who are still waiting to be seen. Although not conclusive, risk-management studies suggest that overcrowding and boarded inpatients pose considerable risk for medical errors.[43] ED overcrowding also has a deleterious effect on the teaching missions of academic medical centers, with more than 90% of teaching hospitals reporting overcrowding.[79]

Adding to the mismatch between a steadily growing patient demand and relatively fixed ED capacity is a shortage of qualified ED staff. Real shortages exist in the supply of residency-trained emergency physicians[80] and subspecialty-trained pediatric emergency physicians. The effects of new residency training rules and the reduction of trainee work hours on both hospital and ED capacity at teaching hospitals are yet to be appreciated. Among all the supply shortages in health care professional groups, the greatest deficiency is found within the ranks of registered nurses. Experienced ED nurses are truly the backbone of emergency care. Nationwide, there is a well-recognized deficiency of nurses, with vacancy rates in some states as high as 18%.[81] Annual turnover rates in high-stress practice settings such as EDs can be 30% or higher. Added to the dilemma of a small workforce is the fact that this workforce is aging steadily. The latest studies indicate an average age of 46 years for the nursing workforce, with only 9% of nurses now younger than 30 years of age, a 40% decrease from 1983 to 1998. One study projects a deficit of nearly 300 000 registered nurses by 2020.[82]

Another notable problem that threatens the viability of our emergency care system and the well-being of the patients it serves is a decreasing number of medical and surgical subspecialists who are willing or available to provide consultative backup to the ED.[83,84] A growing number of hospitals no longer have a "full panel" of on-call specialists who, because of the EMTALA mandate, are expected to provide consultative support to the ED. This problem has grown beyond small rural hospitals to affect large urban hospitals, including trauma centers. This problem will likely spread further in the wake of the November 2003 revisions to EMTALA that relax on-call physician requirements.

Global shortages in key medical subspecialties and surgical specialties and variations in geographic availability are both long-standing contributors to ED overcrowding, particularly for rural hospitals. More recently, 2 pressing issues are driving this growing deficiency. The first is a recent and alarming increase in professional liability insurance premiums. A recent American Medical Association study identified 44 of 50 states as having a current or impending liability crisis, with premiums for some subspecialists increasing as much as 25% to 50% annually.[85] Physicians who provide ED or trauma on-call services typically pay higher liability insurance premiums than those who do not. Many subspecialists have concluded that they can no longer afford to provide ED on-call services. The second issue is the increasing percentage of uninsured or underinsured ED patients and managed care barriers, all of which contribute to poor reimbursement for the mandated emergency services provided by these on-call specialists.

Numerous other factors have contributed to the overcrowding crisis (Table 2). Although some problems are internal to the ED, most are not. Insufficient access to primary and subspecialty care services and barriers to follow-up care each contribute significantly to the problem. The ED has been characterized by some as the proverbial "canary in the coal mine," with ED overcrowding representing a warning sign of growing distress within hospital and primary care delivery systems and a fraying health care safety net.

DELETERIOUS EFFECTS OF ED OVERCROWDING

Overcrowding of EDs produces a series of negative effects. First and foremost is that overcrowding places all involved parties, both patients and health care professionals, at risk. Excessive clinical demands on an already saturated ED often lead to medical errors and poor outcomes.[43] Overcrowding has promoted the expansion of ED facility capacity through increased utilization of hallways and other suboptimal, poorly equipped locations as patient treatment areas, challenging patient comfort, care satisfaction, and confidentiality and adding additional risk for error.[26] The only way busy clinicians faced with too many patients can care for all is to spend less time with each patient. The fine line between a highly efficient assessment and an incomplete assessment is easily crossed, generally at the expense of the patient. In teaching-hospital EDs, effective clinical teaching is an early casualty of excessive patient volumes.[79] The high-stress practice environment of a crowded ED is one that also contributes mightily to staff burnout, higher turnover rates, and worsening deficiencies in clinical staffing.

Lengthy waiting times also promote patient dissatisfaction. More importantly, for patients with acute injuries and other painful conditions, it means prolonged pain and needless suffering. For others, inappropriately long waiting times pose an even greater risk if the acuity of their condition was underassessed during triage or if there has been signif-

TABLE 2.   Causes of ED Overcrowding

Increased ED patient volumes
Increased ED patient acuity
Increased complexity of diseases and associated evaluations
Lack of inpatient hospital beds and related resources
Nursing shortage
Physician shortage
On-call physician/consultant availability
Insufficient physical plant space for the ED
Ancillary service (eg, lab, radiology) delays
Reduced access to primary care services
Reduced access to subspecialty care services
Difficulty in arranging follow-up care
Language and cultural barriers
Increased medical record documentation requirements
Medical liability issues
Managed care issues
Uninsured and underinsured patients
Inadequate funding for emergency services

icant progression of illness during a lengthy stint in the waiting room.

ED patient safety concerns aside, perhaps the most prominent deleterious effect of overcrowding is ambulance diversion. As suggested by survey data, ambulance diversion has become an increasingly common solution pursued by overcrowded EDs. Diversion had previously been confined to large urban teaching hospitals, timed with peak winter influenza outbreaks. Ambulance diversion now has become a year-long phenomenon, affecting more than two thirds of US hospitals in urban, suburban, and rural settings.[16,26,86] It is now fairly common for numerous hospitals within the same city or state EMS region to be on ambulance diversion at the same time. Many EMS systems have reacted to this by eliminating diversion as an option for overcrowded EDs during periods of peak patient volumes or when more than a certain number of institutions are saturated.[16–18,26]

When most or all major hospitals in an area are "on diversion," an entire municipality's EMS system can be paralyzed. This represents failure of the health care safety net at a rudimentary level, one that affects all economic and social strata. With saturated EDs on bypass, ambulance patients with true emergencies are forced to travel to more distant and perhaps less appropriate facilities. For an adult with a myocardial infarction or a stroke or a child with respiratory failure, the additional time to definitive care necessitated by ambulance diversion is a very meaningful factor. For children with special health care needs, this may limit their access to specialized EDs or tertiary care professionals who are familiar with their condition. Once an acutely ill patient is in the back of an ambulance, neither socioeconomic status nor special health care needs may have any bearing on disposition when diversion is in place.

SOLUTIONS TO ED OVERCROWDING: WHAT CAN PEDIATRICIANS DO TO HELP?

The ED overcrowding crisis did not mysteriously appear and, in reality, has been lurking in the shadows for some time. It is attributable, in part, to the absence of a coherent national health policy to create a comprehensive health care and social services delivery system for all Americans. For many adults and children, the ED has become and still remains the access point to health care by default. Intense economic pressure over the past decade has forced a reduction in the capacity of all aspects (primary care through tertiary care) of the American health care system. The result in certain communities is a dangerously overburdened and underfunded EMS system, with our nation's EDs sustaining the brunt of the problem.

The definitive solutions to ED overcrowding are complex, resource intensive, and expensive. Hospitals must improve their inpatient capacity, particularly the number of staffed critical care beds. Hospitals must also become better prepared to manage seasonal variations in acute illness and coordinate elective and nonelective admissions. Existing inpatient beds must be managed in a manner that promotes efficient utilization. Effective use of observa-tion units may help to maximize availability of limited inpatient beds. If the hospital capacity problem can be remedied, one of the root causes of ED overcrowding will have been addressed.

Hospital EDs must also adapt to meet growing patient demand. In the face of steadily growing utilization, there must be a corresponding expansion in the number of ED treatment stations and in the levels of physician and nurse staffing. Of course, this may be easier said than done considering current workforce shortages. Hospital EDs must also strive to improve the efficiency of the care provided to all patient acuity levels, both emergent/urgent and non-urgent groups. Improving ancillary service support will also help to make the ED more effective.

RECOMMENDATIONS

Pediatricians must serve as powerful advocates for improved health care for all children. The problem of ED overcrowding cannot be solved without solutions in our current health care systems that will provide an accessible and comprehensive medical home.[87] There are some specific actions that both primary care pediatricians and pediatric subspecialists can pursue to address this growing problem.

1. Include the management of acute illness or injury and the utilization of emergency services in anticipatory guidance. The best time to educate families about the appropriate use of an ED, calling 911, or calling the regional poison control center is before the emergency occurs. Although parents will continue to view and respond to acute medical problems as laypersons, they may make better-informed decisions if they are prepared.

2. Work with emergency care professionals to make every ED experience an educational opportunity for the patient and family. Components of this education should include: (a) clear instructions for the illness or injury of immediate concern; (b) instructions regarding the management or maintenance of chronic conditions and special health care needs; (c) preventive health education; and (d) guidance about EMS and ED utilization and available sources of primary and specialty care.

3. Connect patients to a fully functional medical home, thereby improving access to office-based acute care and coordinating utilization of after-hours clinical services. Although it would be unreasonable to expect a physician's office to be available 24 hours a day, pediatricians should take a critical look at the accessibility of their practice to patients with acute (nonscheduled) complaints. Hours of operation, same-day appointments, walk-in visits, the function of the practice's answering service, and the application of telephone triage systems should be scrutinized carefully. It might be especially helpful to interview families who have sought emergency care during office hours or those who have visited the ED without first calling the doctor's office to determine if communication or access was an issue in choosing to use the ED. An effective

primary care delivery system may prevent ED visits for low-acuity complaints and may enable timely interventions that prevent low-acuity illnesses from becoming high-acuity illnesses.

4. Coordinate effective follow-up care for ED visits. Even with optimal access to primary care and the medical home, patients will still require access to emergency services. Pediatricians should work closely with local institutions and providers of emergency services to ensure coordination of effective primary and subspecialty follow-up care. This communication and coordination of care is especially important for children with special health care needs.

5. Advocate for improved Medicaid reimbursement. On average, Medicaid reimbursed pediatricians for only 68% of the amount that would be paid under Medicare.[88] Many pediatricians are already doing more than their fair share, devoting a significant amount of their practice to the care of underserved and underfunded populations. In fact, pediatricians' average Medicaid caseload increased from 24.3% in 1983 to 30.0% in 2000, according to American Academy of Pediatrics survey data.[89] Health services research data suggest that we need more pediatricians and other pediatric care professionals to follow suit. We must strongly advocate for fair Medicaid reimbursement rates so that more pediatricians will have the financial incentive to care for these patients. Until then, many Medicaid and uninsured patients will continue to use EDs in the absence of a functional and accessible medical home.

6. Encourage SCHIP enrollment. There is a growing number of children from low-income families who are uninsured or underinsured who would qualify for SCHIP or Medicaid benefits. Because many of these patients have no medical home, pediatricians should partner with their community EDs to identify opportunities to enroll eligible children and families who pass through the ED. Facilitating the enrollment of these children into SCHIP will not be successful in improving their access to a medical home if the SCHIP or Medicaid reimbursement is not sufficient to encourage the participation of pediatric care professionals.

7. Become familiar with local hospital ED and EMS services and their constraints. Pediatricians can play an important role as "consumers" in advocating for expansion of hospital services. Pediatric centers are not immune to overcrowding and now experience many of the same problems as larger adult facilities. This may be an even greater problem for acutely ill or injured children, because many communities are served by a single pediatric tertiary care center. Pediatricians should play a direct role in addressing pediatric inpatient bed (particularly critical care beds) and ED capacity concerns at both their local community hospital and at regional pediatric tertiary care centers.

8. Support advocacy efforts directed toward medical professional liability and tort reform. In states in which tort reform has not occurred, the economic effect is on all health care professionals including pediatricians. Hospital-based specialists and high-risk service providers are affected disproportionately by this burden, which has diminished the availability of key medical subspecialists and surgical specialists for patients when they might need them most. Pediatricians should partner with their state medical society and other professional organizations in this important effort.

9. Conduct and/or advocate for health services research directed toward ED overcrowding. The numerous medical, economic, cultural, and social factors that have led to emergency service saturation are admittedly complex. In sharp contrast to the enormity of this problem is the relative paucity of health services research in this area, particularly regarding pediatric populations. A better understanding of these complex factors might promote a clearer perspective for policy-makers and provide a foundation for effective problem solving. This research agenda also should focus on the unique issues faced by children, including the effect of ED overcrowding and ambulance diversion on the outcome of pediatric emergency care.

10. Advocate for effective reforms in current health care delivery systems. As managers of the pediatric medical home and advocates for children and optimal pediatric health care, there is a very important role for pediatricians in educating citizens, elected officials, and health policy decision-makers about ED overcrowding and effective solutions. This advocacy must be directed toward both optimization of primary care access and improvement of hospital and emergency service capacity. The goal should be for every child to have a fully functional medical home. To maximize the effectiveness of their advocacy, pediatricians should partner with other key stakeholder groups including emergency physicians, emergency nurses, EMS professionals, hospital administrators, legislators, and others in efforts to repair the fraying health care safety net and overburdened emergency services. Organizations such as the ACEP, American Academy of Emergency Medicine, Society for Academic Emergency Medicine, National Association of EMS Physicians, American College of Physicians, Emergency Nurses Association, and others have each engaged in active advocacy programs to address this concern.

APPENDIX: ED Overcrowding Metrics and Definitions (adapted with permission from the American College of Emergency Physicians, Crowding Resources Task Force. *Responding to Emergency Department Crowding: A Guidebook for Chapters.* Dallas, TX: American College of Emergency Physicians; 2002)

ED overcrowding: a situation in which the identified need for emergency services exceeds the available resources in the ED. Evidence of ED overcrowding is typically found when the number of ED patients receiving care exceeds the number of staffed ED beds, which may lead to the use of hallways and other nontreatment areas to assess or monitor patients and is usually associated with lengthy waiting times for treatment.

ED saturation: a situation in which patient needs, including timely evaluation and treatment, as defined by patient acuity or triage level, cannot be met for existing or new patients because of fully committed ED resources.

ED treatment station (ED bed): a gurney or bed in a space designed to be a treatment area in the ED. Beds in such areas as the hallway, waiting room, conference rooms, etc, are not ED beds.

ED boarder: a patient who remains in the ED beyond the time of disposition after the decision has been made for either inpatient admission or transfer to another facility.

ED boarding time: the time interval between the acceptance of an admission or transfer request for an ED patient and the time the patient actually leaves the ED.

Boarding burden: the proportion of the ED functional treatment spaces or beds occupied by boarding patients.

Hospital ED or ambulance diversion: a situation in which a hospital has determined that it does not or will not have the required capacity or capability to accept additional patients from prehospital or EMS ambulance transports. Diversion can be for a specified category of patients (eg, trauma, critical care) or all prehospital or interhospital ambulance transfers.

Left prior to triage: a patient who has been logged as having arrived in the ED requesting medical care yet leaves prior to the triage assessment.

Left without being seen: a patient who has been triaged but leaves the ED prior to receiving an MSE by the ED physician or other qualified personnel.

Refusal of MSE or treatment: a patient presenting to the ED requesting medical evaluation who subsequently declines additional evaluation or treatment prior to the completion of care (also known as leaving against medical advice).

Waiting room time: the time interval between the completion of the triage assessment and placement of that patient in a waiting area and the time at which the patient is placed in a treatment bed.

COMMITTEE ON PEDIATRIC EMERGENCY MEDICINE, 2003–2004
Jane F. Knapp, MD, Chairperson
Thomas Bojko, MD
Margaret A. Dolan, MD
Karen S. Frush, MD
Ronald A. Furnival, MD
Daniel J. Isaacman, MD
*Steven E. Krug, MD
Robert E. Sapien, MD
Kathy N. Shaw, MD, MSCE
Paul E. Sirbaugh, DO

LIAISONS
Jane Ball, RN, DrPH
EMSC National Resource Center

Kathleen Brown, MD
National Association of EMS Physicians
Dan Kavanaugh, MSW
Maternal and Child Health Bureau
Sharon E. Mace, MD
American College of Emergency Physicians
David W. Tuggle, MD
American College of Surgeons

STAFF
Susan Tellez

*Lead author

REFERENCES

1. Shortliffe EC, Hamilton TS, Noroian EH. The emergency room and the changing pattern of medical care. *N Engl J Med.* 1958;258:20–25
2. National Center for Health Statistics. *National Hospital Ambulatory Medical Care Survey. Emergency Department Summary.* Hyattsville, MD: National Center for Health Statistics, Centers for Disease Control and Prevention; 2000. Available at: www.cdc.gov/nchs/about/major/ahcd/ercharts.htm. Accessed December 17, 2003
3. Krug SE. Access and use of emergency services: inappropriate use versus unmet need. *Clin Pediatr Emerg Med.* 1999;1:35–44
4. Richardson LD, Hwang U. Access to care: a review of the emergency medicine literature. *Acad Emerg Med.* 2001;8:1030–1036
5. Clinton WJ. Televised address to the joint session of Congress and the nation [transcript]. September 23, 1993
6. Richardson LD, Asplin BR, Lowe RA. Emergency department crowding as a health policy issue: past development, future directions. *Ann Emerg Med.* 2002;40:388–393
7. Derlet R, Richards J, Kravitz R. Frequent overcrowding in U.S. emergency departments. *Acad Emerg Med.* 2001;8:151–155
8. California Medical Association. *California's Emergency Medical Services: A System in Crisis.* California Medical Association White Paper. San Francisco, CA: California Medical Association; 2001
9. Nordberg M. Overcrowding: the ED's newest predicament. *Emerg Med Serv.* 1990;19:35–38, 40–44
10. McManus M. *Emergency Department Overcrowding in Massachusetts: Making Room in Our Hospitals.* Waltham, MA: Massachusetts Health Policy Forum; 2001. Available at: www.sihp.brandeis.edu/mhpf/Diversions.pdf. Accessed December 17, 2003
11. Taylor TB. *Arizona Emergency Care Crisis: Meeting Summary.* Phoenix, AZ: Arizona College of Emergency Physicians; 2000. Available at: www.azcep.org/er_crowding/summary.pdf. Accessed December 17, 2003
12. Schneider S, Zwemer F, Doniger A, Dick R, Czapranski T, Davis E. Rochester, NY: a decade of emergency department overcrowding. *Acad Emerg Med.* 2001;8:1044–1050
13. Waxman HA. *National Preparedness: Ambulance Diversions Impede Access to Emergency Rooms.* Washington, DC: US House of Representatives, Committee on Government Reform; 2001. Available at: www.house.gov/reform/min/pdfs/pdf_com/pdf_terrorism_diversions_rep.pdf. Accessed December 17, 2003
14. Derlet RW, Richards JR. Overcrowding in the nation's emergency departments: complex causes and disturbing effects. *Ann Emerg Med.* 2000;35:63–68
15. Kellermann AL. Déjà vu. *Ann Emerg Med.* 2000;35:83–85
16. American College of Emergency Physicians, Crowding Resources Task Force. *Responding to Emergency Department Crowding: A Guidebook for Chapters.* Dallas, TX: American College of Emergency Physicians; 2002. Available at: www.acep.org/library/pdf/edCrowdingReport.pdf. Accessed December 17, 2003
17. American College of Emergency Physicians, Safety Net Task Force. *Defending America's Safety Net.* Dallas, TX: American College of Emergency Physicians; 1999. Available at: www.acep.org/library/pdf/safetynet.pdf. Accessed December 17, 2003
18. American College of Emergency Physicians. Measures to deal with emergency department overcrowding. *Ann Emerg Med.* 1990;19:944–945
19. American College of Emergency Physicians. Hospital and emergency department overcrowding. *Ann Emerg Med.* 1990;19:336
20. Emergency Nurses Association. *Emergency Nursing Reference: Use of EMTs and Non-RNs, Diversion, Overcrowding, Observations, Delegation and Holding Patients in the ED.* Des Plaines, IL: Emergency Nurses Association; 2001

21. Emergency Nurses Association. *Position Statement: Hospital and Emergency Department Overcrowding.* Des Plaines, IL: Emergency Nurses Association; 2001. Available at: www.ena.org/publications/statements/positionpdf/hospital&overcrowding.pdf. Accessed December 17, 2003

22. American Hospital Association. *Emergency Department Overload: A Growing Crisis. Results of the AHA Survey of Emergency Department (ED) and Hospital Capacity.* Chicago, IL: American Hospital Association; 2002. Available at: www.hospitalconnect.com/aha/press_room-info/content/EdoCrisisSlides.pdf. Accessed December 17, 2003

23. American Hospital Association. Emergency departments: an essential access point to care. *Trend Watch.* 2001;3:1–8. Available at: www.hospitalconnect.com/ahapolicyforum/trendwatch/content/twmarch2001.pdf. Accessed December 17, 2003

24. American Hospital Association. *Cracks in the Foundation: Averting a Crisis in America's Hospitals.* Chicago, IL: American Hospital Association; 2002. Available at: www.hospitalconnect.com/aha/advocacy-grassroots/advocacy/advocacy/content/cracksreprint08-02.pdf. Accessed December 17, 2003

25. Adams JG, Biros MH. The endangered safety net: establishing a measure of control. *Acad Emerg Med.* 2001;8:1013–1015

26. US General Accounting Office. *Hospital Emergency Departments: Crowded Conditions Vary Among Hospitals and Communities.* Washington, DC: US General Accounting Office; 2003. Publication No. GAO-03-460. Available at: www.gao.gov/highlights/d03460high.pdf. Accessed December 17, 2003

27. Joint Commission on Accreditation of Healthcare Organizations. Emergency department overcrowding standards. Available at: www.jcaho.org/accredited+organizations/hospitals/standards/draft+standards/er_fr_std.pdf. Accessed December 17, 2003

28. Emergency Medical Treatment and Active Labor Act, established under the Consolidated Omnibus Budget Reconciliation Act of 1985. Pub L No. 99-272, 42USC §1395dd (1986)

29. Fields WW, Asplin BR, Larkin GL, et al. The Emergency Medical Treatment and Labor Act as a federal health care safety net program. *Acad Emerg Med.* 2001;8:1064–1069

30. Selbst SM. Emergency Medical Treatment and Active Labor Act: legal concerns about private or managed care patients in the emergency department. *Curr Opin Pediatr.* 1997;9:465–469

31. DeHart KL. Interhospital transfers: the EMTALA provisions of COBRA as amended by OBRA 89 and OBRA 90. In: Salluzzo RF, Mayer TA, Strauss RW, et al, eds. *Emergency Department Management: Principles and Applications.* St Louis, MO: Mosby-Year Book Inc; 1997:550–554

32. Diekema DS. Unwinding the COBRA: new perspectives on EMTALA. *Pediatr Emerg Care.* 1995;11:243–248

33. Institute of Medicine, Committee on the Consequences of Uninsurance. *A Shared Destiny: Community Effects of Uninsurance.* Washington, DC: National Academy of Sciences; 2003. Available at: www.nap.edu/catalog/10602.html. Accessed December 17, 2003

34. Mitchell TA, Remmel RJ. Level of uncompensated care delivered by emergency physicians in Florida. *Ann Emerg Med.* 1992;21:1208–1214

35. Williams RM. The costs of visits to emergency departments. *N Engl J Med.* 1996;334:642–646

36. American Academy of Pediatrics, Division of Health Policy Research. *Medicaid Reimbursement Survey, 2001.* Elk Grove Village, IL: American Academy of Pediatrics; 2001. Available at: www.aap.org/research/medreimPDF01/all_states.pdf. Accessed December 16, 2003

37. Medicaid Statistics Information System. *Statistical Report for Federal Fiscal Year 2000.* Washington, DC: Centers for Medicare and Medicaid Services; 2000

38. American Hospital Association. *Hospital Statistics—2000 Edition.* Chicago, IL: Health Forum LLC; 2000

39. Department of Health and Human Services, Centers for Medicare and Medicaid Services. Medicare program; clarifying policies related to the responsibilities of Medicare-participating hospitals in treating individuals with emergency medical conditions. Final rule. *Fed Regist.* 2003;68:53222–53264.

40. Bonner S. EMTALA guidelines: here's what your ED needs to know. *Emerg Dep Legal Lett.* 1999;10:1–8

41. Levine RJ, Guisto JA, Meislin HW, Spaite DW. Analysis of federally imposed penalties for violations of the Consolidated Omnibus Reconciliation Act. *Ann Emerg Med.* 1996;28:45–50

42. Richardson LD, Hwang U. America's health care safety net: intact or unraveling? *Acad Emerg Med.* 2001;8:1056–1063

43. Gordon JA, Billings J, Asplin BR, Rhodes KV. Safety net research in emergency medicine: proceedings of the Academic Emergency Medicine Consensus Conference on "The Unraveling Safety Net." *Acad Emerg Med.* 2001;8:1024–1029

44. Asplin BR. Tying a knot in the unraveling health care safety net. *Acad Emerg Med.* 2001;8:1075–1079

45. Taylor TB. Threats to the health care safety net. *Acad Emerg Med.* 2001;8:1080–1087

46. Newacheck PW, Pearl M, Hughes DC, Halfon N. The role of Medicaid in ensuring children's access to care. *JAMA.* 1998;280:1789–1793

47. Holl JL, Szilagyi PG, Rodewald LE, Byrd RS, Weitzman ML. Profile of uninsured children in the United States. *Arch Pediatr Adolesc Med.* 1995;149:398–406

48. Malone RE. Whither the almhouse? Overutilization and the role of the emergency department. *J Health Polit Policy Law.* 1998;23:795–832

49. Gordon JA. The hospital emergency department as a social welfare institution. *Ann Emerg Med.* 1999;33:321–325

50. Gordon JA, Chudnofsky CR, Hayward RA. Where health and welfare meet: social deprivation among patients in the emergency department. *J Urban Health.* 2001;78:104–111

51. Muelleman RL, Feighny KM. Effects of an emergency department-based advocacy program for battered women on community resource utilization. *Ann Emerg Med.* 1999;33:62–66

52. Institute of Medicine, Committee on the Changing Market, Managed Care, and the Future Viability of Safety Net Providers. *America's Health Care Safety Net: Intact but Endangered.* Lewin ME, Altman S, eds. Washington, DC: National Academies Press; 2000

53. American Academy of Pediatrics. Children's health insurance status and Medicaid/SCHIP eligibility and enrollment. Characteristics of Medicaid-enrolled and uninsured children. State reports. 2002. Available at: www.aap.org/research/2003cps.pdf. Accessed May 10, 2004

54. D'Amore J, Hung O, Chiang W, Goldfrank L. The epidemiology of the homeless population and its impact on an urban emergency department. *Acad Emerg Med.* 2001;8:1051–1055

55. Berk ML, Schur CL. Access to care: how much difference does Medicaid make? *Health Aff (Millwood).* 1998;17:169–180

56. Berk ML, Schur CL. Measuring access to care: improving information for policymakers. *Health Aff (Millwood).* 1998;17:180–186

57. St Peter RF, Newacheck PW, Halfon N. Access to care for poor children: separate and unequal? *JAMA.* 1992;267:2760–2764

58. Newacheck PW, Hughes DC, Hung YY, Wong S, Stoddard J. The unmet health needs of America's children. *Pediatrics.* 2000;105:989–997

59. US General Accounting Office. *Medicaid: Stronger Efforts Needed to Ensure Children's Access to Health Screening Services. Report to Congressional Requesters.* Washington, DC: US General Accounting Office; 2001. Publication No. GAO-01-749. Available at: www.gao.gov. Accessed December 17, 2003

60. US General Accounting Office. *Medicaid and SCHIP: States Use Varying Approaches to Monitor Children's Access to Care. Report to Congressional Requesters.* Washington, DC: US General Accounting Office; 2003. Publication No. GAO-03-222. Available at: www.gao.gov. Accessed December 17, 2003

61. Shesser R, Kirsch T, Smith J, Hirsch R. An analysis of emergency department use by patients with minor illness. *Ann Emerg Med.* 1991;20:743–748

62. Kelman HR, Lane DS. Use of the hospital emergency room in relation to use of private physicians. *Am J Public Health.* 1976;66:1189–1191

63. Hansagi H, Carlsson B, Brismar B. The urgency of care need and patient satisfaction at a hospital emergency department. *Health Care Manage Rev.* 1992;17:71–75

64. Hilditch JR. Changes in hospital emergency department use associated with increased family physician availability. *J Fam Pract.* 1980;11:91–96

65. Young GP, Wagner MB, Kellermann AL, et al. Ambulatory visits to hospital emergency departments. *JAMA.* 1996;276:460–465

66. Padgett DK, Brodsky B. Psychosocial factors influencing non-urgent use of the emergency room: a review of the literature and recommendations for research and improved service delivery. *Soc Sci Med.* 1992;35:1189–1197

67. Halfon N, Newacheck PW, Wood DL, St Peter RF. Routine emergency department use for sick care by children in the United States. *Pediatrics.* 1996;98:28–34

68. McCaig LF. *National Hospital Ambulatory Medical Care Survey: 1998 Emergency Department Summary.* Hyattsville, MD: National Center for Health Statistics; 2000. Available at: www.cdc.gov/nchs/about/major/ahcd/adata.htm. Accessed December 17, 2003

69. McCaig LF, Burt, CW. *National Hospital Ambulatory Medical Care Survey: 2001 Emergency Department Summary.* Hyattsville, MD: National Center for Health Statistics; 2003. Available at: www.cdc.gov/nchs/about/major/ahcd/adata.htm. Accessed December 17, 2003

70. Luo X, Liu G, Frush K, Hey LA. Children's health insurance status and emergency department utilization in the United States. *Pediatrics.* 2003;112:314–319

71. Orr ST, Charney E, Straus J, et al. Emergency room use by low income children with a regular source of health care. *Med Care.* 1991;29:283–286

72. Petersen LA, Burstin HR, O'Neill AC, Orav EJ, Brennan TA. Nonurgent emergency department visits: the effect of having a regular doctor. *Med Care.* 1998;36:1249–1255

73. Cunningham PJ, May JH. *Insured Americans Drive Surge in Emergency Department Visits.* Washington, DC: Center for Studying Health System Change; 2003. Issue Brief No. 70. Available at: www.hschange.org/CONTENT/613. Accessed December 17, 2003

74. Richards JR. Survey of directors of emergency departments in California on overcrowding. *West J Med.* 2000;172:385–388

75. Reeder TJ, Garrison HG. When the safety net is unsafe: real-time assessment of the overcrowded emergency department. *Acad Emerg Med.* 2001;8:1070–1074

76. Lambe S, Washington DL, Fink A, et al. Trends in the use and capacity of California's emergency departments, 1990–1999. *Ann Emerg Med.* 2002;39:389–396

77. Epstein SK, Slate DH. The Massachusetts College of Emergency Physicians ambulance diversion survey [abstr 306]. *Acad Emerg Med.* 2001;8:526–527

78. American Hospital Association. *Hospital Statistics—1999.* Chicago, IL: American Hospital Association, Health Forum LLC; 1999

79. Derlet RW, Richards JR. Overcrowding in academic emergency departments [abstr 108]. *Acad Emerg Med.* 1999;6:404

80. Moorhead JC, Gallery ME, Hirschkorn C, et al. A study of the workforce in emergency medicine: 1999. *Ann Emerg Med.* 1999;40:3–15

81. Velianoff GD. Overcrowding and diversion in the emergency department: the health care safety net unravels [review]. *Nurs Clin North Am.* 2002;37:59–66, vi

82. Buerhaus PI, Staiger DO, Auerbach DI. Implications of an aging registered nurse workforce. *JAMA.* 2000;283:2948–2954

83. Asplin BR, Knopp RK. A room with a view: on-call specialist panels and other health policy challenges in the emergency department. *Ann Emerg Med.* 2001;37:500–503

84. Johnson LA, Taylor TB, Lev R. The emergency department on-call backup crisis: finding remedies for a serious public health problem. *Ann Emerg Med.* 2001;37:495–499

85. American Medical Association, Council on Medical Service. *Report 12: The Rise in Professional Liability Insurance Premiums.* Chicago, IL: American Medical Association; 2002. Available at: www.ama-assn.org/ama1/pub/upload/mm/372/cms1202.doc. Accessed December 13, 2003

86. Lagoe RJ, Hunt RC, Nadle PA, Kohlbrenner JC. Utilization and impact of ambulance diversion at the community level. *Prehosp Emerg Care.* 2002;6:191–198

87. American Academy of Pediatrics, Medical Home Initiatives for Children With Special Needs Project Advisory Committee. The medical home. *Pediatrics.* 2002;110:184–186

88. Berman S, Dolins J, Tang S, Yudkowsky B. Factors that influence the willingness of primary care pediatricians to accept more Medicaid patients. *Pediatrics.* 2002;110:239–248

89. Tang S, Yudkowsky B, Davis J. Medicaid participation by private and safety net pediatricians, 1993 and 2000. *Pediatrics.* 2003;112:368–372

All policy statements from the American Academy of Pediatrics automatically expire 5 years after publication unless reaffirmed, revised, or retired at or before that time.

Pediatric Fellowship Training

- *Policy Statement*

FEDERATION OF PEDIATRIC ORGANIZATIONS

POLICY STATEMENT
Organizational Principles to Guide and Define the Child Health Care System and/or Improve the Health of All Children

Pediatric Fellowship Training

In 1996, the Federation of Pediatric Organizations revised its 1990 statement on pediatric fellowship training. The following statement represents the current (2004) position of the federation regarding the purpose and objectives of fellowship training.

The goal of subspecialty fellowship training is to advance the health of children by preparing graduates who are competent in clinical care, education, and research. This goal is best achieved by fellowship training that fosters the development of future academic pediatricians, recognizing the diverse roles they now play. This goal requires that graduates of training programs have a keen curiosity about issues in their subspecialty field, a healthy skepticism of their own experience (and the published experience of others), and a working understanding of the analytic tools relevant to exercising critical judgment. Training is best provided in an environment in which there are faculty role models committed to scholarly activities.

Subspecialists may serve as expert clinicians providing direct and consultative care to patients based on their experience and critical evaluation of scientific evidence and research. They may serve as educators helping to guide and facilitate life-long learning of medical students, residents, fellows, and others who provide care for children. They also may be investigators adding to the body of knowledge in their subspecialty. The eventual careers of subspecialists may involve 1 or more of these roles to varying degrees. Therefore, training programs should provide all trainees with experiences that will allow them to develop competence for each of these roles, and applicants must be selected on the basis of their potential to achieve appropriate skills in each of these domains. The following are guidelines for fellowship programs and trainees.

1. Fellowship training must educate trainees to develop and maintain life-long learning skills for themselves, especially the ability to critically evaluate new knowledge to determine its appropriate use in caring for patients.
2. Fellowship training programs must provide the opportunity for trainees to acquire appropriate clinical skills and must incorporate into their curriculum mastery of each of the 6 general competencies identified by the Accreditation Council of

Graduate Medical Education and the American Board of Medical Specialties (medical knowledge, patient care, communication, professionalism, practice-based learning and improvement, and systems-based practice.) Relevant benchmarks and thresholds must be developed to ensure that competency in each area can be verified as achieved by all subspecialty graduates by the conclusion of their training program.

3. To achieve and maintain the goal of subspecialty training, in addition to acquiring appropriate clinical skills and competencies during the period of training, subspecialty trainees must acquire skills that will enable them to provide quality care throughout their professional lifetimes. These skills include the ability to critically analyze and evaluate their own observations and the observations of others; assimilate new knowledge, concepts, and technology; formulate clear and testable questions (hypotheses) from a body of information; and communicate ideas verbally and in writing.

Programs must provide opportunities for trainees to acquire these skills. These opportunities for scholarship may include a variety of activities, but they must result in the acquisition of the skills referred to in the preceding paragraph, and the trainee's participation must be guided by 1 or more mentors.

Scholarly activities, including but not limited to basic, clinical, or translational biomedical research, must be undertaken and successfully completed by trainees. These activities must be integrated into the training experience along with the core curriculum for the subspecialty and any formal coursework that is part of the training experience. Obtaining a graduate degree is not a substitute, per se, for such scholarly activities.

4. Fellowship training must be structured to provide a scholarly experience for every trainee, because it is essential to a successful subspecialty career in clinical care, education, research, or a combination of these activities. The subspecialty training program must have an oversight committee (at least 3 individuals, one of whom should be outside the trainee's subspecialty) for each trainee with appropriate expertise in scholarly endeavors. This committee must assess and confirm the presence of an adequate scholarly experience for each fellowship trainee and evaluate the product of the individual's scholarly experience.
5. Fellowship programs must provide training and experience to ensure that graduates will be effec-

Address correspondence to Richard Behrman, Executive Chair, Pediatric Education Steering Committee, Federation of Pediatric Organizations, 770 Welsh Rd, Ste 350, Palo Alto, CA 94304. E-mail: rbehrman@fopo.org
PEDIATRICS (ISSN 0031 4005). Copyright © 2004 by the American Academy of Pediatrics.

tive teachers for all learners in need of understanding and collaboration in the subspecialist's area(s) of expertise. This training must include the ability to participate effectively in all aspects of the educational process including curriculum development, delivery of information, and assessment of educational outcomes. Graduates should be scholarly and effective in teaching both individuals and groups of learners in clinical settings, classrooms, lectures, and seminars and through electronic and print modalities.

6. Fellowship training programs must provide a career mentor(s) for each trainee who will assist the trainee in developing an individualized learning plan for the entire training period. This mentor must be responsible for providing the ongoing formative feedback that is essential to the trainee's attainment of competence in clinical care, teaching, and scholarship. The mentor may come from a division or department other than the one offering the fellowship.

7. Fellowship training programs must be periodically reviewed and evaluated to improve the quality of the trainee's experiences in clinical care, education, and investigation. Tracking trainee career outcomes must be part of this review. The reports of these evaluations must be used to judge whether a program has met predetermined standards for fellowship training and to identify areas in need of improvement. The reports must be made available to trainee applicants and trainees.

FEDERATION OF PEDIATRIC ORGANIZATIONS
Ambulatory Pediatric Association
American Academy of Pediatrics
American Board of Pediatrics
American Pediatric Society
Association of Medical School Pediatric Department
   Chairs
Association of Pediatric Program Directors
Society of Pediatric Research

All policy statements from the American Academy of Pediatrics automatically expire 5 years after publication unless reaffirmed, revised, or retired at or before that time.

The Pediatrician's Role in the Prevention of Missing Children

- *Clinical Report*

AMERICAN ACADEMY OF PEDIATRICS

CLINICAL REPORT
Guidance for the Clinician in Rendering Pediatric Care

Barbara J. Howard, MD, Daniel D. Broughton, MD, and the Committee on Psychosocial Aspects of Child and Family Health

The Pediatrician's Role in the Prevention of Missing Children

ABSTRACT. In 2002, the *Second National Incidence Studies of Missing, Abducted, Runaway, and Thrownaway Children* report was released by the US Department of Justice, providing new data on a problem that our nation continues to face. This clinical report describes the categories of missing children, the prevalence of each, and prevention strategies that primary care pediatricians can share with parents to increase awareness and education about the safety of their children. *Pediatrics* 2004;114: 1100–1105; *missing children, runaway children, thrownaway children, family abduction, nonfamily abduction.*

ABBREVIATIONS. NISMART-2, Second National Incidence Studies of Missing, Abducted, Runaway, and Thrownaway Children, AMBER, American's Missing: Broadcast Emergency Response.

INTRODUCTION

Missing children are of considerable concern to parents, children, and the nation. In one study, nearly 75% of parents acknowledged worrying about their children being kidnapped, and 35% said they were very concerned.[1] The issue of missing children is complex and needs to be dealt with in the appropriate context. When considering how to counsel parents about this issue, it is important for pediatricians to have a good understanding of the problem.

Of the 837 055 missing persons reported in 2001,[2] it is estimated that 80% of them were children.[3] Fortunately, approximately 99% were found within hours or days by usual law-enforcement response. However, 7115 to 7534 children nationwide were missing for prolonged periods.

There are several categories of missing children. Most children reported missing are runaways and children taken by noncustodial parents, both of which are preventable events. A small but indeterminate number of children are abducted by nonfamily members. Most of these nonfamily abductions occur as a result of direct contact between the perpetrator and the child. However, with the increase in Internet use, an increasing number of children have been reported as missing through contact with people they have met only through this medium. Abduction of newborn infants has been nearly eliminated through additional security and educational measures implemented in hospitals.

Pediatricians have an important role in helping parents put the problem of missing children in perspective, recommending general safety measures to be discussed without frightening children or adults, advocating for services for dysfunctional families and for children after runaway events, and condemning the use of commercial techniques that exploit fears about missing children.

CATEGORIES OF MISSING CHILDREN

In 2002, the US Department of Justice released the *Second National Incidence Studies of Missing, Abducted, Runaway, and Thrownaway Children (NISMART-2)*.[4] Children who had been missing according to their families in 1999 were put into one of several categories: nonfamily abductions; family abductions; runaways or thrownaways (children forced to leave their homes by their parents); missing involuntary, lost, or missing; and missing benign explanation.

Nonfamily Abductions

According to the US Department of Justice, nonfamily abduction occurs when a nonfamily perpetrator takes a child by the use of physical force or threat of bodily harm or detains a child for at least 1 hour in an isolated place by the use of physical force or threat of bodily harm without lawful authority or parental permission or when a child who is younger than 15 years or is mentally incompetent, without lawful authority or parental permission, is taken or detained by or voluntarily accompanies a nonfamily perpetrator who conceals the child's whereabouts, demands ransom, or expresses the intention to keep the child permanently.[5] According to NISMART-2, more than 50 000 children and adolescents were taken in this manner in 1999.[6] Most victims of nonfamily abductions were girls (65%), and most were 12 years old or older (58%). Forty-six percent of the victims were sexually assaulted while missing. Most nonfamily abductions lasted less than 1 day (91%), with 29% lasting 2 hours or less. Less than 1% of children were not yet returned at the time of the study. Although much less common, classic nonfamily kidnappings pose the greatest risk of death or serious harm. According to law-enforcement statis-

The guidance in this report does not indicate an exclusive course of treatment or serve as a standard of medical care. Variations, taking into account individual circumstances, may be appropriate.

doi:10.1542/peds.2004-1397

tics, a few more than 100 children were kidnapped in this sense in 1999.[4] Although these numbers are small, the effects on the child, family, and community are enormous. All nonfamily abductions are part of a continuum. On one end are relatively brief episodes in which there is no physical harm to the victim. At the other extreme are the horrific cases of classic kidnappings that often grab the nation's attention.

The statistics on abductions are powerful reasons for teaching safety principles to older children, especially girls. As an example, the National Center for Missing and Exploited Children has developed a campaign to get kids to "know the rules"[7] when going out:

- Don't go out alone.
- Always tell an adult where you are going.
- Say "no" if you feel threatened.

These are good rules, because they lessen the risk for children and adolescents to develop serious problems from getting into situations in which they are most vulnerable to exploitation and harm, whether with unfamiliar people or as in "date rape."

We all can remember our parents and teachers giving admonitions such as "don't take candy from strangers," hoping to keep us safe. Unfortunately, we now know that most people who perpetrate these crimes on children are not strangers in the eye and mind of the child. A neighbor, a familiar face in a child's daily routine, or someone the child's parents know well enough to speak to or whose name the child knows is probably not viewed as a stranger by the child. The perpetrators usually understand and practice seduction techniques that make themselves appear nonthreatening to children. Such techniques include calling the child by name, becoming familiar with their family or friends to provide a sense of familiarity, and providing toys or sweets for enticement. Often, these perpetrators will ask the child for assistance in looking for something such as an address or a lost puppy, thus becoming a new "friend" or ally. In cases of long-term kidnappings in which the child was found alive, 85% of the victims did not consider the kidnapper to be a stranger. In at least 65% of the cases in which a child was found dead and the perpetrator was identified, it was clear that the child would not have considered the person a stranger.[8] These strategies make it ineffective to give simple instructions to children not to talk to or go with strangers, because these people do not seem to be strangers by the time the abduction occurs. Use of an "appropriate stranger" such as a police officer or a store clerk or manager may be of great assistance to a lost child. Careful supervision of children, screening of references of potential caregivers, and excellent communication between parent and child are the best defense. Children sense unease in inappropriate relationships and can report this as long as parents routinely take all of their concerns in life seriously rather than downplaying or shaming them. Children should also be taught from an early age that they need not kiss, hug, touch, or sit on the lap of anyone, relative or not, if they do not wish to. This

respect for their comfort and wishes translates into self-respect and the ability to differentiate unwanted contacts without generating fear.

Runaways and Thrownaways

Most children reported as missing left of their own accord, often from adverse family or living situations. In fact, leaving home as an impulsive act of protest is very common, occurring in an estimated 1 of 7 children younger than 16 years in England, with 11% being younger than 11 years,[9] with girls leaving twice as often as boys.[10] Traditionally, most of these children were not reported as missing to national authorities, however, and were not included in national statistics from earlier surveys. In 1983, the Inspector General of the Department of Health and Human Services estimated that there were as many as 1 million and possibly more than 2 million runaways annually in the United States.[11] Children who run away commonly live in difficult situations such as poverty or reconstituted homes. Many of them were truant previously.

Runaway or thrownaway children missing for a prolonged time commonly were subject to physical abuse (up to 75%), sexual abuse (up to 20%),[12] or other harsh treatment from which they were seeking escape and felt they had no other way out. A variety of additional risk factors are more common among runaways than among other children and adolescents, including psychological problems, strained family relationships, school difficulties, and adverse peer-group pressure.[13] Up to 30% of runaway children ran away from foster care.[9] Runaways gone for a prolonged time are at risk of many medical and psychological problems including disease, crime (both as victims and perpetrators), injuries, alcohol use, illegal drug use (one third)[10] and selling, sexual contact, and death. They may pose for pornography or prostitute themselves to provide income to survive or be taken into prostitution as a form of "sheltering" relationship. As a result of this activity, they are at high risk of pregnancy and sexually transmitted diseases including human immunodeficiency virus infection. In urban areas, these children often join gangs or are involved in burglary or armed robbery and other crimes. The psychological effect of the coercive parenting they were receiving and their subsequent experiences can be severe. Many have learning disabilities and school failure and belong to deviant peer groups preceding the runaway event, which makes recovery more difficult.

NISMART-2 data about runaways show that 68% of runaways were 15 to 17 years of age, 28% were 12 to 14 years of age, and 4% were 7 to 11 years of age.[14] Runaway episodes are most likely to occur during summer (39%), with the runaway going more than 10 but no more than 50 miles from home (31%), and most were gone from 24 hours to 1 week (58%). Although many such episodes seem minor, 7% of runaways were missing from 1 to 6 months, 23% traveled more than 50 miles from home, and at least 9% traveled out of state. Many of the runaways are harmed during the episode, with 1% having been sexually assaulted or having had someone attempt to do so and 4% having been physically assaulted or having had someone attempt to do so.

Preventing children from becoming runaways and thrownaways lies in detecting family situations that include behavior problems or coercive interactions, especially when discipline is inappropriately harsh. Early and ongoing intervention for these families can promote more positive understanding of their children and better strategies for coexisting. Often, these children are targeted for punishment for the act of running away or for the associated misdeeds of substance use, theft, or prostitution when what is really needed is medical and psychological treatment, family realignment, or foster placement. Pediatricians should support community shelter and hot-line programs for runaways (eg, the National Runaway Switchboard at l-800-621-4000) that provide comprehensive medical and psychological care. Quality follow-up care is also needed to monitor for psychological and family adjustment and long-term sequelae. Problems that warrant treatment include skin, respiratory, gastrointestinal, and genital infections; dental disease; accidental or inflicted trauma; lack of immunizations; poor nutrition; and pregnancy in addition to preexisting and subsequent learning and psychological disorders.[13] On reunion, if it is possible, the entire troubled family needs to be addressed. The pediatrician needs to work as part of a team with the goal of long-term recovery for these children.

Family Abductions

One of the most prevalent categories of missing children is abduction by a noncustodial parent or unauthorized extended visits with family members. NISMART-2 research found that 203 900 children each year were victims of family abduction.[15] Thirty-five percent of these children were 6 to 11 years of age, 23% were 3 to 5 years of age, 21% were younger than 2 years, and 17% were 12 to 14 years of age. Thirty-five percent of abductions occurred in the summer, 26% occurred in the fall, 24% occurred in the winter, and 15% occurred in the spring. Twenty-four percent of these abductions lasted 1 week to 1 month, and less than 1% of children were still absent at the time of the research. Police were contacted in 60% of the cases.

Pediatricians have an important but difficult role to play in preventing family abduction through monitoring for marital difficulties or substance abuse in the family. It is important to offer early advice on ways to protect the child from marital discord and prompt referral to counseling or mediation. In the case of parental separation, the pediatrician may need to give advice on how to manage affected children.[16]

Children abducted by family members may be at increased risk of physical and sexual abuse or neglect.[17] However, data from NISMART-1 indicate that sexual abuse of children may be relatively uncommon in parental kidnapping. Although children abducted by family members can be with familiar and loving caregivers, emotional trauma still occurs. The children are separated from other loved ones and exposed to uncertainty and secrecy, and care is provided by an adult who is usually experiencing his or her own pain or anger. The goal of the adult taking the child generally is revenge or manipulation toward the ex-partner rather than the benefit of the child. In one study[18] of children after family abduction, 16 of 18 had emotional effects including severe fright, mental indoctrination, grief or rage about parental abandonment, rejection of the offending parent, and exaggerated identification with one parent. The 2 children abducted by fathers without any apparent reaction were told the truth, maintained contact with the mother, and came from such lifestyle chaos that this event seemed insignificant.

Missing Benign Explanations

A very large number of children who have not been abducted nor run away end up missing with benign explanations. In fact, this is the second largest category of missing children. "A missing benign explanation episode occurs when a child's whereabouts are unknown to the child's caretaker and this causes the caretaker to 1) be alarmed, 2) try to locate the child, and 3) contact the police about the episode for any reason, as long as the child was not lost, injured, abducted, victimized, or classified as runaway/thrownaway."[5] NISMART-2 data show that 374 000 or 28% of missing children were in this category. NISMART-1 included a category called "otherwise missing" to include those who were missing but did not fit into any of the other categories. There were nearly 440 000 children in this category with one third of the episodes being concerning enough for the parents to have reported them to the police. Children who have wandered off or disappeared in this way are at significant risk even though they have not been abducted or run away. They are vulnerable to abuse and exploitation, may become disoriented, or may be injured unintentionally. One in five suffered some type of physical harm, and 1 in 7 was abused or assaulted while missing, which emphasizes the point that every case in which a child is missing must be taken seriously regardless of the reason or perceived reason the child is gone.

Neonatal Abductions

From 1983 to 2001, the number of neonatal abductions per year ranged from 0 to 12. The perpetrators of this crime were typically females of childbearing age who had had a miscarriage or had been unable to conceive and had carefully planned an abduction to replace the lost child or maintain a relationship with a lover. The infant was usually kept in the area within 25 miles of the hospital[19] and in 95% of cases was returned to the parents.[20] Prevention of infant abductions has been successful through a combination of increased security measures in hospitals, including video cameras and alarm devices, and education of staff and parents about precautions to take while in the hospital. It is critical not to allow anyone without identification to take an infant for any reason and to keep the infant within sight of the parent or nursery staff at all times. These measures should be largely invisible and create a sense of security rather than increasing parental fears about abduction. Apparently as a result of these measures, there were no reported infant abductions from hospitals in the United States in 1999.[21] Infant abductions did occur in 2000 and 2001, but at a lower rate than in previous years. The National Center for Missing and Exploited Children provides free security and training consultations (1-800-843-5678). Pediatricians should support appropriate safeguards in the hospitals they serve but should also reassure parents of the rarity of this crime in a sensitive way so as not to promote a sense of vulnerability at this especially sensitive time of family formation.

Internet Issues

Although still relatively uncommon, the practice of pedophiles and child molesters approaching children on the Internet is occurring more frequently. In some cases, pedophiles and/or child molesters have arranged meetings with children. Nineteen percent of children using the Internet had received unwanted online requests to engage in sexual activities or provide intimate sexual information. Almost half of these solicitations were from other children. However, at least one quarter of them were from adults.[22] The National Center for Missing and Exploited Children reports that approximately 840 cases of people (of unspecified ages) "traveling to or luring" children they had contacted on the Internet are "proven or under investigation." Parents need to be advised to supervise Internet use by their children, discuss Internet experiences with their children, and set clear rules about contacts with people met via the Internet. Any computer with access to the Internet should always be kept in an open place (eg, living room, family room) in any home with children and should not be in a room in which the door can be closed or locked. It is important to monitor where children and adolescents have been surfing on the Internet. Parents may find it desirable to use filtering or censoring devices on the computer or limit access to restricted passwords. Eighty-five percent of parents in a national survey indicated that they had warned their children about the dangers of chats on the Internet, but only one third had used any blocking devices. Children need realistic education about the potential of the Internet as part of their media education but without generating fears for their safety.

IN THE EVENT OF A MISSING CHILD

In the event of a missing child, parents should:

- immediately call local law enforcement.
- provide police and/or the Federal Bureau of Investigation with a detailed description of the child, including clothing or jewelry worn at the time of the disappearance, and medical and dental information.
- be sure that the child is entered into National Crime Information Center logs by their local police.
- report abductions or suspected abductions to the National Center for Missing and Exploited Children (1-800-THE-LOST or www.missingkids.com) by parents or law enforcement.

- report runaways to the hot line (1-800-621-4000) of the federal Runaway and Homeless Youth Program.

PREVENTION

The pediatrician's advice for preventing missing children, as for many other health issues, needs to be a balance of safeguarding children while avoiding generating fear. None of this information needs to be taught specifically as abduction safeguarding, with all its overtones of danger and threat. Instead, it should be taught as developmental achievements to be praised for their own value in the growing child. The appropriate message allows the child to go forward with skill and confidence rather than fear and avoidance.

Pediatricians can help safeguard children older than 5 years by encouraging parents to teach them to memorize their name, address, and phone number, including area code, so that they can be identified readily if separated from their families. Older children can learn numbers for contacting parents at home or at work. Because abductions are rarely conducted by strangers, even in nonfamily abductions, teaching children not to talk to strangers frightens them without any proven benefit. Passive methods of identifying children such as the placement of microchips in the teeth and fingerprinting are primarily techniques for identification of bodies. Their use has become common for fund raising and as a "service to the community" often without considering the potential effect in frightening children and inappropriately raising fears in adults without any perspective provided on the real nature or rareness of abduction.[23,24] On the other hand, keeping recent photographs of children and promptly reporting incidences to the police are extremely helpful measures. Law-enforcement officials consider photographs the number one tool in finding missing children. In addition, photograph campaigns such as direct mail cards and "rogues' galleries" in magazines have resulted in 1 in 6 children being located as a direct result of the photograph. Parents should be instructed to keep a high-quality photograph of each child, updated at least every 6 months. School photographs serve this purpose with only positive connotations.

The importance of a prompt response in missing-children cases is demonstrated in the AMBER (American's Missing: Broadcast Emergency Response) Plan. Patterned after the emergency weather warnings, the AMBER Plan is intended to flood a region with information regarding high-risk missing children when time is of the essence. Strict criteria are in place to initiate an AMBER Plan response. It was introduced in Dallas, Texas, in 1997 and became a national program in 2002. Since its inception, the AMBER Plan has been credited with successfully recovering more than 130 children. When combined with the success of the photograph-distribution campaigns (1 in 6 featured long-term missing children found as a direct result of these programs), we see the value of both a prompt response and persistence in searching in missing-child cases.

Learning about personal safety is an important part of a child's education. Schools should be encouraged to include such a program as part of their K-12 curriculum. Many such programs exist but vary greatly in quality and effectiveness. The National Center for Missing and Exploited Children, in cooperation with the American Academy of Pediatrics and other child-advocacy groups, has developed a tool to help school districts evaluate these programs and select one that best fits their individual needs (*Guidelines for Programs to Reduce Child Victimization: A Resource for Communities When Choosing a Program to Teach Personal Safety to Children*[25]).

ADVICE FOR PEDIATRICIANS

1. Help parents and children put the risk of becoming missing in perspective.
2. Encourage families to teach children self-identifying information without connecting it to a threat of becoming missing.
3. Encourage families to keep a high-quality and current photograph of each child.
4. Encourage families to teach children to accept only touches that are comfortable to them regardless of the toucher's relationship to them.
5. Encourage families to teach older children, especially girls, to "know the rules":

   • When going out, don't go out alone.
   • Always tell an adult where you are going.
   • Say "no" if you feel threatened.

6. Consider advocating for an appropriate personal-safety curriculum to be taught in schools and check its approach.
7. Continually screen for risk factors for missing children (ie, family discord, divorce, coercive parenting, substance abuse, school failure, deviant peer group, etc) and intervene early with appropriate work-up and referrals.
8. Assess whether adolescents consider themselves to have several sources of support, including the pediatrician, so that they need not resort to running away.
9. Be skeptical of new patients presenting with vague stories about absent parents or children who report mysterious parent deaths or separations without contact, because they may represent abductions.
10. Insist on prompt transfer of medical records as a routine practice.
11. Support programs that serve runaways.
12. Consider providing or coordinating comprehensive care to any families who have just had a missing child returned.
13. Expose programs spuriously generating fear of abduction.
14. Look at and encourage others to look at pictures of missing children.

COMMITTEE ON PSYCHOSOCIAL ASPECTS OF CHILD AND FAMILY HEALTH, 2002–2003
Jane Meschan Foy, MD, Chairperson
William L. Coleman, MD
Edward Goldson, MD
Cheryl L. Hausman, MD
Ana Navarro, MD
Thomas J. Sullivan, MD
J. Lane Tanner, MD
Joseph F. Hagan, Jr, MD
  Past Committee Member
Barbara J. Howard, MD
  Past Committee Member

LIAISONS
F. Daniel Armstrong, PhD
  Society of Pediatric Psychology
Janet Mims, MS, CPNP
  National Association of Pediatric Nurse Practitioners
Sally E. A. Longstaffe, MD
  Canadian Paediatric Society
Frances J. Wren, MD
  American Academy of Child and Adolescent Psychiatry

CONSULTANT
George J. Cohen, MD
  National Consortium for Child and Adolescent Mental Health Services

INVITED CONTRIBUTOR
Daniel D. Broughton, MD

STAFF
Karen Smith

REFERENCES

1. Stickler GB, Salter M, Broughton DD, Alario A. Parents' worries about children compared to actual risks. *Clin Pediatr (Phila)*. 1991;30:522–528
2. Federal Bureau of Investigation. *Total NCIC Missing Person Entries by State by Year*. Clarksburg, WV: Criminal Justice Information Services Division, Federal Bureau of Investigation; 2002
3. National Center for Missing and Exploited Children. *June 2003 Review of National Crime Information Center Missing-Person Entries by Age in 2001 and 2002 in the Juvenile, Endangered, and Involuntary Categories*. Alexandria, VA: National Center for Missing and Exploited Children; 2003
4. US Department of Justice, Office of Juvenile Justice and Delinquency Prevention. *Second National Incidence Studies of Missing, Abducted, Runaway, and Thrownaway Children (NISMART-2)*. Washington, DC: US Department of Justice; 2002
5. Sedlack AJ, Finkelhor D, Hammer H, Schultz DJ. *National Estimates of Missing Children: An Overview*. Washington, DC: US Department of Justice; 2002:4–10
6. Finkelhor D, Hammer H, Sedlak AJ. *Nonfamily Abducted Children: National Estimates and Characteristics*. Washington, DC: US Department of Justice; 2002:7, 10
7. National Center for Missing and Exploited Children. *Know the Rules*. Alexandria, VA: National Center for Missing and Exploited Children; 1998. Available at: www.missingkids.com/html/ncmec_default_know_the_rules.html. Accessed October 6, 2003
8. Broughton DD, Allen EE. *How to Keep Your Child Safe: A Message to Every Parent*. Alexandria, VA: National Center for Missing and Exploited Children; 1991
9. Lawrenson F. Runaway children: whose problem? *BMJ*. 1997;314:1064
10. Schmidt WM. Runaway children. *JAMA*. 1975;232:651–652
11. Davidson H. Missing children: a close look at the issue. *Child Today*. 1986;15:26–30
12. Stiffman AR. Physical and sexual abuse in runaway youths. *Child Abuse Negl*. 1989;13:417–426
13. American Medical Association. Missing and exploited children. *R I Med J*. 1986;69:369–376
14. Hammer H, Finkelhor D, Sedlak AJ. *Runaway/Thrownaway Children: National Estimates and Characteristics*. Washington, DC: US Department of Justice; 2002:6–8
15. Hammer H, Finkelhor D, Sedlak AJ. *Children Abducted by Family Members: National Estimates and Characteristics*. Washington, DC: US Department of Justice; 2002:4–8

16. Cohen GJ, American Academy of Pediatrics, Committee on Psychosocial Aspects of Child and Family Health. Helping children and families deal with divorce and separation. *Pediatrics.* 2002;110:1019–1023

17. Abrahms S. *Children in the Crossfire: The Tragedy of Parental Kidnapping.* New York, NY: Atheneum Press; 1984

18. Terr LC. Child snatching: a new epidemic of an ancient malady. *J Pediatr.* 1983;103:151–156

19. Beachy P, Deacon J. Preventing neonatal kidnapping. *J Obstet Gynecol Neonatal Nurs.* 1992;21:12–16

20. Rabun JB Jr. *For Healthcare Professionals: Guidelines on Prevention of and Response to Infant Abductions.* 7th ed. Alexandria, VA: National Center for Missing and Exploited Children; 2003

21. Rabun JB Jr. *National Center for Missing and Exploited Children Quarterly Progress Report.* Alexandria, VA: National Center for Missing and Exploited Children; 2003:10

22. Finkelhor D, Mitchell KJ, Wolak J. *Online Victimization: A Report on the Nation's Youth.* Alexandria, VA: National Center for Missing and Exploited Children; 2000

23. Bergman AB. The business of missing children. *Pediatrics.* 1986;77:119–121

24. Livingston G. Fear of abduction: it's a business now. *San Francisco Examiner.* October 12, 1999:A-19

25. National Center for Missing and Exploited Children. *Guidelines for Programs to Reduce Child Victimization: A Resource for Communities When Choosing a Program to Teach Personal Safety to Children.* Alexandria, VA: National Center for Missing and Exploited Children; 1999. Available at: www.ncmec.org/en_US/publications/NC24.pdf. Accessed October 21, 2003

All clinical reports from the American Academy of Pediatrics automatically expire 5 years after publication unless reaffirmed, revised, or retired at or before that time.

Prenatal Screening and Diagnosis for Pediatricians

• *Clinical Report*

AMERICAN ACADEMY OF PEDIATRICS

CLINICAL REPORT
Guidance for the Clinician in Rendering Pediatric Care

Christopher Cunniff, MD; and the Committee on Genetics

Prenatal Screening and Diagnosis for Pediatricians

ABSTRACT. The pediatrician who cares for a child with a birth defect or genetic disorder may be in the best position to alert the family to the possibility of a recurrence of the same or similar problems in future offspring. The family may wish to know about and may benefit from methods that convert probability statements about recurrence risks into more precise knowledge about a specific abnormality in the fetus. The pediatrician also may be called on to discuss abnormal prenatal test results as a way of understanding the risks and complications that the newborn infant may face. Along with the increase in knowledge brought about by the sequencing of the human genome, there has been an increase in the technical capabilities for diagnosing many chromosome abnormalities, genetic disorders, and isolated birth defects in the prenatal period. The purpose of this report is to update the pediatrician about indications for prenatal diagnosis, current techniques used for prenatal diagnosis, and the status of maternal screenings for detection of fetal abnormalities. *Pediatrics* 2004;114:889–894; *prenatal diagnosis, amniocentesis, chorionic villi sampling, genetic screening, chromosome aberrations, prenatal ultrasonography, neural tube defects, genetic counseling, preimplantation diagnosis, α-fetoproteins.*

ABBREVIATIONS. CVS, chorionic villus sampling; PGD, preimplantation genetic diagnosis; MRI, magnetic resonance imaging; NTD, neural tube defect; MSAFP, maternal serum α-fetoprotein.

INTRODUCTION

When a genetic or potentially genetic disorder is diagnosed prenatally, the pediatrician may assist the family in addressing questions about the natural history of the disorder and in planning for care of the affected newborn. The information gained from prenatal diagnosis is helpful to the obstetrician or family practitioner in the management of pregnancy, labor, and delivery and in some circumstances may improve pregnancy outcome. The availability of prenatal diagnosis gives couples options they might not have otherwise, including preparation for the birth of a child with an abnormality, termination of an affected pregnancy, or use of fetal treatment such as fetal surgery for spina bifida or use of maternal dexamethasone to prevent virilization of affected females with congen-

ital adrenal hyperplasia. These procedures may be important to couples at increased risk of having children with genetic disorders, because without this information they might be unwilling to attempt a pregnancy.

A number of well-studied techniques are used for prenatal diagnosis. For many of these techniques, the accuracy, reliability, and safety of the procedures are positively correlated with operator experience. Procedures such as amniocentesis, chorionic villus sampling (CVS), fetal blood sampling, and preimplantation genetic diagnosis (PGD) allow analysis of embryonic or fetal cells or tissues for chromosomal, genetic, and biochemical abnormalities. Fetal imaging studies such as ultrasonography, magnetic resonance imaging (MRI), and fetal echocardiography identify structural abnormalities and provide definitive diagnostic information or suggest additional evaluation. In addition to these techniques, maternal serum screening is used to identify pregnancies that are at increased risk of adverse outcomes, such as neural tube defects (NTDs), chromosome abnormalities, and fetal abdominal wall defects. This report focuses on the techniques that are most commonly used and provides an outline of pertinent information that the practicing pediatrician may find useful. For more in-depth discussions of these techniques, a number of comprehensive texts are available.[1–3] The GeneTests Web site (www.geneclinics.org) also provides extensive information about testing for many chromosomal and genetic disorders.

INDICATIONS FOR PRENATAL DIAGNOSIS

Prenatal diagnosis is indicated whenever there is a familial, maternal, or fetal condition that confers an increased risk of a malformation, chromosome abnormality, or genetic disorder. Some prenatal diagnostic studies are prompted by abnormal results of tests such as ultrasonographic examinations or maternal serum screening. In other circumstances, parents may be affected with a genetic disorder, may be carriers for autosomal recessive or X-linked recessive disorders, or may be a member of an ethnic group with an increased risk of a specific genetic disease.

Chromosome Analysis

The most commonly cited reason for prenatal diagnosis is advanced maternal age, which in the United States is considered to be 35 years or greater at the time of delivery. Amniocentesis or CVS is

The guidance in this report does not indicate an exclusive course of treatment or serve as a standard of medical care. Variations, taking into account individual circumstances, may be appropriate.

DOI: 10.1542/peds.2004-1368

PEDIATRICS (ISSN 0031 4005). Copyright © 2004 by the American Academy of Pediatrics.

offered to such women because of the increased risk of aneuploidy (an abnormal number of chromosomes in the fetus). Amniocentesis or CVS also is used commonly to evaluate pregnancies in which an ultrasonographic examination or a maternal serum screening result has identified a possible fetal problem. In addition to advanced maternal age or an abnormal screening result, other indications for chromosome analysis include: 1) a chromosome abnormality in a previous offspring, a parent, or a close relative; 2) a previous offspring with multiple malformations in whom no chromosomal study was obtained; and 3) fetal sex determination in pregnancies at risk of a serious X-linked disorder for which specific prenatal diagnostic tests are not available. For the child with a normal prenatal chromosome analysis but with signs of a possible chromosome abnormality such as multiple malformations, growth deficiency, or developmental disabilities, repeat testing should be considered, because the quality of a postnatal study is usually superior to one obtained prenatally, and some cases of chromosome mosaicism may only be diagnosed postnatally.

Biochemical Studies

Biochemical studies are undertaken most often when a known abnormality is present in a family and the disorder can be diagnosed by a specific biochemical test. The number of biochemical disorders that can be diagnosed prenatally is growing rapidly, so that many common inborn errors of metabolism can be diagnosed through biochemical testing for enzyme deficiency or an abnormal metabolite. Conditions such as Tay-Sachs disease, mucopolysaccharidoses, and peroxisomal diseases may be diagnosed by biochemical tests on amniotic fluid, amniocytes, or chorionic villi. Before proceeding to evaluation of the fetus, there should be biochemical confirmation of the diagnosis in the index case, one or both parents should be a confirmed carrier for an autosomal recessive or X-linked recessive disorder, or a family history of a diagnosable disorder and indeterminate carrier status should be established. In a few circumstances, biochemical testing may be used when there is no family history of a disorder but prenatal ultrasonographic findings are suggestive of a biochemical disorder. For example, in a pregnancy in which cleft palate and abnormal genital findings are identified by ultrasonography, biochemical testing for Smith-Lemli-Opitz syndrome, a disorder of cholesterol biogenesis, should be considered, because these are characteristic features of this syndrome.

Molecular Genetic Studies

Similar to biochemical studies, molecular genetic studies almost always are undertaken because there is a positive family history of a specific genetic disease or prenatal findings point to a possible single-gene disorder that can be diagnosed by molecular techniques. The list of available molecular genetic studies has grown dramatically in the last several years, and many of the common single-gene disorders can be diagnosed rapidly and conclusively by

molecular techniques. The description of the methods used to make a molecular diagnosis is beyond the scope of this report, but several useful resources are available for this purpose.[4–6] Examples of disorders that are diagnosed by molecular methods include fragile X syndrome, cystic fibrosis, Duchenne and Becker muscular dystrophy, and hemophilia. In each case, it is important that the clinician first know the specific mutation that is being sought in the case of a positive family history or that the detection rate for the mutation be known if there is no family history. The consultation of a geneticist, genetic counselor, or other clinician familiar with the utility of these prenatal tests may be particularly helpful.

TECHNIQUES FOR PRENATAL DIAGNOSIS BY CELL OR TISSUE SAMPLING

Amniocentesis

Transabdominal amniocentesis is the most commonly used procedure for obtaining fetal cells that can be analyzed for cytogenetic, biochemical, or molecular abnormalities. In addition, amniotic fluid can be analyzed separately for α-fetoprotein and acetylcholinesterase concentrations associated with open NTDs and for other analytes that are diagnostic of specific genetic diseases. The procedure is most commonly performed at 15 to 18 weeks' gestational age. Amniocentesis in the second trimester is associated with a low rate of complications and provides an accurate sample for analysis in more than 99% of cases.[7,8] Fetal chromosome analysis is the most common laboratory study performed on samples obtained by amniocentesis. Results are usually available 1 to 2 weeks after the procedure and sooner in some circumstances. Fluorescence in situ hybridization studies are performed increasingly for rapid detection of fetal aneuploidy or for microdeletion syndromes such as 22q11 deletions in fetuses with conotruncal heart defects. Risks of amniocentesis include fetal loss, chorioamnionitis, fetal injury, and maternal Rh sensitization, each of which is very uncommon. Amniocentesis is performed under ultrasonographic guidance, which minimizes the risk of direct fetal injury. The risk of fetal loss in most large series is less than 0.5%, and many prenatal diagnostic centers have a lower loss rate. To prevent Rh isoimmunization, Rh immune globulin is administered at the time of the procedure to nonsensitized Rh-negative women.

In recent years, amniocentesis performed at 11 to 13 weeks' gestational age has gained increasing attention. Some investigations have suggested that this technique carries similar risks to amniocentesis at 15 to 18 weeks' gestational age.[9] In a large multicenter randomized trial, however, investigators found a higher risk of fetal loss, a greater number of amniotic fluid culture failures, and an increased risk of talipes.[10] Additional investigations have also identified an increased risk of foot deformities in the offspring of women who undergo early amniocentesis.[11,12] Although it is desirable to complete prenatal diagnostic tests as early as possible, the American College of

Obstetricians and Gynecologists does not recommend early amniocentesis because of higher rates of pregnancy loss and other complications compared with amniocentesis after 15 weeks' gestation.[13]

CVS

The advantage of CVS is earlier diagnosis. Earlier diagnosis provides additional time for counseling and decision-making, and in the circumstance in which termination of pregnancy is elected, termination can be performed more safely for the mother. CVS is usually performed at 10 to 12 weeks' gestational age. The procedure involves transcervical placement of a catheter or transabdominal placement of a needle, under ultrasonographic guidance, into the developing placenta. The transcervical and transabdominal approaches seem to have comparable safety and accuracy.[14] A sample of the chorionic villus is removed by aspiration. Once removed, the fetal villi are dissected from the maternal decidual tissue. Cytogenetic, molecular, and some biochemical studies can be performed on CVS samples, but amniotic fluid is not obtained for protein analysis. Therefore, women who have had CVS should also have maternal serum α-fetoprotein (MSAFP) screening at 15 to 20 weeks' gestational age to screen for fetal NTDs.

Although CVS loss rates are slightly higher than those associated with amniocentesis in some clinical trials,[15,16] other studies have suggested that the procedure-related loss rates are comparable between CVS and second-trimester amniocentesis.[17,18] The success of cytogenetic diagnosis is slightly lower for CVS versus amniocentesis. In particular, CVS is associated with an increased frequency of placental mosaicism, which is a cytogenetic abnormality detected in the CVS sample but not found in the fetus or newborn. Placental mosaicism is found in approximately 1% of CVS samples,[19,20] and although the fetus is chromosomally normal, placental mosaicism is associated with an increased risk of non–procedure-related, spontaneous fetal loss. An additional concern for CVS is the reported association of CVS and limb-reduction defects, especially when the procedure is performed before 10 weeks' gestational age; although some investigations have shown an association[21] and others have found none,[22] the American College of Obstetricians and Gynecologists has recommended that CVS not be performed before 10 weeks.[23]

Sampling of Fetal Blood

In some circumstances, it may be useful to obtain a sample of fetal blood. This technique, referred to as cordocentesis or percutaneous umbilical blood sampling, may be used to assess fetal blood disorders, fetal infections, or isoimmunization or may be used for rapid fetal karyotyping. It also has been used to supply fetal treatment such as transfusions. Percutaneous umbilical blood sampling is usually performed with a 20- or 25-gauge spinal needle inserted into the umbilical vein or artery, preferably near the insertion of the cord into the placenta. Fetal loss or spontaneous abortion is reported in approximately 1% to 2% of cases, making the risk associated with this procedure higher than that with amniocentesis or CVS.[24]

PGD

In some circumstances, specific genetic diseases can be diagnosed before implantation of the blastocyst after in vitro fertilization. PGD provides prospective parents the possibility of establishing a pregnancy in which the fetus is unaffected with the disorder for which it is at risk. In this procedure, a single cell is taken from the early embryo and analyzed by molecular techniques after DNA amplification by polymerase chain reaction. For this technique to be useful, it is essential to know the precise abnormality being sought, which usually means that both the genetic locus and the mutation have been identified in a previous child or another family member. PGD is performed in a limited number of prenatal diagnostic centers, and systematic outcome analyses of large groups of patients are not available. It has been used to detect such disorders as cystic fibrosis and Tay-Sachs disease.[25]

TECHNIQUES FOR PRENATAL DIAGNOSIS BY FETAL VISUALIZATION

Ultrasonography

Ultrasonography has become the primary method for fetal anatomic imaging. This technique may be used in pregnancy to monitor fetal growth, movement, position, and morphology; assess amniotic fluid volume; and establish gestational age and placental location. In some countries, it has become standard practice to perform ultrasonographic examination at some time in the second trimester. In many other countries including the United States, ultrasonography is performed at some time during pregnancy for a wide range of clinical indications. During the early second trimester, ultrasonographic examination is used to date the pregnancy, identify twins, diagnose some fetal structural anomalies, and examine the placenta and the amount of amniotic fluid. Improvements in the technical quality of ultrasonographic equipment and increasing skill levels of ultrasonogram operators have led to an ever-increasing identification of fetal structural abnormalities of the genitourinary, gastrointestinal, cardiac, and central nervous systems.

Ultrasonography has become the mainstay for prenatal diagnosis of structural abnormalities, particularly when used in the mid– to late second trimester. As a modality used to follow-up on abnormal maternal screening results, ultrasonographic examination can identify most associated abnormalities such as ventral abdominal wall defects and NTDs. Almost all cases of anencephaly are detectable by ultrasonography, and more than 90% of open spina bifida is detectable when ultrasonography is used for a high-risk population such as those with abnormally high serum α-fetoprotein concentrations.[26,27] With the advent of improved image quality of ultrasonographic examinations, a number of minor abnormalities have been recognized. Studies of these abnormalities in high-risk populations have shown that some of these markers may be seen more commonly in pregnancies with fetal chromosome abnormalities than in unaffected pregnancies. Nuchal translucency, thickened nuchal fold or cystic hygroma, choroid plexus cysts, fetal echogenic bowel, intracardiac echogenic foci, and renal pyelectasis have all been suggested as possible markers for fetal chromosome abnormalities.[28] Although these features are associated with increased fetal risk, they are not used as primary screening methods. When they are identified, however, additional investigation may be warranted on the basis of a number of factors such as maternal age and associated abnormalities. The pediatrician may encounter newborn infants in whom one of these markers has been detected prenatally. Because these infants have an increased risk of aneuploidy such as trisomy 13, 18, or 21, neonatal examination should be directed toward identification of clinical features associated with one of these trisomies. If the clinical examination is not suggestive of one of these conditions and there are no major anomalies, it is reasonable to observe the infant and perform no additional diagnostic testing.

MRI

MRI has received limited use, primarily because fetal movement prevents optimal resolution. Ultrafast MRI scanning has improved its utility. MRI may be especially useful for the evaluation of fetal central nervous system abnormalities, when oligohydramnios is present, or when ultrasonography is difficult.[29] MRI generally is not recommended during the first trimester.

Fetal Echocardiography

Fetal echocardiography is usually performed after 20 weeks' gestation. When used together with duplex and/or color-flow Doppler ultrasonography, it can identify a substantial number of major structural cardiac defects and rhythm disturbances.[30] Fetal echocardiography is considered when there is an increased risk of congenital heart disease because: 1) there is an extracardiac malformation identified by ultrasonographic examination; 2) there has been prenatal exposure to a teratogenic agent; 3) there is a family history of congenital heart defects, especially in a parent or sibling; 4) a fetal chromosome abnormality or genetic disease associated with heart defects is suspected; 5) a maternal disease associated with fetal structural heart defects, such as diabetes or phenylketonuria, or maternal disease associated with fetal cardiac arrhythmia, such as lupus erythematosus, has been identified; 6) a cardiac defect is suspected by findings on routine ultrasonography; or 7) a fetal arrhythmia has been detected on auscultation or examination.

MATERNAL SERUM SCREENING STUDIES

Detection of NTDs

MSAFP concentrations are increased in many abnormal fetal conditions including open NTDs and defects of the genitourinary and gastrointestinal systems. MSAFP screening results are abnormal in approximately 90% of cases of anencephaly and approximately 80% of cases of open spina bifida. It is recommended that MSAFP testing be offered to all prenatal patients, and in some states it is mandated by law.[31] Because elevated MSAFP concentrations have also been associated with adverse pregnancy outcomes such as low birth weight and stillbirth, pregnancies in which concentrations are elevated may be monitored more closely than those with normal concentrations. Most of those who have increased MSAFP concentrations even after repeat testing will have a normal outcome. When concentrations are increased, ultrasonography is used to confirm gestational age, exclude multiple gestation, and assess for recognized causes (primarily NTDs and ventral wall defects) of the increase. A normal result of an ultrasonographic examination performed in a specialized center decreases the probability of a fetal NTD by 95% or more.[32] If ultrasonographic examination does not identify a cause, amniocentesis is offered for measurement of amniotic fluid α-fetoprotein and acetylcholinesterase concentrations, both of which are increased with open NTDs.

Detection of Chromosome Abnormalities

After the advent of MSAFP screening for NTDs, it was recognized that low second-trimester MSAFP concentrations were associated with an increased risk of Down syndrome.[33,34] Since that time, additional serum markers that increase the detection rate for Down syndrome have been identified. When second-trimester MSAFP testing is combined with measurement of human chorionic gonadotropin and unconjugated estriol concentrations (these 3 proteins constitute the "triple screen" for fetal aneuploidy), up to 80% of fetuses with Down syndrome can be identified.[35,36] Decreased concentrations of all 3 analytes are associated with an increased risk of fetal trisomy 18. Some screening programs have added inhibin A to the triple screen to improve the sensitivity and specificity of the test.[37] Clinicians should be aware that MSAFP screening for Down syndrome has a positive screening rate of approximately 5% and a positive predictive value of approximately 3% to 5%, which means that the great majority of those who have a positive screening result have a normal outcome.

Over the last several years, techniques for effective first-trimester screening for Down syndrome have been explored. Although a number of concerns about the appropriateness of adopting these techniques on a population basis have been raised,[38] many perinatologists are already using fetal ultrasonography and/or screening for maternal serum markers in clinical practice.[39] Measurement of nuchal translucency (a sonolucent space at the back of the fetal neck) can be performed between 10 and 13 weeks' gestation. The fetus with Down syndrome tends to have a larger area of translucency when compared with the chromosomally normal fetus. The nuchal translucency measurement is used in combination with 2 serum analytes, pregnancy-associated plasma protein A and the free β subunit of human chorionic gonadotropin, to adjust the risk for Down syndrome based on maternal age alone. The detection rates are comparable to second-trimester serum screening.

Detection of Other Abnormalities

There are a number of conditions associated with high or low MSAFP concentrations. In addition to abdominal wall defects such as omphalocele and gastroschisis, high concentrations are also associated with renal anomalies, congenital nephrosis, gastrointestinal tract obstruction, and low birth weight.[40,41] In addition to these conditions, high MSAFP concentrations may also be seen with multifetal gestation, underestimated gestational age, and some maternal conditions such as low maternal weight. Low MSAFP concentrations are associated with adverse outcomes other than chromosomal trisomies, including fetal death and gestational trophoblastic disease.[42] As with high MSAFP concentrations, low concentrations may be seen in nonpathologic conditions such as overestimated gestational age or high maternal weight.

CONCLUSIONS

Pediatricians may be called on to counsel a family in which prenatal diagnosis is being considered or in which there is a fetus with a genetic disorder. It is important that pediatricians involve themselves at a level appropriate to their training and experience, that they clarify their role in the prenatal diagnostic process with the family, and that they document their discussion and recommendations. In most circumstances, pediatricians will not assume a primary role in performing prenatal diagnostic procedures or counseling the family about their risks and benefits. More frequently, an obstetrician, maternal-fetal medicine specialist, clinical geneticist, and/or a genetic counselor will direct the diagnostic evaluation and provide pretest and posttest counseling. Because of a previous relationship with the family, the pediatrician may be called on to review this information and assist the family in the decision-making process. The pediatrician should be familiar with the principles of prenatal genetic diagnosis and know how to apply them to specific problems in genetic counseling, diagnosis, and management in clinical practice. Pediatricians should be familiar with resources available in their region for obtaining information about whether and how a specific disorder can be diagnosed and when and where to refer patients for prenatal genetic diagnosis. The technology of prenatal diagnosis is changing rapidly, and genetic consultants can assist pediatricians in the appropriate use and interpretation of the diagnostic tests that are available.

COMMITTEE ON GENETICS, 2003–2004
G. Bradley Schaefer, MD, Chairperson
Marilyn J. Bull, MD
Joseph H. Hersh, MD
Celia I. Kaye, MD, PhD
Nancy J. Mendelsohn, MD

John B. Moeschler, MD
Howard M. Saal, MD

LIAISONS
James D. Goldberg, MD
    American College of Obstetricians
    and Gynecologists
James W. Hanson, MD
    National Institute of Child Health
    and Human Development/
    American College of Medical
    Genetics
Michele A. Lloyd-Puryear, MD, PhD
    Health Resources and Services
    Administration
Cynthia A. Moore, MD, PhD
    Centers for Disease Control and
    Prevention

STAFF
Paul Spire

REFERENCES

1. Creasy RK, Resnik R, eds. *Maternal-Fetal Medicine*. 4th ed. Philadelphia, PA: Saunders; 1999
2. Cunningham FG, ed. *Williams Obstetrics*. 21st ed. New York, NY: McGraw-Hill; 2001
3. Simpson JL, Elias S, eds. *Genetics in Obstetrics and Gynecology*. 3rd ed. Philadelphia, PA: Saunders; 2002
4. American Academy of Pediatrics, Committee on Genetics. Molecular genetic testing in pediatric practice: a subject review. *Pediatrics*. 2000; 106:1494–1497
5. Korf B. Molecular diagnosis (1). *N Engl J Med*. 1995;332:1218–1220
6. Korf B. Molecular diagnosis (2) [published correction appears in *N Engl J Med*. 1995;333:331]. *N Engl J Med*. 1995;332:1499–1502
7. National Institute of Child Health and Human Development, National Registry for Amniocentesis Study Group. Midtrimester amniocentesis for prenatal diagnosis. Safety and accuracy. *JAMA*. 1976;236:1471–1476
8. Simpson NE, Dallaire L, Miller JR, et al. Prenatal diagnosis of genetic disease in Canada: report of a collaborative study. *Can Med Assoc J*. 1976;115:739–748
9. Assel BG, Lewis SM, Dickerman LH, Park VM, Jassani MN. Single-operator comparison of early and mid-second-trimester amniocentesis. *Obstet Gynecol*. 1992;79:940–944
10. The Canadian Early and Mid-trimester Amniocentesis Trial (CEMAT) Group. Randomised trial to assess safety and fetal outcome of early and midtrimester amniocentesis. *Lancet*. 1998;351:242–247
11. Nikkila A, Valentin L, Thelin A, Jorgensen C. Early amniocentesis and congenital foot deformities. *Fetal Diagn Ther*. 2002;17:129–132
12. Tredwell SJ, Wilson D, Wilmink MA, Canadian Early and Mid-Trimester Amniocentesis Trial Group (CEMAT), Canadian Orthopedic Review Group. Review of the effect of early amniocentesis on foot deformity in the neonate. *J Pediatr Orthop*. 2001;21:636–641
13. American College of Obstetricians and Gynecologists. ACOG Practice Bulletin. Clinical management guidelines for obstetrician-gynecologists. Prenatal diagnosis of fetal chromosomal abnormalities. *Obstet Gynecol*. 2001;97(5 pt 1):1–12
14. Jackson LG, Zachary JM, Fowler SE, et al. A randomized comparison of transcervical and transabdominal chorionic-villus sampling. The US National Institute of Child Health and Human Development Chorionic-Villus Sampling and Amniocentesis Study Group. *N Engl J Med*. 1992; 327:594–598
15. Medical Research Council European trial of chorion villus sampling. MRC working party on the evaluation of chorion villus sampling. *Lancet*. 1991;337:1491–1499
16. Lippman A, Tomkins DJ, Shime J, Hamerton JL. Canadian multicentre randomized clinical trial of chorion villus sampling and amniocentesis. Final report. *Prenat Diagn*. 1992;12:385–408
17. Smidt-Jensen S, Permin M, Philip J, et al. Randomised comparison of amniocentesis and transabdominal and transcervical chorionic villus sampling. *Lancet*. 1992;340:1237–1244
18. Canadian Collaborative CVS-Amniocentesis Clinical Trial Group. Multicentre randomised clinical trial of chorion villus sampling and amniocentesis. First report. *Lancet*. 1989;1(8628):1–6

19. Johnson A, Wapner RJ, Davis GH, Jackson LG. Mosaicism in chorionic villus sampling: an association with poor perinatal outcome. *Obstet Gynecol.* 1990;75:573–577

20. Wapner RJ, Simpson JL, Golbus MS, et al. Chorionic mosaicism: association with fetal loss but not with adverse perinatal outcome. *Prenat Diagn.* 1992;12:347–355

21. Olney RS, Khoury MJ, Alo CJ, et al. Increased risk for transverse digital deficiency after chorionic villus sampling: results of the United States Multistate Case-Control Study, 1988–1992. *Teratology.* 1995;51:20–29

22. Froster UG, Jackson L. Limb defects and chorionic villus sampling: results from an international registry, 1992–94. *Lancet.* 1996;347:489–494

23. American College of Obstetricians and Gynecologists, Committee on Genetics. Chorionic villus sampling. *ACOG Comm Opin.* 1995;160:1–3

24. Tongsong T, Wanapirak C, Kunavikatikul C, Sirirchotiyakul S, Piyamongkol W, Chanprapaph P. Fetal loss rate associated with cordocentesis at midgestation. *Am J Obstet Gynecol.* 2001;184:719–723

25. Handyside AH, Lesko JG, Tarin JJ, Winston RM, Hughes MR. Birth of a normal girl after in vitro fertilization and preimplantation diagnostic testing for cystic fibrosis. *N Engl J Med.* 1992;327:905–909

26. Limb CJ, Holmes LB. Anencephaly: changes in prenatal detection and birth status, 1972 through 1990. *Am J Obstet Gynecol.* 1994;170:1333–1338

27. Morrow RJ, McNay MB, Whittle MJ. Ultrasound detection of neural tube defects in patients with elevated maternal serum alpha-fetoprotein. *Obstet Gynecol.* 1991;78:1055–1057

28. Sepulveda W, Lopez-Tenorio J. The value of minor ultrasound markers for fetal aneuploidy. *Curr Opin Obstet Gynecol.* 2001;13:183–191

29. American College of Obstetricians and Gynecologists, Committee on Obstetric Practice. Guidelines for diagnostic imaging during pregnancy. *ACOG Comm Opin.* 1995;158:1–4

30. Copel JA, Pilu G, Green J, Hobbins JC, Kleinman CS. Fetal echocardiographic screening for congenital heart disease: the importance of the four-chamber view. *Am J Obstet Gynecol.* 1987;157:648–655

31. American College of Obstetricians and Gynecologists. Maternal serum screening. *ACOG Tech Bull.* 1996;228:1–9

32. Lennon CA, Gray DL. Sensitivity and specificity of ultrasound for the detection of neural tube and ventral wall defects in a high-risk population. *Obstet Gynecol.* 1999;94:562–566

33. Merkatz IR, Nitowsky HM, Macri JN, Johnson WE. An association between low maternal serum alpha-fetoprotein and fetal chromosome abnormalities. *Am J Obstet Gynecol.* 1984;148:886–894

34. Cuckle HS, Wald NJ, Lindenbaum RH. Maternal serum alpha-fetoprotein measurement: a screening test for Down syndrome. *Lancet.* 1984;1:926–929

35. Phillips OP, Elias S, Shulman LP, Andersen RN, Morgan CD, Simpson JL. Maternal serum screening for fetal Down syndrome in women less than 35 years of age using alpha-fetoprotein, hCG, and unconjugated estriol: a prospective 2-year study. *Obstet Gynecol.* 1992;80:353–358

36. Burton BK, Prins GS, Verp MS. A prospective trial of prenatal screening for Down syndrome by means of maternal serum alpha-fetoprotein, human chorionic gonadotropin, and unconjugated estriol. *Am J Obstet Gynecol.* 1993;169:526–530

37. Benn PA. Advances in prenatal screening for Down syndrome: I. General principles and second trimester testing. *Clin Chim Acta.* 2002;323:1–16

38. Malone FD, D'Alton ME, Society for Maternal-Fetal Medicine. First-trimester sonographic screening for Down syndrome. *Obstet Gynecol.* 2003;102:1066–1079

39. Egan JF, Kaminsky LM, DeRoche ME, Barsoom MJ, Borgida AF, Benn PA. Antenatal Down syndrome screening in the United States in 2001: a survey of maternal-fetal medicine specialists. *Am J Obstet Gynecol.* 2002;187:1230–1234

40. Katz VL, Chescheir NC, Cefalo RC. Unexplained elevations of maternal serum alpha-fetoprotein. *Obstet Gynecol Surv.* 1990;45:719–726

41. Simpson JL, Palomaki GE, Mercer B, et al. Associations between adverse perinatal outcome and serially obtained second- and third-trimester maternal serum alpha-fetoprotein measurements. *Am J Obstet Gynecol.* 1995;173:1742–1748

42. Krause TG, Christens P, Wohlfahrt J, et al. Second-trimester maternal serum alpha-fetoprotein and risk of adverse pregnancy outcome (1). *Obstet Gynecol.* 2001;97:277–282

Prescribing Therapy Services for Children With Motor Disabilities

- *Clinical Report*

AMERICAN ACADEMY OF PEDIATRICS

CLINICAL REPORT
Guidance for the Clinician in Rendering Pediatric Care

Linda J. Michaud, MD, and the Committee on Children With Disabilities

Prescribing Therapy Services for Children With Motor Disabilities

ABSTRACT. Pediatricians often are called on to prescribe physical, occupational, and speech-language therapy services for children with motor disabilities. This report defines the context in which rehabilitation therapies should be prescribed, emphasizing the evaluation and enhancement of the child's function and abilities and participation in age-appropriate life roles. The report encourages pediatricians to work with teams including the parents, child, teachers, therapists, and other physicians to ensure that their patients receive appropriate therapy services. *Pediatrics* 2004;113:1836–1838; *children with motor disabilities, physical therapy, occupational therapy, speech-language therapy.*

BACKGROUND

Pediatricians commonly are asked to evaluate children with motor disabilities and to write prescriptions for physical, occupational, and speech-language therapy services. Although many states require a physician's prescription for such services, many physicians have limited formal education about these therapeutic interventions.[1]

The spectrum of motor impairments affecting function in children and adolescents is wide and comprises many congenital and acquired conditions, primarily involving the neurologic and musculoskeletal systems, including but not limited to cerebral palsy, traumatic brain injury, myelomeningocele, spinal cord injury, neuromuscular disease, juvenile rheumatoid arthritis, arthrogryposis, and limb deficiencies. These conditions are associated with motor impairments including muscle weakness, abnormal muscle tone, decreased joint range of motion, and decreased balance and coordination. There are variations in severity within each of these conditions. Many children with impairments attributable to these conditions will have some degree of disability that may limit their participation in age-appropriate activities at home, in school, and in the community and should benefit from physical, occupational, and/or speech-language therapy services.

The pediatrician needs to understand the role of physical, occupational, and speech-language therapists in the overall treatment of children with motor disabilities and the therapeutic interventions that may improve function and participation.[2,3] If the child has motor problems severe enough to interfere with mobility, self-care, or communication, therapists may provide a program to help the child ameliorate, compensate for, or adapt to the impairment or disability. Physical, occupational, and speech-language therapists, working with the family, child, physician, and teacher, promote a positive functional adaptation to impairment or disability in the context of the child's developmental progress.

Physical therapists focus on gross motor skills and functional mobility, including positioning; sitting; transitional movement such as sitting to standing; walking with or without assistive devices (eg, walkers, crutches) and orthoses (braces) or prostheses (artificial limbs); wheelchair propulsion; transfers between the wheelchair and other surfaces such as a desk chair, toilet, or bath; negotiation of stairs, ramps, curbs, and elevators; and problem-solving skills for accessibility of public buildings. Physical therapists often have responsibilities for procuring adaptive equipment related to ambulation, positioning, and mobility.[4–6]

Occupational therapists focus on fine motor, visual-motor, and sensory processing skills needed for basic activities of daily living such as eating, dressing, grooming, toileting, bathing, and written communication (handwriting, keyboard skills).[7] Occupational therapy services may include training in school-related skills and strategies to help children compensate for specific deficits.[7]

Speech-language pathologists address speech, language, cognitive-communication, and swallowing skills in children with disabilities.[8] Speech therapy is the therapy most commonly prescribed by pediatricians.

The services that can be provided by physical and occupational therapists and speech-language pathologists overlap. For example, a physical or occupational therapist can address motor delay or dysfunction in the very young child. Depending on the community, occupational therapists or speech-language pathologists may address deficits in oral motor skills associated with feeding dysfunction related to motor disability. Occupational therapists and/or speech-language pathologists provide expert consultation related to adaptive equipment, environmental modifications, and assistive technology devices such as environmental control units, augmentative communication systems, adapted computers, and adaptive toys.[6]

PEDIATRICS (ISSN 0031 4005). Copyright © 2004 by the American Academy of Pediatrics.

EVALUATING THE EVIDENCE

The therapeutic methods, frequency and duration of service, setting in which the service is delivered, and service delivery system vary.[9] Evaluating the efficacy and effectiveness of therapy for motor disability is difficult, because treatment is not a standardized, readily quantifiable process that can be prescribed in discrete, consistent units. Individualized therapy programs vary in many parameters and incorporate subjective as well as objective elements. Clear documentation of efficacy related to the variable parameters of therapy continues to be elusive. This problem may in part reflect difficult methodologic issues including the measurement of treatment-related change on a background of developmental maturation, the establishment of appropriate outcome criteria, heterogeneity of the populations involved, and the complex nature of the interventions.[10,11]

A recent review of the evidence to support the effectiveness of neurodevelopmental treatment for children with cerebral palsy indicates that this popular method of intervention does not confer an advantage over the alternatives with which it has been compared in altering abnormal motor responses, slowing or preventing contractures, or facilitating more normal motor development or functional motor activities, nor does more intensive neurodevelopmental treatment result in greater benefit.[12] Physical therapy alone was found in 1 well-designed study to be less effective in improving motor development after 1 year than the therapy incorporating developmentally appropriate play and learning skills for children younger than 3 years with motor impairment.[13]

Improvement in motor function is more likely to occur when the goals of therapy are specific and measurable[14] and established in partnership with the child's parents and other caregivers. Intensive amounts of physical therapy may confer no advantage over routine amounts of therapy,[15] and long-term therapy may confer no advantage over short-term therapy. Provision of a home exercise program, with instruction of family members and caregivers in therapeutic exercises and age-appropriate activities to meet the child's goals, is generally indicated. This program can include recommendation of participation in sports to increase endurance, strength, and self-esteem in a natural setting with peers.[16] Aquatic therapy, hippotherapy (horseback-riding therapy), and participation in karate, gymnastics, and dance classes in integrated or special classes also can be considered to meet the child's therapeutic goals. Parent and caregiver education by all therapists is critical in effective partnerships with families for implementation of therapy programs.

Some programs such as patterning have little effect on functional skills and are inappropriate for children with motor disabilities.[17] Scientific legitimacy has also not been established for sensory integration intervention for children with motor disabilities.[18]

Prescribing therapy services for children with motor disabilities clearly cannot be based entirely on sound scientific evidence. As the knowledge base is expanded related to the effectiveness of therapy interventions, evidence-based practice described as using the best available evidence, along with clinical judgment, and taking into consideration the priorities and values of the individual patient and family in a shared decision-making process, as outlined by the Institute of Medicine, is advised.[19]

SERVICE DELIVERY

Therapies for a child with motor impairment are required to be provided by the school if the disability interferes with the educational process.[20] Recently, managed health care has made it more difficult for children with special needs to receive therapy services outside of school, with insurance companies denying services for children who attend school, maintaining that therapy is mandated at school and is partially funded with education and third-party monies.[9] Therapy services at school for students who are eligible for Medicaid and whose disabilities are medically based can be reimbursed by Medicaid if the disability has an adverse effect on the child's ability to benefit from the educational program.[9] Services also may be provided in environments other than the hospital or school, as appropriate for the child's individual circumstances; such other environments include child care, home, or job settings.

THE PEDIATRICIAN'S ROLE

The pediatrician's responsibility in writing a prescription for therapy includes providing an accurate diagnosis when possible. When the exact cause of the disability is not apparent, the physician must provide an accurate description of the medical condition and note whether the child has a transient, static, or progressive impairment. In addition to the primary motor disorder, all potential associated problems such as learning disabilities, mental retardation, sensory impairment, speech disorders, emotional difficulties, and seizure disorders must be identified, and a care plan must be recommended. There are some children with special needs whose medical conditions may be affected adversely by movement or other specific therapeutic activities; therapists and caregivers should be advised to take appropriate precautions with these children.

The physician's prescription for therapy should contain, in addition to the child's diagnosis: age; precautions; type, frequency, and duration of therapy; and designated goals. Goals for physical, occupational, and speech-language therapy do not depend solely on the diagnosis or age of the child, and they are most appropriate when they address the functional capabilities of the individual child and are relevant to the child's age-appropriate life roles (school, play, work).[9] The pediatrician should work with the family, child, therapists, school personnel, developmental diagnostic or rehabilitation team, and other physicians to establish realistic functional goals.[20] The pediatrician can assist families in identifying the short- and long-term goals of treatment, establishing realistic expectations of therapy outcomes, and understanding that therapy will usually help the child adapt to the condition but not change the underlying neuromuscular problem. Pediatricians should be encouraged to seek and use expert consultation as in any other area of medicine. Helpful resources may include local and regional diagnostic and intervention teams, early intervention and developmental evaluation programs, developmental pediatricians, pediatric physiatrists, pediatric neurologists, pediatric orthopedists, and orthotists.

Regular communication among parents and other caregivers, therapists, educators, and prescribing physicians should be ongoing, with periodic reevaluations to assess the achievement of identified goals, to direct therapy toward new objectives, and to determine when therapy is no longer warranted.[21] Changes in the child's status (eg, surgical intervention, school-to-work transition warranting assistive technology intervention) may indicate resumption of specific short-term, goal-directed services.

SUMMARY

Successful therapy programs are individually tailored to meet the child's functional needs and should be comprehensive, coordinated, and integrated with educational and medical treatment plans, with consideration of the needs of parents and siblings. This can be facilitated by primary care pediatricians and tertiary care centers working cooperatively to provide care coordination in the context of a medical home.[22,23]

COMMITTEE ON CHILDREN WITH DISABILITIES, 2003–2004
Adrian D. Sandler, MD, Chairperson
J. Daniel Cartwright, MD
John C. Duby, MD
Chris Plauch Johnson, MD, MEd
Lawrence C. Kaplan, MD
Eric B. Levey, MD
Nancy A. Murphy, MD
Ann Henderson Tilton, MD

PAST COMMITTEE MEMBERS
W. Carl Cooley, MD
Theodore A. Kastner, MD
Marian E. Kummer, MD

LIAISONS
Bev Crider
  Family Voices
Merle McPherson, MD
  Maternal and Child Health Bureau
Linda J. Michaud, MD
  American Academy of Physical Medicine and Rehabilitation
Marshalyn Yeargin-Allsopp, MD
  Centers for Disease Control and Prevention

STAFF
Stephanie Mucha, MPH

REFERENCES

1. Sneed RC, May WL, Stencel CS. Training of pediatricians in care of physical disabilities in children with special health needs: results of a two-state survey of practicing pediatricians and national resident training programs. *Pediatrics.* 2000;105:554–561
2. Consensus statements. *Pediatr Phys Ther.* 1990;2:175–176
3. Piper MC. Efficacy of physical therapy: rate of motor development in children with cerebral palsy. *Pediatr Phys Ther.* 1990;2:126–130
4. Kurtz LA. Rehabilitation: physical therapy and occupational therapy. In: Batshaw ML, ed. *Children With Disabilities.* 5th ed. Baltimore, MD: Paul H. Brookes Publishing; 2002:647–657
5. Carlson SJ, Ramsey C. Assistive technology. In: Campbell SK, Vander Linden DW, Palisano RJ, eds. *Physical Therapy for Children.* 2nd ed. Philadelphia, PA: WB Saunders; 2000:671–708
6. Jump J, Bouwkamp M, Morress C. Assistive technology. In: Rudolph CD, Rudolph AM, Hostetter MK, Lister G, Siegel NJ, eds. *Rudolph's Pediatrics.* 21st ed. New York, NY: McGraw-Hill; 2003:545–547
7. Kurtz LA. Physical therapy and occupational therapy. In: Rudolph CD, Rudolph AM, Hostetter MK, Lister G, Siegel NJ, eds. *Rudolph's Pediatrics.* 21st ed. New York, NY: McGraw-Hill; 2003:544–545
8. Kummer AW. Speech pathology for the child with disability. In: Rudolph CD, Rudolph AM, Hostetter MK, Lister G, Siegel NJ, eds. *Rudolph's Pediatrics.* 21st ed. New York, NY: McGraw-Hill; 2003:545
9. O'Brien MA, Huffman NP. Impact of managed care in the schools. *Lang Speech Hear Serv Sch.* 1998;29:263–269
10. Tirosh E, Rabino S. Physiotherapy for children with cerebral palsy. Evidence for its efficacy. *Am J Dis Child.* 1989;143:552–555
11. Ottenbacher KJ. Efficacy of physical therapy: rate of motor development in children with cerebral palsy. *Pediatr Phys Ther.* 1990;2:131–134
12. Butler C, Darrah J. Effects of neurodevelopmental treatment (NDT) for cerebral palsy: an AACPDM evidence report. *Dev Med Child Neurol.* 2001;43:778–790
13. Palmer FB, Shapiro BK, Wachtel RC, et al. The effects of physical therapy on cerebral palsy: a controlled trial of infants with spastic diplegia. *N Engl J Med.* 1988;318:803–808
14. Bower E, McLellan DL, Arney J, Campbell MJ. A randomised controlled trial of different intensities of physiotherapy and different goal-setting procedures in 44 children with cerebral palsy. *Dev Med Child Neurol.* 1996;38:226–237
15. Bower E, Michell D, Burnett M, Campbell MJ, McLellan DL. Randomized controlled trial of physiotherapy in 56 children with cerebral palsy followed for 18 months. *Dev Med Child Neurol.* 2001;43:4–15
16. Johnstone KS, Perrin JCS. Sports for the handicapped child. *Phys Med Rehabil.* 1991;5:331–350
17. American Academy of Pediatrics, Committee on Children With Disabilities. The treatment of neurologically impaired children using patterning. *Pediatrics.* 1999;104:1149–1151
18. Mulligan S. Advances in sensory integration research. In: Bundy AC, Lane SJ, Murray EA, eds. *Sensory Integration: Theory and Practice.* 2nd ed. Philadelphia, PA: FA Davis; 2002:397–411
19. Committee on Quality of Health Care in America, Institute of Medicine. Improving the 21st-century health care system. In: *Crossing the Quality Chasm: A New Health System for the 21st Century.* Washington, DC: National Academy Press; 2001:39-60
20. American Academy of Pediatrics, Committee on Children With Disabilities. The pediatrician's role in development and implementation of an Individual Education Plan (IEP) and/or an Individual Family Service Plan (IFSP). *Pediatrics.* 1999;104:124–127
21. Levine MS, Kliebhan L. Communication between physician and physical and occupational therapists: a neurodevelopmentally based prescription. *Pediatrics.* 1981;68:208–214
22. American Academy of Pediatrics, Committee on Children With Disabilities. Care coordination: integrating health and related systems of care for children with special health care needs. *Pediatrics.* 1999;104:978–981
23. American Academy of Pediatrics, Medical Home Initiatives for Children With Special Needs Project Advisory Committee. The medical home. *Pediatrics.* 2002;110:184–186

Protective Eyewear for Young Athletes

- *Policy Statement*

AMERICAN ACADEMY OF PEDIATRICS

Committee on Sports Medicine and Fitness

AMERICAN ACADEMY OF OPHTHALMOLOGY

Eye Health and Public Information Task Force

POLICY STATEMENT
Organizational Principles to Guide and Define the Child Health Care System and/or Improve the Health of All Children

Protective Eyewear for Young Athletes

ABSTRACT. The American Academy of Pediatrics and American Academy of Ophthalmology strongly recommend protective eyewear for all participants in sports in which there is risk of eye injury. Protective eyewear should be mandatory for athletes who are functionally 1-eyed and for athletes whose ophthalmologists recommend eye protection after eye surgery or trauma.

ABBREVIATIONS. ASTM, American Society for Testing and Materials; ANSI, American National Standards Institute; CSA, Canadian Standards Association; HECC, Hockey Equipment Certification Council.

BACKGROUND

More than 42 000 sports and recreation-related eye injuries were reported in 2000.[1] Seventy-two percent of the injuries occurred in individuals younger than 25 years, 43% occurred in individuals younger than 15 years, and 8% occurred in children younger than 5 years.[1] Children and adolescents may be particularly susceptible to injuries because of their aggressive play, athletic maturity,[2-4] and poor supervision in some recreational situations.

The sports highlighted in this statement were chosen on the basis of their popularity and/or the high incidence of eye injuries in that sport. Participation rates and information on the severity of the injuries are unavailable; therefore, the relative risk of significant injuries cannot be determined for various sports. Baseball and basketball are associated with the most eye injuries in athletes 5 to 24 years old.[1]

The eye-injury risk of a sport is proportional to the chance of the eye being impacted with sufficient energy to cause injury. The risk is not correlated with the classification of sports into collision, contact, and noncontact categories. Instead, the risk of eye injury to the unprotected player is roughly categorized as high risk, moderate risk, low risk, and eye safe. The sports included in each of these categories are listed in Table 1.

EVALUATION

All athletes and their parents should be made aware of the risks associated with participation in sports and the availability of a variety of certified sports eye protectors. Although eye protectors cannot eliminate the risk of injury, appropriate eye protectors have been found to reduce the risk of significant eye injury by at least 90% when fitted properly.[4-6] It would be ideal if all children and adolescents wore appropriate eye protection for all eye-risk sports and recreational activities.

Physicians should strongly recommend that athletes who are functionally 1-eyed wear appropriate eye protection during all sports, recreational, and work-related activities. Functionally 1-eyed athletes are those who have a best corrected visual acuity of worse than 20/40 in the poorer-seeing eye.[1,4,7] If the better eye is injured, functionally 1-eyed athletes may be handicapped severely and unable to obtain a driver's license in many states.[8]

Athletes who have had eye surgery or trauma to the eye may have weakened eye tissue that is more susceptible to injury.[9] These athletes may need additional eye protection or may need to be restricted from certain sports; they should be evaluated and counseled by an ophthalmologist before sports participation.

PROTECTIVE EYEWEAR OPTIONS

Eye protection and different brands of sports goggles vary significantly in both the way they fit and their capacity to protect the eye from injury. An experienced ophthalmologist, optometrist, optician, physician, or athletic trainer can help an athlete select appropriate protective gear that fits well and provides the maximum amount of protection. Sports programs should assist indigent athletes in evaluating and obtaining protective eyewear.

There are 4 basic types of eyewear. The 2 types that are satisfactory for eye-injury risk sports include:

1. Safety sports eyewear that conforms to the requirements of the American Society for Testing and Materials (ASTM) standard F803 for selected sports (racket sports, baseball fielders, basketball, women's lacrosse, and field hockey).[10]
2. Sports eyewear that is attached to a helmet or for sports in which ASTM standard F803 eyewear is inadequate. Those for which there are standard

PEDIATRICS (ISSN 0031 4005). Copyright © 2004 by the American Academy of Pediatrics.

TABLE 1.   Categories of Sports Eye-Injury Risk to the Unprotected Player*

High Risk	Moderate Risk	Low Risk	Eye Safe
Small, fast projectiles	Tennis	Swimming	Track and field†
Air rifle	Badminton	Diving	Gymnastics
BB gun	Soccer	Skiing (snow and water)	
Paintball	Volleyball	Noncontact martial arts	
Hard projectiles, "sticks," close contact	Water polo	Wrestling	
Basketball	Football	Bicycling	
Baseball/softball	Fishing		
Cricket	Golf		
Lacrosse (men's and women's)			
Hockey (field and ice)			
Squash			
Racquetball			
Fencing			
Intentional injury			
Boxing			
Full-contact martial arts			

* Vinger PF. A practical guide for sports eye protection. *Phys Sports Med.* 2000;28(6). Available at: http://www.physsportsmed.com/issues/2000/06_00/vinger.htm
† Javelin and discus have a small but definite potential for injury. However, good field supervision can reduce the extremely low risk of injury to near-negligible.

specifications include youth baseball batters and base runners (ASTM standard F910), paintball (ASTM standard 1776), skiing (ASTM standard 659), and ice hockey (ASTM standard F513).[10] Other protectors with specific standards are available for football and men's lacrosse.

The 2 types of eyewear that are not satisfactory for eye-injury risk sports include:

1. Streetwear (fashion) spectacles that conform to the requirements of American National Standards Institute (ANSI) standard Z80.3.[11]
2. Safety eyewear that conforms to the requirements of ANSI standard Z87.1,[12] which is mandated by the Occupational Safety and Health Administration for industrial and educational safety eyewear.

Prescription or nonprescription (plano) lenses may be fabricated from any of several types of clear material, including polycarbonate. Polycarbonate is the most shatter-resistant clear lens material and should be used for all safety eyewear.[13]

PROTECTIVE EYEWEAR CERTIFICATION

Protectors that have been tested to an appropriate standard by an independent testing laboratory are often certified and should afford reasonable protection. The Protective Eyewear Certification Council has begun certifying protectors that comply with ASTM standard F803 (racket sports, basketball, baseball, women's lacrosse, and field hockey), ASTM standard F1776 (paintball), and ASTM standard F910 (youth baseball batters and base runners) standards.[10] The Canadian Standards Association (CSA) certifies products that comply with the Canadian racket-sport standard, which is similar to the ASTM standard.[10] The Hockey Equipment Certification Council (HECC) certifies ice hockey equipment including helmets and face shields. The National Operating Committee on Standards in Athletic Equipment certifies baseball and football helmets as well as the face protectors for men's lacrosse and football.

For those sports with certified protectors, it is recommended that products bearing the Protective Eyewear Certification Council, CSA, HECC, or National Operating Committee on Standards for Athletic Equipment seals be used when available.

RECOMMENDATIONS

1. All youths involved in organized sports should be encouraged to wear appropriate eye protection.
2. The recommended sports-protective eyewear as listed in Table 2 should be prescribed. Proper fit is essential. Because some children have narrow facial features, they may be unable to wear even the smallest sports goggles. These children may be fitted with 3-mm polycarbonate lenses in ANSI standard Z87.1 frames designed for children.[12] The parents should be informed that this protection is not optimal, and the choice of eye-safe sports should be discussed.
3. Because contact lenses offer no protection, it is strongly recommended that athletes who wear contact lenses also wear the appropriate eye protection listed in Table 2.
4. An athlete who requires prescription spectacles has 3 options for eye protection: a) polycarbonate lenses in a sports frame that passes ASTM standard F803 for the specific sport; b) contact lenses plus an appropriate protector listed in Table 2; or c) an over-the-glasses eyeguard that conforms to the specifications of ASTM standard F803 for sports in which an ASTM standard F803 protector is sufficient.[10]
5. All functionally 1-eyed athletes should wear appropriate eye protection for all sports.
6. Functionally 1-eyed athletes and those who have had an eye injury or surgery must not participate in boxing or full-contact martial arts. (Eye protection is not practical in boxing or wrestling and is not allowed in full-contact martial arts.) Wrestling has a low incidence of eye injury. Although no standards exist, eye protectors that are firmly

TABLE 2.   Recommended Eye Protectors for Selected Sports

Sport	Minimal Eye Protector	Comment
Baseball/softball (youth batter and base runner)	ASTM standard F910	Face guard attached to helmet
Baseball/softball (fielder)	ASTM standard F803 for baseball	ASTM specifies age ranges
Basketball	ASTM standard F803 for basketball	ASTM specifies age ranges
Bicycling	Helmet plus streetwear/fashion eyewear	
Boxing	None available; not permitted in the sport	Contraindicated for functionally 1-eyed athletes
Fencing	Protector with neck bib	
Field hockey (men and women)	ASTM standard F803 for women's lacrosse (goalie: full face mask)	Protectors that pass for women's lacrosse also pass for field hockey
Football	Polycarbonate eye shield attached to helmet-mounted wire face mask	
Full-contact martial arts	None available; not permitted in the sport	Contraindicated for functionally 1-eyed athletes
Ice hockey	ASTM standard F513 face mask on helmet (goaltenders: ASTM standard F1587)	HECC OR CSA certified Full-face shield
Lacrosse (men)	Face mask attached to lacrosse helmet	
Lacrosse (women)	ASTM standard F803 for women's lacrosse	Should have option to wear helmet
Paintball	ASTM standard F1776 for paintball	
Racquet sports (badminton, tennis, paddle tennis, handball, squash, and racquetball)	ASTM standard F803 for selected sport	
Soccer	ASTM standard F803 for selected sport	
Street hockey	ASTM standard 513 face mask on helmet	Must be HECC or CSA certified
Track and field	Streetwear with polycarbonate lenses/fashion eyewear*	
Water polo/swimming	Swim goggles with polycarbonate lenses	
Wrestling	No standard available	Custom protective eyewear can be made

* Eyewear that passes ASTM standard F803 is safer than streetwear eyewear for all sports activities with impact potential.

fixed to the head have been custom made. The wrestler who has a custom-made eye protector must be aware that the protector design may be insufficient to prevent injury.

7. For sports in which a face mask or helmet with an eye protector or shield must be worn, it is strongly recommended that functionally 1-eyed athletes also wear sports goggles that conform to the requirements of ASTM standard F803 (for any selected sport).[10] This is to maintain some level of protection if the face guard is elevated or removed, such as for hockey or football players on the bench. The helmet must fit properly and have a chinstrap for optimal protection.

8. Athletes should replace sports eye protectors that are damaged or yellowed with age, because they may have become weakened and are, therefore, no longer protective.

COMMITTEE ON SPORTS MEDICINE AND FITNESS, 2003–2004
Reginald L. Washington, MD, Chairperson
David T. Bernhardt, MD
Joel S. Brenner, MD, MPH
Jorge Gomez, MD
Thomas J. Martin, MD
Frederick E. Reed, MD
Stephen G. Rice, MD, PhD, MPH

LIAISONS
Carl Krein, AT, PT
   National Athletic Trainers Association
Claire LeBlanc, MD
   Canadian Paediatric Society

Judith C. Young, PhD
   National Association for Sport and Physical Education

STAFF
Jeanne Christensen Lindros, MPH

EYE HEALTH AND PUBLIC INFORMATION TASK FORCE, 2003–2004
M. Bowes Hamill, MD, Chairperson
Stuart R. Dankner, MD
Roberto Diaz-Rohena, MD
James Garrity, MD
Ana Huaman, MD
Henry Jampel, MD
Terri D. Pickering, MD
Tamara Vrabec, MD

SECRETARIAT
Paul Sternberg, Jr, MD

STAFF
Peggy Kraus
Georgia Alward
Annamarie Harris

REFERENCES

1. US Consumer Product Safety Commission. *Sports and Recreational Eye Injuries.* Washington, DC: US Consumer Product Safety Commission; 2000
2. Nelson LB, Wilson TW, Jeffers JB. Eye injuries in childhood: demography, etiology, and prevention. *Pediatrics.* 1989;84:438–441
3. Grin TR, Nelson LB, Jeffers JB. Eye injuries in childhood. *Pediatrics.* 1987;80:13–17
4. Jeffers JB. An on-going tragedy: pediatric sports-related eye injuries. *Semin Ophthalmol.* 1990;5:216–223
5. Larrison WI, Hersh PS, Kunzweiler T, Shingleton BJ. Sports-related ocular trauma. *Ophthalmology.* 1990;97:1265–1269

6. Strahlman E, Sommer A. The epidemiology of sports-related ocular trauma. *Int Ophthalmol Clin.* 1988;28:199–202

7. Wichmann S, Martin DR. Single-organ patients: balancing sports with safety. *Phys Sportsmed.* 1992;20:176–182

8. Federal Highway Administration. *Manual on Uniform Traffic Control Devices for Streets and Highways.* Washington, DC: US Department of Transportation; 1988

9. Vinger PF. The eye and sports medicine. In: Duane TD, Tasman W, Jaeger EA, eds. *Duane's Clinical Ophthalmology.* Vol 5. Philadelphia, PA: JB Lippincott; 1994:1–103

10. American Society for Testing and Materials. *Annual Book of ASTM Standards: Vol 15.07. Sports Equipment; Safety and Traction for Footwear; Amusement Rides; Consumer Products.* West Conshohocken, PA: American Society for Testing and Materials; 2003

11. American National Standards Institute. Ophthalmics—Nonprescription Sunglasses and Fashion Eyewear—Requirements. Washington, DC: American National Standards Institute; 2001

12. American National Standards Institute. Occupational and Educational Personal Eye and Face Protection Devices. Washington, DC: American National Standards Institute; 2003

13. Vinger PF, Parver L, Alfaro D III, Woods T, Abrams BS. Shatter resistance of spectacle lenses. *JAMA.* 1997;277:142–144

All policy statements from the American Academy of Pediatrics automatically expire 5 years after publication unless reaffirmed, revised, or retired at or before that time.

RESOURCES

American Academy of Ophthalmology, Communications Department, PO Box 7424, San Francisco, CA 94120-7424.

Prevent Blindness America (formerly National Society to Prevent Blindness), 500 E. Remington Rd, Schaumburg, IL 60173.

Providing a Primary Care Medical Home for Children and Youth With Cerebral Palsy

- *Clinical Report*

AMERICAN ACADEMY OF PEDIATRICS

CLINICAL REPORT
Guidance for the Clinician in Rendering Pediatric Care

W. Carl Cooley, MD; and the Committee on Children With Disabilities

Providing a Primary Care Medical Home for Children and Youth With Cerebral Palsy

ABSTRACT. Children and youth with cerebral palsy present pediatricians with complex diagnostic and therapeutic challenges. In most instances, care also requires communication and comanagement with pediatric subspecialists and pediatric surgical specialists, therapists, and community developmental and educational teams. The importance of family resilience to the patient's well-being broadens the ecologic scope of care, which highlights the value of a primary care medical home from which care is initiated, coordinated, and monitored and with which families can form a reliable alliance for information, support, and advocacy from the time of diagnosis through the transition to adulthood. This report reviews the aspects of care specific to cerebral palsy that a medical home should provide beyond the routine health maintenance, preventive care, and anticipatory guidance needed by all children. *Pediatrics* 2004;114:1106–1113; *cerebral palsy, developmental disability, medical home, chronic illness, spasticity.*

INTRODUCTION

Cerebral palsy is the third most common major developmental disability, after autism and mental retardation. More than 100 000 Americans younger than 18 years are affected by cerebral palsy, and the 30-year survival rate is nearly 90%.[1,2] The diversity of individuals with cerebral palsy together with the range of severity and complications makes this condition a challenge for health care systems. Diagnosis may be delayed, care may be fragmented, routine preventive care may be overlooked, and transition to adult health care services may be haphazard at best. In addition to the effects on individuals and families, each new case of cerebral palsy involves an average lifetime cost of $503 000.[3] As such, the primary care management of cerebral palsy provides an opportunity to implement the medical-home model[4] and improve the overall quality of care of affected individuals and their families.

BACKGROUND

Cerebral palsy is a heterogeneous group of neuromotor conditions involving disordered movement or posture and weakness resulting from a nonprogres-sive brain lesion, injury, or malformation occurring prenatally or in the first 2 years of life. In 1843, William Little, MD, pioneered early efforts to classify subtypes of cerebral palsy, which was once called Little's disease.[5] Sigmund Freud, MD, expanded narrow assumptions that cerebral palsy resulted from birth trauma and anoxia by suggesting the possibility of predisposing factors and counseled against classification by causes until evidence for causation was clearly established; this is a challenge that continues today.[6]

Cerebral palsy may be defined further by its topography (quadriplegia, hemiplegia, diplegia) or by its pathophysiology (pyramidal or extrapyramidal). Pyramidal lesions result in predominantly spastic types of cerebral palsy, and extrapyramidal insults cause dyskinetic types including hypotonic, choreoathetoid, and ataxic cerebral palsy. Overlapping or mixed forms of cerebral palsy are common. The overall prevalence of cerebral palsy is between 1.5 and 2.0 cases per 1000 live births and has increased slightly since 1970.[7] However, surviving premature infants with birth weight less than 1500 g experience a risk of cerebral palsy of 90 per 1000 live births, and 50% of new cases of cerebral palsy occur in infants weighing less than 1000 g at birth.[3]

Although the diagnosis of cerebral palsy refers only to the presence of a nonprogressive motor impairment, children with cerebral palsy experience a range of comorbid conditions including mental retardation, sensory impairment, and seizures. They are subject to orthopedic and other functional complications of their primary neuromotor disorder, such as limitations of movement, scoliosis, joint instability, bowel and bladder dysfunction, dysarthria and dysphagia, and altered growth and nutrition. The physical and psychological consequences of compromised mobility and independence, difficulties with communication, altered appearance, and chronic illness may also require identification and intervention.

ETIOLOGY AND RISK

Cerebral palsy may result from a wide range of causes including congenital, genetic, inflammatory, anoxic, traumatic, toxic, and metabolic. Only 6% or 7% of cases result from asphyxia at birth, and as many as 80% seem to be prenatal in origin.[8] Preterm birth is the most common antecedent event, but cau-

The guidance in this report does not indicate an exclusive course of treatment or serve as a standard of medical care. Variations, taking into account individual circumstances, may be appropriate.

doi:10.1542/peds.2004-1409

sality and coincidence are not always clearly distinguished. Although significant postnatal intraventricular hemorrhage is likely to have neurologic sequelae, most hypoxic-ischemic injuries associated with cerebral palsy are prenatal.[3,9,10] The cause of prenatal brain injury usually eludes identification, but recent studies have suggested that prenatal maternal chorioamnionitis may play a significant role, accounting for as many as 12% of cases of spastic cerebral palsy in term infants and more than twice that among preterm infants.[11] Nevertheless, a specific cause for cerebral palsy often cannot be determined, and an interplay of multiple factors is likely in many instances.

A variety of risk factors has been associated with cerebral palsy. Perinatal events such as preterm birth, low birth weight, asphyxia, intracranial hemorrhage, infection, seizures, hypoglycemia, and hyperbilirubinemia would warrant careful developmental and neurologic screening during subsequent primary care office visits. Prenatal risk factors are more nonspecific and harder to identify but include intrauterine infections, teratogenic exposures, placental complications, multiple births, and maternal conditions such as mental retardation, seizures, or hyperthyroidism. Socioeconomic factors may increase risk but also may be linked to other pathophysiologic factors such as low birth weight or preterm birth.

DIAGNOSIS AND INITIAL COUNSELING OF FAMILIES

The diagnosis of cerebral palsy is a clinical determination made through neurologic and developmental surveillance and an awareness of risk factors. Early brain development results in a gradual and variable pattern of emergence of signs of cerebral palsy, complicating the diagnosis. Spasticity may be preceded by hypotonia, which, although associated with delayed motor milestones, may be less obvious to parents and clinicians. On the other hand, early alterations in movement and tone may subsequently attenuate or disappear. Efforts to standardize or formalize such observations are helpful in infants at high risk or those who have suspicious findings from developmental screening during well-child care. Clues during well-child visits include the persistence of infantile reflexes, delayed appearance of postural and protective reflexes, asymmetrical movements or reflexes, variations in muscle tone, and delays in the emergence of motor milestones.[12] Primary care physicians can enhance their assessment through the use of a more rigorous neuromotor examination such as that of Milani-Comparetti and Gidoni.[13] Standardized instruments such as the Bayley Scales of Infant Development, Bayley Infant Neurodevelopmental Screener, or the Movement Assessment of Infants provide scores that may be predictive of long-term motor impairment.[14]

The consideration of specific underlying causes of motor delays and impairments found on neurologic examination may be important. Conditions for which an intervention might prove crucial, such as a treatable metabolic disorder or child abuse ("shaken-baby

syndrome"), must not be overlooked. Other identifiable syndromes and conditions may have prognostic significance or associated complications or recurrence risks. A dysmorphology or genetics consultation may be useful to rule out specific conditions in which cerebral palsy is one of the characteristics. Brain imaging, usually by magnetic resonance imaging, may be performed to identify such causes as intracranial hemorrhage/infarction or cerebral dysgenesis.[12]

When the primary care physician becomes suspicious of cerebral palsy, it is important to share those concerns with parents. Parents may understand and cope better with the eventual diagnosis of cerebral palsy if they feel involved in the diagnostic process from the beginning. Furthermore, the symptoms and signs themselves, before they are sufficient for a diagnosis, may already be worrisome to parents and will usually justify a referral for early-intervention services. The motor delays alone may also confer eligibility for Supplemental Security Income, which in turn may (in most states) provide Medicaid eligibility.

The average child with cerebral palsy is not diagnosed until approximately 12 months of age,[3,15] and some experts have suggested that a definitive diagnosis should be deferred until 2 years of age.[3] When it becomes clear that a fixed pattern of altered movement, muscle tone, and reflexes is associated with weakness and delayed motor milestones, then a diagnosis of cerebral palsy is warranted. As with other developmental disabilities, care should be taken in the process of informing parents. The diagnosis might be framed in provisional terms for a mildly affected child younger than 2 years because of the possibility of improvement. The term "cerebral palsy" must be presented and discussed carefully with parents to avoid misunderstanding of its meaning and range of implications. The prognosis is uncertain in nearly all children at the time of diagnosis, particularly with respect to specific outcomes such as independent ambulation, language, or cognitive ability. Children with the most severe motor involvement (not rolling over or persistent infantile reflexes at 12 months of age or not sitting by 24 months of age) are less likely to be independent walkers, although this may vary with the type of cerebral palsy.[16] The Gross Motor Function Classification System provides a valid tool for the classification of severity of cerebral palsy and prognostication about motor skills.[17]

Plans need to be made with the family for a definitive diagnostic evaluation.[12] Most children and families will benefit from referral to a multidisciplinary neuromotor clinic or team when available. This team may include a pediatric orthopedist, pediatric physiatrist, developmental pediatrician, pediatric neurologist, pediatric neurosurgeon, nurse coordinator and/or social worker, pediatric physical therapist, and orthotist. Other therapeutic clinicians such as psychologists, occupational and speech therapists, therapeutic recreation specialists, dietitians or nutritionists, and assistive technology technicians may also be members of such teams.

ONGOING CARE IN THE MEDICAL HOME

High-quality care for most children with cerebral palsy is exemplified by the primary care medical home working in collaboration with parents, medical specialists, and community agencies.[4] The primary care medical home should provide proactive care coordination, including monitoring, interpreting, and orchestrating comanagement with specialists and specialty teams while communicating from the health care perspective with therapeutic, educational, family-support, and other resources in the community. The medical home also provides advocacy with payers and providers such as local school districts.

Associated factors and complications of cerebral palsy require initial assessment and ongoing vigilance. Hearing and vision may be vulnerable to the same insults that caused the neuromotor impairment. As a result, all children suspected of having cerebral palsy should undergo audiologic and pediatric ophthalmologic consultation. Seizures occur in more than 25% of individuals with cerebral palsy, with the greatest risk among those with spastic quadriplegia and hemiplegia.[18,19]

Managing Spasticity

Seventy-five percent of children with cerebral palsy have spasticity.[20] Active and careful management of spasticity is important to decrease or prevent deformity, promote function, alleviate pain, and increase the ease of caregiving.[19] A plan for spasticity management may integrate physical therapy, orthopedic and orthotic management, and systemically or regionally administered medication. Most patients require daily range-of-motion exercises with regular monitoring and supervision by a physical therapist.[21] These exercises should be supplemented by periodic pediatric orthopedic, pediatric neurosurgical, and/or physiatric consultation for the consideration and implementation of more specialized interventions. The unopposed, deforming forces of increased muscle tone may be altered by casting and orthotic devices or by soft-tissue or bony surgery. Furthermore, osteoporosis may result from diminished weight-bearing, compromised nutritional status, and use of some anticonvulsants and may lead to pathologic fractures.[22]

Direct treatments of spasticity involve a progressive and proactive approach moving from less invasive to more invasive modalities. Traditional therapeutic and orthotic management may be supplemented with oral medication if spasticity is generalized.[23] Benzodiazepines, including diazepam, clonazepam, and clorazepate dipotassium, provide general relaxation and antispasticity effects, but use may be limited by sedation. These drugs demonstrate a benefit for athetosis as well as spasticity and may have enhanced benefit in combination with other drugs such as dantrolene sodium.

Baclofen is most effective for spasticity associated with spinal cord lesions but equals diazepam in improving tone and movement in cerebral palsy with somewhat less sedation.[23,24] Baclofen and benzodiazepines act centrally on synaptic neurotransmission, and dantrolene directly affects muscle contractility and has proven useful in treating the spasticity of cerebral palsy.[25] Hepatoxicity is a serious issue with long-term use of dantrolene in 1% of cases, and adverse effects include excessive weakness and gastrointestinal distress.[26] The α_2-agonist tizanidine hydrochloride may induce less reduction in strength than baclofen and diazepam but may cause more sedation.[27] Dry mouth and hypotension also may occur with tizanidine.

If oral medications prove insufficient or if spasticity is focal, more invasive methods including specific nerve and motor blocks and botulinum-toxin injections can be considered.[26] The latter are useful for the treatment of focal spasticity in a specific muscle group.[28] A single set of injections will produce clinical results in 1 to 3 days, peak after 4 weeks, and provide benefit for 3 or 4 months with rare adverse effects. Injections may be repeated every 3 to 6 months, sometimes delaying or obviating the need for surgery.

By using a pump placed in the lower abdomen and an intrathecal catheter, baclofen can be delivered continuously into the intrathecal space.[29] This technique decreases systemic adverse effects and the dose of baclofen required, thereby increasing the efficacy for a subgroup of significantly involved children with cerebral palsy. For appropriate candidates with severe spasticity, a baclofen pump may increase functionality or improve the quality of caregiving and may be particularly useful in the treatment of dystonia when oral medication has failed or resulted in unacceptable adverse effects. However, intrathecal baclofen may be associated with complications and adverse effects including drug-related (hypotonia, weakness, nausea, vomiting, alteration in bowel and bladder function) and device-related (seroma, infection, catheter problems) complications. The most serious complication may result from overinfusion, usually related to programming errors, which may cause respiratory suppression and reversible coma.[30,31] With both oral and intrathecal baclofen, rapid withdrawal should be avoided.

Dorsal rhizotomy is a surgical approach to spasticity aimed at decreasing the stimulatory afferent input from spastic muscles by severing lumbosacral dorsal rootlets.[32,33] The greatest benefit is seen in young children (3-7 years of age) with spastic diplegia but stable trunk control and good lower extremity strength.

Associated Care Issues

Cerebral palsy imposes an extraordinary metabolic burden associated with spasticity and disordered movement. Increased fluid and caloric needs may be compromised further by problems with the mechanics of chewing and swallowing and with gastroesophageal reflux. Nearly half of all children with cerebral palsy have evidence of significant undernutrition.[34] Particular attention should be given to ensuring adequate calcium and vitamin D intake. The recognition and early treatment of undernutrition may require skilled nutritional and dietary assessment, the involvement of a feeding or dysphagia team, and consultation with a pediatric gastroenterologist for assistance in the treatment of reflux or decision-making about gastrostomy tube feeding.[35] Excessive weight gain, particularly associated with gastrostomy tube feeding, must also be avoided because of its effects on health, mobility, caregiving, and adaptive equipment.

Altered smooth muscle and sphincter tone together with the effects of medications, diminished activity, and variable hydration contribute to the high incidence of constipation in children with cerebral palsy.[36] Many individuals with cerebral palsy require regular interventions including oral stool softeners and bowel stimulants, rectal suppositories, and occasionally enemas. For children for whom constipation is a recurring problem, a regular program should be followed. Pediatric gastroenterologic consultation may be helpful in some cases. Children with cerebral palsy experience a greater likelihood of neurogenic bladder dysfunction complicating the achievement of independence with toileting and increasing the risk of urinary tract complications.[37] Pediatric urologic consultation and appropriate studies of bladder function may be required.

Dental care may require special attention to the consequences of altered oral motor tone, enamel dysplasia, bruxism, tongue movements, mouth breathing, anticonvulsant medications, and challenges to dental hygiene maintenance.[38] Drooling is a problem for approximately 10% of children with cerebral palsy and presents health and cosmetic issues. Interventions may include oral motor stimulation therapy, behavioral modification, stylish scarves, medications (eg, glycopyrrolate), botulinum-toxin injections, oral appliances, or surgery.[39]

Pain can be a challenge to assess in an individual with cerebral palsy, particularly if there is significant impairment of communication skills, cognitive functioning, or both. Pain may be suspected when there is a persistent change in mood, temperament, appetite, sleep behavior, or tolerance of movement. Evaluation may require a thoughtful but systematic review of potential causes including dental pain, gastroesophageal reflux, constipation, orthopedic pain, and urinary tract problems, including kidney stones.

Brain injury or dysgenesis resulting in cerebral palsy also may affect higher cognitive functioning, resulting in evidence of learning disability, language and communication impairment, autism, and, in approximately 50% of cases, mental retardation.[19] Appropriate neuropsychological and psychoeducational assessments may facilitate a better understanding of learning style and more appropriate educational programming and future planning.

As with many chronic conditions associated with constant and variable manifestations, complementary and alternative methods of treatment for cerebral palsy are common. Many of these interventions are promoted by enthusiastic advocates but have little more than testimonial evidence of efficacy. Some, such as "hippotherapy" (therapeutic horseback riding), have few risks and intuitively logical benefits in terms of self-esteem and confidence building as well as possible improvements in balance, tone, and range of motion.[40] On the other hand, hyperbaric oxygen therapy, advocated as a method of reviving injured brain tissue, has far more cost and risk in the face of no evidence of improvement in function.[41] Nutritional supplements have been promoted for many developmental disabilities including Down syndrome, autism, and cerebral palsy, but beyond what is needed to maintain normal nutrition, there is no scientific evidence of benefit. Variations on methods of motor treatment associated with the "patterning" technique continue to be offered to families with no evidence of usefulness despite a high cost and time commitment for families.[42] The primary care medical home can partner with families in their exploration of therapeutic alternatives by assisting in the collection of information, offering review of scientific claims and evidence, and maintaining a supportive, nonjudgmental approach.

Care Over the Long-Term

All office visits for children with cerebral palsy should be anticipated as requiring extra time and scheduled as such. The regular schedule of visits for well-child care and anticipatory guidance will require supplementation with additional periodic chronic condition management visits. It is the responsibility of the medical home to ensure that routine preventive care goals are met and additional preventive care requirements associated with cerebral palsy are fulfilled in a timely way. A written care plan should be developed together with the child and family and reviewed at each office encounter. Care planning for children with particularly complex medical issues may include an emergency information form for use when care is provided in an emergency department or by health care professionals who are less familiar with the child and family (available at www.medicalhomeinfo.org/tools/assess.html). Physical access to the office, examination rooms, and toilets should be evaluated starting from the parking lot for a typical office visit. Inviting a child in a wheelchair or with other assistive equipment on a "ride or walk-through" of the office will highlight obstacles and supplement the regulatory provisions of the Americans With Disabilities Act (Pub L No. 101–336 [1990]). The periodic solicitation of parental and patient input about ways in which medical-home office systems could be changed to improve the care experience can be obtained through mini-surveys, focus groups, or suggestion boxes.

A complete review of the coding and reimbursement options in the provision of a medical home for a child with cerebral palsy is beyond the scope of this report. Chronic condition management may be provided as an extension of a preventive medicine visit by adding the -25 modifier to a separately reported office or other outpatient services code. In this instance, the procedures involved with the preventive medicine visit and those involved in follow-up of cerebral palsy need to be documented clearly and separately in the medical record. Alternatively, chronic condition management visits may be scheduled separately from preventive-medicine visits and reported as time-related office or other outpatient visits from among the series of codes from 99212 to 99215. The medical record must provide appropriate documentation of the time involved for the visit, including a statement that more than half of the visit was devoted to counseling and discussion of issues related to the child's diagnosis. Team conferences or "wrap-around" meetings with early intervention or school staff or with an interdisciplinary team for planning or coordination do not need to include the child and can be coded as 99361 or 99362 for 30 and 60 minutes, respectively. For children receiving home health services or those in skilled nursing settings, care plan oversight time can be coded and billed as 99374 and 99375 for less than or more than 30 minutes, respectively. When services are prolonged beyond the time frames provided by the original code, there are a number of "prolonged physician services" codes to account for the extra time involved with or without direct patient contact (codes range from 99354 to 99359). Some medical-home settings are experimenting with drop-in group medical appointments ("DIGMA" visits), in which several children with cerebral palsy and their parents or guardians are seen simultaneously for the purpose of parent education on topics related to cerebral palsy, entitlements and benefits, patient and parent education, and family support. The 99078 code can be used for these physician educational services rendered in group settings. Unfortunately, the latter code as well as a number of others relevant to medical home services for children with cerebral palsy may frequently be denied by public, and especially private, payers. Medical home staff members should be aware of the codes covered by individual payers and consider advocating with individual health plans for coverage of codes such as those described above.

SUPPORTING CHILDREN, YOUTH, AND FAMILIES

Although there have been controversies about the effects of specific therapies on the achievement of specific developmental outcomes for children with cerebral palsy, there is little doubt that the prevention of orthopedic complications, the achievement of alternative means of communication, the optimization of motor skills, and the close monitoring of nutrition and growth have positive effects on the well-being and realization of potential in most children with cerebral palsy. In addition, early responses to family-support needs may enhance resilience and coping and equip families with some of the "marathon skills" that caring for their child may require.[43] With this in mind, prompt referral to an early-intervention professional is important for children from birth to 3 years of age.[44] The diagnosis of cerebral palsy need not be confirmed; suspicion of motor delays or altered tone and movement are sufficient to justify such a referral. After 3 years of age, the child with cerebral palsy is likely to be eligible for special-education services from the local educational agency serving the child's neighborhood or community.[45]

Among the most important roles for the medical home are being aware of the broad array of family needs and facilitating the family's access to support.[46] Many parents will benefit from parent-to-parent contact with a more experienced family as a source of information, perspective, and self-esteem. The daily demands of home care may gradually exhaust families, and child care may not be available from conventional community providers. Parents can be encouraged to use respite care to offset the fatigue of ongoing care. The medical home should be prepared to provide advocacy for public and private educational and financial entitlements including participation in the development of individualized education programs (formerly called individual education plans) or Section 504 plans in school settings.[45] Many health insurance plans do not have benefit packages that favor children with chronic conditions, and thus letters of medical necessity, contacts with health plan medical directors, and other forms of advocacy may be necessary. The medical home is ideally positioned to monitor the needs of siblings at times when children with cerebral palsy demand and receive much of the parents' energy and attention. In addition to their own routine health needs, siblings may have milder challenges that do not receive sufficient attention or more specific fears and conflicts about their chronically affected brother or sister. Finally, a family's cultural heritage can affect the style and content of their support for their child with cerebral palsy because of language or educational barriers or because of less obvious cultural differences in beliefs about a condition such as cerebral palsy.[47] A culturally effective medical home will recognize these barriers, anticipate their possible implications, and actively attempt to ameliorate their consequences.

Cerebral palsy poses life-long challenges for those affected, and more than 90% of individuals with cerebral palsy survive to adulthood. It is important that the pediatric primary care medical home opens an early dialogue with families about planning for the transition to adulthood.[48,49] Financial and estate planning may be important to begin in very early childhood, and educational, vocational, and guardianship planning should begin in early adolescence. The medical home will need to devote specific time and attention to transitions to adult health care including primary and specialty care. The pediatrician can provide specific longitudinal knowledge about an individual child as well as a current care plan, characterizing recent issues and plans for addressing them to the adult primary care setting.

OUTCOMES AND QUALITY OF LIFE FOR INDIVIDUALS WITH CEREBRAL PALSY

Using the World Health Organization and National Center for Medical Rehabilitation Research models, the severity of cerebral palsy can be assessed at the cellular (pathophysiology), organ (impairment), or whole-person (disability) level.[50–52] However, according to the National Center for Medical Rehabilitation Research model, quality of life for individuals with cerebral palsy cannot be determined simply by measures at any of these levels. Instead, quality of life depends on a complex interplay between the individual's functional limitations, the family's assets and challenges, and the resources and limitations of the society in which the individual and his or her family are immersed. Just as simply surviving the pathophysiologic events causing cerebral palsy does not ensure a high quality of life, the presence of severe organic impairment does not predict a uniformly dismal outcome.

Most children with cerebral palsy live at home with their families, attend regular classrooms at their neighborhood schools, and participate in a variety of natural community activities. As adults, most continue to live in community settings, but one third live at home with their parents, whose ability to continue caregiving may decrease as they age. Twenty percent of adults with cerebral palsy are ambulatory, and 40% can walk with assistance; the remaining 40% are nonambulatory.

The horizon of opportunity for individuals with cerebral palsy has continued to expand with improvements in health care, developmental and educational services, and support for individuals and families in community settings. The primary care medical home is an organizing force for the provision of appropriate preventive health care and for the integration of care into the fabric of other important supports and services.

IMPORTANT POINTS FOR THE PEDIATRICIAN

1. Be aware of risk factors associated with cerebral palsy and incorporate neuromotor screening into routine developmental surveillance.
2. Provide prompt referral for early-intervention services for all children with alterations in motor development without waiting for diagnostic confirmation of cerebral palsy.
3. Partner with parents in the pursuit of a diagnosis and a culturally effective discussion of its implications for health, development, and family life.
4. Include screening for sensory impairments in the care plan for all newly identified children with cerebral palsy; brain imaging should be performed when appropriate.
5. Consider referral to a geneticist or pediatric neurologist in the presence of dysmorphic features, positive family history, or any atypical clinical characteristics.
6. Make your office a medical home that includes services such as care coordination, a written care plan, patient and family education, parent-to-parent referral, and advocacy.
7. After the definitive diagnosis of cerebral palsy, begin comanagement with a multidisciplinary neuromotor team and schedule regular chronic condition management visits in addition to regular preventive medical care.
8. Manage spasticity by using a "ladder" approach, starting with the least invasive interventions and adding treatments as needed.
9. Maintain vigilance for the new onset of comorbid conditions such as seizures, cognitive or learning disabilities, nutritional complications, etc.
10. Advocate with parents to school personnel about appropriate educational and therapeutic strate-

gies including: physical, occupational, and speech therapy; nursing; and adaptive and assistive technology.[44,45,53–55]
11. Be aware of and make timely referrals to community and state agencies providing support and services to which the child and family may be entitled.
12. Be a sensitive and useful resource for families in their exploration of complementary and alternative interventions for cerebral palsy.
13. Solicit feedback from families of children with cerebral palsy about the care and services provided in your office and how they could be improved.
14. Assess the quality of your medical home services for children with cerebral palsy and engage in systematic, incremental efforts to improve them.
15. Begin planning for the transition to adulthood with the child and family as early as possible but no later than 12 years of age.

COMMITTEE ON CHILDREN WITH DISABILITIES,
2003–2004
Adrian D. Sandler, MD, Chairperson
J. Daniel Cartwright, MD
John C. Duby, MD
Chris Plauche Johnson, MD, MEd
Lawrence C. Kaplan, MD
Eric B. Levey, MD
Nancy A. Murphy, MD
Ann Henderson Tilton, MD
W. Carl Cooley, MD
    Past Committee Member
Theodore A. Kastner, MD, MS
    Past Committee Member
Marian E. Kummer, MD
    Past Committee Member

LIAISONS
Beverly Crider
    Family Voices
Merle McPherson, MD, MPH
    Maternal and Child Health Bureau
Linda Michaud, MD
    American Academy of Physical Medicine and
    Rehabilitation
Marshalyn Yeargin-Allsopp, MD
    Centers for Disease Control and Prevention

STAFF
Stephanie Mucha, MPH

REFERENCES

1. Crichton JU, Mackinnon M, White CP. The life-expectancy of persons with cerebral palsy. *Dev Med Child Neurol.* 1995;37:567–576
2. Newacheck PW, Taylor WR. Childhood chronic illness: prevalence, severity, and impact. *Am J Public Health.* 1992;82:364–371
3. Kuban KC, Leviton A. Cerebral palsy. *N Engl J Med.* 1994;330:188–195
4. American Academy of Pediatrics, Medical Home Initiatives for Children With Special Needs Project Advisory Committee. The medical home. *Pediatrics.* 2002;110:184–186
5. Little W. Course of lectures on the deformities of the human frame. *Lancet.* 1843;1:318–322
6. Freud S. *Infantile Cerebral Paralysis.* Coral Gables, FL: University of Miami Press; 1968
7. Murphy CC, Yeargin-Allsopp M, Decoufle P, Drews CD. Prevalence of cerebral palsy among 10-year-old children in metropolitan Atlanta, 1985 through 1987. *J Pediatr.* 1993;123:S13–S20
8. Nelson KB, Ellenberg JH. Antecedents of cerebral palsy: multivariate analysis of risk. *N Engl J Med.* 1986;315:81–86

9. American Academy of Pediatrics, American College of Obstetricians and Gynecologists. *Neonatal Encephalopathy and Cerebral Palsy: Defining the Pathogenesis and Pathophysiology.* Elk Grove Village, IL: American Academy of Pediatrics; 2003

10. Gaffney G, Sellers S, Flavell V, Squier M, Johnson A. Case-control study of intrapartum care, cerebral palsy, and perinatal death. *BMJ.* 1994;308: 743–750

11. Wu YW, Colford JM Jr. Chorioamnionitis as a risk factor for cerebral palsy: a meta-analysis. *JAMA.* 2000;284:1417–1424

12. Ashwal S, Russman B, Blasco P, et al. Practice parameter: diagnostic assessment of the child with cerebral palsy: report of the quality standards subcommittee of the American Academy of Neurology and the Practice Committee of the Child Neurology Society. *Neurology.* 2004;62: 851–863.

13. Milani-Comparetti A, Gidoni EA. Routine developmental examination in normal and retarded children. *Dev Med Child Neurol.* 1976;9:631–638

14. Morgan AM, Aldag JC. Early identification of cerebral palsy using a profile of abnormal motor patterns. *Pediatrics.* 1996;98:692–697

15. Palfrey JS, Singer JD, Walker DK, Butler JA. Early identification of children's special needs: a study of five metropolitan communities. *J Pediatr.* 1987;111:651–659

16. Molnar GE. Cerebral palsy: prognosis and how to judge it. *Pediatr Ann.* 1979;8:596–605

17. Rosenbaum PL, Walter SD, Hanna SE, et al. Prognosis for gross motor function in cerebral palsy: creation of motor development curves. *JAMA.* 2002;288:1357–1363

18. Rosenbloom L. Diagnosis and management of cerebral palsy. *Arch Dis Child.* 1995;72:350–354

19. Tilton AH, Butterbaugh G. Mental retardation and cerebral palsy. In: Noseworthy JH, ed. *Neurological Therapeutics: Principles and Practice.* New York, NY: Martin Dunitz; 2003:1617–1629

20. Wilson GN, Cooley WC. Cerebral palsy and congenital brain defects. In: *Preventive Management of Children With Congenital Anomalies and Syndromes.* Cambridge, MA: Cambridge University Press; 2000:49–58

21. Barry M. Physical therapy interventions for patients with movement disorders due to cerebral palsy. *J Child Neurol.* 1996;11(suppl 1):S51–S60

22. Shaw NJ, White CP, Fraser WD, Rosenbloom L. Osteopenia in cerebral palsy. *Arch Dis Child.* 1994;71:235–238

23. Pranzatelli M. Oral pharmacotherapy for the movement disorders of cerebral palsy. *J Child Neurol.* 1996;11(suppl 1):S13–S22

24. Milla PJ, Jackson AD. A controlled trial of baclofen in children with cerebral palsy. *J Int Med Res.* 1977;5:398–404

25. Joynt RL, Leonard JA Jr. Dantrolene sodium suspension in treatment of spastic cerebral palsy. *Dev Child Neurol.* 1980;22:755–767

26. Katz RT. Management of spasticity. *Am J Phys Med Rehabil.* 1988;1988: 108–116

27. Lataste X, Emre M, Davis C, Groves L. Comparative profile of tizanidine in the management of spasticity. *Neurology.* 1994;44(suppl 9):S53–S59

28. Koman L, Mooney J, Smith B. Management of cerebral palsy with botulinum-A toxin: preliminary investigation. *J Pediatr Orthop.* 1993;13: 489–495

29. Wiens HD. Spasticity in children with cerebral palsy: a retrospective review of the effects of intrathecal baclofen. *Issues Compr Pediatr Nurs.* 1998;21:49–61

30. Albright AL, Cervi A, Singletary J. Intrathecal baclofen for spasticity in cerebral palsy. *JAMA.* 1991;265:1418–1422

31. Gilmartin F, Bruce D, Storrs BB, et al. Intrathecal baclofen for the management of spastic cerebral palsy: multicenter trial. *J Child Neurol.* 2000;15:71–77

32. Wong AM, Chen CL, Hong WH, Tang FT, Lui TN, Chou SW. Motor control assessment for rhizotomy in cerebral palsy. *Am J Phys Med Rehabil.* 2000;79:441–450

33. Bloom KK, Nazar GB. Functional assessment following selective posterior rhizotomy in spastic cerebral palsy. *Childs Nerv Syst.* 1994;10:84–86

34. Samson-Fang L, Fung E, Stallings VA, et al. Relationship of nutritional status to health and societal participation in children with cerebral palsy. *J Pediatr.* 2002;141:637–643

35. McGrath SJ, Splaingard ML, Alba HM, Kaufman BH, Glicklick M. Survival and functional outcome of children with severe cerebral palsy following gastrostomy. *Arch Phys Med Rehabil.* 1992;73:133–137

36. Eicher P. Nutrition and feeding. In: Dormans J, Pellegrino L, eds. *Caring for Children With Cerebral Palsy.* Baltimore, MD: Paul H. Brookes Publishing Co; 1998:243–279

37. Reid CJ, Borzyskowski M. Lower urinary tract dysfunction in cerebral palsy. *Arch Dis Child.* 1993;68:739–742

38. Helpin ML, Rosenberg HM. Dental care: beyond brushing and flossing. In: Batshaw M, ed. *Children With Disabilities.* 4th ed. Baltimore, MD: Paul H. Brookes Publishing Co; 1997:643–656

39. Matthews DJ, Wilson P. Cerebral palsy. In: Molnar GE, Alexander MA, eds. *Pediatric Rehabilitation.* 3rd ed. Philadelphia, PA: Hanley & Belfus; 1999:193–217

40. Deitz-Curry JE. Promoting functional mobility. In: Dormans JP, Pellagrino L, eds. *Caring for Children With Cerebral Palsy.* Baltimore, MD: Paul H. Brookes Publishing Co; 1998:283–322

41. Collet J, Vanasse M, Marois P. Hyperbaric oxygen for children with cerebral palsy: a randomised multicenter trial. *Lancet.* 2001;357:582–586

42. American Academy of Pediatrics, Committee on Children With Disabilities. The treatment of neurologically impaired children using patterning. *Pediatrics.* 1999;104:1149–1151

43. Patterson JM. Understanding family resilience. *J Clin Psychol.* 2002;58: 233–246

44. American Academy of Pediatrics, Committee on Children With Disabilities. Role of the pediatrician in family-centered early intervention services. *Pediatrics.* 2001;107:1155–1157

45. American Academy of Pediatrics, Committee on Children With Disabilities. The pediatrician's role in development and implementation of an Individual Education Plan (IEP) and/or an Individual Family Service Plan (IFSP). *Pediatrics.* 1999;104:124–127

46. Liptak GS, Revell GM. Community physician's role in the case management of children with chronic illnesses. *Pediatrics.* 1989;84:465–471

47. Harkness S, Super CM, Keffer CH. Culture and ethnicity. In: Levine MD, Carey WB, Crocker AC, eds. *Developmental-Behavioral Pediatrics.* 2nd ed. Philadelphia, PA: WB Saunders; 1992:103–108

48. Cathels BA, Reddihough DS. The health care of young adults with cerebral palsy. *Med J Aust.* 1993;159:444–446

49. American Academy of Pediatrics, Committee on Children With Disabilities and Committee on Adolescence. Transition of care provided for adolescents with special health care needs. *Pediatrics.* 1996;98:1203–1206

50. Dossa PA. Quality of life: individualism or holism? A critical review of the literature. *Int J Rehabil Res.* 1989;12:121–136

51. Goldberg MJ. Measuring outcomes in cerebral palsy. *J Pediatr Orthop.* 1991;11:682–685

52. Campo SF, Sharpton WR, Thompson B, Sexton D. Correlates of the quality of life of adults with severe or profound mental retardation. *Ment Retard.* 1997;35:329–337

53. American Academy of Pediatrics, Committee on Children With Disabilities. The role of the pediatrician in prescribing therapy services for children with motor disabilities. *Pediatrics* 1996;98:308–310

54. American Academy of Pediatrics, Committee on Children With Disabilities. Provision of educationally-related services for children and adolescents with chronic diseases and disabling conditions. *Pediatrics.* 2000; 105:448–451

55. American Academy of Pediatrics, Committee on School Health and Committee on Bioethics. Do not resuscitate orders in schools. *Pediatrics.* 2000;105:878–879

RESOURCES FOR THE MEDICAL HOME

American Academy of Pediatrics. Coding and reimbursement. AAP coding hot line and fax-back service: 1-800-433-9016, extension 4022

American Academy of Pediatrics. Coding for Pediatrics (available annually from the American Academy of Pediatrics: provides easy reference to pediatric codes including clinical examples for children with special health care needs)

American Academy of Pediatrics, National Center of Medical Home Initiatives for Children With Special Needs (information and tools for developing and providing a medical home for children with special health care needs). Available at: www.medicalhomeinfo.org

Center for Medical Home Improvement. Available at: www.medicalhomeimprovement.org

Family Voices. Available at: www.familyvoices.org

Geralis E, ed. *Children with Cerebral Palsy: A Parents' Guide.* Baltimore, MD: Woodbine House; 1998

Kids as Self Advocates. Available at: www.fvkasa.org

United Cerebral Palsy. Available at: www.ucp.org

ADDITIONAL RELEVANT AMERICAN ACADEMY OF PEDIATRICS POLICY STATEMENTS/CLINICAL REPORTS

American Academy of Pediatrics, Committee on Children With Disabilities. A consensus statement on health care transitions for young adults with special health care needs. *Pediatrics.* 2002;110:1304–1306

American Academy of Pediatrics, Committee on Children With Disabilities. Care coordination: integrating health and related systems of care for children with special health care needs. *Pediatrics*. 1999;104:978–981

American Academy of Pediatrics, Committee on Children With Disabilities. Counseling families who choose complementary and alternative medicine for their child with chronic illness or disability. *Pediatrics*. 2001;107:598–601

American Academy of Pediatrics, Committee on Children With Disabilities. Developmental surveillance and screening of infants and young children. *Pediatrics*. 2001;108:192–195

American Academy of Pediatrics, Committee on Children With Disabilities. General principles in the care of children and adolescents with genetic disorders and other chronic health conditions. *Pediatrics*. 1997;99:643–644

American Academy of Pediatrics, Committee on Children With Disabilities. The continued importance of Supplemental Security Income (SSI) for children and adolescents with disabilities. *Pediatrics*. 2001;107:790–793

American Academy of Pediatrics, Committee on Children With Disabilities. The role of the pediatrician in transitioning children and adolescents with developmental disabilities and chronic illnesses from school to work or college. *Pediatrics*. 2000;106:854–856

Greer FR, American Academy of Pediatrics, Committee on Nutrition. Reimbursement for foods for special dietary use. *Pediatrics*. 2003;111:1117–1119

All clinical reports from the American Academy of Pediatrics automatically expire 5 years after publication unless reaffirmed, revised, or retired at or before that time.

Recommendations for Influenza Immunization of Children

- *Policy Statement*

AMERICAN ACADEMY OF PEDIATRICS

POLICY STATEMENT
Organizational Principles to Guide and Define the Child Health Care System and/or Improve the Health of All Children

Committee on Infectious Diseases

Recommendations for Influenza Immunization of Children

ABSTRACT. Epidemiologic studies indicate that children of all ages with certain chronic conditions and otherwise healthy children younger than 24 months of age are hospitalized for influenza infection and its complications at high rates similar to those experienced by the elderly. Annual influenza immunization is recommended for all children with high-risk conditions who are 6 months of age and older. Young, healthy children are at high risk of hospitalization for influenza infection; therefore, the American Academy of Pediatrics recommends influenza immunization for healthy children 6 through 24 months of age, for household contacts and out-of-home caregivers of all children younger than 24 months of age, and for health care professionals. To protect these children more fully against the complications of influenza, increased efforts are needed to identify all high-risk children and inform their parents when annual immunization is due. The purposes of this statement are to update recommendations for routine use of influenza vaccine in children and to review the indications for use of trivalent inactivated influenza vaccine and live-attenuated influenza vaccine. *Pediatrics* 2004; 113:1441–1447; *influenza, vaccine, immunization, children.*

ABBREVIATIONS. AOM, acute otitis media; TIV, trivalent inactivated influenza vaccine; LAIV, live-attenuated influenza vaccine; GBS, Guillain-Barré syndrome; HIV, human immunodeficiency virus; CI, confidence interval.

BACKGROUND INFORMATION

In community studies, school-aged children have had the highest rates of influenza infection. Prospective surveillance of influenza illness demonstrates annual attack rates of between 15% and 42% in preschool- and school-aged children.[1,2] During various influenza seasons, rates of annual outpatient visits attributable to influenza vary from 6 to 29 per 100 children.[2,3] Influenza also may be important in the pathogenesis of acute otitis media (AOM) during influenza seasons[4]; 3% to 5% of children annually are estimated to experience AOM associated with influenza.[2,5,6] Influenza and its complications have been reported to result in a 10% to 30% increase in the number of antimicrobial courses prescribed to children during the influenza season.[7] Antecedent influenza infection is sometimes associated with development of severe pneumococcal and staphylococcal pneumonia in children.[8]

The risk of influenza-associated hospitalization in healthy children younger than 24 months of age has

been shown to be equal to or greater than the risk in previously recognized high-risk groups. Young children also seem to be at higher risk of hospitalization for influenza infection than are healthy 50- to 64-year-old adults, for whom routine immunization has been recommended since 2000 (Table 1). High rates of hospitalization of the young during influenza seasons have been appreciated for decades,[3,9,10] but it has been difficult to determine the proportion of hospitalizations during influenza season attributable to respiratory syncytial virus and other respiratory tract viruses. Several published studies have made reasonable attempts to separate the relative contributions of respiratory syncytial virus and influenza to the hospitalization rate.[2,7,11] Influenza hospitalization rates vary among studies (190–480 per 100 000 population) because of differences in methodology and severity of influenza seasons. However, children younger than 24 months of age are consistently at substantially higher risk of hospitalization than are older children, and the risk of hospitalization attributable to influenza infection is highest in the youngest children. Of 182 patients hospitalized at Montreal Children's Hospital with laboratory-proven influenza between 1999 and 2002, 34% were younger than 6 months of age.[12] Seventy percent of these 182 children had no underlying medical disorder. Suspected sepsis was the admission diagnosis for 31% of these hospitalized children.

Although serious morbidity and mortality can result from influenza infection in any person, the risk of complications is increased among pregnant women,[13] individuals with underlying chronic cardiopulmonary conditions,[14,15] and immunocompromised persons.[16,17] Persons with renal, metabolic, and hematologic diseases are presumed to be at higher risk of severe influenza and its complications.

More severe outcomes of influenza, such as encephalopathy and death, have not been well studied, although deaths attributable to influenza are far less common in children than in the elderly. The fatality rate in children has been estimated to be 3.8 per 100 000 population.[9] Cases of encephalopathy and sudden unexplained death have been reported in US children,[18] but population-based rates are not known. The Centers for Disease Control and Prevention began to actively solicit reports of influenza-associated deaths and encephalopathy in individuals younger than 18 years of age during the 2003–2004 influenza season.[19]

PEDIATRICS (ISSN 0031 4005). Copyright © 2004 by the American Academy of Pediatrics.

TABLE 1.   Estimated Influenza-Associated Hospitalization Rates (Per 100 000 Persons) From Selected Studies

Study Years	Population	Age Group	Persons in Previously Recognized High-Risk Group	Persons Not in Previously Recognized High-Risk Group
1973–1993[7,15]	Tennessee Medicaid	0–11 mo	1900	496 (0–5 mo) 1038 (6–11 mo)
		1–2 y	800	186
		3–4 y	320	86
		5–14 y	92	41
1974–1999[2]	Vaccine clinic	<2 y		200–300
1992–1997[11]	Health maintenance organizations	0–23 mo		144–187
		2–4 y		0–25
		5–17 y		8–12
1968–1973[68]	Health maintenance organization	15–44 y	56–110	23–25
		45–64 y	392–635	13–23
		≥65 y	399–518	—
1969–1995[69]	National hospital discharge data	<65 y		20–42
		≥65 y		125–228

Adapted from *MMWR Recomm Rep.* 2001;50(RR-4):1–44.

VACCINES

The only influenza vaccine licensed for use in children younger than 5 years of age and for children 6 months of age and older with high-risk medical conditions is the trivalent inactivated influenza vaccine (TIV). A live-attenuated influenza vaccine (LAIV), which is administered intranasally, was licensed by the Food and Drug Administration for use in healthy individuals between 5 and 49 years of age. Current formulations of both these vaccines contain 3 virus strains representing influenza A subtypes H1N1 and H3N2 and influenza B. The strains to be included in the vaccine are selected annually on the basis of the viruses anticipated to be circulating during the upcoming influenza season.

TIV

Manufacturing, Handling, and Administration

TIV viruses are grown in embryonated hen eggs, inactivated, and then (in most instances) preserved with thimerosal (1:10 000). Manufacturers currently distributing TIV in the United States are Aventis Pasteur (Swiftwater, PA) (Fluzone) and Evans Vaccines (Liverpool, England) (Fluvirin). Fluzone and Fluvirin can be obtained thimerosal-preservative–free. Fluvirin is not licensed for children younger than 4 years of age, because efficacy has not been established in this age group. Removal of thimerosal from TIV results in wastage of one third of doses produced. Most experts view the protection of more children against the known risks of influenza more important than the theoretic risk of small amounts of thimerosal in influenza vaccine. Children younger than 9 years of age receiving any influenza vaccine for the first time should be given 2 doses 1 month apart. TIV vaccines licensed in the United States consist of disrupted virus particles and are termed split-virus vaccines.

Safety of TIV

The most common symptoms associated with TIV administration are soreness at the injection site and fever. Fever, usually occurring 6 to 24 hours after immunization, is more common in children younger than 2 years of age (10%–35% of recipients).[20,21] Mild systemic symptoms such as nausea, lethargy, headache, muscle aches, and chills are reported also. A retrospective "self-control" analysis of 251 000 children 6 months to 17 years of age who received influenza immunization in 1 of 5 managed care settings did not reveal any evidence of increased occurrence of important medically attended events associated with immunization.[22] Immunization of children who have asthma with TIV does not increase bronchial hyperactivity.[23]

During the "swine flu" vaccine program in 1976, an increase in the number of cases of Guillain-Barré syndrome (GBS) was reported in adults within 10 weeks after immunization. Additional investigations have revealed that there may be a slight increase in the risk of GBS (approximately 1 additional case of GBS per 1 million vaccine recipients) among adults after influenza immunization, at least in some years.[24–27] It is unknown whether influenza immunization of individuals with a history of GBS increases the rate of recurrence of GBS. History of GBS is considered a relative contraindication to immunization with TIV. The Institute of Medicine evaluated the association of demyelinating diseases and influenza vaccine and concluded that there is no evidence bearing on a causal relationship between influenza vaccines and demyelinating neurologic disorders in children 6 to 23 months of age.[28] Health care professionals should promptly report all clinically significant adverse events after influenza immunization to the Vaccine Adverse Events Reporting System (www.vaers.org) even if it is uncertain that the vaccine caused the event. The Institute of Medicine has specifically recommended reporting of neurologic events.

A newly described syndrome, oculorespiratory syndrome, was described during 2000–2001 among 3.4% of adult recipients of an influenza vaccine distributed in Canada by Shire Biologics (Fluviral S/F). Symptoms occurred within 24 hours of immunization and included bilateral red eyes and/or facial edema, respiratory complaints (coughing, wheezing, tightness of chest, difficulty breathing), difficulty swallowing, or sore throat. Symptoms were generally mild, and all resolved. The implicated vaccine contained large clumps of unsplit virus particles as evidenced by electron microscopy.[29,30] It is not known with certainty whether this reaction follows immunization with other influenza vaccines or whether it occurs in children. Only split-virus influenza vaccine is available in the United States.

Studies of the safety of TIV immunization of children and adults with human immunodeficiency virus (HIV) infection have yielded conflicting results. Some studies have demonstrated a transient (2- to 8-week) increase in HIV-1 replication and/or a decrease in CD4+ T-lymphocyte cell counts,[31–34] and other studies have reported no significant effects.[33–40] Most experts believe that the benefits of influenza immunization with TIV far outweigh the risks in children with HIV infection.

Allergic Reactions to TIV

Because influenza vaccine is grown in embryonated hen eggs, children demonstrating anaphylactic reactions to chicken or egg proteins may rarely experience a similar reaction to influenza vaccine and therefore should not be given TIV unless they undergo desensitization. Inactivated influenza vaccine containing thimerosal should not be given to individuals with hypersensitivity to thimerosal. Urticarial reactions to TIV have been reported.

Efficacy of TIV

Efficacy estimates vary depending on the age group, season, degree of antigenic match between the circulating viruses and the vaccine strains, and end points studied. Protective efficacy against influenza illness confirmed by positive culture varies between 30% and 95% depending on season and population studied.[41–45] Studies in the United States and Japan raise the possibility that immunization of a high proportion of school-aged children may result in diminished incidence of disease in all age groups including the elderly.[46,47]

Studies of the efficacy of influenza immunization against AOM have produced conflicting results. The incidence of AOM attributable to all causes in a group child care center was 36% less among 187 children immunized with TIV than among 187 children not immunized in other child care centers.[42] In that same evaluation, there was an 83% decrease in influenza-associated AOM in immunized versus nonimmunized children. In a second child care center study, 186 children 6 to 30 months of age were assigned randomly to receive TIV or no influenza vaccine and then were followed biweekly by blinded observers. Influenza vaccine was slightly protective against AOM during the influenza season (odds ratio: 0.69; 95% confidence interval [CI]: 0.49–0.98).[48] However, a randomized, placebo-controlled study of TIV among more than 750 children 6 to 24 months of age failed to show decreases in the incidence of AOM or in duration of middle-ear effusion among vaccine recipients, compared with placebo recipients.[45]

TIV Vaccine Coverage

Despite recommendations to immunize all children with asthma, only 10% to 31% of this population receives the TIV vaccine each year.[49–51] In 4 health maintenance organizations, 40% of patients with asthma attending an allergy clinic were given influenza vaccine; however, only 1% of all children with asthma made a visit to an allergy clinic.[49] A survey of parents of all children hospitalized during the influenza season revealed that the most important determinant of immunization was the physician's recommendation for influenza vaccine.[51]

Costs of TIV Influenza Immunization

Whether universal immunization of young children would result in a net cost or a net savings to society depends on the influenza attack rate, the rates of health outcomes (ie, outpatient visits, hospitalizations, and deaths), and the cost of immunization. The attack rate and rates of health outcomes can vary considerably from year to year, and regional variation in both these factors is possible within a given season. These variations make it impossible to generate a single, precise estimate of the cost-effectiveness or cost-benefit of universal immunization of children.

The total cost of immunizing a single child includes direct and indirect costs. The direct costs include supplies (eg, syringe and vaccine), personnel, and administrative expenses. Indirect costs can be a significant component of the total cost of immunization. One of the most important factors is the time lost from work by caregivers of children to be immunized. Three studies have suggested that universal childhood immunization may be cost-saving if immunizations could be performed in a group-based setting such as an after-hours or weekend immunization clinic that would not require a parent to miss work.[52–54] A subcommittee of the Advisory Committee on Immunization Practices, after a review of the major economic studies of influenza immunization,[52–56] concluded that universal influenza immunization of young children may generate savings, from a societal perspective, if the total costs of immunization are less than $30 per child immunized (M. Meltzer, oral presentation at Advisory Committee on Immunization Practices Influenza Workshop, October 15, 2003, Atlanta, GA).

Public and private insurers should be responsible for payment of costs for the influenza vaccine for children. Transferring financial responsibility to intermediate risk-bearing entities such as independent practice associations or other physician groups, individual physicians, or hospitals will result in children not being immunized and should not be allowed. Physicians incur significant administrative expenses associated with ensuring that children are fully immunized in a timely fashion, including explaining the benefits and risks of immunization to parents; ordering, purchasing, storing, and administering vaccines; recording immunizations in patients' charts; tracking immunization schedules and notifying patients; and other activities. Therefore, they should receive reimbursement for the expenses associated with these tasks for each vaccine administration.

It has been estimated that between 46% and 74% of

children 6 to 23 months of age will require at least 1 additional visit to a health care professional to receive influenza immunization. Suggested strategies to minimize the strain on practices include 1) beginning immunization as early in the season as possible, 2) using all visits (not just well-child visits) for immunizations, and 3) and scheduling specific clinic times for influenza immunizations.[57]

Availability of TIV

In recent years, approximately 70 to 90 million doses of TIV, which generally meet national vaccine demands, have been available annually. Vaccine demand may be increasing, and therefore preordering of vaccine is recommended. If vaccine supplies are limited, visit the American Academy of Pediatrics web site (www.aap.org) for suggestions for prioritization of use.

LAIV

Viral Strains and Manufacturing

Cold-adapted, live-attenuated influenza A and B strains were developed by passaging the viruses at successively lower temperatures in tissue culture.[58] These LAIV strains grow at 25°C, and their replication is restricted at 38°C to 39°C. LAIV strains, similar to influenza A strains contained in TIV, are produced through genetic reassortment. Because LAIV is grown in embryonated hen eggs, it should not be given to anyone who has had an anaphylactic reaction to chicken or egg proteins. The LAIV licensed for use in the United States (FluMist) is manufactured by MedImmune Inc (Gaithersburg, MD).

Storage, Administration, and Schedule of LAIV

The current LAIV formulation licensed in the United States must be stored frozen (refer to the FluMist package insert for specific requirements of each lot of vaccine). Once the vaccine is warmed to room temperature, it must be used within 30 minutes. Each 0.5-mL dose of vaccine contains approximately 10^7 tissue culture infectivity doses of influenza strains A subtype H1N1, A subtype H3N2, and B. It is administered intranasally (0.25 mL in each nostril) by a Becton Dickinson (Franklin Lakes, NJ) AccuSpray device, which resembles a tuberculin syringe. Children younger than 9 years of age being immunized against influenza for the first time should receive 2 doses of LAIV given 6 weeks apart before the start of the influenza season.

Safety of LAIV in Healthy Children

An analysis of solicited events combined across the 4 placebo-controlled trials in the subset of healthy children 60 to 71 months of age was performed (see the FluMist package insert). The largest absolute differences between LAIV and placebo after dose 1 were increases in headache (18% with FluMist vs 12% with placebo) and runny nose or nasal congestion (48% with LAIV vs 44% with placebo). These differences were not statistically significant. No differences were observed for fever. After dose 2, the largest absolute differences between FluMist and placebo were runny nose or nasal congestion (46%

with FluMist vs 32% with placebo) and cough (39% with FluMist vs 31% with placebo). A randomized (vaccine to placebo, 2:1), double-blind trial in healthy children 1 to 17 years of age was conducted in the Northern California Kaiser Permanente health maintenance organization to assess the rate of medically attended events within 42 days of immunization. In an unplanned retrospective analysis, a statistically significant increase in asthma or reactive airway disease was observed for children 12 to 59 months of age after dose 1 (relative risk: 3.53; 90% CI: 1.1, 15.7). There was no clustering of wheezing events. However, because of this finding, FluMist currently is not licensed by the Food and Drug Administration for children younger than 60 months of age. Additional evaluation of safety data within this age group is needed.

Efficacy of LAIV in Healthy Children

All prelicensure studies were performed in healthy children. There are no data on the effectiveness of LAIV when given to children with rhinitis attributable to infection or allergy. Vaccine efficacy against influenza A (H3N2) and B outbreaks was demonstrated in a US pediatric, multicenter trial of Flu-Mist.[59] The wild-type strains that circulated the first season after immunization were influenza A (H3N2) and B. Efficacy of 2 doses of LAIV against influenza illness confirmed by positive culture was 96.0% (95% CI: 89.4–98.5) for influenza A (H3N2) and 90.5% (95% CI: 78.0–95.9) for influenza B. Protective efficacy in children who received only 1 dose of vaccine also was high; it was 86.9% (95% CI: 46.6–96.8) against influenza A (H3N2) and 91.3% (95% CI: 45.6–98.6) against influenza B. Eighty-five percent of the children who participated in the US multicenter study returned for reimmunization before the next influenza season and received vaccine or placebo as they had previously. The influenza A/Sydney/H3N2 that circulated in year 2 was a drifted strain that did not match the vaccine strain influenza A/Wuhan. Despite the strain differences, the LAIV was 85.9% (95% CI: 75.3–91.9) efficacious in preventing influenza illness confirmed by positive culture attributable to influenza A/Sydney, indicating good heterotypic protection against this strain.[60] The efficacy of LAIV against influenza A (H1N1) infection could not be determined in the multicenter US trial, because influenza A (H1N1) did not circulate during either season. Therefore, a challenge study with the influenza H1N1 vaccine strain was performed in 222 randomly chosen previous vaccine and placebo recipients. Previous immunization was 82.9% (95% CI: 60.2–92.7) efficacious in preventing shedding of influenza A (H1N1) vaccine strain virus after challenge.[61]

Efficacy of LAIV Against AOM

In the US multicenter LAIV efficacy study, vaccine efficacy against otitis media associated with influenza illness confirmed by positive culture was 97.5% (95% CI: 85.5–99.6). The decrease in all episodes of otitis media attributable to all causes during the influenza season among vaccine recipients compared with placebo recipients was 8.7% (95% CI: −5.5–20.8), and the decrease in episodes of febrile otitis media attributable to any cause was 30.1% (95% CI: 11.3–45.0).[60]

Transmissibility of LAIV

Studies of transmission of LAIV strains to nonimmunized contacts have included nasal secretion cultures and serologic evaluation. Several studies have failed to document transmission.[62] However, in a child care trial in which 80% of 98 vaccine recipients shed vaccine virus, 1 of 99 placebo recipients shed type B vaccine virus on a single day.[63]

The proposed explanation for the uncommon occurrence of transmission is that the vaccine virus is shed for a shorter duration and in a much smaller quantity than are wild-type strains. In seronegative children, virus shedding usually occurs from day 2 to day 9 after immunization, and the average peak virus titers approach 10^3 plaque-forming units/mL. The maximal virus shedding observed has been 10^4 to 10^5 plaque-forming units/mL, which is 10- to 100-fold less than that typically seen with natural infection.[64]

Coadministration of LAIV With Other Vaccines

No data about concurrent administration of LAIV and recommended childhood vaccines are available currently. According to the general recommendations on immunization, inactivated vaccines can be given simultaneously with LAIV. Live vaccines also can be administered at the same time. However, if live vaccines are not administered on the same day, they should be separated by 4 weeks.

Genetic Stability of LAIV

In multiple studies conducted over 20 years, no reversion of the LAIV strains to a virulent phenotype in vaccine recipients has been detected. The stability of LAIV is attributed to the fact that the donor strains contain attenuating mutations in at least 3 genes and that the overall replication of the vaccine virus in the human mucosa is low. Consequently, the probability of generating mutants that have lost the attenuated phenotype is small.[65,66]

ANTIVIRAL MEDICATION

For a discussion of the use of antiviral medications in influenza illness, refer to the *Red Book*.[67]

RECOMMENDATIONS

TIV Indications

1. Health care professionals should be diligent with their efforts, through tracking and reminder systems, to ensure that children traditionally considered at high risk of severe disease and complications from influenza infection receive annual influenza immunization. High-risk children and adolescents who should receive priority for influenza immunization are those with the following (evidence grade II-3 [see Appendix 1]):
   - Asthma or other chronic pulmonary diseases such as cystic fibrosis;
   - Hemodynamically significant cardiac disease;
   - Immunosuppressive disorders or therapy;
   - HIV infection;
   - Sickle cell anemia and other hemoglobinopathies;
   - Diseases requiring long-term aspirin therapy, such as rheumatoid arthritis or Kawasaki disease;
   - Chronic renal dysfunction;
   - Chronic metabolic disease such as diabetes mellitus.

   Other individuals who should receive priority for influenza immunization include:
   - Women who will be in their second or third trimester of pregnancy during influenza season (evidence grade II-3), and
   - Persons who are in close contact with high-risk children, including 1) all health care professionals in contact with pediatric patients in hospital and outpatient settings and 2) household contacts and out-of-home caregivers of high-risk individuals of any age (evidence grade II-3).

2. Young, healthy children are at high risk of hospitalization for influenza infection; therefore, the American Academy of Pediatrics recommends influenza immunization of healthy children between 6 and 24 months of age (evidence grade II-3). This recommendation applies to any child who will be from 6 through 23 months of age at any time during the influenza season, which extends from the beginning of October through March. Children should not be immunized before they reach 6 months of age. Influenza immunization of household contacts and out-of-home caregivers of children younger than 24 months of age is recommended also (evidence grade III). Immunization of close contacts of children younger than 6 months may be particularly important, because these infants will not be immunized.

3. TIV may be given to any person older than 6 months of age who (or whose parent) wishes to prevent influenza. Persons who should not receive TIV include individuals who have had anaphylactic reaction to chicken or egg proteins or any other component of the vaccine, such as thimerosal.

LAIV Indications

LAIV is indicated for healthy individuals 5 to 49 years of age who want to be protected against influenza. TIV is preferred for close contacts of immunosuppressed individuals.

Persons should not receive LAIV if any of the following criteria are present:
- Age <5 years;
- History of anaphylactic reaction to egg or chicken protein;
- Receiving salicylates;
- Known or suspected immunodeficiency;
- History of GBS;
- Reactive airway disease or asthma;
- Other conditions traditionally considered high risk for severe influenza (chronic pulmonary disorders

or cardiac disorders, pregnancy, chronic metabolic disease, renal dysfunction, hemoglobinopathies, immunodeficiency, or immunosuppressive therapy).

COMMITTEE ON INFECTIOUS DISEASES, 2003–2004
Margaret B. Rennels, MD, Chairperson
H. Cody Meissner, MD, Vice Chairperson
Carol J. Baker, MD
Robert S. Baltimore, MD
Joseph A. Bocchini, Jr, MD
Penelope H. Dennehy, MD
Robert W. Frenck, Jr, MD
Caroline B. Hall, MD
Sarah S. Long, MD
Julia A. McMillan, MD
Keith R. Powell, MD
Lorry G. Rubin, MD
Thomas N. Saari, MD

EX OFFICIO
Larry K. Pickering, MD
    Red Book Editor

LIAISONS
Richard D. Clover, MD
    American Academy of Family Physicians
Steven Cochi, MD
    Centers for Disease Control and Prevention
Joanne Embree, MD
    Canadian Paediatric Society
Marc A. Fischer, MD
    Centers for Disease Control and Prevention
Bruce G. Gellin, MD, MPH
    National Vaccine Program Office
Mamodikoe Makhene, MD
    National Institutes of Health
Douglas R. Pratt, MD
    Food and Drug Administration
Jeffrey R. Starke, MD
    American Thoracic Society
Jack Swanson, MD
    American Academy of Pediatrics Practice Action
    Group
Walter A. Orenstein, MD (Past Liaison)
    Centers for Disease Control and Prevention

CONSULTANT
Edgar O. Ledbetter, MD

STAFF
Martha Cook, MS

APPENDIX 1. US Preventive Services Task Force Rating System of Quality of Scientific Evidence[70]

I	Evidence obtained from at least 1 properly designed, randomized, controlled trial
II-1	Evidence obtained from well-designed controlled trials without randomization
II-2	Evidence obtained from well-designed cohort or case-control analytic studies, preferentially from >1 center or group
II-3	Evidence obtained from multiple time series with or without the intervention or dramatic results in uncontrolled experiments (such as the results of the introduction of penicillin treatment in the 1940s)
III	Opinions of respected authorities, based on clinical experience, descriptive studies, or reports of expert committees

REFERENCES

1. Glezen WP, Couch RB. Interpandemic influenza in the Houston area, 1974–76. *N Engl J Med.* 1978;298:587–592
2. Neuzil KM, Zhu Y, Griffin MR, et al. Burden of interpandemic influenza in children younger than 5 years: a 25-year prospective study. *J Infect Dis.* 2002;185:147–152
3. Glezen WP, Decker M, Joseph SW, Mercready RG Jr. Acute respiratory disease associated with influenza epidemics in Houston, 1981–1983. *J Infect Dis.* 1987;155:1119–1126
4. Heikkinen T, Thint M, Chonmaitree T. Prevalence of various respiratory viruses in the middle ear during acute otitis media. *N Engl J Med.* 1999;340:260–264
5. Ruuskanen O, Arola M, Putto-Laurila A, et al. Acute otitis media and respiratory virus infections. *Pediatr Infect Dis J.* 1989;8:94–99
6. Chonmaitree T, Owen MJ, Patel JA, Hedgpeth D, Horlick D, Howie VM. Effect of viral respiratory tract infection on outcome of acute otitis media. *J Pediatr.* 1992;120:856–862
7. Neuzil KM, Mellen BG, Wright PF, Mitchel EF Jr, Griffin MR. The effect of influenza on hospitalizations, outpatient visits, and courses of antibiotics in children. *N Engl J Med.* 2000;342:225–231
8. O'Brien KL, Walters MI, Sellman J, et al. Severe pneumococcal pneumonia in previously healthy children: the role of preceding influenza infection. *Clin Infect Dis.* 2000;30:784–789
9. Glezen WP. Serious morbidity and mortality associated with influenza epidemics. *Epidemiol Rev.* 1982;4:25–44
10. Mullooly JP, Barker WH. Impact of type A influenza on children: a retrospective study. *Am J Public Health.* 1982;72:1008–1016
11. Izurieta HS, Thompson WW, Kramarz P, et al. Influenza and the rates of hospitalization for respiratory disease among infants and young children. *N Engl J Med.* 2000;342:232–239
12. Quach C, Piché-Walker L, Platt R, Moore D. Risk factors associated with severe influenza infections in childhood: implication for vaccine strategy. *Pediatrics.* 2003;112(3). Available at: www.pediatrics.org/cgi/content/full/112/3/e197
13. Neuzil KM, Reed GW, Mitchel EF, Simonsen L, Griffin MR. Impact of influenza on acute cardiopulmonary hospitalizations in pregnant women. *Am J Epidemiol.* 1998;148:1094–1102
14. Ferson MJ, Morton JR, Robertson PW. Impact of influenza on morbidity in children with cystic fibrosis. *J Paediatr Child Health.* 1991;27:308–311
15. Neuzil KM, Wright PF, Mitchel EF Jr, Griffin MR. The burden of influenza illness in children with asthma and other chronic medical conditions. *J Pediatr.* 2000;137:856–864
16. Neuzil KM, Reed GW, Mitchel EF Jr, Griffin MR. Influenza-associated morbidity and mortality in young and middle-aged women. *JAMA.* 1999;281:901–907
17. Lin JC, Nichol KL. Excess mortality due to pneumonia or influenza during influenza seasons among persons with acquired immunodeficiency syndrome. *Arch Intern Med.* 2001;161:441–446
18. Centers for Disease Control and Prevention. Severe morbidity and mortality associated with influenza in children and young adults—Michigan, 2003. *MMWR Morb Mortal Wkly Rep.* 2003;52:837–840
19. Centers for Disease Control and Prevention. Update: influenza-associated deaths reported among children aged <18 years—United States, 2003–04 influenza season. *MMWR Morb Mortal Wkly Rep.* 2004;52:1286–1288
20. Bernstein DI, Zahradnik JM, DeAngelis CJ, Cherry JD. Clinical reactions and serologic responses after vaccination with whole-virus or split-virus influenza vaccines in children aged 6 to 36 months. *Pediatrics.* 1982;69:404–408
21. Hall CB, Lee H, Alexson C, Meagher MP, Manning JA. Trial of bivalent influenza A vaccine in high-risk infants. *J Infect Dis.* 1977;136(suppl):S648–S651
22. France EK, Xu S, Davis RL, et al. Safety of the trivalent inactivated influenza vaccine among children: a population based study [abstract]. *Pediatr Res.* 2003;53(4 pt 2):164A
23. Kramarz P, Destefano F, Gargiullo PM, et al. Does influenza vaccination prevent asthma exacerbations in children? *J Pediatr.* 2001;138:306–310
24. Hurwitz ES, Schonberger LB, Nelson DB, Holman RC. Guillain-Barré syndrome and the 1978–1979 influenza vaccine. *N Engl J Med.* 1981;304:1557–1561
25. Kaplan JE, Katona P, Hurwitz ES, Schonberger LB. Guillain-Barré syndrome in the United States, 1979–1980 and 1980–1981. Lack of an association with influenza vaccination. *JAMA.* 1982;248:698–700
26. Chen R, Kent J, Rhodes P, Simon P, Schoenberger L. Investigation of a possible association between influenza vaccination and Guillian-Barré in the United States, 1990–1991 [abstract 040]. *Post Mark Surveill.* 1992;6:5–6

27. Lasky T, Terracciano GJ, Magder L, et al. The Guillain-Barré syndrome and the 1992–1993 and 1993–1994 influenza vaccines. *N Engl J Med.* 1998;339:1797–1802

28. Institute of Medicine. *Immunization Safety Review Committee Meeting: Influenza Vaccines and Neurological Complications.* Washington, DC: National Academies Press; 2003

29. Sowronski, DM, Struass B, De Serres G, et al. Oculo-respiratory syndrome: a new influenza vaccine-associated adverse event? *Clin Infect Dis.* 2003;36:705–713

30. Scheifele DW, Duval B, Russell ML, et al. Ocular and respiratory symptoms attributable to inactivated split influenza vaccine: evidence from a controlled trial involving adults. *Clin Infect Dis.* 2003;36:850–857

31. Staprans SI, Hamilton BL, Follansbee SE, et al. Activation of virus replication after vaccination of HIV-1-infected individuals. *J Exp Med.* 1995;182:1727–1737

32. O'Brien WA, Grovit-Ferbas K, Namazi A, et al. Human immunodeficiency virus-type 1 replication can be increased in peripheral blood of seropositive patients after influenza vaccination. *Blood.* 1995;86:1082–1089

33. Gunthard HF, Wong JK, Spina CA, et al. Effect of influenza vaccination on viral replication and immune response in persons infected with human immunodeficiency virus receiving potent antiretroviral therapy. *J Infect Dis.* 2000;181:522–531

34. Tasker SA, O'Brien WA, Treanor JJ, et al. Effects of influenza vaccination in HIV-infected adults: a double-blind, placebo-controlled trial. *Vaccine.* 1998;16:1039–1042

35. Glesby MJ, Hoover DR, Farzadegan H, Margolick JB, Saah AJ. The effect of influenza vaccination on human immunodeficiency virus type 1 load: a randomized, double-blind, placebo-controlled study. *J Infect Dis.* 1996;174:1332–1336

36. Fowke KR, D'Amico R, Chernoff DN, et al. Immunologic and virologic evaluation after influenza vaccination of HIV-1-infected patients. *AIDS.* 1997;11:1013–1021

37. Fuller JD, Craven DE, Steger KA, Cox N, Heeren TC, Chernoff D. Influenza vaccination of human immunodeficiency virus (HIV)-infected adults: impact on plasma levels of HIV type 1 RNA and determinants of antibody response. *Clin Infect Dis.* 1999;28:541–547

38. Jackson CR, Vavro CL, Valentine ME, et al. Effect of influenza immunization on immunologic and virologic characteristics of pediatric patients infected with human immunodeficiency virus. *Pediatr Infect Dis J.* 1997;16:200–204

39. Sullivan PS, Hanson DL, Dworkin MS, Jones JL, Ward JW. Effect of influenza vaccination on disease progression among HIV-infected persons. *AIDS.* 2000;14:2781–2785

40. King JC Jr, Fast PE, Zangwill KM, et al. Safety, vaccine virus shedding and immunogenicity of trivalent, cold-adapted, live attenuated influenza vaccine administered to human immunodeficiency virus-infected and noninfected children. *Pediatr Infect Dis J.* 2001;20:1124–1131

41. Gruber WC, Taber LH, Glezen WP, et al. Live attenuated and inactivated influenza vaccine in school-age children. *Am J Dis Child.* 1990;144:595–600

42. Heikkinen T, Ruuskanen O, Waris M, Ziegler T, Arola M, Halonen P. Influenza vaccination in the prevention of acute otitis media in children. *Am J Dis Child.* 1991;145:445–448

43. Hurwitz ES, Haber M, Chang A, et al. Studies of the 1996–1997 inactivated influenza vaccine among children attending day care: immunologic response, protection against infection, and clinical effectiveness. *J Infect Dis.* 2000;182:1218–1221

44. Neuzil KM, Dupont WD, Wright PF, Edwards KM. Efficacy of inactivated and cold-adapted vaccines against influenza A infection, 1985 to 1990: the pediatric experience. *Pediatr Infect Dis J.* 2001;20:733–740

45. Hoberman A, Greenberg DP, Paradise JL, et al. Effectiveness of inactivated influenza vaccine in preventing acute otitis media in young children: a randomized controlled trial. *JAMA.* 2003;290:1608–1616

46. Monto AS, Davenport FM, Napier JA, Francis T Jr. Effect of vaccination of a school-age population upon the course of an A2-Hong Kong influenza epidemic. *Bull World Health Organ.* 1969;41:537–542

47. Reichert TA, Sugaya N, Fedson DS, Glezen WP, Simonsen L, Tashiro M. The Japanese experience with vaccinating schoolchildren against influenza. *N Engl J Med.* 2001;344:889–896

48. Clements DA, Langdon L, Bland C, Walter E. Influenza A vaccine decreases the incidence of otitis media in 6- to 30-month-old children in day care. *Arch Pediatr Adolesc Med.* 1995;149:1113–1117

49. Kramarz P, DeStefano F, Gargiullo PM, et al. Influenza vaccination in children with asthma in health maintenance organizations. Vaccine Safety Datalink Team. *Vaccine.* 2000;18:2288–2294

50. Hall CB. Influenza: a shot or not? *Pediatrics.* 1987;79:564–566

51. Poehling KA, Speroff T, Dittus RS, Griffin MR, Hickson GB, Edwards KM. Predictors of influenza virus vaccination status in hospitalized children. *Pediatrics.* 2001;108(6). Available at: www.pediatrics.org/cgi/content/full/108/6/e99

52. White T, Lavoie S, Nettleman MD. Potential cost savings attributable to influenza vaccination of school-aged children. *Pediatrics.* 1999;103(6). Available at: www.pediatrics.org/cgi/content/full/103/6/e73

53. Cohen GM, Nettleman MD. Economic impact of influenza vaccination in preschool children. *Pediatrics.* 2000;106:973–976

54. Luce BR, Zangwill KM, Palmer CS, et al. Cost-effectiveness analysis of an intranasal influenza vaccine for the prevention of influenza in healthy children. *Pediatrics.* 2001;108(2). Available at: www.pediatrics.org/cgi/content/full/108/2/e24

55. Riddiough MA, Sisk JE, Bell JC. Influenza vaccination. *JAMA.* 1983;249:3189–3195

56. Meltzer MI, Cox NJ, Fukuda K. The economic impact of pandemic influenza in the United States: priorities for intervention. *Emerg Infect Dis.* 1999;5:659–671

57. Szilagyi PG, Iwane MK, Schaffer S, et al. Potential burden of universal influenza vaccination of young children on visits to primary care practices. *Pediatrics.* 2003;112:821–828

58. Maassab HF, Cox NJ, Murphy BR, Kendal AP. Biological, genetic and biochemical characterization of a cold-adapted recombinant A/Victoria/3/75 virus and its evaluation in volunteers. *Dev Biol Stand.* 1977;39:25–31

59. Belshe RB, Mendelman PM, Treanor J, et al. The efficacy of live attenuated, cold-adapted, trivalent, intranasal influenzavirus vaccine in children. *N Engl J Med.* 1998;338:1405–1412

60. Belshe RB, Gruber WC, Mendelman PM, et al. Efficacy of vaccination with live attenuated, cold-adapted, trivalent, intranasal influenza virus vaccine against a variant (A/Sydney) not contained in the vaccine. *J Pediatr.* 2000;136:168–175

61. Belshe RB, Gruber WC, Mendelman PM, et al. Correlates of immune protection induced by live, attenuated, cold-adapted, trivalent, intranasal influenza virus vaccine. *J Infect Dis.* 2000;181:1133–1137

62. Wright PF, Karzon DT. Live attenuated influenza vaccines. *Prog Med Virol.* 1987;34:70–88

63. Vesikari T, Karvonen A, Korhonen I, et al. A randomized double-blind placebo-controlled trial of the safety, transmissibility and phenotypic stability of a live attenuated cold-adapted influenza virus vaccine (CAIV) in children attending day care [abstract 37359]. Paper presented at: 41st Interscience Conference on Antimicrobial Agents and Chemotherapy; December 16–19, 2001; Chicago, IL

64. Wright PF, Johnson PR, Karzon DT. Clinical experience with live, attenuated vaccines in children. In: Kendal AP, Patriarca PA, eds. *Options for the Control of Influenza: Proceedings of a Viratek-UCLA Symposium.* New York, NY: Alan R. Liss; 1986:243–254

65. Belshe R. A review of attenuation of influenza viruses by genetic manipulation. *Am J Respir Crit Care Med.* 1995;152(4 Pt 2):S72–S75

66. Cha TA, Kao K, Zhao J, Fast PE, Mendelman PM, Arvin A. Genotypic stability of cold-adapted influenza virus vaccine in an efficacy clinical trial. *J Clin Microbiol.* 2000;38:839–845

67. American Academy of Pediatrics. *Red Book: 2003 Report of the Committee on Infectious Diseases.* Pickering LK, ed. 26th ed. Elk Grove Village, IL: American Academy of Pediatrics; 2003

68. Barker WH, Mullooly JP. Impact of epidemic type A influenza in a defined adult population. *Am J Epidemiol.* 1980;112:798–811

69. Simonsen L, Fukuda K, Schoenberger LB, Cox NJ. The impact of influenza epidemics on hospitalizations. *J Infect Dis.* 2000;181:831–837

70. US Preventive Services Task Force. Appendix A: task force ratings. In: *Guide to Clinical Preventive Services.* 2nd ed. Alexandria, VA: International Medical Publishing; 1996:861–865

All policy statements from the American Academy of Pediatrics automatically expire 5 years after publication unless reaffirmed, revised, or retired at or before that time.

Recommended Childhood and Adolescent Immunization Schedule—United States, July–December 2004

• *Policy Statement*

AMERICAN ACADEMY OF PEDIATRICS

POLICY STATEMENT
Organizational Principles to Guide and Define the Child Health Care System and/or Improve the Health of All Children

Committee on Infectious Diseases

Recommended Childhood and Adolescent Immunization Schedule—United States, July–December 2004

The mid-year recommended childhood and adolescent immunization schedule of the American Academy of Pediatrics, the Advisory Committee on Immunization Practices of the Centers for Disease Control and Prevention, and the American Academy of Family Physicians is issued for July to December 2004.

Changes in the mid-year schedule include the following:

1. The range of recommendations bar for influenza vaccine for children 6 through 23 months of age is moved above the dotted line, indicating that these children should be immunized annually.
2. The influenza vaccine footnote has been updated to highlight the recommendation that healthy children 6 through 23 months of age and close contacts of healthy children aged 0 through 23 months should receive the influenza vaccine, because children in this age group are at substantially increased risk of influenza-related hospitalizations.
3. The influenza vaccine footnote has been updated to highlight the recommendation that health care workers and other persons (including household members) in close contact with persons at high risk should be immunized annually.

COMMITTEE ON INFECTIOUS DISEASES, 2003–2004
Margaret B. Rennels, MD, Chairperson
Carol J. Baker, MD
Robert S. Baltimore, MD
Joseph A. Bocchini, Jr, MD
Penelope H. Dennehy, MD
Robert W. Frenck, Jr, MD
Caroline B. Hall, MD
Sarah S. Long, MD
Julia A. McMillan, MD

H. Cody Meissner, MD
Keith R. Powell, MD
Lorry G. Rubin, MD
Thomas N. Saari, MD

LIAISONS
Jack Swanson, MD
    Pediatric Practice Action Group
Joanne Embree, MD
    Canadian Paediatric Society
Marc A. Fischer, MD
    Centers for Disease Control and Prevention
Richard Clover, MD
    American Academy of Family Physicians
Bruce Gellin, MD
    Centers for Disease Control and Prevention
Mamodikoe Makhene, MD
    National Institutes of Health
Walter A. Orenstein, MD
    Centers for Disease Control and Prevention
Douglas R. Pratt
    Food and Drug Administration
Jeffrey R. Starke, MD
    American Thoracic Society

EX OFFICIO
Larry K. Pickering, MD
    Red Book Editor

CONSULTANT
Edgar O. Ledbetter, MD

STAFF
Martha Cook, MS

Recommended childhood and adolescent immunization schedule[1] — United States, July-December 2004

| Range of Recommended Ages | | | | Catch-up Immunization | | | | Preadolescent Assessment | | | |

Vaccine ▼ / Age ▶	Birth	1 mo	2 mo	4 mo	6 mo	12 mo	15 mo	18 mo	24 mo	4-6 y	11-12 y	13-18 y
Hepatitis B[2]	HepB #1	only if mother HBsAg (-)									HepB series	
		HepB #2				HepB #3						
Diphtheria, Tetanus, Pertussis[3]			DTaP	DTaP	DTaP		DTaP			DTaP	Td	Td
Haemophilus influenzae Type b[4]			Hib	Hib	Hib[4]	Hib						
Inactivated Poliovirus			IPV	IPV		IPV				IPV		
Measles, Mumps, Rubella[5]						MMR #1				MMR #2	MMR #2	
Varicella[6]						Varicella					Varicella	
Pneumococcal[7]			PCV	PCV	PCV	PCV				PCV	PPV	
Influenza[8]						Influenza (yearly)				Influenza (yearly)		
Vaccines below this line are for selected populations												
Hepatitis A[9]										Hepatitis A series		

1. Indicates the recommended ages for routine administration of currently licensed childhood vaccines, as of April 1, 2004, for children through age 18 years. Any dose not given at the recommended age should be given at any subsequent visit when indicated and feasible. ▨ Indicates age groups that warrant special effort to administer those vaccines not given previously. Additional vaccines may be licensed and recommended during the year. Licensed combination vaccines may be used whenever any components of the combination are indicated and the vaccine's other components are not contraindicated. Providers should consult the manufacturers' package inserts for detailed recommendations. Clinically significant adverse events that follow vaccination should be reported to the Vaccine Adverse Event Reporting System (VAERS). Guidance about how to obtain and complete a VAERS form is available at http://www.vaers.org/ or by telephone, 1-800-822-7967.

2. Hepatitis B vaccine (HepB). All infants should receive the first dose of HepB vaccine soon after birth and before hospital discharge; the first dose may also be given by age 2 months if the infant's mother is HBsAg-negative. Only monovalent HepB vaccine can be used for the birth dose. Monovalent or combination vaccine containing HepB may be used to complete the series; 4 doses of vaccine may be administered when a birth dose is given. The second dose should be given at least 4 weeks after the first dose except for combination vaccines, which cannot be administered before age 6 weeks. The third dose should be given at least 16 weeks after the first dose and at least 8 weeks after the second dose. The last dose in the vaccination series (third or fourth dose) should not be administered before age 24 weeks. Infants born to HBsAg-positive mothers should receive HepB vaccine and 0.5 mL hepatitis B immune globulin (HBIG) within 12 hours of birth at separate sites. The second dose is recommended at age 1-2 months. The last dose in the vaccination series should not be administered before age 24 weeks. These infants should be tested for HBsAg and anti-HBs at 9-15 months of age. Infants born to mothers whose HBsAg status is unknown should receive the first dose of the HepB vaccine series within 12 hours of birth. Maternal blood should be drawn as soon as possible to determine the mother's HBsAg status; if the HBsAg test is positive, the infant should receive HBIG as soon as possible (no later than age 1 week). The second dose is recommended at age 1-2 months. The last dose in the vaccination series should not be administered before age 24 weeks.

3. Diphtheria and tetanus toxoids and acellular pertussis vaccine (DTaP). The fourth dose of DTaP may be administered at age 12 months provided that 6 months have elapsed since the third dose and the child is unlikely to return at age 15-18 months. The final dose in the series should be given at age ≥4 years. Tetanus and diphtheria toxoids (Td) is recommended at age 11-12 years if at least 5 years have elapsed since the last dose of tetanus and diphtheria toxoid-containing vaccine. Subsequent routine Td boosters are recommended every 10 years.

4. Haemophilus influenzae type b (Hib) conjugate vaccine. Three Hib conjugate vaccines are licensed for infant use. If PRP-OMP (PedvaxHIB® or ComVax® [Merck]) is administered at ages 2 and 4 months, a dose at age 6 months is not required. DTaP/Hib combination products should not be used for primary vaccination in infants at ages 2, 4, or 6 months but can be used as boosters after any Hib vaccine. The final dose in the series should be given at age ≥12 months.

5. Measles, mumps, and rubella vaccine (MMR). The second dose of MMR is recommended routinely at age 4-6 years but may be administered during any visit, provided at least 4 weeks have elapsed since the first dose and both doses are administered beginning at or after age 12 months. Those who have not received the second dose previously should complete the schedule by the visit at age 11-12 years.

6. Varicella vaccine (VAR). Varicella vaccine is recommended at any visit at or after age 12 months for susceptible children (i.e., those who lack a reliable history of chickenpox). Susceptible persons aged ≥13 years should receive 2 doses given at least 4 weeks apart.

7. Pneumococcal vaccine. The heptavalent pneumococcal conjugate vaccine (PCV) is recommended for all children aged 2-23 months. It is also recommended for certain children aged 24-59 months. The final dose in the series should be given at age ≥12 months. Pneumococcal polysaccharide vaccine (PPV) is recommended in addition to PCV for certain high-risk groups. See MMWR 2000;49(No. RR-9):1-35.

8. Influenza vaccine. Influenza vaccine is recommended annually for children aged ≥6 months with certain risk factors (including but not limited to asthma, cardiac disease, sickle cell disease, HIV, and diabetes), health care workers, and other persons (including household members) in close contact with persons in groups at high-risk (see MMWR 2004;53[in press]) and can be administered to all others wishing to obtain immunity. In addition, healthy children aged 6-23 months and close contacts of healthy children aged 0-23 months are recommended to receive influenza vaccine, because children in this age group are at substantially increased risk of influenza-related hospitalizations. For healthy persons aged 5-49 years, the intranasally administered live, attenuated influenza vaccine (LAIV) is an acceptable alternative to the intramuscular trivalent inactivated influenza vaccine (TIV). See MMWR 2003;52(No. RR-13):1-8. Children receiving TIV should be administered a dosage appropriate for their age (0.25 mL if 6-35 months or 0.5 mL if ≥3 years). Children aged ≤8 years who are receiving influenza vaccine for the first time should receive 2 doses (separated by at least 4 weeks for TIV and at least 6 weeks for LAIV).

9. Hepatitis A vaccine. Hepatitis A vaccine is recommended for children and adolescents in selected states and regions and for certain high-risk groups. Consult your local public health authority and MMWR 1999;48(No.RR-12):1-37. Children and adolescents in these states, regions, and high-risk groups who have not been immunized against hepatitis A can begin the hepatitis A vaccination series during any visit. The two doses in the series should be administered at least 6 months apart.

Additional information about vaccines, including precautions and contraindications for vaccination and vaccine shortages is available at http://www.cdc.gov/nip or from the National Immunization Information Hotline, 800-232-2522 (English) or 800-232-0233 (Spanish). Approved by the Advisory Committee on Immunization Practices (http://www.cdc.gov/nip/acip), the American Academy of Pediatrics (http://www.aap.org), and the American Academy of Family Physicians (http://www.aafp.org).

For Children and Adolescents Who Start Late or Who Are >1 Month Behind

Tables 1 and 2 give catch-up schedules and minimum intervals between doses for children who have delayed immunizations. There is no need to restart a vaccine series regardless of the time that has elapsed between doses. Use the chart appropriate for the child's age.

Catch-up schedule for children age 4 months through 6 years

Dose 1 (Minimum Age)	Minimum Interval Between Doses			
	Dose 1 to Dose 2	Dose 2 to Dose 3	Dose 3 to Dose 4	Dose 4 to Dose 5
DTaP (6 wk)	4 wk	4 wk	6 mo	6 mo[1]
IPV (6 wk)	4 wk	4 wk	4 wk[2]	
HepB[3] (birth)	4 wk	8 wk (and 16 wk after first dose)		
MMR (12 mo)	4 wk[4]			
Varicella (12 mo)				
Hib[5] (6 wk)	**4 wk:** if first dose given at age <12 mo **8 wk (as final dose):** if first dose given at age 12-14 mo **No further doses needed:** if first dose given at age ≥15 mo	**4 wk[6]:** if current age <12 mo **8 wk (as final dose)[6]:** if current age ≥12 mo and second dose given at age <15 mo **No further doses needed:** if previous dose given at age ≥15 mo	**8 wk (as final dose):** this dose only necessary for children age 12 mo–5 yr who received 3 doses before age 12 mo	
PCV[7]: (6 wk)	**4 wk:** if first dose given at age <12 mo and current age <24 mo **8 wk (as final dose):** if first dose given at age ≥12 mo or current age 24-59 mo **No further doses needed:** for healthy children if first dose given at age >24 mo	**4 wk:** if current age <12 mo **8 wk (as final dose):** if current age ≥12 mo **No further doses needed:** for healthy children if previous dose given at age ≥24 mo	**8 wk (as final dose):** this dose only necessary for children age 12 mo–5 y who received 3 doses before age 12 mo	

Catch-up schedule for children age 7 through 18 years

Minimum Interval Between Doses		
Dose 1 to Dose 2	Dose 2 to Dose 3	Dose 3 to Booster Dose
Td: 4 wk	**Td:** 6 mo	**Td[8]:** **6 mo:** if first dose given at age <12 mo and current age <11 y **5 y:** if first dose given at age ≥12 mo and third dose given at age <7 y and current age ≥11 y **10 y:** if third dose given at age ≥7 y
IPV[9]: 4 wk	**IPV[9]:** 4 wk	**IPV[2,9]**
HepB: 4 wk	**HepB:** 8 wk (and 16 wk after first dose)	
MMR: 4 wk		
Varicella[10]: 4 wk		

1. **DTaP:** The fifth dose is not necessary if the fourth dose was given after the fourth birthday.
2. **IPV:** For children who received an all-IPV or all-oral poliovirus (OPV) series, a fourth dose is not necessary if third dose was given at age ≥4 years. If both OPV and IPV were given as part of a series, a total of 4 doses should be given, regardless of the child's current age.
3. **HepB:** All children and adolescents who have not been immunized against hepatitis B should begin the HepB immunization series during any visit. Providers should make special efforts to immunize children who were born in, or whose parents were born in, areas of the world where hepatitis B virus infection is moderately or highly endemic.
4. **MMR:** The second dose of MMR is recommended routinely at age 4 to 6 years but may be given earlier if desired.
5. **Hib:** Vaccine is not generally recommended for children age ≥5 years.
6. **Hib:** If current age <12 months and the first 2 doses were PRP-OMP (PedvaxHIB or ComVax [Merck]), the third (and final) dose should be given at age 12-15 months and at least 8 weeks after the second dose.
7. **PCV:** Vaccine is not generally recommended for children age ≥5 years.
8. **Td:** For children age 7 to 10 years, the interval between the third and booster dose is determined by the age when the first dose was given. For adolescents age 11 to 18 years, the interval is determined by the age when the third dose was given.
9. **IPV:** Vaccine is not generally recommended for persons age ≥18 years.
10. **Varicella:** Give 2-dose series to all susceptible adolescents age ≥13 years.

Reporting Adverse Reactions
Report adverse reactions to vaccines through the federal Vaccine Adverse Event Reporting System. For information on reporting reactions following immunization, please visit www.vaers.org or call the 24-hour national toll-free information line (800) 822-7967.

Disease Reporting
Report suspected cases of vaccine-preventable diseases to your state or local health department.

For additional information about vaccines, including precautions and contraindications for immunization and vaccine shortages, please visit the National Immunization Program Web site at www.cdc.gov/nip or call the National Immunization Information Hotline at 800-232-2522 (English) or 800-232-0233 (Spanish).

Relief of Pain and Anxiety in Pediatric Patients in Emergency Medical Systems

- *Clinical Report*

AMERICAN ACADEMY OF PEDIATRICS

CLINICAL REPORT
Guidance for the Clinician in Rendering Pediatric Care

William T. Zempsky, MD; Joseph P. Cravero, MD; and the Committee on Pediatric Emergency Medicine and Section on Anesthesiology and Pain Medicine

Relief of Pain and Anxiety in Pediatric Patients in Emergency Medical Systems

ABSTRACT. Whether a component of a disease process, the result of acute injury, or a product of a diagnostic or therapeutic procedure, pain should be relieved and stress should be decreased for pediatric patients. Control of pain and stress for children who enter into the emergency medical system, from the prehospital arena to the emergency department, is a vital component of emergency care. Any barriers that prevent appropriate and timely administration of analgesia to the child who requires emergency medical treatment should be eliminated. Although more research and innovation are needed, every opportunity should be taken to use available methods of pain control. A systematic approach to pain management and anxiolysis, including staff education and protocol development, can have a positive effect on providing comfort to children in the emergency setting. *Pediatrics* 2004;114:1348–1356; *pain, stress, anxiety, analgesia, opiates, topical anesthesia.*

ABBREVIATIONS. ED, emergency department, EMS, emergency medical services, EMLA, eutectic mixture of local anesthetics, LMX$_4$, liposomal 4% lidocaine cream, LET, lidocaine, epinephrine, and tetracaine, AAP, American Academy of Pediatrics, ASA, American Society of Anesthesiologists, NPO, nil per os.

BACKGROUND

A systematic approach to pain management is required to ensure pain relief for children who enter into the emergency medical system, which includes all emergency medical transport systems as well as the emergency department (ED). Over the past 20 years, improvements in the recognition and treatment of pain in children have led to changes in the approach to pain management for acutely ill and injured pediatric patients. Studies have shown an increase in opiate use in children with fractures.[1-3] However, there is still progress to be made; the administration of analgesia in children varies by age and lags behind adults, and our youngest patients are at the highest risk of receiving inadequate analgesia.[1-4] There is also wide variation in pain management practice by different EDs and health care professionals; in some settings, analgesics are underused in the care of children with pain.[2,5]

Inadequate sedation and pain control has negative implications for pediatric patients. Neonates who undergo procedures with inadequate analgesia have long-standing alterations in their response to and perceptions of painful experiences.[6-10] Inadequate pain control during oncology procedures leads to significantly increased pain scores for subsequent painful procedures.[11] Posttraumatic stress disorder can occur after procedures or stressful medical experiences that are not accompanied by appropriate pain control or sedation.[12,13]

Ethnicity affects pain management from both a patient and health care professional perspective. It is clear that ethnicity is an important contributor to an individual's pain perception as well as to manifested behavioral distress and anxiety.[14-17] However, no predictable patterns have emerged in regard to a consistent pain experience within ethnic groups. Studies have noted that Hispanic and black individuals with long-bone fractures were less likely to receive analgesics than were non-Hispanic white individuals.[18,19] A review of the National Hospital Ambulatory Medical Care Survey from 1992 to 1997 demonstrated that among patients with fractures, black children covered by Medicaid were least likely to receive parenteral sedation and analgesia.[20] However, in other studies, analgesic administration was not associated with ethnicity.[21,22] From a health care professional perspective, the clinician's own cultural background and bias may affect the decision of whether to administer analgesics.

A system-wide approach to pain management is required for children who enter into the emergency medical system. Pain management awareness and techniques should be woven into the fabric of the emergency medical system through education, protocol development, and changes in attitudes. The purpose of this report is to provide information to optimize the comfort of children whether they are cared for in the emergency setting or other environments.

STATEMENT OF THE PROBLEM

Barriers in general, as well as those intrinsic to the emergency setting, can affect the provision of ade-

The guidance in this report does not indicate an exclusive course of treatment or serve as a standard of medical care. Variations, taking into account individual circumstances, may be appropriate.

doi:10.1542/peds.2004-1752

PEDIATRICS (ISSN 0031 4005). Copyright © 2004 by the American Academy of Pediatrics.

quate analgesia.[23-28] The myths that children do not feel pain the same way adults do and that pain has no untoward consequences in children still exist.[28] Children's pain is underestimated because of a lack of adequate assessment tools and the inability to account for the wide range of children's developmental stages. Pain is often undermedicated because of fears of oversedation, respiratory depression, addiction, and unfamiliarity with use of sedative and analgesic agents in children.

In the ED, children often present with a constellation of symptoms but no final diagnosis; they are usually unknown to the treating clinician, have a wide range of medical or surgical problems, and are unlikely to be fasting on arrival.[24] These factors make their assessment and the selection of appropriate analgesic intervention more complicated. As well, the emergency setting can be a busy, fast-paced environment in which heightened patient and parental anxiety increases the perception of pain and makes its treatment more difficult.[25]

Analgesic agents typically used for pain in other settings might not be used in the ED because of concerns regarding masking of symptoms and prevention of appropriate diagnoses. Topical anesthetics may be underused because of concerns regarding delay in definitive treatment, cost, or lack of availability.

Until recently, education in pain management was not emphasized for clinical staff.[29,30] Optimal pain management requires a thorough understanding of pain assessment and management strategies.[25,26] Prehospital providers typically receive inadequate pain management instruction,[31,32] and pain management has received little emphasis in undergraduate or graduate medical education.[33-37]

NEW INFORMATION

Prehospital Care

The development of pain assessment and management protocols specifically for prehospital providers, along with educational initiatives, can improve pain management in the field.[31,38] Several adult studies[39-41] and 1 pediatric trial[42] show that analgesics such as opiates and tramadol hydrochloride can be used in prehospital protocols to decrease pain scores without causing respiratory depression. Alternative delivery systems, such as inhaled nitrous oxide, could offer pain control without requiring intravenous access, providing advantages in the field as well as in the hospital setting.[43-47] Some systems have implemented a "toolbox" of distraction equipment on emergency medical services (EMS) units as an adjunct to providing pain relief in the anxious, uncomfortable child.

Assessment and Management of Pain, Stress, and Anxiety in the ED

The Environment

The creation of an appropriate environment is essential to minimize the pain and distress of a child's ED visit.[25] Ideally, each child should be placed in a private room.[25] This room should provide a child-friendly, calming environment.[24] Colorful walls, pictures on the ceiling, and a collection of toys and games will minimize fear induced by this strange setting.[25]

Nonpharmacologic or stress management and emotional support are essential to providing a comfortable environment for the child. Distraction can range from simple techniques, such as a bubble blower or pinwheel used by the child during a painful injection, to structural changes, such as outfitting each procedure room with video cassette players to provide music and distraction stations equipped with bubble columns, light wands, and imagery projectors.[48-52] Training the staff in distraction and imagery increases the use of these techniques.[53]

A child life specialist based in the ED has the ability to (1) decrease anxiety and pain perception, (2) teach the child and staff simple distraction techniques, and (3) support family involvement in the child's care.[54,55] The child life specialist has an important role; he or she is one of a few professionals in the emergency setting who is not in a position to cause emotional or physical pain to the child.[56,57]

Allowing (but not requiring) family presence during painful procedures will also be of benefit. Although there is no evidence that family presence decreases pain, their presence for procedures does decrease parental and child distress.[58-61] Family presence does not increase anxiety of the child or decrease the procedure success rate of experienced clinicians.[58,59]

Pain Assessment in the ED

Assessment is the first step in the recognition and treatment of pain.[26,30] Assessment should begin at the triage desk, the entry point to all EDs, allowing triage to become the focal point for improving pain management.[25,26] The Joint Commission on Accreditation of Healthcare Organizations standards include mandatory pain assessments for all hospital patients.[30] Pain should be assessed routinely, along with vital signs, and reassessed during the ED stay. Pain should be monitored, and intervention should be begun and modified as the clinical situation demands.

The clinical standard for pain assessment is a self-report scale. Several well-validated scales exist for children as young as 3 years to report their own pain level.[62-64] The Wong-Baker Faces scale and the 10-cm Visual Analog Scale have been used successfully in many EDs caring for children.[62,64] For those who are unable to use self-report scales, behavioral scales can be combined with an evaluation of the patient's history and physical findings to assess the level of a child's pain.[65-67]

Children with severe pain require immediate triage, pain assessment, and pain treatment.[68] Patients with less acute conditions should also receive analgesia.[69] Treating pain in patients with less acute conditions does not interfere with physical examination or diagnosis. Protocols should be developed to allow for the delivery of appropriate medications such as acetaminophen, ibuprofen, or oral opiates to these patients (Table 1).

TABLE 1. Triage Oral Analgesic Administration Guidelines

Purpose
    To provide analgesic therapy to patients presenting to triage
    with a complaint of pain
Procedure
    1. Pain assessment
    2. Immediate triage to department for all those with severe
       pain as assessed by triage nurse and consideration of pain
       score
    3. For those not requiring immediate evaluation with pain
       score >3 (0–10 scale) or chief complaint consistent with
       pain, consider administration of oral analgesic
    4. Assess recent analgesic use
Contraindications
    1. Allergy to analgesic (consider alternative)
    2. NPO status (if patient may require procedural sedation or
       general anesthesia, consult with a physician before
       analgesic administration)
Medications
    1. Ibuprofen (avoid if the patient has an aspirin allergy,
       anticipated surgery, bleeding disorder, hemorrhage, or
       renal disease)
    2. Acetaminophen (avoid if the patient has hepatic disease or
       dysfunction)
    3. Acetaminophen with codeine or other oral opiate

TABLE 2. Guidelines for Use of EMLA/LMX$_4$ in the ED

EMLA/LMX$_4$ use should be considered in any patient who has
    a high likelihood of undergoing a nonemergent invasive
    procedure on intact skin in the ED. These include:
    Intravenous line placement or venipuncture
    Lumbar puncture
    Abscess drainage
    Joint aspiration

Discussion with parents should bring up these issues:
    EMLA/LMX$_4$ does not provide complete pain relief
    Some patients may require a procedure before EMLA/LMX$_4$
    reaches its full effectiveness (see below)

Contraindications
    Emergent need for intravenous access
    Allergy to amide anesthetics
    Nonintact skin
    Recent sulfonamide antibiotic use (trimethoprim-
       sulfamethoxazole, erythromycin-sulfisoxazole) (EMLA only)
    Congenital or idiopathic methemoglobinemia (EMLA only)

The EMLA dose should be lower for patients <12 months old
    or weighing <10 kg

Placement of EMLA/LMX$_4$
    Intravenous line placement
       EMLA/LMX$_4$ should be placed in at least 2 sites over veins
          amenable to placement of an intravenous line as judged
          by the triage nurse.
       EMLA reaches full effectiveness in 1 h; LMX$_4$ reaches full
          effectiveness in 30 min
       Care should be taken to avoid mucous membrane contact
          or ingestion
    Lumbar Puncture
       Placement of EMLA/LMX$_4$ for lumbar puncture should be
          considered at triage; accurate placement requires
          consultation with the attending physician

TABLE 3. Triage Guidelines for Use of LET (a Topical Anesthetic for Open Wounds)

Eligibility
    Simple lacerations of the head, neck, extremities, or trunk <5
       cm in length
Contraindications
    Allergy to amide anesthetics
    Gross contamination of wound
    Involvement of mucous membranes, digits, genitalia, ear, or
       nose
Procedure
    LET should be placed according to standard ED procedure;
       time of placement should be documented on triage sheet

Maximum wound length: 5 cm; maximum dose: 3 mL

(1) Place 3 mL of LET mixed with cellulose on open wound
    and cover with occlusive dressing or (2) place cotton ball
    soaked with LET solution into wound

Triage should be used as an opportunity to predict the future pain medication needs of the ED patient. For example, in 1 inner city pediatric ED, 90% of patients requiring intravenous access did not undergo this procedure until at least 60 minutes after triage.[70] A prediction model could be developed whereby the patient's chief complaint and medical history, combined with an experienced triage nurse assessment, could determine with some accuracy which patients have a high probability of needing intravenous access, and these patients could receive topical anesthetic application at triage.[71] These findings could be adapted to develop topical anesthetic protocols for painful procedures in other emergency centers, taking into account their patient volume, acuity, and flow characteristics (Table 2). Similar protocols should be developed for topical anesthetic placement for laceration repair at triage (Table 3).

Controlling Pain Related to Minor Procedures

Topical anesthetics can be placed proactively as described previously to control the pain associated with minor procedures. Procedures can be delayed in some cases in which topical anesthetic is not placed proactively. Some topical anesthetics have been developed that produce anesthesia more rapidly than eutectic mixture of local anesthetics (EMLA [AstraZeneca, Wilmington, DE]). A topical liposomal 4% lidocaine cream (LMX$_4$ [Ferndale Labs, Ferndale, MI]) provides anesthesia in approximately 30 minutes.[72,73] Lidocaine iontophoresis provides superior anesthesia to EMLA in 10 minutes or less; however, approximately 5% of children find the sensation caused by iontophoretic drug delivery to be unpleasant.[74,75] Vapocoolant sprays that have immediate onset of action can be used successfully for injection pain in children; however, they are not effective for intravenous line placement.[76,77]

Laceration repair should be completed with an emphasis on minimizing pain and anxiety. Several topical anesthetic/vasoconstrictor combinations such as lidocaine, epinephrine, and tetracaine (LET), which can be made by the in-hospital pharmacy as a liquid or gel preparation, provide excellent wound anesthesia in 20 to 30 minutes.[78,79] EMLA cream also provides topical anesthesia for laceration repair, although it is not approved by the US Food and Drug Administration for this purpose.[80,81] Tissue adhesives such as octyl cyanoacrylate provide essentially painless closure for low-tension wounds.[82,83] Steri-Strips (3M, St Paul, MN) provide similar painless closure and are less expensive than currently available tissue adhesives.[84] In general, absorbable sutures should be considered for facial wounds that must be sutured to avoid the pain and anxiety produced by suture removal.[85,86]

Lidocaine can be used alone in urgent situations or as an adjunct to topical anesthetics. Lidocaine can be injected in an almost painless manner.[87] This technique includes buffering the anesthetic with bicarbonate, warming the lidocaine before injection, and injecting slowly with a small-gauge needle.[88–92] Lidocaine buffered with bicarbonate made by a pharmacy in advance can be stocked in the ED and will remain stable for up to 30 days.[93,94] Lidocaine injection decreases the pain of venous cannulation without affecting procedural success rate.[87]

Neonatal Pain Management in the ED

Simple changes in practice can minimize painful stimuli for infants. Protocols for topical anesthetic placement should include neonates. Use of EMLA for procedures ranging from circumcision to venipuncture is safe in newborns and even preterm infants.[95–97]

Recent studies have suggested methods by which neonatal distress during painful procedures can be minimized. Sucrose has been found to decrease the response to noxious stimuli such as heel sticks and injections in neonates.[98–101] This effect seems to be strongest in the newborn infant and decreases gradually over the first 6 months of life.[98–101] Nursing protocols that allow for the use of sucrose before painful procedures are in place at many hospitals (Table 4). A 12% to 25% sucrose solution that is made by the pharmacy or is available commercially can be used (Sweet-Ease, Children's Medical Ventures, Norwell, MA). The use of a pacifier alone or in conjunction with sucrose also has been shown to have analgesic effects in neonates undergoing routine venipuncture.[102] Skin-to-skin contact of an infant with his or her mother and breastfeeding during a procedure decrease pain behaviors associated with painful stimuli.[103,104]

Available evidence supports the use of local and topical anesthetic for lumbar puncture in neonates.[105,106] Protocols can allow for the timely placement of topical anesthetic, or injected buffered lidocaine can be used at the site of needle insertion before the procedure. Concerns over the increased difficulty

of lumbar puncture after local anesthetic use have proved to be unfounded.[105,107]

Pain can be decreased in neonates by the elimination of heel sticks and intramuscular injections. Venipuncture seems to be less painful than heel lancing for obtaining blood for diagnostic testing.[108] When the intramuscular route is necessary, topical anesthetic should be used if time permits.[109] Use of distraction techniques discussed previously, ice, and less painful injection techniques can also be efficacious.[110–113] The use of lidocaine as the diluent for ceftriaxone can decrease the pain of intramuscular injection.[114]

Does the Appropriate Use of Analgesics Make Evaluation More Difficult?

There is no evidence that pain management masks symptoms or clouds mental status, preventing adequate assessment and diagnosis. For patients with abdominal pain, several adult studies have shown that pain medications such as morphine can be used without affecting diagnostic accuracy.[115–117] A recent pediatric study demonstrates similar findings.[118] Clinical experience suggests that the use of pain medication makes children more comfortable and the examination of the patient's abdomen and diagnostic testing (such as ultrasonography) easier, thus aiding in diagnosis. In the child who has suffered multisystem trauma, small titrated doses of opiates can be used to provide pain relief without affecting the clinical examination or the ability to perform neurologic assessments.[119,120] The development of pain protocols can improve the management of children who suffer major trauma.[121] Regional anesthesia should also be considered for patients who have injuries that are amenable to these techniques.[122,123] Additional studies evaluating these practices in pediatric patients are necessary but should not delay the development of protocols for the use of analgesics in patients with acute abdominal pain and multisystem trauma.

Administration of Pain Medications

Optimal pain management requires expeditious pain assessment and the rapid administration of systemic opioid pain medication to patients in severe pain. This may occur through the intravenous route, which allows for rapid relief of pain and drug titration as necessary and provides a route for other medications. Delivery of pain medications through the intramuscular route is painful both at the time of delivery and for days afterward and does not allow for titration of drug dose. Adjunctive pain medications such as nonsteroidal antiinflammatory drugs (NSAIDS) can be used judiciously in children with pain, acknowledging their known adverse effects such as antiplatelet activity and gastrointestinal and renal toxicity. Oral opiates and NSAIDs are appropriate for mild to moderate pain if the patient has no contraindications to receiving oral medications (ie, potential to require sedation or anesthesia).

Alternative routes of medication administration including oral, intranasal, transdermal, and inhaled should be used whenever possible. Nitrous oxide is a

---

TABLE 4.　　Guidelines for Use of Sucrose in the ED

Indications
　　Use as an adjunct for limiting the pain associated with procedures such as heel sticks, venipuncture, intravenous line insertion, arterial puncture, insertion of a Foley catheter, and lumbar puncture in neonates and infants younger than 6 months
Procedure
　　1. Administer 2 mL of 25% sucrose solution by syringe into the infant's mouth (1 mL in each cheek) or allow infant to suck solution from a nipple (pacifier) no more than 2 min before the start of the painful procedure
　　2. Sucrose may be given for >1 procedure within a relatively short period of time but should not be administered more than twice in 1 h
　　3. Sucrose seems to be more effective when given in combination with a pacifier; nonnutritive suck also contributes to calming the infant and decreasing pain-elicited distress
Contraindications
　　Avoid use if patient is under NPO restrictions

potent analgesic that does not require venous access and is available in some EDs and EMS systems.[43-47] Nitrous oxide should be used in conjunction with appropriate sedation guidelines and avoided in patients with pneumothorax, bowel obstruction, intracranial injury, and cardiovascular compromise.[46,47] Nitrous oxide has many potential applications including anxiolysis for procedures such as intravenous access and laceration repair and pain control for burn debridement and fracture and dislocation reduction.

Pain medication should be provided in the ED as well as on discharge even for those with mild to moderate pain. Patients should get specific instructions in regard to dose and duration of use. Pain medication should be recommended on an around-the-clock basis for anyone in whom moderate pain is anticipated.

Need for Sedation Policies and Protocols in the ED

The use of sedative hypnotic medication may be required to bring pain and stress levels under adequate control for many procedures in the emergency medical system. Unfortunately, pain and anxiety are often difficult to differentiate in infants and toddlers.

Although many procedures are not intrinsically painful or can be performed painlessly with the use of a topical or local anesthetic, this does not obviate the use of pharmacologic agents to decrease the anxiety and stress in children undergoing procedures in the ED.

Excellent reviews have been published that describe the safe and effective use of sedation in the ED.[124,125] Procedural sedation is generally combined with analgesia to minimize pain whenever the procedure is uncomfortable or painful. Analgesia may take the form of local anesthetics or systemic analgesics. Combinations of medications, particularly the addition of opiates to sedative medications, may increase the risk of respiratory depression and should only be used by individuals trained in airway management and resuscitation.[126]

Although the incidence of serious complications is low, it is imperative to develop ongoing policies that establish close monitoring of these patients. Current guidelines from the American Academy of Pediatrics (AAP), American Society of Anesthesiologists (ASA), and American College of Emergency Physicians[127-130] all recommend a structured evaluation of children that allows risk stratification before beginning sedation. This evaluation should include issues such as preexisting medical conditions, focused airway examination, and consideration of nil per os (NPO) status. Recent data have confirmed the concept that adherence to a structured AAP/ASA-based sedation model can significantly decrease the risk of complications in the pediatric age group.[131]

A critical component of any sedation protocol is to require a trained observer to be solely responsible for monitoring the patient while the procedure is being performed.[128,129,132] In addition, physicians who administer sedation and analgesia should have proven training and skills and ongoing training in the management of pediatric airways and resuscitation.

NPO guidelines for children receiving sedation in the ED are controversial. Many children who receive procedural sedation for emergencies have not fasted in accordance with published guidelines for elective procedures.[133-136] Currently, there are insufficient data to determine the length of time that constitutes safety in regard to NPO status.[134-140] Given the low incidence of adverse events during procedural sedation, larger studies are required to clearly define appropriate NPO duration.

Decisions regarding sedation of a child should be balanced by considering the urgency of the procedure, the effects of prolonged pain and anxiety, the depth and type of sedative and analgesic agents required, inconvenience to the patient and family, and the expenditure of finite ED resources as well as individual patient characteristics. A collaborative pediatric sedation database should be developed to help define the complications associated with these procedures.

Quality Improvement Programs

Any emergency medical system that provides treatment for children should have a demonstrated quality improvement program in which review of sedation and pain management practices in pediatric patients takes place at regular intervals. Transport and prehospital providers are essential components of this ongoing review. Indicators that should be evaluated include compliance with the use of validated pain scores, use of appropriate analgesics for specific disease states (whether severe or mild to moderate pain), use of topical anesthetics and other nonnoxious routes of analgesia and anesthesia, monitoring for adverse outcomes, and the use of discharge instructions that outline the indications, dose, and duration of analgesic to be used.[141-143]

Implementation

A systematic approach to pain management in emergency medical systems requires an implementation strategy advocated by leadership, which should include (1) a comprehensive evaluation of current pain management practices, (2) an educational program regarding pain assessment and management techniques for all clinical staff, (3) the development of protocols to allow the universal and efficient application of pain management strategies and medications, and (4) a quality improvement process to evaluate the ongoing success of the program.[24,26]

CONCLUSIONS

Health care professionals have a duty to provide compassionate care to all children. Pain and sedation management are an important yet complex aspect of emergency care for children. Multiple modalities are now available that allow pain and anxiety control for all age groups. Health care professionals should be aware of all the available analgesic options. Adequate pain assessment is essential for pain relief and should begin on entry into the emergency medical system and continue through discharge of the child from the ED. As medications and technologies evolve, it is more important than ever that safe sedation protocols and practices are in place for children receiving emergency care.

SUMMARY OF KEY POINTS

1. Training and education in pediatric pain assessment and management should be provided to all participants in emergency medical systems for children.
2. Simple methods for creating favorable environmental conditions for pediatric patients in the EMS setting should be advocated by caregivers.
3. Incorporation of child life specialists and others trained in nonpharmacologic stress reduction should be encouraged.
4. Family presence should be offered as an option during painful procedures.
5. Pain assessment for children should begin at admission to EMS and continue until discharge from the ED. On discharge, patients should receive detailed instruction regarding analgesic administration.
6. Painless administration of analgesics and anesthetics should be practiced when possible.
7. Neonates and young infants should receive appropriate pain relief.
8. Administration of pain medication has not been shown to hinder the evaluation of a possible surgical patient in the ED, and pain medication should not be withheld on this account.
9. Sedation should be provided for patients undergoing painful or stressful procedures in the ED. A structured protocol for pediatric sedation, based on AAP, ASA, American College of Emergency Physicians, and Emergency Medical Services for Children recommendations, should be followed for all children who receive sedative medications in EMS.

COMMITTEE ON PEDIATRIC EMERGENCY MEDICINE, 2003–2004
Jane F. Knapp, MD, Chairperson
Thomas Bojko, MD
Margaret A. Dolan, MD
Karen S. Frush, MD
Ronald A. Furnival, MD
Steven E. Krug, MD
Daniel J. Isaacman, MD
Robert E. Sapien, MD
Kathy N. Shaw, MD, MSCE
Paul E. Sirbaugh, DO

LIAISONS
Jane Ball, RN, DrPH
    EMSC National Resource Center
Kathleen Brown, MD
    National Association of EMS Physicians
Dan Kavanaugh, MSW
    Maternal and Child Health Bureau
Sharon E. Mace, MD
    American College of Emergency Physicians
David W. Tuggle, MD
    American College of Surgeons

STAFF
Susan Tellez

SECTION ON ANESTHESIOLOGY AND PAIN MEDICINE, 2003–2004
Thomas J. Mancuso, MD, Chairperson
Joseph P. Cravero, MD, Chairperson-elect
Rita Agarwal, MD
Constance S. Houck, MD
Zeev Kain, MD
Lynne G. Maxwell, MD
Robert D. Valley, MD, Immediate Past
    Chairperson
Patricia J. Davidson, MD

LIAISON
Carolyn Fleming Bannister, MD
    American Society of Anesthesiologists,
    Committee on Pediatrics

STAFF
Kathleen Kuk Ozmeral

REFERENCES

1. Selbst SM, Clark M. Analgesic use in the emergency department. *Ann Emerg Med*. 1990,19:1010–1013
2. Petrack EM, Christopher NC, Kriwinsky J. Pain management in the emergency department: patterns of analgesic utilization. *Pediatrics*. 1997,99:711–714
3. Alexander J, Manno M. Underuse of analgesia in very young pediatric patients with isolated painful injuries. *Ann Emerg Med*. 2003,41:617–622
4. Lewis LM, Lasater LC, Brooks CB. Are emergency physicians too stingy with analgesics? *South Med J*. 1994,87:7–9
5. Krauss B, Zurakowski D. Sedation patterns in pediatric and general community hospital emergency departments. *Pediatr Emerg Care*. 1998,14:99–103
6. Taddio A, Goldbach M, Ipp M, Stevens B, Koren G. Effect of neonatal circumcision on pain response during vaccination in boys. *Lancet*. 1995,345:291–292
7. Taddio A, Katz J, Ilersich AL, Koren G. Effect of neonatal circumcision on pain response during subsequent routine vaccination. *Lancet*. 1997,349:599–603
8. Grunau RE, Whitfield MF, Petrie J. Children's judgments about pain at age 8–10 years: do extremely low birthweight (≤1000 g) children differ from full birthweight peers? *J Child Psychol Psychiatry*. 1998,39:587–594
9. Johnston CC, Stevens BJ. Experience in a neonatal intensive care unit affects pain response. *Pediatrics*. 1996,98:925–930
10. Grunau RV, Whitfield MF, Petrie JH. Pain sensitivity and temperament in extremely low-birth-weight premature toddlers and preterm and full-term controls. *Pain*. 1994,58:341–346
11. Weisman SJ, Bernstein B, Schechter NL. Consequences of inadequate analgesia during painful procedures in children. *Arch Pediatr Adolesc Med*. 1998,152:147–149
12. Wintgens A, Boileau B, Robaey P. Posttraumatic stress symptoms and medical procedures in children. *Can J Psychiatry*. 1997,42:611–616
13. Kain ZN, Mayes LC, Wang SM, Hofstadter MB. Postoperative behavioral outcomes in children: effects of sedative premedication. *Anesthesiology*. 1999,90:758–765
14. Lipton J, Marbach J. Ethnicity and the pain experience. *Soc Sci Med*. 1984,19:1279–1298
15. Wolff BB. Ethnocultural factors influencing pain and illness behavior. *Clin J Pain*. 1985,1:23–30
16. Martinelli AM. Pain and ethnicity: how people of different cultures experience pain. *AORN J*. 1987,46:273–274, 276, 278
17. Bernstein BA, Pachter LM. Cultural considerations in children's pain. In: Schechter NL, Berde CB, Yaster M, eds. *Pain in Infants, Children, and Adolescents*. Philadelphia, PA: Lippincott, Williams, and Wilkins; 2003: 142–156
18. Todd KH, Deaton C, D'Adamo AP, Goe L. Ethnicity and analgesic practice. *Ann Emerg Med*. 2000,35:11–16
19. Todd KH, Samaroo N, Hoffman JR. Ethnicity as a risk factor for inadequate emergency department analgesia. *JAMA*. 1993,269: 1537–1539

20. Hoestetler MA, Auinger P, Szilagyi PG. Parenteral analgesic and sedative use among ED patients in the United States: combined results from the national hospital ambulatory medical care survey (NHAMCS) 1992–1997. *Am J Emerg Med.* 2002,20:139–143

21. Karpman RR, Del Mar N, Bay C. Analgesia for emergency centers' orthopaedic patients: does an ethnic bias exist? *Clin Orthop.* 1997,334:270–275

22. Fuentes EF, Kohn MA, Neighbor ML. Lack of association between patient ethnicity or race and fracture analgesia. *Acad Emerg Med.* 2002,9:910–915

23. McGrath PJ, Frager G. Psychological barriers to optimal pain management in infants and children. *Clin J Pain.* 1996,12:135–141

24. Craig KD, Lilley CM, Gilbert CA. Social barriers to optimal pain management in infants and children. *Clin J Pain.* 1996,12:232–242

25. Zempsky WT. Developing the painless emergency department: a systematic approach to change. *Clin Pediatr Emerg Med.* 2000,1:253–259

26. Ducharme J. Acute pain and pain control: state of the art. *Ann Emerg Med.* 2000,35:592–603

27. Kelly AM. A process approach to improving pain management in the emergency department: development and evaluation. *J Accid Emerg Med.* 2000,17:185–187

28. American Academy of Pediatrics, Committee on Psychosocial Aspects of Child and Family Health and American Pain Society, Task Force on Pain in Infants, Children, and Adolescents. The assessment and management of acute pain in infants, children, and adolescents. *Pediatrics.* 2001,108:793–797

29. Twycross A. Education about pain: a neglected area? *Nurse Educ Today.* 2000,20:244–253

30. Joint Commission on Accreditation of Healthcare Organizations. *Comprehensive Accreditation Manual for Hospitals.* Oakbrook Terrace, IL: Joint Commission on Accreditation of Healthcare Organizations; 2001

31. Ricard-Hibbon A, Chollet C, Saada S, Loridant B, Marty J. A quality control program for acute pain management in out-of-hospital critical care medicine. *Ann Emerg Med.* 1999,34:738–744

32. Dieckmann R, Brownstein D, Gausche-Hill M, eds. *Pediatric Education for Prehospital Professionals.* Sudbury, MA: Jones and Bartlett; 2000: 151–152

33. Accreditation Council for Graduate Medical Education. *Program Requirements for Residency Education in Emergency Medicine.* Chicago, IL: Accreditation Council for Graduate Medical Education; 2001

34. Accreditation Council for Graduate Medical Education. *Program Requirements for Residency Education in Pediatrics.* Chicago, IL: Accreditation Council for Graduate Medical Education; 2001

35. Bennedetti C, Dickerson ED, Nichols LL. Medical education: a barrier to pain therapy and palliative care. *J Pain Symptom Manage.* 2001,21:360–362

36. Weinstein SM, Laux LF, Thornby JI, et al. Medical students' attitudes toward pain and the use of opioid analgesics: implications for changing medical school curriculum. *South Med J.* 2000,93:472–478

37. Phillips DM. JCAHO pain management standards are unveiled. Joint Commission on Accreditation of Healthcare Organizations. *JAMA.* 2000,284:428–429

38. Baskett PJ. Acute pain management in the field. *Ann Emerg Med.* 1999,34:784–785

39. Ward ME, Radburn J, Morant S. Evaluation of intravenous tramadol for use in the prehospital situation by ambulance patients. *Prehospital Disaster Med.* 1997,12:158–162

40. Vergnion M, Degesves S, Garcet L, Magotteaux V. Tramadol, an alternative to morphine for treating posttraumatic pain in the prehospital situation. *Anesth Analg.* 2001,92:1543–1546

41. Bruns BM, Dieckmann R, Shagoury C, Dingerson A, Swartzell C. Safety of pre-hospital therapy with morphine sulfate. *Am J Emerg Med.* 1992,10:53–57

42. Devellis P, Thomas SH, Wedel SK, Stein JP, Vinci RJ. Prehospital fentanyl analgesia in air-transported pediatric trauma patients. *Pediatr Emerg Care.* 1998,14:321–323

43. National Association of Emergency Medical Services Physicians. Use of nitrous oxide: oxygen mixtures in prehospital emergency medical care. *Prehospital Disaster Med.* 1990,5:273–274

44. Baskett PJ. Nitrous oxide in pre-hospital care. *Acta Anaesthesiol Scand.* 1994,38:775–776

45. Burton JH, Auble TE, Fuchs SM. Effectiveness of 50% nitrous oxide/50% oxygen during laceration repair in children. *Acad Emerg Med.* 1998,5:112–117

46. Luhmann JD, Kennedy RM, Jaffe DM, McAllister JD. Continuous-flow delivery of nitrous oxide and oxygen: a safe and cost-effective technique for inhalation analgesia and sedation of pediatric patients. *Pediatr Emerg Care.* 1999,15:388–392

47. Luhmann JD, Kennedy RM, Porter FL, Miller JP, Jaffe DM. A randomized clinical trial of continuous-flow nitrous oxide and midazolam for sedation of young children during laceration repair. *Ann Emerg Med.* 2001,37:20–27

48. French GM, Painter EC, Coury DL. Blowing away shot pain: a technique for pain management during immunization. *Pediatrics.* 1994, 93:384–388

49. Fowler-Kerry S, Lander JR. Management of injection pain in children. *Pain.* 1987,30:169–175

50. Megel ME, Houser CW, Gleaves LS. Children's responses to immunizations: lullabies as distraction. *Issues Compr Pediatr Nurs.* 1998,21:129–145

51. Fratianne RB, Prensner JD, Huston MJ, Super DM, Yowler CJ, Standley JM. The effect of music-based imagery and musical alternate engagement on the burn debridement process. *J Burn Care Rehabil.* 2001,22:47–53

52. Favara-Scacco C, Smirne G, Schiliro G, DiCataldo A. Art therapy as support for children with leukemia during painful procedures. *Med Pediatr Oncol.* 2001,36:474–480

53. Kutner L. *No Fears No Tears: Children With Cancer Coping With Pain* [videotape]. Vancouver, BC, Canada: Canadian Cancer Society; 1986

54. Alcock DS, Feldman W, Goodman JT, McGrath PJ, Park JM. Evaluation of child life intervention in emergency department suturing. *Pediatr Emerg Care.* 1985,1:111–115

55. American Academy of Pediatrics, Committee on Hospital Care. Child life services. *Pediatrics.* 2000,106:1156–1159

56. Rothenberg MB. The unique role of the child life worker in children's health care settings. *Child Health Care.* 1982,10:121–124

57. Rae WA, Worchel FF, Upchurch J, Sanner JH, Daniel CA. The psychosocial impact of play on hospitalized children. *J Pediatr Psychol.* 1989,14:617–627

58. Bauchner H, Waring C, Vinci R. Parental presence during procedures in an emergency room: results from 50 observations. *Pediatrics.* 1991,87:544–588

59. Wolfram RW, Turner ED, Philput C. Effects of parental presence during young children's venipuncture. *Pediatr Emerg Care.* 1997,13: 325–328

60. Bordreaux ED, Francis JL, Loyacano T. Family presence during invasive procedures and resuscitations in the emergency department: a critical review and suggestions for future research. *Ann Emerg Med.* 2002,40:193–205

61. Emergency Nurses Association. Emergency Nurses Association position statements: family presence at the bedside during invasive procedures and resuscitation. 2001. Available at: www.ena.org/about/position/familypresence.asp. Accessed April 28, 2004

62. Wong DL, Hockenberry-Eaton M, Winkelstein ML, et al, eds. Pain assessment. In: *Whaley and Wong's Nursing Care of Infants and Children.* 6th ed. St Louis, MO: Mosby; 1999:1148–1159

63. Beyer JE, Aradine CR. Content validity of an instrument to measure young children's perceptions of the intensity of their pain. *J Pediatr Nurs.* 1986,1:386–395

64. Scott J, Huskisson EC. Graphic representation of pain. *Pain.* 1976,2: 175–184

65. McGrath PA, Johnson G, Goodman JT, et al. CHEOPS: a behavioral scale for rating postoperative pain in children. *Adv Pain Res Ther.* 1985,9:395–402

66. Grunau RV, Craig KD. Pain expression in neonates: facial action and cry. *Pain.* 1987,28:395–410

67. McGrath PJ. Behavioral measures of pain. In: Finley GA, McGrath PJ, eds. *Measurement of Pain in Infants and Children.* Seattle, WA: IASP Press; 1998:83–102

68. Fry M, Holdgate A. Nurse-initiated intravenous morphine in the emergency department: efficacy, rate of adverse events and impact on time to analgesia. *Emerg Med (Fremantle).* 2002,14:249–254

69. Michalewski TG, Zempsky WT, Schechter NL. Pain in low-severity emergency department visits: frequency and management [abstract]. *Ann Emerg Med.* 2001,38:S21

70. Fein JA, Callahan JM, Boardman CR. Intravenous catheterization in the ED: is there a role for topical anesthesia? *Am J Emerg Med.* 1999,17:624–625

71. Fein JA, Callahan JM, Boardman CR, Gorelick MH. Predicting the need for topical anesthetic in the pediatric emergency department. *Pediatrics.* 1999,104(2). Available at: www.pediatrics.org/cgi/content/full/104/2/e19

72. Kleiber C, Sorenson M, Whiteside K, Gronstal BA, Tannous R. Topical anesthetics for intravenous insertion in children: a randomized equivalency study. *Pediatrics.* 2002,110:758–761

73. Eichenfield LF, Funk A, Fallon-Friedlander S, Cunnigham BB. A clinical study to evaluate the efficacy of ELA-Max (4% liposomal lidocaine) as compared with eutectic mixture of local anesthetics cream for pain reduction of venipuncture in children. *Pediatrics*. 2002,109: 1093–1099

74. Zempsky WT, Anand KJ, Sullivan KM, Fraser D, Cucina K. Lidocaine iontophoresis for topical anesthesia before intravenous line placement in children. *J Pediatr*. 1998,132:1061–1063

75. Squire SJ, Kirchhoff KT, Hissong K. Comparing two methods of topical anesthesia used before intravenous cannulation in pediatric patients. *J Pediatr Health Care*. 2000,14:68–72

76. Cohen Reis E, Holobukov R. Vapocoolant spray is equally effective as EMLA cream in reducing immunization pain in school-aged children. *Pediatrics*. 1997,100(6). Available at: www.pediatrics.org/cgi/content/full/100/6/e5

77. Ramsook CA, Kozinetz C, Moro-Sutherland D. The efficacy of ethyl chloride as a local anesthetic for venipuncture in an emergency room setting. Paper presented at: 39th Annual Meeting of the Ambulatory Pediatric Association; May 3, 1999; San Francisco, CA

78. Schilling CG, Bank DE, Borchert BA, Klatzko MD, Uden DL. Tetracaine, epinephrine and cocaine (TAC) versus lidocaine, epinephrine, and tetracaine (LET) for anesthesia of lacerations in children. *Ann Emerg Med*. 1995,25:203–208

79. Ernst AA, Marvez E, Nick TG, Chin E, Wood E, Gonzaba WT. Lidocaine adrenaline tetracaine gel versus tetracaine adrenaline cocaine gel for topical anesthesia in linear scalp and facial lacerations in children aged 5 to 17 years. *Pediatrics*. 1995,95:255–258

80. Zempsky WT, Karasic RB. EMLA versus TAC for topical anesthesia of extremity wounds in children. *Ann Emerg Med*. 1997,30:163–166

81. Singer AJ, Stark MJ. LET versus EMLA for pretreating lacerations: a randomized trial. *Acad Emerg Med*. 2001,8:223–230

82. Simon HK, McLario DJ, Bruns TJ, Zempsky WT, Wood RJ, Sullivan KM. Long-term appearance of lacerations repaired using a tissue adhesive. *Pediatrics*. 1997,99:193–195

83. Quinn J, Wells G, Sutcliffe T, et al. A randomized trial comparing octylcyanoacrylate tissue adhesive and sutures in the management of lacerations. *JAMA*. 1997,277:1527–1530

84. Zempsky WT, Parrotti D, Grem C, Nichols J. Randomized controlled comparison of cosmetic outcomes of simple facial lacerations closed with SteriStrip Skin Closures or Dermabond tissue adhesive. *Pediatr Emerg Care*. 2004;20:519–524

85. Holger JS, Wandersee SC, Hale DB. Cosmetic outcomes in facial lacerations closed with rapid absorbing gut, octylcyanoacrylate or nylon [abstract]. *Acad Emerg Med*. 2002,9:447–448

86. Karounis H, Gouin S, Eisman H, Chalut D, Pelletier H, Williams B. A randomized, controlled trial comparing long-term cosmetic outcomes of traumatic pediatric lacerations repaired with absorbable plain gut versus nonabsorbable nylon sutures. *Acad Emerg Med*. 2004;11:730–735

87. Klein EJ, Shugerman RP, Leigh-Taylor K, Schneider C, Portscheller D, Koepsell T. Buffered lidocaine: analgesia for intravenous line placement in children. *Pediatrics*. 1995,95:709–712

88. Bartfield JM, Gennis P, Barbera J, Breuer B, Gallagher EJ. Buffered versus plain lidocaine as a local anesthetic for simple laceration repair. *Ann Emerg Med*. 1990,19:1387–1390

89. Davidson JA, Boom SJ. Warming lignocaine to reduce pain associated with injection. *BMJ*. 1992,305:617–618

90. Krause RS, Moscati R, Filice M, Lerner EB, Hughes D. The effect of injection speed on the pain of lidocaine infiltration. *Acad Emerg Med*. 1997,4:1032–1035

91. Scarfone RJ, Jasani M, Gracely EJ. Pain of local anesthetics: rate of administration and buffering. *Ann Emerg Med*. 1998,31:36–40

92. Bartfield JM, Sokaris SJ, Raccio-Robak N. Local anesthesia for lacerations: pain of infiltration inside versus outside the wound. *Acad Emerg Med*. 1998,5:100–104

93. Bartfield JM, Homer PJ, Ford DT, Sternklar P. Buffered lidocaine as a local anesthetic: an investigation of shelf life. *Ann Emerg Med*. 1992,21:16–19

94. Meyer G, Henneman PL, Fu P. Buffered lidocaine [letter]. *Ann Emerg Med*. 1991,20:218–219

95. Taddio A, Ohlsson A, Einarson TR, Stevens B, Koren G. A systematic review of lidocaine-prilocaine cream (EMLA) in the treatment of acute pain in neonates. *Pediatrics*. 1998,101(2). Available at: www.pediatrics.org/cgi/content/full/101/2/e1

96. Essink-Tebbes CM, Wuis EW, Liem KD, van Dongen RT, Hekster YA. Safety of lidocaine-prilocaine cream application four times a day in premature neonates: a pilot study. *Eur J Pediatr*. 1999,158:421–423

97. Brisman M, Ljung BM, Otterbom I, Larsson LE, Andreasson SE. Methaemoglobin formation after the use of EMLA cream in term neonates. *Acta Paediatr*. 1998,87:1191–1194

98. Blass E, Fitzgerald E, Kehoe P. Interactions between sucrose, pain and isolation distress. *Pharmacol Biochem Behav*. 1987,26:483–489

99. Barr RG, Young SN, Wright JH, et al. "Sucrose analgesia" and diphtheria-tetanus-pertussis immunizations at 2 and 4 months. *J Dev Behav Pediatr*. 1995,16:220–225

100. Lewindon PJ, Harkness L, Lewindon N. Randomised controlled trial of sucrose by mouth for the relief of infant crying after immunisation. *Arch Dis Child*. 1998,78:453–456

101. Stevens B, Taddio A, Ohlsson A, Einarson T. The efficacy of sucrose for relieving procedural pain in neonates—a systematic review and meta-analysis. *Acta Paediatr*. 1997,86:837–842

102. Carbajal R, Chauvet X, Couderc S, Olivier-Martin M. Randomised trial of analgesic effects of sucrose, glucose, and pacifiers in term neonates. *BMJ*. 1999,319:1393–1397

103. Gray L, Watt L, Blass EM. Skin-to-skin contact is analgesic in healthy newborns. *Pediatrics*. 2000,105(1). Available at: www.pediatrics.org/cgi/content/full/105/1/e14

104. Gray L, Miller LW, Philipp BL, Blass EM. Breastfeeding is analgesic in healthy newborns. *Pediatrics*. 2002,109:590–593

105. Pinheiro JM, Furdon S, Ochoa LF. Role of local anesthesia during lumbar puncture in neonates. *Pediatrics*. 1993,91:379–382

106. Kaur G, Gupta P, Kumar A. A randomized trial of eutectic mixture of local anesthetics during lumbar puncture in newborns. *Arch Pediatr Adolesc Med*. 2003,157:1065–1070

107. Carraccio C, Feinberg P, Hart LS, Quinn M, King J, Lichenstein R. Lidocaine for lumbar punctures. A help not a hindrance. *Arch Pediatr Adolesc Med*. 1996,150:1044–1046

108. Larsson BA, Tannfeldt G, Lagercrantz H, Olsson GL. Venipuncture is more effective and less painful than heel lancing for blood tests in neonates. *Pediatrics*. 1998,101:882–886

109. Uhari M. A eutectic mixture of lidocaine and prilocaine for alleviating vaccination pain in infants. *Pediatrics*. 1993,92:719–722

110. Holmes HS. Options for painless local anesthesia. *Postgrad Med*. 1991,89:71–72

111. Keen MF. Comparison of intramuscular injection techniques to reduce site discomfort and lesions. *Nursing Res*. 1986,35:207–210

112. Main KM, Jorgensen JT, Hertel NT, Jensen S, Jakobsen L. Automatic needle insertion diminishes pain during growth hormone injection. *Acta Pediatr*. 1995,84:331–334

113. Ipp MM, Gold R, Goldbach M, et al. Adverse reactions to diphtheria, tetanus, pertussis-polio vaccination at 18 months of age: effect of injection site and needle length. *Pediatrics*. 1989,83:679–682

114. Schichor A, Bernstein B, Weinerman H, Fitzgerald J, Yordan E, Schechter N. Lidocaine as a diluent for ceftriaxone in the treatment of gonorrhea: does it reduce the pain of injection? *Arch Pediatr Adolesc Med*. 1994,148:72–75

115. LoVecchio F, Oster N, Sturmann K, Nelson LS, Flashner S, Finger R. The use of analgesics in patients with acute abdominal pain. *J Emerg Med*. 1997,15:775–779

116. Pace S, Burke TF. Intravenous morphine for early pain relief in patients with acute abdominal pain. *Acad Emerg Med*. 1996,3:1086–1092

117. Attard AR, Corlett MJ, Kidner NJ, et al. Safety of early pain relief for acute abdominal pain. *BMJ*. 1992,305:554–556

118. Kim MK, Strait RT, Sato TT, Hennes HM. A randomized clinical trial of analgesia in children with acute abdominal pain. *Acad Emerg Med*. 2002,9:281–287

119. Hedderich R, Ness TJ. Analgesia for trauma and burns. *Crit Care Clin*. 1999,15:167–184

120. Joseph MH, Brill J, Zeltzer LK. Pediatric pain relief in trauma. *Pediatr Rev*. 1999,20:75–83

121. Zohar Z, Eitan A, Halperin P, et al. Pain relief in major trauma patients: an Israeli perspective. *J Trauma*. 2001,51:767–772

122. Fletcher AK, Rigby AS, Heyes FL. Three-in-one femoral nerve block as analgesia for fractured neck of femur in the emergency department: a randomized, controlled trial. *Ann Emerg Med*. 2003,41:227–233

123. Blasier RD, White R. Intravenous regional anesthesia for management of children's extremity fractures in the emergency department. *Pediatr Emerg Care*. 1996,12:404–406

124. Krauss B. Managing acute pain and anxiety in children undergoing procedures in the emergency department. *Emerg Med (Fremantle)*. 2001,13:293–304

125. Kennedy RM, Luhmann JD. The "ouchless emergency department." Getting closer: advances in decreasing distress during painful procedures in the emergency department [review]. *Pediatr Clin North Am*. 1999,46:1215–1247, vii–viii

126. Yaster M, Nichols DG, Deshpande JK, Wetzel RC. Midazolam-fentanyl intravenous sedation in children: case report of respiratory arrest. *Pediatrics.* 1990,86:463–466

127. American Academy of Pediatrics, Committee on Drugs. Guidelines for monitoring and management of pediatric patients during and after sedation for diagnostic and therapeutic procedures. *Pediatrics.* 1992,89:1110–1115

128. American Academy of Pediatrics, Committee on Drugs. Guidelines for monitoring and management of pediatric patients during and after sedation for diagnostic and therapeutic procedures: addendum. *Pediatrics.* 2002,110:836–838

129. American Society of Anesthesiologists, Task Force on Sedation and Analgesia by Non-Anesthesiologists. Practice guidelines for sedation and analgesia by non-anesthesiologists. *Anesthesiology.* 2002,96: 1004–1017

130. American College of Emergency Physicians. Clinical policy for procedural sedation and analgesia in the emergency department. *Ann Emerg Med.* 1998,31:663–677

131. Hoffman GM, Nowakowski R, Troshynski TJ, Berens RJ, Weisman SJ. Risk reduction in pediatric procedural sedation by application of an American Academy of Pediatrics/American Society of Anesthesiologists process model. *Pediatrics.* 2002,109:236–243

132. Cote CJ, Notterman DA, Karl HW, Weinberg JA, McCloskey C. Adverse sedation events in pediatrics: a critical incident analysis of contributing factors. *Pediatrics.* 2000,105:805–814

133. McDevit DC, Perry H, Tucker J, Zempsky W. Sedation in the pediatric emergency department: a survey of emergency department directors' adherence to sedation guidelines [abstract]. *Ann Emerg Med.* 2000,36:S28. Abstract 106

134. Roback MG, Wathen J, Bajaj L. Effect of NPO time on adverse events in pediatric procedural sedation and analgesia [abstract]. *Pediatr Res.* 2003,53:109A. Abstract 620

135. Phrampus ED, Pitetti RD, Singh S. Duration of fasting and occurrence of adverse events during procedural sedation in a pediatric emergency department [abstract]. *Pediatr Res.* 2003,53:109A. Abstract 621

136. Agrawal D, Manzi SF, Gupta R, Krauss B. Preprocedural fasting state and adverse events in children undergoing procedural sedation and analgesia in a pediatric emergency department. *Ann Emerg Med.* 2003,42:636–646

137. Pena BM, Krauss B. Adverse events of procedural sedation and analgesia in a pediatric emergency department. *Ann Emerg Med.* 1999,34:483–491

138. Green SM, Kupperman N, Rothrock SG, Hummel CB, Ho M. Predictors of adverse events with intramuscular ketamine sedation in children. *Ann Emerg Med.* 2000,35:35–42

139. Green SM, Krauss B. Pulmonary aspiration risk during emergency department procedural sedation—an examination of the role of fasting and sedation depth. *Acad Emerg Med.* 2002,9:35–42

140. American Society of Anesthesiologists, Task Force on Preoperative Fasting. Practice guidelines for preoperative fasting and the use of pharmacologic agents to reduce the risk of pulmonary aspiration: application to healthy patients undergoing elective procedures. *Anesthesiology.* 1999,90:896–905

141. Miaskowski C. Monitoring and improving pain management practices. A quality improvement approach. *Crit Care Nurs Clin North Am.* 2001,13:311–317

142. Gordon DB, Pellino TA, Miaskowski C, et al. A 10-year review of quality improvement monitoring in pain management: recommendations for standardized outcome measures. *Pain Manag Nurs.* 2002,3:116–130

143. American Pain Society, Quality of Care Committee. Quality improvement guidelines for the treatment of acute pain and cancer pain. *JAMA.* 1995,274:1874–1880

All clinical reports from the American Academy of Pediatrics automatically expire 5 years after publication unless reaffirmed, revised, or retired at or before that time.

Role of Pediatricians in Advocating Life Support Training Courses for Parents and the Public

• *Policy Statement*

AMERICAN ACADEMY OF PEDIATRICS

POLICY STATEMENT
Organizational Principles to Guide and Define the Child Health Care System and/or Improve the Health of All Children

Committee on Pediatric Emergency Medicine

Role of Pediatricians in Advocating Life Support Training Courses for Parents and the Public

ABSTRACT. Available literature suggests a need for both initial cardiopulmonary resuscitation basic life support training and refresher courses for parents and the public as well as health care professionals. The promotion of basic life support training courses that establish a pediatric chain of survival spanning from prevention of cardiac arrest and trauma to rehabilitative and follow-up care for victims of cardiopulmonary arrest is advocated in this policy statement and is the focus of an accompanying technical report. Immediate bystander cardiopulmonary resuscitation for victims of cardiac arrest improves survival for out-of-hospital cardiac arrest. Pediatricians will improve the chance of survival of children and adults who experience cardiac arrest by advocating for cardiopulmonary resuscitation training and participating in basic life support training courses as participants and instructors. *Pediatrics* 2004;114:1676; *basic life support training courses, cardiopulmonary resuscitation, CPR, cardiac arrest, community education, parents, school children, automated external defibrillator, chain of survival.*

INTRODUCTION

Childhood out-of-hospital cardiac arrest is a traumatic event for the entire community. Outcome is determined by timeliness of implementation of cardiopulmonary resuscitation. The establishment of a pediatric chain of survival for victims of cardiopulmonary arrest is advocated in this policy statement. Pediatricians are asked to advocate for basic life support training whenever possible in their local community.

RECOMMENDATIONS

1. Pediatricians should promote parental education in pediatric basic life support. Families of children with special health care needs, neonatal intensive care unit graduates, children who have ready access to water, or children who are active in water sports should be especially encouraged to undergo training and should be assisted in obtaining access to the training.

2. Pediatricians should encourage and collaborate with parents to promote basic life support training for adolescents, parents, caregivers, school personnel, youth leaders, and coaches to build the "chain of survival" in the community.

3. Basic life support training for the aforementioned groups should be advocated in policy advisory discussions at all governmental levels with a goal of making the training readily available and affordable.

4. Pediatricians and pediatric subspecialty providers should lead by example by taking and teaching basic life support training courses.

COMMITTEE ON PEDIATRIC EMERGENCY MEDICINE, 2002–2003
*Jane F. Knapp, MD, Chairperson
Thomas Bojko, MD
Margaret A. Dolan, MD
Ronald A. Furnival, MD
Steven E. Krug, MD
Deborah Mulligan-Smith, MD
Richard M. Ruddy, MD
Kathy N. Shaw, MD, MSCE
*Lee A. Pyles, MD, Past Committee Member

LIAISONS
Jane Ball, RN, DrPH
    EMSC National Resource Center
Kathleen Brown, MD
    National Association of EMS Physicians
Dan Kavanaugh, MSW
    Maternal and Child Health Bureau
Sharon E. Mace, MD
    American College of Emergency Physicians
David W. Tuggle, MD
    American College of Surgeons

STAFF
Susan Tellez

* Lead authors

doi:10.1542/peds.2004-2020
PEDIATRICS (ISSN 0031 4005). Copyright © 2004 by the American Academy of Pediatrics.

School-Based Mental Health Services

- *Policy Statement*

AMERICAN ACADEMY OF PEDIATRICS

POLICY STATEMENT
Organizational Principles to Guide and Define the Child Health Care System and/or Improve the Health of All Children

Committee on School Health

School-Based Mental Health Services

ABSTRACT. More than 20% of children and adolescents have mental health problems. Health care professionals for children and adolescents must educate key stakeholders about the extent of these problems and work together with them to increase access to mental health resources. School-based programs offer the promise of improving access to diagnosis of and treatment for the mental health problems of children and adolescents. Pediatric health care professionals, educators, and mental health specialists should work in collaboration to develop and implement effective school-based mental health services. *Pediatrics* 2004;113:1839–1845; *school, mental health, school-based health center, SBHC, medical home, adolescent, prevention, intervention, confidentiality, assessment, referral, evaluation, school counselor, risk behavior, resilience, individualized education program, IEP, therapy, special education, special needs, curricular, managed care, emotional disorder.*

ABBREVIATIONS. SBHC, school-based health center; AAP, American Academy of Pediatrics; IEP, individualized education program.

"The burden of suffering experienced by children with mental health needs and their families has created a health crisis in this country."[1]

David Satcher, MD, PhD

Pediatric health care professionals increasingly are becoming aware of the high level of mental health needs of children. School violence, high dropout rates, bullying, high suicide and homicide rates, and increased levels of high-risk behaviors are reported commonly across the United States. The human and economic toll of inadequately addressing these mental health problems is significant. Untreated mental health disorders lead to higher rates of juvenile incarcerations, school dropout, family dysfunction, drug abuse, and unemployment.

The proportion of pediatric patients in which psychosocial problems are seen in primary care has increased from 7% to 19% over the past 20 years.[2] According to the 2001 US Surgeon General's report on children's mental health,[1] 20% of children need active mental health interventions, 11% have significant functional impairment, and 5% have extreme functional impairment. These data were derived from the Methodology for Epidemiology of Mental Disorders in Children and Adolescents study, which also found that 13% of children and adolescents have anxiety disorders, 6.2% have mood disorders, 10.3% have disruptive disorders, and 2% have substance abuse disorders, for a total of 20.9% having 1 or more mental health disorders. The Great Smoky Mountain Study of Youth found that 27% of children 9, 11, and 13 years of age have mental health impairment and 20% have a diagnosable mental health condition. This study also found that only 21% of children with mental health problems receive mental health services.[3] Similarly, the Ontario Child Health Study found that only 20% of children with emotional disorders had received mental or social services during the 6 months before the survey despite existence of universal health insurance in Canada.[4] Mental health and substance abuse issues are the most common reasons for visits to school-based health centers (SBHCs).[5]

Another potential indicator of the mental health of our children and adolescents may be the prevalence of risk behaviors. In the 2001 Youth Risk Behavior Survey coordinated by the Centers for Disease Control and Prevention, 30% of youth reported episodic heavy drinking, 14% reported frequent cigarette use, 24% reported using marijuana within the last month, and 9% reported a suicide attempt during the past 12 months.[6] In the United States, suicide is the third leading cause of death in youth 10 to 19 years of age. Homicide is the fourth leading cause of death for children 5 to 14 years of age and the second leading cause of death for youth 15 to 19 years of age.[7]

Acknowledging that mental health needs are significant, physicians must identify and address the barriers to mental health services. A recent American Academy of Pediatrics (AAP) policy statement addressed insurance and managed care barriers.[8] Many families will not address their mental health needs if their health insurance does not offer adequate coverage. Additional barriers include lack of transportation, financial constraints, child mental health professional shortages, and stigmas related to mental health problems. These barriers may help to explain why 40% to 60% of families who begin therapy terminate prematurely[9] and why most people attend only 1 to 2 sessions before terminating services.[10] Another significant barrier is the paucity of training in medical school and primary care residency programs. Pediatricians often are professionally unprepared and usually have inadequate appointment

PEDIATRICS (ISSN 0031 4005). Copyright © 2004 by the American Academy of Pediatrics.

time to address the mental health needs of children and adolescents. As a result, pediatricians may not uncover significant mental health problems. The medical home model does not require that pediatricians personally provide all services required by the families and children that they treat. This can be accomplished through collaboration and coordination with other agencies, such as mental health agencies, or mental health services provided in schools. Pediatricians can enhance the medical home model by improving communication with schools on mental health concerns of their patients and can improve access to mental health services by encouraging and supporting school-based mental health services.

School-based mental health services are evolving as a strategy to address these concerns by removing barriers to accessing mental health services and improving coordination of those services. School-based mental health services offer the potential for prevention efforts as well as intervention strategies. More than 75% of pediatricians support the provision of psychological and counseling services in schools, which include assessments, interventions, and referrals.[11] Schools are the primary providers of mental health services for many children.[3,12,13] School-based mental health services range from minimal support services provided by a school counselor to a comprehensive, integrated program of prevention, identification, and treatment within a school. In some schools, comprehensive mental health services are provided in an SBHC. There are now more than 1300 SBHCs, with most providing mental health services.[14]

SCHOOL-BASED MENTAL HEALTH SERVICES

One way to categorize components of a school or district's mental health program is to consider a 3-tiered model of services and needs. The first tier is an array of preventive mental health programs and services. Activities in this tier need to be ubiquitous so that they target all children in all school settings. Preventive programs are those that focus on decreasing risk factors and building resilience, including providing a positive, friendly, and open social environment at school and ensuring that each student has access to community and family supports that are associated with healthy emotional development. A sense of student "connectedness" to schools has been found to have positive effects on academic achievement and to decrease risky behaviors.[15] For example, schools should provide students with multiple and varied curricular and extracurricular activities, thereby increasing the chances that each student will feel successful in some aspect of school life. Schools also should provide numerous opportunities for positive individual interactions with adults at school so that each student has positive adult role models and opportunities to develop a healthy adult relationship outside his or her family. Schools can provide families with support services and should implement "prevention" curricula (eg, curricula that decrease risk-taking behaviors). Behavioral expectations, rules, and discipline plans should be well publicized and enforced school-wide. A recent review of

effective programs is available for schools and those who advise schools on development of their preventive programs.[16]

The second tier consists of targeted mental health services that are designed to assist students who have 1 or more identified mental health needs but who function well enough to engage successfully in many social, academic, and other daily activities. Services in this tier would include the provision of group or individual therapy to students. For students in special education for learning problems who also have behavioral problems, this tier also may consist of the behavioral components of these students' individualized education programs (IEPs) or individual health service plans that address these students' behavioral issues.

The third tier of health services targets the smallest population of students and addresses needs of children with severe mental health diagnoses and symptoms. These students require the services of a multidisciplinary team of professionals, usually including special education services, individual and family therapy, pharmacotherapy, and school and social agency coordination.[17]

Outcome studies on school-based mental health models are limited, as are outcome studies on typical delivery methods of outpatient mental health services. The Bridges Project is a model that uses the 3-tiered model in schools and has demonstrated positive outcomes with improved school attendance, improved school grades, and improved scores on the Child Behavior Checklist and the Behavior and Emotional Rating Scale.[18]

Preventive Strategies

As they develop the first tier of services (a comprehensive mental health prevention program), each school and district should involve school nurses; pediatricians and other primary care physicians; mental health, social services, and other community agencies; and parents. The program should include: 1) multiple opportunities for students to build developmental assets and resilience to other stresses[19]; 2) behavior and discipline plans; and 3) mental health curricula (eg, violence prevention[20]) that are incorporated into other health education curricula (refer to Fig 1 for a visual description of these tiers of mental health in schools).

Behavior and discipline plans should be school-wide and provide clear and consistent behavior expectations and consequences. School staff training should teach educators, administrators, and support staff specific fundamentals: 1) building a supportive school environment; 2) the essential components of behavior management techniques; and 3) early recognition of mental health problems. Many schools have prepared teachers, school nurses, and other staff members successfully to volunteer in student assistance programs, whereby these staff members lead after-school support groups designed to help students express themselves to their peers and adults within a safe, comfortable environment.

Schools should have multidisciplinary student-support teams that include school nurses, school

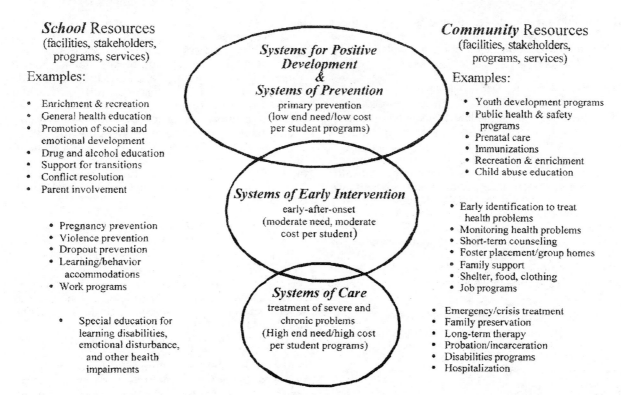

Fig 1. A comprehensive, multifaceted, and integrated approach to addressing barriers to learning and promoting healthy development. Adapted from various public domain documents written by H.S. Adelman and L. Taylor and circulated through the Center for Mental Health in Schools at the University of California (Los Angeles).

personnel, mental health consultants, and school physicians to review and plan evaluations and intervention strategies for students experiencing problems at school or otherwise identified as having potential mental health problems.

Schools can develop relationships with agencies that assist them with external stressors for students, including but not limited to housing, nutrition, clothing, employment, safety in their neighborhood, and after-school care. Support services for families can be established through the development of collaborative relationships with family resource centers. Other social agencies, public health departments, and providers of community-based services are also important partners.

Advantages of Basing Mental Health Services at School

Unlike preventive mental health services and those related to special education, the provision of other mental health services such as individual, group, or family counseling is optional for schools, yet many schools realize the value of helping families meet mental health needs and recognize distinct advantages to providing these services within the school system. One advantage of the familiar setting of school for provision of mental health services is that students and families avoid the stigma and intimidation they may feel when they go to an unfamiliar and perhaps less culturally compatible mental health settings. Of course, receiving services at school may put students at risk of another form of stigmatization, that is, stigmatization by their peers.

This issue must be addressed on both a programmatic level (eg, discretion, strategic scheduling of appointments, private waiting areas) and individually with each student receiving services. Providing school-based mental health services eliminates the need for transportation of students to and from off-site appointments and facilitates parent participation in mental health appointments, because many parents live within walking distance of neighborhood schools. These advantages may encourage more parents to seek mental health care for their children and more students to self-refer for treatment. Kaplan et al[21] showed that adolescents with access to SBHCs with mental health services were 10 times more likely than students without such access to initiate a visit for a mental health or substance abuse concern (98% of such visits were at an SBHC). The convenience and comfort of having school-based mental health services also may promote a longer-lasting commitment to following through with all recommended therapy.

In addition to eliminating barriers to access to care, school-based mental health services offer the potential to improve accuracy of diagnosis as well as assessment of progress. One of the major challenges to providing mental health services to students is gaining access to information concerning the functionality of the student in various environments. Schools have a wealth of opportunities to acquire information on how children deal with physical and social stresses and challenges and on how they perform in the academic setting, on community-related roles in which children engage (eg, in sports, with younger children as a mentor, etc), and on the nature and extent of many sorts of interpersonal relationships (eg, adults, peers).

Mental Health Service Delivery Models

Schools have a convoluted history of involvement in mental health since the late 1890s, when psychology clinics were placed in some schools in Philadelphia, Pennsylvania.[22] Today, some schools have mental health curricula and offer students the services of a wide array of social and mental health professionals, including social workers; guidance counselors; school psychologists; mental health therapists providing group, child, and/or family therapy; and mental health units within SBHCs. These services may be provided by schools or public or private mental health professionals or agencies. The following 3 models are not mutually exclusive. Many schools offer components of more than 1 of these models.

1. School-supported mental health models
   - Social workers, guidance counselors, and school psychologists are employed directly by the school system.
   - Separate mental health units exist within the school system.
   - School nurses serve as a major portal of entry for students with mental health concerns.
2. Community connections models
   - A mental health agency or individual delivers direct services in the school part-time or full-time under contract.
   - Mental health professionals are available within an SBHC or are invited into after-school programs.
   - There is a formal linkage to an off-site mental health professional and/or to a managed care organization.
3. Comprehensive, integrated models
   - A comprehensive and integrated mental health program addresses prevention strategies, school environment, screening, referral, special education, and family and community issues and delivers direct mental health services.
   - SBHCs provide comprehensive and integrated health and mental health services within the school environment.

A recent pilot study[23] on cost of care reported that school-based mental health services were less expensive than private or community-based mental health services. Therefore, cost of providing mental health services at school, versus traditional settings, should not be an inhibiting factor for health insurers (private or Medicaid) and managed care organizations that are already resolved to providing these services somewhere.

Currently, there is great diversity in the scope of mental health services delivered in the school setting. Unfortunately, there is no comprehensive report available on the extent of mental health services offered in schools across the country. Although some schools may not offer any clearly defined mental health programs, most of them offer at least a school guidance counselor. Some schools have specific mental health programs offered on campus through local mental health agencies (multiprofessional groups, outpatient clinics of hospitals, agencies that provide mental health services under Medicaid), local mental health professionals, or arrangements with managed care organizations. Other schools have mental health programs through an SBHC. In a survey of SBHCs performed by Making the Grade,[14] 25% of visits to SBHCs were for mental health reasons. Almost 60% of all SBHCs offer mental health services, averaging 33 hours per week of coverage by a mental health professional.[14]

SPECIAL EDUCATION AND MENTAL HEALTH SERVICES

When providing a mental health service is an integral part of the child's education, the mental health service is mandated by law to be provided by schools. Severe conduct disorders, psychoses, and severe emotional problems are examples of mental health disorders that often impede the student's ability to be educated in a general education program. Rarely, when attention-deficit disorders are not readily treated by medications and the severity precludes students from benefiting from even a modified regular educational program and environment, students with this disorder are placed in a special education program. Services for students with these diagnoses who qualify for special education on the basis of their mental health status may include provision of classrooms with a high teacher-to-student ratio, special education teachers who have been trained to deal with disordered conduct and emotional problems, availability of child psychiatrists and/or psychologists who can help teachers troubleshoot difficult situations, IEPs that include detailed behavior management plans, and ability of the school to deliver multiple medications and monitor the benefits and adverse effects of these medications at school. These services may be provided in either separate or integrated schools. Often, these students attend their neighborhood school but are placed in special classrooms. Other students can be completely integrated with regular education students. Some schools or classrooms operate as day-treatment programs, but they are located on school campuses and have an educational component. As with other services, mental health services provided as part of a student's IEP should allow the student to be in the least restrictive school setting, have clear goals and objectives that are individualized to each student's particular needs, have well-outlined activities that are specifically designed to meet educational program goals, and have designated personnel to carry out the activities. If the school provides transportation to school or school-sponsored extracurricular activities or field trips, accommodations need to be considered so that students do not miss mental health appointments and yet can participate to the fullest extent possible in extracurricular activities. Many of the services that schools provide to these students may be reimbursed through Medicaid programs for students who are eligible for and enrolled in Medicaid.

CHALLENGES IN SCHOOL-BASED MENTAL HEALTH PROGRAMS

Several challenges exist in school-based mental health care. First, services must be coordinated with the medical home (usually this will be a primary care physician), mental health professionals, and social agencies. Otherwise, services may be duplicated or crucial patient needs may be overlooked. Second, services must be integrated within the school environment so that school personnel view the mental health services as an integral part of the educational system. Integration necessitates gaining the support of the school administration and staff, obtaining confidential space, working with school schedules to minimize missed class time, and avoiding turf issues. Third, because parents are a vital element in mental health treatment for children, creative strategies must be devised to solicit parental involvement in school-based intervention services, not merely parental consent. Finally, because confidentiality of mental health information is mandated by law, a well-defined system must be developed. There must be written, informed consent that is designed to protect confidential information but allow sharing of information that pertains to a student's education and socialization at school or that needs to be shared to ensure the safety of students and staff. School staff members must understand and honor confidentiality, and students and parents should be encouraged to allow sharing of information that would improve the student's success at school. Breaking confidentiality should never be taken lightly but would be necessary when a student is thought to be likely to harm himself or herself or others. Without these confidentiality policies, students and their parents will not trust the mental health care system and may undermine the intent of the services. Specific issues regarding adolescent confidentiality are discussed in the AAP policy statement "Confidentiality in Adolescent Health Care."[24]

School staff members and mental health professionals need to be sensitive to the appropriateness of dealing with certain health issues. It may be determined, for example, that for certain students who are victims of sexual abuse, services are more confidentially provided at a site off the school campus.

Screening for mental health illness differs significantly from early identification of mental illness. A screening program, for example, might evaluate all students in a 6th-grade class for mental illness, whereas an early-identification program would educate staff to recognize early signs and symptoms of illness. Many screening tools have been established for mental health and have been shown to be effective when used in physicians' offices. There is not any scientific evidence yet to support performing school-based screening programs using these tools.

RECOMMENDATIONS FOR SCHOOLS

1. The mental health program (preventive strategies and mental health services) should be coordinated with educational programs and other school-based health services. School social workers, guidance counselors, school psychologists, school nurses, and all mental health therapists should plan preventive and intervention strategies together with school administrators and teachers as well as with families and community members.

2. Preventive mental health programs should be developed that include a healthy social environment, clear rules, and expectations that are well publicized. Staff members should be trained to recognize stresses that may lead to mental health problems as well as early signs of mental illness and refer these students to trained professionals within the school setting.

3. Mental health referrals (within the school system as well as to community-based professionals and agencies) should be coordinated by using written protocols, should be monitored for adherence, and should be evaluated for effectiveness.

4. School-based specific diagnostic screenings, such as for depression, should be implemented at school only if they have been supported by peer-reviewed evidence of their effectiveness in that setting.

5. Roles of all the various mental health professionals who work on campus with students should be defined so that they are understood by students, families, all school staff members, and the mental health professionals themselves.

6. Group, individual, and family therapies should be included as schools arrange for direct services to be provided at school sites. Alternatively, referral systems should be available for each of these modes of therapy so that students and families receive the mode of therapy most appropriate to their needs.

7. It should be documented that mental health professionals providing services on site in school (whether hired, contracted, or invited to school sites to provide services) have training specifically in child and adolescent mental health (appropriate for students' ages) and are competent to provide mental health services in the school setting.

8. Private, confidential, and comfortable physical space should be provided at the school site. Often, this is not difficult for schools if mental health services are provided after school hours. Having school-based services should not preclude the opportunity for mental health services to be provided at nonschool sites for situations in which therapy at school for a student may be ill advised (eg, a student who feels uncomfortable discussing a history of sexual abuse at the school setting). During extended school breaks, schools must provide continued access to mental health services.

9. Staff members should be provided with opportunities to consult with a child psychiatrist or clinical psychologist (on or off the school site) so that they may explore specific difficult situations or student behaviors and review school policies,

programs, and protocols related to mental health.

10. Quality-assurance strategies should be developed for mental health services provided at school, and all aspects of the school health program should be evaluated, including satisfaction of the parent, student, third-party payers, and mental health professionals.

11. Confidentiality of health information should be maintained, as mandated by law.

RECOMMENDATIONS FOR PEDIATRICIANS AND OTHER PROVIDERS OF PRIMARY CARE FOR CHILDREN AND ADOLESCENTS

The following recommendations are targeted to individual pediatricians and/or groups of physicians such as local chapters of the AAP:

1. An ecologic view of mental health should be taken, and support structures should be built not just for individual patients but also for the community. Pediatricians should advocate for schools to develop comprehensive mental health programs with a strong preventive component that focuses on building strengths and resilience, not just on problems, and that involves students' families.

2. Pediatricians should develop a relationship with local schools, serve on school health advisory councils, and promote school-based mental health services (as outlined in "Recommendations for Schools").

3. Management of one's own patients with mental health problems should be coordinated with school-based mental health professionals.

4. Mental health services should be included in IEPs for patients enrolled in a special education program.

5. Pediatricians should advocate for financial and institutional changes that are likely to provide medical homes and families with the option of access to mental health services through school settings, such as coverage of school-based mental health services by health insurers and school billing of Medicaid for school-based mental health services payable under this program.

6. Pediatricians should work with schools to help identify strategies and community resources that will augment school-based mental health programs.

7. Outcomes-based research should be performed on the effectiveness of various school-based mental health models that are designed to improve psychosocial and academic outcomes.

8. Pediatricians, through enhanced collaboration and communication with school mental health service professionals, can strengthen the medical-home model and improve the mental health of their patients.

COMMITTEE ON SCHOOL HEALTH, 2002–2003
*Howard L. Taras, MD, Chairperson
Barbara L. Frankowski, MD, MPH
Jane W. McGrath, MD
Cynthia J. Mears, DO

Robert D. Murray, MD
*Thomas L. Young, MD

LIAISONS
Janet Long, MEd
    American School Health Association
Jerald L. Newberry, MEd
    National Education Association, Health Information Network
Mary Vernon-Smiley, MD, MPH
    Centers for Disease Control and Prevention
Janis Hootman, RN, PhD
    National Association of School Nurses

STAFF
Su Li, MPA

Lead authors

REFERENCES

1. US Public Health Service. *Report of the Surgeon General's Conference on Children's Mental Health: A National Action Agenda.* Washington, DC: US Department of Health and Human Services; 2000. Available at: www.surgeongeneral.gov/topics/cmh/childreport.htm. Accessed July 15, 2003

2. Kelleher KJ, McInerny TK, Gardner WP, Childs GE, Wasserman RC. Increasing identification of psychosocial problems: 1979–1996. *Pediatrics.* 2000;105:1313–1321

3. Burns BJ, Costello EJ, Angold A, et al. Children's mental health service use across service sectors. *Health Aff (Millwood).* 1995;14:147–159

4. Links PS, Boyle MH, Offord DR. The prevalence of emotional disorders in children. *J Nerv Ment Dis.* 1989;177:85–91

5. Anglin TM, Naylor KE, Kaplan DW. Comprehensive school-based health care: high school students' use of medical, mental health, and substance abuse services. *Pediatrics.* 1996;97:318–330

6. Centers for Disease Control and Prevention. Youth risk behavior surveillance—United States, 1999. *MMWR CDC Surveill Summ.* 2000;49(5): 1–32

7. Hoyert DL, Freedman MA, Strobino D, Guyer B. Annual summary of vital statistics: 2000. *Pediatrics.* 2001;108:1241–1255

8. American Academy of Pediatrics. Insurance coverage of mental health and substance abuse services for children and adolescents: a consensus statement. *Pediatrics.* 2000;106:860–862

9. Kazdin AE, Holland L, Crowley M. Family experience of barriers to treatment and premature termination from child therapy. *J Consult Clin Psychol.* 1997;65:453–463

10. Armbruster P, Fallon T. Clinical, sociodemographic, and systems risk factors for attrition in a children's mental health clinic. *Am J Orthopsychiatry.* 1994;64:577–585

11. Barnett S, Duncan P, O'Conner KG. Pediatricians' response to the demand for school health programming. *Pediatrics.* 1999;103(4). Available at: www.pediatrics.org/cgi/content/full/103/4/e45

12. Hoagwood K, Erwin HD. Effectiveness of school-based mental health services for children: a 10 year research review. *J Child Fam Stud.* 1997;6:435–451

13. Catron T, Weiss B. The Vanderbilt School-Based Counseling Program: an interagency, primary-care model of mental health services. *J Emot Behav Disord.* 1994;2:247–253

14. Center for Health and Healthcare in Schools. *School-Based Health Centers: Results From a 50 State Survey. School Year 1999–2000.* Washington, DC: George Washington University; 2001

15. Resnick MD, Bearman PS, Blum RW, et al. Protecting adolescents from harm. Findings from the National Longitudinal Study on Adolescent Health. *JAMA.* 1997;278:823–832

16. Greenberg MT, Domitrovich C, Bumbarger B. *Preventing Mental Health Disorders in School-Age Children: A Review of the Effectiveness of Prevention Programs.* University Park, PA: Prevention Research Center, Penn State University; 1999. Available at: www.prevention.psu.edu. Accessed July 15, 2003

17. Policy Leadership Cadre for Mental Health in Schools. *Mental Health in Schools: Guidelines, Models, Resources, and Policy Considerations.* Los Angeles, CA: University of California-Los Angeles, Center for Mental Health in Schools; 2001

18. Robbins V, Armstrong B, Collins K. The Bridges Project: closing the gap between schools, families, and mental health services for all children and youth. *Community Mental Health Report.* July 2002:67–70

19. Starkman W, Scales P, Roberts C. *Great Places to Learn: How Asset Building Schools Help Students Succeed.* Minneapolis, MN: Search Institute; 1999

20. Grossman DC, Neckerman HJ, Koepsell TD, et al. Effectiveness of a violence prevention curriculum among children in elementary school. A randomized controlled trial. *JAMA.* 1997;277:1605–1611

21. Kaplan DW, Calonge BN, Guernsey BP, Hanrahan MB. Managed care and school-based health centers. Use of health services. *Arch Pediatr Adolesc Med.* 1998;152:25–33

22. Sedlak MW. The uneasy alliance of mental health services and the schools: an historical perspective. *Am J Orthopsychiatry.* 1997;67:349–362

23. Nabors LA, Leff SS, Mettrick JE. Assessing the costs of school-based mental health services. *J Sch Health.* 2001;71:199–200

24. American Academy of Pediatrics. Confidentiality in adolescent health care. *AAP News.* April 1989;5:9

All policy statements from the American Academy of Pediatrics automatically expire 5 years after publication unless reaffirmed, revised, or retired at or before that time.

Sexual Orientation and Adolescents

• *Clinical Report*

AMERICAN ACADEMY OF PEDIATRICS

CLINICAL REPORT
Guidance for the Clinician in Rendering Pediatric Care

Barbara L. Frankowski, MD, MPH; and the Committee on Adolescence

Sexual Orientation and Adolescents

ABSTRACT. The American Academy of Pediatrics issued its first statement on homosexuality and adolescents in 1983, with a revision in 1993. This report reflects the growing understanding of youth of differing sexual orientations. Young people are recognizing their sexual orientation earlier than in the past, making this a topic of importance to pediatricians. Pediatricians should be aware that some youths in their care may have concerns about their sexual orientation or that of siblings, friends, parents, relatives, or others. Health care professionals should provide factual, current, nonjudgmental information in a confidential manner. All youths, including those who know or wonder whether they are not heterosexual, may seek information from physicians about sexual orientation, sexually transmitted diseases, substance abuse, or various psychosocial difficulties. The pediatrician should be attentive to various potential psychosocial difficulties, offer counseling or refer for counseling when necessary and ensure that every sexually active youth receives a thorough medical history, physical examination, immunizations, appropriate laboratory tests, and counseling about sexually transmitted diseases (including human immunodeficiency virus infection) and appropriate treatment if necessary.

Not all pediatricians may feel able to provide the type of care described in this report. Any pediatrician who is unable to care for and counsel nonheterosexual youth should refer these patients to an appropriate colleague. *Pediatrics* 2004;113:1827–1832; *sexual orientation, adolescents, homosexuality, gay, lesbian, bisexual.*

ABBREVIATIONS. STD, sexually transmitted disease; HIV, human immunodeficiency virus; AAP, American Academy of Pediatrics; AIDS, acquired immunodeficiency syndrome.

INTRODUCTION

Pediatricians are being asked with increasing frequency to address questions about sexual behavior and sexual orientation. It is important that pediatricians be able to discuss the range of sexual orientation with all adolescents and be competent in dealing with the needs of patients who are gay, lesbian, bisexual, or transgendered or who may not identify themselves as such but who are experiencing confusion with regard to their sexual orientation. Young people whose sexual orientation is not heterosexual can have risks to their physical, emo-

tional, and social health, primarily because of societal stigma, which can result in isolation.[1,2] Because self-awareness of sexual orientation commonly occurs during adolescence, the pediatrician should be available to youth who are struggling with sexual orientation issues and support a healthy passage through the special challenges of the adolescent years. Pediatricians may be called on to help parents, siblings, and extended families of nonheterosexual youth. Also, nonheterosexual youth and adults are part of peer groups with whom all pediatric patients and their parents spend time in the neighborhood, at school, or at work. Thus, pediatricians may be called on to help promote better understanding of issues involving nonheterosexual youth.

Gay, lesbian, and bisexual people in the United States have unique health risks. The US Department of Health and Human Services has identified 29 *Healthy People 2010* objectives in which disparities exist between homosexual or bisexual persons and heterosexual persons. These focus areas include access to care, educational and community-based programs, family planning, immunization and infectious disease, sexually transmitted diseases (STDs) including human immunodeficiency virus (HIV) infection, injury and violence prevention, mental health and mental disorders, substance abuse, and tobacco use.[3]

DEFINITIONS

Sexual orientation[4,5] refers to an individual's pattern of physical and emotional arousal toward other persons. Heterosexual individuals are attracted to persons of the opposite sex, homosexual individuals are attracted to persons of the same sex, and bisexual individuals are attracted to persons of both sexes. Homosexual males are often referred to as "gay"; homosexual females are often referred to as "lesbian." In contrast, gender identity is the knowledge of oneself as being male or female, and gender role is the outward expression of maleness or femaleness. Gender identity and gender role usually conform to anatomic sex in both heterosexual and homosexual individuals. Exceptions to this are transgendered individuals and transvestites. Transgendered individuals feel themselves to be of a gender different from their biological sex; their gender identity does not match their anatomic or chromosomal sex. Transvestites are individuals who dress in the clothing of the opposite gender and derive pleasure from such ac-

The guidance in this report does not indicate an exclusive course of treatment or serve as a standard of medical care. Variations, taking into account individual circumstances, may be appropriate.
PEDIATRICS (ISSN 0031 4005). Copyright © 2004 by the American Academy of Pediatrics.

tions; their gender role does not match societal norms. Transgendered individuals and transvestites can be heterosexual, homosexual, or bisexual.

Sexual orientation is not synonymous with sexual activity or sexual behavior (the way one chooses to express one's sexual feelings). Certain sexual behaviors can put individuals of any sexual orientation at risk of pregnancy (penile-vaginal sexual intercourse) and/or certain diseases (penile-vaginal, oral, and anal sexual intercourse). Especially during adolescence, individuals may participate in a variety of sexual behaviors. Many homosexual adults report having relationships and sexual activity with persons of the opposite sex as adolescents,[6,7] and many adults who identify themselves as heterosexual report sexual activity with persons of the same sex during adolescence.[8-10] Also, many youth label themselves as gay, lesbian, or bisexual years after labeling their attractions as such.[11] In addition, adolescents may also self-identify as nonheterosexual without ever being sexually active. Pediatricians need to understand that they should inquire about sexual attraction or orientation even when youth do not report being gay or lesbian.

ETIOLOGY AND PREVALENCE

Homosexuality has existed in most societies for as long as recorded descriptions of sexual beliefs and practices have been available.[4] Societal attitudes toward homosexuality have had a decisive effect on the extent to which individuals have hidden or made known their sexual orientation.

Human sexual orientation most likely exists as a continuum from solely heterosexual to solely homosexual. In 1973, the American Psychiatric Association reclassified homosexuality as a sexual orientation or expression and not a mental disorder.[12] The mechanisms for the development of a particular sexual orientation remain unclear, but the current literature and most scholars in the field state that one's sexual orientation is not a choice; that is, individuals do not choose to be homosexual or heterosexual.[8,11]

A variety of theories about the influences on sexual orientation have been proposed.[5] Sexual orientation probably is not determined by any one factor but by a combination of genetic, hormonal, and environmental influences.[2] In recent decades, biologically based theories have been favored by experts. The high concordance of homosexuality among monozygotic twins and the clustering of homosexuality in family pedigrees support biological models. There is some evidence that prenatal androgen exposure influences development of sexual orientation, but postnatal sex steroid concentrations do not vary with sexual orientation. The reported association in males between homosexual orientation and loci on the X chromosome remains to be replicated. Some research has shown neuroanatomic differences between homosexual and heterosexual persons in sexually dimorphic regions of the brain.[5] Although there continues to be controversy and uncertainty as to the genesis of the variety of human sexual orientations, there is no scientific evidence that abnormal parenting, sexual abuse, or other adverse life events influence sexual orientation.[4,5] Current knowledge suggests that sexual orientation is usually established during early childhood.[1,2,4,5]

The estimated proportion of Americans who are homosexual is imprecise at best, because surveys are hampered by the stigmatization and the climate of fear that still surround homosexuality. Past studies asked more often about sexual behavior and not sexual orientation. Kinsey et al,[9,13] from their studies in the 1930s and 1940s, reported that 37% of adult men and 13% of adult women had at least 1 sexual experience resulting in orgasm with a person of the same sex and that 4% of adult men and 2% of adult women are exclusively homosexual in their behavior and fantasies. A more recent review of various US studies estimated that 2% of men are exclusively homosexual and 3% are bisexual.[14] Other current studies conclude that somewhere between 3% and 10% of the adult population is gay or lesbian, and perhaps a larger percentage is bisexual.[4,5] Sorenson[15] surveyed a group of 16- to 19-year-olds and reported that 6% of females and 17% of males had at least 1 sexual experience with a person of the same sex. Remafedi et al,[10] in a large, population-based study of junior and senior high school students performed in the late 1980s that measured sexual fantasy, emotional attraction, and sexual behavior, found that more than 25% of 12-year-old students felt uncertain about their sexual orientation. This uncertainty decreased with the passage of time and increasing sexual experience to only 5% of 18-year-old students. Only 1.1% of students reported themselves as predominantly homosexual or bisexual. However, 4.5% reported primary sexual attractions to persons of the same sex, which better reflects actual sexual orientation. The Garofalo et al study,[16] based on the 1995 Massachusetts Youth Risk Behavior Survey, found that 2.5% of youth self-identified as gay, lesbian, or bisexual.

These data illustrate the complexity of labeling sexual orientation in adolescents. Health care professionals should be aware that a large number of adolescents have questions about their sexual feelings; some are attracted to and may have sexual relations with people of the same sex, and a small number may know themselves to be gay or lesbian.

SPECIAL NEEDS OF NONHETEROSEXUAL AND QUESTIONING YOUTH

The overall goal in caring for youth who are or think they might be gay, lesbian, or bisexual is the same as for all youth: to promote normal adolescent development, social and emotional well-being, and physical health. If their environment is critical of their emerging sexual orientation, these adolescents may experience profound isolation and fear of discovery, which interferes with achieving developmental tasks of adolescence related to self-esteem, identity, and intimacy.[17,18] Nonheterosexual youth often are subjected to harassment and violence; 45% of gay men and 20% of lesbians surveyed were victims of verbal and physical assaults in secondary school specifically because of their sexual orientation.[1,19]

Nonheterosexual youth are at higher risk of dropping out of school, being kicked out of their homes, and turning to life on the streets for survival. Some of these youth engage in substance use, and they are more likely than heterosexual peers to start using tobacco, alcohol, and illegal drugs at an earlier age.[20] Nonheterosexual youth are more likely to have had sexual intercourse, to have had more partners, and to have experienced sexual intercourse against their will,[20] putting them at increased risk of STDs including HIV infection. In a recent study of HIV seroprevalence, 7% of 3492 15- to 22-year-old males who have sex with males living in 7 US cities were HIV-seropositive. Among adolescent males who have sex with males, HIV seroprevalence rates in descending order were highest among black adolescents, then "mixed race or other" adolescents, and then Hispanic adolescents and were lowest among Asian and white adolescents.[21] Women having sex with women have the lowest risk of any STD, but lesbian adolescents remain at significant risk because they are likely to have had sexual intercourse with males. Youth in high school who identify themselves as gay, lesbian, or bisexual; engage in sexual activity with persons of the same sex; or report same-sex romantic attractions or relationships are more likely to attempt suicide, be victimized, and abuse substances.[20,22] Although only representing a portion of youth who someday will self-identify as gay, lesbian, or bisexual, school-based studies have found that these adolescents, compared with heterosexual peers, are 2 to 7 times more likely to attempt suicide,[16,19,23,24] are 2 to 4 times more likely to be threatened with a weapon at school,[16,23] and are more likely to engage in frequent and heavy use of alcohol, marijuana, and cocaine. It is important to note that these psychosocial problems and suicide attempts in nonheterosexual youth are neither universal nor attributable to homosexuality per se, but they are significantly associated with stigmatization of gender nonconformity, stress, violence, lack of support, dropping out of school, family problems, acquaintances' suicide attempts, homelessness, and substance abuse.[2,25] In addition to suicidality, young gay and bisexual men might also suffer body image dissatisfaction and disordered eating behaviors for some of the same reasons.[26]

Nonheterosexual youth are represented within all populations of adolescents, all social classes, and all racial and ethnic groups. Ethnic minority youth who are nonheterosexual are required to manage more than one stigmatized identity, which increases their level of vulnerability and stress.[27] They retain their minority status when they seek help in the predominately white gay and lesbian support communities. In addition, sexual minority youth are represented among handicapped adolescents, homeless adolescents, and incarcerated youth.[1]

Most nonheterosexual youths are "invisible" and will pass through pediatricians' offices without raising the issue of sexual orientation on their own. Therefore, health care professionals should raise issues of sexual orientation and sexual behavior with all adolescent patients or refer them to a colleague who can. Such discussions normalize the notion that

there is a range of sexual orientation. The portrayal of openly gay or lesbian characters in media is starting to change how adolescents view these differences. Even adolescents who are quite sure of their own heterosexuality are likely to have friends, relatives, teachers, etc whom they know or suspect to be gay or lesbian or who are struggling with questions about their sexual orientation. Rather than asking patients whether they have a "boyfriend" or "girlfriend," pediatricians could ask, "Have you ever had a romantic relationship with a boy or a girl?" or "When you think of people to whom you are sexually attracted, are they men, women, both, neither, or are you not sure yet?" By doing so, pediatricians open the door to additional communication and start to break down stereotypes and stigmatization. It implies that any of the options is possible and that an adolescent may not be sure of his or her sexual orientation. If these issues are addressed, specifically targeted medical screening, medical treatment, and anticipatory guidance can be provided to adolescents who need it. Pediatricians can have an important positive effect on young people and their families by addressing sexual orientation and sexual behavior on several levels: office and hospital policies, clinical care, and community advocacy.[2]

OFFICE PRACTICE: ENSURE A SAFE AND SUPPORTIVE ENVIRONMENT

A pediatric encounter may give adolescents a rare opportunity to discuss their concerns about their sexual orientation and/or activities. Adolescents' level of comfort in the pediatric office sets the tone for their other health care interactions. The way sexuality and other important personal issues are discussed also sets an example for all adolescents and their parents. In the office, pediatricians are encouraged to[28]:

1. Assure the patient that his or her confidentiality is protected.[29]
2. Implement policies against insensitive or inappropriate jokes and remarks by office staff.
3. Be sure that information forms use gender-neutral, nonjudgmental language.
4. Consider displaying posters, brochures, and information on bulletin boards that demonstrate support of issues important to nonheterosexual youth and their families (eg, the American Academy of Pediatrics [AAP] brochure "Gay, Lesbian, and Bisexual Teens: Facts for Teens and their Parents").
5. Provide information about support groups and other resources to nonheterosexual youth and their friends and families if requested.

COMPREHENSIVE HEALTH CARE FOR ALL ADOLESCENTS

Pediatricians are not responsible for labeling or even identifying nonheterosexual youth. Instead, the pediatrician should create a clinical environment in which clear messages are given that sensitive personal issues including sexual orientation can be discussed whenever the adolescent feels ready to do so. A major obstacle to effective medical care is adolescents' misunderstanding of their right to confidential care.[30] The pediatrician should be ready to raise and discuss issues of sexual orientation with all adolescents, particularly those in distress or engaged in high-risk behaviors. The pediatrician should be able to explore the adolescent's understanding and concerns about sexual orientation, dispel any misconceptions, provide appropriate medical care and anticipatory guidance, and connect the adolescent to appropriate supportive community resources. Pediatricians are encouraged to[29,31]:

1. Be aware of the special issues surrounding the development of sexual orientation.[29]
2. Assure the patient that his or her confidentiality is protected.[29]
3. Discuss emerging sexuality with all adolescents.[32]
   - Be knowledgeable that many heterosexual youth also may have sexual experiences with people of their own sex. Labeling as homosexual an adolescent who has had sexual experiences with persons of the same sex or is questioning his or her sexual orientation could be premature, inappropriate, and counterproductive.
   - Use gender-neutral language in discussing sexuality; use the word "partner" rather than "boyfriend" or "girlfriend," and talk about "protection" rather than just "birth control."
   - Give evidence of support and acceptance to adolescents questioning their sexual orientation.
   - Provide information and resources regarding gay, lesbian, and bisexual issues to all interested adolescents.
   - Ask all adolescents about risky behaviors, depression, and suicidal thoughts.
   - Encourage abstinence, discourage multiple partners, and provide "safer sex" guidelines to all adolescents.[33] Discuss the risks associated with anal intercourse for those who choose to engage in this behavior, and teach them ways to decrease risk.
   - Counsel all adolescents about the link between substance use (alcohol, marijuana, and other drugs) and unsafe sexual intercourse.
   - Ask all adolescents about personal experience with violence including sexual or intimate-partner violence.

   Provide additional screening and education as indicated for each adolescent's sexual activity:
   - STD testing from appropriate sites[34]
   - HIV testing with appropriate support and counseling[35]
   - Pregnancy testing and counseling[36,37]
   - Papanicolaou testing
   - Hepatitis B and, when appropriate, hepatitis A immunization
4. Ensure that colleagues to whom adolescents are referred or with whom you consult are respectful of the range of adolescents' sexual orientation.

SPECIAL CONSIDERATIONS FOR NONHETEROSEXUAL YOUTH

For adolescents who self-identify as gay, lesbian, or bisexual, pediatricians should be particularly aware of several points:

1. Be prepared to refer adolescents' care if you have personal barriers to providing such care. Many individuals have strong negative attitudes about homosexuality or may simply feel uncomfortable with the subject. Even discomfort expressed through body language can send a very damaging message to nonheterosexual youth. It is an ethical and professional obligation to make an appropriate referral in these situations for the good of the child or adolescent.
2. Assure the patient that his or her confidentiality is protected.[29] Discuss with adolescents and, if appropriate, their parents whether they wish to have their sexual orientation recorded in office and hospital charts. Many nonheterosexual adults prefer to have this information recorded so that health care professionals will not assume heterosexuality.
3. Help the adolescent think through his or her feelings carefully; strong same-sex feelings and even sexual experiences can occur at this age and do not define sexual orientation.
4. Carefully identify all risky behaviors (sexual behaviors; use of tobacco, alcohol, and drugs; etc) and offer advice and treatment if indicated.
5. Ask about mental health concerns and evaluate or refer patients with identified problems.
6. Offer support and advice to adolescents faced with or anticipating conflicts with families and/or friends.
7. Encourage transition to adult health care when age-appropriate.

Pediatricians should be aware that the revelation of an adolescent's homosexuality (also called disclosure or "coming out") has the potential for intense family discord.[1,2,28] In many families, it precipitates physical and/or emotional abuse or even expulsion. The pediatrician can advise the adolescent to use certain language that may be helpful at the time of disclosure, such as "I am the same person, you just know one more thing about me now." However, there is no one disclosure technique that will preclude negative reactions. Parents, siblings, and other family members may require professional help to deal with their confusion, anger, guilt, and feelings of loss, and professionals who work with adolescents may be required to intervene on the adolescent's behalf. If the pediatrician has a relationship with the parents from ongoing primary care, he or she can be an important initial source of support and information. However, adolescents should be counseled to think carefully about the consequences of disclosure and to take their time in sharing information that could have many repercussions.[1]

With regard to parents of nonheterosexual adolescents, pediatricians are encouraged to:

1. Advise adolescents about whether, when, and how to disclose their nonheterosexuality to their parents. If unsure, assist the adolescent in finding a knowledgeable professional who can help.
2. Be knowledgeable about the process of disclosure.

3. Be supportive of parents of adolescents who have disclosed that they are not heterosexual. Most states have chapters of Parents and Friends of Lesbians and Gays (PFLAG) to which interested families may be referred.
4. Remind parents and adolescents that gay and lesbian individuals can be successful parents themselves.[38-41]
5. Be prepared to refer parents if you do not feel personally comfortable accepting this responsibility.

COMMUNITY ADVOCACY

Despite AAP statements issued in 1983[42] and 1993[43] urging excellent clinical care for nonheterosexual adolescents, these patients still experience many risks to their physical and mental health and safety that occur outside the scope of usual office practice. Some pediatricians may wish to take a broader role in their communities to help decrease these risks. Pediatricians could model and provide opportunities for increasing awareness and knowledge of homosexuality and bisexuality among school staff, mental health professionals, and other community leaders. They can make themselves available as resources for community HIV and acquired immunodeficiency syndrome (AIDS) education and prevention activities. It is critical that schools find a way to create safe and supportive environments for students who are or wonder about being nonheterosexual or who have a parent or other family member who is nonheterosexual. Support from respected pediatricians can facilitate these efforts greatly. Pediatricians who choose to be active on these issues may wish to[2,28]:

1. Help raise awareness among school and community leaders of issues relevant to nonheterosexual youth.
2. Help with the discussion of when and how factual materials about sexual orientation should be included in school curricula and in school and community libraries.
3. Support the development and maintenance of school- and community-based support groups for nonheterosexual students and their friends and parents.
4. Support HIV and AIDS prevention and education efforts.
5. Develop and/or request continuing education opportunities for health care professionals related to issues of sexual orientation, nonheterosexual youth, and their families.

SUMMARY OF PHYSICIAN GUIDELINES

The AAP reaffirms the physician's responsibility to provide comprehensive health care and guidance in a safe and supportive environment for all adolescents, including nonheterosexual adolescents and young people struggling with issues of sexual orientation. Some pediatricians might choose to assume the additional role of advocating for nonheterosexual youth and their families in their communities. The deadly consequences of HIV and AIDS, the damaging effects of violence and ostracism, and the increased prevalence of adolescent suicidal behavior underscore the critical need to address and seek to prevent the major physical and mental health problems that confront nonheterosexual youths in their transition to a healthy adulthood.

COMMITTEE ON ADOLESCENCE, 2002–2003
David W. Kaplan, MD, MPH, Chairperson
Angela Diaz, MD
Ronald A. Feinstein, MD
Martin M. Fisher, MD
Jonathan D. Klein, MD, MPH
W. Samuel Yancy, MD

PAST COMMITTEE MEMBERS
Luis F. Olmedo, MD
Ellen S. Rome, MD, MPH

LIAISONS
S. Paige Hertweck, MD
    American College of Obstetricians and
    Gynecologists
Glen Pearson, MD
    American Academy of Child and Adolescent
    Psychiatry
Miriam E. Kaufman, MD
    Canadian Paediatric Society

Barbara L. Frankowski, MD, MPH
    Past Liaison to Section on School Health
Diane G. Sacks, MD
    Past Liaison From Canadian Paediatric Society

CONSULTANT
Ellen C. Perrin, MD

STAFF
Karen S. Smith

REFERENCES

1. Ryan C, Futterman D. *Lesbian and Gay Youth: Care and Counseling.* New York, NY: Columbia University Press; 1998
2. Perrin EC. *Sexual Orientation in Child and Adolescent Health Care.* New York, NY: Kluwer Academic/Plenum Publishers; 2002
3. Sell RL, Becker JB. Sexual orientation data collection and progress toward Healthy People 2010. *Am J Public Health.* 2001;91:876–882
4. Friedman RC, Downey JI. Homosexuality. *N Engl J Med.* 1994;331:923–930
5. Stronski Huwiler SM, Remafedi G. Adolescent homosexuality. *Adv Pediatr.* 1998;45:107–144
6. Bell AP, Weinberg MS. *Homosexualities: A Study of Diversity Among Men and Women.* New York, NY: Simon and Shuster; 1978
7. Jay K, Young A. *The Gay Report: Lesbians and Gay Men Speak Out About Their Sexual Experiences and Lifestyles.* New York, NY: Summitt Books; 1979
8. Rowlett JD, Patel D, Greydanus DE. Homosexuality. In: Greydanus DE, Wolraich ML, eds. *Behavioral Pediatrics.* New York, NY: Springer-Verlag; 1992:37–54
9. Kinsey AC, Pomeroy WB, Martin CE. *Sexual Behavior in the Human Male.* Philadelphia, PA: WB Saunders Co; 1948
10. Remafedi G, Resnick M, Blum R, Harris L. Demography of sexual orientation in adolescents. *Pediatrics.* 1992;89:714–721
11. Savin-Williams RC. Theoretical perspectives accounting for adolescent homosexuality. *J Adolesc Health Care.* 1988;9:95–104
12. American Psychiatric Association. *Diagnostic and Statistical Manual of Mental Disorders.* 3rd ed. Revised. Washington, DC: American Psychiatric Association; 1987
13. Kinsey AC, Pomeroy WB, Martin CE. *Sexual Behavior in the Human Female.* Philadelphia, PA: WB Saunders Co; 1953
14. Seidman SN, Reider RO. A review of sexual behavior in the United States. *Am J Psychiatry.* 1994;151:330–341
15. Sorenson RC. *Adolescent Sexuality in Contemporary America.* New York, NY: World Publishing; 1973

16. Garofalo R, Wolf RC, Wissow LS, Woods ER, Goodman E. Sexual orientation and risk of suicide attempts among a representative sample of youth. *Arch Pediatr Adolesc Med.* 1999;153:487–493

17. Kreiss JL, Patterson DL. Psychosocial issues in primary care of lesbian, gay, bisexual, and transgender youth. *J Pediatr Health Care.* 1997;11:266–274

18. Remafedi G. Adolescent homosexuality: psychosocial and medical implications. *Pediatrics.* 1987;79:331–337

19. Russell ST, Franz BT, Driscoll AK. Same-sex romantic attraction and experiences of violence in adolescence. *Am J Public Health.* 2001;91:903–906

20. Garofalo R, Wolf RC, Kessel S, Palfrey SJ, DuRant RH. The association between health risk behaviors and sexual orientation among a school-based sample of adolescents. *Pediatrics.* 1998;101:895–902

21. Valleroy LA, MacKellar DA, Karon JM, et al. HIV prevalence and associated risks in young men who have sex with men. *JAMA.* 2000;284:198–204

22. Remafedi G, Farrow JA, Deisher RW. Risk factors for attempted suicide in gay and bisexual youth. *Pediatrics.* 1991;87:869–875

23. Faulkner AH, Cranston K. Correlates of same-sex sexual behavior in a random sample of Massachusetts high school students. *Am J Public Health.* 1998;88:262–266

24. Remafedi G, French S, Story M, Resnick MD, Blum R. The relationship between suicide risk and sexual orientation: results of a population-based study. *Am J Public Health.* 1998;88:57–60

25. Remafedi G. Sexual orientation and youth suicide. *JAMA.* 1999;282:1291–1292

26. French SA, Story M, Remafedi G, Resnick MD, Blum RW. Sexual orientation and prevalence of body dissatisfaction and eating disordered behaviors: a population-based study of adolescents. *Int J Eat Disord.* 1996;19:119–126

27. Savin-Williams RC, Cohen KM. *The Lives of Lesbians, Gays, and Bisexuals: Children to Adults.* Fort Worth, TX: Harcourt Brace College Publishing; 1996

28. Perrin EC. Pediatricians and gay and lesbian youth. *Pediatr Rev.* 1996;17:311–318

29. American Academy of Pediatrics. Confidentiality in adolescent health care. *AAP News.* April 1989:9. Reaffirmed January 1993

30. Allen LB, Glicken AD, Beach RK, Naylor KE. Adolescent health care experience of gay, lesbian, and bisexual young adults. *J Adolesc Health.* 1998;23:212–220

31. Ryan C, Futterman D. Caring for gay and lesbian teens. *Contemp Pediatr.* 1998;15:107–130

32. American Academy of Pediatrics, Committee on Psychosocial Aspects of Child and Family Health and Committee on Adolescence. Sexuality education for children and adolescents. *Pediatrics.* 2001;108:498–502

33. American Academy of Pediatrics, Committee on Adolescence. Condom use by adolescents. *Pediatrics.* 2001;107:1463–1469

34. American Academy of Pediatrics, Committee on Adolescence. Sexually transmitted diseases. *Pediatrics.* 1994;94:568–572

35. American Academy of Pediatrics, Committee on Pediatric AIDS and Committee on Adolescence. Adolescents and human immunodeficiency virus infection: the role of the pediatrician in prevention and intervention. *Pediatrics.* 2001;107:188–190

36. American Academy of Pediatrics, Committee on Adolescence. Counseling the adolescent about pregnancy options. *Pediatrics.* 1998;101:938–940

37. American Academy of Pediatrics, Committee on Adolescence. Adolescent pregnancy—current trends and issues: 1998. *Pediatrics.* 1999;103:516–520

38. Gold MA, Perrin EC, Futterman D, Friedman SB. Children of gay or lesbian parents. *Pediatr Rev.* 1994;15:354–358

39. Perrin EC. Children whose parents are lesbian or gay. *Contemp Pediatr.* 1998;15:113–130

40. American Academy of Pediatrics, Committee on Psychosocial Aspects of Child and Family Health. Coparent or second-parent adoption by same-sex parents. *Pediatrics.* 2002;109:339–340

41. Benkov L. *Reinventing the Family: The Emerging Story of Lesbian and Gay Parents.* New York, NY: Crown Publishers; 1994

42. American Academy of Pediatrics, Committee on Adolescence. Homosexuality and adolescence. *Pediatrics.* 1983;72:249–250

43. American Academy of Pediatrics, Committee on Adolescence. Homosexuality and adolescence. *Pediatrics.* 1993;92:631–634

Soft Drinks in Schools

• *Policy Statement*

AMERICAN ACADEMY OF PEDIATRICS

POLICY STATEMENT
Organizational Principles to Guide and Define the Child Health Care System and/or Improve the Health of All Children

Committee on School Health

Soft Drinks in Schools

ABSTRACT. This statement is intended to inform pediatricians and other health care professionals, parents, superintendents, and school board members about nutritional concerns regarding soft drink consumption in schools. Potential health problems associated with high intake of sweetened drinks are 1) overweight or obesity attributable to additional calories in the diet; 2) displacement of milk consumption, resulting in calcium deficiency with an attendant risk of osteoporosis and fractures; and 3) dental caries and potential enamel erosion. Contracts with school districts for exclusive soft drink rights encourage consumption directly and indirectly. School officials and parents need to become well informed about the health implications of vended drinks in school before making a decision about student access to them. A clearly defined, district-wide policy that restricts the sale of soft drinks will safeguard against health problems as a result of overconsumption.

BACKGROUND AND INFORMATION

Overweight

Overweight is now the most common medical condition of childhood, with the prevalence having doubled over the past 20 years. Nearly 1 of every 3 children is at risk of overweight (defined as body mass index [BMI] between the 85th and 95th percentiles for age and sex), and 1 of every 6 is overweight (defined as BMI at or above the 95th percentile).[1] Complications of the obesity epidemic include high cholesterol, high blood pressure, type 2 diabetes mellitus, coronary plaque formation, and serious psychosocial implications.[2–6] Annually, obesity-related diseases in adults and children account for more than 300 000 deaths and more than $100 billion per year in treatment costs.[7–9]

Soft Drinks and Fruit Drinks

In the United States, children's daily food selections are excessively high in discretionary, or added, fat and sugar.[10–15] This category of fats and sugars accounts for 40% of children's daily energy intake.[10] Soft drink consumers have a higher daily energy intake than nonconsumers at all ages.[16] Sweetened drinks (fruitades, fruit drinks, soft drinks, etc) constitute the primary source of added sugar in the daily diet of children.[17] High-fructose corn syrup, the principle nutrient in sweetened drinks, is not a problem food when consumed in smaller amounts, but each 12-oz serving of a carbonated, sweetened soft drink contains the equivalent of 10 teaspoons of sugar and 150 kcal. Soft drink consumption increased by 300% in 20 years,[12] and serving sizes have increased from 6.5 oz in the 1950s to 12 oz in the 1960s and 20 oz by the late 1990s. Between 56% and 85% of children in school consume at least 1 soft drink daily, with the highest amounts ingested by adolescent males. Of this group, 20% consume 4 or more servings daily.[16]

Each 12-oz sugared soft drink consumed daily has been associated with a 0.18-point increase in a child's BMI and a 60% increase in risk of obesity, associations not found with "diet" (sugar-free) soft drinks.[18] Sugar-free soft drinks constitute only 14% of the adolescent soft drink market.[19] Sweetened drinks are associated with obesity, probably because overconsumption is a particular problem when energy is ingested in liquid form[20] and because these drinks represent energy added to, not displacing, other dietary intake.[21–23] In addition to the caloric load, soft drinks pose a risk of dental caries because of their high sugar content and enamel erosion because of their acidity.[24]

Calcium

Milk consumption decreases as soft drinks become a favorite choice for children, a transition that occurs between the third and eighth grades.[12,15] Milk is the principle source of calcium in the typical American diet.[11] Dairy products contain substantial amounts of several nutrients, including 72% of calcium, 32% of phosphorus, 26% of riboflavin, 22% of vitamin B_{12}, 19% of protein, and 15% of vitamin A in the US food supply.[25] The percent daily value for milk is considered either "good" or "excellent" for 9 essential nutrients depending on age and gender. Intake of protein and micronutrients is decreased in diets low in dairy products.[19,26] The resulting diminished calcium intake jeopardizes the accrual of maximal peak bone mass at a critical time in life, adolescence.[27] Nearly 100% of the calcium in the body resides in bone.[27] Nearly 40% of peak bone mass is accumulated during adolescence. Studies suggest that a 5% to 10% deficit in peak bone mass may result in a 50% greater lifetime prevalence of hip fracture,[28] a problem certain to worsen if steps are not taken to improve calcium intake among adolescents.[29]

PEDIATRICS (ISSN 0031 4005). Copyright © 2004 by the American Academy of Pediatrics.

STATEMENT OF PROBLEM

Soft drinks and fruit drinks are sold in vending machines, in school stores, at school sporting events, and at school fund drives. "Exclusive pouring rights" contracts, in which the school agrees to promote one brand exclusively in exchange for money, are being signed in an increasing number of school districts across the country,[30] often with bonus incentives tied to sales.[31] Although they are a new phenomenon, such contracts already have provided schools with more than $200 million in unrestricted revenue.

Some superintendents, school board members, and principals claim that the financial gain from soft drink contracts is an unquestioned "win" for students, schools, communities, and taxpayers.[31,32] Parents and school authorities generally are uninformed about the potential risk to the health of their children that may be associated with the unrestricted consumption of soft drinks. The decision regarding which foods will be sold in schools more often is made by school district business officers alone rather than with input from local health care professionals.

Subsidized school lunch programs are associated with a high intake of dietary protein, complex carbohydrates, dairy products, fruits, and vegetables.[16] The US Department of Agriculture, which oversees the National School Lunch Program, is concerned that foods with high sugar content (especially foods of minimal nutritional value, such as soft drinks) are displacing nutrients within the school lunch program, and there is evidence to support this.[26]

There are precedents for using optimal nutrition standards to create a model district-wide school nutrition policy,[33] but this is not yet a routine practice in most states. The discussion engendered by the creation of such a policy would be an important first step in establishing an ideal nutritional environment for students.

RECOMMENDATIONS

1. Pediatricians should work to eliminate sweetened drinks in schools. This entails educating school authorities, patients, and patients' parents about the health ramifications of soft drink consumption. Offerings such as real fruit and vegetable juices, water, and low-fat white or flavored milk provide students at all grade levels with healthful alternatives. Pediatricians should emphasize the notion that every school in every district shares a responsibility for the nutritional health of its student body.

2. Pediatricians should advocate for the creation of a school nutrition advisory council comprising parents, community and school officials, food service representatives, physicians, school nurses, dietitians, dentists, and other health care professionals. This group could be one component of a school district's health advisory council. Pediatricians should ensure that the health and nutritional interests of students form the foundation of nutritional policies in schools.

3. School districts should invite public discussion before making any decision to create a vended food or drink contract.

4. If a school district already has a soft drink contract in place, it should be tempered such that it does not promote overconsumption by students.
   - Soft drinks should not be sold as part of or in competition with the school lunch program, as stated in regulations of the US Department of Agriculture.[34]
   - Vending machines should not be placed within the cafeteria space where lunch is sold. Their location in the school should be chosen by the school district, not the vending company.
   - Vending machines with foods of minimal nutritional value, including soft drinks, should be turned off during lunch hours and ideally during school hours.
   - Vended soft drinks and fruit-flavored drinks should be eliminated in all elementary schools.
   - Incentives based on the amount of soft drinks sold per student should not be included as part of exclusive contracts.
   - Within the contract, the number of machines vending sweetened drinks should be limited. Schools should insist that the alternative beverages listed in recommendation 1 be provided in preference over sweetened drinks in school vending machines.
   - Schools should preferentially vend drinks that are sugar-free or low in sugar to lessen the risk of overweight.

5. Consumption or advertising of sweetened soft drinks within the classroom should be eliminated.

COMMITTEE ON SCHOOL HEALTH, 2002–2003
Howard L. Taras, MD, Chairperson
Barbara L. Frankowski, MD, MPH
Jane W. McGrath, MD
Cynthia J. Mears, DO
*Robert D. Murray, MD
Thomas L. Young, MD

LIAISONS
Janis Hootman, RN, PhD
    National Association of School Nurses
Janet Long, MEd
    American School Health Association
Jerald L. Newberry, MEd
    National Education Association, Health Information
Mary Vernon-Smiley, MD, MPH
    Centers for Disease Control and Prevention

STAFF
Su Li, MPA

*Lead author

REFERENCES

1. American Academy of Pediatrics, Committee on Nutrition. Prevention of pediatric overweight and obesity. *Pediatrics*. 2003;112:424–430

2. Freedman DS, Dietz WH, Srinivasan SR, Berenson GS. The relation of overweight to cardiovascular risk factors among children and adolescents: the Bogalusa Heart Study. *Pediatrics*. 1999;103:1175–1182

3. Pinhas-Hamiel O, Dolan LM, Daniels SR, Standiford D, Khoury PR, Zeitler P. Increased incidence of non-insulin-dependent diabetes mellitus among adolescents. *J Pediatr*. 1996;128:608–615

4. Ludwig DS, Ebbeling CB. Type 2 diabetes mellitus in children: primary care and public health considerations. *JAMA*. 2001;286:1427–1430

5. Dietz W. Health consequences of obesity in youth: childhood predictors of adult disease. *Pediatrics*. 1998;101:518–525

6. Davison KK, Birch LL. Weight status, parent reaction, and self-concept in five-year-old girls. *Pediatrics*. 2001;107:46–53

7. Allison DB, Fontaine KR, Manson JE, Stevens J, VanItallie TB. Annual deaths attributable to obesity in the United States. *JAMA*. 1999;282: 1530–1538

8. Must A, Spadano J, Coakley EH, Field AE, Colditz G, Dietz WH. The disease burden associated with overweight and obesity. *JAMA*. 1999; 282:1523–1529

9. Blumenthal D. Controlling health care expenditures. *N Engl J Med*. 2001;344:766–769

10. Muñoz KA, Krebs-Smith SM, Ballard-Barbash R, Cleveland LE. Food intakes of US children and adolescents compared with recommendations. *Pediatrics*. 1997;100:323–329

11. Subar AF, Krebs-Smith SM, Cook A, Kahle LL. Dietary sources of nutrients among US children, 1989–1991. *Pediatrics*. 1998;102:913–923

12. Calvadini C, Siega-Riz AM, Popkin BM. US adolescent food intake trends from 1965 to 1996. *Arch Dis Child*. 2000;83:18–24

13. Borrud LG, Enns CW, Mickle S. What we eat in America: USDA surveys food consumption changes. *Food Rev*. 1996;19:14–19. Available at: http://www.ers.usda.gov/publications/foodreview/sep1996/sept96d.pdf. Accessed February 12, 2003

14. Borrud LG, Mickle S, Nowverl A, Tippett K. *Eating Out in America: Impact on Food Choices and Nutrient Profiles*. Beltsville, MD: Food Surveys Research Group, US Department of Agriculture; 1998. Available at: http://www.barc.usda.gov/bhnrc/foodsurvey/Eatout95.html. Accessed February 12, 2003

15. Lytle LA, Seifert S, Greenstein J, McGovern P. How do children's eating patterns and food choices change over time? Results from a cohort study. *Am J Health Promot*. 2000;14:222–228

16. Gleason P, Suitor C. *Children's Diets in the Mid-1990s: Dietary Intake and Its Relationship with School Meal Participation*. Alexandria, VA: US Department of Agriculture, Food and Nutrition Service, Office of Analysis, Nutrition and Evaluation; 2001. Available at: http://www.fns.usda.gov/oane/menu/published/cnp/files/childiet.pdf. Accessed February 12, 2003

17. Guthrie JF, Morton JF. Food sources of added sweeteners in the diets of Americans. *J Am Diet Assoc*. 2000;100:43–51

18. Ludwig DS, Peterson KE, Gortmaker SL. Relation between consumption of sugar-sweetened drinks and childhood obesity: a prospective observational analysis. *Lancet*. 2001;357:505–508

19. Harnack L, Stang J, Story M. Soft drink consumption among US children and adolescents: nutritional consequences. *J Am Diet Assoc*. 1999; 99:436–441

20. Mattes RD. Dietary compensation by humans for supplemental energy provided as ethanol or carbohydrates in fluids. *Physiol Behav*. 1996;59: 179–187

21. Bellisle F, Rolland-Cachera M-F. How sugar-containing drinks might increase adiposity in children. *Lancet*. 2001;357:490–491

22. Tordoff MG, Alleva AM. Effect of drinking soda sweetened with aspartame or high-fructose corn syrup on food intake and body weight. *Am J Clin Nutr*. 1990;51:963–969

23. De Castro JM, Orozco S. Moderate alcohol intake and spontaneous eating patterns of humans: evidence of unregulated supplementation. *Am J Clin Nutr*. 1990;52:246–253

24. Heller K, Burt BA, Eklund SA. Sugared soda consumption and dental caries in the United States. *J Dent Res*. 2001;80:1949–1953

25. Gerrior S, Bente L. *Nutrient Content of the US Food Supply, 1909–97*. Home Economics Research Report No. 54. Washington, DC: Center for Nutrition Policy and Promotion, US Department of Agriculture; 2001. Available at: http://www.usda.gov/cnpp/Pubs/Food%20Supply/foodsupplyrpt.pdf. Accessed February 12, 2003

26. Johnson RK, Panely C, Wang MQ. The association between noon beverage consumption and the diet quality of school-age children. *J Child Nutr Manage*. 1998;22:95–100

27. American Academy of Pediatrics, Committee on Nutrition. Calcium requirements of infants, children, and adolescents. *Pediatrics*. 1999;104: 1152–1157

28. Wyshak G. Teenaged girls, carbonated beverage consumption, and bone fractures. *Arch Pediatr Adolesc Med*. 2000;154:610–613

29. NIH Consensus Development Panel on Osteoporosis Prevention, Diagnosis, and Therapy. Osteoporosis: prevention, diagnosis, and therapy. *JAMA*. 2001;285:785–795

30. Henry T. Coca-cola rethinks school contracts. Bottlers asked to fall in line. *USA Today*. March 14, 2001:A01

31. Nestle M. Soft drink "pouring rights": marketing empty calories to children. *Public Health Rep*. 2000;115:308–319

32. Zorn RL. The great cola wars: how one district profits from the competition for vending machines. *Am Sch Board J*. 1999;186:31–33

33. Stuhldreher WL, Koehler AN, Harrison MK, Deel H. The West Virginia Standards for School Nutrition. *J Child Nutr Manage*. 1998;22:79–86

34. National School Lunch Program Regulations. 7 CFR §210.11 (2002). Competitive food services

---

All policy statements from the American Academy of Pediatrics automatically expire 5 years after publication unless reaffirmed, revised, or retired at or before that time.

Telemedicine: Pediatric Applications

- *Technical Report*

AMERICAN ACADEMY OF PEDIATRICS

TECHNICAL REPORT

S. Andrew Spooner, MD, MS; Edward M. Gotlieb, MD; and the Steering Committee on
Clinical Information Technology and Committee on Medical Liability

Telemedicine: Pediatric Applications

ABSTRACT. The newly developing field of telemedicine has the potential to benefit pediatric care by increasing access to pediatric specialists and services. This report explores the current uses and limitations of telemedicine in pediatrics. *Pediatrics* 2004;113:e639–e643. URL: http://www.pediatrics.org/cgi/content/full/113/6/e639; *telemedicine, pediatrics, access to care.*

ABBREVIATION. CMS, Centers for Medicaid and Medicare Services.

INTRODUCTION

This report defines telemedicine in pediatrics as the use of electronic communications technology to provide and support health care for infants, children, adolescents, and young adults when distance separates the practitioner from the patient, parent, guardian, or referring practitioner. This definition specifically excludes from discussion the use of ordinary telephone communication between practitioners and patients and the use of communications technology for education of practitioners. This discussion includes what some have termed "e-health," meaning use of the Internet (with or without using videoconference functions) to provide health care.[1]

The information transferred in a telemedicine exchange may include live bidirectional audio or video, recorded audio or video sent after the encounter (so-called "store-and-forward" technology), medical records, medical images, sounds, or output from medical devices such as pulmonary function instruments, electrocardiographs, and ultrasonography devices.

Much has been written about the potential for telemedicine to increase access to care, but applications in pediatrics are sparse. Nevertheless, when telemedicine researchers and application developers apply their efforts to pediatric applications, one would expect that there would be significant benefits to children with special needs or children residing in underserved areas. This report explores the special pediatric needs that may be met by telemedicine. By understanding these needs and the efforts made thus far to develop telemedicine applications to meet those needs, pediatricians and the American Academy of Pediatrics are in a position to develop priorities and agendas for child health advocacy and telemedicine research.[2]

SCOPE OF TELEMEDICINE

It is worth stressing that there is not universal agreement on the scope of the new field of telemedicine. Field[3] defines telemedicine as the use of electronic information and communications to provide and support health care when distance separates the participants. The American Telemedicine Association defines it as the use of medical information exchanged from one site to another via electronic communication for the health and education of the patient or practitioner and for the purpose of improving patient care.[4] This definition of telemedicine would seem to include ordinary telephone communications with patients for the purpose of diagnosis and treatment. Although the use of the telephone to implement care is telemedicine, it usually is not included in telemedicine discussions. The scope of reimbursable telemedicine described under the Medicare Reimbursement for Telehealth Services legislation is much narrower.[5] Within this legislation, the Centers for Medicaid and Medicare Services (CMS [formerly the Health Care Financing Administration]) defines reimbursable telemedicine encounters as "interactive audio and video telecommunications...permitting real-time communication between the distant site physician or practitioner and the Medicare beneficiary." This narrower view specifically excludes store-and-forward methods. In addition, CMS limits reimbursement by Medicare for telemedicine services to beneficiaries who are treated in rural health practice shortage areas. The CMS has not formally defined telemedicine for the Medicaid program, and federal Medicaid law does not recognize telemedicine as a distinct service, but reimbursement is available at a state's option as a cost-effective alternative to traditional care.[2]

CURRENT STATE OF THE FIELD OF TELEMEDICINE

Telemedicine holds considerable promise for pediatrics and pediatricians. Virtually any service can be provided via telecommunications technology, but a rigorous evaluation of telemedicine's potential is

---

PEDIATRICS (ISSN 0031 4005). Copyright © 2004 by the American Academy of Pediatrics.

hampered by a lack of high-quality studies[6] and cost-benefit analyses, especially in pediatrics.[6,7]

Certain pediatric services seem well adapted to telemedicine, including the following.

Radiology

Effective teleradiology programs have been in existence for the last 30 years. Over this period, the profession has developed extensive standards for how images should be stored and displayed to ensure accurate representations.[8,9] Radiology reports are forwarded easily by using secure, low-bandwidth messaging systems. The electronic transmission of images to meet the needs of pediatric care has been well researched[10] and is routine in most medical centers. The implications for providing high-quality pediatric radiology services over broad areas (and concomitant health care workforce redistribution issues) are immense.

Mental Health

Evidence suggests that patients are highly satisfied with psychiatric counseling delivered via telemedicine,[11,12] and this is true also for children.[13,14] Diagnostic accuracy seems to be excellent.[14] Before applying telemedicine applications in mental health, it is important to consider the setting, staff capabilities, and access to information sharing.

Dermatology

Many diagnostic dermatologic evaluations can be performed by using high-quality still images. Although standard video cameras used in teleconferencing systems may not provide enough detail to make a dermatologic diagnosis, special peripheral cameras termed "dermatoscopes" have proved adequate. Remote "teledermatology" consultations have become commonplace at many medical centers.[15]

Cardiology

Cardiology has already widely embraced telemedicine.[16–19] Electronic stethoscopes can facilitate the transmission of heart sounds with excellent fidelity.[20] Echocardiograms, ultrasonographic images, electrocardiograms, and other images can readily be transmitted electronically and evaluated accurately as part of established telecardiology programs.[18]

Emergency and Transport Services

According to one study, teleconferencing provides a way by which practitioners in a remote area can receive real-time emergency consultations with acceptable diagnostic sensitivity and specificity.[21] Emergency teleconferencing may be particularly beneficial for infants and children in rural general emergency departments, in which complex pediatric disease is seen only rarely, giving these patients the benefit of pediatric consultants where none were available previously. One of the most immediately visible cost savings of telemedicine is the decreased need to transport patients to pediatric centers for critical care.[17,18,21]

Hospital Care and Family Communication

The Infant Carelink Program, initially developed at Beth Israel Deaconess Medical Center (Boston, MA), allows families separated from their infants to keep updated on their infants' condition and to view images of their infants while they are in the neonatal intensive care unit.[22,23] Data show that parental satisfaction with care is enhanced by this system. One study showed an increase in the rate of direct discharge home from the neonatal intensive care unit, as opposed to a costly intermediate transfer to a community hospital. Media reports suggest that similar projects are in place at other hospitals.[24]

Pathology

Similar to dermatology and radiology, this visually intensive discipline is readily amenable to telemedicine consultation, especially in developing or rural areas.[25] Telepathology may offer some financial benefits over physical transportation of specimens, and there may be a financial model for pediatric pathology services.[26]

Child Abuse

Expertise in child abuse and neglect and the interdisciplinary communication that often must take place for an adequate child-maltreatment investigation present challenges that telemedicine could help to address.[27] One pilot study on the use of teleconference facilities in the evaluation of child abuse in Florida showed that teleconferencing was acceptable to patients.[28] No evaluation data were provided. There is at least one software package (Second Opinion Software, Gardenia, CA) specifically marketed for the sharing of still photographs in child abuse consultations.

Patient Education and Chronic Disease

Some evidence exists that children who depend on medical equipment have access to improved care by use of telemedicine monitoring.[29] The efficacy of telemedicine in patient education via teleconferencing to teach the proper use of asthma medications has been demonstrated, as has patient satisfaction.[30,31] Similar results have been reported for childhood diabetes teaching.[32]

School Health

Some school systems are experimenting with telemedicine links to extend the range of services in school-based clinics and decrease absenteeism for illness or disease-management encounters.[33–38]

Home Health

Health care professionals can remotely monitor a patient's vital signs, pulmonary function, or glucose concentration and then communicate with the patient to direct care by telephone, computer, or television monitor. Technology for this type of monitoring requires only a conventional telephone line. Communication technology has helped enable patients to remain at home while being monitored for congestive heart failure, diabetic control, arrhythmias, or metabolic stability.[6,39] Research suggests that homebound patients are pleased with this type of home health care service.[40] Some data suggest that telemedicine-mediated home care of children with chronic disease can save money while preserving care quality.[41,42]

Other Services

Although not extensively studied, there also have been some promising results using telemedicine for pediatric dentistry (assessment of tooth decay),[43] neonatal ophthalmology (retinopathy assessment),[44] and interpretation of radiographs by neonatologists.[45]

RESEARCH AND POLICY QUESTIONS

Research into telemedicine's usefulness has a long way to go. The American Academy of Pediatrics recognizes the need for additional research on the appropriate and effective use of telemedicine, including exploration of the following issues specifically related to pediatrics.

Medical Home

Does a telemedicine relationship change the concept of the traditional medical home? Telemedicine may have an increasing role in ensuring continuously available ambulatory and inpatient pediatric care. Telemedicine in the medical home will require that safeguards be built into insurance-contracting procedures, which will help to preserve the medical home when health services are available from telemedicine practitioners.

Incarcerated Youth

The provision of health care to prison inmates and children incarcerated in juvenile detention facilities presents special challenges. It is expensive and cumbersome to transport incarcerated individuals to health care facilities. The need for the transport of patients has resulted in delayed access to care. Telecommunication technologies have enabled adult prisoners to access care more rapidly and have minimized the potential danger to those at nonsecure facilities to which prisoners might otherwise be transported. Studies have shown acceptance of this technology by both prisoners and practitioners and reasonable cost-effectiveness.[46,47] This technology has not been studied yet in incarcerated children. Can it be demonstrated that standards of care delivered by telemedicine for the incarcerated child population are at least equivalent to those accepted in the local community?[48]

Genetics and Dysmorphology

It is remarkable how little telemedicine has been used in genetics and dysmorphology, considering that telemedicine's strengths (visual diagnosis and counseling) would seem to have obvious application to this specialty.[49] Given the scarcity of practitioners in genetics and dysmorphology, it would seem that telemedicine would afford a tremendous increase in patient access to these services. Application of tele-

medicine to this area of pediatrics should be considered well suited for effectiveness studies.

Subspecialty Distribution and Access Issues

The most natural use of telemedicine in pediatrics is the use of teleconferencing facilities to connect patients to pediatric subspecialists. There are a growing number of reports that suggest this is feasible and well accepted by patients.[13,50–52] The ability of pediatric subspecialists to provide telemedicine care in areas now served only by adult medical specialists should increase the options and quality of services available to patients.[53] Studies still need to be performed to demonstrate that subspecialty consultation by telemedicine improves access for children located in rural areas and that such programs are economically sustainable without grant support. Health care workforce studies need to be performed to evaluate assumptions about the effectiveness and penetration of telemedicine into pediatric practice.

Ethical Issues

It is possible that telemedicine could create a 2-tiered system in which patients who are able to pay are granted in-person access and poor children are treated by telemedicine. On the other hand, will off-hours telemedicine consultation become available only to those who can pay while poorer patients wait for an in-person encounter?

Educational Issues

There are several educational considerations related to teaching telemedicine as a technique in pediatric residency. For example, should proficiency with telemedicine equipment be assessed to determine an understanding of telemedicine applications and technologies? An assessment could be done at telecommunications facilities used in telemedicine to provide supervision for residents and students in, for example, rural or other underserved communities. Special educational training programs for pediatric subspecialists would provide the preparation needed to assist patients via telemedicine. Residency training programs that incorporate a multidisciplinary approach may provide an additional benefit. A multidisciplinary telemedical program might include primary care pediatricians, pediatric medical subspecialists, pediatric surgical specialists, primary care physicians, and other midlevel practitioners. As the need for telemedicine increases, medical schools and residency training must prepare to train physicians using the latest techniques in the 21st century.

REIMBURSEMENT ISSUES

Physicians have been relatively slow to adopt telemedicine. Where telemedicine has been used, it has frequently been a demonstration or research project and has been supported by grants and contracts. Without the widespread agreement by insurers on reimbursement issues surrounding telemedicine, the adoption of this technology may be delayed. There is little solid research examining how reimbursement for physician telemedicine services has developed in real-world settings. There is no literature on the need for parity with other specialties of pediatric reimbursement for telemedicine care. Such evaluations need to be performed before a long-term commitment by the pediatric community is likely to occur.

CONCLUSIONS

Research is limited on the clinical usage of telemedicine in pediatrics.[6] The few studies cited here seem to indicate that telemedicine has important implications for accessing pediatric subspecialty services, determining future health care workforce requirements and their distribution, improving communications with parents of sick and chronically ill children, and extending the boundaries of the medical home.

STEERING COMMITTEE ON CLINICAL INFORMATION
TECHNOLOGY, 2002–2003
S. Andrew Spooner, MD, MS, Chairperson
Jan E. Berger, MD
Robert S. Gerstle, MD
Edward M. Gotlieb, MD
Kevin B. Johnson, MD
Christoph U. Lehmann, MD
Joseph H. Schneider, MD
Mark M. Simonian, MD
Douglas M. Stetson, MD

LIAISONS
David C. Stockwell, MD
    American Academy of Pediatrics Section on
    Residents
Loren G. Yamamoto, MD, MPH
    National Conference and Exhibition Planning
    Group Representative

STAFF
Aiysha Johnson, MA

COMMITTEE ON MEDICAL LIABILITY, 2002–2003
Charles H. Deitschel, Jr, MD, Chairperson
C. Morrison Farish, MD
Gary N. McAbee, DO, JD
Robert A. Mendelson, MD
Sally L. Reynolds, MD
Steven M. Donn, MD

LIAISON
Larry Veltman, MD
    American College of Obstetricians and
    Gynecologists

CONSULTANT
Holly Myers, JD

STAFF
Julie Kersten Ake

REFERENCES

1. Eng TR, ed. *The eHealth Landscape: A Terrain Map of Emerging Information and Communication Technologies in Health and Health Care.* Princeton, NJ: The Robert Wood Johnson Foundation; 2001
2. Centers for Medicare and Medicaid Services. *Medicaid And Telemedicine.* Baltimore, MD: Centers for Medicare and Medicaid Services, Department of Health and Human Services; 2002. Available at: http://cms.hhs.gov/states/telemed.asp. Accessed February 5, 2003
3. Field MJ, ed. *Telemedicine: A Guide to Assessing Telecommunications for Health Care.* Washington, DC: National Academy Press; 1996
4. Linkous JD. *Toward A Rapidly Evolving Definition of Telemedicine.* Washington, DC: American Telemedicine Association; 2001. Available at: www.atmeda.org/news/definition.html. Accessed February 5, 2003
5. Centers for Medicare and Medicaid Services. *Program Memorandum: Intermediaries/Carriers.* Transmittal AB-02-052. Baltimore, MD: Centers for Medicare and Medicaid Services, Department of Health and Human Services; 2002. Available at: http://cms.hhs.gov/manuals/pm_trans/AB02052.pdf. Accessed February 5, 2003
6. Hersh WR, Wallace JA, Patterson PK, et al. *Telemedicine for the Medicare Population: Pediatric, Obstetric, and Clinician-Indirect Home Interventions.* Rockville, MD: Agency for Healthcare Research and Quality; 2001. Evidence Report/Technology Assessment No. 24, Supplement, AHRQ Publication No. 01-E060. Available at: www.ahrq.gov/clinic/epcsums/telmedsup.htm. Accessed February 5, 2003
7. Hersh WR, Patterson PK, Kraemer DF. Telehealth: the need for evaluation redux. *J Am Med Inform Assoc.* 2002,9:89–91
8. Kuzmak PM, Dayhoff RE. The use of digital imaging and communications in medicine (DICOM) in the integration of imaging into the electronic patient record at the Department of Veterans Affairs. *J Digit Imaging.* 2000,13(2 suppl 1):133–137
9. The DICOM standard. Understanding the benefits, recognizing the limitations. *Health Devices.* 2000,29:398
10. Slovis TL, Guzzardo-Dobson PR. The clinical usefulness of teleradiology of neonates: expanded services without expanded staff. *Pediatr Radiol.* 1991,21:333–335
11. Simpson J, Doze S, Urness D, Hailey D, Jacobs P. Telepsychiatry as a routine service—the perspective of the patient. *J Telemed Telecare.* 2001,7:155–160
12. Gelber H, Alexander M. An evaluation of an Australian videoconferencing project for child and adolescent telepsychiatry. *J Telemed Telecare.* 1999,5(suppl 1):S21–S23
13. Ermer DJ. Experience with a rural telepsychiatry clinic for children and adolescents. *Psychiatr Serv.* 1999,50:260–261
14. Elford R, White H, Bowering R, et al. A randomized, controlled trial of child psychiatric assessments conducted using videoconferencing. *J Telemed Telecare.* 2000,6:73–82
15. Whited JD. Teledermatology. Current status and future directions. *Am J Clin Dermatol.* 2001,2:59–64
16. Casey F, Brown D, Craig BG, Rogers J, Mulholland HC. Diagnosis of neonatal congenital heart defects by remote consultation using a low-cost telemedicine link. *J Telemed Telecare.* 1996,2:165–169
17. Finley JP, Sharratt GP, Nanton MA, et al. Paediatric echocardiography by telemedicine—nine years' experience. *J Telemed Telecare.* 1997,3:200–204
18. Sable C, Roca T, Gold J, Gutierrez A, Gulotta E, Culpepper W. Live transmission of neonatal echocardiograms from underserved areas: accuracy, patient care, and cost. *Telemed J.* 1999,5:339–347
19. Sable CA, Cummings SD, Pearson GD, et al. Impact of telemedicine on the practice of pediatric cardiology in community hospitals. *Pediatrics.* 2002,109(1). Available at: www.pediatrics.org/cgi/content/full/109/1/e3
20. Belmont JM, Mattioli LF, Goertz KK, Ardinger RH Jr, Thomas CM. Evaluation of remote stethoscopy for pediatric telecardiology. *Telemed J.* 1995,1:133–149
21. Kofos D, Pitetti R, Orr R, Thompson A. Telemedicine in pediatric transport: a feasibility study. *Pediatrics.* 1998,102(5). Available at: www.pediatrics.org/cgi/content/full/102/5/e58
22. Gray J, Pompilio-Weitzner G, Jones PC, Wang Q, Coriat M, Safran C. Baby CareLink: development and implementation of a WWW-based system for neonatal home telemedicine. *Proc AMIA Symp.* 1998:351–355
23. Gray JE, Safran C, Davis RB, et al. Baby Carelink: using the Internet and telemedicine to improve care for high-risk infants. *Pediatrics.* 2000,106:1318–1324
24. Hopkins-Koglin O. Loved ones are only a click away for kids with cancer.Oregonian. September 2, 2000:C1, C5
25. Bilalovic N, Paties C, Mason A. Benefits of using telemedicine and first results in Bosnia and Herzegovina. *J Telemed Telecare.* 1998,4(suppl 1):S91–S93
26. Della Mea V, Cortolezzis D, Beltrami CA. The economics of telepathology—a case study. *J Telemed Telecare.* 2000,6(suppl 1):S168–S169
27. Kellogg ND, Lamb JL, Lukefahr JL. The use of telemedicine in child sexual abuse evaluations. *Child Abuse Negl.* 2000,24:1601–1612
28. Pammer W, Haney M, Wood BM, et al. Use of telehealth technology to extend child protection team services. *Pediatrics.* 2001,108:584–590
29. Miyasaka K, Suzuki Y, Sakai H, Kondo Y. Interactive communication in high-technology home care: videophones for pediatric ventilatory care. *Pediatrics.* 1997,99(1). Available at: www.pediatrics.org/cgi/content/full/99/1/e1

30. Bynum A, Hopkins D, Thomas A, Copeland N, Irwin C. The effect of telepharmacy counseling on metered-dose inhaler technique among adolescents with asthma in rural Arkansas. *Telemed J E Health.* 2001,7:207–217

31. Romano MJ, Hernandez J, Gaylor A, Howard S, Knox R. Improvement in asthma symptoms and quality of life in pediatric patients through specialty care delivered via telemedicine. *Telemed J E Health.* 2001,7:281–286

32. Marrero DG, Vandagriff JL, Kronz K, et al. Using telecommunication technology to manage children with diabetes: the Computer-Linked Outpatient Clinic (CLOC) Study. *Diabetes Educ.* 1995,21:313–319

33. Miller TW, Miller JM. Telemedicine: new directions for health care delivery in Kentucky schools [letter]. *J Ky Med Assoc.* 1999,97:170–172

34. Wheeler T. Urban kids receive telemedical care at school. *Telemed Today.* 1998,6:6

35. Wheeler T. West Texas community gets school-based telemedicine clinic. *Telemed Today.* 1998,6:29

36. Whitten P, Cook DJ, Shaw P, Ermer D, Goodwin J. Tele-Kid Care: Bringing health care into schools. *Telemed J.* 1998,4:335–343

37. Whitten P, Cook D. School-based telemedicine: teachers', nurses' and administrators' perceptions. *J Telemed Telecare.* 2000,6(suppl 1):S129–S132

38. Mair F, Whitten P. Systematic review of students of patient satisfaction with telemedicine. *BMJ.* 2000,320:1517–1520

39. Johnston B, Wheeler L, Deuser J, Sousa KH. Outcomes of the Kaiser Permanente Tele-Home Health Research Project. *Arch Fam Med.* 2000,9:40–45

40. Agrell H, Dahlberg S, Jerant AF. Patients' perceptions regarding home telecare. *Telemed J E Health.* 2000,6:409–415

41. Rylander E, Fagerberg M, Bergius H, et al. Hospital managed care of children in their homes by integrating advanced medical treatment, telemedicine, and health management: an approach by the pediatric clinics at Karolinska Hospital in Stockholm, Sweden. *Telemed J.* 2000,6:295

42. Bergius H, Eng A, Fagerberg M, et al. Hospital-managed advanced care of children in their homes. *J Telemed Telecare.* 2001,7(suppl 1):S32–S34

43. Patterson S, Botchway C. Dental screenings using telehealth technology: a pilot study. *J Can Dent Assoc.* 1998,64:806–810

44. Schwartz SD, Harrison SA, Ferrone PJ, Trese MT. Telemedical evaluation and management of retinopathy of prematurity using a fiberoptic digital fundus camera. *Ophthalmology.* 2000,107:25–28

45. Yamamoto LG, Ash KM, Boychuk RB, et al. Personal computer teleradiology interhospital image transmission of neonatal radiographs to facilitate tertiary neonatology telephone consultation and patient transfer. *J Perinatol.* 1996,16:292–298

46. Brecht RM, Gray CL, Peterson C, Youngblood B. The University of Texas Medical Branch—Texas Department of Criminal Justice Telemedicine Project: findings from the first year of operation. *Telemed J.* 1996,2:25–35

47. Zollo S, Kienzle M, Loeffelholz P, Sebille S. Telemedicine to Iowa's correctional facilities: initial clinical experience and assessment of program costs. *Telemed J.* 1999,5:291–301

48. American Academy of Pediatrics, Committee on Adolescence. Health care for children and adolescents in the juvenile correctional care system. *Pediatrics.* 2001,107:799–803

49. Gattas MR, MacMillan JC, Meinecke I, Loane M, Wootton R. Telemedicine and clinical genetics: establishing a successful service. *J Telemed Telecare.* 2001,7(suppl 2):S68–S70

50. Murdison KA. Telemedicine: a useful tool for the pediatric cardiologist. *Telemed J.* 1997,3:179–184

51. Woods KF, Johnson JA, Kutlar A, Daitch L, Stachura ME. Sickle cell disease telemedicine network for rural outreach. *J Telemed Telecare.* 2000,6:285–290

52. Karp WB, Grigsby RK, McSwiggan-Hardin M, et al. Use of telemedicine for children with special health care needs. *Pediatrics.* 2000,105:843–847

53. Gruskin A, Williams RG, McCabe ER, et al. Final report of the FOPE II Pediatric Subspecialists of the Future Workgroup. *Pediatrics.* 2000,106:1224–1244

All technical reports from the American Academy of Pediatrics automatically expire 5 years after publication unless reaffirmed, revised, or retired at or before that time.

Section 4

Current Policies

From the American Academy of Pediatrics

• •

(Through December 2004)

- • *Policy Statements*
  *ORGANIZATIONAL PRINCIPLES TO GUIDE AND DEFINE THE CHILD HEALTH CARE SYSTEM
  AND/OR IMPROVE THE HEALTH OF ALL CHILDREN*

- • *Clinical Reports*
  GUIDANCE FOR THE CLINICIAN IN RENDERING PEDIATRIC CARE

- • *Technical Reports*
  BACKGROUND INFORMATION TO SUPPORT AMERICAN ACADEMY OF PEDIATRICS POLICY

AMERICAN ACADEMY OF PEDIATRICS

Policy Statements, Clinical Reports, Technical Reports

Current through December 2004

Full text of all titles listed below is available on the *Pediatric Clinical Practice Guidelines & Policies* CD-ROM included with this publication.

ACCESS TO PEDIATRIC EMERGENCY MEDICAL CARE

Committee on Pediatric Emergency Medicine

ABSTRACT. Hundreds of thousands of pediatric patients require some level of emergency care annually, and significant barriers limit access to appropriate services for large numbers of children. The American Academy of Pediatrics has a strong commitment to identify barriers to access to emergency care, work to surmount these obstacles, and encourage through education increased levels of emergency care available to all children. It is also crucial to involve and incorporate the child's medical home into emergency care, both during acute presentation when the medical home is identified and by assisting in locating a medical home for follow-up when none previously exists. (3/00)

ACETAMINOPHEN TOXICITY IN CHILDREN

Committee on Drugs

ABSTRACT. Acetaminophen is widely used in children, because its safety and efficacy are well established. Although the risk of developing toxic reactions to acetaminophen appears to be lower in children than in adults, such reactions occur in pediatric patients from intentional overdoses. Less frequently, acetaminophen toxicity is attributable to unintended inappropriate dosing or the failure to recognize children at increased risk in whom standard acetaminophen doses have been administered. Because the symptoms of acetaminophen intoxication are nonspecific, the diagnosis and treatment of acetaminophen intoxication are more likely to be delayed in unintentional cases of toxicity. This statement describes situations and conditions that may contribute to acetaminophen toxicity not associated with suicidal intentions. (10/01)

ADMISSION AND DISCHARGE GUIDELINES FOR THE PEDIATRIC PATIENT REQUIRING INTERMEDIATE CARE (CLINICAL REPORT)

American Academy of Pediatrics Committee on Hospital Care and Section on Critical Care and Society of Critical Care Medicine

See full text on page 261. (5/04)

ADOLESCENT PREGNANCY—CURRENT TRENDS AND ISSUES: 1998

Committee on Adolescence

ABSTRACT. Although the prevention of unintended adolescent pregnancy is a primary goal of the American Academy of Pediatrics and society, many adolescents continue to become pregnant. Since the last statement on adolescent pregnancy was issued by the Academy in 1989, new observations have been recorded in the literature. The purpose of this new statement is to review current trends and issues on adolescent pregnancy to update practitioners on this topic. (2/99)

THE ADOLESCENT'S RIGHT TO CONFIDENTIAL CARE WHEN CONSIDERING ABORTION

Committee on Adolescence

ABSTRACT. In this statement, the American Academy of Pediatrics (AAP) reaffirms its position that the rights of adolescents to confidential care when considering abortion should be protected. The AAP supports the recommendations presented in the report on mandatory parental consent to abortion by the Council on Ethical and Judicial Affairs of the American Medical Association. Adolescents should be strongly encouraged to involve their parents and other trusted adults in decisions regarding pregnancy termination, and the majority of them voluntarily do so. Legislation mandating parental involvement does not achieve the intended benefit of promoting family communication, but it does increase the risk of harm to the adolescent by delaying access to appropriate medical care. The statement presents a summary of pertinent current information related to the benefits and risks of legislation requiring mandatory parental involvement in an adolescent's decision to obtain an abortion. The AAP acknowledges and respects the diversity of beliefs about abortion and affirms the value of voluntary parental involvement in decision making by adolescents. (5/96, reaffirmed 5/99, 11/02)

ADOLESCENTS AND ANABOLIC STEROIDS: A SUBJECT REVIEW (CLINICAL REPORT)

Committee on Sports Medicine and Fitness

ABSTRACT. This revision of a previous statement by the American Academy of Pediatrics provides current information on anabolic steroid use by young athletes. It provides the information needed to enable pediatricians to discuss the benefits and risks of anabolic steroids in a well-informed, nonjudgmental fashion. (6/97, reaffirmed 5/00)

ADOLESCENTS AND HUMAN IMMUNODEFICIENCY VIRUS INFECTION: THE ROLE OF THE PEDIATRICIAN IN PREVENTION AND INTERVENTION

Committee on Pediatric AIDS and Committee on Adolescence

ABSTRACT. Half of all new human immunodeficiency virus (HIV) infections in the United States occur among young people between the ages of 13 and 24. Sexual transmission accounts for most cases of HIV during adolescence. Pediatricians can play an important role in educating adolescents about HIV prevention, transmission, and testing, with an emphasis on risk reduction, and in advocating for the special needs of adolescents for access to information about HIV. (1/01, reaffirmed 10/03)

ADVANCED PRACTICE IN NEONATAL NURSING
Committee on Fetus and Newborn
ABSTRACT. The advanced practice neonatal nurse's participation in newborn care continues to be accepted and supported by the American Academy of Pediatrics. Recognized categories of advanced practice neonatal nurse are the neonatal clinical nurse specialist and the neonatal nurse practitioner. Training and credentialing requirements have been updated recently and are endorsed in this revised statement. (6/03)

AGE LIMITS OF PEDIATRICS
Child and Adolescent Health Action Group (5/88, reaffirmed 9/92, 1/97, 3/02)

AGE FOR ROUTINE ADMINISTRATION OF THE SECOND DOSE OF MEASLES-MUMPS-RUBELLA VACCINE
Committee on Infectious Diseases
ABSTRACT. The purpose of this statement is to inform physicians of a modification in the recommendation of the appropriate age for routine administration of the second dose of measles-mumps-rubella (MMR) vaccine. The implementation of the two-dose measles vaccine schedule has improved the control of measles, but some outbreaks continue to occur in school children, although ≥95% of children in school have received one dose of vaccine. Because most measles vaccine failures are attributable to failure to respond to the first dose, that all children receive two doses of measles-containing vaccine is essential for the control of measles. Routine administration of the second dose of MMR vaccine at school entry (4 to 6 years of age) will help prevent school-based outbreaks. Physicians should continue to review the records of all children 11 to 12 years of age to be certain that they have received two doses of MMR vaccine after their first birthday. Documenting that all school children have received two doses of measles-containing vaccine by the year 2001 will help ensure the elimination of measles in the United States and contribute to the global effort to control and possibly eradicate measles. (1/98, reaffirmed 8/04)

AGE TERMINOLOGY DURING THE PERINATAL PERIOD
Committee on Fetus and Newborn
See full text on page 267. (11/04)

ALCOHOL USE AND ABUSE: A PEDIATRIC CONCERN
Committee on Substance Abuse
ABSTRACT. Alcohol use and abuse by children and adolescents continue to be a major problem. Pediatricians should interview their patients regularly about alcohol use within the family, by friends, and by themselves. A comprehensive substance abuse curriculum should be integrated into every pediatrician's training. Advertising of alcohol in the media, on the Internet, and during sporting events is a powerful force that must be addressed. Availability of alcohol to minors must be controlled, and interventions for the child and adolescent drinker and punitive action for the purveyor are encouraged. (7/01)

ALL-TERRAIN VEHICLE INJURY PREVENTION: TWO-, THREE-, AND FOUR-WHEELED UNLICENSED MOTOR VEHICLES
Committee on Injury and Poison Prevention
ABSTRACT. Since 1987, the American Academy of Pediatrics (AAP) has had a policy about the use of motorized cycles and all-terrain vehicles (ATVs) by children. The purpose of this policy statement is to update and strengthen previous policy. This statement describes the various kinds of motorized cycles and ATVs and outlines the epidemiologic characteristics of deaths and injuries related to their use by children in light of the 1987 consent decrees entered into by the US Consumer Product Safety Commission and the manufacturers of ATVs. Recommendations are made for public, patient, and parent education by pediatricians; equipment modifications; the use of safety equipment; and the development and improvement of safer off-road trails and responsive emergency medical systems. In addition, the AAP strengthens its recommendation for passage of legislation in all states prohibiting the use of 2- and 4-wheeled off-road vehicles by children younger than 16 years, as well as a ban on the sale of new and used 3-wheeled ATVs, with a recall of all used 3-wheeled ATVs. (6/00, reaffirmed 5/04)

ALTERNATIVE DISPUTE RESOLUTION IN MEDICAL MALPRACTICE (TECHNICAL REPORT)
Committee on Medical Liability
ABSTRACT. The purpose of this technical report is to provide pediatricians with an understanding of past crises within the professional liability insurance industry, the difficulties of the tort system, and alternative strategies for resolving malpractice disputes that have been applied to medical malpractice actions. Through this report, pediatricians will gain a technical understanding of common alternative dispute resolution (ADR) strategies. The report explains the distinctions between various ADR methods in terms of process and outcome, risks and benefits, appropriateness to the nature of the dispute, and long-term ramifications. By knowing these concepts, pediatricians faced with malpractice claims will be better-equipped to participate in the decision-making with legal counsel on whether to settle, litigate, or explore ADR options. (3/01)

ALTERNATIVE ROUTES OF DRUG ADMINISTRATION— ADVANTAGES AND DISADVANTAGES (SUBJECT REVIEW) (CLINICAL REPORT)
Committee on Drugs
ABSTRACT. During the past 20 years, advances in drug formulations and innovative routes of administration have been made. Our understanding of drug transport across tissues has increased. These changes have often resulted in improved patient adherence to the therapeutic regimen and pharmacologic response. The administration of drugs by transdermal or transmucosal routes offers the advantage of being relatively painless. Also, the potential for greater flexibility in a variety of clinical situations exists, often precluding the need to establish intravenous access, which is a particular benefit for children.

This statement focuses on the advantages and disadvantages of alternative routes of drug administration. Issues of particular importance in the care of pediatric patients, especially factors that could lead to drug-related toxicity or adverse responses, are emphasized. (7/97, reaffirmed 10/00, 11/03)

ALUMINUM TOXICITY IN INFANTS AND CHILDREN
Committee on Nutrition (3/96, reaffirmed 4/00, 4/03)

AMBIENT AIR POLLUTION: HEALTH HAZARDS TO CHILDREN
Committee on Environmental Health
See full text on page 273. (12/04)

APNEA, SUDDEN INFANT DEATH SYNDROME, AND HOME MONITORING
Committee on Fetus and Newborn
ABSTRACT. More than 25 years have elapsed since continuous cardiorespiratory monitoring at home was suggested to decrease the risk of sudden infant death syndrome (SIDS). In the ensuing interval, multiple studies have been unable to establish the alleged efficacy of its use. In this statement, the most recent research information concerning extreme limits for a prolonged course of apnea of prematurity is reviewed. Recommendations regarding the appropriate use of home cardiorespiratory monitoring after hospital discharge emphasize limiting use to specific clinical indications for a predetermined period, using only monitors equipped with an event recorder, and counseling parents that monitor use does not prevent sudden, unexpected death in all circumstances. The continued implementation of proven SIDS prevention measures is encouraged. (4/03)

APPLICATION OF THE RESOURCE-BASED RELATIVE VALUE SCALE SYSTEM TO PEDIATRICS
Committee on Coding and Nomenclature
See full text on page 285. (5/04)

APPROPRIATE BOUNDARIES IN THE PEDIATRICIAN-FAMILY-PATIENT RELATIONSHIP
Committee on Bioethics
ABSTRACT. All professionals are concerned about maintaining the appropriate limits in their relationships with those they serve. Romantic and sexual involvement between physicians and patients is unacceptable. Pediatricians also must strive to maintain appropriate professional boundaries in their relationships with the family members of their patients. Pediatricians should avoid behavior that patients and parents might misunderstand as having sexual or inappropriate social meaning. The acceptance of gifts or nonmonetary compensation for medical services has the potential to affect adversely the professional relationship. (8/99, reaffirmed 11/02)

ASSESSMENT OF MALTREATMENT OF CHILDREN WITH DISABILITIES
Committee on Child Abuse and Neglect and Committee on Children With Disabilities
ABSTRACT. Widespread efforts are continuously being made to increase awareness and provide education to pediatricians regarding risk factors of child abuse and neglect. The purpose of this statement is to ensure that children with disabilities are recognized as a population that is also at risk for maltreatment. The need for early recognition and intervention of child abuse and neglect in this population, as well as the ways that a medical home can facilitate the prevention and early detection of child maltreatment, should be acknowledged. (8/01)

THE ASSESSMENT AND MANAGEMENT OF ACUTE PAIN IN INFANTS, CHILDREN, AND ADOLESCENTS
American Academy of Pediatrics Committee on Psychosocial Aspects of Child and Family Health and American Pain Society Task Force on Pain in Infants, Children, and Adolescents
ABSTRACT. Acute pain is one of the most common adverse stimuli experienced by children, occurring as a result of injury, illness, and necessary medical procedures. It is associated with increased anxiety, avoidance, somatic symptoms, and increased parent distress. Despite the magnitude of effects that acute pain can have on a child, it is often inadequately assessed and treated. Numerous myths, insufficient knowledge among caregivers, and inadequate application of knowledge contribute to the lack of effective management. The pediatric acute pain experience involves the interaction of physiologic, psychologic, behavioral, developmental, and situational factors. Pain is an inherently subjective multifactorial experience and should be assessed and treated as such. Pediatricians are responsible for eliminating or assuaging pain and suffering in children when possible. To accomplish this, pediatricians need to expand their knowledge, use appropriate assessment tools and techniques, anticipate painful experiences and intervene accordingly, use a multimodal approach to pain management, use a multidisciplinary approach when possible, involve families, and advocate for the use of effective pain management in children. (9/01)

ATHLETIC PARTICIPATION BY CHILDREN AND ADOLESCENTS WHO HAVE SYSTEMIC HYPERTENSION
Committee on Sports Medicine and Fitness
ABSTRACT. Children and adolescents who have systemic hypertension may be at risk for complications when exercise causes their blood pressures to rise even higher. The purpose of this statement is to make recommendations concerning the athletic participation of individuals with hypertension using the 26th Bethesda Conference on heart disease and athletic participation and of the Second Task Force on Blood Pressure Control in Children as a basis. (4/97, reaffirmed 5/00, 5/04)

ATLANTOAXIAL INSTABILITY IN DOWN SYNDROME: SUBJECT REVIEW (CLINICAL REPORT)
Committee on Sports Medicine and Fitness (7/95, reaffirmed 11/98, 5/00, 5/04)

AUDITORY INTEGRATION TRAINING AND FACILITATED COMMUNICATION FOR AUTISM
Committee on Children With Disabilities
ABSTRACT. This statement reviews the basis for two new therapies for autism—auditory integration training and facilitative communication. Both therapies seek to improve communication skills. Currently available information does not support the claims of proponents that these treatments are efficacious. Their use does not appear warranted at this time, except within research protocols. (8/98, reaffirmed 5/02)

BICYCLE HELMETS
Committee on Injury and Poison Prevention

ABSTRACT. Bicycling remains one of the most popular recreational sports among children in America and is the leading cause of recreational sports injuries treated in emergency departments. An estimated 23 000 children younger than 21 years sustained head injuries (excluding the face) while bicycling in 1998. The bicycle helmet is a very effective device that can prevent the occurrence of up to 88% of serious brain injuries. Despite this, most children do not wear a helmet each time they ride a bicycle, and adolescents are particularly resistant to helmet use. Recently, a group of national experts and government agencies renewed the call for all bicyclists to wear helmets. This policy statement describes the role of the pediatrician in helping attain universal helmet use among children and teens for each bicycle ride. (10/01, reaffirmed 11/04)

BREASTFEEDING AND THE USE OF HUMAN MILK
Provisional Section on Breastfeeding

ABSTRACT. This policy statement on breastfeeding replaces the previous policy statement of the American Academy of Pediatrics, reflecting the considerable advances that have occurred in recent years in the scientific knowledge of the benefits of breastfeeding, in the mechanisms underlying these benefits, and in the practice of breastfeeding. This document summarizes the benefits of breastfeeding to the infant, the mother, and the nation, and sets forth principles to guide the pediatrician and other health care providers in the initiation and maintenance of breastfeeding. The policy statement also delineates the various ways in which pediatricians can promote, protect, and support breastfeeding, not only in their individual practices but also in the hospital, medical school, community, and nation. (12/97)

CALCIUM REQUIREMENTS OF INFANTS, CHILDREN, AND ADOLESCENTS
Committee on Nutrition

ABSTRACT. This statement is intended to provide pediatric caregivers with advice about the nutritional needs of calcium of infants, children, and adolescents. It will review the physiology of calcium metabolism and provide a review of the data about the relationship between calcium intake and bone growth and metabolism. In particular, it will focus on the large number of recent studies that have identified a relationship between childhood calcium intake and bone mineralization and the potential relationship of these data to fractures in adolescents and the development of osteoporosis in adulthood. The specific needs of children and adolescents with eating disorders are not considered. (11/99)

CAMPHOR REVISITED: FOCUS ON TOXICITY
Committee on Drugs (7/94, reaffirmed 6/97, 5/00)

CARDIAC DYSRHYTHMIAS AND SPORTS
Committee on Sports Medicine and Fitness (5/95, reaffirmed 11/98, 5/00, 5/04)

CARE OF ADOLESCENT PARENTS AND THEIR CHILDREN
Committee on Adolescence and Committee on Early Childhood, Adoption, and Dependent Care

ABSTRACT. Many children live with their adolescent parents, alone, or as part of an extended family. This statement updates a previous statement on adolescent parents and addresses specific medical and psychosocial risks specific to adolescent parents and their children. Challenges unique to the adolescent mother and her partner, as well as mitigating circumstances and protective factors that have been identified in the recent literature, are reviewed, along with suggestions for the pediatrician on models for intervention and care. (2/01)

CARE OF THE ADOLESCENT SEXUAL ASSAULT VICTIM
Committee on Adolescence

ABSTRACT. Sexual assault is a broad-based term that encompasses a wide range of sexual victimizations, including rape. Since the American Academy of Pediatrics published its last policy statement on this topic in 1994, additional information and data have emerged about sexual assault and rape in adolescents, the adolescent's perception of sexual assault, and the treatment and management of the adolescent who has been a victim of sexual assault. This new information mandates an updated knowledge base for pediatricians who care for adolescent patients. This statement provides that update, focusing on sexual assault and rape in the adolescent population. (6/01)

CARE OF CHILDREN IN THE EMERGENCY DEPARTMENT: GUIDELINES FOR PREPAREDNESS
American Academy of Pediatrics Committee on Pediatric Emergency Medicine and American College of Emergency Physicians Pediatric Committee

ABSTRACT. Children requiring emergency care have unique and special needs. This is especially so for those with serious and life-threatening emergencies. There are a variety of components of the emergency care system that provide emergency care to children that are not limited to children. With regard to hospitals, most children are brought to community hospital emergency departments (EDs) by virtue of their availability rather than to facilities designed and operated solely for children. Emergency medical services (EMS) agencies, similarly, provide the bulk of out-of-hospital emergency care to children. It is imperative that all hospital EDs and EMS agencies have the appropriate equipment, staff, and policies to provide high quality care for children. This statement provides guidelines for necessary resources to ensure that children receive quality emergency care and to facilitate, after stabilization, timely transfer to a facility with specialized pediatric services when appropriate. It is important to realize that some hospitals and local EMS systems will have difficulty in meeting these guidelines, and others will develop more comprehensive guidelines based on local resources. It is hoped, however, that hospital ED staff and administrators and local EMS systems administrators will seek to meet these guidelines to best ensure that their facilities or systems provide the resources necessary for the care of children. This statement has been reviewed by and is supported in concept by the Ambulatory Pediatric Association, American Association of Poison Control Centers, American College of Surgeons, American Hospital Association, American Medical Association, American Pediatric Surgical Association, American Trauma Society, Brain Injury Association Inc, Emergency Nurses Association, Joint Commission on Accreditation of Healthcare Organizations, National Association of Children's Hospitals and Related Institutions, National Association of EMS Physicians, National Association of EMTs, National Association of School Nurses, National Association of State EMS Directors, National Committee for Quality Assurance, and Society for Academic Emergency Medicine. (4/01, reaffirmed 5/04)

CARE COORDINATION: INTEGRATING HEALTH AND RELATED SYSTEMS OF CARE FOR CHILDREN WITH SPECIAL HEALTH CARE NEEDS
Committee on Children With Disabilities
ABSTRACT. *Care coordination* is a process that links children with special health care needs and their families to services and resources in a coordinated effort to maximize the potential of the children and provide them with optimal health care. Care coordination often is complicated because there is no single entry point to multiple systems of care, and complex criteria determine the availability of funding and services among public and private payers. Economic and sociocultural barriers to coordination of care exist and affect families and health care professionals. In their important role of providing a medical home for all children, primary care pediatricians have a vital role in the process of care coordination, in concert with the family. (10/99)

CHANGING CONCEPTS OF SUDDEN INFANT DEATH SYNDROME: IMPLICATIONS FOR INFANT SLEEPING ENVIRONMENT AND SLEEP POSITION
Task Force on Infant Sleep Position and Sudden Infant Death Syndrome
ABSTRACT. The American Academy of Pediatrics has recommended since 1992 that infants be placed to sleep on their backs to reduce the risk of sudden infant death syndrome (SIDS). Since that time, the frequency of prone sleeping has decreased from >70% to ~20% of US infants, and the SIDS rate has decreased by >40%. However, SIDS remains the highest cause of infant death beyond the neonatal period, and there are still several potentially modifiable risk factors. Although some of these factors have been known for many years (eg, maternal smoking), the importance of other hazards, such as soft bedding and covered airways, has been demonstrated only recently. The present statement is intended to review the evidence about prone sleeping and other risk factors and to make recommendations about strategies that may be effective for further reducing the risk of SIDS. This statement is intended to consolidate and supplant previous statements made by this Task Force. (3/00)

CHEMICAL-BIOLOGICAL TERRORISM AND ITS IMPACT ON CHILDREN: A SUBJECT REVIEW (CLINICAL REPORT)
Committee on Environmental Health and Committee on Infectious Diseases
ABSTRACT. There is an increasing threat that chemical and biological weapons will be used on a civilian population in an act of domestic terrorism. Casualties among adults and children could be significant in such an event. Federal, state, and local authorities have begun extensive planning to meet a chemical-biological incident by developing methods of rapid identification of potential agents and protocols for management of victims without injury to health care personnel. Because children would be disproportionately affected by a chemical or biological weapons release, pediatricians must assist in planning for a domestic chemical-biological incident. Government agencies should seek input from pediatricians and pediatric subspecialists to ensure that the situations created by multiple pediatric casualties after a chemical-biological incident are considered. This statement reviews key aspects of chemical-biological agents, the consequences of their use, the potential impact of a chemical-biological attack on children, and issues to consider in disaster planning and management for pediatric patients. (3/00)

THE CHILD IN COURT: A SUBJECT REVIEW (CLINICAL REPORT)
Committee on Psychosocial Aspects of Child and Family Health
ABSTRACT. When children come to court as witnesses, or when their needs are decided in a courtroom, they face unique stressors from the legal proceeding and from the social predicament that resulted in court action. Effective pediatric support and intervention requires an understanding of the situations that bring children to court and the issues that will confront children and child advocates in different court settings. (11/99, reaffirmed 11/02)

CHILD LIFE SERVICES
Committee on Hospital Care
ABSTRACT. Child life programs have become the standard in large pediatric settings to address the psychosocial concerns that accompany hospitalization and other health care experiences. Child life programs facilitate coping and the adjustment of children and families in 3 primary service areas: 1) providing play experiences; 2) presenting developmentally appropriate information about events and procedures; and 3) establishing therapeutic relationships with children and parents to support family involvement in each child's care. Although other members of the health care team share these responsibilities for the psychosocial concerns of the child and the family, for the child life specialist, this is the primary role. The child life specialist focuses on the strengths and sense of well-being of children while promoting their optimal development and minimizing the adverse effects of children's experiences in a hospital setting. (11/00)

CHILDREN, ADOLESCENTS, AND ADVERTISING
Committee on Public Education (2/95)

CHILDREN, ADOLESCENTS, AND TELEVISION
Committee on Public Education
ABSTRACT. This statement describes the possible negative health effects of television viewing on children and adolescents, such as violent or aggressive behavior, substance use, sexual activity, obesity, poor body image, and decreased school performance. In addition to the television ratings system and the v-chip (electronic device to block programming), media education is an effective approach to mitigating these potential problems. The American Academy of Pediatrics offers a list of recommendations on this issue for pediatricians and for parents, the federal government, and the entertainment industry. (2/01)

CHILDREN IN PICKUP TRUCKS
Committee on Injury and Poison Prevention
ABSTRACT. Pickup trucks have become increasingly popular in the United States. A recent study found that in crashes involving fatalities, cargo area passengers were 3 times more likely to die than were occupants in the cab. Compared with restrained cab occupants, the risk of death for those in the cargo area was 8 times higher. Furthermore, the increased use of extended-cab pickup trucks and air bag-equipped front passenger compartments creates concerns about the safe transport of children. The most effective preventive strategies are the legislative prohibition of travel in the cargo area and requirements for age-appropriate restraint use and seat selection in the cab. Parents should select vehicles that are appropriate for the safe transportation needs of the family. Physicians have an important role in counseling families and advocating public policy measures to reduce the number of deaths and injuries to occupants of pickup trucks. (10/00, reaffirmed 5/04)

CHOLESTEROL IN CHILDHOOD
Committee on Nutrition
ABSTRACT. This updated statement reviews the scientific justification for the recommendations of dietary changes in all healthy children (a population approach) and a strategy to identify and treat children who are at highest risk for the development of accelerated atherosclerosis in early adult life (an individualized approach). Although the precise fraction of risk for future coronary heart disease conveyed by elevated cholesterol levels in childhood is unknown, clear epidemiologic and experimental evidence indicates that the risk is significant. Diet changes that lower fat, saturated fat, and cholesterol intake in children and adolescents can be applied safely and acceptably, resulting in improved plasma lipid profiles that, if carried into adult life, have the potential to reduce atherosclerotic vascular disease. (1/98, reaffirmed 4/01)

CIRCUMCISION POLICY STATEMENT
Task Force on Circumcision
ABSTRACT. Existing scientific evidence demonstrates potential medical benefits of newborn male circumcision; however, these data are not sufficient to recommend routine neonatal circumcision. In circumstances in which there are potential benefits and risks, yet the procedure is not essential to the child's current well-being, parents should determine what is in the best interest of the child. To make an informed choice, parents of all male infants should be given accurate and unbiased information and be provided the opportunity to discuss this decision. If a decision for circumcision is made, procedural analgesia should be provided. (3/99)

CLASSIFYING RECOMMENDATIONS FOR CLINICAL PRACTICE GUIDELINES
Steering Committee on Quality Improvement and Management
See full text on page 291. (9/04)

CLIMATIC HEAT STRESS AND THE EXERCISING CHILD AND ADOLESCENT
Committee on Sports Medicine and Fitness
ABSTRACT. For morphologic and physiologic reasons, exercising children do not adapt as effectively as adults when exposed to a high climatic heat stress. This may affect their performance and well-being, as well as increase the risk for heat-related illness. This policy statement summarizes approaches for the prevention of the detrimental effects of children's activity in hot or humid climates, including the prevention of exercise-induced dehydration. (7/00, reaffirmed 5/04)

CLIOQUINOL (IODOCHLORHYDROXYQUIN, VIOFORM) AND IODOQUINOL (DIIODOHYDROXYQUIN): BLINDNESS AND NEUROPATHY
Committee on Drugs (11/90, reaffirmed 2/94, 2/97, 2/00, 4/03)

COMBINATION VACCINES FOR CHILDHOOD IMMUNIZATION: RECOMMENDATIONS OF THE ADVISORY COMMITTEE ON IMMUNIZATION PRACTICES (ACIP), THE AMERICAN ACADEMY OF PEDIATRICS (AAP), AND THE AMERICAN ACADEMY OF FAMILY PHYSICIANS (AAFP)
American Academy of Pediatrics Committee on Infectious Diseases, Advisory Committee on Immunization Practices, and American Academy of Family Physicians
SUMMARY. An increasing number of new and improved vaccines to prevent childhood diseases are being introduced. Combination vaccines represent one solution to the problem of increased numbers of injections during single clinic visits. This statement provides general guidance on the use of combination vaccines and related issues and questions.

To minimize the number of injections children receive, parenteral combination vaccines should be used, if licensed and indicated for the patient's age, instead of their equivalent component vaccines. Hepatitis A, hepatitis B, and *Haemophilus influenzae* type b vaccines, in either monovalent or combination formulations from the same or different manufacturers, are interchangeable for sequential doses in the vaccination series. However, using acellular pertussis vaccine product(s) from the same manufacturer is preferable for at least the first three doses, until studies demonstrate the interchangeability of these vaccines. Immunization providers should stock sufficient types of combination and monovalent vaccines needed to vaccinate children against all diseases for which vaccines are recommended, but they need not stock all available types or brand-name products. When patients have already received the recommended vaccinations for some of the components in a combination vaccine, administering the extra antigen(s) in the combination is often permissible if doing so will reduce the number of injections required.

To overcome recording errors and ambiguities in the names of vaccine combinations, improved systems are needed to enhance the convenience and accuracy of transferring vaccine-identifying information into medical records and immunization registries. Further scientific and programmatic research is needed on specific questions related to the use of combination vaccines. (5/99, reaffirmed 3/02)

CONDOM USE BY ADOLESCENTS
Committee on Adolescence
ABSTRACT. The use of condoms as part of the prevention of unintended pregnancies and sexually transmitted diseases (STDs) in adolescents is evaluated in this policy statement. Sexual activity and pregnancies decreased slightly among adolescents in the 1990s, reversing trends that were present in the 1970s and 1980s, while condom use among adolescents increased significantly. These trends likely reflect initial success of primary and secondary prevention messages aimed at adolescents. Rates of acquisition of STDs and human immunodeficiency virus (HIV) among adolescents remain unacceptably high, highlighting the need for continued prevention efforts and reflecting the fact that improved condom use can decrease, but never eliminate, the risk of acquisition of STDs and HIV as well as unintended pregnancies. While many condom education and availability programs have been shown to have modest effects on condom use, there is no evidence that these programs contribute to increased sexual activity among adolescents. These trends highlight the progress that has been made and the large amount that still needs to be accomplished. (6/01, reaffirmed 5/04)

CONFIDENTIALITY IN ADOLESCENT HEALTH CARE
Committee on Adolescence (4/89, reaffirmed 1/93, 11/97, 5/00, 5/04)

CONGENITAL ADRENAL HYPERPLASIA
(TECHNICAL REPORT)
Section on Endocrinology and Committee on Genetics
ABSTRACT. The Section on Endocrinology and the Committee on Genetics of the American Academy of Pediatrics, in collaboration with experts from the field of pediatric endocrinology and genetics, developed this policy statement as a means of providing up-to-date information for the practicing pediatrician about current practice and controversial issues in congenital adrenal hyperplasia (CAH), including the current status of prenatal diagnosis and treatment, the benefits and problem areas of neonatal screening programs, and the management of children with nonclassic CAH. The reference list is designed to allow physicians who wish more information to research the topic more thoroughly. (12/00, reaffirmed 12/03)

A CONSENSUS STATEMENT ON HEALTH CARE TRANSITIONS FOR YOUNG ADULTS WITH SPECIAL HEALTH CARE NEEDS
American Academy of Pediatrics, American Academy of Family Physicians, and American College of Physicians-American Society of Internal Medicine
ABSTRACT. This policy statement represents a consensus on the critical first steps that the medical profession needs to take to realize the vision of a family-centered, continuous, comprehensive, coordinated, compassionate, and culturally competent health care system that is as developmentally appropriate as it is technically sophisticated. The goal of transition in health care for young adults with special health care needs is to maximize lifelong functioning and potential through the provision of high-quality, developmentally appropriate health care services that continue uninterrupted as the individual moves from adolescence to adulthood. This consensus document has now been approved as policy by the boards of the American Academy of Pediatrics, the American Academy of Family Physicians, and the American College of Physicians-American Society of Internal Medicine. (12/02)

CONSENT FOR EMERGENCY MEDICAL SERVICES FOR CHILDREN AND ADOLESCENTS
Committee on Pediatric Emergency Medicine
ABSTRACT. Pediatric patients frequently seek medical treatment in the emergency department (ED) unaccompanied by a legal guardian. Current state and federal laws and medical ethics recommendations support the ED treatment of minors with an identified emergency medical condition, regardless of consent issues. Financial reimbursement should not limit the minor patient's access to emergency medical care or result in a breach of patient confidentiality. Every clinic, office practice, and ED should develop policies and guidelines regarding consent for the treatment of minors. The physician should document all discussions of consent and attempt to seek consent for treatment from the family or legal guardian and assent from the pediatric patient. Appropriate medical care for the pediatric patient with an urgent or emergent condition should never be withheld or delayed because of problems with obtaining consent. *This statement has been endorsed by the American College of Surgeons, the Society of Pediatric Nurses, the Society of Critical Care Medicine, the American College of Emergency Physicians, the Emergency Nurses Association, and the National Association of EMS Physicians.* (3/03)

CONSENT BY PROXY FOR NONURGENT PEDIATRIC CARE (CLINICAL REPORT)
Committee on Medical Liability
ABSTRACT. Minor-aged patients are often brought to the pediatrician for nonurgent acute medical care or health supervision visits by someone other than their custodial parent or guardian. These surrogates can be members of the child's extended family, such as a grandparent or aunt. In cases of divorce and remarriage, a noncustodial parent or stepparent may accompany the patient. Sometimes, children are brought for care by adults living in the home who are not biologically or legally related to the child. In

some instances, a child care professional (eg, au pair, nanny) brings the pediatric patient for medical care. This report identifies common situations in which pediatricians may encounter "consent by proxy" for nonurgent medical care for minors and explains the potential for liability exposure associated with these circumstances. The report suggests practical steps that balance the need to minimize the physician's liability exposure with the patient's access to health care. Key issues to be considered when creating or updating office policies for obtaining and documenting consent by proxy are offered. (11/03)

THE CONTINUED IMPORTANCE OF SUPPLEMENTAL SECURITY INCOME (SSI) FOR CHILDREN AND ADOLESCENTS WITH DISABILITIES
Committee on Children With Disabilities
ABSTRACT. In 1996, as part of the Personal Responsibility and Work Opportunity Reconciliation (Welfare Reform) Act, Congress redefined the Supplemental Security Income (SSI) definition of disability for children and removed the individual functional assessment (IFA) step from the disability determination process. As a result, an estimated 100 000 SSI child beneficiaries have lost or will lose their SSI benefits. The publicity associated with this Congressionally mandated change might also have reduced the number of families applying for SSI benefits on behalf of their children because of a widely held belief that the eligibility criteria for disability benefits are now so restrictive that almost no children are determined to be eligible. The purpose of this statement is to provide updated information about the SSI Program's disability and financial eligibility criteria and disability determination process. This statement also discusses how pediatricians can help to ensure that all eligible children receive the SSI monies and associated benefits to which they are entitled. (4/01)

CONTRACEPTION AND ADOLESCENTS
Committee on Adolescence
ABSTRACT. The risks and negative consequences of adolescent sexual intercourse are of national concern, and promoting sexual abstinence is an important goal of the American Academy of Pediatrics. In previous publications, the American Academy of Pediatrics has addressed important issues of adolescent sexuality, pregnancy, sexually transmitted diseases, and contraception. The development of new contraceptive technologies mandates a revision of this policy statement, which provides the pediatrician with an updated review of adolescent sexuality and use of contraception by adolescents and presents current guidelines for counseling adolescents on sexual activity and contraceptive methods. (11/99)

CONTROVERSIES CONCERNING VITAMIN K AND THE NEWBORN
Committee on Fetus and Newborn
ABSTRACT. Prevention of early vitamin K deficiency bleeding (VKDB) of the newborn, with onset at birth to 2 weeks of age (formerly known as classic hemorrhagic disease of the newborn), by oral or parenteral administration of vitamin K is accepted practice. In contrast, late VKDB, with onset from 2 to 12 weeks of age, is most effectively prevented by parenteral administration of vitamin K. Earlier concern regarding a possible causal association between parenteral vitamin K and childhood cancer has not been substantiated. This revised statement presents updated recommendations for the use of vitamin K in the prevention of early and late VKDB. (7/03)

COPARENT OR SECOND-PARENT ADOPTION BY SAME-SEX PARENTS
Committee on Psychosocial Aspects of Child and Family Health
ABSTRACT. Children who are born to or adopted by 1 member of a same-sex couple deserve the security of 2 legally recognized parents. Therefore, the American Academy of Pediatrics supports legislative and legal efforts to provide the possibility of adoption of the child by the second parent or coparent in these families. (2/02)

COPARENT OR SECOND-PARENT ADOPTION BY SAME-SEX PARENTS (TECHNICAL REPORT)
Committee on Psychosocial Aspects of Child and Family Health
ABSTRACT. A growing body of scientific literature demonstrates that children who grow up with 1 or 2 gay and/or lesbian parents fare as well in emotional, cognitive, social, and sexual functioning as do children whose parents are heterosexual. Children's optimal development seems to be influenced more by the nature of the relationships and interactions within the family unit than by the particular structural form it takes. (2/02)

CORD BLOOD BANKING FOR POTENTIAL FUTURE TRANSPLANTATION: SUBJECT REVIEW (CLINICAL REPORT)
Work Group on Cord Blood Banking
ABSTRACT. In recent years, umbilical cord blood, which contains a large number of hematopoietic stem cells, has been used successfully for allogeneic transplantation to treat a variety of pediatric genetic, hematologic, and oncologic disorders. It is a potential alternative when autologous or allogeneic transplantation with HLA-matched marrow is unavailable for children. This advance has resulted in the establishment of not-for-profit and for-profit cord blood banking programs for autologous and allogeneic transplantation. Many issues confront institutions that wish to establish such a program. Parents also seek information from their physicians about this new modality. This document is intended to provide information to guide physicians in responding to parents' questions about cord blood banking. The document also makes recommendations about appropriate ethical and operational standards, including informed consent policies, for the institutions that operate a program. (7/99)

CORPORAL PUNISHMENT IN SCHOOLS
Committee on School Health
ABSTRACT. The American Academy of Pediatrics recommends that corporal punishment in schools be abolished in all states by law and that alternative forms of student behavior management be used. (8/00, reaffirmed 6/03)

COUNSELING THE ADOLESCENT ABOUT PREGNANCY OPTIONS
Committee on Adolescence
ABSTRACT. When consulted by a pregnant adolescent, pediatricians should be able to make a timely diagnosis and to help the adolescent understand her options and act on her decision to continue or terminate her pregnancy. Pediatricians may not impose their values on the decision-making process and should be prepared to support the adolescent in her decision or refer her to a physician who can. (5/98, reaffirmed 1/01)

COUNSELING FAMILIES WHO CHOOSE COMPLEMENTARY AND ALTERNATIVE MEDICINE FOR THEIR CHILD WITH CHRONIC ILLNESS OR DISABILITY
Committee on Children With Disabilities
ABSTRACT. The use of complementary and alternative medicine (CAM) to treat chronic illness or disability is increasing in the United States. This is especially evident among children with autism and related disorders. It may be challenging to the practicing pediatrician to distinguish among accepted biomedical treatments, unproven therapies, and alternative therapies. Moreover, there are no published guidelines regarding the use of CAM in the care of children with chronic illness or disability. To best serve the interests of children, it is important to maintain a scientific perspective, to provide balanced advice about therapeutic options, to guard against bias, and to establish and maintain a trusting relationship with families. This statement provides information and guidance for pediatricians when counseling families about CAM. (3/01)

DEALING WITH THE PARENT WHOSE JUDGMENT IS IMPAIRED BY ALCOHOL OR DRUGS: LEGAL AND ETHICAL CONSIDERATIONS (CLINICAL REPORT)
Committee on Medical Liability
See full text on page 297. (9/04)

DEATH OF A CHILD IN THE EMERGENCY DEPARTMENT: JOINT STATEMENT OF THE AMERICAN ACADEMY OF PEDIATRICS AND THE AMERICAN COLLEGE OF EMERGENCY PHYSICIANS
American Academy of Pediatrics Committee on Pediatric Emergency Medicine and the American College of Emergency Physicians (10/02)

DEVELOPMENTAL DYSPLASIA OF THE HIP PRACTICE GUIDELINE (TECHNICAL REPORT)
Steering Committee on Quality Improvement and Management
See summary on page 47. (4/00)

DEVELOPMENTAL ISSUES FOR YOUNG CHILDREN IN FOSTER CARE
Committee on Early Childhood, Adoption, and Dependent Care
ABSTRACT. Greater numbers of young children with complicated, serious physical health, mental health, or developmental problems are entering foster care during the early years when brain growth is most active. Every effort should be made to make foster care a positive experience and a healing process for the child. Threats to a child's development from abuse and neglect should be understood by all participants in the child welfare system. Pediatricians have an important role in assessing the child's needs, providing comprehensive services, and advocating on the child's behalf.

The developmental issues important for young children in foster care are reviewed, including: 1) the implications and consequences of abuse, neglect, and placement in foster care on early brain development; 2) the importance and challenges of establishing a child's attachment to caregivers; 3) the importance of considering a child's changing sense of time in all aspects of the foster care experience; and 4) the child's response to stress. Additional topics addressed relate to parental roles and kinship care, parent-child contact, permanency decision-making, and the components of comprehensive assessment and treatment of a child's development and mental health needs. (11/00)

DEVELOPMENTAL SURVEILLANCE AND SCREENING OF INFANTS AND YOUNG CHILDREN
Committee on Children With Disabilities
ABSTRACT. Early identification of children with developmental delays is important in the primary care setting. The pediatrician is the best-informed professional with whom many families have contact during the first 5 years of a child's life. Parents look to the pediatrician to be the expert not only on childhood illnesses but also on development. Early intervention services for children from birth to 3 years of age and early childhood education services for children 3 to 5 years of age are widely available for children with developmental delays or disabilities in the United States. Developmental screening instruments have improved over the years, and instruments that are accurate and easy to use in an office setting are now available to the pediatrician. This statement provides recommendations for screening infants and young children and intervening with families to identify developmental delays and disabilities. (7/01)

DIAGNOSIS AND MANAGEMENT OF CHILDHOOD OBSTRUCTIVE SLEEP APNEA SYNDROME (TECHNICAL REPORT)
Steering Committee on Quality Improvement and Management and Section on Pediatric Pulmonology
See summary on page 213. (4/02)

DIAGNOSTIC IMAGING OF CHILD ABUSE
Section on Radiology
ABSTRACT. The role of imaging in cases of child abuse is to identify the extent of physical injury when abuse occurs, as well as to elucidate all imaging findings that point to alternative diagnoses. Diagnostic imaging of child abuse is based on both advances in imaging technology, as well as a better understanding of the subject based on scientific data obtained during the past 10 years. The initial recommendation was published in *Pediatrics* (1991;87:262–264). (6/00)

DISCLOSURE OF ILLNESS STATUS TO CHILDREN AND ADOLESCENTS WITH HIV INFECTION
Committee on Pediatric AIDS
ABSTRACT. Many children with human immunodeficiency virus (HIV) infection and acquired immunodeficiency syndrome are surviving to middle childhood and adolescence. Studies suggest that children who know their HIV status have higher self-esteem than children who are unaware of their status. Parents who have disclosed the status to their children experience less depression than those who do not. This statement addresses our current knowledge and recommendations for disclosure of HIV infection status to children and adolescents. (1/99, reaffirmed 2/02)

DISTINGUISHING SUDDEN INFANT DEATH SYNDROME FROM CHILD ABUSE FATALITIES
Committee on Child Abuse and Neglect
ABSTRACT. In most cases, when a healthy infant younger than 1 year dies suddenly and unexpectedly, the cause is sudden infant death syndrome (SIDS). SIDS is more common than infanticide. Parents of SIDS victims typically are anxious to provide unlimited information to professionals involved in death investigation or research. They also want and deserve to be approached in a nonaccusatory manner. This statement provides professionals with information and guidelines to avoid distressing or stigmatizing families of SIDS victims while allowing accumulation of appropriate evidence in potential cases of death by infanticide. (2/01)

DISTINGUISHING SUDDEN INFANT DEATH SYNDROME FROM CHILD ABUSE FATALITIES (ADDENDUM)
Committee on Child Abuse and Neglect (9/01)

DO NOT RESUSCITATE ORDERS IN SCHOOLS
Committee on School Health and Committee on Bioethics
ABSTRACT. Increased medical knowledge and technology have led to the survival of many children who previously would have died of a variety of conditions. As these children with continuing life-threatening problems reach school age, families, professionals, and paraprofessionals have to deal with the challenges involved in their care. Some children may be at high risk of dying while in school. When families have chosen to limit resuscitative efforts, school officials should understand the medical, emotional, and legal issues involved. (4/00, reaffirmed 6/03)

DO-NOT-RESUSCITATE ORDERS FOR PEDIATRIC PATIENTS WHO REQUIRE ANESTHESIA AND SURGERY (CLINICAL REPORT)
Section on Surgery, Section on Anesthesia and Pain Medicine, and Committee on Bioethics
See full text on page 305. (12/04)

DRUGS FOR PEDIATRIC EMERGENCIES
Committee on Drugs
ABSTRACT. This statement provides current recommendations about the use of emergency drugs for acute pediatric problems that require pharmacologic intervention. At each clinical setting, physicians and other providers should evaluate drug, equipment, and training needs. The information provided here is not all-inclusive and is not intended to be appropriate to every health care setting. When possible, dosage recommendations are consistent with those in standard references, such as the *Advanced Pediatric Life Support* (APLS) and *Pediatric Advanced Life Support* (PALS) textbooks. Additional guidance is available in the manual *Emergency Medical Services for Children: The Role of the Primary Care Provider*, published by the American Academy of Pediatrics, as well as in the PALS and APLS textbooks. (1/98)

ECHOCARDIOGRAPHY IN INFANTS AND CHILDREN
Section on Cardiology
ABSTRACT. It is the intent of this statement to inform pediatric providers on the appropriate use of echocardiography. Although on-site consultation may be impossible, methods should be established to ensure timely review of echocardiograms by a pediatric cardiologist. With advances in data transmission, echocardiography information can be exchanged, in some cases eliminating the need for a costly patient transfer. By cooperating through training, education, and referral, complete and cost-effective echocardiographic services can be provided to all children. (6/97, reaffirmed 3/03)

EDUCATION OF CHILDREN WITH HUMAN IMMUNODEFICIENCY VIRUS INFECTION
Committee on Pediatric AIDS
ABSTRACT. Treatment for human immunodeficiency virus (HIV) infection has enabled more children and youths to attend school and participate in school activities. Children and youths with HIV infection should receive the same education as those with other chronic illnesses. They may require special services, including home instruction, to provide continuity of education. Confidentiality about HIV infection status should be maintained with parental consent required for disclosure. Youths also should assent or consent as is appropriate for disclosure of their diagnosis. (6/00, reaffirmed 3/03)

E-MAIL COMMUNICATION BETWEEN PEDIATRICIANS AND THEIR PATIENTS (CLINICAL REPORT)
Steering Committee on Clinical Information Technology
See full text on page 315. (7/04)

EMERGENCY PREPAREDNESS FOR CHILDREN WITH SPECIAL HEALTH CARE NEEDS
Committee on Pediatric Emergency Medicine
ABSTRACT. Children with special health care needs are those who have, or are at risk for, chronic physical, developmental, behavioral, or emotional conditions and who also require health and related services of a type or amount not usually required by typically developing children. Formulation of an emergency care plan has been advocated by the Emergency Medical Services for Children (EMSC) program through its Children With Special Heath Care Needs Task Force. Essential components of a program of providing care plans include use of a standardized form, a method of identifying at-risk children, completion of a data set by the child's physicians

and other health care professionals, education of families, other caregivers, and health care professionals in use of the emergency plan, regular updates of the information, 24-hour access to the information by authorized emergency health care professionals, and maintenance of patient confidentiality. (10/99, reaffirmed 8/02)

ENHANCING THE RACIAL AND ETHNIC DIVERSITY OF THE PEDIATRIC WORKFORCE
Committee on Pediatric Workforce
ABSTRACT. *Purpose.* This statement seeks to increase the awareness of the importance of diversity; to encourage the incorporation of principles of cultural competence into all aspects of pediatric education, training, and practice, as exemplified by practitioners, educators, and our national leadership; and finally to identify strategies for implementing this incorporation.

Key Concepts. The increasing cultural diversity of the population has significant implications for the pediatric workforce and for the provision of pediatric health services. Diversity within the pediatric workforce will enhance the potential for pediatricians to acquire the knowledge and practice skills needed to effectively address the health and wellness needs of children and families. Support from this diversity should be integrated into all aspects of education, including providing quality education for minority students and attracting and retaining minority faculty; and should be sought through collaboration locally, regionally, and nationally with organizations and community leaders.

Anticipated Outcomes. The Policy Statement recommendations will be used to inform educators, administrators, practitioners, and others in the development of curricula, programs, and initiatives to enhance the diversity of the pediatric workforce and increase the cultural competence of practitioners. (1/00)

ENSURING CULTURALLY EFFECTIVE PEDIATRIC CARE: IMPLICATIONS FOR EDUCATION AND HEALTH POLICY
Committee on Pediatric Workforce
See full text on page 323. (12/04)

ENVIRONMENTAL TOBACCO SMOKE: A HAZARD TO CHILDREN
Committee on Environmental Health
ABSTRACT. Results of epidemiologic studies provide strong evidence that exposure of children to environmental tobacco smoke is associated with increased rates of lower respiratory illness and increased rates of middle ear effusion, asthma, and sudden infant death syndrome. Exposure during childhood may also be associated with development of cancer during adulthood. This statement reviews the health effects of environmental tobacco smoke on children and offers pediatricians a strategy for promoting a smoke-free environment. (4/97, reaffirmed 10/00)

ETHICAL CONSIDERATIONS IN RESEARCH WITH SOCIALLY IDENTIFIABLE POPULATIONS
Committee on Native American Child Health and Committee on Community Health Services
See full text on page 335. (1/04)

ETHICAL ISSUES WITH GENETIC TESTING IN PEDIATRICS
Committee on Bioethics
ABSTRACT. Advances in genetic research promise great strides in the diagnosis and treatment of many childhood diseases. However, emerging genetic technology often enables testing and screening before the development of definitive treatment or preventive measures. In these circumstances, careful consideration must be given to testing and screening of children to ensure that use of this technology promotes the best interest of the child. This statement reviews considerations for the use of genetic technology for newborn screening, carrier testing, and testing for susceptibility to late-onset conditions. Recommendations are made promoting informed participation by parents for newborn screening and limited use of carrier testing and testing for late-onset conditions in the pediatric population. Additional research and education in this developing area of medicine are encouraged. (6/01, reaffirmed 4/04)

ETHICS AND THE CARE OF CRITICALLY ILL INFANTS AND CHILDREN
Committee on Bioethics
ABSTRACT. The ability to provide life support to ill children who, not long ago, would have died despite medicine's best efforts challenges pediatricians and families to address profound moral questions. Our society has been divided about extending the life of some patients, especially newborns and older infants with severe disabilities. The American Academy of Pediatrics (AAP) supports individualized decision making about life-sustaining medical treatment for all children, regardless of age. These decisions should be jointly made by physicians and parents, unless good reasons require invoking established child protective services to contravene parental authority. At this time, resource allocation (rationing) decisions about which children should receive intensive care resources should be made clear and explicit in public policy, rather than be made at the bedside. (7/96, reaffirmed 10/99, 6/03)

EVALUATION OF THE NEWBORN WITH DEVELOPMENTAL ANOMALIES OF THE EXTERNAL GENITALIA
Committee on Genetics, Section on Endocrinology, and Section on Urology
ABSTRACT. The newborn with abnormal genital development presents a difficult diagnostic and treatment challenge for the primary care pediatrician. It is important that a definitive diagnosis be determined as quickly as possible so that an appropriate treatment plan can be established to minimize medical, psychological, and social complications. The purpose of this review is to identify which newborns among those with abnormal genital development need to be screened for intersexuality, to outline the investigations necessary, and to suggest indications for referral to a center with experience in the diagnosis and management of these disorders. An outline is also presented of the embryology of the external genitalia indicating where errors can arise to provide a framework for pediatricians

to use when counseling families. Although the focus of this review is on newborns with what has been termed "ambiguous genitalia," it should be recognized that most genital abnormalities in newborns do not result in an ambiguous appearance. These anomalies include hypospadias, in which the genitalia are clearly malformed, although the sex is unquestionably male. (7/00)

EVALUATION AND PREPARATION OF PEDIATRIC PATIENTS UNDERGOING ANESTHESIA
Section on Anesthesiology and Pain Medicine (9/96)

EVALUATION AND TREATMENT OF THE HUMAN IMMUNODEFICIENCY VIRUS-1–EXPOSED INFANT (CLINICAL REPORT)
American Academy of Pediatrics Committee on Pediatric AIDS and Canadian Paediatric Society
See full text on page 341. (8/04)

EVIDENCE FOR THE DIAGNOSIS AND TREATMENT OF ACUTE UNCOMPLICATED SINUSITIS IN CHILDREN: A SYSTEMATIC OVERVIEW (TECHNICAL REPORT)
Steering Committee on Quality Improvement and Management
See summary on page 193. (9/01)

AN EVIDENCE-BASED REVIEW OF IMPORTANT ISSUES CONCERNING NEONATAL HYPERBILIRUBINEMIA (TECHNICAL REPORT)
Steering Committee on Quality Improvement and Management
See summary on page 125. (7/04)

EYE EXAMINATION IN INFANTS, CHILDREN, AND YOUNG ADULTS BY PEDIATRICIANS
American Academy of Pediatrics Committee on Practice and Ambulatory Medicine and Section on Ophthalmology, American Association of Certified Orthoptists, American Association for Pediatric Ophthalmology and Strabismus, and American Academy of Ophthalmology
ABSTRACT. Early detection and prompt treatment of ocular disorders in children is important to avoid lifelong visual impairment. Examination of the eyes should be performed beginning in the newborn period and at all well-child visits. Newborns should be examined for ocular structural abnormalities, such as cataract, corneal opacity, and ptosis, which are known to result in visual problems. Vision assessment beginning at birth has been endorsed by the American Academy of Pediatrics, the American Association for Pediatric Ophthalmology and Strabismus, and the American Academy of Ophthalmology. All children who are found to have an ocular abnormality or who fail vision assessment should be referred to a pediatric ophthalmologist or an eye care specialist appropriately trained to treat pediatric patients. (4/03)

FACILITIES AND EQUIPMENT FOR THE CARE OF PEDIATRIC PATIENTS IN A COMMUNITY HOSPITAL (CLINICAL REPORT)
Committee on Hospital Care
ABSTRACT. Many children who require hospitalization are admitted to community hospitals that are more accessible for families and their primary care physicians but vary substantially in their pediatric resources. The intent of this clinical report is to provide basic guidelines for furnishing and equipping a pediatric area in a community hospital. (5/03)

FALLS FROM HEIGHTS: WINDOWS, ROOFS, AND BALCONIES
Committee on Injury and Poison Prevention
ABSTRACT. Falls of all kinds represent an important cause of child injury and death. In the United States, approximately 140 deaths from falls occur annually in children younger than 15 years. Three million children require emergency department care for fall-related injuries. This policy statement examines the epidemiology of falls from heights and recommends preventive strategies for pediatricians and other child health care professionals. Such strategies involve parent counseling, community programs, building code changes, legislation, and environmental modification, such as the installation of window guards and balcony railings. (5/01, reaffirmed 5/04)

FAMILIES AND ADOPTION: THE PEDIATRICIAN'S ROLE IN SUPPORTING COMMUNICATION (CLINICAL REPORT)
Committee on Early Childhood, Adoption, and Dependent Care
ABSTRACT. Each year, more children join families through adoption. Pediatricians have an important role in assisting adoptive families in the various challenges they may face with respect to adoption. The acceptance of the differences between families formed through birth and those formed through adoption is essential in promoting positive emotional growth within the family. It is important for pediatricians to be informed about adoption and to share this knowledge with adoptive families. Parents need ongoing advice with respect to adoption issues and need to be supported in their communication with their adopted children. (12/03)

FAMILY-CENTERED CARE AND THE PEDIATRICIAN'S ROLE
American Academy of Pediatrics Committee on Hospital Care and Institute for Family-Centered Care
ABSTRACT. Drawing on several decades of work with families, pediatricians, other health care professionals, and policy makers, the American Academy of Pediatrics provides a definition of family-centered care. In pediatrics, family-centered care is based on the understanding that the family is the child's primary source of strength and support. Further, this approach to care recognizes that the perspectives and information provided by families, children, and young adults are important in clinical decision making. This policy statement outlines the core principles of family-centered care, summarizes the recent literature linking family-centered care to improved health outcomes, and lists various other benefits to be expected when engaging in family-centered pediatric practice. The statement concludes with specific recommendations for how pediatricians can integrate family-centered care in hospitals, clinics, and community settings as well as in more broad systems of care. (9/03)

FATHERS AND PEDIATRICIANS: ENHANCING MEN'S ROLES IN THE CARE AND DEVELOPMENT OF THEIR CHILDREN (CLINICAL REPORT)
Committee on Psychosocial Aspects of Child and Family Health
See full text on page 353. (5/04)

FEMALE GENITAL MUTILATION
Committee on Bioethics
ABSTRACT. The traditional custom of ritual cutting and alteration of the genitalia of female infants, girls, and adolescents, referred to as female genital mutilation (FGM), persists primarily in Africa and among certain communities in the Middle East and Asia. Immigrants in the United States from areas where FGM is endemic may have daughters who have undergone a ritual genital procedure or may request that such a procedure be performed by a physician. The American Academy of Pediatrics (AAP) believes that pediatricians and pediatric surgical specialists should be aware that this practice has serious, life-threatening health risks for children and women. The AAP opposes all forms of FGM, counsels its members not to perform such ritual procedures, and encourages the development of community educational programs for immigrant populations. (7/98, reaffirmed 11/02)

FETAL ALCOHOL SYNDROME AND ALCOHOL-RELATED NEURODEVELOPMENTAL DISORDERS
Committee on Substance Abuse and Committee on Children With Disabilities
ABSTRACT. Prenatal exposure to alcohol is one of the leading preventable causes of birth defects, mental retardation, and neurodevelopmental disorders. In 1973, a cluster of birth defects resulting from prenatal alcohol exposure was recognized as a clinical entity called *fetal alcohol syndrome.* More recently, alcohol exposure in utero has been linked to a variety of other neurodevelopmental problems, and the terms *alcohol-related neurodevelopmental disorder* and *alcohol-related birth defects* have been proposed to identify infants so affected. This statement is an update of a previous statement by the American Academy of Pediatrics and reflects the current thinking about alcohol exposure in utero and the revised nosology. (8/00)

FETAL THERAPY—ETHICAL CONSIDERATIONS
Committee on Bioethics
ABSTRACT. Decisions to undertake fetal therapy involve a complex assessment of the best interests of the fetus and a pregnant woman's interest in her own health and freedom from unwanted invasion of her body. Pregnant women almost always accept a recommendation for fetal therapy that is approached collaboratively, especially if the therapy is of proven efficacy and has a low maternal risk. Fetal therapy of unproven efficacy should only be undertaken as part of an approved research protocol. In recommending fetal therapy of proven efficacy, physicians should respect maternal choice and assessment of risk. Under limited circumstances when fetal therapy would be effective in preventing irrevocable and substantial fetal harm with negligible risk to the health and well-being of the pregnant woman, should the pregnant woman be opposed to the intervention, physicians should engage in a process of communication and conflict resolution that may require consultation from an ethics committee and, in rare cases, require judicial review. A physician should never intervene without the woman's explicit consent before judicial review. (5/99, reaffirmed 11/02)

FIREARM-RELATED INJURIES AFFECTING THE PEDIATRIC POPULATION
Committee on Injury and Poison Prevention
ABSTRACT. This statement reaffirms the 1992 position of the American Academy of Pediatrics that the absence of guns from children's homes and communities is the most reliable and effective measure to prevent firearm-related injuries in children and adolescents. A number of specific measures are supported to reduce the destructive effects of guns in the lives of children and adolescents, including the regulation of the manufacture, sale, purchase, ownership, and use of firearms; a ban on handguns and semiautomatic assault weapons; and expanded regulations of handguns for civilian use. In addition, this statement reviews recent data, trends, prevention, and intervention strategies of the past 5 years. (4/00, reaffirmed 5/04)

FIREWORKS-RELATED INJURIES TO CHILDREN
Committee on Injury and Poison Prevention
ABSTRACT. An estimated 8500 individuals, approximately 45% of them children younger than 15 years, were treated in US hospital emergency departments during 1999 for fireworks-related injuries. The hands (40%), eyes (20%), and head and face (20%) are the body areas most often involved. Approximately one third of eye injuries from fireworks result in permanent blindness. During 1999, 16 people died as a result of injuries associated with fireworks. Every type of legally available consumer (so-called "safe and sane") firework has been associated with serious injury or death. In 1997, 20 100 fires were caused by fireworks, resulting in $22.7 million in direct property damage. Fireworks typically cause more fires in the United States on the Fourth of July than all other causes of fire combined on that day. Pediatricians should educate parents, children, community leaders, and others about the dangers of fireworks. Fireworks for individual private use should be banned. Children and their families should be encouraged to enjoy fireworks at public fireworks displays conducted by professionals rather than purchase fireworks for home or private use. (7/01, reaffirmed 11/04)

FOLIC ACID FOR THE PREVENTION OF NEURAL TUBE DEFECTS
Committee on Genetics
ABSTRACT. The American Academy of Pediatrics endorses the US Public Health Service (USPHS) recommendation that all women capable of becoming pregnant consume 400 μg of folic acid daily to prevent neural tube defects (NTDs). Studies have demonstrated that periconceptional folic acid supplementation can prevent 50% or more of NTDs such as spina bifida and anencephaly. For women who have previously had an NTD-affected pregnancy, the Centers for Disease Control and Prevention (CDC) recommends increasing the intake of folic acid to 4000 μg per day beginning at least 1 month before conception and continuing through the first trimester. Implementation of these recommendations is essential for the primary prevention of these serious and disabling birth

defects. Because fewer than 1 in 3 women consume the amount of folic acid recommended by the USPHS, the Academy notes that the prevention of NTDs depends on an urgent and effective campaign to close this prevention gap. (8/99, reaffirmed 11/02)

FOLLOW-UP MANAGEMENT OF CHILDREN WITH TYMPANOSTOMY TUBES

Section on Otolaryngology and Bronchoesophagology

ABSTRACT. The follow-up care of children in whom tympanostomy tubes have been placed is shared by the pediatrician and the otolaryngologist. Guidelines are provided for routine follow-up evaluation, perioperative hearing assessment, and the identification of specific conditions and complications that warrant urgent otolaryngologic consultation. These guidelines have been developed by a consensus of expert opinions. (2/02)

FORGOING LIFE-SUSTAINING MEDICAL TREATMENT IN ABUSED CHILDREN

Committee on Child Abuse and Neglect and Committee on Bioethics

ABSTRACT. A decision to forgo life-sustaining medical treatment (LSMT) for a critically ill child injured as the result of abuse should be made using the same criteria as those used for any critically ill child. The parent or guardian of an abused child may have a conflict of interest when a decision to forgo LSMT risks changing the legal charge faced by a parent, guardian, relative, or acquaintance from assault to manslaughter or homicide. If a physician suspects that a parent or guardian is not acting in a child's best interest, further review and consultation should be sought in hopes of resolving the conflict. A guardian ad litem who will represent the child's interests regarding LSMT should be appointed in all cases in which a parent or guardian may have a conflict of interest. (11/00, reaffirmed 6/03)

GENERIC PRESCRIBING, GENERIC SUBSTITUTION, AND THERAPEUTIC SUBSTITUTION

Committee on Drugs (5/87, reaffirmed 6/93, 5/96, 6/99, 5/01)

GRADUATE MEDICAL EDUCATION AND PEDIATRIC WORKFORCE ISSUES AND PRINCIPLES

Task Force on Graduate Medical Education Reform (6/94)

GUIDANCE FOR EFFECTIVE DISCIPLINE

Committee on Psychosocial Aspects of Child and Family Health

ABSTRACT. When advising families about discipline strategies, pediatricians should use a comprehensive approach that includes consideration of the parent-child relationship, reinforcement of desired behaviors, and consequences for negative behaviors. Corporal punishment is of limited effectiveness and has potentially deleterious side effects. The American Academy of Pediatrics recommends that parents be encouraged and assisted in the development of methods other than spanking for managing undesired behavior. (4/98, reaffirmed 5/04)

GUIDELINES FOR THE ADMINISTRATION OF MEDICATION IN SCHOOL

Committee on School Health

ABSTRACT. Many children who take medications require them during the school day. This policy statement is designed to guide prescribing physicians as well as school administrators and health staff on the administration of medications to children at school. The statement addresses over-the-counter products, herbal medications, experimental drugs that are administered as part of a clinical trial, emergency medications, and principles of student safety. (9/03)

GUIDELINES FOR DEVELOPING ADMISSION AND DISCHARGE POLICIES FOR THE PEDIATRIC INTENSIVE CARE UNIT

American Academy of Pediatrics Committee on Hospital Care and Section on Critical Care and the Society of Critical Care Medicine Pediatric Section Admission Criteria Task Force

ABSTRACT. These guidelines were developed to provide a reference for preparing policies on admission to and discharge from pediatric intensive care units. They represent a consensus opinion of physicians, nurses, and allied health care professionals. By using this document as a framework for developing multidisciplinary admission and discharge policies, use of pediatric intensive care units can be optimized and patients can receive the level of care appropriate for their condition. (4/99)

GUIDELINES FOR EMERGENCY MEDICAL CARE IN SCHOOL

Committee on School Health

ABSTRACT. Minor and major illnesses and injuries can occur in children during the school day. This statement provides recommendations for emergency health care for children in school, including information about procedures, staff and their education, documentation, and parental notification. (2/01)

GUIDELINES FOR THE ETHICAL CONDUCT OF STUDIES TO EVALUATE DRUGS IN PEDIATRIC POPULATIONS

Committee on Drugs (2/95, reaffirmed 3/98, 5/01)

GUIDELINES FOR THE EVALUATION OF SEXUAL ABUSE OF CHILDREN: SUBJECT REVIEW (CLINICAL REPORT)

Committee on Child Abuse and Neglect

ABSTRACT. This statement serves to update guidelines for the evaluation of child sexual abuse first published in 1991. The role of the physician is outlined with respect to obtaining a history, physical examination, and appropriate laboratory data and in determining the need to report sexual abuse. (1/99)

GUIDELINES FOR EXPERT WITNESS TESTIMONY IN MEDICAL MALPRACTICE LITIGATION

Committee on Medical Liability

ABSTRACT. The interests of the public and the medical profession are best served when scientifically sound and unbiased expert witness testimony is readily available to plaintiffs and defendants in medical negligence suits. As members of the physician community, as patient advocates, and as private citizens, pediatricians have ethical and professional obligations to assist in the administration of justice, particularly in matters concerning potential medical malpractice. The American Academy of Pediatrics believes that the adoption of the recommendations outlined in this statement will improve the quality of medical expert witness testimony in such proceedings and thereby increase the probability of achieving equitable outcomes. Strategies to enforce ethical guidelines should be monitored for efficacy before offering policy recommendations on disciplining physicians for providing biased, false, or unscientific medical expert witness testimony. (5/02)

GUIDELINES ON FORGOING LIFE-SUSTAINING MEDICAL TREATMENT
Committee on Bioethics (3/94, reaffirmed 11/97, 10/00, 1/04)

GUIDELINES FOR HOME CARE OF INFANTS, CHILDREN, AND ADOLESCENTS WITH CHRONIC DISEASE
Committee on Children With Disabilities (7/95, reaffirmed 4/00)

GUIDELINES AND LEVELS OF CARE FOR PEDIATRIC INTENSIVE CARE UNITS (CLINICAL REPORT)
American Academy of Pediatrics Committee on Hospital Care and Section on Critical Care and Society of Critical Care Medicine
See full text on page 361. (10/04)

GUIDELINES FOR MONITORING AND MANAGEMENT OF PEDIATRIC PATIENTS DURING AND AFTER SEDATION FOR DIAGNOSTIC AND THERAPEUTIC PROCEDURES
Committee on Drugs (6/92, reaffirmed 6/95, 6/98, 5/02)

GUIDELINES FOR MONITORING AND MANAGEMENT OF PEDIATRIC PATIENTS DURING AND AFTER SEDATION FOR DIAGNOSTIC AND THERAPEUTIC PROCEDURES: ADDENDUM
Committee on Drugs
ABSTRACT. The purpose of this addendum to the 1992 policy statement is to clarify some of the terms used in that document and to more thoroughly delineate the responsibilities of the practitioner when sedating children. (10/02)

GUIDELINES FOR OPHTHALMOLOGIC EXAMINATIONS IN CHILDREN WITH JUVENILE RHEUMATOID ARTHRITIS
Section on Ophthalmology and Section on Rheumatology (8/93, reaffirmed 8/99)

GUIDELINES FOR PEDIATRIC CANCER CENTERS
Section on Hematology/Oncology
See full text on page 375. (6/04)

GUIDELINES FOR PEDIATRIC CARDIOVASCULAR CENTERS
Section on Cardiology and Cardiac Surgery
ABSTRACT. Pediatric cardiovascular centers should aim to provide high-quality therapeutic outcomes for infants and children with congenital and acquired heart diseases. This policy statement describes critical elements and organizational features of centers in which high-quality outcomes have the greatest likelihood of occurring. Center elements include noninvasive diagnostic modalities, cardiac catheterization, cardiovascular surgery, and cardiovascular intensive care. These elements should be organizationally united in centers in which pediatric cardiac physician specialists and specialized pediatric staff work together to achieve and surpass existing quality-of-care benchmarks. (3/02)

GUIDELINES FOR THE PEDIATRIC PERIOPERATIVE ANESTHESIA ENVIRONMENT
Section on Anesthesiology and Pain Medicine
ABSTRACT. The American Academy of Pediatrics proposes the following guidelines for the pediatric perioperative anesthesia environment. Essential components are identified that make the perioperative environment satisfactory for the anesthesia care of infants and children. Such an environment promotes the safety and well-being of infants and children by reducing the risk for adverse events. (2/99, reaffirmed 10/02)

GUIDELINES FOR REFERRAL TO PEDIATRIC SURGICAL SPECIALISTS
Surgical Advisory Panel (7/02)

GUIDING PRINCIPLES, ATTRIBUTES, AND PROCESS TO REVIEW MEDICAL MANAGEMENT GUIDELINES
Task Force on Medical Management Guidelines
ABSTRACT. Few issues are more central to the ongoing debate about health care in the United States than concerns about cost and quality of medical care. The recent development and implementation of medical management guidelines that include recommendations for diagnostic and therapeutic interventions, hospital length of stay, intensity of service, home care, and access to specialists have often focused this debate on the potential trade-off between cost reductions and quality of care. The American Academy of Pediatrics recognizes that cost and quality are integrally related and that it is possible to reduce costs while maintaining and improving quality. The purpose of this statement is to help pediatricians and other health care providers interpret, evaluate, and improve medical management guidelines. (12/01)

GUIDING PRINCIPLES FOR MANAGED CARE ARRANGEMENTS FOR THE HEALTH CARE OF NEWBORNS, INFANTS, CHILDREN, ADOLESCENTS, AND YOUNG ADULTS
Committee on Child Health Financing
ABSTRACT. By including the precepts of primary care in the delivery of services, managed care can be a tool to increase access to a full range of health care clinicians and services. On the other hand, managed care can result in underutilization of appropriate services and reduced quality of care. Therefore, the American Academy of Pediatrics urges the use of the principles outlined in this statement in designing and implementing managed care for newborns, infants, children, adolescents, and young adults for several reasons. This policy statement replaces the 1995 policy statement, "Guiding Principles for Managed Care Arrangements for the Health Care of Infants, Children, Adolescents and Young Adults," and outlines the key principles of managed care for newborns, infants, children, adolescents, and young adults. (1/00)

THE HAZARDS OF CHILD LABOR
Committee on Environmental Health (2/95, reaffirmed 11/98)

HEAD LICE (CLINICAL REPORT)
Committee on Infectious Diseases and Committee
   on School Health
ABSTRACT. Head lice infestation is associated with little morbidity but causes a high level of anxiety among parents of school-aged children. This statement attempts to clarify issues of diagnosis and treatment of head lice and makes recommendations for dealing with head lice in the school setting. (9/02)

HEALTH APPRAISAL GUIDELINES FOR DAY CAMPS AND RESIDENT CAMPS
Committee on School Health
ABSTRACT. The American Academy of Pediatrics recommends that specific guidelines be established for pre-camp health appraisals of young people in day and resident camps. Camp guidelines also should include reference to health maintenance, storage and administration of medication, and emergency medical services.

Although camps have diverse environments, there are general guidelines that apply to all situations, and specific recommendations are appropriate under special conditions. (3/00)

HEALTH CARE FOR CHILDREN AND ADOLESCENTS IN THE JUVENILE CORRECTIONAL CARE SYSTEM
Committee on Adolescence
ABSTRACT. Over the past decade, there has been a dramatic increase in the population of juvenile offenders in the United States. Juveniles detained or confined in correctional care facilities have been shown to have numerous health problems. Such conditions may have existed before incarceration; may be closely associated with legal problems; may have resulted from parental neglect, mental health disorders, or physical, drug, or sexual abuse; or may develop within the institutional environment. Delinquent youths are often disenfranchised from traditional health care services in the community. For these adolescents, health care provided through correctional services may be their major source of health services. Pediatricians and correctional health care systems have an opportunity and responsibility to help improve the health of this underserved and vulnerable group of adolescents. (4/01)

HEALTH CARE SUPERVISION FOR CHILDREN WITH WILLIAMS SYNDROME
Committee on Genetics
ABSTRACT. This set of guidelines is designed to assist the pediatrician to care for children with Williams syndrome diagnosed by clinical features and with regional chromosomal microdeletion confirmed by fluorescence in situ hybridization. (5/01)

HEALTH CARE OF YOUNG CHILDREN IN FOSTER CARE
Committee on Early Childhood, Adoption, and Dependent Care
ABSTRACT. Greater numbers of infants and young children with increasingly complicated and serious physical, mental health, and developmental problems are being placed in foster care. All children in foster care need to receive initial health screenings and comprehensive assessments of their medical, mental, dental health, and developmental status. Results of these assessments must be included in the court-approved social services plan and should be linked to the provision of individualized comprehensive care that is continuous and part of a medical home. Pediatricians have an important role in all aspects of the foster care system. (3/02)

HEALTH SUPERVISION FOR CHILDREN WITH ACHONDROPLASIA
Committee on Genetics (3/95, reaffirmed 10/98)

HEALTH SUPERVISION FOR CHILDREN WITH DOWN SYNDROME
Committee on Genetics
ABSTRACT. These guidelines are designed to assist the pediatrician in caring for the child in whom the diagnosis of Down syndrome has been confirmed by karyotype. Although the pediatrician's initial contact with the child is usually during infancy, occasionally the pregnant woman who has been given the prenatal diagnosis of Down syndrome will be referred for counseling. Therefore, these guidelines offer advice for this situation as well. (2/01)

HEALTH SUPERVISION FOR CHILDREN WITH FRAGILE X SYNDROME
Committee on Genetics (8/96, reaffirmed 10/99)

HEALTH SUPERVISION FOR CHILDREN WITH MARFAN SYNDROME
Committee on Genetics
ABSTRACT. This set of guidelines is designed to assist the pediatrician in caring for children with Marfan syndrome confirmed by clinical criteria. Although pediatricians usually first see children with Marfan syndrome during infancy, occasionally they will be called on to advise the pregnant woman who has been informed of the prenatal diagnosis of Marfan syndrome. Therefore, these guidelines offer advice for this situation as well. (11/96, reaffirmed 10/99, 11/02)

HEALTH SUPERVISION FOR CHILDREN WITH NEUROFIBROMATOSIS
Committee on Genetics (8/95, reaffirmed 10/98)

HEALTH SUPERVISION FOR CHILDREN WITH SICKLE CELL DISEASE
Section on Hematology/Oncology and Committee on Genetics
ABSTRACT. Sickle cell disease (SCD) is a group of complex genetic disorders with multisystem manifestations. This statement provides pediatricians in primary care and subspecialty practice with an overview of the genetics, diagnosis, clinical manifestations, and treatment of SCD. Specialized comprehensive medical care decreases morbidity and mortality during childhood. The provision of comprehensive care is a time-intensive endeavor that includes ongoing patient and family education, periodic comprehensive evaluations and other disease-specific health maintenance services, psychosocial care, and genetic counseling. Timely and appropriate treatment of acute illness is critical, because life-threatening complica-

tions develop rapidly. It is essential that every child with SCD receive comprehensive care that is coordinated through a medical home with appropriate expertise. (3/02)

HEALTH SUPERVISION FOR CHILDREN WITH TURNER SYNDROME (CLINICAL REPORT)

Committee on Genetics and Section on Endocrinology

ABSTRACT. This report is designed to assist the pediatrician in caring for the child in whom the diagnosis of Turner syndrome has been confirmed by karyotyping. The report is meant to serve as a supplement to the American Academy of Pediatrics' "Recommendations for Preventive Pediatric Health Care" and emphasizes the importance of continuity of care and the need to avoid its fragmentation by ensuring a medical home for every girl with Turner syndrome. The pediatrician's first contact with a child with Turner syndrome may occur during infancy or childhood. This report also discusses interactions with expectant parents who have been given the prenatal diagnosis of Turner syndrome and have been referred for advice. (3/03)

HEARING ASSESSMENT IN INFANTS AND CHILDREN: RECOMMENDATIONS BEYOND NEONATAL SCREENING (CLINICAL REPORT)

Committee on Practice and Ambulatory Medicine and Section on Otolaryngology and Bronchoesophagology

ABSTRACT. Congenital or acquired hearing loss in infants and children has been linked with lifelong deficits in speech and language acquisition, poor academic performance, personal-social maladjustments, and emotional difficulties. Identification of hearing loss through neonatal hearing screening as well as objective hearing screening of all infants and children can prevent or reduce many of these adverse consequences. This report outlines the risk indicators for hearing loss, provides guidance for when and how to assess hearing loss, and addresses hearing referral resources for children of all ages. (2/03)

HELPING CHILDREN AND FAMILIES DEAL WITH DIVORCE AND SEPARATION (CLINICAL REPORT)

Committee on Psychosocial Aspects of Child and Family Health

ABSTRACT. More than 1 million children each year experience their parents' divorce. For these children and their parents, this process can be emotionally traumatic from the beginning of parental disagreement and rancor, through the divorce, and often for many years thereafter. Pediatricians are encouraged to be aware of behavioral changes in their patients that might be signals of family dysfunction so they can help parents and children understand and deal more positively with the issue. Age-appropriate explanation and counseling is important so children realize that they are not the cause of, and cannot be the cure for, the divorce. Pediatricians can offer families guidance in dealing with their children through the troubled time as well as appropriate lists of reading material and, if indicated, can refer them to professionals with expertise in the emotional, social, and legal aspects of divorce and its aftermath. (11/02)

HOME, HOSPITAL, AND OTHER NON–SCHOOL-BASED INSTRUCTION FOR CHILDREN AND ADOLESCENTS WHO ARE MEDICALLY UNABLE TO ATTEND SCHOOL

Committee on School Health

ABSTRACT. The American Academy of Pediatrics recommends that school-aged children and adolescents obtain their education in school in the least restrictive setting, that is, the setting most conducive to learning for the particular student. However, at times, acute illness or injury and chronic medical conditions preclude school attendance. This statement is meant to assist evaluation and planning for children to receive non–school-based instruction and to return to school at the earliest possible date. (11/00, reaffirmed 6/03)

HOSPITAL DISCHARGE OF THE HIGH-RISK NEONATE— PROPOSED GUIDELINES

Committee on Fetus and Newborn

ABSTRACT. This policy statement is the first formal statement of the American Academy of Pediatrics on the issue of hospital discharge of the high-risk neonate. It has been developed, to the extent possible, on the basis of published, scientifically derived information. Four categories of high risk are identified: 1) the preterm infant, 2) the infant who requires technological support, 3) the infant primarily at risk because of family issues, and 4) the infant whose irreversible condition will result in an early death. The unique home care issues for each are reviewed within a common framework. Recommendations are given for four areas of readiness for hospital discharge: infant, home care planning, family and home environment, and the community and health care system. The need for individualized planning and physician judgment is emphasized. (8/98, reaffirmed 6/01)

THE HOSPITAL RECORD OF THE INJURED CHILD AND THE NEED FOR EXTERNAL CAUSE-OF-INJURY CODES

Committee on Injury and Poison Prevention

ABSTRACT. Proper record-keeping of emergency department visits and hospitalizations of injured children is vital for appropriate patient management. Determination and documentation of the circumstances surrounding the injury event are essential. This information not only is the basis for preventive counseling, but also provides clues about how similar injuries in other youth can be avoided. The hospital records have an important secondary purpose; namely, if sufficient information about the cause and mechanism of injury is documented, it can be subsequently coded, electronically compiled, and retrieved later to provide an epidemiologic profile of the injury, the first step in prevention at the population level. To be of greatest use, hospital records should indicate the "who, what, when, where, why, and how" of the injury occurrence and whether protective equipment (eg, a seat belt) was used. The pediatrician has two important roles in this area: to document fully the injury event and to advocate the use of standardized external cause-of-injury codes, which allow such data to be compiled and analyzed. (2/99, reaffirmed 5/02)

HOSPITAL STAY FOR HEALTHY TERM NEWBORNS
Committee on Fetus and Newborn
See full text on page 386. (5/04)

HOW PEDIATRICIANS CAN RESPOND TO THE PSYCHOSOCIAL IMPLICATIONS OF DISASTERS
Committee on Psychosocial Aspects of Child and Family Health
ABSTRACT. Natural and human-caused disasters, violence with weapons, and terrorist acts have touched directly the lives of thousands of families with children in the United States. Media coverage of disasters has brought images of floods, hurricanes, and airplane crashes into the living rooms of most American families, with limited censorship for vulnerable young children. Therefore, children may be exposed to disastrous events in ways that previous generations never or rarely experienced. Pediatricians should serve as important resources to the community in preparing for disasters, as well as acting in its behalf during and after such events. (2/99)

HUMAN EMBRYO RESEARCH
Committee on Pediatric Research and Committee on Bioethics
ABSTRACT. In 1996, a ban on the use of US Department of Health and Human Services funds for research on the creation of human embryos and research that involved the injury or destruction of human embryos was signed into law. This ban was partially reversed in 2000 when the National Institutes of Health announced it would fund selective research on human pluripotent stem cells. Given the potential benefits to society, research using human embryos is an issue that deserves additional consideration. The American Academy of Pediatrics believes that, under certain conditions, research using human embryos and pluripotent stem cells is of sufficient scientific importance that the National Institutes of Health should fund it and that federal oversight is morally preferable to the currently unregulated private sector approach. (9/01, reaffirmed 4/04)

HUMAN IMMUNODEFICIENCY VIRUS AND OTHER BLOOD-BORNE VIRAL PATHOGENS IN THE ATHLETIC SETTING
Committee on Sports Medicine and Fitness
ABSTRACT. Because athletes and the staff of athletic programs can be exposed to blood during athletic activity, they have a very small risk of becoming infected with human immunodeficiency virus, hepatitis B virus, or hepatitis C virus. This statement, which updates a previous position statement of the American Academy of Pediatrics, discusses sports participation for athletes infected with these pathogens and the precautions needed to reduce the risk of infection to others in the athletic setting. Each of the recommendations in this statement is dependent upon and intended to be considered with reference to the other recommendations in this statement and not in isolation. (12/99, reaffirmed 5/04)

HUMAN IMMUNODEFICIENCY VIRUS SCREENING
American Academy of Pediatrics Committee on Fetus and Newborn and Committee on Pediatric AIDS and American College of Obstetricians and Gynecologists (7/99, reaffirmed 6/02)

HUMAN MILK, BREASTFEEDING, AND TRANSMISSION OF HUMAN IMMUNODEFICIENCY VIRUS IN THE UNITED STATES
Committee on Pediatric AIDS (11/95, reaffirmed 11/99, 11/03)

HUMAN MILK, BREASTFEEDING, AND TRANSMISSION OF HUMAN IMMUNODEFICIENCY VIRUS TYPE 1 IN THE UNITED STATES (TECHNICAL REPORT)
Committee on Pediatric AIDS
ABSTRACT. Transmission of human immunodeficiency virus type 1 (HIV-1) through breastfeeding has been conclusively demonstrated. The risk of such transmission has been quantified, the timing has been clarified, and certain risk factors for breastfeeding transmission have been identified. In areas where infant formula is accessible, affordable, safe, and sustainable, avoidance of breastfeeding has represented one of the main components of mother-to-child HIV-1 transmission prevention efforts for many years. In areas where affordable and safe alternatives to breastfeeding may not be available, interventions to prevent breastfeeding transmission are being investigated. Complete avoidance of breastfeeding by HIV-1-infected women has been recommended by the American Academy of Pediatrics and the Centers for Disease Control and Prevention and remains the only means by which prevention of breastfeeding transmission of HIV-1 can be absolutely ensured. This technical report summarizes the information available regarding breastfeeding transmission of HIV-1. (11/03)

HYPOALLERGENIC INFANT FORMULAS
Committee on Nutrition
ABSTRACT. The American Academy of Pediatrics is committed to breastfeeding as the ideal source of nutrition for infants. For those infants who are formula-fed, either as a supplement to breastfeeding or exclusively during their infancy, it is common practice for pediatricians to change the formula when symptoms of intolerance occur. Decisions about when the formula should be changed and which formula should be used vary significantly, however, among pediatric practitioners. This statement clarifies some of these issues as they relate to protein hypersensitivity (protein allergy), one of the causes of adverse reactions to feeding during infancy. (8/00)

IDENTIFICATION AND CARE OF HIV-EXPOSED AND HIV-INFECTED INFANTS, CHILDREN, AND ADOLESCENTS IN FOSTER CARE
Committee on Pediatric AIDS
ABSTRACT. As a consequence of the expanding human immunodeficiency virus (HIV) epidemic and major advances in medical management of HIV-exposed and HIV-infected persons, revised recommendations are provided for HIV testing of infants, children, and adolescents

in foster care. Updated recommendations also are provided for the care of HIV-exposed and HIV-infected persons who are in foster care. (7/00, reaffirmed 3/03)

IDENTIFYING AND TREATING EATING DISORDERS
Committee on Adolescence
ABSTRACT. Pediatricians are called on to become involved in the identification and management of eating disorders in several settings and at several critical points in the illness. In the primary care pediatrician's practice, early detection, initial evaluation, and ongoing management can play a significant role in preventing the illness from progressing to a more severe or chronic state. In the subspecialty setting, management of medical complications, provision of nutritional rehabilitation, and coordination with the psychosocial and psychiatric aspects of care are often handled by pediatricians, especially those who have experience or expertise in the care of adolescents with eating disorders. In hospital and day program settings, pediatricians are involved in program development, determining appropriate admission and discharge criteria, and provision and coordination of care. Lastly, primary care pediatricians need to be involved at local, state, and national levels in preventive efforts and in providing advocacy for patients and families. The roles of pediatricians in the management of eating disorders in the pediatric practice, subspecialty, hospital, day program, and community settings are reviewed in this statement. (1/03)

IMMUNIZATION OF PRETERM AND LOW BIRTH WEIGHT INFANTS (CLINICAL REPORT)
Committee on Infectious Diseases
ABSTRACT. Preterm (PT) infants are at increased risk of experiencing complications of vaccine-preventable diseases but are less likely to receive immunizations on time. Medically stable PT and low birth weight (LBW) infants should receive full doses of diphtheria, tetanus, acellular pertussis, Haemophilus influenzae type b, hepatitis B, poliovirus, and pneumococcal conjugate vaccines at a chronologic age consistent with the schedule recommended for full-term infants. Infants with birth weight less than 2000 g may require modification of the timing of hepatitis B immunoprophylaxis depending on maternal hepatitis B surface antigen status. All PT and LBW infants benefit from receiving influenza vaccine beginning at 6 months of age before the beginning of and during the influenza season. All vaccines routinely recommended during infancy are safe for use in PT and LBW infants. The occurrence of mild vaccine-attributable adverse events are similar in both full-term and PT vaccine recipients. Although the immunogenicity of some childhood vaccines may be decreased in the smallest PT infants, antibody concentrations achieved usually are protective. (7/03)

IMPACT OF MUSIC LYRICS AND MUSIC VIDEOS ON CHILDREN AND YOUTH
Committee on Public Education (12/96)

IMPLEMENTATION OF THE IMMUNIZATION POLICY
Committee on Practice and Ambulatory Medicine (8/95)

IMPLEMENTATION PRINCIPLES AND STRATEGIES FOR THE STATE CHILDREN'S HEALTH INSURANCE PROGRAM
Committee on Child Health Financing
ABSTRACT. This policy statement presents principles and implementation and evaluation strategies recommended for the State Children's Health Insurance Program (SCHIP). The statement summarizes the current status of SCHIP, the needs of uninsured children, and the potential benefits of SCHIP programs. Principles and recommended strategies include expanding eligibility, maximizing funding, providing comprehensive benefits, including pediatricians in program design and evaluation, providing adequate reimbursement and access to pediatricians, ensuring choices for families and pediatricians, and establishing simple administrative procedures. (5/01)

IMPROVING SUBSTANCE ABUSE PREVENTION, ASSESSMENT, AND TREATMENT FINANCING FOR CHILDREN AND ADOLESCENTS
Committee on Child Health Financing and Committee on Substance Abuse
ABSTRACT. The numbers of children, adolescents, and families affected by substance abuse have sharply increased since the early 1990s. The American Academy of Pediatrics recognizes the scope and urgency of this problem and has developed this policy statement for consideration by Congress, federal and state agencies, employers, national organizations, health care professionals, health insurers, managed care organizations, advocacy groups, and families. (10/01)

THE INAPPROPRIATE USE OF SCHOOL "READINESS" TESTS
Committee on Early Childhood, Adoption, and Dependent Care and Committee on School Health (3/95, reaffirmed 4/98, 1/04)

INCREASING IMMUNIZATION COVERAGE
Committee on Community Health Services and Committee on Practice and Ambulatory Medicine
ABSTRACT. Despite many recent advances in vaccine delivery, the goal for universal immunization set in 1977 has not been reached. In 2001, only 77.2% of US toddlers 19 to 35 months of age had received their basic immunization series of 4 doses of diphtheria and tetanus toxoids and acellular pertussis (DTaP) vaccine, 3 doses of inactivated poliovirus vaccine, 1 dose of measles-mumps-rubella (MMR) vaccine, and 3 doses of Haemophilus influenzae type b (Hib) vaccine. Children who are members of a racial or ethnic minority, who are poor, or who live in inner-city or rural areas have lower immunization rates than do children in the general population. Additional challenges to vaccine delivery include the introduction of new childhood vaccines, ensuring a dependable supply of vaccines, bolstering public confidence in vaccine safety, and sufficient compensation for vaccine administration.

Recent research has demonstrated specific and practical changes physicians can make to improve their practices' effectiveness in immunizing children, including the following: 1) sending parent reminders for upcoming visits and recall notices; 2) using prompts during all office visits to remind parents and staff about immunizations needed at that visit; 3) repeatedly measuring practice-wide immunization rates over time as part of a quality improvement effort; and 4) having in place standing orders for registered nurses, physician assistants, and medical assistants to identify opportunities to administer vaccines. Pediatricians should work individually and collectively at local and national levels to ensure that all children receive all childhood immunizations on time. Pediatricians also can proactively communicate with parents to ensure they understand the overall safety and efficacy of vaccines. (10/03)

INDICATIONS FOR MANAGEMENT AND REFERRAL OF PATIENTS INVOLVED IN SUBSTANCE ABUSE
Committee on Substance Abuse

ABSTRACT. This statement addresses the challenge of evaluating and managing the various stages of substance use by children and adolescents in the context of pediatric practice. Approaches are suggested that would assist the pediatrician in differentiating highly prevalent experimental and occasional use from more severe use with adverse consequences that affect emotional, behavioral, educational, or physical health. Comorbid psychiatric conditions are common and should be evaluated and treated simultaneously by child and adolescent mental health specialists. Guidelines for referral based on severity of involvement using established patient treatment-matching criteria are outlined. Pediatricians need to become familiar with treatment professionals and facilities in their communities and to ensure that treatment for adolescent patients is appropriate based on their developmental, psychosocial, medical, and mental health needs. The family should be encouraged to participate actively in the treatment process. (7/00)

INFANT METHEMOGLOBINEMIA: THE ROLE OF DIETARY NITRATE
Committee on Nutrition (9/70, reaffirmed 4/94, 6/97, 4/00)

INFANTS WITH ANENCEPHALY AS ORGAN SOURCES: ETHICAL CONSIDERATIONS
Committee on Bioethics (6/92, reaffirmed 11/95, 11/98, 11/02)

INFECTION CONTROL IN PHYSICIANS' OFFICES
Committee on Infectious Diseases and Committee on Practice and Ambulatory Medicine

ABSTRACT. Infection control is an integral part of pediatric practice in outpatient settings as well as in hospitals. All employees should be educated regarding the routes of transmission and techniques used to prevent transmission of infectious agents. Policies for infection control and prevention should be written, readily available, updated annually, and enforced. The Centers for Disease Control and Prevention standard precautions for hospitalized patients with modifications from the American Academy of Pediatrics are appropriate for most patient encounters.

As employers, pediatricians are required by the Occupational Safety and Health Administration (OSHA) to take precautions to protect staff likely to be exposed to blood or other potentially infectious materials while on the job. Key principles of infection control include the following: hand-washing before and after every patient contact, separation of infected, contagious children from uninfected children, safe handling and disposal of needles and other sharp medical devices, appropriate use of personal protection equipment such as gloves, appropriate sterilization, disinfection and antisepsis, and judicious use of antibiotics. (6/00)

INFORMED CONSENT, PARENTAL PERMISSION, AND ASSENT IN PEDIATRIC PRACTICE
Committee on Bioethics (2/95, reaffirmed 11/98, 11/02)

INHALANT ABUSE
Committee on Native American Child Health and Committee on Substance Abuse (3/96, reaffirmed 5/99)

INITIAL MEDICAL EVALUATION OF AN ADOPTED CHILD
Committee on Early Childhood, Adoption, and Dependent Care (9/91)

THE INITIATION OR WITHDRAWAL OF TREATMENT FOR HIGH-RISK NEWBORNS
Committee on Fetus and Newborn (8/95, reaffirmed 10/98, 6/01)

INJURIES ASSOCIATED WITH INFANT WALKERS
Committee on Injury and Poison Prevention

ABSTRACT. In 1999, an estimated 8800 children younger than 15 months were treated in hospital emergency departments in the United States for injuries associated with infant walkers. Thirty-four infant walker-related deaths were reported from 1973 through 1998. The vast majority of injuries occur from falls down stairs, and head injuries are common. Walkers do not help a child learn to walk; indeed, they can delay normal motor and mental development. The use of warning labels, public education, adult supervision during walker use, and stair gates have all been demonstrated to be insufficient strategies to prevent injuries associated with infant walkers. To comply with the revised voluntary standard (ASTM F977-96), walkers manufactured after June 30, 1997, must be wider than a 36-in doorway or must have a braking mechanism designed to stop the walker if 1 or more wheels drop off the riding surface, such as at the top of a stairway. Because data indicate a considerable risk of major and minor injury and even death from the use of infant walkers, and because there is no clear benefit from their use, the American Academy of Pediatrics recommends a ban on the manufacture and sale of mobile infant walkers. If a parent insists on using a mobile infant walker, it is vital that they choose a walker that meets the performance standards of ASTM F977-96 to prevent falls down stairs. Stationary activity centers should be promoted as a safer alternative to mobile infant walkers. (9/01, reaffirmed 11/04)

INJURIES IN YOUTH SOCCER: A SUBJECT REVIEW (CLINICAL REPORT)
Committee on Sports Medicine and Fitness
ABSTRACT. The current literature on injuries in youth soccer, known as football worldwide, has been reviewed to assess the frequency, type, and causes of injuries in this sport. The information in this review serves as a basis for encouraging safe participation in soccer for children and adolescents. (3/00)

INJURY RISK OF NONPOWDER GUNS (TECHNICAL REPORT)
Committee on Injury, Violence, and Poison Prevention
See full text on page 387. (11/04)

IN-LINE SKATING INJURIES IN CHILDREN AND ADOLESCENTS
Committee on Injury and Poison Prevention and Committee on Sports Medicine and Fitness
ABSTRACT. In-line skating has become one of the fastest-growing recreational sports in the United States. Recent studies emphasize the value of protective gear in reducing the incidence of injuries. Recommendations are provided for parents and pediatricians, with special emphasis on the novice or inexperienced skater. (4/98, reaffirmed 1/02)

INSTITUTIONAL ETHICS COMMITTEES
Committee on Bioethics
ABSTRACT. In hospitals throughout the United States, institutional ethics committees (IECs) have become a standard vehicle for the education of health professionals about biomedical ethics, for the drafting and review of hospital policy, and for clinical ethics case consultation. In addition, there is increasing interest in a role for the IEC in organizational ethics. Recommendations are made about the membership and structure of an IEC, and guidelines are provided for those serving on an ethics committee. (1/01, reaffirmed 1/04)

INSURANCE COVERAGE OF MENTAL HEALTH AND SUBSTANCE ABUSE SERVICES FOR CHILDREN AND ADOLESCENTS: A CONSENSUS STATEMENT
Joint Statement (10/00)

INTENSIVE TRAINING AND SPORTS SPECIALIZATION IN YOUNG ATHLETES
Committee on Sports Medicine and Fitness
ABSTRACT. Children involved in sports should be encouraged to participate in a variety of different activities and develop a wide range of skills. Young athletes who specialize in just one sport may be denied the benefits of varied activity while facing additional physical, physiologic, and psychologic demands from intense training and competition.

This statement reviews the potential risks of high-intensity training and sports specialization in young athletes. Pediatricians who recognize these risks can have a key role in monitoring the health of these young athletes and helping reduce risks associated with high-level sports participation. (7/00, reaffirmed 11/04)

INVESTIGATION AND REVIEW OF UNEXPECTED INFANT AND CHILD DEATHS
Committee on Child Abuse and Neglect and Committee on Community Health Services
ABSTRACT. Although there is a continuing need for timely review of child deaths, no uniform system exists for investigation in the United States. Investigation of a death that is traumatic, unexpected, obscure, suspicious, or otherwise unexplained in a child younger than 18 years requires a scene investigation and an autopsy. Review of these deaths requires the participation of pediatricians and other professionals, usually as a child death review team. An appropriately constituted team should evaluate the death investigation process, review difficult cases, and compile child death statistics. (11/99, reaffirmed 10/02)

IRON FORTIFICATION OF INFANT FORMULAS
Committee on Nutrition
ABSTRACT. Despite the American Academy of Pediatrics' (AAP) strong endorsement for breastfeeding, most infants in the United States are fed some infant formula by the time they are 2 months old. The AAP Committee on Nutrition has strongly advocated iron fortification of infant formulas since 1969 as a way of reducing the prevalence of iron-deficiency anemia and its attendant sequelae during the first year. The 1976 statement titled "Iron Supplementation for Infants" delineated the rationale for iron supplementation, proposed daily dosages of iron, and summarized potential sources of iron in the infant diet. In 1989, the AAP Committee on Nutrition published a statement that addressed the issue of iron-fortified infant formulas and concluded that there was no convincing contraindication to iron-supplemented formulas and that continued use of "low-iron" formulas posed an unacceptable risk for iron deficiency during infancy. The current statement represents a scientific update and synthesis of the 1976 and 1989 statements with recommendations about the use of iron-fortified and low-iron formulas in term infants. (7/99, reaffirmed 11/02)

ISSUES RELATED TO HUMAN IMMUNODEFICIENCY VIRUS TRANSMISSION IN SCHOOLS, CHILD CARE, MEDICAL SETTINGS, THE HOME, AND COMMUNITY
Committee on Pediatric AIDS and Committee on Infectious Diseases
ABSTRACT. Current recommendations of the American Academy of Pediatrics (AAP) for infection control practices to prevent transmission of blood-borne pathogens, including human immunodeficiency virus (HIV) in hospitals, other medical settings, schools, and child care facilities, are reviewed and explained. Hand-washing is essential, whether or not gloves are used, and gloves should be used when contact with blood or blood-containing body fluids may occur. In hospitalized children, the 1996 recommendations of the Centers for Disease Control and Prevention (CDC) should be implemented as modified in the *1997 Red Book*. The generic principles of Standard Precautions in the CDC guidelines generally are applicable to children in all health care settings, schools, child care facilities, and the home. However, gloves are not required for routine changing of diapers or

for wiping nasal secretions of children in most circumstances. This AAP recommendation differs from that in the CDC guidelines.

Current US Public Health Service guidelines for the management of potential occupational exposures of health care workers to HIV are summarized. As previously recommended by the AAP, HIV-infected children should be admitted without restriction to child care centers and schools and allowed to participate in all activities to the extent that their health and other recommendations for management of contagious diseases permit. Because it is not required that the school be notified of HIV infection, it may be helpful if the pediatrician notify the school that he or she is operating under a policy of nondisclosure of infection with blood-borne pathogens. Thus, it is possible that the pediatrician will not report the presence of such infections on the form. Because HIV infection occurs in persons throughout the United States, these recommendations for prevention of HIV transmission should be applied universally. (8/99, reaffirmed 2/02)

KNEE BRACE USE IN THE YOUNG ATHLETE (TECHNICAL REPORT)
Committee on Sports Medicine and Fitness
ABSTRACT. This statement is a revision of a previous statement on prophylactic knee bracing and provides information for pediatricians regarding the use of various types of knee braces, indications for the use of knee braces, and the background knowledge necessary to prescribe the use of knee braces for children. (8/01)

LAWN MOWER-RELATED INJURIES TO CHILDREN
Committee on Injury and Poison Prevention
ABSTRACT. Lawn mower-related injuries to children are relatively common and can result in severe injury or death. Many amputations during childhood are caused by power mowers. Pediatricians have an important role as advocates and educators to promote the prevention of these injuries. (6/01, reaffirmed 5/04)

LAWN MOWER-RELATED INJURIES TO CHILDREN (TECHNICAL REPORT)
Committee on Injury and Poison Prevention
ABSTRACT. In the United States, approximately 9400 children younger than 18 years receive emergency treatment annually for lawn mower-related injuries. More than 7% of these children require hospitalization, and power mowers cause a large proportion of the amputations during childhood. Prevention of lawn mower-related injuries can be achieved by design changes of lawn mowers, guidelines for mower operation, and education of parents, child caregivers, and children. Pediatricians have an important role as advocates and educators to promote the prevention of these injuries. (6/01, reaffirmed 5/04)

LEARNING DISABILITIES, DYSLEXIA, AND VISION: A SUBJECT REVIEW (CLINICAL REPORT)
American Academy of Pediatrics Committee on Children With Disabilities, American Academy of Ophthalmology, and American Association for Pediatric Ophthalmology and Strabismus
ABSTRACT. Learning disabilities are common conditions in pediatric patients. The etiology of these difficulties is multifactorial, reflecting genetic influences and abnormalities of brain structure and function. Early recognition and referral to qualified educational professionals is critical for the best possible outcome. Visual problems are rarely responsible for learning difficulties. No scientific evidence exists for the efficacy of eye exercises ("vision therapy") or the use of special tinted lenses in the remediation of these complex pediatric developmental and neurologic conditions. (11/98, reaffirmed 5/02)

LEGALIZATION OF MARIJUANA: POTENTIAL IMPACT ON YOUTH
Committee on Substance Abuse and Committee on Adolescence
See full text on page 395. (6/04)

LEGALIZATION OF MARIJUANA: POTENTIAL IMPACT ON YOUTH (TECHNICAL REPORT)
Committee on Substance Abuse and Committee on Adolescence
See full text on page 399. (6/04)

LEVELS OF NEONATAL CARE
Committee on Fetus and Newborn
See full text on page 407. (11/04)

MANAGED CARE AND CHILDREN WITH SPECIAL HEALTH CARE NEEDS (CLINICAL REPORT)
Committee on Children With Disabilities
See full text on page 417. (12/04)

MARIJUANA: A CONTINUING CONCERN FOR PEDIATRICIANS
Committee on Substance Abuse
ABSTRACT. Marijuana, the common name for products derived from the plant *Cannabis sativa*, is the most common illicit drug used by children and adolescents in the United States. Despite growing concerns by the medical profession about the physical and psychological effects of its active ingredient, Δ-9-tetrahydrocannabinol, survey data continue to show that increasing numbers of young people are using the drug as they become less concerned about its dangers. (10/99, reaffirmed 4/03)

MATERNAL PHENYLKETONURIA
Committee on Genetics
ABSTRACT. Elevated maternal phenylalanine levels during pregnancy are teratogenic and may result in growth retardation, significant psychomotor handicaps, and birth defects in the offspring of unmonitored and untreated pregnancies. Women of childbearing age with all forms of phenylketonuria, including mild variants such as hyperphenylalaninemia, should receive counseling concerning their risks for adverse fetal effects optimally before con-

ceiving. The best outcomes occur when strict control of maternal phenylalanine levels is achieved before conception and continued throughout the pregnancy. (2/01)

MEASLES IMMUNIZATION IN HIV-INFECTED CHILDREN
Committee on Infectious Diseases and Committee on Pediatric AIDS
ABSTRACT. Children infected with human immunodeficiency virus (HIV) have had high rates of mortality attributable to measles, but until recently, measles vaccine was assumed to be safe for these children. A single fatal case of pneumonia attributable to vaccine type-measles virus has been documented in a young adult with acquired immunodeficiency syndrome. Because a protective immune response often does not develop in severely immunocompromised HIV-infected patients after immunization and some risk of severe complications exists, HIV-infected children, adolescents, and young adults who are severely immunocompromised (based on age-specific CD4 lymphocyte enumeration) attributable to HIV infection should not receive measles vaccine. All other HIV-infected children, adolescents, and young adults who are not severely immunocompromised should receive measles-mumps-rubella vaccine. (5/99, reaffirmed 10/01 COID)

MEDIA EDUCATION
Committee on Public Education
ABSTRACT. The American Academy of Pediatrics recognizes that exposure to mass media (ie, television, movies, video and computer games, the Internet, music lyrics and videos, newspapers, magazines, books, advertising, etc) presents both health risks and benefits for children and adolescents. Media education has the potential to reduce the harmful effects of media. By understanding and supporting media education, pediatricians can play an important role in reducing the risk of exposure to mass media for children and adolescents. (8/99)

MEDIA VIOLENCE
Committee on Public Education
ABSTRACT. The American Academy of Pediatrics recognizes exposure to violence in media, including television, movies, music, and video games, as a significant risk to the health of children and adolescents. Extensive research evidence indicates that media violence can contribute to aggressive behavior, desensitization to violence, nightmares, and fear of being harmed. Pediatricians should assess their patients' level of media exposure and intervene on media-related health risks. Pediatricians and other child health care providers can advocate for a safer media environment for children by encouraging media literacy, more thoughtful and proactive use of media by children and their parents, more responsible portrayal of violence by media producers, and more useful and effective media ratings. (11/01)

MEDICAID POLICY STATEMENT
Committee on Child Health Financing
ABSTRACT. This policy statement replaces the 1994 Medicaid Policy Statement. The new policy statement incorporates federal legislative changes and policy recommendations related to eligibility, outreach and enrollment, Medicaid managed care, covered benefits, access to pediatric care, and quality improvement plans. (8/99)

MEDICAL CONCERNS IN THE FEMALE ATHLETE
Committee on Sports Medicine and Fitness
ABSTRACT. Female children and adolescents who participate regularly in sports may develop certain medical conditions, including disordered eating, menstrual dysfunction, and decreased bone mineral density. The pediatrician can play an important role in monitoring the health of young female athletes. This revised policy statement provides updated and expanded information for pediatricians on these health concerns as well as recommendations for evaluation, treatment, and ongoing assessments of female athletes. (9/00, reaffirmed 5/04)

MEDICAL CONDITIONS AFFECTING SPORTS PARTICIPATION
Committee on Sports Medicine and Fitness
ABSTRACT. Children and adolescents with medical conditions present special issues with respect to participation in athletic activities. The pediatrician can play an important role in determining whether a child with a health condition should participate in certain sports by assessing the child's health status, suggesting appropriate equipment or modifications of sports to decrease the risk of injury, and educating the athlete and parents on the risks of injury as they relate to the child's condition. This statement updates a previous policy statement and provides information for pediatricians on sports participation for children and adolescents with medical conditions. (5/01)

THE MEDICAL HOME
Medical Home Initiatives for Children With Special Needs Project Advisory Committee (7/02)

MEDICAL NECESSITY FOR THE HOSPITALIZATION OF THE ABUSED AND NEGLECTED CHILD
Committee on Hospital Care and Committee on Child Abuse and Neglect
ABSTRACT. The child suspected of being abused or neglected demands prompt evaluation in a protective environment where knowledgeable consultants are readily available. In communities without specialized centers for the care of abused children, the hospital inpatient unit becomes an appropriate setting for their initial management. Medical, psychosocial, and legal concerns may be assessed expeditiously while the child is housed in a safe haven awaiting final disposition by child protective services. The American Academy of Pediatrics recommends that hospitalization of abused and neglected children, when medically indicated or for their protection/diagnosis when there are no specialized facilities in the community for their care, should be viewed as medically necessary by both health professionals and third-party payors. (4/98, reaffirmed 5/01, 5/04 COHC, 10/01, 8/04 COCAN)

MEDICAL STAFF APPOINTMENT AND DELINEATION OF PEDIATRIC PRIVILEGES IN HOSPITALS (CLINICAL REPORT)
Committee on Hospital Care

ABSTRACT. The review and verification of credentials and the granting of clinical privileges are required of every hospital to ensure that members of the medical staff are competent and qualified to provide specified levels of patient care. The credentialing process involves the following: 1) assessment of the professional and personal background of each practitioner seeking privileges; 2) assignment of privileges appropriate for the clinician's training and experience; 3) ongoing monitoring of the professional activities of each staff member; and 4) periodic reappointment to the medical staff on the basis of objectively measured performance. This statement examines the essential elements of a credentials review for initial and renewed medical staff appointments along with suggested criteria for the delineation of clinical privileges. Sample forms for the delineation of privileges can be found on the American Academy of Pediatrics Web site (http://www.aap.org/visit/cmte19.htm). Because of the differences in individual hospitals, no one method for credentialing is universally applicable. The medical staff of each hospital must, therefore, establish its own process based on the general principles reviewed in this statement. The issues of medical staff membership and credentialing have become very complex, and institutions and medical staffs are vulnerable to legal action. Consequently, it is advisable for hospitals and medical staffs to obtain expert legal advice when medical staff bylaws are constructed or revised. (8/02)

MENINGOCOCCAL DISEASE PREVENTION AND CONTROL STRATEGIES FOR PRACTICE-BASED PHYSICIANS (ADDENDUM: RECOMMENDATIONS FOR COLLEGE STUDENTS)
Committee on Infectious Diseases

ABSTRACT. The numbers of reported cases of meningococcal disease in 15- to 24-year-olds and outbreaks of meningococcal serogroup C disease, including outbreaks in schools and other institutions, have increased during the past decade. In response to outbreaks on college campuses, the American College Health Association has taken an increasingly proactive role in alerting college students and their parents to the risk of this disease and informing them about the availability of an effective vaccine. Recent epidemiologic studies have demonstrated an increased risk of disease in college students living in dormitories, particularly among freshmen, compared with similarly aged persons in the general population. At least 60% of these cases are potentially preventable by vaccination with the quadrivalent meningococcal A, C, Y, and W-135 polysaccharide vaccine. These findings support immunization of college students, particularly freshmen living in dormitories. Hence, college students and their parents should be informed by health care professionals at routine prematriculation visits and during college matriculation of the risk of meningococcal disease and potential benefits of immunization. Vaccine should be made available to those requesting immunization. College and university health services also should facilitate implementation of educational programs concerning meningococcal disease and availability of immunization services. (12/00, reaffirmed 10/01)

MERCURY IN THE ENVIRONMENT: IMPLICATIONS FOR PEDIATRICIANS (TECHNICAL REPORT)
Committee on Environmental Health

ABSTRACT. Mercury is a ubiquitous environmental toxin that causes a wide range of adverse health effects in humans. Three forms of mercury (elemental, inorganic, and organic) exist, and each has its own profile of toxicity. Exposure to mercury typically occurs by inhalation or ingestion. Readily absorbed after its inhalation, mercury can be an indoor air pollutant, for example, after spills of elemental mercury in the home; however, industry emissions with resulting ambient air pollution remain the most important source of inhaled mercury. Because fresh-water and ocean fish may contain large amounts of mercury, children and pregnant women can have significant exposure if they consume excessive amounts of fish. The developing fetus and young children are thought to be disproportionately affected by mercury exposure, because many aspects of development, particularly brain maturation, can be disturbed by the presence of mercury. Minimizing mercury exposure is, therefore, essential to optimal child health. This review provides pediatricians with current information on mercury, including environmental sources, toxicity, and treatment and prevention of mercury exposure. (7/01)

MINOR HEAD INJURY IN CHILDREN (TECHNICAL REPORT)
Steering Committee on Quality Improvement and Management
See summary on page 95. (12/99)

MOLECULAR GENETIC TESTING IN PEDIATRIC PRACTICE: A SUBJECT REVIEW (CLINICAL REPORT)
Committee on Genetics

ABSTRACT. Although many types of diagnostic and carrier testing for genetic disorders have been available for decades, the use of molecular methods is a relatively recent phenomenon. Such testing has expanded the range of disorders that can be diagnosed and has enhanced the ability of clinicians to provide accurate prognostic information and institute appropriate health supervision measures. However, the proper application of these tests may be difficult because of their scientific complexity and the potential for negative, sometimes unexpected, consequences for many patients. The purposes of this subject review are to provide background information on molecular genetic tests, to describe specific testing modalities, and to discuss some of the benefits and risks specific to the pediatric population. It is likely that pediatricians will use these testing methods increasingly for their patients and will need to evaluate critically their diagnostic and prognostic implications. (12/00)

NEONATAL DRUG WITHDRAWAL
Committee on Drugs
ABSTRACT. Maternal drug use during pregnancy may result in neonatal withdrawal. This statement presents current information about the clinical presentation, differential diagnosis, therapeutic options, and outcome for the offspring associated with intrauterine drug exposure. (6/98, reaffirmed 5/01)

THE NEURODIAGNOSTIC EVALUATION OF THE CHILD WITH A FIRST SIMPLE FEBRILE SEIZURE (TECHNICAL REPORT)
Steering Committee on Quality Improvement and Management
See summary on page 75. (5/96)

THE NEW MORBIDITY REVISITED: A RENEWED COMMITMENT TO THE PSYCHOSOCIAL ASPECTS OF PEDIATRIC CARE
Committee on Psychosocial Aspects of Child and Family Health
ABSTRACT. In 1993, the American Academy of Pediatrics adopted the policy statement "The Pediatrician and the 'New Morbidity.'" Since then, social difficulties, behavioral problems, and developmental difficulties have become a main part of the scope of pediatric practice, and recognition of the importance of these areas has increased. This statement reaffirms the Academy's commitment to prevention, early detection, and management of behavioral, developmental, and social problems as a focus in pediatric practice. (11/01)

NEWBORN SCREENING FOR CONGENITAL HYPOTHYROIDISM: RECOMMENDED GUIDELINES
American Academy of Pediatrics Committee on Genetics and Section on Endocrinology and American Thyroid Association Committee on Public Health (6/93, reaffirmed 10/96, 10/99 COG)

NEWBORN SCREENING FACT SHEETS
Committee on Genetics (9/96, reaffirmed 10/99)

NOISE: A HAZARD FOR THE FETUS AND NEWBORN
Committee on Environmental Health
ABSTRACT. Noise is ubiquitous in our environment. High intensities of noise have been associated with numerous health effects in adults, including noise-induced hearing loss and high blood pressure. The intent of this statement is to provide pediatricians and others with information on the potential health effects of noise on the fetus and newborn. The information presented here supports a number of recommendations for both pediatric practice and government policy. (10/97, reaffirmed 10/00)

NONDISCRIMINATION IN PEDIATRIC HEALTH CARE
Committee on Pediatric Workforce
ABSTRACT. This policy statement reaffirms and consolidates the positions of the American Academy of Pediatrics relative to nondiscrimination in pediatric health care. It addresses pediatricians who provide health care and the infants, children, adolescents, and young adults who are entitled to optimal pediatric care. (11/01)

NONTHERAPEUTIC USE OF ANTIMICROBIAL AGENTS IN ANIMAL AGRICULTURE: IMPLICATIONS FOR PEDIATRICS (TECHNICAL REPORT)
Committee on Environmental Health and Committee on Infectious Diseases
See full text on page 425. (9/04)

OFFICE-BASED COUNSELING FOR INJURY PREVENTION
Committee on Injury and Poison Prevention (10/94, reaffirmed 10/98)

ORAL AND DENTAL ASPECTS OF CHILD ABUSE AND NEGLECT
American Academy of Pediatrics Committee on Child Abuse and Neglect and the American Academy of Pediatric Dentistry Ad Hoc Work Group on Child Abuse and Neglect
ABSTRACT. In all states, physicians and dentists recognize their responsibility to report suspected cases of abuse and neglect. The purpose of this statement is to review the oral and dental aspects of physical and sexual abuse and dental neglect and the role of physicians and dentists in evaluating such conditions. This statement also addresses the oral manifestations of sexually transmitted diseases and bite marks, including the collection of evidence and laboratory documentation of these injuries. (8/99)

ORAL HEALTH RISK ASSESSMENT TIMING AND ESTABLISHMENT OF THE DENTAL HOME
Section on Pediatric Dentistry
ABSTRACT. Early childhood dental caries has been reported by the Centers for Disease Control and Prevention to be perhaps the most prevalent infectious disease of our nation's children. Early childhood dental caries occurs in all racial and socioeconomic groups; however, it tends to be more prevalent in low-income children, in whom it occurs in epidemic proportions. Dental caries results from an overgrowth of specific organisms that are a part of normally occurring human flora. Human dental flora is site specific, and an infant is not colonized until the eruption of the primary dentition at approximately 6 to 30 months of age. The most likely source of inoculation of an infant's dental flora is the mother or another intimate care provider, through shared utensils, etc. Decreasing the level of cariogenic organisms in the mother's dental flora at the time of colonization can significantly impact the child's predisposition to caries. To prevent caries in children, high-risk individuals must be identified at an early age (preferably high-risk mothers during prenatal care), and aggressive strategies should be adopted, including anticipatory guidance, behavior modifications (oral hygiene and feeding practices), and establishment of a dental home by 1 year of age for children deemed at risk. (5/03)

ORGANIZED SPORTS FOR CHILDREN AND PREADOLESCENTS
Committee on Sports Medicine and Fitness and Committee on School Health
ABSTRACT. Participation in organized sports provides an opportunity for young people to increase their physical activity and develop physical and social skills. However, when the demands and expectations of organized sports exceed the maturation and readiness of the participant, the positive aspects of participation can be negated. The

nature of parental or adult involvement can also influence the degree to which participation in organized sports is a positive experience for preadolescents. This updates a previous policy statement on athletics for preadolescents and incorporates guidelines for sports participation for preschool children. Recommendations are offered on how pediatricians can help determine a child's readiness to participate, how risks can be minimized, and how child-oriented goals can be maximized. (6/01, reaffirmed 11/04)

OUT-OF-SCHOOL SUSPENSION AND EXPULSION
Committee on School Health
ABSTRACT. Suspension and expulsion from school are used to punish students, alert parents, and protect other students and school staff. Unintended consequences of these practices require more attention from health care professionals. Suspension and expulsion may exacerbate academic deterioration, and when students are provided with no immediate educational alternative, student alienation, delinquency, crime, and substance abuse may ensue. Social, emotional, and mental health support for students at all times in all schools can decrease the need for expulsion and suspension and should be strongly advocated by the health care community. This policy statement, however, highlights aspects of expulsion and suspension that jeopardize children's health and safety. Recommendations are targeted at pediatricians, who can help schools address the root causes of behaviors that lead to suspension and expulsion and can advocate for alternative disciplinary policies. Pediatricians can also share responsibility with schools to provide students with health and social resources. (11/03)

OVERCROWDING CRISIS IN OUR NATION'S EMERGENCY DEPARTMENTS: IS OUR SAFETY NET UNRAVELING?
Committee on Pediatric Emergency Medicine
See full text on page 435. (9/04)

PALLIATIVE CARE FOR CHILDREN
Committee on Bioethics and Committee on Hospital Care
ABSTRACT. This statement presents an integrated model for providing palliative care for children living with a life-threatening or terminal condition. Advice on the development of a palliative care plan and on working with parents and children is also provided. Barriers to the provision of effective pediatric palliative care and potential solutions are identified. The American Academy of Pediatrics recommends the development and broad availability of pediatric palliative care services based on child-specific guidelines and standards. Such services will require widely distributed and effective palliative care education of pediatric health care professionals. The Academy offers guidance on responding to requests for hastening death, but does not support the practice of physician-assisted suicide or euthanasia for children. (8/00, reaffirmed 6/03)

PARENTAL LEAVE FOR RESIDENTS AND PEDIATRIC TRAINING PROGRAMS
Committee on Early Childhood, Adoption, and Dependent Care and Section on Residents (11/95, reaffirmed 4/98)

PARTICIPATION IN BOXING BY CHILDREN, ADOLESCENTS, AND YOUNG ADULTS
Committee on Sports Medicine and Fitness
ABSTRACT. Because boxing may result in serious brain and eye injuries, the American Academy of Pediatrics opposes this sport. This policy statement summarizes the reasons. (1/97, reaffirmed 5/00)

PEDIATRIC CARE RECOMMENDATIONS FOR FREESTANDING URGENT CARE FACILITIES
Committee on Pediatric Emergency Medicine
ABSTRACT. Freestanding urgent care centers are increasing as a source of after-hours pediatric care. These facilities may be used as an alternative to hospital emergency departments for the care and stabilization of serious and critically ill and injured children. The purpose of this policy statement is to provide recommendations for assuring appropriate stabilization in pediatric emergency situations and timely transfer to a hospital for definitive care when necessary. (5/99)

PEDIATRIC EXPOSURE AND POTENTIAL TOXICITY OF PHTHALATE PLASTICIZERS (TECHNICAL REPORT)
Committee on Environmental Health
ABSTRACT. Phthalates are plasticizers that are added to polyvinyl chloride (PVC) products to impart flexibility and durability. They are produced in high volume and generate extensive though poorly defined human exposures and unique childhood exposures. Phthalates are animal carcinogens and can cause fetal death, malformations, and reproductive toxicity in laboratory animals. Toxicity profiles and potency vary by specific phthalate. The extent of these toxicities and their applicability to humans remains incompletely characterized and controversial. Two phthalates, diethylhexyl phthalate (DEHP) and diisononyl phthalate (DINP), have received considerable attention recently because of specific concerns about pediatric exposures. Like all phthalates, DEHP and DINP are ubiquitous contaminants in food, indoor air, soils, and sediments. DEHP is used in toys and medical devices. DINP is a major plasticizer used in children's toys.

Scientific panels, advocacy groups, and industry groups have analyzed the literature on DEHP and DINP and have come to different conclusions about their safety. The controversy exists because risk to humans must be extrapolated from animal data that demonstrate differences in toxicity by species, route of exposure, and age at exposure and because of persistent uncertainties in human exposure data. This report addresses sensitive endpoints of reproductive and developmental toxicity and the unique aspects of pediatric exposures to phthalates that generate concern. DEHP and DINP are used as specific examples to illustrate the controversy. (6/03)

PEDIATRIC FELLOWSHIP TRAINING
Federation of Pediatric Organizations
See full text on page 449. (7/04)

PEDIATRIC ORGAN DONATION AND TRANSPLANTATION
Committee on Hospital Care and Section on Surgery
ABSTRACT. Pediatric organ donation and organ transplantation can have a significant life-extending benefit to the young recipients of these organs and a high emotional impact on donor and recipient families. Pediatricians should become better acquainted with evolving national strategies involving organ procurement and organ transplantation to help acquaint families with the benefits of organ donation and to help shape public policies that will aid in efforts to provide a system of procurement, distribution, and finance that is fair and equitable to children and adults. Major issues of concern are availability and access; oversight and control; pediatric medical and surgical consultation throughout the organ donation and transplantation process; ethical, social, financial, and follow-up issues; insurance coverage issues; and public awareness of the need for organ donors of all ages. (5/02)

PEDIATRIC PHYSICIAN PROFILING
Committee on Practice and Ambulatory Medicine and
   Committee on Medical Liability
ABSTRACT. Employers, insurers, and other purchasers of health care services collect data to profile the practice habits of pediatricians and other physicians. This policy statement delineates a series of recommendations that should be adopted by health care purchasers to guide the development and implementation of physician profiling systems. (10/99)

PEDIATRIC PRIMARY HEALTH CARE
Committee on Pediatric Workforce (11/93, reaffirmed 6/01
   AAP News)

PEDIATRIC WORKFORCE STATEMENT
Committee on Pediatric Workforce
ABSTRACT. This statement reviews current physician workforce projections, and identifies the factors that will have the most impact on future pediatric workforce projections. It discusses the key issues relating to the pediatric workforce: utilization of services, provision of care by both pediatricians and nonpediatricians, pediatric subspecialization, ethnic composition of the population and of the pediatric workforce, indebtedness, and geographic distribution. In a concluding series of recommendations, the statement addresses the steps that must be taken to ensure that all of America's infants, children, adolescents, and young adults have access to appropriate pediatric health care. (8/98)

THE PEDIATRICIAN AND CHILDHOOD BEREAVEMENT
Committee on Psychosocial Aspects of Child and Family
   Health
ABSTRACT. Pediatricians should understand and evaluate children's reactions to the death of a person important to them by using age-appropriate and culturally sensitive guidance while being alert for normal and complicated

grief responses. Pediatricians also should advise and assist families in responding to the child's needs. Sharing, family support, and communication have been associated with positive long-term bereavement adjustment. (2/00, reaffirmed 1/04)

THE PEDIATRICIAN'S ROLE IN COMMUNITY PEDIATRICS
Committee on Community Health Services
ABSTRACT. This policy statement offers pediatricians a concise definition of community pediatrics and provides a set of specific recommendations that underscore the critical nature of this important dimension of the profession. (6/99)

THE PEDIATRICIAN'S ROLE IN DEVELOPMENT AND IMPLEMENTATION OF AN INDIVIDUAL EDUCATION PLAN (IEP) AND/OR AN INDIVIDUAL FAMILY SERVICE PLAN (IFSP)
Committee on Children With Disabilities
ABSTRACT. The Individual Education Plan and Individual Family Service Plan are legally mandated documents developed by a multidisciplinary team assessment that specifies goals and services for each child eligible for special educational services or early intervention services. Pediatricians need to be knowledgeable of federal, state, and local requirements; establish linkages with early intervention, educational professionals, and parent support groups; and collaborate with the team working with individual children. (7/99, reaffirmed 11/02)

THE PEDIATRICIAN'S ROLE IN THE DIAGNOSIS AND MANAGEMENT OF AUTISTIC SPECTRUM DISORDER IN CHILDREN
Committee on Children With Disabilities
ABSTRACT. Primary care physicians have the opportunity, especially within the context of the medical home, to be the first point of contact when parents have concerns about their child's development or behavior. The goal of this policy statement is to help the pediatrician recognize the early symptoms of autism and participate in its diagnosis and management. This statement and the accompanying technical report will serve to familiarize the pediatrician with currently accepted criteria defining the spectrum of autism, strategies used in making a diagnosis, and conventional and alternative interventions. (5/01)

THE PEDIATRICIAN'S ROLE IN THE DIAGNOSIS AND MANAGEMENT OF AUTISTIC SPECTRUM DISORDER IN CHILDREN (TECHNICAL REPORT)
Committee on Children With Disabilities
ABSTRACT. Primary care physicians have the opportunity, especially within the context of the medical home, to be the first point of contact when parents have concerns about their child's development or behavior. The goal of this policy statement is to help the pediatrician recognize the early symptoms of autism and participate in its diagnosis and management. This statement and the accompanying technical report will serve to familiarize the pediatrician with currently accepted criteria defining the spectrum of autism, strategies used in making a diagnosis, and conventional and alternative interventions. (5/01)

THE PEDIATRICIAN'S ROLE IN FAMILY SUPPORT PROGRAMS
Committee on Early Childhood, Adoption, and
  Dependent Care

ABSTRACT. Children's brain growth, general health, and development are directly influenced by emotional relationships during early childhood. Contemporary American life challenges families' abilities to promote successful developmental outcomes and emotional health for their children. Pediatricians are positioned to serve as family advisors and community partners in supporting the well-being of children and families. This statement recommends opportunities for pediatricians to develop their expertise in assessing the strengths and stresses in families, in counseling families about strategies and resources, and in collaborating with others in their communities to support family relationships. (1/01)

THE PEDIATRICIAN'S ROLE IN THE PREVENTION OF MISSING CHILDREN (CLINICAL REPORT)
Committee on Psychosocial Aspects of Child and
  Family Health
See full text on page 453. (10/04)

PEDIATRICIANS' LIABILITY DURING DISASTERS
Committee on Pediatric Emergency Medicine and Committee
  on Medical Liability

ABSTRACT. This statement addresses the need for professional liability insurance coverage for pediatricians during disasters and suggests measures to ensure adequate coverage. (12/00, reaffirmed 1/04)

PERINATAL CARE AT THE THRESHOLD OF VIABILITY (CLINICAL REPORT)
Committee on Fetus and Newborn

ABSTRACT. In the United States, an increase in the number of births of extremely preterm infants and in their survival potential has occurred over the last decade. Determining the survival prognosis for the infant of a pregnancy with threatened preterm delivery between 22 and 25 completed weeks of gestation remains problematic. Many physicians and families encounter the difficulty of making decisions regarding the institution and continuation of life support for an infant born within this threshold period. This report addresses the process of counseling, assisting, and supporting families faced with the dilemma of an extremely preterm delivery. (11/02)

PERINATAL HUMAN IMMUNODEFICIENCY VIRUS TESTING
Committee on Pediatric AIDS (2/95, reaffirmed 10/96, 11/99,
  3/03)

PERINATAL HUMAN IMMUNODEFICIENCY VIRUS TESTING AND PREVENTION OF TRANSMISSION (TECHNICAL REPORT)
Committee on Pediatric AIDS

ABSTRACT. In 1994, the US Public Health Service published guidelines for the use of zidovudine to decrease the risk of perinatal transmission of human immunodeficiency virus (HIV). In 1995, the American Academy of Pediatrics and the US Public Health Service recommended documented, routine HIV education and testing with consent for all pregnant women in the United States. Widespread incorporation of these guidelines into clinical practice has resulted in a dramatic decrease in the rate of perinatal HIV transmission and has contributed to more than a 75% decrease in reported cases of pediatric acquired immunodeficiency syndrome (AIDS) since 1992. Substantial advances have been made in the treatment and monitoring of HIV infection; combination antiretroviral regimens that maximally suppress virus replication are now available. These regimens are recommended for pregnant and nonpregnant individuals who require treatment. Risk factors associated with perinatal HIV transmission are now better understood, and recent results from trials to decrease the rate of mother-to-child HIV transmission have contributed new strategies with established efficacy. However, perinatal HIV transmission still occurs; the Centers for Disease Control and Prevention estimates that 300 to 400 infected infants are born annually. Full implementation of recommendations for universal, routine prenatal HIV testing and evaluation of missed prevention opportunities will be critical to further decrease the incidence of pediatric HIV infection in the United States. This technical report summarizes recent advances in the prevention of perinatal transmission of HIV relevant to screening of pregnant women and their infants. (12/00, reaffirmed 3/03)

PERSONAL WATERCRAFT USE BY CHILDREN AND ADOLESCENTS
Committee on Injury and Poison Prevention

ABSTRACT. The use of personal watercraft (PWC) has increased dramatically during the past decade as have the speed and mobility of the watercraft. A similar dramatic increase in PWC-related injury and death has occurred simultaneously. No one younger than 16 years should operate a PWC. The operator and all passengers must wear US Coast Guard-approved personal flotation devices. Other safety recommendations are suggested for parents and pediatricians. (2/00, reaffirmed 5/04)

PHYSICAL FITNESS AND ACTIVITY IN SCHOOLS
Committee on Sports Medicine and Fitness and Committee on
  School Health

ABSTRACT. Schools are in a uniquely favorable position to increase physical activity and fitness among their students. This policy statement reaffirms the American Academy of Pediatrics' support for the efforts of schools to include increased physical activity in the curriculum, suggests ways in which schools can meet their goals in physical fitness, and encourages pediatricians to offer their assistance. The recommendations in this statement are consistent with those published in 1997 by the Centers for Disease Control and Prevention. (5/00)

PHYSICIANS' ROLES IN COORDINATING CARE OF HOSPITALIZED CHILDREN (CLINICAL REPORT)
Committee on Hospital Care
ABSTRACT. The care of hospitalized children has become increasingly complex and intense and often involves multiple physicians beyond the traditional primary care attending physician. Pediatric and adult subspecialists and surgeons, teaching attending physicians, and hospitalists may all participate in the care of hospitalized children. This report summarizes the responsibilities of the primary care physician, attending physician, and other involved physicians to ensure that children receive appropriate, coordinated, and comprehensive inpatient care that is delivered within the context of their medical home and is appropriately continued on an outpatient basis. (3/03)

PLANNING FOR CHILDREN WHOSE PARENTS ARE DYING OF HIV/AIDS
Committee on Pediatric AIDS
ABSTRACT. Although the character of acquired immunodeficiency syndrome is changing into a chronic illness, it is estimated that by the end of this century, 80 000 children and adolescents in the United States will be orphaned by parental death caused by human immunodeficiency virus infection. Plans for these children need to be made to ensure not only a stable, consistent environment that provides love and nurturing, but also the medical and social interventions necessary to cope with the tragic loss. Pediatricians should become aware of local laws and community resources and initiate discussion early in the course of parental illness to facilitate planning for the future care and custody of the children. States need to adopt laws and regulations that provide flexible approaches to guardianship and placement of children orphaned by acquired immunodeficiency syndrome. (2/99, reaffirmed 2/02)

POISON TREATMENT IN THE HOME
Committee on Injury, Violence, and Poison Prevention
ABSTRACT. The ingestion of a potentially poisonous substance by a young child is a common event, with the American Association of Poison Control Centers reporting approximately 1.2 million such events in the United States in 2001. The American Academy of Pediatrics (AAP) has long concerned itself with this issue and has made poison prevention an integral component of its injury prevention initiatives. A key AAP recommendation has been to keep a 1-oz bottle of syrup of ipecac in the home to be used only on the advice of a physician or poison control center. Recently, there has been interest regarding activated charcoal in the home as a poison treatment strategy. After reviewing the evidence, the AAP believes that ipecac should no longer be used routinely as a home treatment strategy, that existing ipecac in the home should be disposed of safely, and that it is premature to recommend the administration of activated charcoal in the home. The first action for a caregiver of a child who may have ingested a toxic substance is to consult with the local poison control center. (11/03)

POLICY ON THE DEVELOPMENT OF IMMUNIZATION TRACKING SYSTEMS
Committee on Practice and Ambulatory Medicine (6/96)

POSTEXPOSURE PROPHYLAXIS IN CHILDREN AND ADOLESCENTS FOR NONOCCUPATIONAL EXPOSURE TO HUMAN IMMUNODEFICIENCY VIRUS (CLINICAL REPORT)
Committee on Pediatric AIDS
ABSTRACT. Exposure to human immunodeficiency virus (HIV) can occur in a number of situations unique to, or more common among, children and adolescents. Guidelines for postexposure prophylaxis (PEP) for occupational and nonoccupational (eg, sexual, needle-sharing) exposures to HIV have been published by the US Public Health Service, but they do not directly address nonoccupational HIV exposures unique to children (such as accidental exposure to human milk from a woman infected with HIV or a puncture wound from a discarded needle on a playground), and they do not provide antiretroviral drug information relevant to PEP in children.

This clinical report reviews issues of potential exposure of children and adolescents to HIV and gives recommendations for PEP in those situations. The risk of HIV transmission from nonoccupational, nonperinatal exposure is generally low. Transmission risk is modified by factors related to the source and extent of exposure. Determination of the HIV infection status of the exposure source may not be possible, and data on transmission risk by exposure type may not exist. Except in the setting of perinatal transmission, no studies have demonstrated the safety and efficacy of postexposure use of antiretroviral drugs for the prevention of HIV transmission in nonoccupational settings. Antiretroviral therapy used for PEP is associated with significant toxicity. The decision to initiate prophylaxis needs to be made in consultation with the patient, the family, and a clinician with experience in treatment of persons with HIV infection. If instituted, therapy should be started as soon as possible after an exposure— no later than 72 hours—and continued for 28 days. Many clinicians would use 3 drugs for PEP regimens, although 2 drugs may be considered in certain circumstances. Instruction for avoiding secondary transmission should be given. Careful follow-up is needed for psychologic support, encouragement of medication adherence, toxicity monitoring, and serial HIV antibody testing. (6/03)

POSTNATAL CORTICOSTEROIDS TO TREAT OR PREVENT CHRONIC LUNG DISEASE IN PRETERM INFANTS
American Academy of Pediatrics Committee on Fetus and Newborn and Canadian Paediatric Society Fetus and Newborn Committee
ABSTRACT. This statement is intended for health care professionals caring for neonates and young infants. The objectives of this statement are to review the short- and long-term effects of systemic and inhaled postnatal corticosteroids for the prevention or treatment of evolving or established chronic lung disease and to make recommendations for the use of corticosteroids in infants with very low birth weight. The routine use of systemic dex-

amethasone for the prevention or treatment of chronic lung disease in infants with very low birth weight is not recommended. (2/02)

THE PRACTICAL SIGNIFICANCE OF LACTOSE INTOLERANCE IN CHILDREN
Committee on Nutrition (8/78, reaffirmed 12/93, 6/97, 4/00)

PRACTICAL SIGNIFICANCE OF LACTOSE INTOLERANCE IN CHILDREN: SUPPLEMENT
Committee on Nutrition (10/90, reaffirmed 12/93, 6/97, 4/00)

PRECAUTIONS CONCERNING THE USE OF THEOPHYLLINE
Committee on Drugs (4/92, reaffirmed 6/95, 6/98, 5/01)

PRECAUTIONS REGARDING THE USE OF AEROSOLIZED ANTIBIOTICS (TECHNICAL REPORT)
Committee on Infectious Diseases and Committee on Drugs
ABSTRACT. In 1998, the Food and Drug Administration (FDA) approved the licensure of tobramycin solution for inhalation (TOBI). Although a number of additional antibiotics, including other aminoglycosides, ß-lactams, antibiotics in the polymyxin class, and vancomycin, have been administered as aerosols for many years, none are approved by the FDA for administration by inhalation.

TOBI was approved by the FDA for the maintenance therapy of patients 6 years or older with cystic fibrosis (CF) who have between 25% and 75% of predicted forced expiratory volume in 1 second (FEV1), are colonized with *Pseudomonas aeruginosa*, and are able to comply with the prescribed medical regimen. TOBI was not approved for the therapy of acute pulmonary exacerbations in patients with CF nor was it approved for use in patients without CF. Currently, no other antibiotics are approved for administration by inhalation to patients with or without CF.

The purpose of this statement is to briefly summarize the data that supported approval for licensure of TOBI and to provide recommendations for its safe use. The pharmacokinetics of inhaled aminoglycosides and problems associated with aerosolized antibiotic treatment, including environmental contamination, selection of resistant microbes, and airway exposure to excipients in intravenous formulations, will be discussed. (12/00, reaffirmed 1/04)

PRECERTIFICATION PROCESS
Committee on Hospital Care
ABSTRACT. Precertification is a process still used by health insurance companies to control health care costs. Although we believe precertification is unnecessary and not cost-effective, in those instances where precertification is still being utilized, we suggest that the following procedures be adopted. This statement suggests guidelines that should help achieve this goal while allowing optimal access to care for children. (8/00)

PRENATAL GENETIC DIAGNOSIS FOR PEDIATRICIANS
Committee on Genetics (6/94, reaffirmed 10/97)

PRENATAL SCREENING AND DIAGNOSIS FOR PEDIATRICIANS (CLINICAL REPORT)
Committee on Genetics
See full text on page 461. (9/04)

THE PRENATAL VISIT
Committee on Psychosocial Aspects of Child and Family Health
ABSTRACT. In their role as advocates for children and families, pediatricians are in an excellent position to support and guide parents during the prenatal period. Prenatal visits allow the pediatrician to gather basic information from parents, provide information and advice to them, and identify high-risk situations in which parents may need to be referred to appropriate resources for help. In addition, prenatal visits are the first step in establishing a relationship between the pediatrician and parents and help parents develop parenting skills. The prenatal visit may take several possible forms depending on the experience and preferences of the parents, competence and availability of the pediatrician, and provisions of the health care plan. (6/01)

PRESCRIBING THERAPY SERVICES FOR CHILDREN WITH MOTOR DISABILITIES (CLINICAL REPORT)
Committee on Children With Disabilities
See full text on page 469. (6/04)

PREVENTION OF AGRICULTURAL INJURIES AMONG CHILDREN AND ADOLESCENTS
Committee on Injury and Poison Prevention and Committee on Community Health Services
ABSTRACT. Although the annual number of farm deaths to children and adolescents has decreased since publication of the 1988 American Academy of Pediatrics statement, "Rural Injuries," the rate of nonfatal farm injuries has increased. Approximately 100 unintentional injury deaths occur annually to children and adolescents on US farms, and an additional 22 000 injuries to children younger than 20 years occur on farms. Relatively few adolescents are employed on farms compared with other types of industry, yet the proportion of fatalities in agriculture is higher than that for any other type of adolescent employment. The high mortality and severe morbidity associated with farm injuries require continuing and improved injury-control strategies. This statement provides recommendations for pediatricians regarding patient and community education as well as public advocacy related to agricultural injury prevention in childhood and adolescence. (10/01)

PREVENTION OF DROWNING IN INFANTS, CHILDREN, AND ADOLESCENTS
Committee on Injury, Violence, and Poison Prevention
ABSTRACT. Drowning is a leading cause of injury-related death in children. In 2000, more than 1400 US children younger than 20 years drowned. A number of strategies are available to prevent these tragedies. Pediatricians play an important role in prevention of drownings as educators and advocates. (8/03)

PREVENTION OF DROWNING IN INFANTS, CHILDREN, AND ADOLESCENTS (TECHNICAL REPORT)

Committee on Injury, Violence, and Poison Prevention

ABSTRACT. Drowning is a leading cause of injury-related death in children. In 2000, more than 1400 US children younger than 20 years drowned. Most (91%) of these deaths were unintentional and were not related to boating. For each drowning death, it is estimated that at least 1 to 4 children suffer a serious nonfatal submersion event, many of which leave children with permanent disabilities. Environmental strategies, such as installation of 4-sided fences around swimming pools, and behavioral strategies, such as increased supervision of children while around water, are needed to prevent these tragedies. (8/03)

PREVENTION AND MANAGEMENT OF PAIN AND STRESS IN THE NEONATE

American Academy of Pediatrics Committee on Fetus and
Newborn, Committee on Drugs, Section on Anesthesiology
and Pain Medicine, and Section on Surgery and Canadian
Paediatric Society Fetus and Newborn Committee

ABSTRACT. This statement is intended for health care professionals caring for neonates (preterm to 1 month of age). The objectives of this statement are to:
1. Increase awareness that neonates experience pain;
2. Provide a physiological basis for neonatal pain and stress assessment and management by health care professionals;
3. Make recommendations for reduced exposure of the neonate to noxious stimuli and to minimize associated adverse outcomes; and
4. Recommend effective and safe interventions that relieve pain and stress. (2/00, reaffirmed 4/03)

PREVENTION AND MANAGEMENT OF POSITIONAL SKULL DEFORMITIES IN INFANTS (CLINICAL REPORT)

Committee on Practice and Ambulatory Medicine, Section on
Plastic Surgery, and Section on Neurological Surgery

ABSTRACT. Cranial asymmetry may be present at birth or may develop during the first few months of life. Over the past several years, pediatricians have seen an increase in the number of children with cranial asymmetry, particularly unilateral flattening of the occiput. This increase likely is attributable to parents following the American Academy of Pediatrics "Back to Sleep" positioning recommendations aimed at decreasing the risk of sudden infant death syndrome. Although associated with some risk of deformational plagiocephaly, healthy young infants should be placed down for sleep on their backs. This practice has been associated with a dramatic decrease in the incidence of sudden infant death syndrome. Pediatricians need to be able to properly diagnose skull deformities, educate parents on methods to proactively decrease the likelihood of the development of occipital flattening, initiate appropriate management, and make referrals when necessary. This report provides guidelines for the prevention, diagnosis, and management of positional skull deformity in an otherwise normal infant without evidence of associated anomalies, syndromes, or spinal disease. (7/03)

PREVENTION OF MEDICATION ERRORS IN THE PEDIATRIC INPATIENT SETTING

Committee on Drugs and Committee on Hospital Care

ABSTRACT. Although medication errors in hospitals are common, medication errors that result in death or serious injury occur rarely. Even before the Institute of Medicine reported on medical errors in 1999, the American Academy of Pediatrics and its members had been committed to improving the health care system to provide the best and safest health care for infants, children, adolescents, and young adults. This commitment includes designing health care systems to prevent errors and emphasizing the pediatrician's role in this system. Human and device errors can lead to preventable morbidity and mortality. National and state legislative actions have heightened public awareness of these events. All involved persons, beginning with the physician and including every member of the health care team, must be better educated about and engaged in the several steps recommended to decrease these errors. The safe administration of medications to hospitalized infants and children requires additional specific safeguards that are above and beyond those for adult patients. Pediatricians should help hospitals develop effective programs for safely providing medications, reporting medication errors, and creating an environment of medication safety for all hospitalized pediatric patients. (8/03)

PREVENTION OF PEDIATRIC OVERWEIGHT AND OBESITY

Committee on Nutrition

ABSTRACT. The dramatic increase in the prevalence of childhood overweight and its resultant comorbidities are associated with significant health and financial burdens, warranting strong and comprehensive prevention efforts. This statement proposes strategies for early identification of excessive weight gain by using body mass index, for dietary and physical activity interventions during health supervision encounters, and for advocacy and research. (8/03)

PREVENTION OF RICKETS AND VITAMIN D DEFICIENCY: NEW GUIDELINES FOR VITAMIN D INTAKE (CLINICAL REPORT)

Section on Breastfeeding and Committee on Nutrition

ABSTRACT. Rickets in infants attributable to inadequate vitamin D intake and decreased exposure to sunlight continues to be reported in the United States. It is recommended that all infants, including those who are exclusively breastfed, have a minimum intake of 200 IU of vitamin D per day beginning during the first 2 months of life. In addition, it is recommended that an intake of 200 IU of vitamin D per day be continued throughout childhood and adolescence, because adequate sunlight exposure is not easily determined for a given individual. These new vitamin D intake guidelines for healthy infants and children are based on the recommendations of the National Academy of Sciences. (4/03)

PREVENTION OF SEXUAL HARASSMENT IN THE WORKPLACE AND EDUCATIONAL SETTINGS
Committee on Pediatric Workforce

ABSTRACT. The American Academy of Pediatrics is committed to all its constituents supporting workplaces and educational settings free of sexual harassment. The purpose of this statement is to heighten awareness and sensitivity to this important issue, recognizing that institutions may have existing policies. (12/00)

PREVENTION AND TREATMENT OF TYPE 2 DIABETES MELLITUS IN CHILDREN, WITH SPECIAL EMPHASIS ON AMERICAN INDIAN AND ALASKA NATIVE CHILDREN (CLINICAL REPORT)
Committee on Native American Child Health and Section on Endocrinology

ABSTRACT. The emergence of type 2 diabetes mellitus in the American Indian/Alaska Native pediatric population presents a new challenge for pediatricians and other health care professionals. This chronic disease requires preventive efforts, early diagnosis, and collaborative care of the patient and family within the context of a medical home. (10/03)

THE PREVENTION OF UNINTENTIONAL INJURY AMONG AMERICAN INDIAN AND ALASKA NATIVE CHILDREN: A SUBJECT REVIEW (CLINICAL REPORT)
Committee on Native American Child Health and Committee on Injury and Poison Prevention

ABSTRACT. Among ethnic groups in the United States, American Indian and Alaska Native (AI/AN) children experience the highest rates of injury mortality and morbidity. Injury mortality rates for AI/AN children have decreased during the past quarter century, but remain almost double the rate for all children in the United States. The Indian Health Service (IHS), the federal agency with the primary responsibility for the health care of AI/AN people, has sponsored an internationally recognized injury prevention program designed to reduce the risk of injury death by addressing community-specific risk factors. Model programs developed by the IHS and tribal governments have led to successful outcomes in motor vehicle occupant safety, drowning prevention, and fire safety. Injury prevention programs in tribal communities require special attention to the sovereignty of tribal governments and the unique cultural aspects of health care and communication. Pediatricians working with AI/AN children on reservations or in urban environments are strongly urged to collaborate with tribes and the IHS to create community-based coalitions and develop programs to address highly preventable injury-related mortality and morbidity. Strong advocacy also is needed to promote childhood injury prevention as an important priority for federal agencies and tribes. (12/99, reaffirmed 12/02 COIVPP, 5/03 CONACH)

PRINCIPLES OF CHILD HEALTH CARE FINANCING
Committee on Child Health Financing

ABSTRACT. Child health care financing must maximize access to quality, comprehensive pediatric and prenatal health care. This policy statement replaces the 1998 policy statement by the same title. Changes reflect recent state and federal legislation that affect child health care financing. The principles outlined in the statement will be used to evaluate the changing structure of child health care financing. (10/03)

PRINCIPLES OF PATIENT SAFETY IN PEDIATRICS
National Initiative for Children's Health Care Quality Project Advisory Committee

ABSTRACT. The American Academy of Pediatrics and its members are committed to improving the health care system to provide the best and safest health care for infants, children, adolescents, and young adults. In response to a 1999 Institute of Medicine report on building a safer health system, a set of principles was established to guide the profession in designing a health care system that maximizes quality of care and minimizes medical errors through identification and resolution. This set of principles provides direction on setting up processes to identify and learn from errors, developing performance standards and expectations for safety, and promoting leadership and knowledge. (6/01)

PRIVACY PROTECTION OF HEALTH INFORMATION: PATIENT RIGHTS AND PEDIATRICIAN RESPONSIBILITIES
Pediatric Practice Action Group and Task Force on Medical Informatics

ABSTRACT. Pediatricians and pediatric medical and surgical subspecialists should know their legal responsibilities to protect the privacy of identifiable patient health information. Although paper and electronic medical records have the same privacy standards, health data that are stored or transmitted electronically are vulnerable to unique security breaches. This statement describes the privacy and confidentiality needs and rights of pediatric patients and suggests appropriate security strategies to deter unauthorized access and inappropriate use of patient data. Limitations to physician liability are discussed for transferred data. Any new standards for patient privacy and confidentiality must balance the health needs of the community and the rights of the patient without compromising the ability of pediatricians to provide quality care. (10/99)

PROFESSIONAL LIABILITY COVERAGE FOR RESIDENTS AND FELLOWS
Committee on Medical Liability

ABSTRACT. The American Academy of Pediatrics first developed a policy on professional liability coverage for pediatricians-in-training in 1989 and subsequently reaffirmed its basic position with slight modification in 1993. In this latest iteration of the statement, the original positions have been strengthened to address changes in the professional liability insurance industry, the structure and settings of residency training, and mandated reporting to health provider data banks. The new policy emphasizes the need to provide pediatricians in training with adequate professional liability insurance coverage and to educate residents and fellows on the importance of adequate and uninterrupted professional liability coverage—both during and after residency. (9/00)

PROMOTING EDUCATION, MENTORSHIP, AND SUPPORT FOR PEDIATRIC RESEARCH
Committee on Pediatric Research
ABSTRACT. Pediatricians have an important role to play in the advancement of child health research and should be encouraged and supported to pursue research activities. Education and training in child health research should be part of every level of pediatric training. Continuing education and access to research advisors should be available to practitioners and academic faculty. Recommendations to promote additional research education and support at all levels of pediatric training, from premedical to continuing medical education, as well as suggestions for means to increase support and mentorship for research activities, are outlined in this statement. (6/01)

PROMOTION OF HEALTHY WEIGHT-CONTROL PRACTICES IN YOUNG ATHLETES
Committee on Sports Medicine and Fitness (5/96, reaffirmed 10/99)

PROTECTIVE EYEWEAR FOR YOUNG ATHLETES
American Academy of Pediatrics Committee on Sports Medicine and Fitness and American Academy of Ophthalmology
See full text on page 475. (3/04)

PROVIDING A PRIMARY CARE MEDICAL HOME FOR CHILDREN AND YOUTH WITH CEREBRAL PALSY (CLINICAL REPORT)
Committee on Children With Disabilities
See full text on page 481. (10/04)

PROVISION OF EDUCATIONALLY-RELATED SERVICES FOR CHILDREN AND ADOLESCENTS WITH CHRONIC DISEASES AND DISABLING CONDITIONS
Committee on Children With Disabilities
ABSTRACT. Children and adolescents with chronic diseases and disabling conditions often need related services. As medical home professionals, pediatricians can assist children, adolescents, and their families with the complex federal, state, and local laws, regulations, and systems associated with these services. Expanded roles for pediatricians in Individual Family Service Plan, Individualized Education Plan, and 504 Plan development and implementation are recommended.

The complex range of federal, state, and local laws, regulations, and systems for special education and related services for children and adolescents in public schools is beyond the scope of this statement. Readers are referred to the policy statement "The Pediatrician's Role in Development and Implementation of an Individual Education Plan (IEP) and/or an Individual Family Services Plan" by the American Academy of Pediatrics for additional background materials. (2/00)

THE PSYCHOLOGICAL MALTREATMENT OF CHILDREN (TECHNICAL REPORT)
Committee on Child Abuse and Neglect
ABSTRACT. Psychological maltreatment is a common consequence of physical and sexual abuse but also may occur as a distinct entity. Until recently, there has been controversy regarding the definition and consequences of psychological maltreatment. Sufficient research and consensus now exist about the incidence, definition, risk factors, and consequences of psychological maltreatment to bring this form of child maltreatment to the attention of pediatricians. This technical report provides practicing pediatricians with definitions and risk factors for psychological maltreatment and details how pediatricians can prevent, recognize, and report psychological maltreatment. Contemporary references and resources are provided for pediatricians and parents. (4/02)

PSYCHOSOCIAL RISKS OF CHRONIC HEALTH CONDITIONS IN CHILDHOOD AND ADOLESCENCE
Committee on Children With Disabilities and Committee on Psychosocial Aspects of Child and Family Health (12/93, reaffirmed 10/96)

PUBLIC DISCLOSURE OF PRIVATE INFORMATION ABOUT VICTIMS OF ABUSE
Committee on Child Abuse and Neglect (2/91, reaffirmed 5/94, 9/00)

RACE/ETHNICITY, GENDER, SOCIOECONOMIC STATUS—RESEARCH EXPLORING THEIR EFFECTS ON CHILD HEALTH: A SUBJECT REVIEW (CLINICAL REPORT)
Committee on Pediatric Research
ABSTRACT. Data on research participants and populations frequently include race, ethnicity, and gender as categorical variables, with the assumption that these variables exert their effects through innate or genetically determined biologic mechanisms. There is a growing body of research that suggests, however, that these variables have strong social dimensions that influence health. Socioeconomic status, a complicated construct in its own right, interacts with and confounds analyses of race/ethnicity and gender. The Academy recommends that research studies include race/ethnicity, gender, and socioeconomic status as explanatory variables only when data relevant to the underlying social mechanisms have been collected and included in the analyses. (6/00)

RADIATION DISASTERS AND CHILDREN
Committee on Environmental Health
ABSTRACT. The special medical needs of children make it essential that pediatricians be prepared for radiation disasters, including 1) the detonation of a nuclear weapon; 2) a nuclear power plant event that unleashes a radioactive cloud; and 3) the dispersal of radionuclides by conventional explosive or the crash of a transport vehicle. Any of these events could occur unintentionally or as an act of terrorism. Nuclear facilities (eg, power plants, fuel processing centers, and food irradiation facilities) are often located in highly populated areas, and as they age, the risk of mechanical failure increases. The short- and long-term consequences of a radiation disaster are significantly greater in children for several reasons. First, children have a disproportionately higher minute ventilation, leading to greater internal exposure to radioactive gases. Children have a significantly greater risk of developing cancer even when they are exposed to radiation in utero. Finally, children and the parents of young children are more likely than are adults to develop enduring psycho-

logic injury after a radiation disaster. The pediatrician has a critical role in planning for radiation disasters. For example, potassium iodide is of proven value for thyroid protection but must be given before or soon after exposure to radioiodines, requiring its placement in homes, schools, and child care centers. Pediatricians should work with public health authorities to ensure that children receive full consideration in local planning for a radiation disaster. (6/03)

REAPPRAISAL OF LYTIC COCKTAIL/DEMEROL, PHENERGAN, AND THORAZINE (DPT) FOR THE SEDATION OF CHILDREN
Committee on Drugs (4/95, reaffirmed 3/98, 5/01)

RECOMMENDATIONS FOR INFLUENZA IMMUNIZATION OF CHILDREN
Committee on Infectious Diseases
See full text on page 491. (5/04)

RECOMMENDATIONS FOR PREVENTIVE PEDIATRIC HEALTH CARE
Committee on Practice and Ambulatory Medicine (3/00)

RECOMMENDATIONS FOR THE USE OF LIVE ATTENUATED VARICELLA VACCINE
Committee on Infectious Diseases (5/95, reaffirmed 6/98)

RECOMMENDED CHILDHOOD AND ADOLESCENT IMMUNIZATION SCHEDULE—UNITED STATES, JULY–DECEMBER 2004
Committee on Infectious Diseases
See full text on page 501. (5/04)

RED REFLEX EXAMINATION IN INFANTS
Section on Ophthalmology
ABSTRACT. Red reflex examination is recommended for all infants. This statement describes the indications for and the technique to perform this examination, including indications for dilation of the pupils before examination and indications for referral to an ophthalmologist. (5/02)

REDUCING THE NUMBER OF DEATHS AND INJURIES FROM RESIDENTIAL FIRES
Committee on Injury and Poison Prevention
ABSTRACT. Smoke inhalation, severe burns, and death from residential fires are devastating events, most of which are preventable. In 1998, approximately 381 500 residential structure fires resulted in 3250 non-firefighter deaths, 17 175 injuries, and approximately $4.4 billion in property loss. This statement reviews important prevention messages and intervention strategies related to residential fires. It also includes recommendations for pediatricians regarding office anticipatory guidance, work in the community, and support of regulation and legislation that could result in a decrease in the number of fire-related injuries and deaths to children. (6/00)

REDUCING THE RISK OF HUMAN IMMUNODEFICIENCY VIRUS INFECTION ASSOCIATED WITH ILLICIT DRUG USE
Committee on Pediatric AIDS (12/94, reaffirmed 1/98)

REDUCTION OF THE INFLUENZA BURDEN IN CHILDREN (TECHNICAL REPORT)
Committee on Infectious Diseases
ABSTRACT. Epidemiologic studies have shown that children of all ages with certain chronic conditions, such as asthma, and otherwise healthy children younger than 24 months (6 through 23 months) are hospitalized for influenza and its complications at high rates similar to those experienced by the elderly. Annual influenza immunization is already recommended for all children 6 months and older with high-risk conditions. By contrast, influenza immunization has not been recommended for healthy young children. To protect children against the complications of influenza, increased efforts are needed to identify and recall high-risk children. In addition, immunization of children between 6 through 23 months of age and their close contacts is now encouraged to the extent feasible. Children younger than 6 months may be protected by immunization of their household contacts and out-of-home caregivers. The ultimate goal is universal immunization of children 6 to 24 months of age. Issues that need to be addressed before institution of routine immunization of healthy young children include education of physicians and parents about the morbidity caused by influenza, adequate vaccine supply, and appropriate reimbursement of practitioners for influenza immunization. This report contains a summary of the influenza virus, protective immunity, disease burden in children, diagnosis, vaccines, and antiviral agents. (12/02)

REIMBURSEMENT FOR FOODS FOR SPECIAL DIETARY USE
Committee on Nutrition
ABSTRACT. Foods for special dietary use are recommended by physicians for chronic diseases or conditions of childhood, including inherited metabolic diseases. Although many states have created legislation requiring reimbursement for foods for special dietary use, legislation is now needed to mandate consistent coverage and reimbursement for foods for special dietary use and related support services with accepted medical benefit for children with designated medical conditions. (5/03)

RELIEF OF PAIN AND ANXIETY IN PEDIATRIC PATIENTS IN EMERGENCY MEDICAL SYSTEMS (CLINICAL REPORT)
Committee on Pediatric Emergency Medicine and Section on Anesthesiology and Pain Medicine
See full text on page 507. (11/04)

RELIGIOUS OBJECTIONS TO MEDICAL CARE
Committee on Bioethics
ABSTRACT. Parents sometimes deny their children the benefits of medical care because of religious beliefs. In some jurisdictions, exemptions to child abuse and neglect laws restrict government action to protect children or seek legal redress when the alleged abuse or neglect has

occurred in the name of religion. The American Academy of Pediatrics (AAP) believes that all children deserve effective medical treatment that is likely to prevent substantial harm or suffering or death. In addition, the AAP advocates that all legal interventions apply equally whenever children are endangered or harmed, without exemptions based on parental religious beliefs. To these ends, the AAP calls for the repeal of religious exemption laws and supports additional efforts to educate the public about the medical needs of children. (2/97, reaffirmed 10/00, 6/03)

RESIDENCY TRAINING AND CONTINUING MEDICAL EDUCATION IN SCHOOL HEALTH
Section on School Health (9/93)

RESTRAINT USE ON AIRCRAFT
Committee on Injury and Poison Prevention
ABSTRACT. Occupant protection policies for children younger than 2 years on aircraft are inconsistent with all other national policies on safe transportation. Children younger than 2 years are not required to be restrained or secured on aircraft during takeoff, landing, and conditions of turbulence. They are permitted to be held on the lap of an adult. Preventable injuries and deaths have occurred in children younger than 2 years who were unrestrained in aircraft during survivable crashes and conditions of turbulence. The American Academy of Pediatrics recommends a mandatory federal requirement for restraint use for children on aircraft. The Academy further recommends that parents ensure that a seat is available for all children during aircraft transport and follow current recommendations for restraint use for all children. Physicians play a significant role in counseling families, advocating for public policy mandates, and encouraging technologic research that will improve protection of children in aircraft. (11/01)

RETINOID THERAPY FOR SEVERE DERMATOLOGICAL DISORDERS
Committee on Drugs (7/92, reaffirmed 6/95, 6/98)

REVISED INDICATIONS FOR THE USE OF PALIVIZUMAB AND RESPIRATORY SYNCYTIAL VIRUS IMMUNE GLOBULIN INTRAVENOUS FOR THE PREVENTION OF RESPIRATORY SYNCYTIAL VIRUS INFECTIONS
Committee on Infectious Diseases and Committee on Fetus and Newborn
ABSTRACT. Palivizumab and Respiratory Syncytial Virus Immune Globulin Intravenous (RSV-IGIV) are licensed by the Food and Drug Administration for use in preventing severe lower respiratory tract infections caused by respiratory syncytial virus (RSV) in high-risk infants, children younger than 24 months with chronic lung disease (formerly called bronchopulmonary dysplasia), and certain preterm infants. This statement provides revised recommendations for administering RSV prophylaxis to infants and children with congenital heart disease, for identifying infants with a history of preterm birth and chronic lung disease who are most likely to benefit from immunoprophylaxis, and for reducing the risk of RSV exposure and infection in high-risk children. On the basis of results of a recently completed clinical trial, prophylaxis with palivizumab is appropriate for infants and young children with hemodynamically significant congenital heart disease. RSV-IGIV should not be used in children with hemodynamically significant heart disease. Palivizumab is preferred for most highrisk infants and children because of ease of intramuscular administration. Monthly administration of palivizumab during the RSV season results in a 45% to 55% decrease in the rate of hospitalization attributable to RSV. Because of the large number of infants born after 32 to 35 weeks' gestation and because of the high cost, immunoprophylaxis should be considered for this category of preterm infants only if 2 or more risk factors are present. High-risk infants should not attend child care during the RSV season when feasible, and exposure to tobacco smoke should be eliminated. (12/03)

REVISED INDICATIONS FOR THE USE OF PALIVIZUMAB AND RESPIRATORY SYNCYTIAL VIRUS IMMUNE GLOBULIN INTRAVENOUS FOR THE PREVENTION OF RESPIRATORY SYNCYTIAL VIRUS INFECTIONS (TECHNICAL REPORT)
Committee on Infectious Diseases and Committee on Fetus and Newborn
ABSTRACT. Palivizumab and Respiratory Syncytial Virus Immune Globulin Intravenous (RSV-IGIV) are licensed by the Food and Drug Administration for use in preventing severe respiratory syncytial virus (RSV) infections in high-risk infants, children younger than 24 months with chronic lung disease (formerly called bronchopulmonary dysplasia), and certain preterm infants. This report summarizes the clinical trial information on which the guidance in the accompanying policy statement for administering RSV prophylaxis to certain children with a history of preterm birth, chronic lung disease, or congenital heart disease is based. On the basis of results of a recently completed clinical trial, palivizumab is appropriate for infants and young children with hemodynamically significant congenital heart disease. RSV-IGIV should not be used in children with hemodynamically significant heart disease. Palivizumab is preferred for most high-risk infants and children because of ease of intramuscular administration. Monthly administration of palivizumab during the RSV season results in a 45% to 55% decrease in the rate of hospitalization attributable to RSV. Because of the large number of infants born after 32 to 35 weeks' gestation and because of the high cost, immunoprophylaxis should be considered for this category of preterm infants only if 2 or more risk factors are present. (12/03)

RISK OF INJURY FROM BASEBALL AND SOFTBALL IN CHILDREN
Committee on Sports Medicine and Fitness
ABSTRACT. This statement updates the 1994 American Academy of Pediatrics policy statement on baseball and softball injuries in children. Current studies on acute, overuse, and catastrophic injuries are reviewed with emphasis on the causes and mechanisms of injury. This information serves as a basis for recommending safe training practices and the appropriate use of protective equipment. (4/01)

THE ROLE OF HOME-VISITATION PROGRAMS IN IMPROVING HEALTH OUTCOMES FOR CHILDREN AND FAMILIES
Council on Child and Adolescent Health

ABSTRACT. Traditional pediatric care is often based on the assumption that parents have the basic knowledge and resources to provide a nurturing, safe environment and to provide for the emotional, physical, developmental, and health care needs of their infants and young children. Unfortunately, many families have insufficient knowledge of parenting skills and an inadequate support system of friends, extended family, or professionals to help with these vital tasks. Home-visitation programs offer an effective mechanism to ensure ongoing parental education, social support, and linkage with public and private community services. This statement reviews the history and current research on home-visitation programs and provides recommendations about the pediatrician's role in supporting and using home visitation. (3/98, reaffirmed 5/01)

THE ROLE OF THE NURSE PRACTITIONER AND PHYSICIAN ASSISTANT IN THE CARE OF HOSPITALIZED CHILDREN
Committee on Hospital Care

ABSTRACT. The positions of nurse practitioner and physician assistant were created approximately 30 years ago. Since then, the role and responsibilities of these individuals have developed and grown and now may include involvement in the care of hospitalized patients. The intent of this statement is to suggest a manner in which nurse practitioners and physician's assistants may participate in and contribute to the care of the hospitalized child on the general inpatient unit, among other areas. (5/99, reaffirmed 11/01)

ROLE OF THE PEDIATRICIAN IN FAMILY-CENTERED EARLY INTERVENTION SERVICES
Committee on Children With Disabilities

ABSTRACT. There is growing evidence that early intervention services have had a positive influence on the developmental outcome of children with established disabilities or those considered "at risk" for disabilities and their families. Various federal and state statutes now mandate that community-based, coordinated, multidisciplinary, family-centered programs be established, which are accessible to serve children and families in need. The pediatrician, in close collaboration with the family and the early intervention team, plays a critical role in guiding the clinical and developmental aspects of the early intervention services provided. This role can be best served in the context of providing a medical home for children with special health care needs. The purpose of this statement is to assist the pediatrician in assuming a proactive role on the multidisciplinary team providing early intervention services. (5/01)

THE ROLE OF THE PEDIATRICIAN IN IMPLEMENTING THE AMERICANS WITH DISABILITIES ACT: SUBJECT REVIEW (CLINICAL REPORT)
Committee on Children With Disabilities

ABSTRACT. In this statement, the American Academy of Pediatrics reaffirms the importance of the Americans With Disabilities Act (ADA), which guarantees people with disabilities certain rights to enable them to participate more fully in their communities. Pediatricians need to know about the ADA provisions to be able to educate and counsel their patients and patients' families appropriately. The ADA mandates changes to our environment, including reasonable accommodation to the needs of individuals with disabilities, which has application to schools, hospitals, physician offices, community businesses, and recreational programs. Pediatricians should be a resource to their community by providing information about the ADA and the special needs of their patients, assisting with devising reasonable accommodation, and counseling adolescents about their expanded opportunities under the ADA. (7/96, reaffirmed 10/00, 1/04)

THE ROLE OF THE PEDIATRICIAN IN RECOGNIZING AND INTERVENING ON BEHALF OF ABUSED WOMEN
Committee on Child Abuse and Neglect

ABSTRACT. Pediatricians are in a position to recognize abused women in pediatric settings. Intervening on behalf of battered women is an active form of child abuse prevention. Knowledge of local resources and state laws for reporting abuse are emphasized. (6/98, reaffirmed 10/01, 5/04)

THE ROLE OF THE PEDIATRICIAN IN RURAL EMSC
Committee on Pediatric Emergency Medicine

ABSTRACT. In rural America pediatricians can play a key role in the development, implementation, and ongoing supervision of emergency medical services for children (EMSC). Often the only pediatric resource for a large region, rural access pediatricians are more likely to treat pediatric emergencies in their own offices, and are a vital resource for rural physicians, or other rural health care professionals (physician assistants, nurse practitioners), and emergency medical technicians (EMTs) to improve system-wide EMSC by providing education about issues from prevention to rehabilitation, technical assistance in protocol writing, hospital care, and data accumulation, and as advocates for community and state legislation to support the goals of EMSC. (5/98, reaffirmed 6/00)

THE ROLE OF THE PEDIATRICIAN IN TRANSITIONING CHILDREN AND ADOLESCENTS WITH DEVELOPMENTAL DISABILITIES AND CHRONIC ILLNESSES FROM SCHOOL TO WORK OR COLLEGE
Committee on Children With Disabilities

ABSTRACT. The role of the pediatrician in transitioning children with disabilities and chronic illnesses from school to work or college is to provide anticipatory guidance and to promote self-advocacy and self-determination. Knowledge of the provisions of the key federal laws affecting vocational education is essential for the pediatrician's successful advocacy for patients. (10/00, reaffirmed 1/04)

THE ROLE OF THE PEDIATRICIAN IN YOUTH VIOLENCE PREVENTION IN CLINICAL PRACTICE AND AT THE COMMUNITY LEVEL

Task Force on Violence

ABSTRACT. Violence and violent injuries are a serious threat to the health of children and youth in the United States. It is crucial that pediatricians define their role and develop the appropriate skills to address this threat effectively. From a clinical perspective, pediatricians should incorporate into their practices preventive education, screening for risk, and linkages to necessary intervention and follow-up services. As advocates, pediatricians should become involved at the local and national levels to address key risk factors and assure adequacy of preventive and treatment programs. There are also educational and research needs central to the development of effective clinical strategies. This policy statement defines the emerging role of pediatricians in youth violence prevention and management. It reflects the importance of this issue in the strategic agenda of the American Academy of Pediatrics for promoting optimal child health and development. (1/99, reaffirmed 5/02)

ROLE OF PEDIATRICIANS IN ADVOCATING LIFE SUPPORT TRAINING COURSES FOR PARENTS AND THE PUBLIC

Committee on Pediatric Emergency Medicine
See full text on page 519. (12/04)

THE ROLE OF THE PRIMARY CARE PEDIATRICIAN IN THE MANAGEMENT OF HIGH-RISK NEWBORN INFANTS

*Committee on Practice and Ambulatory Medicine and
Committee on Fetus and Newborn*

ABSTRACT. Quality care for high-risk newborns can best be provided by coordinating the efforts of the primary care pediatrician and the neonatologist. This ideally occurs in the newborn period, during the critical care and convalescing periods, and through the time of discharge. This statement offers guidelines for the primary care pediatrician involved in providing neonatal care, and discusses his/her individual and shared responsibilities, roles, and relationships with the neonatologist and the neonatal intensive care unit. (10/96)

THE ROLE OF THE SCHOOL NURSE IN PROVIDING SCHOOL HEALTH SERVICES

Committee on School Health

ABSTRACT. The school nurse has a crucial role in the provision of school health services. This statement describes the school nurse as a member of the school health services team and its relation to children with special health care needs. Recommendations for the professional preparation and education of school nurses also are provided. (11/01)

THE ROLE OF SCHOOLS IN COMBATTING SUBSTANCE ABUSE

Committee on Substance Abuse (5/95, reaffirmed 5/99)

SAFE TRANSPORTATION OF NEWBORNS AT HOSPITAL DISCHARGE

Committee on Injury and Poison Prevention

ABSTRACT. All hospitals should set policies that require the discharge of every newborn in a car safety seat that is appropriate for the infant's maturity and medical condition. Discharge policies for newborns should include a parent education component, regular review of educational materials, and periodic in-service education for responsible staff. Appropriate child restraint systems should become a benefit of coverage by Medicaid, managed care organizations, and other third-party insurers. (10/99, reaffirmed 12/02)

SAFE TRANSPORTATION OF PREMATURE AND LOW BIRTH WEIGHT INFANTS

Committee on Injury and Poison Prevention and Committee on Fetus and Newborn

ABSTRACT. Special considerations are essential to ensure the safe transportation of premature and low birth weight infants. Both physical and physiologic issues must be considered in the proper positioning of these infants. This statement discusses current recommendations based on the latest research and provides guidelines for physicians who counsel parents of very small infants on the choice of the best car safety seats for their infants. (5/96, reaffirmed 4/99)

SAFETY IN YOUTH ICE HOCKEY: THE EFFECTS OF BODY CHECKING

Committee on Sports Medicine and Fitness

ABSTRACT. Ice hockey is a sport enjoyed by many young people. The occurrence of injury can offset what may otherwise be a positive experience. A high proportion of injuries in hockey appear to result from intentional body contact or the practice of checking. The American Academy of Pediatrics recommends limiting checking in hockey players 15 years of age and younger as a means to reduce injuries. Strategies such as the fair play concept can also help decrease injuries that result from penalties or unnecessary contact. (3/00, reaffirmed 5/04)

SCHOOL BUS TRANSPORTATION OF CHILDREN WITH SPECIAL HEALTH CARE NEEDS

Committee on Injury and Poison Prevention (8/01, reaffirmed 11/04)

SCHOOL HEALTH ASSESSMENTS

Committee on School Health

ABSTRACT. Comprehensive health assessments often are performed in school-based clinics or public health clinics by health professionals other than pediatricians. Pediatricians or other physicians skilled in child health care should participate in such evaluations. This statement provides guidance on the scope of in-school health assessments and the roles of the pediatrician, school nurse, school, and community. (4/00, reaffirmed 6/03)

SCHOOL HEALTH CENTERS AND OTHER INTEGRATED SCHOOL HEALTH SERVICES
Committee on School Health
ABSTRACT. This statement offers guidelines on the integration of expanded school health services, including school-based and school-linked health centers, into community-based health care systems. Expanded school health services should be integrated so that they enhance accessibility, provide high-quality health care, link children to a medical home, are financially sustainable, and address both long- and short-term needs of children and adolescents. (1/01)

SCHOOL TRANSPORTATION SAFETY
Committee on School Health and Committee on Injury and Poison Prevention
ABSTRACT. The following policy statement is a revision of the American Academy of Pediatrics' 1985 statement entitled "School Bus Safety." It provides updated information regarding relevant federal regulations and outlines recommendations that can enhance community systems for addressing school bus safety education, awareness, and practices. Pediatricians can assist in this process by sharing these recommendations at both the community and state levels. (5/96, reaffirmed 4/99)

SCHOOL-BASED MENTAL HEALTH SERVICES
Committee on School Health
See full text on page 523. (6/04)

SCOPE OF HEALTH CARE BENEFITS FOR NEWBORNS, INFANTS, CHILDREN, ADOLESCENTS, AND YOUNG ADULTS THROUGH AGE 21 YEARS
Committee on Child Health Financing
ABSTRACT. The optimal health of children can best be achieved by providing access to comprehensive health care benefits. This policy statement replaces the 1993 statement, "Scope of Health Care Benefits for Infants, Children, and Adolescents Through Age 21 Years." Changes involve services and procedures specific to the delivery of comprehensive preventive, prenatal, postnatal, and mental health care. These services should be delivered by appropriately trained and board-eligible/certified pediatric providers, including primary care pediatricians, pediatric medical subspecialists, and pediatric surgical specialists. (12/97)

SCOPE OF PRACTICE ISSUES IN THE DELIVERY OF PEDIATRIC HEALTH CARE
Committee on Pediatric Workforce
ABSTRACT. In recent years, there has been an increase in the number of nonphysician pediatric clinicians and an expansion in their respective scopes of practice. This raises critical public policy and child health advocacy concerns. The American Academy of Pediatrics (AAP) believes that optimal pediatric health care depends on a team-based approach with coordination by a physician leader, preferably a pediatrician. The pediatrician is uniquely suited to manage, coordinate, and supervise the entire spectrum of pediatric care, from diagnosis through all stages of treatment, in all practice settings. The AAP recognizes the valuable contributions of nonphysician clinicians, including nurse practitioners and physician assistants, in delivering optimal pediatric care. The AAP also believes that nonphysician clinicians who provide health care services in underserved areas should be supported by consulting pediatricians and other physicians using technologies including telemedicine. Pediatricians should serve as advocates for optimal pediatric care in state legislatures, public policy forums, and the media and should pursue opportunities to resolve scope of practice conflicts outside state legislatures. The AAP affirms that as nonphysician clinicians seek to expand their scopes of practice as providers of pediatric care, standards of education, training, examination, regulation, and patient care are needed to ensure patient safety and quality health care for all infants, children, adolescents, and young adults. (2/03)

SCREENING FOR ELEVATED BLOOD LEAD LEVELS
Committee on Environmental Health
ABSTRACT. Although recent data continue to demonstrate a decline in the prevalence of elevated blood lead levels (BLLs) in children, lead remains a common, preventable, environmental health threat. Because recent epidemiologic data have shown that lead exposure is still common in certain communities in the United States, the Centers for Disease Control and Prevention recently issued new guidelines endorsing universal screening in areas with ≥27% of housing built before 1950 and in populations in which the percentage of 1- and 2-year-olds with elevated BLLs is ≥12%. For children living in other areas, the Centers for Disease Control and Prevention recommends targeted screening based on risk-assessment during specified pediatric visits. In this statement, the American Academy of Pediatrics supports these new guidelines and provides an update on screening for elevated BLLs. The American Academy of Pediatrics recommends that pediatricians continue to provide anticipatory guidance to parents in an effort to prevent lead exposure (primary prevention). Additionally, pediatricians should increase their efforts to screen children at risk for lead exposure to find those with elevated BLLs (secondary prevention). (6/98)

SCREENING EXAMINATION OF PREMATURE INFANTS FOR RETINOPATHY OF PREMATURITY
American Academy of Pediatrics Section on Ophthalmology, American Association for Pediatric Ophthalmology and Strabismus, and American Academy of Ophthalmology
ABSTRACT. This statement revises a previous statement on screening of premature infants for retinopathy of prematurity originally published in 1997. (9/01)

SCREENING FOR RETINOPATHY IN THE PEDIATRIC PATIENT WITH TYPE 1 DIABETES MELLITUS
Section on Endocrinology and Section on Ophthalmology (2/98)

SELECTING APPROPRIATE TOYS FOR YOUNG CHILDREN: THE PEDIATRICIAN'S ROLE (CLINICAL REPORT)
Committee on Early Childhood, Adoption, and Dependent Care
ABSTRACT. Play is essential for learning in children. Toys are the tools of play. Which play materials are provided and how they are used are equally important. Adults caring for children can be reminded that toys facilitate but do

not substitute for the most important aspect of nurture—warm, loving, dependable relationships. Toys should be safe, affordable, and developmentally appropriate. Children do not need expensive toys. Toys should be appealing to engage the child over a period of time. Information and resources are provided in this report so pediatricians can give parents advice about selecting toys. (4/03)

SELECTING AND USING THE MOST APPROPRIATE CAR SAFETY SEATS FOR GROWING CHILDREN: GUIDELINES FOR COUNSELING PARENTS

Committee on Injury and Poison Prevention

ABSTRACT. Despite the existence of laws in all 50 states requiring the use of car safety seats or child restraint devices for young children, more children are still killed as passengers in car crashes than from any other type of injury. Pediatricians and other health care professionals need to provide up-to-date, appropriate information for parents regarding car safety seat choices and proper use. Although the American Academy of Pediatrics is not a testing or standard-setting organization, this policy statement discusses the Academy's current recommendations based on the peer-reviewed literature available at the time of publication and sets forth some of the factors that parents should consider before selecting and using a car safety seat. (3/02)

SEXUAL ORIENTATION AND ADOLESCENTS (CLINICAL REPORT)

Committee on Adolescence

See full text on page 533. (6/04)

SEXUALITY, CONTRACEPTION, AND THE MEDIA

Committee on Public Education

ABSTRACT. Early sexual intercourse among American adolescents represents a major public health problem. Although early sexual activity may be caused by a variety of factors, the media are believed to play a significant role. In film, television, and music, sexual messages are becoming more explicit in dialogue, lyrics, and behavior. In addition, these messages contain unrealistic, inaccurate, and misleading information that young people accept as fact. Teens rank the media second only to school sex education programs as a leading source of information about sex. Recommendations are presented to help pediatricians address the effects of the media on sexual attitudes, beliefs, and behaviors of their patients. (1/01)

SEXUALITY EDUCATION FOR CHILDREN AND ADOLESCENTS

Committee on Psychosocial Aspects of Child and Family Health and Committee on Adolescence

ABSTRACT. Children and adolescents need accurate and comprehensive education about sexuality to practice healthy sexual behavior as adults. Early, exploitative, or risky sexual activity may lead to health and social problems, such as unintended pregnancy and sexually transmitted diseases, including human immunodeficiency virus infection and acquired immunodeficiency syndrome. This statement reviews the role of the pediatrician in providing sexuality education to children, adolescents, and their families. Pediatricians should integrate sexuality education into the confidential and longitudinal relationship they develop with children, adolescents, and families to complement the education children obtain at school and at home. Pediatricians must be aware of their own attitudes, beliefs, and values so their effectiveness in discussing sexuality in the clinical setting is not limited. (8/01, reaffirmed 5/04)

SEXUALITY EDUCATION OF CHILDREN AND ADOLESCENTS WITH DEVELOPMENTAL DISABILITIES

Committee on Children With Disabilities (2/96, reaffirmed 4/00)

SHAKEN BABY SYNDROME: ROTATIONAL CRANIAL INJURIES (TECHNICAL REPORT)

Committee on Child Abuse and Neglect

ABSTRACT. Shaken baby syndrome is a serious and clearly definable form of child abuse. It results from extreme rotational cranial acceleration induced by violent shaking or shaking/impact, which would be easily recognizable by others as dangerous. More resources should be devoted to prevention of this and other forms of child abuse. (7/01)

SKATEBOARD AND SCOOTER INJURIES

Committee on Injury, Violence, and Poison Prevention

ABSTRACT. Skateboard-related injuries account for an estimated 50 000 emergency department visits and 1500 hospitalizations among children and adolescents in the United States each year. Nonpowered scooter-related injuries accounted for an estimated 9400 emergency department visits between January and August 2000, and 90% of these patients were children younger than 15 years. Many such injuries can be avoided if children and youth do not ride in traffic, if proper protective gear is worn, and if, in the absence of close adult supervision, skateboards and scooters are not used by children younger than 10 and 8 years, respectively. (3/02)

SMALLPOX VACCINE

Committee on Infectious Diseases

ABSTRACT. After an extensive worldwide eradication program, the last nonlaboratory case of smallpox occurred in 1977 in Somalia. In 1972, routine smallpox immunization was discontinued in the United States, and since 1983, vaccine production has been halted. Stockpiled vaccine has been used only for laboratory researchers working on orthopoxviruses. In recent years, there has been concern that smallpox virus stocks may be in the hands of bioterrorists, and this concern has been heightened by the terrorist attack on the World Trade Center and the Pentagon on September 11, 2001. Because most of the population is considered to be nonimmune, there is debate as to whether smallpox immunization should be resumed. This statement reviews the current status of smallpox vaccine, the adverse effects that were associated with smallpox vaccine in the past, and the major proposals for vaccine use. The statement provides the rationale for a policy based on the so-called ring vaccination strategy recommended by the Centers for Disease Control and Prevention, in which cases of smallpox are rapidly identified, infected individuals are isolated, and contacts of the infected individuals as well as their contacts are immunized immediately. (10/02)

SNOWMOBILING HAZARDS
Committee on Injury and Poison Prevention
ABSTRACT. Snowmobiles continue to pose a significant risk to children younger than 15 years and adolescents and young adults 15 through 24 years of age. Head injuries remain the leading cause of mortality and serious morbidity, arising largely from snowmobilers colliding, falling, or overturning during operation. Children also were injured while being towed in a variety of conveyances by snowmobiles. No uniform code of state laws governs the use of snowmobiles by children and youth. Because evidence is lacking to support the effectiveness of operator safety certification and because many children and adolescents do not have the required strength and skills to operate a snowmobile safely, the recreational operation of snowmobiles by persons younger than 16 years is not recommended. Snowmobiles should not be used to tow persons on a tube, tire, sled, or saucer. Furthermore, a graduated licensing program is advised for snowmobilers 16 years and older. Both active and passive snowmobile injury prevention strategies are suggested, as well as recommendations for manufacturers to make safer equipment for snowmobilers of all ages. (11/00, reaffirmed 5/04)

SOFT DRINKS IN SCHOOLS
Committee on School Health
See full text on page 541. (1/04)

SOY PROTEIN-BASED FORMULAS: RECOMMENDATIONS FOR USE IN INFANT FEEDING
Committee on Nutrition
ABSTRACT. The American Academy of Pediatrics is committed to the use of maternal breast milk as the ideal source of nutrition for infant feeding. Even so, by 2 months of age, most infants in North America are formula-fed. Despite limited indications, the use of soy protein-based formula has nearly doubled during the past decade to achieve 25% of the market in the United States. Because an infant formula provides the largest, if not sole, source of nutrition for an extended interval, the nutritional adequacy of the formula must be confirmed and the indications for its use well understood. This statement updates the 1983 Committee on Nutrition review and contains some important recommendations on the appropriate use of soy protein-based formulas. (1/98, reaffirmed 4/01)

SPECIAL REQUIREMENTS FOR ELECTRONIC MEDICAL RECORD SYSTEMS IN PEDIATRICS
Task Force on Medical Informatics
ABSTRACT. Electronic medical record (EMR) systems, which are usually designed for adult care, must perform certain functions to be useful in pediatric care. This statement outlines these functions (eg, immunization tracking and pediatric dosing calculations) to assist vendors and standards organizations with software design for pediatric systems. The description of these functions should also provide pediatricians with a set of requirements or desirable features to use when evaluating EMR systems. Particular attention is paid to special aspects of pediatric clinical care and privacy issues unique to pediatrics. (8/01)

STERILIZATION OF MINORS WITH DEVELOPMENTAL DISABILITIES
Committee on Bioethics
ABSTRACT. Sterilization of persons with developmental disabilities has often been performed without appropriate regard for their decision-making capacities, abilities to care for children, feelings, or interests. In addition, sterilization sometimes has been performed with the mistaken belief that it will prevent expressions of sexuality, diminish the chances of sexual exploitation, or reduce the likelihood of acquiring sexually transmitted diseases. A decision to pursue sterilization of someone with developmental disabilities requires a careful assessment of the individual's capacity to make decisions, the consequences of reproduction for the person and any child that might be born, the alternative means available to address the consequences of sexual maturation, and the applicable local, state, and federal laws. Pediatricians can facilitate good decision-making by raising these issues at the onset of puberty. (8/99, reaffirmed 11/02)

STRENGTH TRAINING BY CHILDREN AND ADOLESCENTS
Committee on Sports Medicine and Fitness
ABSTRACT. Pediatricians are often asked to give advice on the safety and efficacy of strength training programs for children and adolescents. This review, a revision of a previous American Academy of Pediatrics policy statement, defines relevant terminology and provides current information on risks and benefits of strength training for children and adolescents. (6/01)

SUICIDE AND SUICIDE ATTEMPTS IN ADOLESCENTS
Committee on Adolescence
ABSTRACT. Suicide is the third leading cause of death for adolescents 15 to 19 years old. Pediatricians can help prevent adolescent suicide by knowing the symptoms of depression and other presuicidal behavior. This statement updates the previous statement by the American Academy of Pediatrics and assists the pediatrician in the identification and management of the adolescent at risk for suicide. The extent to which pediatricians provide appropriate care for suicidal adolescents depends on their knowledge, skill, comfort with the topic, and ready access to appropriate community resources. All teenagers with suicidal symptoms should know that their pleas for assistance are heard and that pediatricians are willing to serve as advocates to help resolve the crisis. (4/00)

SURFACTANT REPLACEMENT THERAPY FOR RESPIRATORY DISTRESS SYNDROME
Committee on Fetus and Newborn
ABSTRACT. Respiratory failure secondary to surfactant deficiency is a major cause of morbidity and mortality in low birth weight immature infants. Surfactant therapy substantially reduces mortality and respiratory morbidity for this population. The statement summarizes the indications for surfactant replacement therapy. Because respira-

tory insufficiency may be a component of multiorgan dysfunction in sick infants, surfactant should be administered only at institutions with qualified personnel and facilities for the comprehensive care of sick infants. (3/99)

SURVEILLANCE OF PEDIATRIC HIV INFECTION
Committee on Pediatric AIDS
ABSTRACT. Pediatric human immunodeficiency virus (HIV)/acquired immunodeficiency syndrome (AIDS) surveillance should expand to include perinatal HIV exposure and HIV infection as well as AIDS to delineate completely the extent and impact of HIV infection on children and families, accurately assess the resources necessary to provide services to this population, evaluate the efficacy of public health recommendations, and determine any potential long-term consequences of interventions to prevent perinatal transmission to children ultimately determined to be uninfected as well as for those who become infected. Ensuring the confidentiality of information collected in the process of surveillance is critical. In addition, expansion of surveillance must not compromise the established, ongoing surveillance system for pediatric AIDS. An expanded pediatric HIV surveillance program provides an important counterpart to existing American Academy of Pediatrics and American College of Obstetricians and Gynecologists recommendations for HIV counseling and testing in the prenatal setting. (2/98, reaffirmed 2/02)

SWIMMING PROGRAMS FOR INFANTS AND TODDLERS
Committee on Sports Medicine and Fitness and Committee on Injury and Poison Prevention
ABSTRACT. Infant and toddler aquatic programs provide an opportunity to introduce young children to the joy and risks of being in or around water. Generally, children are not developmentally ready for swimming lessons until after their fourth birthday. Aquatic programs for infants and toddlers have not been shown to decrease the risk of drowning, and parents should not feel secure that their child is safe in water or safe from drowning after participating in such programs. Young children should receive constant, close supervision by an adult while in and around water. (4/00, reaffirmed 5/04)

THE TEENAGE DRIVER
Committee on Injury and Poison Prevention and Committee on Adolescence
ABSTRACT. Motor vehicle-related injuries continue to be of paramount importance to adolescents. This statement describes why teenagers are at particularly great risk, suggests topics suitable for office-based counseling, describes innovative programs, and proposes steps for prevention for pediatricians, legislators, educators, and other child advocates. (11/96, reaffirmed 11/99)

TELEMEDICINE: PEDIATRIC APPLICATIONS (TECHNICAL REPORT)
Steering Committee on Clinical Information Technology and Committee on Medical Liability
See full text on page 547. (6/04)

TESTING FOR DRUGS OF ABUSE IN CHILDREN AND ADOLESCENTS
Committee on Substance Abuse
ABSTRACT. The American Academy of Pediatrics (AAP) recognizes the abuse of psychoactive drugs as one of the greatest problems facing children and adolescents and condemns all such use. Diagnostic testing for drugs of abuse is frequently an integral part of the pediatrician's evaluation and management of those suspected of such use. "Voluntary screening" is the term applied to many mass non–suspicion-based screening programs, yet such programs may not be truly voluntary as there are often negative consequences for those who choose not to take part. Participation in such programs should not be a prerequisite to participation in school activities. Involuntary testing is not appropriate in adolescents with decisional capacity—even with parental consent—and should be performed only if there are strong medical or legal reasons to do so. The AAP reaffirms its position that the appropriate response to the suspicion of drug abuse in a young person is the referral to a qualified health care professional for comprehensive evaluation. (8/96, reaffirmed 5/99)

THERAPY FOR CHILDREN WITH INVASIVE PNEUMOCOCCAL INFECTIONS
Committee on Infectious Diseases
ABSTRACT. This statement provides guidelines for therapy of children with serious infections possibly caused by *Streptococcus pneumoniae*. Resistance of invasive pneumococcal strains to penicillin, cefotaxime, and ceftriaxone has increased over the past few years. Reports of failures of cefotaxime or ceftriaxone in the treatment of children with meningitis caused by resistant *S pneumoniae* necessitates a revision of Academy recommendations. For nonmeningeal infections, modifications of the initial therapy need to be considered only for patients who are critically ill and those who have a severe underlying or potentially immunocompromising condition or patients from whom a highly resistant strain is isolated. Because vancomycin is the only antibiotic to which all *S pneumoniae* strains are susceptible, its use should be restricted to minimize the emergence of vancomycin-resistant organisms. Patients with probable aseptic (viral) meningitis should not be treated with vancomycin. These recommendations are subject to change as new information becomes available. (2/97, reaffirmed 10/99, 1/04)

TIMING OF ELECTIVE SURGERY ON THE GENITALIA OF MALE CHILDREN WITH PARTICULAR REFERENCE TO THE RISKS, BENEFITS, AND PSYCHOLOGICAL EFFECTS OF SURGERY AND ANESTHESIA
Section on Urology (4/96)

TOBACCO, ALCOHOL, AND OTHER DRUGS: THE ROLE OF THE PEDIATRICIAN IN PREVENTION AND MANAGEMENT OF SUBSTANCE ABUSE
Committee on Substance Abuse
ABSTRACT. During the past three decades, the responsibility of pediatricians to their patients and their patients' families regarding the prevention of substance abuse and the diagnosis and management of problems related to substance abuse has increased. The American Academy of

Pediatrics (AAP) has highlighted the importance of such issues in a variety of ways, including its guidelines for preventive services. Nonetheless, many pediatricians remain reluctant to address this issue. The harmful consequences of tobacco, alcohol, and other drug use are a concern of medical professionals who care for infants, children, adolescents, and young adults. Thus, pediatricians should include discussion of substance abuse as a part of routine health care, starting with the prenatal visit and as a part of ongoing anticipatory guidance. Knowledge of the extent and nature of the consequences of tobacco, alcohol, and other drug use as well as the physical, psychological, and social consequences is important for pediatricians. Pediatricians should incorporate substance abuse prevention into daily practice, acquire the skills necessary to identify young people at risk for substance abuse, and provide or obtain assessment, intervention, and treatment as necessary. (1/98)

TOBACCO'S TOLL: IMPLICATIONS FOR THE PEDIATRICIAN
Committee on Substance Abuse
ABSTRACT. The disease of tobacco addiction, which is pervasive in the United States, begins in childhood and adolescence. Twenty-five percent of the population regularly uses tobacco, despite evidence that such use is the leading preventable cause of death in the United States. Tobacco use reportedly kills 2.5 times as many people each year as alcohol and drug abuse combined. According to 1998 data from the World Health Organization, there were 1.1 billion smokers worldwide and 10 000 tobacco-related deaths per day. Furthermore, in the United States, 43% of children aged 2 to 11 years are exposed to environmental tobacco smoke, which has been implicated in sudden infant death syndrome, low birth weight, asthma, middle ear disease, pneumonia, cough, and upper respiratory infection. Pediatricians play a crucial role in reducing both tobacco use (by children, adolescents, and their parents) and exposure to tobacco smoke and should rank this among their highest health prevention priorities. (4/01)

TOXIC EFFECTS OF INDOOR MOLDS
Committee on Environmental Health
ABSTRACT. This statement describes molds, their toxic properties, and their potential for causing toxic respiratory problems in infants. Guidelines for pediatricians are given to help reduce exposures to mold in homes of infants. This is a rapidly evolving area and more research is ongoing. (4/98, reaffirmed 4/02)

TRAMPOLINES AT HOME, SCHOOL, AND RECREATIONAL CENTERS
Committee on Injury and Poison Prevention and Committee on Sports Medicine and Fitness
ABSTRACT. The latest available data indicate that an estimated 83 400 trampoline-related injuries occurred in 1996 in the United States. This represents an annual rate 140% higher than was reported in 1990. Most injuries were sustained on home trampolines. In addition, 30% of trampoline-related injuries treated in an emergency department were fractures often resulting in hospitalization and surgery. These data support the American Academy of Pediatrics' reaffirmation of its recommendation that trampolines should never be used in the home environment, in routine physical education classes, or in outdoor playgrounds. Design and behavioral recommendations are made for the limited use of trampolines in supervised training programs. (5/99, reaffirmed 12/02)

THE TRANSFER OF DRUGS AND OTHER CHEMICALS INTO HUMAN MILK
Committee on Drugs
ABSTRACT. The American Academy of Pediatrics places emphasis on increasing breastfeeding in the United States. A common reason for the cessation of breastfeeding is the use of medication by the nursing mother and advice by her physician to stop nursing. Such advice may not be warranted. This statement is intended to supply the pediatrician, obstetrician, and family physician with data, if known, concerning the excretion of drugs into human milk. Most drugs likely to be prescribed to the nursing mother should have no effect on milk supply or on infant well-being. This information is important not only to protect nursing infants from untoward effects of maternal medication but also to allow effective pharmacologic treatment of breastfeeding mothers. Nicotine, psychotropic drugs, and silicone implants are 3 important topics reviewed in this statement. (9/01)

TRANSMISSIBLE SPONGIFORM ENCEPHALOPATHIES: A REVIEW FOR PEDIATRICIANS (TECHNICAL REPORT)
Committee on Infectious Diseases
ABSTRACT. Transmissible spongiform encephalopathies (TSEs) are a family of rare, slowly progressive, and universally fatal neurodegenerative syndromes affecting animals and humans. Until recently, TSEs were of little interest to pediatricians. However, since the outbreak in adolescents and the association of TSEs with new-variant Creutzfeldt-Jakob disease (nvCJD), interest among pediatricians and the general public has increased. Even before bovine spongiform encephalopathy and nvCJD were linked, the recognition that iatrogenic Creutzfeldt-Jakob disease (CJD) had been acquired from administration of cadaveric human growth and gonadotropic hormones and from corneal and dura mater transplants prompted medical vigilance. Furthermore, recent concern about the potential for transmission of CJD by blood and blood products has raised awareness among public health and regulatory agencies, pediatricians, and the public, although no epidemiologic data support this concern. Because of worldwide concern (although no cases have been reported in North America), this review focuses on the potential impact of TSEs, particularly CJD and nvCJD, on the pediatric population. (11/00, reaffirmed 1/04)

TRANSPORTING CHILDREN WITH SPECIAL HEALTH CARE NEEDS
Committee on Injury and Poison Prevention
ABSTRACT. Children with special health care needs should have access to proper resources for safe transportation. This statement reviews important considerations for transporting children with special health care needs and provides current guidelines for the protection of children with specific health care needs, including those with

a tracheostomy, a spica cast, challenging behaviors, or muscle tone abnormalities as well as those transported in wheelchairs. (10/99, reaffirmed 12/02)

TREATMENT OF THE CHILD WITH SIMPLE FEBRILE SEIZURES (TECHNICAL REPORT)
Steering Committee on Quality Improvement and Management
See summary on page 63. (6/99)

TREATMENT GUIDELINES FOR LEAD EXPOSURE IN CHILDREN
Committee on Drugs (7/95, reaffirmed 10/98, 11/01)

THE TREATMENT OF NEUROLOGICALLY IMPAIRED CHILDREN USING PATTERNING
Committee on Children With Disabilities
ABSTRACT. This statement reviews patterning as a treatment for children with neurologic impairments. This treatment is based on an outmoded and oversimplified theory of brain development. Current information does not support the claims of proponents that this treatment is efficacious, and its use continues to be unwarranted. (11/99, reaffirmed 11/02)

ULTRAVIOLET LIGHT: A HAZARD TO CHILDREN
Committee on Environmental Health (8/99, reaffirmed 10/02)

UNIVERSAL ACCESS TO GOOD-QUALITY EDUCATION AND CARE OF CHILDREN FROM BIRTH TO 5 YEARS
Committee on Early Childhood, Adoption, and Dependent Care (3/96)

URINARY TRACT INFECTIONS IN FEBRILE INFANTS AND YOUNG CHILDREN (TECHNICAL REPORT)
Steering Committee on Quality Improvement and Management
See summary on page 239. (4/99)

USE AND ABUSE OF THE APGAR SCORE
American Academy of Pediatrics Committee on Fetus and Newborn and American College of Obstetricians and Gynecologists Committee on Obstetric Practice
ABSTRACT. This is a revised statement published jointly with the American College of Obstetricians and Gynecologists that emphasizes the appropriate use of the Apgar Score. The highlights of the statement include: (1) the Apgar Score is useful in assessing the condition of the infant at birth; (2) the Apgar score alone should not be used as evidence that neurologic damage was caused by hypoxia that results in neurologic injury or from inappropriate intrapartum treatment; and (3) an infant who has had "asphyxia" proximate to delivery that is severe enough to result in acute neurologic injury should demonstrate all of the following: (a) profound metabolic or mixed acidemia (pH <7.00) on an umbilical arterial blood sample, if obtained, (b) an Apgar score of 0 to 3 for longer than 5 minutes, (c) neurologic manifestation, eg, seizure, coma, or hypotonia, and (d) evidence of multiorgan dysfunction. (7/96, reaffirmed 10/97, 10/00)

THE USE OF CHAPERONES DURING THE PHYSICAL EXAMINATION OF THE PEDIATRIC PATIENT
Committee on Practice and Ambulatory Medicine (12/96, reaffirmed 11/99, 2/00)

USE OF CODEINE- AND DEXTROMETHORPHAN-CONTAINING COUGH REMEDIES IN CHILDREN
Committee on Drugs
ABSTRACT. Numerous prescription and nonprescription medications are currently available for suppression of cough, a common symptom in children. Because adverse effects and overdosage associated with the administration of cough and cold preparations in children have been reported, education of patients and parents about the lack of proven antitussive effects and the potential risks of these products is needed. (6/97, reaffirmed 5/00, 6/03)

USE OF INHALED NITRIC OXIDE
Committee on Fetus and Newborn
ABSTRACT. Approval of inhaled nitric oxide by the US Food and Drug Administration for hypoxic respiratory failure of the term and near-term newborn provides an important new therapy for this serious condition. This statement addresses the conditions under which inhaled nitric oxide should be administered to the neonate with hypoxic respiratory failure. (8/00, reaffirmed 4/03)

THE USE AND MISUSE OF FRUIT JUICE IN PEDIATRICS
Committee on Nutrition
ABSTRACT. Historically, fruit juice was recommended by pediatricians as a source of vitamin C and an extra source of water for healthy infants and young children as their diets expanded to include solid foods with higher renal solute. Fruit juice is marketed as a healthy, natural source of vitamins and, in some instances, calcium. Because juice tastes good, children readily accept it. Although juice consumption has some benefits, it also has potential detrimental effects. Pediatricians need to be knowledgeable about juice to inform parents and patients on its appropriate uses. (5/01)

USE OF PHOTOSCREENING FOR CHILDREN'S VISION SCREENING
Committee on Practice and Ambulatory Medicine and Section on Ophthalmology
ABSTRACT. This statement asserts that all children should be screened for risk factors associated with amblyopia. Guidelines are suggested for the use of photoscreening as a technique for the detection of amblyopia and strabismus in children of various age groups. The American Academy of Pediatrics favors additional research of the efficacy and cost-effectiveness of photoscreening as a vision screening tool. (3/02)

USE OF PSYCHOACTIVE MEDICATION DURING PREGNANCY AND POSSIBLE EFFECTS ON THE FETUS AND NEWBORN
Committee on Drugs
ABSTRACT. Psychoactive drugs are those psychotherapeutic drugs used to modify emotions and behavior in the treatment of psychiatric illnesses. This statement will limit its scope to drug selection guidelines for those psychoac-

tive agents used during pregnancy for prevention or treatment of the following common psychiatric disorders: schizophrenia, major depression, bipolar disorder, panic disorder, and obsessive-compulsive disorder. The statement assumes that pharmacologic therapy is needed to manage the psychiatric disorder. This decision requires thoughtful psychiatric and obstetric advice. (4/00, reaffirmed 4/03)

USES OF DRUGS NOT DESCRIBED IN THE PACKAGE INSERT (OFF-LABEL USES)
Committee on Drugs
ABSTRACT. New regulatory initiatives have been designed to ensure that new drugs and biologicals include adequate pediatric labeling for the claimed indications at the time of, or soon after, approval. However, because such labeling may not immediately be available, off-label use (or use that is not included in the approved label) of therapeutic agents is likely to remain common in the practice of pediatrics. This policy statement was written to address questions practitioners have regarding off-label use. The purpose of off-label use is to benefit the individual patient. Practitioners may use their professional judgment to determine these uses. Practitioners should understand that the Food and Drug Administration does not regulate off-label use. (7/02)

VARICELLA VACCINE UPDATE
Committee on Infectious Diseases
ABSTRACT. Recommendations for routine varicella vaccination were published by the American Academy of Pediatrics in May 1995, but many eligible children remain unimmunized. This update provides additional information on the varicella disease burden before the availability of varicella vaccine, potential barriers to immunization, efforts to increase the level of coverage, new safety data, and new recommendations for use of the varicella vaccine after exposure and in children with human immunodeficiency virus infections. Pediatricians are strongly encouraged to support public health officials in the development and implementation of varicella immunization requirements for child care and school entry. (1/00)

WHEN INFLICTED SKIN INJURIES CONSTITUTE CHILD ABUSE
Committee on Child Abuse and Neglect
ABSTRACT. Child abuse should be considered as the most likely explanation for inflicted skin injuries if they are nonaccidental and there is any injury beyond temporary reddening of the skin. Minor forms of abuse may lead to severe abuse unless abusive skin injuries are identified and labeled as such and interventions are made. (9/02)

WIC PROGRAM
Provisional Section on Breastfeeding
ABSTRACT. This policy statement highlights the important collaboration between pediatricians and local Special Supplemental Nutrition Program for Women, Infants, and Children (WIC) programs to ensure that infants and children receive high-quality, cost-effective health care and nutrition services. Specific recommendations are provided for pediatricians and WIC personnel to help children and their families receive optimum services through a medical home. (11/01)

SECTION 5

Endorsed Policies

· ·

*The American Academy of Pediatrics endorses
and accepts as its policy the following
documents from other organizations*

AMERICAN ACADEMY OF PEDIATRICS

Endorsed Policies

CONCUSSION IN SPORTS
American Orthopaedic Society for Sports Medicine (1999)

DIAGNOSIS, TREATMENT, AND LONG-TERM MANAGE-MENT OF KAWASAKI DISEASE: A STATEMENT FOR HEALTH PROFESSIONALS (CLINICAL REPORT)
American Heart Association (12/04)

FOSTER CARE MENTAL HEALTH VALUES
American Academy of Child and Adolescent Psychiatry and the Child Welfare League of America (2002)

GIFTS TO PHYSICIANS FROM INDUSTRY
American Medical Association (8/01)

GUIDELINES FOR REFERRAL OF CHILDREN AND ADOLESCENTS TO PEDIATRIC RHEUMATOLOGISTS
American College of Rheumatology (6/02)

HELPING THE STUDENT WITH DIABETES SUCCEED: A GUIDE FOR SCHOOL PERSONNEL
National Diabetes Education Program (6/03)

IDENTIFYING AND RESPONDING TO DOMESTIC VIOLENCE: CONSENSUS RECOMMENDATIONS FOR CHILD AND ADOLESCENT HEALTH
Family Violence Prevention Fund (9/02)

LIGHTNING SAFETY FOR ATHLETICS AND RECREATION (POSITION STATEMENT)
National Athletic Trainers' Association
ABSTRACT. *Objective:* To educate athletic trainers and others about the dangers of lightning, provide lightning-safety guidelines, define safe structures and locations, and advocate prehospital care for lightning-strike victims.

Background: Lightning may be the most frequently encountered severe-storm hazard endangering physically active people each year. Millions of lightning flashes strike the ground annually in the United States, causing nearly 100 deaths and 400 injuries. Three quarters of all lightning casualties occur between May and September, and nearly four fifths occur between 10:00 AM and 7:00 PM, which coincides with the hours for most athletic or recreational activities. Additionally, lightning casualties from sports and recreational activities have risen alarmingly in recent decades.

Recommendations: The National Athletic Trainers' Association recommends a proactive approach to lightning safety, including the implementation of a lightning-safety policy that identifies safe locations for shelter from the lightning hazard. Further components of this policy are monitoring local weather forecasts, designating a weather watcher, and establishing a chain of command. Additionally, a flash-to-bang count of 30 seconds or more should be used as a minimal determinant of when to suspend activities. Waiting 30 minutes or longer after the last flash of lightning or sound of thunder is recommended before athletic or recreational activities are resumed. Lightning safety strategies include avoiding shelter under trees, avoiding open fields and spaces, and suspending the use of land-line telephones during thunderstorms. Also outlined in this document are the prehospital care guidelines for triaging and treating lightning-strike victims. It is important to evaluate victims quickly for apnea, asystole, hypothermia, shock, fractures, and burns. Cardiopulmonary resuscitation is effective in resuscitating pulseless victims of lightning strike. Maintenance of cardiopulmonary resuscitation and first-aid certification should be required of all persons involved in sports and recreational activities. (12/00)

MENTAL HEALTH AND SUBSTANCE USE SCREENING AND ASSESSMENT OF CHILDREN IN FOSTER CARE
American Academy of Child and Adolescent Psychiatry and the Child Welfare League of America (2003)

PEDIATRIC CARE IN THE EMERGENCY DEPARTMENT
Society for Academic Emergency Medicine
ABSTRACT. Physicians who have successfully completed an accredited Emergency Medicine residency and are certified in emergency medicine by the American Board of Emergency Medicine (ABEM) or the American Osteopathic Board of Emergency Medicine (AOBEM) ABEM/AOBEM or those who are certified in pediatric emergency medicine by ABEM or the American Board of Pediatrics (ABP) possess the knowledge and skills required to provide quality emergency medical care to children of all ages for a wide variety of illnesses, injuries or poisonings. To provide quality care, the emergency physician must have all necessary and age-appropriate medical equipment readily available. The emergency physician must also have access via consultation, admission, or transfer, to appropriate specialty and sub-specialty physicians, to who will provide any needed patient care after emergency department treatment. Physically separated care areas for children are not mandatory in order to provide high-quality care to patients of all ages. Although physically separate care areas for children are ideal, they are not mandatory to provide high-quality care. (11/03)

PRINCIPLES AND GUIDELINES FOR EARLY HEARING DETECTION AND INTERVENTION PROGRAMS (YEAR 2000 POSITION STATEMENT)
Joint Committee on Infant Hearing (10/00)

RESPONSE TO CARDIAC ARREST AND SELECTED LIFE-THREATENING MEDICAL EMERGENCIES: THE MEDICAL EMERGENCY RESPONSE PLAN FOR SCHOOLS. A STATEMENT FOR HEALTHCARE PROVIDERS, POLICYMAKERS, SCHOOL ADMINISTRATORS, AND COMMUNITY LEADERS
American Heart Association (1/04)

TARGETED TUBERCULIN TESTING AND TREATMENT OF LATENT TUBERCULOSIS INFECTION
American Thoracic Society and Centers for Disease Control and Prevention (4/00) (The AAP endorses and accepts as its policy the sections of this statement as they relate to infants and children.)

TYPE 2 DIABETES IN CHILDREN AND ADOLESCENTS
American Diabetes Association (3/00)

Policies by Committee

AMERICAN ACADEMY OF PEDIATRICS

Policies by Committee

CHILD AND ADOLESCENT HEALTH ACTION GROUP (FORMERLY COUNCIL ON CHILD AND ADOLESCENT HEALTH)

Age Limits of Pediatrics, 5/88, reaffirmed 9/92, 1/97, 3/02

The Role of Home-Visitation Programs in Improving Health Outcomes for Children and Families, 3/98, reaffirmed 5/01

COMMITTEE ON ADOLESCENCE

Adolescent Pregnancy—Current Trends and Issues: 1998, 2/99

The Adolescent's Right to Confidential Care When Considering Abortion, 5/96, reaffirmed 5/99, 11/02

Adolescents and Human Immunodeficiency Virus Infection: The Role of the Pediatrician in Prevention and Intervention (joint with Committee on Pediatric AIDS), 1/01, reaffirmed 10/03

Care of Adolescent Parents and Their Children (joint with Committee on Early Childhood, Adoption, and Dependent Care), 2/01

Care of the Adolescent Sexual Assault Victim, 6/01

Condom Use by Adolescents, 6/01, reaffirmed 5/04

Confidentiality in Adolescent Health Care, 4/89, reaffirmed 1/93, 11/97, 5/00, 5/04

Contraception and Adolescents, 11/99

Counseling the Adolescent About Pregnancy Options, 5/98, reaffirmed 1/01

Health Care for Children and Adolescents in the Juvenile Correctional Care System, 4/01

Identifying and Treating Eating Disorders, 1/03

Legalization of Marijuana: Potential Impact on Youth (joint with Committee on Substance Abuse), 6/04

Legalization of Marijuana: Potential Impact on Youth (Technical Report) (joint with Committee on Substance Abuse), 6/04

Sexual Orientation and Adolescents (Clinical Report), 6/04

Sexuality Education for Children and Adolescents (joint with Committee on Psychosocial Aspects of Child and Family Health), 8/01, reaffirmed 5/04

Suicide and Suicide Attempts in Adolescents, 4/00

The Teenage Driver (joint with Committee on Injury and Poison Prevention), 11/96, reaffirmed 11/99

COMMITTEE ON BIOETHICS

Appropriate Boundaries in the Pediatrician-Family-Patient Relationship, 8/99, reaffirmed 11/02

Do Not Resuscitate Orders in Schools (joint with Committee on School Health), 4/00, reaffirmed 6/03

Do-Not-Resuscitate Orders for Pediatric Patients Who Require Anesthesia and Surgery (Clinical Report) (joint with Section on Surgery and Section on Anesthesia and Pain Medicine), 12/04

Ethical Issues With Genetic Testing in Pediatrics, 6/01, reaffirmed 4/04

Ethics and the Care of Critically Ill Infants and Children, 7/96, reaffirmed 10/99, 6/03

Female Genital Mutilation, 7/98, reaffirmed 11/02

Fetal Therapy—Ethical Considerations, 5/99, reaffirmed 11/02

Forgoing Life-Sustaining Medical Treatment in Abused Children (joint with Committee on Child Abuse and Neglect), 11/00, reaffirmed 6/03

Guidelines on Forgoing Life-Sustaining Medical Treatment, 3/94, reaffirmed 11/97, 10/00, 1/04

Human Embryo Research (joint with Committee on Pediatric Research), 9/01, reaffirmed 4/04

Infants With Anencephaly as Organ Sources: Ethical Considerations, 6/92, reaffirmed 11/95, 11/98, 11/02

Informed Consent, Parental Permission, and Assent in Pediatric Practice, 2/95, reaffirmed 11/98, 11/02

Institutional Ethics Committees, 1/01, reaffirmed 1/04

Palliative Care for Children (joint with Committee on Hospital Care), 8/00, reaffirmed 6/03

Religious Objections to Medical Care, 2/97, reaffirmed 10/00, 6/03

Sterilization of Minors With Developmental Disabilities, 8/99, reaffirmed 11/02

COMMITTEE ON CHILD ABUSE AND NEGLECT

Assessment of Maltreatment of Children With Disabilities (joint with Committee on Children With Disabilities), 8/01

Distinguishing Sudden Infant Death Syndrome From Child Abuse Fatalities, 2/01

Distinguishing Sudden Infant Death Syndrome From Child Abuse Fatalities (Addendum), 9/01

Forgoing Life-Sustaining Medical Treatment in Abused Children (joint with Committee on Bioethics), 11/00, reaffirmed 6/03

Guidelines for the Evaluation of Sexual Abuse of Children: Subject Review (Clinical Report), 1/99

Investigation and Review of Unexpected Infant and Child Deaths (joint with Committee on Community Health Services), 11/99, reaffirmed 10/02

Medical Necessity for the Hospitalization of the Abused and Neglected Child (joint with Committee on Hospital Care), 4/98, reaffirmed 10/01, 8/04

Oral and Dental Aspects of Child Abuse and Neglect (joint with American Academy of Pediatric Dentistry), 8/99

The Psychological Maltreatment of Children (Technical Report), 4/02, *Pediatrics electronic pages* (pediatrics.aappublications.org/cgi/reprint/109/4/e68)

Public Disclosure of Private Information About Victims of Abuse, 2/91, reaffirmed 5/94, 9/00

The Role of the Pediatrician in Recognizing and Intervening on Behalf of Abused Women, 6/98, reaffirmed 10/01, 5/04

Shaken Baby Syndrome: Rotational Cranial Injuries (Technical Report), 7/01

When Inflicted Skin Injuries Constitute Child Abuse, 9/02

COMMITTEE ON CHILD HEALTH FINANCING

Guiding Principles for Managed Care Arrangements for the Health Care of Newborns, Infants, Children, Adolescents, and Young Adults, 1/00

Implementation Principles and Strategies for the State Children's Health Insurance Program, 5/01

Improving Substance Abuse Prevention, Assessment, and Treatment Financing for Children and Adolescents (joint with Committee on Substance Abuse), 10/01

Medicaid Policy Statement, 8/99

Principles of Child Health Care Financing, 10/03

Scope of Health Care Benefits for Newborns, Infants, Children, Adolescents, and Young Adults Through Age 21 Years, 12/97

COMMITTEE ON CHILDREN WITH DISABILITIES

Assessment of Maltreatment of Children With Disabilities (joint with Committee on Child Abuse and Neglect), 8/01

Auditory Integration Training and Facilitated Communication for Autism, 8/98, reaffirmed 5/02

Care Coordination: Integrating Health and Related Systems of Care for Children With Special Health Care Needs, 10/99

The Continued Importance of Supplemental Security Income (SSI) for Children and Adolescents With Disabilities, 4/01

Counseling Families Who Choose Complementary and Alternative Medicine for Their Child With Chronic Illness or Disability, 3/01

Developmental Surveillance and Screening of Infants and Young Children, 7/01

Fetal Alcohol Syndrome and Alcohol-Related Neurodevelopmental Disorders (joint with Committee on Substance Abuse), 8/00

Guidelines for Home Care of Infants, Children, and Adolescents With Chronic Disease, 7/95, reaffirmed 4/00

Learning Disabilities, Dyslexia, and Vision: A Subject Review (Clinical Report) (joint with American Academy of Ophthalmology and American Association for Pediatric Ophthalmology and Strabismus), 11/98, reaffirmed 5/02

Managed Care and Children With Special Health Care Needs (Clinical Report), 12/04

The Pediatrician's Role in Development and Implementation of an Individual Education Plan (IEP) and/or an Individual Family Service Plan (IFSP), 7/99, reaffirmed 11/02

The Pediatrician's Role in the Diagnosis and Management of Autistic Spectrum Disorder in Children, 5/01

The Pediatrician's Role in the Diagnosis and Management of Autistic Spectrum Disorder in Children (Technical Report), 5/01, *Pediatrics electronic pages* (pediatrics.aappublications.org/cgi/content/full/107/5/e85)

Prescribing Therapy Services for Children With Motor Disabilities (Clinical Report), 6/04

Providing a Primary Care Medical Home for Children and Youth With Cerebral Palsy (Clinical Report), 10/04

Provision of Educationally-Related Services for Children and Adolescents With Chronic Diseases and Disabling Conditions, 2/00

Psychosocial Risks of Chronic Health Conditions in Childhood and Adolescence (joint with Committee on Psychosocial Aspects of Child and Family Health), 12/93, reaffirmed 10/96

Role of the Pediatrician in Family-Centered Early Intervention Services, 5/01

The Role of the Pediatrician in Implementing the Americans With Disabilities Act: Subject Review (Clinical Report), 7/96, reaffirmed 10/00, 1/04

The Role of the Pediatrician in Transitioning Children and Adolescents With Developmental Disabilities and Chronic Illnesses From School to Work or College, 10/00, reaffirmed 1/04

Sexuality Education of Children and Adolescents With Developmental Disabilities, 2/96, reaffirmed 4/00

The Treatment of Neurologically Impaired Children Using Patterning, 11/99, reaffirmed 11/02

STEERING COMMITTEE ON CLINICAL INFORMATION TECHNOLOGY (FORMERLY SECTION ON COMPUTERS AND OTHER TECHNOLOGIES AND TASK FORCE ON MEDICAL INFORMATICS)

E-mail Communication Between Pediatricians and Their Patients (Clinical Report), 7/04

Privacy Protection of Health Information: Patient Rights and Pediatrician Responsibilities (joint with Pediatric Practice Action Group), 10/99

Special Requirements for Electronic Medical Record Systems in Pediatrics, 8/01

Telemedicine: Pediatric Applications (Technical Report) (joint with Committee on Medical Liability), 6/04

COMMITTEE ON CODING AND NOMENCLATURE (FORMERLY COMMITTEE ON CODING AND REIMBURSEMENT)

Application of the Resource-Based Relative Value Scale System to Pediatrics, 5/04

COMMITTEE ON COMMUNICATIONS (FORMERLY COMMITTEE ON PUBLIC EDUCATION)

Children, Adolescents, and Advertising, 2/95

Children, Adolescents, and Television, 2/01

Impact of Music Lyrics and Music Videos on Children and Youth, 12/96

Media Education, 8/99

Media Violence, 11/01

Sexuality, Contraception, and the Media, 1/01

COMMITTEE ON COMMUNITY HEALTH SERVICES

Ethical Considerations in Research With Socially Identifiable Populations (joint with Committee on Native American Child Health), 1/04

Increasing Immunization Coverage (joint with Committee on Practice and Ambulatory Medicine), 10/03

Investigation and Review of Unexpected Infant and Child Deaths (joint with Committee on Child Abuse and Neglect), 11/99, reaffirmed 10/02

The Pediatrician's Role in Community Pediatrics, 6/99

Prevention of Agricultural Injuries Among Children and Adolescents (joint with Committee on Injury and Poison Prevention), 10/01

COMMITTEE ON DRUGS

Acetaminophen Toxicity in Children, 10/01

Alternative Routes of Drug Administration—Advantages and Disadvantages (Subject Review) (Clinical Report), 7/97, reaffirmed 10/00, 11/03

Camphor Revisited: Focus on Toxicity, 7/94, reaffirmed 6/97, 5/00

Clioquinol (Iodochlorydroxyquin, Vioform) and Iodoquinol (Diiodohydroxyquin): Blindness and Neuropathy, 11/90, reaffirmed 2/94, 2/97, 2/00, 4/03

Drugs for Pediatric Emergencies, 1/98, *Pediatrics electronic pages* (pediatrics.aappublications.org/cgi/reprint/101/1/e13)

Generic Prescribing, Generic Substitution, and Therapeutic Substitution, 5/87, reaffirmed 6/93, 5/96, 6/99, 5/01

Guidelines for the Ethical Conduct of Studies to Evaluate Drugs in Pediatric Populations, 2/95, reaffirmed 3/98, 5/01

Guidelines for Monitoring and Management of Pediatric Patients During and After Sedation for Diagnostic and Therapeutic Procedures, 6/92, reaffirmed 6/95, 6/98, 5/02

Guidelines for Monitoring and Management of Pediatric Patients During and After Sedation for Diagnostic and Therapeutic Procedures: Addendum, 10/02

Neonatal Drug Withdrawal, 6/98, reaffirmed 5/01

Precautions Concerning the Use of Theophylline, 4/92, reaffirmed 6/95, 6/98, 5/01

Precautions Regarding the Use of Aerosolized Antibiotics (Technical Report) (joint with Committee on Infectious Diseases), 12/00, reaffirmed 1/04, *Pediatrics electronic pages* (pediatrics.aappublications.org/cgi/reprint/106/6/e89)

Prevention and Management of Pain and Stress in the Neonate (joint with American Academy of Pediatrics Committee on Fetus and Newborn, Section on Anesthesiology and Pain Medicine, and Section on Surgery and Canadian Paediatric Society), 2/00, reaffirmed 4/03

Prevention of Medication Errors in the Pediatric Inpatient Setting (joint with Committee on Hospital Care), 8/03

Reappraisal of Lytic Cocktail/Demerol, Phenergan, and Thorazine (DPT) for the Sedation of Children, 4/95, reaffirmed 3/98, 5/01

Retinoid Therapy for Severe Dermatological Disorders, 7/92, reaffirmed 6/95, 6/98

The Transfer of Drugs and Other Chemicals Into Human Milk, 9/01

Treatment Guidelines for Lead Exposure in Children, 7/95, reaffirmed 10/98, 11/01

Use of Codeine- and Dextromethorphan-Containing Cough Remedies in Children, 6/97, reaffirmed 5/00, 6/03

Use of Psychoactive Medication During Pregnancy and Possible Effects on the Fetus and Newborn, 4/00, reaffirmed 4/03

Uses of Drugs Not Described in the Package Insert (Off-Label Uses), 7/02

COMMITTEE ON EARLY CHILDHOOD, ADOPTION, AND DEPENDENT CARE

Care of Adolescent Parents and Their Children (joint with Committee on Adolescence), 2/01

Developmental Issues for Young Children in Foster Care, 11/00

Families and Adoption: The Pediatrician's Role in Supporting Communication (Clinical Report), 12/03

Health Care of Young Children in Foster Care, 3/02

The Inappropriate Use of School "Readiness" Tests (joint with Committee on School Health), 3/95, reaffirmed 4/98, 1/04

Initial Medical Evaluation of an Adopted Child, 9/91

Parental Leave for Residents and Pediatric Training Programs (joint with Section on Residents), 11/95, reaffirmed 4/98

The Pediatrician's Role in Family Support Programs, 1/01

Selecting Appropriate Toys for Young Children: The Pediatrician's Role (Clinical Report), 4/03

Universal Access to Good-quality Education and Care of Children From Birth to 5 Years, 3/96

COMMITTEE ON ENVIRONMENTAL HEALTH

Ambient Air Pollution: Health Hazards to Children, 12/04

Chemical-Biological Terrorism and Its Impact on Children: A Subject Review (Clinical Report) (joint with Committee on Infectious Diseases), 3/00

Environmental Tobacco Smoke: A Hazard to Children, 4/97, reaffirmed 10/00

The Hazards of Child Labor, 2/95, reaffirmed 11/98

Mercury in the Environment: Implications for Pediatricians (Technical Report), 7/01

Noise: A Hazard for the Fetus and Newborn, 10/97, reaffirmed 10/00

Nontherapeutic Use of Antimicrobial Agents in Animal Agriculture: Implications for Pediatrics (Technical Report) (joint with Committee on Infectious Diseases), 9/04

Pediatric Exposure and Potential Toxicity of Phthalate Plasticizers (Technical Report), 6/03

Radiation Disasters and Children, 6/03

Screening for Elevated Blood Lead Levels, 6/98

Toxic Effects of Indoor Molds, 4/98, reaffirmed 4/02

Ultraviolet Light: A Hazard to Children, 8/99, reaffirmed 10/02

COMMITTEE ON FETUS AND NEWBORN

Advanced Practice in Neonatal Nursing, 6/03

Age Terminology During the Perinatal Period, 11/04

Apnea, Sudden Infant Death Syndrome, and Home Monitoring, 4/03

Controversies Concerning Vitamin K and the Newborn, 7/03

Hospital Discharge of the High-Risk Neonate— Proposed Guidelines, 8/98, reaffirmed 6/01

Hospital Stay for Healthy Term Newborns, 5/04

Human Immunodeficiency Virus Screening (joint with American Academy of Pediatrics Committee on Pediatric AIDS and American College of Obstetricians and Gynecologists), 7/99, reaffirmed 6/02

The Initiation or Withdrawal of Treatment for High-Risk Newborns, 8/95, reaffirmed 10/98, 6/01

Levels of Neonatal Care, 11/04

Perinatal Care at the Threshold of Viability (Clinical Report), 11/02

Postnatal Corticosteroids to Treat or Prevent Chronic Lung Disease in Preterm Infants (joint with Canadian Paediatric Society), 2/02

Prevention and Management of Pain and Stress in the Neonate (joint with American Academy of Pediatrics Committee on Drugs, Section on Anesthesiology and Pain Medicine, and Section on Surgery and Canadian Paediatric Society), 2/00, reaffirmed 4/03

Revised Indications for the Use of Palivizumab and Respiratory Syncytial Virus Immune Globulin Intravenous for the Prevention of Respiratory Syncytial Virus Infections (joint with Committee on Infectious Diseases), 12/03

Revised Indications for the Use of Palivizumab and Respiratory Syncytial Virus Immune Globulin Intravenous for the Prevention of Respiratory Syncytial Virus Infections (Technical Report) (joint with Committee on Infectious Diseases), 12/03

The Role of the Primary Care Pediatrician in the Management of High-risk Newborn Infants (joint with Committee on Practice and Ambulatory Medicine), 10/96

Safe Transportation of Premature and Low Birth Weight Infants (joint with Committee on Injury and Poison Prevention), 5/96, reaffirmed 4/99

Surfactant Replacement Therapy for Respiratory Distress Syndrome, 3/99

Use and Abuse of the Apgar Score (joint with American College of Obstetricians and Gynecologists), 7/96, reaffirmed 10/97, 10/00

Use of Inhaled Nitric Oxide, 8/00, reaffirmed 4/03

COMMITTEE ON GENETICS

Congenital Adrenal Hyperplasia (Technical Report) (joint with Section on Endocrinology), 12/00, reaffirmed 12/03

Evaluation of the Newborn With Developmental Anomalies of the External Genitalia (joint with Section on Endocrinology and Section on Urology), 7/00

Folic Acid for the Prevention of Neural Tube Defects, 8/99, reaffirmed 11/02

Health Care Supervision for Children With Williams Syndrome, 5/01

Health Supervision for Children With Achondroplasia, 3/95, reaffirmed 10/98

Health Supervision for Children With Down Syndrome, 2/01

Health Supervision for Children With Fragile X Syndrome, 8/96, reaffirmed 10/99

Health Supervision for Children With Marfan Syndrome, 11/96, reaffirmed 10/99, 11/02

Health Supervision for Children With Neurofibromatosis, 8/95, reaffirmed 10/98

Health Supervision for Children With Sickle Cell Disease (joint with Section on Hematology/Oncology), 3/02

Health Supervision for Children With Turner Syndrome (Clinical Report) (joint with Section on Endocrinology), 3/03

Maternal Phenylketonuria, 2/01

Molecular Genetic Testing in Pediatric Practice: A Subject Review (Clinical Report), 12/00

Newborn Screening for Congenital Hypothyroidism: Recommended Guidelines (joint with American Academy of Pediatrics Section on Endocrinology and American Thyroid Association Committee on Public Health), 6/93, reaffirmed 10/96, 10/99

Newborn Screening Fact Sheets, 9/96, reaffirmed 10/99

Prenatal Genetic Diagnosis for Pediatricians, 6/94, reaffirmed 10/97

Prenatal Screening and Diagnosis for Pediatricians (Clinical Report), 9/04

COMMITTEE ON HOSPITAL CARE

Admission and Discharge Guidelines for the Pediatric Patient Requiring Intermediate Care (Clinical Report) (joint with American Academy of Pediatrics Section on Critical Care and Society of Critical Care Medicine), 5/04

Child Life Services, 11/00

Facilities and Equipment for the Care of Pediatric Patients in a Community Hospital (Clinical Report), 5/03

Family-Centered Care and the Pediatrician's Role (joint with Institute for Family-Centered Care), 9/03

Guidelines for Developing Admission and Discharge Policies for the Pediatric Intensive Care Unit (joint with American Academy of Pediatrics Section on Critical Care and Society of Critical Care Medicine), 4/99

Guidelines and Levels of Care for Pediatric Intensive Care Units (Clinical Report) (joint with American Academy of Pediatrics Section on Critical Care and Society of Critical Care Medicine), 10/04

Medical Necessity for the Hospitalization of the Abused and Neglected Child (joint with Committee on Child Abuse and Neglect), 4/98, reaffirmed 5/01, 5/04

Medical Staff Appointment and Delineation of Pediatric Privileges in Hospitals (Clinical Report), 8/02

Palliative Care for Children (joint with Committee on Bioethics), 8/00, reaffirmed 6/03

Pediatric Organ Donation and Transplantation (joint with Section on Surgery), 5/02

Physicians' Roles in Coordinating Care of Hospitalized Children (Clinical Report), 3/03

Precertification Process, 8/00

Prevention of Medication Errors in the Pediatric Inpatient Setting (joint with Committee on Drugs), 8/03

The Role of the Nurse Practitioner and Physician Assistant in the Care of Hospitalized Children, 5/99, reaffirmed 11/01

COMMITTEE ON INFECTIOUS DISEASES

Age for Routine Administration of the Second Dose of Measles-Mumps-Rubella Vaccine, 1/98, reaffirmed 8/04

Chemical-Biological Terrorism and Its Impact on Children: A Subject Review (Clinical Report) (joint with Committee on Environmental Health), 3/00

Combination Vaccines for Childhood Immunization: Recommendations of the Advisory Committee on Immunization Practices (ACIP), the American Academy of Pediatrics (AAP), and the American Academy of Family Physicians (AAFP) (joint with Advisory Committee on Immunization Practices and American Academy of Family Physicians), 5/99, reaffirmed 3/02

Head Lice (Clinical Report) (joint with Committee on School Health), 9/02

Immunization of Preterm and Low Birth Weight Infants (Clinical Report), 7/03

Infection Control in Physicians' Offices (joint with Committee on Practice and Ambulatory Medicine), 6/00

Issues Related to Human Immunodeficiency Virus Transmission in Schools, Child Care, Medical Settings, the Home, and Community (joint with Committee on Pediatric AIDS), 8/99, reaffirmed 2/02

Measles Immunization in HIV-Infected Children (joint with Committee on Pediatric AIDS), 5/99, reaffirmed 10/01

Meningococcal Disease Prevention and Control Strategies for Practice-Based Physicians (Addendum: Recommendations for College Students), 12/00, reaffirmed 10/01

Nontherapeutic Use of Antimicrobial Agents in Animal Agriculture: Implications for Pediatrics (Technical Report) (joint with Committee on Environmental Health), 9/04

Precautions Regarding the Use of Aerosolized Antibiotics (Technical Report) (joint with Committee on Drugs), 12/00, reaffirmed 1/04, *Pediatrics electronic pages* (pediatrics.aappublications.org/cgi/reprint/106/6/e89)

Recommendations for Influenza Immunization of Children, 5/04

Recommendations for the Use of Live Attenuated Varicella Vaccine, 5/95, reaffirmed 6/98

Recommended Childhood and Adolescent Immunization Schedule—United States, July–December 2004, 5/04

Reduction of the Influenza Burden in Children (Technical Report), 12/02, *Pediatrics electronic pages* (pediatrics.aappublications.org/cgi/content/full/110/6/e80)

Revised Indications for the Use of Palivizumab and Respiratory Syncytial Virus Immune Globulin Intravenous for the Prevention of Respiratory Syncytial Virus Infections (joint with Committee on Fetus and Newborn), 12/03

Revised Indications for the Use of Palivizumab and Respiratory Syncytial Virus Immune Globulin Intravenous for the Prevention of Respiratory Syncytial Virus Infections (Technical Report) (joint with Committee on Fetus and Newborn), 12/03

Smallpox Vaccine, 10/02

Therapy for Children With Invasive Pneumococcal Infections, 2/97, reaffirmed 10/99, 1/04

Transmissible Spongiform Encephalopathies: A Review for Pediatricians (Technical Report), 11/00, reaffirmed 1/04

Varicella Vaccine Update, 1/00

COMMITTEE ON INJURY, VIOLENCE, AND POISON PREVENTION

All-Terrain Vehicle Injury Prevention: Two-, Three-, and Four-Wheeled Unlicensed Motor Vehicles, 6/00, reaffirmed 5/04

Bicycle Helmets, 10/01, reaffirmed 11/04

Children in Pickup Trucks, 10/00, reaffirmed 5/04

Falls From Heights: Windows, Roofs, and Balconies, 5/01, reaffirmed 5/04

Firearm-Related Injuries Affecting the Pediatric Population, 4/00, reaffirmed 5/04

Fireworks-Related Injuries to Children, 7/01, reaffirmed 11/04

The Hospital Record of the Injured Child and the Need for External Cause-of-Injury Codes, 2/99, reaffirmed 5/02

Injuries Associated With Infant Walkers, 9/01, reaffirmed 11/04

Injury Risk of Nonpowder Guns (Technical Report), 11/04

In-line Skating Injuries in Children and Adolescents (joint with Committee on Sports Medicine and Fitness), 4/98, reaffirmed 1/02

Lawn Mower-Related Injuries to Children, 6/01, reaffirmed 5/04

Lawn Mower-Related Injuries to Children (Technical Report), 6/01, reaffirmed 5/04, *Pediatrics electronic pages* (pediatrics.aappublications.org/cgi/content/full/107/6/e106)

Office-Based Counseling for Injury Prevention, 10/94, reaffirmed 10/98

Personal Watercraft Use by Children and Adolescents, 2/00, reaffirmed 5/04

Poison Treatment in the Home, 11/03

Prevention of Agricultural Injuries Among Children and Adolescents (joint with Committee on Community Health Services), 10/01

Prevention of Drowning in Infants, Children, and Adolescents, 8/03

Prevention of Drowning in Infants, Children, and Adolescents (Technical Report), 8/03

The Prevention of Unintentional Injury Among American Indian and Alaska Native Children: A Subject Review (Clinical Report) (joint with Committee on Native American Child Health), 12/99, reaffirmed 12/02

Reducing the Number of Deaths and Injuries From Residential Fires, 6/00

Restraint Use on Aircraft, 11/01

Safe Transportation of Newborns at Hospital Discharge, 10/99, reaffirmed 12/02

Safe Transportation of Premature and Low Birth Weight Infants (joint with Committee on Fetus and Newborn), 5/96, reaffirmed 4/99

School Bus Transportation of Children With Special Health Care Needs, 8/01, reaffirmed 11/04

School Transportation Safety (joint with Committee on School Health), 5/96, reaffirmed 4/99

Selecting and Using the Most Appropriate Car Safety Seats for Growing Children: Guidelines for Counseling Parents, 3/02

Skateboard and Scooter Injuries, 3/02

Snowmobiling Hazards, 11/00, reaffirmed 5/04

Swimming Programs for Infants and Toddlers (joint with Committee on Sports Medicine and Fitness), 4/00, reaffirmed 5/04

The Teenage Driver (joint with Committee on Adolescence), 11/96, reaffirmed 11/99

Trampolines at Home, School, and Recreational Centers (joint with Committee on Sports Medicine and Fitness), 5/99, reaffirmed 12/02

Transporting Children With Special Health Care Needs, 10/99, reaffirmed 12/02

COMMITTEE ON MEDICAL LIABILITY

Alternative Dispute Resolution in Medical Malpractice (Technical Report), 3/01

Consent by Proxy for Nonurgent Pediatric Care (Clinical Report), 11/03

Dealing With the Parent Whose Judgment Is Impaired by Alcohol or Drugs: Legal and Ethical Considerations (Clinical Report), 9/04

Guidelines for Expert Witness Testimony in Medical Malpractice Litigation, 5/02

Pediatric Physician Profiling (joint with Committee on Practice and Ambulatory Medicine), 10/99

Pediatricians' Liability During Disasters (joint with Committee on Pediatric Emergency Medicine), 12/00, reaffirmed 1/04

Professional Liability Coverage for Residents and Fellows, 9/00

Telemedicine: Pediatric Applications (Technical Report) (joint with Steering Committee on Clinical Information Technology), 6/04

COMMITTEE ON NATIVE AMERICAN CHILD HEALTH

Ethical Considerations in Research With Socially Identifiable Populations (joint with Committee on Community Health Services), 1/04

Inhalant Abuse (joint with Committee on Substance Abuse), 3/96, reaffirmed 5/99

Prevention and Treatment of Type 2 Diabetes Mellitus in Children, With Special Emphasis on American Indian and Alaska Native Children (Clinical Report) (joint with Section on Endocrinology), 10/03, *Pediatrics electronic pages* (pediatrics.aappublications.org/cgi/reprint/112/4/e328)

The Prevention of Unintentional Injury Among American Indian and Alaska Native Children: A Subject Review (Clinical Report) (joint with Committee on Injury and Poison Prevention), 12/99, reaffirmed 5/03

COMMITTEE ON NUTRITION

Aluminum Toxicity in Infants and Children, 3/96, reaffirmed 4/00, 4/03

Calcium Requirements of Infants, Children, and Adolescents, 11/99

Cholesterol in Childhood, 1/98, reaffirmed 4/01

Hypoallergenic Infant Formulas, 8/00

Infant Methemoglobinemia: The Role of Dietary Nitrate, 9/70, reaffirmed 4/94, 6/97, 4/00

Iron Fortification of Infant Formulas, 7/99, reaffirmed 11/02

The Practical Significance of Lactose Intolerance in Children, 8/78, reaffirmed 12/93, 6/97, 4/00

Practical Significance of Lactose Intolerance in Children: Supplement, 10/90, reaffirmed 12/93, 6/97, 4/00

Prevention of Pediatric Overweight and Obesity, 8/03

Prevention of Rickets and Vitamin D Deficiency: New Guidelines for Vitamin D Intake (Clinical Report) (joint with Section on Breastfeeding), 4/03

Reimbursement for Foods for Special Dietary Use, 5/03

Soy Protein-based Formulas: Recommendations for Use in Infant Feeding, 1/98, reaffirmed 4/01

The Use and Misuse of Fruit Juice in Pediatrics, 5/01

COMMITTEE ON PEDIATRIC AIDS

Adolescents and Human Immunodeficiency Virus Infection: The Role of the Pediatrician in Prevention and Intervention (joint with Committee on Adolescence), 1/01, reaffirmed 10/03

Disclosure of Illness Status to Children and Adolescents With HIV Infection, 1/99, reaffirmed 2/02

Education of Children With Human Immunodeficiency Virus Infection, 6/00, reaffirmed 3/03

Evaluation and Treatment of the Human Immunodeficiency Virus-1–Exposed Infant (Clinical Report) (joint with Canadian Paediatric Society), 8/04

Human Immunodeficiency Virus Screening (joint with American Academy of Pediatrics Committee on Fetus and Newborn and American College of Obstetricians and Gynecologists), 7/99, reaffirmed 6/02

Human Milk, Breastfeeding, and Transmission of Human Immunodeficiency Virus in the United States, 11/95, reaffirmed 11/99, 11/03

Human Milk, Breastfeeding, and Transmission of Human Immunodeficiency Virus Type 1 in the United States (Technical Report), 11/03

Identification and Care of HIV-Exposed and HIV-Infected Infants, Children, and Adolescents in Foster Care, 7/00, reaffirmed 3/03

Issues Related to Human Immunodeficiency Virus Transmission in Schools, Child Care, Medical Settings, the Home, and Community (joint with Committee on Infectious Diseases), 8/99, reaffirmed 2/02

Measles Immunization in HIV-Infected Children (joint with Committee on Infectious Diseases), 5/99

Perinatal Human Immunodeficiency Virus Testing, 2/95, reaffirmed 10/96, 11/99, 3/03

Perinatal Human Immunodeficiency Virus Testing and Prevention of Transmission (Technical Report), 12/00, reaffirmed 3/03, *Pediatrics electronic pages* (pediatrics.aappublications.org/cgi/reprint/106/6/e88)

Planning for Children Whose Parents Are Dying of HIV/AIDS, 2/99, reaffirmed 2/02

Postexposure Prophylaxis in Children and Adolescents for Nonoccupational Exposure to Human Immunodeficiency Virus (Clinical Report), 6/03

Reducing the Risk of Human Immunodeficiency Virus Infection Associated With Illicit Drug Use, 12/94, reaffirmed 1/98

Surveillance of Pediatric HIV Infection, 2/98, reaffirmed 2/02

COMMITTEE ON PEDIATRIC EMERGENCY MEDICINE

Access to Pediatric Emergency Medical Care, 3/00

Care of Children in the Emergency Department: Guidelines for Preparedness (joint with American College of Emergency Physicians), 4/01, reaffirmed 5/04

Consent for Emergency Medical Services for Children and Adolescents, 3/03

Death of a Child in the Emergency Department: Joint Statement of the American Academy of Pediatrics and the American College of Emergency Physicians (joint with American College of Emergency Physicians), 10/02

Emergency Preparedness for Children With Special Health Care Needs, 10/99, reaffirmed 8/02, *Pediatrics electronic pages* (pediatrics.aappublications.org/cgi/reprint/104/4/e53)

Overcrowding Crisis in Our Nation's Emergency Departments: Is Our Safety Net Unraveling?, 9/04

Pediatric Care Recommendations for Freestanding Urgent Care Facilities, 5/99

Pediatricians' Liability During Disasters (joint with Committee on Medical Liability), 12/00, reaffirmed 1/04

Relief of Pain and Anxiety in Pediatric Patients in Emergency Medical Systems (Clinical Report) (joint with Section on Anesthesiology and Pain Medicine), 11/04

The Role of the Pediatrician in Rural EMSC, 5/98, reaffirmed 6/00

Role of Pediatricians in Advocating Life Support Training Courses for Parents and the Public, 12/04

COMMITTEE ON PEDIATRIC RESEARCH

Human Embryo Research (joint with Committee on Bioethics), 9/01, reaffirmed 4/04

Promoting Education, Mentorship, and Support for Pediatric Research, 6/01

Race/Ethnicity, Gender, Socioeconomic Status—Research Exploring Their Effects on Child Health: A Subject Review (Clinical Report), 6/00

COMMITTEE ON PEDIATRIC WORKFORCE

Enhancing the Racial and Ethnic Diversity of the Pediatric Workforce, 1/00

Ensuring Culturally Effective Pediatric Care: Implications for Education and Health Policy, 12/04

Nondiscrimination in Pediatric Health Care, 11/01

Pediatric Primary Health Care, 11/93, reaffirmed 6/01

Pediatric Workforce Statement, 8/98

Prevention of Sexual Harassment in the Workplace and Educational Settings, 12/00

Scope of Practice Issues in the Delivery of Pediatric Health Care, 2/03

COMMITTEE ON PRACTICE AND AMBULATORY MEDICINE

Eye Examination in Infants, Children, and Young Adults by Pediatricians (joint with American Academy of Pediatrics Section on Ophthalmology, American Association of Certified Orthoptists, American Association for Pediatric Ophthalmology and Strabismus, and American Academy of Ophthalmology), 4/03

Hearing Assessment in Infants and Children: Recommendations Beyond Neonatal Screening (Clinical Report) (joint with Section on Otolaryngology and Bronchoesophagology), 2/03

Implementation of the Immunization Policy, 8/95

Increasing Immunization Coverage (joint with Committee on Community Health Services), 10/03

Infection Control in Physicians' Offices (joint with Committee on Infectious Diseases), 6/00

Pediatric Physician Profiling (joint with Committee on Medical Liability), 10/99

Policy on the Development of Immunization Tracking Systems, 6/96

Prevention and Management of Positional Skull Deformities in Infants (Clinical Report) (joint with Section on Plastic Surgery and Section on Neurological Surgery), 7/03

Recommendations for Preventive Pediatric Health Care, 3/00

The Role of the Primary Care Pediatrician in the Management of High-risk Newborn Infants (joint with Committee on Fetus and Newborn), 10/96

The Use of Chaperones During the Physical Examination of the Pediatric Patient, 12/96, reaffirmed 11/99, 2/00

Use of Photoscreening for Children's Vision Screening (joint with Section on Ophthalmology), 3/02

COMMITTEE ON PSYCHOSOCIAL ASPECTS OF CHILD AND FAMILY HEALTH

The Assessment and Management of Acute Pain in Infants, Children, and Adolescents (joint with American Pain Society), 9/01

The Child in Court: A Subject Review (Clinical Report), 11/99, reaffirmed 11/02

Coparent or Second-Parent Adoption by Same-Sex Parents, 2/02

Coparent or Second-Parent Adoption by Same-Sex Parents (Technical Report), 2/02

Fathers and Pediatricians: Enhancing Men's Roles in the Care and Development of Their Children (Clinical Report), 5/04

Guidance for Effective Discipline, 4/98, reaffirmed 5/04

Helping Children and Families Deal With Divorce and Separation (Clinical Report), 11/02

How Pediatricians Can Respond to the Psychosocial Implications of Disasters, 2/99

The New Morbidity Revisited: A Renewed Commitment to the Psychosocial Aspects of Pediatric Care, 11/01

The Pediatrician and Childhood Bereavement, 2/00, reaffirmed 1/04

The Pediatrician's Role in the Prevention of Missing Children (Clinical Report), 10/04

The Prenatal Visit, 6/01

Psychosocial Risks of Chronic Health Conditions in Childhood and Adolescence (joint with Committee on Children With Disabilities), 12/93, reaffirmed 10/96

Sexuality Education for Children and Adolescents (joint with Committee on Adolescence), 8/01, reaffirmed 5/04

STEERING COMMITTEE ON QUALITY IMPROVEMENT AND MANAGEMENT

Classifying Recommendations for Clinical Practice Guidelines, 9/04

Developmental Dysplasia of the Hip Practice Guideline (Technical Report), 4/00, *Pediatrics electronic pages* (pediatrics.aappublications.org/cgi/reprint/105/4/e57)

Diagnosis and Evaluation of the Child With Attention-Deficit/Hyperactivity Disorder (Clinical Practice Guideline), 5/00

Diagnosis and Management of Acute Otitis Media (Clinical Practice Guideline) (joint with American Academy of Family Physicians), 5/04

Diagnosis and Management of Childhood Obstructive Sleep Apnea Syndrome (Clinical Practice Guideline) (joint with Section on Pediatric Pulmonology), 4/02

Diagnosis and Management of Childhood Obstructive Sleep Apnea Syndrome (Technical Report) (joint with Section on Pediatric Pulmonology), 4/02

The Diagnosis, Treatment, and Evaluation of the Initial Urinary Tract Infection in Febrile Infants and Young Children (Clinical Practice Guideline), 4/99

Early Detection of Developmental Dysplasia of the Hip (Clinical Practice Guideline), 4/00

Evidence for the Diagnosis and Treatment of Acute Uncomplicated Sinusitis in Children: A Systematic Overview (Technical Report), 9/01, *Pediatrics electronic pages* (pediatrics.aappublications.org/cgi/reprint/108/3/e57)

An Evidence-Based Review of Important Issues Concerning Neonatal Hyperbilirubinemia (Technical Report), 7/04, *Pediatrics electronic pages* (pediatrics.aappublications.org/cgi/content/full/114/1/e130)

Long-term Treatment of the Child With Simple Febrile Seizures (Clinical Practice Guideline), 6/99

Management of Hyperbilirubinemia in the Newborn Infant 35 or More Weeks of Gestation (Clinical Practice Guideline), 7/04

The Management of Minor Closed Head Injury in Children (Clinical Practice Guideline) (joint with American Academy of Family Physicians), 12/99

Management of Sinusitis (Clinical Practice Guideline), 9/01

Minor Head Injury in Children (Technical Report), 12/99, *Pediatrics electronic pages* (pediatrics.aappublications.org/cgi/reprint/104/6/e78)

The Neurodiagnostic Evaluation of the Child With a First Simple Febrile Seizure (Clinical Practice Guideline), 5/96

The Neurodiagnostic Evaluation of the Child With a First Simple Febrile Seizure (Technical Report), 5/96

Otitis Media With Effusion (Clinical Practice Guideline), 5/04

Treatment of the Child With Simple Febrile Seizures (Technical Report), 6/99, *Pediatrics electronic pages* (pediatrics.aappublications.org/cgi/reprint/103/6/e86)

Treatment of the School-Aged Child With Attention-Deficit/Hyperactivity Disorder (Clinical Practice Guideline), 10/01

Urinary Tract Infections in Febrile Infants and Young Children (Technical Report), 4/99, *Pediatrics electronic pages* (pediatrics.aappublications.org/cgi/reprint/103/4/e54)

COMMITTEE ON SCHOOL HEALTH

Corporal Punishment in Schools, 8/00, reaffirmed 6/03

Do Not Resuscitate Orders in Schools (joint with Committee on Bioethics), 4/00, reaffirmed 6/03

Guidelines for the Administration of Medication in School, 9/03

Guidelines for Emergency Medical Care in School, 2/01

Head Lice (Clinical Report) (joint with Committee on Infectious Diseases), 9/02

Health Appraisal Guidelines for Day Camps and Resident Camps, 3/00

Home, Hospital, and Other Non–School-based Instruction for Children and Adolescents Who Are Medically Unable to Attend School, 11/00, reaffirmed 6/03

The Inappropriate Use of School "Readiness" Tests (joint with Committee on Early Childhood, Adoption, and Dependent Care), 3/95, reaffirmed 4/98, 1/04

Organized Sports for Children and Preadolescents (joint with Committee on Sports Medicine and Fitness), 6/01, reaffirmed 11/04

Out-of-School Suspension and Expulsion, 11/03

Physical Fitness and Activity in Schools (joint with Committee on Sports Medicine and Fitness), 5/00

The Role of the School Nurse in Providing School Health Services, 11/01

School Health Assessments, 4/00, reaffirmed 6/03

School Health Centers and Other Integrated School Health Services, 1/01

School Transportation Safety (joint with Committee on Injury and Poison Prevention), 5/96, reaffirmed 4/99

School-Based Mental Health Services, 6/04

Soft Drinks in Schools, 1/04

COMMITTEE ON SPORTS MEDICINE AND FITNESS

Adolescents and Anabolic Steroids: A Subject Review (Clinical Report), 6/97, reaffirmed 5/00

Athletic Participation by Children and Adolescents Who Have Systemic Hypertension, 4/97, reaffirmed 5/00, 5/04

Atlantoaxial Instability in Down Syndrome: Subject Review (Clinical Report), 7/95, reaffirmed 11/98, 5/00, 5/04

Cardiac Dysrhythmias and Sports, 5/95, reaffirmed 11/98, 5/00, 5/04

Climatic Heat Stress and the Exercising Child and Adolescent, 7/00, reaffirmed 5/04

Human Immunodeficiency Virus and Other Blood-borne Viral Pathogens in the Athletic Setting, 12/99, reaffirmed 5/04

Injuries in Youth Soccer: A Subject Review (Clinical Report), 3/00

In-line Skating Injuries in Children and Adolescents (joint with Committee on Injury and Poison Prevention), 4/98, reaffirmed 1/02

Intensive Training and Sports Specialization in Young Athletes, 7/00, reaffirmed 11/04

Knee Brace Use in the Young Athlete (Technical Report), 8/01

Medical Concerns in the Female Athlete, 9/00, reaffirmed 5/04

Medical Conditions Affecting Sports Participation, 5/01

Organized Sports for Children and Preadolescents (joint with Committee on School Health), 6/01, reaffirmed 11/04

Participation in Boxing by Children, Adolescents, and Young Adults, 1/97, reaffirmed 5/00

Physical Fitness and Activity in Schools (joint with Committee on School Health), 5/00

Promotion of Healthy Weight-control Practices in Young Athletes, 5/96, reaffirmed 10/99

Protective Eyewear for Young Athletes (joint with American Academy of Ophthalmology), 3/04

Risk of Injury From Baseball and Softball in Children, 4/01

Safety in Youth Ice Hockey: The Effects of Body Checking, 3/00, reaffirmed 5/04

Strength Training by Children and Adolescents, 6/01

Swimming Programs for Infants and Toddlers (joint with Committee on Injury and Poison Prevention), 4/00, reaffirmed 5/04

Trampolines at Home, School, and Recreational Centers (joint with Committee on Injury and Poison Prevention), 5/99, reaffirmed 12/02

COMMITTEE ON SUBSTANCE ABUSE

Alcohol Use and Abuse: A Pediatric Concern, 7/01

Fetal Alcohol Syndrome and Alcohol-Related Neurodevelopmental Disorders (joint with Committee on Children With Disabilities), 8/00

Improving Substance Abuse Prevention, Assessment, and Treatment Financing for Children and Adolescents (joint with Committee on Child Health Financing), 10/01

Indications for Management and Referral of Patients Involved in Substance Abuse, 7/00

Inhalant Abuse (joint with Committee on Native American Child Health), 3/96, reaffirmed 5/99

Legalization of Marijuana: Potential Impact on Youth (joint with Committee on Adolescence), 6/04

Legalization of Marijuana: Potential Impact on Youth (Technical Report) (joint with Committee on Adolescence), 6/04

Marijuana: A Continuing Concern for Pediatricians, 10/99, reaffirmed 4/03

The Role of Schools in Combatting Substance Abuse, 5/95, reaffirmed 5/99

Testing for Drugs of Abuse in Children and Adolescents, 8/96, reaffirmed 5/99

Tobacco, Alcohol, and Other Drugs: The Role of the Pediatrician in Prevention and Management of Substance Abuse, 1/98

Tobacco's Toll: Implications for the Pediatrician, 4/01

MEDICAL HOME INITIATIVES FOR CHILDREN WITH SPECIAL NEEDS PROJECT ADVISORY COMMITTEE

The Medical Home, 7/02

NATIONAL INITIATIVE FOR CHILDREN'S HEALTH CARE QUALITY PROJECT ADVISORY COMMITTEE

Principles of Patient Safety in Pediatrics, 6/01

PEDIATRIC PRACTICE ACTION GROUP

Privacy Protection of Health Information: Patient Rights and Pediatrician Responsibilities (joint with Task Force on Medical Informatics), 10/99

SECTION ON ANESTHESIOLOGY AND PAIN MEDICINE

Do-Not-Resuscitate Orders for Pediatric Patients Who Require Anesthesia and Surgery (Clinical Report) (joint with Section on Surgery and Committee on Bioethics), 12/04

Evaluation and Preparation of Pediatric Patients Undergoing Anesthesia, 9/96

Guidelines for the Pediatric Perioperative Anesthesia Environment, 2/99, reaffirmed 10/02

Prevention and Management of Pain and Stress in the Neonate (joint with American Academy of Pediatrics Committee on Drugs, Committee on Fetus and Newborn, and Section on Surgery and Canadian Paediatric Society), 2/00, reaffirmed 4/03

Relief of Pain and Anxiety in Pediatric Patients in Emergency Medical Systems (Clinical Report) (joint with Committee on Pediatric Emergency Medicine), 11/04

SECTION ON BREASTFEEDING

Breastfeeding and the Use of Human Milk, 12/97

Prevention of Rickets and Vitamin D Deficiency: New Guidelines for Vitamin D Intake (Clinical Report) (joint with Committee on Nutrition), 4/03

WIC Program, 11/01

SECTION ON CARDIOLOGY AND CARDIAC SURGERY

Echocardiography in Infants and Children, 6/97, reaffirmed 3/03

Guidelines for Pediatric Cardiovascular Centers, 3/02

SECTION ON CRITICAL CARE

Admission and Discharge Guidelines for the Pediatric Patient Requiring Intermediate Care (Clinical Report) (joint with American Academy of Pediatrics Committee on Hospital Care and Society of Critical Care Medicine), 5/04

Guidelines for Developing Admission and Discharge Policies for the Pediatric Intensive Care Unit (joint with American Academy of Pediatrics Committee on Hospital Care and Society of Critical Care Medicine), 4/99

Guidelines and Levels of Care for Pediatric Intensive Care Units (Clinical Report) (joint with American Academy of Pediatrics Committee on Hospital Care and Society of Critical Care Medicine), 10/04

SECTION ON ENDOCRINOLOGY

Congenital Adrenal Hyperplasia (Technical Report) (joint with Committee on Genetics), 12/00, reaffirmed 12/03

Evaluation of the Newborn With Developmental Anomalies of the External Genitalia (joint with Committee on Genetics and Section on Urology), 7/00

Health Supervision for Children With Turner Syndrome (Clinical Report) (joint with Committee on Genetics), 3/03

Newborn Screening for Congenital Hypothyroidism: Recommended Guidelines (joint with American Academy of Pediatrics Committee on Genetics and American Thyroid Association Committee on Public Health), 6/93, reaffirmed 10/96

Prevention and Treatment of Type 2 Diabetes Mellitus in Children, With Special Emphasis on American Indian and Alaska Native Children (Clinical Report) (joint with Committee on Native American Child Health), 10/03, *Pediatric electronic pages* (pediatrics.aappublications.org/cgi/reprint/112/4/e328)

Screening for Retinopathy in the Pediatric Patient With Type 1 Diabetes Mellitus (joint with Section on Ophthalmology), 2/98

SECTION ON HEMATOLOGY/ONCOLOGY

Guidelines for Pediatric Cancer Centers, 6/04

Health Supervision for Children With Sickle Cell Disease (joint with Committee on Genetics), 3/02

SECTION ON NEUROLOGICAL SURGERY

Prevention and Management of Positional Skull Deformities in Infants (Clinical Report) (joint with Committee on Practice and Ambulatory Medicine and Section on Plastic Surgery), 7/03

SECTION ON OPHTHALMOLOGY

Eye Examination in Infants, Children, and Young Adults by Pediatricians (joint with American Academy of Pediatrics Committee on Practice and Ambulatory Medicine, American Association of Certified Orthoptists, American Association for Pediatric Ophthalmology and Strabismus, and American Academy of Ophthalmology), 4/03

Guidelines for Ophthalmologic Examinations in Children With Juvenile Rheumatoid Arthritis (joint with Section on Rheumatology), 8/93, reaffirmed 8/99

Red Reflex Examination in Infants, 5/02

Screening Examination of Premature Infants for Retinopathy of Prematurity (joint with American Association for Pediatric Ophthalmology and Strabismus and American Academy of Ophthalmology), 9/01

Screening for Retinopathy in the Pediatric Patient With Type 1 Diabetes Mellitus (joint with Section on Endocrinology), 2/98

Use of Photoscreening for Children's Vision Screening (joint with Committee on Practice and Ambulatory Medicine), 3/02

SECTION ON OTOLARYNGOLOGY—HEAD & NECK SURGERY

Follow-up Management of Children With Tympanostomy Tubes, 2/02

Hearing Assessment in Infants and Children: Recommendations Beyond Neonatal Screening (Clinical Report) (joint with Committee on Practice and Ambulatory Medicine), 2/03

SECTION ON PEDIATRIC DENTISTRY

Oral Health Risk Assessment Timing and Establishment of the Dental Home, 5/03

SECTION ON PEDIATRIC PULMONOLOGY

Diagnosis and Management of Childhood Obstructive Sleep Apnea Syndrome (Clinical Practice Guideline) (joint with Steering Committee on Quality Improvement and Management), 4/02

Diagnosis and Management of Childhood Obstructive Sleep Apnea Syndrome (Technical Report) (joint with Steering Committee on Quality Improvement and Management), 4/02

SECTION ON PLASTIC SURGERY

Prevention and Management of Positional Skull Deformities in Infants (Clinical Report) (joint with Committee on Practice and Ambulatory Medicine and Section on Neurological Surgery), 7/03

SECTION ON RADIOLOGY

Diagnostic Imaging of Child Abuse, 6/00

SECTION ON RESIDENTS

Parental Leave for Residents and Pediatric Training Programs (joint with Committee on Early Childhood, Adoption, and Dependent Care), 11/95, reaffirmed 4/98

SECTION ON RHEUMATOLOGY

Guidelines for Ophthalmologic Examinations in Children With Juvenile Rheumatoid Arthritis (joint with Section on Ophthalmology), 8/93, reaffirmed 8/99

SECTION ON SCHOOL HEALTH

Residency Training and Continuing Medical Education in School Health, 9/93

SECTION ON SURGERY

Do-Not-Resuscitate Orders for Pediatric Patients Who Require Anesthesia and Surgery (Clinical Report) (joint with Section on Anesthesia and Pain Medicine and Committee on Bioethics), 12/04

Pediatric Organ Donation and Transplantation (joint with Committee on Hospital Care), 5/02

Prevention and Management of Pain and Stress in the Neonate (joint with American Academy of Pediatrics Committee on Drugs, Committee on Fetus and Newborn, and Section on Anesthesiology and Pain Medicine and Canadian Paediatric Society), 2/00, reaffirmed 4/03

SECTION ON UROLOGY

Evaluation of the Newborn With Developmental Anomalies of the External Genitalia (joint with Committee on Genetics and Section on Endocrinology), 7/00

Timing of Elective Surgery on the Genitalia of Male Children With Particular Reference to the Risks, Benefits, and Psychological Effects of Surgery and Anesthesia, 4/96

SURGICAL ADVISORY PANEL

Guidelines for Referral to Pediatric Surgical Specialists, 7/02

TASK FORCE ON CIRCUMCISION

Circumcision Policy Statement, 3/99

TASK FORCE ON GRADUATE MEDICAL EDUCATION REFORM

Graduate Medical Education and Pediatric Workforce Issues and Principles, 6/94

TASK FORCE ON INFANT SLEEP POSITION AND SUDDEN INFANT DEATH SYNDROME

Changing Concepts of Sudden Infant Death Syndrome: Implications for Infant Sleeping Environment and Sleep Position, 3/00

TASK FORCE ON MEDICAL MANAGEMENT GUIDELINES

Guiding Principles, Attributes, and Process to Review Medical Management Guidelines, 12/01

TASK FORCE ON VIOLENCE

The Role of the Pediatrician in Youth Violence Prevention in Clinical Practice and at the Community Level, 1/99, reaffirmed 5/02

WORK GROUP ON CORD BLOOD BANKING

Cord Blood Banking for Potential Future Transplantation: Subject Review (Clinical Report), 7/99

JOINT STATEMENTS

Joint Statement of the American Academy of Pediatrics, the Advisory Committee on Immunization Practices, and the American Academy of Family Physicians

Combination Vaccines for Childhood Immunization: Recommendations of the Advisory Committee on Immunization Practices (ACIP), the American Academy of Pediatrics (AAP), and the American Academy of Family Physicians (AAFP), 5/99, reaffirmed 3/02

Joint Statement of the American Academy of Pediatrics and the American Academy of Family Physicians

Diagnosis and Management of Acute Otitis Media (Clinical Practice Guideline), 5/04

The Management of Minor Closed Head Injury in Children (Clinical Practice Guideline), 12/99

Joint Statement of the American Academy of Pediatrics, the American Academy of Family Physicians, and the American College of Physicians-American Society of Internal Medicine

A Consensus Statement on Health Care Transitions for Young Adults With Special Health Care Needs, 12/02

Joint Statement of the American Academy of Pediatrics and the American Academy of Ophthalmology

Protective Eyewear for Young Athletes, 3/04

Joint Statement of the American Academy of Pediatrics and the American Academy of Pediatric Dentistry

Oral and Dental Aspects of Child Abuse and Neglect, 8/99

Joint Statement of the American Academy of Pediatrics, the American Association of Certified Orthoptists, the American Association for Pediatric Ophthalmology and Strabismus, and the American Academy of Ophthalmology

Eye Examination in Infants, Children, and Young Adults by Pediatricians, 4/03

Joint Statement of the American Academy of Pediatrics, the American Association for Pediatric Ophthalmology and Strabismus, and the American Academy of Ophthalmology

Learning Disabilities, Dyslexia, and Vision: A Subject Review (Clinical Report), 11/98, reaffirmed 5/02

Screening Examination of Premature Infants for Retinopathy of Prematurity, 9/01

Joint Statement of the American Academy of Pediatrics and the American College of Emergency Physicians
Care of Children in the Emergency Department: Guidelines for Preparedness, 4/01, reaffirmed 5/04
Death of a Child in the Emergency Department: Joint Statement of the American Academy of Pediatrics and the American College of Emergency Physicians, 10/02

Joint Statement of the American Academy of Pediatrics and the American College of Obstetricians and Gynecologists
Human Immunodeficiency Virus Screening, 7/99, reaffirmed 6/02
Use and Abuse of the Apgar Score, 7/96, reaffirmed 10/97, 10/00

Joint Statement of the American Academy of Pediatrics and the American Pain Society
The Assessment and Management of Acute Pain in Infants, Children, and Adolescents, 9/01

Joint Statement of the American Academy of Pediatrics and the American Thyroid Association Committee on Public Health
Newborn Screening for Congenital Hypothyroidism: Recommended Guidelines, 6/93, reaffirmed 10/96

Joint Statement of the American Academy of Pediatrics and the Canadian Paediatric Society
Evaluation and Treatment of the Human Immuno-deficiency Virus-1–Exposed Infant (Clinical Report), 8/04
Postnatal Corticosteroids to Treat or Prevent Chronic Lung Disease in Preterm Infants, 2/02
Prevention and Management of Pain and Stress in the Neonate, 2/00, reaffirmed 4/03

Joint Statement of the American Academy of Pediatrics and the Institute for Family-Centered Care
Family-Centered Care and the Pediatrician's Role, 9/03

Joint Statement of the American Academy of Pediatrics and Others
Insurance Coverage of Mental Health and Substance Abuse Services for Children and Adolescents: A Consensus Statement, 10/00

Joint Statement of the American Academy of Pediatrics and the Society of Critical Care Medicine
Admission and Discharge Guidelines for the Pediatric Patient Requiring Intermediate Care, 5/04
Guidelines for Developing Admission and Discharge Policies for the Pediatric Intensive Care Unit, 4/99
Guidelines and Levels of Care for Pediatric Intensive Care Units (Clinical Report), 10/04

Joint Statement of the Federation of Pediatric Organizations
Pediatric Fellowship Training, 7/04

ENDORSED CLINICAL PRACTICE GUIDELINES AND POLICIES
(The AAP endorses and accepts as its policy the following clinical practice guidelines and policies that have been published by other organizations.)

American Academy of Allergy, Asthma, and Immunology and American College of Allergy, Asthma, and Immunology
Allergen Immunotherapy: A Practice Parameter (Clinical Practice Guideline), 1/03

American Academy of Child and Adolescent Psychiatry and the Child Welfare League of America
Foster Care Mental Health Values, 2002
Mental Health and Substance Use Screening and Assessment of Children in Foster Care, 2003

American College of Rheumatology
Guidelines for Referral of Children and Adolescents to Pediatric Rheumatologists, 6/02

American Diabetes Association
Type 2 Diabetes in Children and Adolescents, 3/00

American Heart Association
Diagnosis, Treatment, and Long-Term Management of Kawasaki Disease: A Statement for Health Professionals (Clinical Report), 12/04
Response to Cardiac Arrest and Selected Life-Threatening Medical Emergencies: The Medical Emergency Response Plan for Schools. A Statement for Healthcare Providers, Policymakers, School Administrators, and Community Leaders, 1/04

American Medical Association
Gifts to Physicians From Industry, 8/01

American Orthopaedic Society for Sports Medicine
Concussion in Sports, 1999

American Thoracic Society and Centers for Disease Control and Prevention
(The AAP endorses and accepts as its policy the sections of this statement as they relate to infants and children.)
Targeted Tuberculin Testing and Treatment of Latent Tuberculosis Infection, 4/00

American Urological Association
Report on the Management of Primary Vesicoureteral Reflux in Children (Clinical Practice Guideline), 5/97

Centers for Disease Control and Prevention
Managing Acute Gastroenteritis Among Children: Oral Rehydration, Maintenance, and Nutritional Therapy (Clinical Practice Guideline), 11/03
Prevention of Perinatal Group B Streptococcal Disease (Clinical Practice Guideline), 8/02
Recommendations for Using Fluoride to Prevent and Control Dental Caries in the United States (Clinical Practice Guideline), 8/01

Centers for Disease Control and Prevention, Infectious Diseases Society of America, and the American Society of Blood and Marrow Transplantation
Guidelines for Preventing Opportunistic Infections Among Hematopoietic Stem Cell Transplant Recipients (Clinical Practice Guideline), 10/00

Family Violence Prevention Fund
Identifying and Responding to Domestic Violence:
Consensus Recommendations for Child and
Adolescent Health, 9/02

Infectious Diseases Society of America
Practice Guidelines for the Treatment of Lyme Disease
(Clinical Practice Guideline), 9/00

Inter-Association Task Force for Appropriate Care of the Spine-Injured Athlete
Prehospital Care of the Spine-Injured Athlete (Clinical
Practice Guideline), 2001

Joint Committee on Infant Hearing
Principles and Guidelines for Early Hearing Detection
and Intervention Programs (Year 2000 Position
Statement), 10/00

National Asthma Education and Prevention Program
Guidelines for the Diagnosis and Management of
Asthma—Update on Selected Topics (Clinical
Practice Guideline), 2002

National Athletic Trainers' Association
Lightning Safety for Athletics and Recreation (Position
Statement), 12/00

National Consensus Project for Quality Palliative Care
Clinical Practice Guidelines for Quality Palliative Care
(Clinical Practice Guideline), 5/04

National Diabetes Education Program
Helping the Student with Diabetes Succeed: A Guide
for School Personnel, 6/03

North American Society of Pediatric Gastroenterology, Hepatology, and Nutrition
Constipation in Infants and Children: Evaluation and
Treatment (Clinical Practice Guideline), 3/00
Guidelines for Evaluation and Treatment of
Gastroesophageal Reflux in Infants and Children
(Clinical Practice Guideline), 2001
Helicobacter pylori Infection in Children: Recommenda-
tions for Diagnosis and Treatment (Clinical Practice
Guideline), 11/00

Quality Standards Subcommittee of the American Academy of Neurology and the Child Neurology Society
Diagnostic Assessment of the Child with Cerebral Palsy
(Clinical Practice Guideline), 3/04
Neuroimaging of the Neonate (Clinical Practice
Guideline), 6/02
Pharmacological Treatment of Migraine Headache in
Children and Adolescents (Clinical Practice
Guideline), 12/04
Screening and Diagnosis of Autism (Clinical Practice
Guideline), 8/00
Treatment of the Child With a First Unprovoked Seizure
(Clinical Practice Guideline), 1/03

Quality Standards Subcommittee of the American Academy of Neurology, the Child Neurology Society, and the American Epilepsy Society
Evaluating a First Nonfebrile Seizure in Children
(Clinical Practice Guideline), 8/00

Society for Academic Emergency Medicine
Pediatric Care in the Emergency Department, 11/03

Society of Critical Care Medicine, Infectious Diseases Society of America, Society for Healthcare Epidemiology of America, Surgical Infection Society, American College of Chest Physicians, American Thoracic Society, American Society of Critical Care Anesthesiologists, Association for Professionals in Infection Control and Epidemiology, Infusion Nurses Society, Oncology Nursing Society, Society of Cardiovascular and Interventional Radiology, American Academy of Pediatrics, and the Healthcare Infection Control Practices Advisory Committee of the Centers for Disease Control and Prevention
Guidelines for the Prevention of Intravascular Catheter-
Related Infections (Clinical Practice Guideline), 2002

US Department of Health and Human Services
Treating Tobacco Use and Dependence (Clinical Practice
Guideline), 6/00

Subject Index

· · · · · · · · · · · · · · · · · · ·

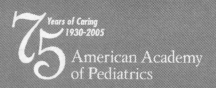
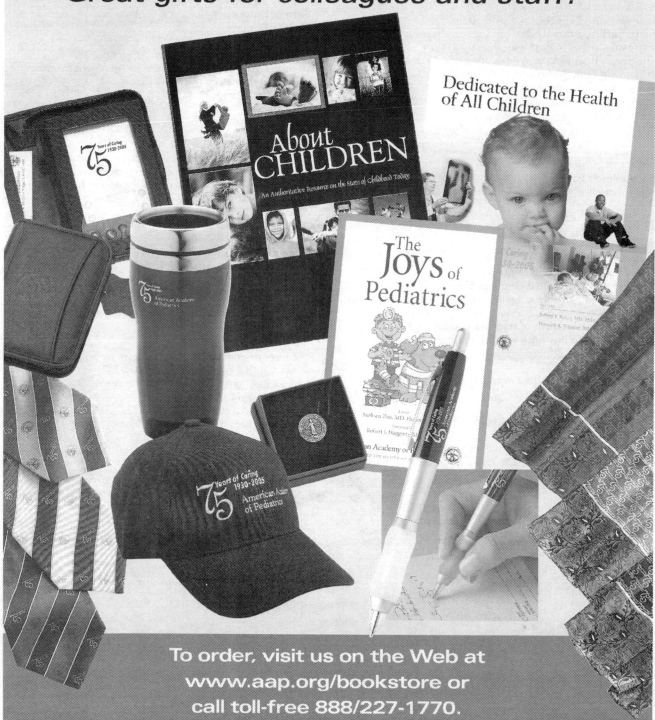